Massachusetts General Hospital

HANDBOOK *of* GENERAL HOSPITAL PSYCHIATRY

Seventh Edition

Massachusetts General Hospital

HANDBOOK *of* GENERAL HOSPITAL PSYCHIATRY

Seventh Edition

Theodore A. Stern, M.D.
Psychiatrist and Chief Emeritus, Avery D. Weisman Psychiatry Consultation Service,
Director, Thomas P. Hackett Center for Scholarship in Psychosomatic Medicine,
Director, Office for Clinical Careers,
Massachusetts General Hospital;
Ned H. Cassem Professor of Psychiatry in the field of Psychosomatic Medicine/Consultation,
Harvard Medical School,
Boston, MA, USA

Oliver Freudenreich, M.D.
Co-Director, Massachusetts General Hospital Schizophrenia Clinical and Research Program,
Erich Lindemann Mental Health Center;
Associate Professor of Psychiatry,
Harvard Medical School,
Boston, MA, USA

Felicia A. Smith, M.D.
Psychiatrist and Chief, Avery D. Weisman Psychiatry Consultation Service,
Director, Division of Psychiatry and Medicine,
Massachusetts General Hospital;
Assistant Professor of Psychiatry,
Harvard Medical School,
Boston, MA, USA

Gregory L. Fricchione, M.D.
Director, Benson-Henry Institute for Mind Body Medicine,
Director Emeritus, Division of Psychiatry and Medicine,
Massachusetts General Hospital;
Mind Body Medical Professor of Psychiatry,
Harvard Medical School,
Boston, MA, USA

Jerrold F. Rosenbaum, M.D.
Chief of Psychiatry,
Massachusetts General Hospital;
Stanley Cobb Professor of Psychiatry,
Harvard Medical School,
Boston, MA, USA

ELSEVIER

Edinburgh London New York Oxford Philadelphia St Louis Sydney Toronto 2018

ELSEVIER

First edition 1978
Second edition 1987
Third edition 1991
Fourth edition 1997
Fifth edition 2004
Sixth edition 2010
Seventh edition 2018

Notices

Knowledge and best practice in this field are constantly changing. As new research and experience broaden our understanding, changes in research methods, professional practices, or medical treatment may become necessary.

Practitioners and researchers must always rely on their own experience and knowledge in evaluating and using any information, methods, compounds, or experiments described herein. In using such information or methods they should be mindful of their own safety and the safety of others, including parties for whom they have a professional responsibility.

With respect to any drug or pharmaceutical products identified, readers are advised to check the most current information provided (i) on procedures featured or (ii) by the manufacturer of each product to be administered, to verify the recommended dose or formula, the method and duration of administration, and contraindications. It is the responsibility of practitioners, relying on their own experience and knowledge of their patients, to make diagnoses, to determine dosages and the best treatment for each individual patient, and to take all appropriate safety precautions.

To the fullest extent of the law, neither the Publisher nor the authors, contributors, or editors, assume any liability for any injury and/or damage to persons or property as a matter of products liability, negligence or otherwise, or from any use or operation of any methods, products, instructions, or ideas contained in the material herein.

ISBN: 978-0-323-48411-4
E-ISBN: 978-0-323-49643-8
Inkling ISBN: 978-0-323-49644-5

Senior Content Strategist: Charlotta Kryhl/Sharon Nash
Senior Content Development Specialist: Sharon Nash
Senior Project Manager: Beula Christopher
Design Specialist: Paula Catalano
Illustration Manager: Karen Giacomucci
Marketing Manager: Rachael Pignotti

Printed in India

Last digit is the print number: 9 8 7

To our patients, our students, our colleagues, and our mentors …

Preface

This seventh edition, revised, updated, and substantially expanded, was put together by a stalwart group of general hospital psychiatrists. Our collective efforts culminated in this book, with 54 chapters written by over 100 authors, most from the Massachusetts General Hospital. It was designed to help busy practitioners care for patients on medical and surgical floors and in outpatient practices filled by co-morbid medical and psychiatric illness. The chapters, which cover specific illnesses and care settings, were crafted for readability. Moreover, clinical vignettes strategically placed throughout the book were meant to act as a nidus upon which clinical pearls would grow.

Consultation psychiatry, now a subspecialty called *psychosomatic medicine*, involves the rapid recognition, evaluation, and treatment of psychiatric problems in the medical setting. Practitioners of psychosomatic medicine must also manage psychiatric reactions to medical illness, psychiatric complications of medical illness and its treatment, and psychiatric illness in those who suffer from medical or surgical illness. Because clinicians who work in general hospitals face problems related to the affective, behavioral, and cognitive (the "ABCs") realms of dementia, depression, anxiety, substance abuse, disruptive personalities, and critical illness, emphasis has been placed on successful strategies for their management by the consultant and by the physician of record.

This book would not have been possible were it not for the steady hands of our acquisitions editor at Elsevier, Charlotta Kryhl, and senior content development specialist, Sharon Nash, and to them we owe our gratitude.

On behalf of the patients who suffer, we hope this edition improves the detection and treatment of psychiatric problems and brings much needed relief.

Theodore A. Stern
Oliver Freudenreich
Felicia A. Smith
Gregory L. Fricchione
Jerrold F. Rosenbaum

Contents

Contributing Authors xiii

1. Beginnings: Psychosomatic Medicine and Consultation Psychiatry in the General Hospital 1
Theodore A. Stern, M.D.
Gregory L. Fricchione, M.D.
Nicholas Kontos, M.D.

2. Approach to Psychiatric Consultations in the General Hospital 7
John Querques, M.D.
Theodore A. Stern, M.D.

3. The Doctor–Patient Relationship 15
Christopher Gordon, M.D.
Gene V. Beresin, M.D., M.A.

4. The Psychiatric Interview 23
Gene V. Beresin, M.D., M.A.
Christopher Gordon, M.D.

5. Functional Neuroanatomy and the Neurologic Examination 37
Joel Salinas, M.D., M.B.A., M.Sc.
Joan A. Camprodon, M.D., M.P.H., Ph.D.

6. Limbic Music: The Band Plays On 43
Nicholas Kontos, M.D.
Anna R. Weissman, M.D.
John B. Taylor, M.D., M.B.A.

7. Psychological and Neuropsychological Assessment 51
Mary K. Colvin, Ph.D., A.B.P.P.
Mark A. Blais, Psy.D.
Sheila M. O'Keefe, Ed.D.
Dennis K. Norman, Ed.D., A.B.P.P.
Janet Sherman, Ph.D.

8. Diagnostic Rating Scales and Laboratory Tests 59
Joshua L. Roffman, M.D., M.M.sc.
David Mischoulon, M.D., Ph.D.
Theodore A. Stern, M.D.

9. Depressed Patients 69
Benjamin G. Shapero, Ph.D.
Paolo Cassano, M.D., Ph.D.
George I. Papakostas, M.D.
Maurizio Fava, M.D.
Theodore A. Stern, M.D.

10. Delirious Patients 83
Jason P. Caplan, M.D.

11. Patients With Neurocognitive Disorders 95
Franklin King IV, M.D.
Ilse R. Wiechers, M.D., M.P.P., M.H.S.

12. Psychotic Patients 109
Oliver Freudenreich, M.D.
Daphne J. Holt, M.D., Ph.D.
Donald C. Goff, M.D.

13. Anxious Patients 123
Sean P. Glass, M.D.
Mark H. Pollack, M.D.
Michael W. Otto, Ph.D.
Curtis W. Wittmann, M.D.
Jerrold F. Rosenbaum, M.D.

14. Patients With Alcohol Use Disorder 141
Mladen Nisavic, M.D.
Shamim H. Nejad, M.D.

15. Patients With Substance Use Disorders 149
Mladen Nisavic, M.D.
Shamim H. Nejad, M.D.

16. Psychosomatic Conditions: Somatic Symptom and Related Disorders, Functional Somatic Syndromes, and Deception Syndromes 161
Nicholas Kontos, M.D.
Scott R. Beach, M.D., F.A.P.M.
Felicia A. Smith, M.D.
Donna B. Greenberg, M.D.

17. Patients With an Eating Disorder 177
Jennifer J. Thomas, Ph.D.
Esther Jacobowitz Israel, M.D.
Lazaro V. Zayas, M.D.
Kristin Russell, M.D., M.B.A.
Kathryn Coniglio, B.A.
Rosanna Fox, M.B.B.S.

18. Pain Patients 189
Shamim H. Nejad, M.D.
Menekse Alpay, M.D.

19. Patients With Seizure Disorders 213
Taha Gholipour, M.D.
Felicia A. Smith, M.D.
Jeff C. Huffman, M.D.
Theodore A. Stern, M.D.

20. Patients With Cerebrovascular Disease and Traumatic Brain Injury 223
Felicia A. Smith, M.D.
Jeff C. Huffman, M.D.
Theodore A. Stern, M.D.

21. Patients With Abnormal Movements 231
Oliver Freudenreich, M.D.
Alice W. Flaherty, M.D., Ph.D.

22. Patients With Infectious or Inflammatory Neuropsychiatric Impairment 241
Jenny J. Linnoila, M.D., Ph.D.

23. Catatonia, Neuroleptic Malignant Syndrome, and Serotonin Syndrome 253
Gregory L. Fricchione, M.D.
Scott R. Beach, M.D., F.A.P.M.
Anne F. Gross, M.D.
Jeff C. Huffman, M.D.
George Bush, M.D., M.M.Sc.
Theodore A. Stern, M.D.

24. Patients With Disordered Sleep 267
Matt T. Bianchi, M.D., Ph.D., M.M.Sc.
Patrick Smallwood, M.D.
Davin K. Quinn, M.D.
Theodore A. Stern, M.D.

25. Sexual Disorders or Sexual Dysfunction 279
Linda C. Shafer, M.D.

26. The Psychiatric Management of Patients With Cardiac Disease 291
Scott R. Beach, M.D., F.A.P.M.
Christopher M. Celano, M.D.
Jeff C. Huffman, M.D.
James L. Januzzi, Jr., M.D., FACC, FESC
Theodore A. Stern, M.D.

27. Patients With Renal Disease 303
Ana Ivkovic, M.D.
Kassem Safa, M.D.
Sean P. Glass, M.D.
Mary C. Vance, M.D.
Theodore A. Stern, M.D.

28. Patients With Gastrointestinal Disease 313
Sean P. Glass, M.D.

29. Organ Failure and Transplantation 327
Laura M. Prager, M.D.

30. Patients With Human Immunodeficiency Virus Infection and Acquired Immunodeficiency Syndrome 335
Scott R. Beach, M.D., F.A.P.M.
BJ Beck, M.S.N., M.D.
Jacqueline T. Chu, M.D.
Oliver Freudenreich, M.D.

31. Patients With Cancer 349
Carlos G. Fernandez-Robles, M.D.
Kelly E. Irwin, M.D.
William F. Pirl, M.D., M.P.H.
Donna B. Greenberg, M.D.

32. Burn Patients 359
Sean P. Glass, M.D.
Shamim H. Nejad, M.D.
Gregory L. Fricchione, M.D.
Frederick J. Stoddard, Jr., M.D.

33. Chronic Medical Illness and Rehabilitation 371
Nasser Karamouz, M.D.
John B. Levine, M.D., Ph.D.
Gregory L. Fricchione, M.D.

34. Intensive Care Unit Patients 381
John Querques, M.D.
Theodore A. Stern, M.D.

35. Patients With Genetic Syndromes 385
Tamar C. Katz, M.D., Ph.D.
Christine T. Finn, M.D.
Joan M. Stoler, M.D.

36. Coping With Illness and Psychotherapy of the Medically Ill 397
Steven C. Schlozman, M.D.
James E. Groves, M.D.
Anne F. Gross, M.D.

37. Electroconvulsive Therapy and Neurotherapeutics ... 405
Aura M. Hurtado-Puerto, M.D.
Carlos G. Fernandez-Robles, M.D.
Michael E. Henry, M.D.
Cristina Cusin, M.D.
Sheri Berg, M.D.
Joan A. Camprodon, M.D., M.P.H., Ph.D.

38. Psychopharmacology in the Medical Setting ... 413
Jonathan R. Stevens, M.D., M.P.H.
Theodore A. Stern, M.D.
Maurizio Fava, M.D.
Jerrold F. Rosenbaum, M.D.
Jonathan E. Alpert, M.D., Ph.D.

39. Psychopharmacologic Management of Children and Adolescents ... 437
Jonathan R. Stevens, M.D., M.P.H.
Amy F. Vyas, M.D.
Boris A. Lorberg, M.D.
Jefferson B. Prince, M.D.
Theodore A. Stern, M.D.

40. Mind–Body Medicine ... 455
Micaela B. Owusu, M.D., M.Sc.
Deanna C. Chaukos, M.D.
Elyse R. Park, Ph.D., M.P.H.
Gregory L. Fricchione, M.D.

41. Chronic Disease and Unhealthy Habits: Behavioral Management ... 461
Elizabeth Pegg Frates, M.D.
Elyse R. Park, Ph.D., M.P.H.
A. Eden Evins, M.D., M.P.H.
Gregory L. Fricchione, M.D.

42. Complementary Medicine and Natural Medications ... 471
Felicia A. Smith, M.D.
David Mischoulon, M.D., Ph.D.

43. Difficult Patients ... 477
Franklin King IV, M.D.
James E. Groves, M.D.

44. Care of the Suicidal Patient ... 491
Rebecca Weintraub Brendel, M.D., J.D.
Katherine A. Koh, M.D., M.Sc.
Roy H. Perlis, M.D., M.Sc.
Theodore A. Stern, M.D.

45. Emergency Psychiatry ... 501
Abigail L. Donovan, M.D.
Laura M. Prager, M.D.
Suzanne A. Bird, M.D.

46. Care at the End of Life ... 513
M. Cornelia Cremens, M.D., M.P.H.
Ellen M. Robinson, R.N., Ph.D.
Keri O. Brenner, M.D., M.P.A.
Thomas H. McCoy, M.D.
Rebecca Weintraub Brendel, M.D., J.D.

47. Pediatric Consultation ... 521
Kenny A. Lin, M.D.
Eric P. Hazen, M.D.
Annah N. Abrams, M.D.

48. Care of the Geriatric Patient ... 539
M. Cornelia Cremens, M.D., M.P.H.
James M. Wilkins, M.D., D.Phil.
Ilse R. Wiechers, M.D., M.P.P., M.H.S.

49. Psychiatric Illness During Pregnancy and the Postpartum Period ... 547
Charlotte Hogan, M.D.
Betty Wang, M.D.
Marlene P. Freeman, M.D.
Ruta Nonacs, M.D., Ph.D.
Lee S. Cohen, M.D.

50. Culture and Psychiatry ... 559
Justin A. Chen, M.D., M.P.H.
Michelle P. Durham, M.D., M.P.H., F.A.P.A.
Andrea Madu, B.A.
Nhi-Ha Trinh, M.D., M.P.H.
Gregory L. Fricchione, M.D.
David C. Henderson, M.D.

51. Legal Aspects of Consultation ... 569
Ronald Schouten, M.D., J.D.
Rebecca Weintraub Brendel, M.D., J.D.

52. Approaches to Collaborative Care and Behavioral Health Integration ... 581
Andrew D. Carlo, M.D.
BJ Beck, M.S.N., M.D.
Eric M. Weil, M.D.
Jonathan E. Alpert, M.D., Ph.D.

53. Physician Well-Being and Coping With the Rigors of Psychiatric Practice ... 591
Deanna C. Chaukos, M.D.
Abigail L. Donovan, M.D.
Theodore A. Stern, M.D.

54. Management of a Psychiatric Consultation Service ... 599
John B. Taylor, M.D., M.B.A.
Felicia A. Smith, M.D.
Theodore A. Stern, M.D.

Index ... 605

Contributing Authors

The editor(s) would like to acknowledge and offer grateful thanks for the input of all previous editions' contributors, without whom this new edition would not have been possible.

Annah N. Abrams, M.D.
Chief, Division of Pediatric Psychooncology, Department of Pediatric Hematology and Oncology,
Massachusetts General Hospital;
Staff, Pediatric Psychiatry Consultation Liaison Service, Child and Adolescent Psychiatry,
Massachusetts General Hospital;
Assistant Professor of Psychiatry,
Harvard Medical School,
Boston, MA, USA
47 Pediatric Consultation

Menekse Alpay, M.D.
Clinical Assistant in Psychiatry,
Massachusetts General Hospital;
Instructor in Psychiatry,
Harvard Medical School,
Boston, MA, USA
18 Pain Patients

Jonathan E. Alpert, M.D., Ph.D.
Psychiatrist-in-Chief,
Montefiore Medical Center;
Dorothoy and Marty Silverman University Chair, Department of Psychiatry and Behavioral Science,
Professor of Psychiatry, Neuroscience, and Pediatrics,
Albert Einstein College of Medicine,
Bronx, MA, USA
38 Psychopharmacology in the Medical Setting
52 Approaches to Collaborative Care and Behavioral Health Integration

Scott R. Beach, M.D., F.A.P.M
Psychiatrist, Avery D. Weisman Psychiatric Consultation Service,
Program Director, MGH/McLean Adult Psychiatry Residency Training Program,
Assistant Professor of Psychiatry,
Boston, MA, USA
16 Psychosomatic Conditions: Somatic Symptom and Related Disorders, Functional Somatic Syndromes, and Deception Syndromes
23 Catatonia, Neuroleptic Malignant Syndrome, and Serotonin Syndrome
26 The Psychiatric Management of Patients with Cardiac Disease
30 Patients with Human Immunodeficiency Virus Infection and Acquired Immunodeficiency Syndrome

BJ Beck, M.S.N., M.D.
Psychiatrist, Robert B. Andrews Unit,
Massachusetts General Hospital,
Boston, MA, USA;
President and Chief Medical Officer,
College Health IPA,
Cypress, CA, USA;
Assistant Professor (Part-Time) of Psychiatry,
Harvard Medical School,
Boston, MA, USA
30 Patients with Human Immunodeficiency Virus Infection and Acquired Immunodeficiency Syndrome
52 Approaches to Collaborative Care and Behavioral Health Integration

Gene V. Beresin, M.D., M.A.
Executive Director, The Clay Center for Young Healthy Minds at the Massachusetts General Hospital;
Senior Educator in Child and Adolescent Psychiatry, Department of Psychiatry,
Massachusetts General Hospital;
Professor of Psychiatry,
Harvard Medical School,
Boston, MA, USA
3 The Doctor–Patient Relationship
4 The Psychiatric Interview

Sheri Berg, M.D.
Medical Director, Post Anesthesia Care Units, Anesthesia, Critical Care, and Pain Medicine,
Massachusetts General Hospital;
Instructor in Anesthesiology,
Harvard Medical School,
Boston, MA, USA
37 Electroconvulsive Therapy and Neurotherapeutics

Matt T. Bianchi, M.D., Ph.D., MMSc.
Director, Sleep Division, Neurology,
Massachusetts General Hospital;
Assistant Professor of Neurology,
Harvard Medical School,
Boston, MA, USA
24 Patients with Disordered Sleep

Suzanne A. Bird, M.D.
Director, Acute Psychiatry Service,
Massachusetts General Hospital;
Assistant Professor of Psychiatry,
Harvard Medical School,
Boston, MA, USA
45 Emergency Psychiatry

Mark A. Blais, Psy.D.
Director, Psychological Evaluation and Research Laboratory, Department of Psychiatry,
Massachusetts General Hospital;
Associate Professor of Psychology,
Harvard Medical School,
Boston, MA, USA
7 Psychological and Neuropsychological Assessment

Rebecca Weintraub Brendel, M.D., J.D.
Associate Psychiatrist,
Massachusetts General Hospital;
Director, Master of Bioethics Degree Program,
Assistant Professor of Psychiatry,
Harvard Medical School,
Boston, MA, USA
44 Care of the Suicidal Patient
46 Care at the End of Life
51 Legal Aspects of Consultation

Keri O. Brenner, M.D., M.P.A.
Attending in Palliative Care and Psychiatry,
Massachusetts General Hospital;
Instructor in Psychiatry,
Harvard Medical School,
Boston, MA, USA
46 Care at the End of Life

George Bush, M.D., M.M.Sc.
Director, MGH Cingulate Cortex Research Laboratory,
MGH/MIT/HMS Athinoula A. Martinos Center for Functional and Structural Biomedical Imaging,
Massachusetts General Hospital,
Charlestown, MA, USA;
Associate Professor of Psychiatry,
Harvard Medical School,
Boston, MA, USA
23 Catatonia, Neuroleptic Malignant Syndrome, and Serotonin Syndrome

Joan A. Camprodon, M.D., M.P.H., Ph.D.
Director, Division of Neuropsychiatry,
Director, Laboratory for Neuropsychiatry and Neuromodulation,
Director, Transcranial Magnetic Stimulation (TMS) clinical service,
Massachusetts General Hospital;
Assistant Professor of Psychiatry,
Harvard Medical School,
Boston, MA, USA
5 Functional Neuroanatomy and the Neurologic Examination
37 Electroconvulsive Therapy and Neurotherapeutics

Jason P. Caplan, M.D.
Chair, Department of Psychiatry,
Creighton University School of Medicine at St. Joseph's Hospital and Medical Center,
Phoenix, AZ, USA
10 Delirious Patients

Andrew D. Carlo, M.D.
Acting Instructor and Senior Fellow,
University of Washington School of Medicine,
Seattle, WA, USA
52 Approaches to Collaborative Care and Behavioral Health Integration

Paolo Cassano, M.D., Ph.D.
Director of Photobiomodulation, Depression Clinical and Research Program, Department of Psychiatry,
Massachusetts General Hospital;
Assistant Professor of Psychiatry,
Harvard Medical School,
Boston, MA, USA
9 Depressed Patients

Christopher M. Celano, M.D.
Assistant Psychiatrist, Department of Psychiatry,
Massachusetts General Hospital;
Assistant Professor of Psychiatry,
Harvard Medical School,
Boston, MA, USA
26 The Psychiatric Management of Patients with Cardiac Disease

Deanna C. Chaukos, M.D.
Psychiatrist, Consultation-Liaison Psychiatry and Geriatric Psychiatry,
Mount Sinai Hospital;
Department of Psychiatry, University of Toronto Faculty of Medicine,
Toronto, Ontario, Canada
40 Mind–Body Medicine
53 Physician Well-being and Coping with the Rigors of Psychiatric Practice

Justin A. Chen, M.D., M.P.H.
Executive Director, MGH Center for Cross-Cultural Student Emotional Wellness,
Psychiatrist, MGH Depression Clinical and Research Program,
Massachusetts General Hospital;
Associate Director of Medical Student Education in Psychiatry,
Assistant Professor of Psychiatry,
Harvard Medical School,
Boston, MA, USA
50 Culture and Psychiatry

Jacqueline T. Chu, M.D.
Attending Physician,
Assistant in Medicine, Division of Infectious Diseases,
Massachusetts General Hospital,
Boston, MA, USA
30 Patients with Human Immunodeficiency Virus Infection and Acquired Immunodeficiency Syndrome

Lee S. Cohen, M.D.
Director, Ammon-Pinizzotto Center for Women's Mental Health,
Massachusetts General Hospital;
Edmund and Carroll Carpenter Professor of Psychiatry,
Harvard Medical School,
Boston, MA, USA
49 Psychiatric Illness during Pregnancy and the Postpartum Period

Mary K. Colvin, Ph.D., A.B.P.P.
Clinical Neuropsychologist, Department of Psychiatry,
Massachusetts General Hospital;
Assistant Professor of Psychology,
Harvard Medical School,
Boston, MA, USA
7 Psychological and Neuropsychological Assessment

Kathryn Coniglio, B.A.
Clinical Research Coordinator, Eating Disorders Clinical and Research Program,
Massachusetts General Hospital,
Boston, MA, USA
17 Patients with an Eating Disorder

M. Cornelia Cremens, M.D., M.P.H.
Psychiatrist,
Massachusetts General Hospital;
Co-Chair, Edwin H. Cassem Optimum Care (Ethics) Committee,
Assistant Professor of Psychiatry,
Harvard Medical School,
Boston, MA, USA
46 Care at the End of Life
48 Care of the Geriatric Patient

Cristina Cusin, M.D.
Psychiatrist,
Massachusetts General Hospital;
Assistant Professor of Psychiatry,
Harvard Medical School,
Boston, MA, USA
37 Electroconvulsive Therapy and Neurotherapeutics

Abigail L. Donovan, M.D.
Director, First Episode and Early Psychosis Program,
Associate Director, Acute Psychiatry Service,
Massachusetts General Hospital;
Assistant Professor of Psychiatry,
Harvard Medical School,
Boston, MA, USA
45 Emergency Psychiatry
53 Physician Well-being and Coping with the Rigors of Psychiatric Practice

Michelle P. Durham, M.D., M.P.H., F.A.P.A.
Residency Training Director, General Psychiatry Residency,
Associate Director, Global and Local Center for Mental Health Disparities,
Attending Adult, Child and Adolescent Psychiatrist,
Boston Medical Center;
Assistant Professor of Psychiatry,
Boston University School of Medicine,
Boston, MA, USA
50 Culture and Psychiatry

A. Eden Evins, M.D., M.P.H.
Director, Center for Addiction Medicine,
Massachusetts General Hospital;
William Cox Family Professor of Psychiatry in the Field of Addiction Medicine,
Harvard Medical School,
Boston, MA, USA
41 Chronic Disease and Unhealthy Habits: Behavioral Management

Maurizio Fava, M.D.
Director of the Division of Clinical Research of the MGH Research Institute,
Executive Vice Chair, Department of Psychiatry,
Executive Director, Clinical Trials Network and Institute (CTNI),
Massachusetts General Hospital;
Associate Dean for Clinical and Translational Research and Slater Family Professor of Psychiatry,
Harvard Medical School,
Boston, MA, USA
9 Depressed Patients
38 Psychopharmacology in the Medical Setting

Carlos G. Fernandez-Robles, M.D.
Clinical Director, Center for Psychiatric Oncology and Behavioral Sciences,
Associate Director, Somatic Therapies Service,
Psychiatrist, The Avery D. Weisman Psychiatric Consultation Service,
Massachusetts General Hospital;
Assistant Professor of Psychiatry,
Harvard Medical School,
Boston, MA, USA
31 Patients with Cancer
37 Electroconvulsive Therapy and Neurotherapeutics

Christine T. Finn, M.D.
Vice Chair for Education, Psychiatry,
Dartmouth Hitchcock Medical Center;
Assistant Professor of Psychiatry,
Geisel School of Medicine,
Lebanon, NH, USA
35 Patients with Genetic Syndromes

Alice W. Flaherty, M.D., Ph.D.
Attending Physician, Neurology and Psychiatry,
Massachusetts General Hospital;
Associate Professor of Neurology and Psychiatry,
Harvard Medical School,
Boston, MA, USA
21 Patients with Abnormal Movements

Rosanna Fox, M.B.B.S.
Medical Student,
University College London,
London, UK
17 Patients with an Eating Disorder

Elizabeth Pegg Frates, M.D.
Director, Wellness Programming,
Stroke Institute for Research and Recovery,
Spaulding Rehabilitation Hospital,
Charlestown, MA, USA;
Assistant Professor (Part-Time), Department of Physical Medicine and Rehabilitation,
Harvard Medical School,
Boston, MA, USA
41 Chronic Disease and Unhealthy Habits: Behavioral Management

Marlene P. Freeman, M.D.
Associate Director, Perinatal and Reproductive Psychiatry Program,
Massachusetts General Hospital;
Associate Professor of Psychiatry,
Harvard Medical School,
Boston, MA, USA
49 Psychiatric Illness during Pregnancy and the Postpartum Period

Oliver Freudenreich, M.D.
Co-Director, Massachusetts General Hospital Schizophrenia Clinical and Research Program,
Erich Lindemann Mental Health Center;
Associate Professor of Psychiatry,
Harvard Medical School,
Boston, MA, USA
12 Psychotic Patients
21 Patients with Abnormal Movements
30 Patients with Human Immunodeficiency Virus Infection and Acquired Immunodeficiency Syndrome

Gregory L. Fricchione, M.D.
Director, Benson-Henry Institute for Mind Body Medicine,
Director Emeritus, Division of Psychiatry and Medicine,
Massachusetts General Hospital;
Mind Body Medical Professor of Psychiatry,
Harvard Medical School,
Boston, MA, USA
1 Beginnings: Psychosomatic Medicine and Consultation Psychiatry in the General Hospital
23 Catatonia, Neuroleptic Malignant Syndrome, and Serotonin Syndrome
32 Burn Patients
33 Chronic Medical Illness and Rehabilitation
40 Mind–Body Medicine
41 Chronic Disease and Unhealthy Habits: Behavioral Management
50 Culture and Psychiatry

Taha Gholipour, M.D.
Neurologist, Department of Neurology, Division of Epilepsy,
Brigham and Women's Hospital;
Instructor in Neurology,
Harvard Medical School,
Boston, MA, USA
19 Patients with Seizure Disorders

Sean P. Glass, M.D.
Assistant in Psychiatry,
Massachusetts General Hospital;
Instructor in Psychiatry,
Harvard Medical School,
Boston, MA, USA
13 Anxious Patients
27 Patients with Renal Disease
28 Patients with Gastrointestinal Disease
32 Burn Patients

Donald C. Goff, M.D.
Director,
Nathan Kline Institute for Psychiatric Research;
Vice Chair for Research in Psychiatry,
NYU Langone Medical Center;
Marvin Stern Professor of Psychiatry,
NYU School of Medicine,
New York, NY, USA
12 Psychotic Patients

Christopher Gordon, M.D.
Medical Director, Senior Vice President,
Advocates,
Framingham, MA, USA;
Associate Professor (Part-Time) of Psychiatry,
Harvard Medical School,
Boston, MA, USA
3 The Doctor–Patient Relationship
4 The Psychiatric Interview

Donna B. Greenberg, M.D.
Psychiatrist,
Director Education Psychiatric Oncology and Medical Student Teaching
Massachusetts General Hospital;
Associate Professor of Psychiatry,
Harvard Medical School,
Boston, MA, USA
16 Psychosomatic Conditions: Somatic Symptom and Related Disorders, Functional Somatic Syndromes, and Deception Syndromes
31 Patients with Cancer

Anne F. Gross, M.D.
Medical Director, Psychiatric Emergency Service,
Unity Behavioral Health;
Director, Psychosomatic Medicine Fellowship,
Associate Professor of Psychiatry,
Oregon Health and Science University,
Portland, OR, USA
23 Catatonia, Neuroleptic Malignant Syndrome, and Serotonin Syndrome
36 Coping with Illness and Psychotherapy of the Medically Ill

James E. Groves, M.D.
Psychiatrist,
Massachusetts General Hospital;
Associate Professor of Psychiatry,
Harvard Medical School,
Boston, MA, USA
36 Coping with Illness and Psychotherapy of the Medically Ill
43 Difficult Patients

Eric P. Hazen, M.D.
Director, Pediatric Psychiatry Consultation Service, Child and Adolescent Psychiatry,
Massachusetts General Hospital;
Assistant Professor of Psychiatry,
Harvard Medical School,
Boston, MA, USA
47 Pediatric Consultation

David C. Henderson, M.D.
Professor and Chair, Psychiatry,
Boston University School of Medicine;
Psychiatrist-in-Chief, Psychiatry,
Boston Medical Center,
Boston, MA, USA
50 Culture and Psychiatry

Michael E. Henry, M.D.
Director, Somatic Therapy, Psychiatry,
Massachusetts General Hospital;
Lecturer in Psychiatry,
Harvard Medical School,
Boston, MA, USA
37 Electroconvulsive Therapy and Neurotherapeutics

Charlotte Hogan, M.D.
Assistant in Psychiatry, Department of Psychiatry,
Massachusetts General Hospital;
Instructor in Psychiatry
Harvard Medical School,
Boston, MA, USA
49 Psychiatric Illness during Pregnancy and the Postpartum Period

Daphne J. Holt, M.D., Ph.D.
Co-Director, MGH Schizophrenia Clinical and Research Program, Department of Psychiatry,
Massachusetts General Hospital;
Associate Professor of Psychiatry,
Harvard Medical School,
Boston, MA, USA
12 Psychotic Patients

Jeff C. Huffman, M.D.
Director, Cardiac Psychiatry Research Program,
Clinical Director, Department of Psychiatry,
Massachusetts General Hospital;
Associate Professor of Psychiatry,
Harvard Medical School,
Boston, MA, USA
19 Patients with Seizure Disorders
20 Patients with Cerebrovascular Disease and Traumatic Brain Injury
23 Catatonia, Neuroleptic Malignant Syndrome, and Serotonin Syndrome
26 The Psychiatric Management of Patients with Cardiac Disease

Aura M. Hurtado-Puerto, M.D.
Post-Doctoral Research Fellow, Laboratory for Neuropsychiatry and Neuromodulation, Transcranial Magnetic Stimulation Clinical Service, Department of Psychiatry, Division of Neurotherapeutics,
Massachusetts General Hospital,
Boston, MA, USA
37 Electroconvulsive Therapy and Neurotherapeutics

Kelly E. Irwin, M.D.
Director, Collaborative Care and Community Engagement Program,
Center for Psychiatric Oncology and Behavioral Sciences,
Massachusetts General Hospital;
Instructor in Psychiatry,
Harvard Medical School,
Boston, MA, USA
31 Patients with Cancer

Esther Jacobowitz Israel, M.D.
Associate Unit Chief, Department of Pediatric Gastroenterology and Nutrition,
Massachusetts General Hospital;
Assistant Professor of Pediatrics,
Harvard Medical School,
Boston, MA, USA
17 Patients with an Eating Disorder

Ana Ivkovic, M.D.
Psychiatrist,
Director, Transplant Psychiatry Service,
Massachusetts General Hospital;
Instructor in Psychiatry,
Harvard Medical School,
Boston, MA, USA
27 Patients with Renal Disease

James L. Januzzi, Jr., M.D., FACC, FESC
Physician, Cardiology Division,
Massachusetts General Hospital;
Hutter Family Professor of Medicine,
Harvard Medical School,
Boston, MA, USA
26 The Psychiatric Management of Patients with Cardiac Disease

Nasser Karamouz, M.D.
Assistant Professor (Part-Time) of Psychiatry,
Harvard Medical School,
Boston, MA, USA;
Consultant Psychiatrist,
Spaulding Rehabilitation Hospital,
Charlestown, MA, USA
33 Chronic Medical Illness and Rehabilitation

Tamar C. Katz, M.D., Ph.D.
Clinical Fellow, Pediatric Neuropsychiatry, Department of Psychiatry,
Boston Childrens' Hospital;
Clinical Fellow of Psychiatry,
Harvard Medical School,
Boston, MA, USA
35 Patients with Genetic Syndromes

Franklin King IV, M.D.
Fellow in Psychosomatic Medicine,
Massachusetts General Hospital;
Clinical Fellow in Psychiatry,
Harvard Medical School,
Boston, MA, USA
11 Patients with Neurocognitive Disorders
43 Difficult Patients

Katherine A. Koh, M.D., M.Sc.
Fellow in Psychiatry,
Massachusetts General Hospital;
Clinical Fellow in Psychiatry,
Harvard Medical School,
Boston, MA, USA
44 Care of the Suicidal Patient

Nicholas Kontos, M.D.
Director, Fellowship in Psychosomatic Medicine,
Massachusetts General Hospital;
Assistant Professor of Psychiatry,
Harvard Medical School,
Boston, MA, USA
1 Beginnings: Psychosomatic Medicine and Consultation Psychiatry in the General Hospital
6 Limbic Music: The Band Plays On
18 Psychosomatic Conditions: Somatic Symptom and Related Disorders, Functional Somatic Syndromes, and Deception Syndromes

John B. Levine, M.D., Ph.D.
Clinical Associate, Psychiatry,
Massachusetts General Hospital;
Consultant Psychiatrist,
Spaulding Rehabilitation Hospital,
Charlestown, MA, USA;
Assistant Professor (Part-Time) of Psychiatry,
Harvard Medical School,
Boston, MA, USA
33 Chronic Medical Illness and Rehabilitation

Kenny A. Lin, M.D.
Child and Adolescent Psychiatry Fellow,
Massachusetts General Hospital;
Clinical Fellow in Psychiatry,
Harvard Medical School,
Boston, MA, USA
47 Pediatric Consultation

Jenny J. Linnoila, M.D., Ph.D.
Assistant in Neurology and Associate Director of Autoimmune Neurology,
Massachusetts General Hospital;
Instructor in Neurology,
Harvard Medical School,
Boston, MA, USA
22 Patients with Infectious or Inflammatory Neuropsychiatric Impairment

Boris A. Lorberg, M.D.
Associate Medical Director, Adolescent Psychiatric Continuing Care Units,
Worcester Recovery Centre and Hospital;
Assistant Professor of Psychiatry and Pediatrics,
University of Massachusetts Medical School,
Worcester, MA, USA
39 Psychopharmacologic Management of Children and Adolescents

Andrea Madu, B.A.
Senior Research Assistant Disparities Solutions Center,
Massachusetts General Hospital,
Boston, MA, USA
50 Culture and Psychiatry

Thomas H. McCoy, M.D.
Assistant Psychiatrist,
Massachusetts General Hospital;
Member of the Faculty,
Harvard Medical School,
Boston, MA, USA
46 Care at the End of Life

David Mischoulon, M.D., Ph.D.
Director, Depression Clinical and Research Program,
Massachusetts General Hospital;
Associate Professor of Psychiatry,
Harvard Medical School,
Boston, MA, USA
8 Diagnostic Rating Scales and Laboratory Tests
42 Complementary Medicine and Natural Medications

Shamim H. Nejad, M.D.
Medical Director, Division of Psycho-Oncology,
Swedish Cancer Institute, Swedish Medical Center,
Seattle, WA, USA
14 Patients with Alcohol Use Disorder
15 Patients with Substance Use Disorders
18 Pain Patients
32 Burn Patients

Mladen Nisavic, M.D.
Assistant in Psychiatry,
Massachusetts General Hospital;
Instructor in Psychiatry,
Harvard Medical School,
Boston, MA, USA
14 Patients with Alcohol Use Disorder
15 Patients with Substance Use Disorders

Ruta Nonacs, M.D., Ph.D.
Assistant in Psychiatry Department of Psychiatry,
Massachusetts General Hospital;
Instructor in Psychiatry,
Harvard Medical School,
Boston, MA, USA
49 Psychiatric Illness during Pregnancy and the Postpartum Period

Dennis K. Norman, Ed.D., A.B.P.P.
Senior Psychologist, Department of Psychiatry,
Massachusetts General Hospital,
Boston, MA, USA;
Faculty Chair, Harvard University Native American Program,
Harvard University,
Cambridge, MA, USA
7 Psychological and Neuropsychological Assessment

Sheila M. O'Keefe, Ed.D.
Director of Psychology Training,
Director of Clinical Operations, Learning and Emotional Assessment Program, Department of Psychiatry,
Massachusetts General Hospital;
Assistant Professor of Psychology,
Harvard Medical School,
Boston, MA, USA
7 Psychological and Neuropsychological Assessment

Michael W. Otto, Ph.D.
Director, Translational Research Program,
Center for Anxiety and Related Disorders;
Boston University Professor, Department of Psychological and Brain Sciences,
Boston University,
Boston, MA, USA
13 Anxious Patients

Micaela B. Owusu, M.D., M.Sc.
Fellow in Psychiatry,
Massachusetts General Hospital;
Clinical Fellow in Psychiatry,
Harvard Medical School,
Boston, MA, USA
40 Mind–Body Medicine

George I. Papakostas, M.D.
Scientific Director, Clinical Trial Network and Institute,
Massachusetts General Hospital;
Associate Professor of Psychiatry,
Harvard Medical School,
Boston, MA, USA
9 Depressed Patients

Elyse R. Park, Ph.D., M.P.H.
Director of Behavioral Health Research, MGH Benson Henry Institute for Mind Body Medicine,
Director of Behavioral Sciences, MGH Tobacco Treatment and Research Center,
Massachusetts General Hospital;
Associate Professor of Psychiatry,
Harvard Medical School,
Boston, MA, USA
40 Mind–Body Medicine
41 Chronic Disease and Unhealthy Habits: Behavioral Management

Roy H. Perlis, M.D., M.Sc.
Medical Director, Bipolar Clinic and Research Program,
Massachusetts General Hospital;
Professor of Psychiatry,
Harvard Medical School,
Boston, MA, USA
44 Care of the Suicidal Patient

William F. Pirl, M.D., M.P.H.
Associate Director,
Sylvester Comprehensive Cancer Center Cancer Support Services,
Associate Professor of Psychiatry,
Miller School of Medicine, University of Miami,
Coral Gables, FL, USA
31 Patients with Cancer

Mark H. Pollack, M.D.
Chairperson, Department of Psychiatry,
Rush Medical College;
Director, Road Home Program: Center for Veterans and Their Families,
Director, Center for Anxiety and Traumatic Stress,
Grainger Professor of Psychiatry,
Rush University Medical Center,
Chicago, IL, USA
13 Anxious Patients

Laura M. Prager, M.D.
Director, Child Psychiatry Emergency Consult Service,
Director, Transitional Age Youth Clinic,
Psychiatrist, Lung Transplant Team,
Massachusetts General Hospital;
Associate Professor of Psychiatry,
Harvard Medical School,
Boston, MA, USA
29 Organ Failure and Transplantation
45 Emergency Psychiatry

Jefferson B. Prince, M.D.
Vice-Chair, Department of Psychiatry, North Shore Medical Center,
Director, Child Psychiatry MassGeneral for Children at North Shore Medical Center,
Medical Director, Inpatient Pediatric Psychiatry, MassGeneral for Children at North Shore Medical Center,
Medical Co-Director, Massachusetts Child Psychiatry Access Project, Eastern Team,
Salem, MA, USA;
Staff, Child Psychiatry,
Massachusetts General Hospital;
Instructor in Psychiatry,
Harvard Medical School,
Boston, MA, USA
39 Psychopharmacologic Management of Children and Adolescents

John Querques, M.D.
Chief, Inpatient Services,
Associate Director, Psychiatry Residency Program, Department of Psychiatry,
Tufts Medical Center;
Associate Professor of Psychiatry,
Tufts University School of Medicine,
Boston, MA, USA
2 Approach to Psychiatric Consultations in the General Hospital
34 Intensive Care Unit Patients

Davin K. Quinn, M.D.
Chief, Division of Behavioral Health Consultation and Integration,
Chief, Division of Psychiatric Neuromodulation, Department of Psychiatry and Behavioral Sciences,
Associate Professor of Psychiatry,
University of New Mexico School of Medicine,
Albuquerque, NM, USA
24 Patients with Disordered Sleep

Ellen M. Robinson, R.N., Ph.D.
Nurse Ethicist and Co-Chair, Edwin H. Cassem Optimum Care (Ethics) Committee,
Massachusetts General Hospital,
Boston, MA, USA
46 Care at the End of Life

Joshua L. Roffman, M.D., M.M.sc.
Co-Director, Division of Psychiatric Neuroimaging,
Director of Research, Schizophrenia Clinical and Research Program, Department of Psychiatry,
Massachusetts General Hospital;
Associate Professor of Psychiatry,
Harvard Medical School,
Charlestown, MA, USA
8 Diagnostic Rating Scales and Laboratory Tests

Jerrold F. Rosenbaum, M.D.
Chief of Psychiatry,
Massachusetts General Hospital;
Stanley Cobb Professor of Psychiatry,
Harvard Medical School,
Boston, MA, USA
13 Anxious Patients
38 Psychopharmacology in the Medical Setting

Kristin Russell, M.D., M.B.A.
Psychiatrist, Department of Psychiatry,
Massachusetts General Hospital;
Instructor in Psychiatry,
Harvard Medical School,
Boston, MA, USA
17 Patients with an Eating Disorder

Kassem Safa, M.D.
Transplant Nephrologist, Transplant Center and Division of Nephrology,
Massachusetts General Hospital;
Instructor in Medicine,
Harvard Medical School,
Boston, MA, USA
27 Patients with Renal Disease

Joel Salinas, M.D., M.B.A., M.Sc.
Instructor in Cognitive Behavioral Neurology and Neuropsychiatry, Neurology,
Massachusetts General Hospital;
Instructor in Neurology,
Harvard Medical School,
Boston, MA, USA
5 Functional Neuroanatomy and the Neurologic Examination

Steven C. Schlozman, M.D.
Associate Director, The Clay Center for Young Healthy Minds,
Course Director, Psychiatry and Psychopathology, Health Science And Technology Program at Harvard Medical School and MIT,
Staff Psychiatrist and Consultant, Pediatric Solid Organ Transplant Team,
Massachusetts General Hospital;
Assistant Professor of Psychiatry,
Harvard Medical School,
Boston, MA, USA
36 Coping with Illness and Psychotherapy of the Medically Ill

Ronald Schouten, M.D., J.D.
Director, Law and Psychiatry Service,
Massachusetts General Hospital;
Associate Professor of Psychiatry,
Harvard Medical School,
Boston, MA, USA
51 Legal Aspects of Consultation

Linda C. Shafer, M.D.
Psychiatrist,
Massachusetts General Hospital;
Assistant Professor of Psychiatry,
Harvard Medical School,
Boston, MA, USA
25 Sexual Disorders or Sexual Dysfunction

Benjamin G. Shapero, Ph.D.
Assistant in Psychology, Department of Psychiatry,
Massachusetts General Hospital;
Member of Faculty,
Harvard Medical School,
Boston, MA, USA
9 Depressed Patients

Janet Sherman, Ph.D.
Clinical Director, Psychology Assessment Center, Department of Psychiatry,
Massachusetts General Hospital;
Assistant Professor of Psychology,
Harvard Medical School,
Boston, MA, USA
7 Psychological and Neuropsychological Assessment

Patrick Smallwood, M.D.
Vice Chair, Adult Clinical Services,
UMass Memorial Healthcare;
Assistant Professor of Psychiatry,
University of Massachusetts School of Medicine,
Worcester, MA, USA
24 Patients with Disordered Sleep

Felicia A. Smith, M.D.
Psychiatrist and Chief, Avery D. Weisman Psychiatry Consultation Service,
Director, Division of Psychiatry and Medicine,
Massachusetts General Hospital;
Assistant Professor of Psychiatry,
Harvard Medical School,
Boston, MA, USA
16 Psychosomatic Conditions: Somatic Symptom and Related Disorders, Functional Somatic Syndromes, and Deception Syndromes
19 Patients with Seizure Disorders
20 Patients with Cerebrovascular Disease and Traumatic Brain Injury
42 Complementary Medicine and Natural Medications
54 Management of a Psychiatric Consultation Service

Theodore A. Stern, M.D.
Psychiatrist and Chief Emeritus, Avery D. Weisman Psychiatry Consultation Service,
Director, Thomas P. Hackett Center for Scholarship in Psychosomatic Medicine,
Director, Office for Clinical Careers,
Massachusetts General Hospital;
Ned H. Cassem Professor of Psychiatry in the field of Psychosomatic Medicine/Consultation,
Harvard Medical School,
Boston, MA, USA
1 Beginnings: Psychosomatic Medicine and Consultation Psychiatry in the General Hospital
2 Approach to Psychiatric Consultations in the General Hospital
8 Diagnostic Rating Scales and Laboratory Tests
9 Depressed Patients
19 Patients with Seizure Disorders
20 Patients with Cerebrovascular Disease and Traumatic Brain Injury
23 Catatonia, Neuroleptic Malignant Syndrome, and Serotonin Syndrome
24 Patients with Disordered Sleep
26 The Psychiatric Management of Patients with Cardiac Disease
27 Patients with Renal Disease
34 Intensive Care Unit Patients
38 Psychopharmacology in the Medical Setting
39 Psychopharmacologic Management of Children and Adolescents
44 Care of the Suicidal Patient
53 Physician Well-being and Coping with the Rigors of Psychiatric Practice
54 Management of a Psychiatric Consultation Service

Jonathan R. Stevens, M.D., M.P.H.
Chief, Child and Adolescent Psychiatry,
Chief, Outpatient Services,
The Menninger Clinic;
Assistant Professor of Psychiatry and Behavioral Sciences,
Baylor College of Medicine,
Houston, TX, USA
38 Psychopharmacology in the Medical Setting
39 Psychopharmacologic Management of Children and Adolescents

Frederick J. Stoddard, Jr., M.D.
Chief of Psychiatry, Emeritus,
Shriners Hospital for Children;
Psychiatrist, Department of Psychiatry,
Massachusetts General Hospital;
Professor (Part-Time) of Psychiatry,
Harvard Medical School,
Boston, MA, USA
32 Burn Patients

Joan M. Stoler, M.D.
Clinical Geneticist, Division of Genetics and Genomics,
Boston Children's Hospital;
Assistant Professor of Pediatrics,
Harvard Medical School,
Boston, MA, USA
35 Patients with Genetic Syndromes

John B. Taylor, M.D., M.B.A.
Associate Fellowship Director, MGH Psychosomatic Medicine Fellowship,
Assistant Training Director, MGH/McLean Adult Psychiatry Residency,
Instructor in Psychiatry,
Harvard Medical School,
Massachusetts General Hospital,
Boston, MA, USA
6 Limbic Music: The Band Plays On
54 Management of a Psychiatric Consultation Service

Jennifer J. Thomas, Ph.D.
Co-Director, Eating Disorders Clinical and Research Program,
Massachusetts General Hospital;
Associate Professor of Psychology, Department of Psychiatry,
Harvard Medical School,
Boston, MA, USA
17 Patients with an Eating Disorder

Nhi-Ha Trinh, M.D., M.P.H.
Director, Department of Psychiatry Center for Diversity,
Director of Multicultural Studies, Depression Clinical and Research Program, Department of Psychiatry,
Massachusetts General Hospital;
Assistant Professor of Psychiatry,
Harvard Medical School,
Boston, MA, USA
50 Culture and Psychiatry

Mary C. Vance, M.D.
Psychiatry Resident, MGH-McLean Residency Program,
Clinical Fellow in Psychiatry,
Harvard Medical School,
Boston, MA, USA
27 Patients with Renal Disease

Amy F. Vyas, M.D.
Staff Psychiatrist,
The Menninger Clinic;
Assistant Professor of Psychiatry and Behavioral Sciences,
Baylor College of Medicine,
Houston, TX, USA
39 Psychopharmacologic Management of Children and Adolescents

Betty Wang, M.D.
Assistant in Psychiatry, Department of Psychiatry,
Massachusetts General Hospital;
Instructor in Psychiatry,
Harvard Medical School,
Boston, MA, USA
49 Psychiatric Illness during Pregnancy and the Postpartum Period

Eric M. Weil, M.D.
Chief Medical Officer, Primary Care,
Center for Population Health, Partners Healthcare;
General Internist,
Massachusetts General Hospital;
Assistant Professor of Medicine,
Harvard Medical School,
Boston, MA, USA
52 Approaches to Collaborative Care and Behavioral Health Integration

Anna R. Weissman, M.D.
Resident in Psychiatry,
Massachusetts General Hospital and McLean Hospital;
Clinical Fellow in Psychiatry,
Harvard Medical School,
Boston, MA, USA
6 Limbic Music: The Band Plays On

Ilse R. Wiechers, M.D., M.P.P., M.H.S.
Assistant Professor, Psychiatry,
Yale University School of Medicine,
New Haven, CT, USA;
National Program Director, Psychotropic Drug Safety Initiative,
Office of Mental Health and Suicide Prevention, Department of Veterans Affairs,
West Haven, CT, USA
11 Patients with Neurocognitive Disorders
48 Care of the Geriatric Patient

James M. Wilkins, M.D., D.Phil.
Assistant Medical Director, Cognitive Neuropsychiatry Unit,
McLean Hospital,
Belmont, MA, USA;
Instructor in Psychiatry,
Harvard Medical School,
Boston, MA, USA
48 Care of the Geriatric Patient

Curtis W. Wittmann, M.D.
Associate Director, Acute Psychiatry Services,
Massachusetts General Hospital;
Instructor in Psychiatry,
Harvard Medical School,
Boston, MA, USA
13 Anxious Patients

Lazaro V. Zayas, M.D.
Staff Psychiatrist, Eating Disorders Clinical and Research Program,
Assistant in Psychiatry,
Massachusetts General Hospital;
Instructor in Psychiatry,
Harvard Medical School,
Boston, MA, USA
17 Patients with an Eating Disorder

Beginnings: Psychosomatic Medicine and Consultation Psychiatry in the General Hospital

1

Theodore A. Stern, M.D.
Gregory L. Fricchione, M.D.
Nicholas Kontos, M.D.

PSYCHOSOMATIC MEDICINE

A keen interest in the relationship between the psyche and the soma has been maintained in medicine since early times, and certain ancient physicians (such as Hippocrates) have been eloquent on the subject. A search for the precise origins of psychosomatic medicine is, however, a difficult undertaking unless one chooses to focus on the first use of the term itself. Johann Heinroth appears to have coined the term *psychosomatic* in reference to certain causes of insomnia in 1818.[1] The word *medicine* was added to *psychosomatic* first by the psychoanalyst Felix Deutsch in the early 1920s.[2] Deutsch later emigrated to the United States with his wife Helene, and both worked at Massachusetts General Hospital (MGH) for a time in the 1930s and 1940s.

Three streams of thought flowed into the area of psychosomatic medicine, providing fertile ground for the growth of general hospital and consultation psychiatry.[3,4] The psychophysiologic school, perhaps represented by the Harvard physiologist, Walter B. Cannon, emphasized the effects of stress on the body.[5] The psychoanalytic school, best personified by the psychoanalyst Franz Alexander, focused on the effects that psychodynamic conflicts had on the body.[6] The organic synthesis point of view, ambitiously pursued by Helen Flanders Dunbar, tried with limited success to unify the physiologic and psychoanalytic approaches.[7] George Engel's biopsychosocial model[8] sought and seeks to apply not just these approaches, but all branches of knowledge to health-related considerations. It has perhaps had more impact on medical education than practice.[9] More recently, a higher overall profile for mind–body investigations practices is evident in mainstream medicine. These latter two trends affiliate themselves with medicine more broadly than these earlier approaches. While often championed by, and important to psychosomatic medicine, they are not its "property," *per se*.

HISTORY

The history of general hospital psychiatry in the United States in general,[10] and consultation–liaison (C-L) psychiatry in particular,[11] has been extensively reviewed elsewhere. For those interested in a more detailed account of both historic trends and conceptual issues of C-L psychiatry, the writings of Lipowski[12–17] are highly recommended.

In years gone by, controversy surrounded the use of the term *liaison* in C-L psychiatry. We believe that using the term *liaison* has been confusing and unnecessary. It has been confusing because no other service in the practice of medicine employed the term for its consultation activities. In addition, the activity it referred to—to teach non-psychiatrists psychiatric and interpersonal skills—is undertaken as a matter of course during the routine consultation. The term *liaison*, although still used, has come to be associated with educational and outreach efforts that run far afield of the original meaning of the word.

In March 2003, the American Board of Medical Specialties unanimously approved the American Board of Psychiatry and Neurology's (ABPN's) issuance of Subspecialty Certification in psychosomatic medicine. The first certifying examinations were administered in 2005. As of 2009, the completion of an American Board of Medical Specialties-certified fellowship in psychosomatic medicine became mandatory for all who wish to sit for that examination. The achievement of subspecialty status for psychosomatic medicine was the product of nearly 75 years of clinical work by psychiatrists on medical–surgical units, an impressive accumulation of scholarly work contributing to the psychiatric care of general medical patients, and determined intellectual and organizational efforts by the Academy of Psychosomatic Medicine (APM). The latter's efforts included settling on the name psychosomatic medicine after *C-L Psychiatry* met with resistance from the ABPN during the first application for subspecialty status in 1992.[18] Psychosomatic medicine was ultimately felt to best capture the field's heritage and work on mind–body relationships, though there remains controversy and continued deliberation over its nebulous boundaries and linguistic awkwardness.[19]

When the history of consultation psychiatry is examined, 1975 seems to be the watershed year. Before 1975, scant attention was given to the work of psychiatrists in general medicine. Consultation topics were seldom presented at the national meetings of the American Psychiatric Association. Even the American Psychosomatic Society, which has many strong links to consultation work, rarely gave more than a nod of acknowledgment to presentations or panels discussing this aspect of psychiatry. Residency training programs on the whole were no better. In 1966, Mendel[20] surveyed training programs in the United States to determine the extent to which residents were exposed to a training experience in consultation psychiatry. He found that 75% of the 202 programs surveyed offered some training in consultation psychiatry, but most of it was informal and poorly organized. Ten years later, Schubert and McKegney[21] found only "a slight increase" in the amount of time devoted to C-L training in residency programs. Today, C-L training is mandated by the ABPN as part of general adult psychiatry training.

Several factors account for the growth of C-L psychiatry in the last quarter of the 20th century. One was the leadership of Dr. James Eaton, former director of the Psychiatric Education Branch of the National Institute of Mental Health (NIMH). Eaton provided the support and encouragement that enabled the creation of C-L programs throughout the United States. Another reason for this growth was the burgeoning interest in primary care, which required skills in psychiatric diagnosis and treatment. Finally, parallel yet related threats to the viability of the psychiatric profession from third-party payers and non-physician providers were an incentive to (re-)medicalize the field. Although creation of the *Diagnostic and Statistical Manual of Mental Disorders* (3rd edition; DSM-III), and increased pharmacotherapy were the two most obvious upshots of this trend,[22,23] an elevated profile for C-L psychiatry also emerged as uniquely tailored to the psychiatrist's skill set. For these reasons, and because of expanding knowledge in neuropsychiatry, consultation work enjoyed a renaissance.

The origins of organized interest in the mental life of patients at the MGH dates back to 1873, when James Jackson Putnam, a young Harvard neurologist, returned from his grand tour of German Departments of Medicine to practice his specialty. He was awarded a small office under the arch of one of the famous twin flying staircases of the Bulfinch Building. The office was the size of a cupboard and was designed to house electrical equipment. Putnam was given the title of "electrician." One of his duties was to ensure the proper function of various galvanic and faradic devices then used to treat nervous and muscular disorders. It is no coincidence that his office came to be called the "cloaca maxima" by Professor of Medicine George Shattuck. This designation stemmed from the fact that patients whose maladies defied diagnosis and treatment—in short, referred to as the "crocks"—were referred to young Putnam. With such a beginning, it is not difficult for today's consultation psychiatrist to relate to Putnam's experience and mission. Putnam eventually became a Professor of Neuropathology and practiced both neurology and psychiatry, treating medical and surgical patients who developed mental disorders. Putnam's distinguished career, interwoven with the acceptance of Freudian psychology in the United States, is chronicled elsewhere.[24]

In the late 1920s, Dr. Howard Means, Chief of Medicine, appointed Boston psychiatrist William Herman to study patients who developed mental disturbances in conjunction with endocrine disorders. Herman's studies are hardly remembered today, although he was honored by having a conference room at the MGH named after him.

In 1934, the Department of Psychiatry took shape when Stanley Cobb was given the Bullard Chair of Neuropathology and granted sufficient money by the Rockefeller Foundation to establish a ward for the study of psychosomatic conditions. Under Cobb's tutelage, the Department expanded and became known for its eclecticism and for its interest in the mind–brain relationship. A number of European emigrants fled Nazi tyranny and were welcomed to the department by Cobb. Felix and Helene Deutsch, Edward and Grete Bibring, and Hans Sachs were early arrivals from the continent. Erich Lindemann came in the mid-1930s and worked with Cobb on a series of projects, the most notable being his study of grief, which came as a result of his work with victims of the 1942 Cocoanut Grove nightclub fire.

When Lindemann became Chief of the Psychiatric Service in 1954, the Consultation Service had not yet been established. Customarily, the resident assigned to night call in the Emergency Department saw all medical and surgical patients in need of psychiatric evaluation. This was regarded as an onerous task, and such calls were often set aside until after supper in the hope that the disturbance might quiet in the intervening hours. Notes in the chart were terse and often impractical. Seldom was there any follow-up. As a result, animosity toward psychiatry grew. To remedy this, Lindemann officially established the Psychiatric Consultation Service under the leadership of Avery Weisman in 1956. Weisman's resident, Thomas Hackett, divided his time between doing consultations and learning outpatient psychotherapy. During the first year of the consultation service, 130 consultations were performed. In 1958, the number of consultations increased to 370, and an active research program was organized that later became one of the cornerstones of the overall operation and part of its legacy of scholarship.

By 1960, a rotation through the Consultation Service had become a mandatory part of the MGH residency in psychiatry. Second-year residents were each assigned two wards. Each resident spent 20 to 30 hours a week on the Consultation Service for 6 months. Between 1956 and 1960, the service attracted the interest of fellowship students, who contributed postgraduate work on psychosomatic topics. Medical students also began to choose the Consultation Service as part of their elective in psychiatry during this period. From our work with these fellows and medical students, collaborative research studies were initiated with other services. Examples of these early studies are the surgical treatment of intractable pain,[25,26] the compliance of duodenal ulcer patients with their medical regimen,[27] post-amputation depression in the elderly patient,[28] emotional maladaptation in the surgical patient,[29–32] and the psychological aspects of acute myocardial infarction.[33,34]

By 1970, Hackett, then Chief of the Consultation Service, had one full-time (postgraduate year [PGY]-IV) chief resident and six half-time (PGY-III) residents to see consultations from the approximately 400 house beds. A private Psychiatric Consultation Service was begun, to systematize consultations for the 600 private beds of the hospital. A Somatic Therapies Service was created and it offered electroconvulsive therapy to treat refractory conditions. Three fellows and a full-time faculty member were added to the roster in 1976. Edwin (Ned) Cassem became Chief of the Consultation Service, and George Murray was appointed director of a new fellowship program in psychosomatic medicine. In 1995, Theodore Stern was named Chief of the Avery Weisman

Psychiatric Consultation Service. Now both fellows and residents take consultations in rotation from throughout the hospital. Our Child Psychiatry Division, composed of residents, fellows, and attending physicians, provides full consultation to the 50 beds of the MGH Hospital for Children.

In July 2002, Gregory Fricchione was appointed director of the new Division of Psychiatry and Medicine, with a mission to integrate the various inpatient and outpatient medical–psychiatry services at the MGH and its affiliates, while maintaining the diverse characteristics and strengths of each unit. The Division includes the Avery D. Weisman Psychiatry Consultation Service; the MGH Center for Psychiatric Oncology and Behavioral Sciences at the Massachusetts General Hospital Cancer Center; the Transplant Psychiatry Consultation Service; the Trauma and Burns Psychiatry Service; the HIV and Infectious Disease Psychiatry Service; the Primary Care Psychiatry Service; the Pain Center Psychiatry Service; the Cardiovascular Disease Prevention Center Service; the Behavioral Medicine Service; and the Spaulding Rehabilitation Hospital's Behavioral and Mental Health Service.

THE CONSULTATION SERVICE

The three functions provided by any consultation service are: patient care, teaching, and research.

Patient Care

At the MGH, between 11% and 13% of all admitted patients are followed by the Psychiatric Consultation Service psychiatrist; more than 3500 initial consultations are performed each year. An additional 5% of inpatients with substance-related problems are seen by our newly created Addictions Consultation Team (ACT). The problems discovered reflect the gamut of conditions listed in the DSM-5;[35] however, the most common reasons for consultation are related to depression, delirium, anxiety, substance abuse, character pathology, dementia, somatic symptom disorders, or medically unexplained symptoms, and the evaluation of capacity.

Patients are seen in consultation only at the request of another physician, who must write an order for the consultation. When performing a consultation, the psychiatrist, like any other physician, is expected to provide a diagnosis and treatment recommendations. This includes defining the reason for the consultation; reading the chart; gathering information from nurses and family members when indicated; interviewing the patient; performing the appropriate physical and neurologic examinations; writing a clear consultation note in the electronic medical record with a clinical impression and treatment plan; ordering or suggesting laboratory tests, procedures, and medications; speaking with the referring physician when indicated; and making follow-up visits until the patient's problems are resolved, the patient is discharged, or the patient dies.

Interviewing style, individual to begin with, is further challenged and refined in the consultation arena, where the psychiatrist is presented with a patient who typically did not ask to be seen and who is often put off by the very idea that a psychiatrist has been called. In addition, the hospital room setting and the threat of acute illness might cause the patient to be either more or less forthcoming than under usual circumstances. The stigma of mental illness and the fear of any illness are universal; they are part of every physician's territory, and each psychiatrist learns to deal with them in a unique way. Residents learn to coax cooperation from such patients by trial and error, by self-understanding, and by observing role models, rather than by observing formulas. Essential, however, are interest in the patient's medical situation and an approach that is comparable with that used by a rigorous and caring physician in any specialty. Each consultation can thus be viewed as an opportunity to provide care, to de-stigmatize mental illness, and to de-stigmatize psychiatry by personally representing it, via manner, tone, and examination, as a proper medical specialty.

Teaching

Teaching psychiatry to medical and surgical house officers on a formal basis can be challenging. More than 50 years ago, Lindemann, in an attempt to educate medical house officers about the emotional problems of their patients, enlisted the help of several psychiatric luminaries from the Boston area. A series of biweekly lectures was announced, in which Edward and Grete Bibring, Felix and Helene Deutsch, Stanley Cobb, and Carl Binger, among others, shared their knowledge and skills. In the beginning, approximately one-fifth of the medical house officers attended. Attendance steadily dwindled in subsequent sessions until finally the psychiatry residents were required to attend, so as to infuse the lecturers with enough spirit to continue. This might be alleged to illustrate disinterest or intimidation on the part of the non-psychiatric staff, but we think that such didactics were simply too far removed (geographically and philosophically) from their day-to-day work.

We believe that teaching, to be most effective and reliable, is best done at the bedside on a case-by-case basis. Each resident is paired with an attending physician for bedside supervision, and all new patients are interviewed by our consultation attending staff. Residents teach as well. Medical students, neurology residents, and other visiting trainees are supervised by PGY-III residents, the chief resident, the fellows, and our attending staff. Twice weekly, rounds are held with Stern, the chief resident, and the rest of the service. In 90 to 120 minutes, new and ongoing cases are discussed in significant depth, with a focus as much on habits of thought as on medical knowledge and problem-solving.

Before each group of residents begin their 4-month half-time rotation (in July, November, and March), they receive 25 introductory lectures on practical topics (e.g., how to perform a consultation; how to write the note; how to perform the neurologic or neuropsychological examination; the nature of normal and maladaptive coping; ruling out organic causes of psychiatric symptoms; the interface of psychiatry and oncology; diagnosing delirium and dementia; using psychotropic medications in the medically ill; assessing decisional capacity; geriatric psychiatry; performing hypnosis; identifying factitious disorders and malingering; assessment and management of depression; anxiety; post-traumatic stress disorder; pain; substance use/abuse/withdrawal; and managing functional somatic symptoms). In concert with the orientation lecture series, we provide residents with relevant articles, with an annotated bibliography,[36] and with updates in psychosomatic medicine.[37] The overall curriculum we provide is quite similar to that recommended by the APM's Task Force on Residency Training in C-L Psychiatry.[38]

Fellows also attend the rounds with Fricchione (Director Emeritus) and Nicholas Kontos (Director), as well as a "deep bench" of former fellows who preside three times per week. In addition to routine staffing of cases, fellows see patients at the bedside with senior attending staff, including Kontos and Fricchione, weekly. Fellows have an additional 2 hours per week of didactic sessions on advanced topics of psychosomatic medicine, neuropsychiatry, leadership, service delivery, and guided readings in psychodynamics, as well as attend the Department's monthly Morbidity and Mortality Conference; they also have individual supervision with Kontos or Fricchione each week. The Fellowship Program in psychosomatic medicine, largely under the leadership of Murray, is entering its 40th year; it has trained 118 fellows as of this writing. Many graduates have gone on to direct C-L programs and Departments of Psychiatry across the United States.

Each resident and fellow makes two formal presentations (i.e., 45-minute reviews of the literature on topics chosen by the resident, and elaborated on by a senior discussant for 45 minutes). These weekly Psychosomatic Conferences not only produce presentations of high quality but also lead to improved speaking skills, occasional publications, and the beginning of specialized interests and expertise for the resident.[39–86]

Research

Research activity by the Consultation Service, besides answering important questions, builds bridges between medical specialties. When physicians from other services are involved in research planning and when there is dual authorship of published accounts, friendships are firmly bonded, and differences fade. Eventually, multisite collaborations become possible. The general hospital population provides such a cornucopia of academic material that a consultation service would be lax or unresponsive not to take advantage of it. Examples ranging from multisite studies, to reviews, to case reports, and conceptual papers are cited here and in the chapters that follow.[80–115]

Small projects are the cornerstone of larger ones. So long as generativity is held as a value, research need not be funded through federal or state agencies, and scholarliness need not be confined to research. Projects can be assigned as such to medical students during their month on the service. They can also be suggested to fellows for more extensive development over the course of the year. What begins as a project to be presented at psychiatric grand rounds can, over a year, develop into a fully fledged publication. This, in turn, might be the starting point for a larger investigation, and, sometimes, a career.

A filing system should be designed to keep potential research materials readily accessible through a shared hard drive. While journals are increasingly digitizing their back catalogs, the use of computerized file systems can be supplemented by a well-curated, non-virtual file of classic articles in the field.

Once the direction of the consultation team has been pointed toward research, scholarship, and publication, the results usually fall into line. One of the distressing roadblocks en route to publication is the poor writing skills of many physicians. One or two resource people who can serve as editors and teachers can be of great help. For almost four decades, we have held a biweekly writing seminar, in which members submit manuscripts that are reviewed by the seminar group and Dr. Stern. The late Eleanor Hackett was pivotal in co-founding and co-running this group. All efforts seem worthwhile once the printed or digital page ends up before the authors' eyes. When a service begins to develop a file of publications authored by various members of the team, a pride of accomplishment exists, and this compounds the excitement of the research and stimulates renewed academic effort. This intramural effort also builds the outside profile of the service, through publication in a broad array of journals, especially when this also involves non-psychiatric journals.

RECENT DIRECTIONS

The approval of psychosomatic medicine as a psychiatric subspecialty brings with it changes in many domains of our service. Interestingly, some of these are revivals of older patterns of service provision to various medical domains. Perhaps inevitably, subspecialization invites sub-subspecialization. Over the past decades, particular staff members carved out sectors of the hospital as areas of interest/work (e.g., burns, surgery, medical intensive care, rehabilitation, cardiology, dermatology, oncology, orthopedics, obstetrics, and gynecology). After a while, the pendulum swung toward a more global, general consultation service. In more recent years, the pendulum has swung back, with more formalized re-entry of staff into many of these areas, as well as into some others (e.g., infectious disease, gastroenterology).

Connected with this trend, fueled by a robust literature,[116–118] and codified in the Accreditation Council for Graduate Medical Education requirements for psychosomatic medicine fellowship training, is the provision of "outpatient consultation" to primary care settings. Recognizing the importance of this latter approach, MGH is developing collaborative and integrated care systems, supplemented by telemedicine/video-conferencing for our satellite clinics, to be of help to our primary care colleagues and to better serve our system's population of patients in need of psychiatric assistance. These endeavors expand potential training experiences and academic opportunities and introduce new logistical challenges to the administration of consultation psychiatry and psychosomatic medicine services.

Psychosomatic medicine, by virtue of the premium it places on effective communication with other specialties and systems, and its understanding of the interface between medical illnesses and psychiatric disorders, is well suited to participate in global mental health, an important undertaking given the enormous global burden of disease secondary to neuropsychiatric disorders. Psychosomatic medicine also has a large role to play in population health promotion and illness prevention. The knowledge base we use to help manage acute illnesses in the general hospital can be exploited to reduce stress and enhance resilience, leading to a field called *mind–body medicine*, which links up clinical medicine and public health. At MGH, these principles are keynotes of the Chester M. Pierce, M.D., Division of Global Psychiatry and of the Benson-Henry Institute for Mind Body Medicine.

SUMMARY

From early in medical history, curious physicians have investigated the mysteries of the mind–body relationship, developing a field of study called psychosomatic medicine. The energy of this intellectual enterprise has led to the growth of general hospital psychiatry, initially aided by Rockefeller Foundation funding in 1934, as well as the development of consultation psychiatry, supported through the funding of Eaton's NIMH program in the 1970s and 1980s. The subspecialty of psychiatry called psychosomatic medicine has recently been approved, which recognizes the maturation of the field and the growth that lies ahead.

At each step of the way, the MGH Psychiatric Consultation Service has played an important role. This book, which reviews the essentials of general hospital psychiatry, is a testimony to the caring, creativity, and diligence of those who have come before us.

REFERENCES

Access the reference list online at https://expertconsult.inkling.com/.

Approach to Psychiatric Consultations in the General Hospital

2

John Querques, M.D.
Theodore A. Stern, M.D.

My emphasis to the residents is: 'Now that you've learned a lot about compassion and human dignity … you must learn to be competent,' adding 'or else.' The goals for the trainee are specialty-competence, that is, some specific things about consultation: accountability, commitment, industry, discipline; these are the components that go into the make-up of a professional.

— Ned H. Cassem, M.D.[1]

This chapter provides a practical approach to the assessment of affective, behavioral, and cognitive problems of patients in the general hospital. We first survey the landscape of consultation psychiatry and then identify six broad domains of psychiatric problems commonly encountered in the medical setting. Next, we describe the differences in clinical approach, environment, interactive style, and use of language that distinguish psychiatry in the general hospital from practice in other venues. Then we offer a step-by-step guide to the conduct of a psychiatric consultation. The chapter concludes with a review of treatment principles critical to caring for the medically ill. Throughout this chapter, we emphasize the hallmarks of competence identified by Cassem[1] more than three decades ago: accountability, commitment, industry, and discipline.

CATEGORIES OF PSYCHIATRIC DIFFERENTIAL DIAGNOSIS IN THE GENERAL HOSPITAL

The borderland between psychiatry and medicine, in which consultation psychiatrists ply their trade can be visualized as the area shared by two intersecting circles in a Venn diagram (Figure 2-1). As depicted in the figure and consistent with the fundamental tenet of psychosomatic medicine (i.e., that mind and body are indivisible), the likelihood that either a psychiatric or a medical condition will have no impact on the other is incredibly slim. Within the broad region of bi-directional influence (the area of overlap in the Venn diagram), the problems most commonly encountered on a consultation–liaison (C-L) service can be grouped into six categories (modified from Lipowski;[2] see Figure 2-1). Examples of each classification follow.

Psychiatric Presentations of Medical Conditions

CASE 1

An elderly man underwent neurosurgery for clipping of an aneurysm of the anterior communicating artery. A few days after surgery, he became diaphoretic, confused, and agitated and was tachycardic and hypertensive. Because of a history of alcoholism, a diagnosis of alcohol withdrawal delirium was made. He remained confused, despite aggressive benzodiazepine treatment. When he later became febrile, a lumbar puncture was done and the cerebrospinal fluid (CSF) analysis was consistent with herpes simplex virus (HSV) infection. His sensorium cleared after a course of acyclovir.

In this case, infection of the central nervous system (CNS) by HSV was heralded by delirium.

Psychiatric Complications of Medical Conditions or Treatments

CASE 2

Newly diagnosed with human immunodeficiency virus (HIV) infection with a high viral load, a young man without a history of psychiatric illness began treatment with efavirenz, a non-nucleoside reverse transcriptase inhibitor. Within a few days, he experienced vivid nightmares; a known side effect of efavirenz. Over the next several weeks, the nightmares resolved. He continued antiretroviral treatment, but became increasingly despondent with a full complement of neurovegetative symptoms of major depression.

A chronic, incurable viral illness—the treatment of which caused a neuropsychiatric complication—precipitated a depressive episode.

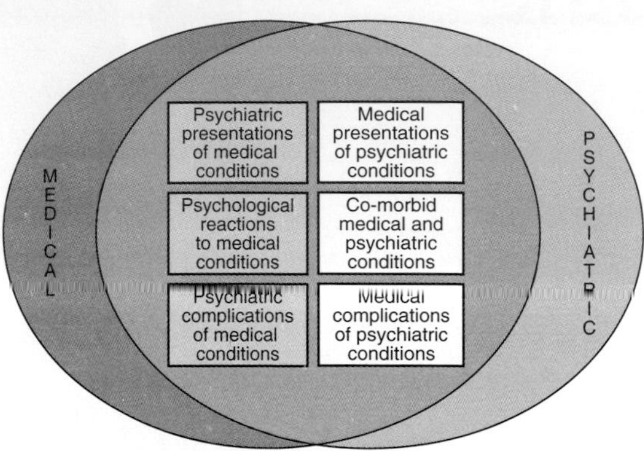

Figure 2-1. A representation of the overlap between medical and psychiatric care.

Psychological Reactions to Medical Conditions or Treatments

CASE 3

A woman with a history of pre-eclampsia during her first pregnancy was admitted with hypertension in the 38th week of her second pregnancy. Pre-eclampsia was diagnosed, and she delivered a healthy baby. As she prepared for discharge, and despite her obstetrician's reassurance, she fretted that a hypertensive catastrophe was going to befall her at home.

Pathologic anxiety resulting from an acute obstetric condition.

Medical Presentations of Psychiatric Conditions

CASE 4

A young female graduate student from another country, who for several years had habitually induced vomiting to relieve persistent abdominal pain, presented with generalized weakness and was found to have low serum potassium. She had long since been diagnosed with bulimia nervosa, but the psychiatric consultant found no evidence for this disorder and instead diagnosed conversion disorder, construing her chronic abdominal pain as a converted symptom of psychological distress over leaving her family to study abroad.

Conversion disorder presenting as persistent abdominal pain.

Medical Complications of Psychiatric Conditions or Treatments

CASE 5

An obese man with schizophrenia treated with olanzapine gained 30 pounds in 6 months. Repeated measurements of fasting serum glucose were consistent with a diagnosis of diabetes mellitus.

Treatment with an atypical antipsychotic complicated by an endocrine condition.

Co-morbid Medical and Psychiatric Conditions

CASE 6

A middle-aged man with long-standing obsessive–compulsive disorder (OCD), effectively treated with high-dose fluoxetine, presented with cough, dyspnea, and fever. Chest radiography showed a left lower-lobe infiltrate, consistent with pneumonia. He defervesced after a few doses of intravenous (IV) antibiotics and was discharged to complete the antibiotic course at home. His OCD remained in remission.

Infectious and psychiatric conditions existed independently.

THE ART OF PSYCHIATRIC CONSULTATION IN THE GENERAL HOSPITAL

Determining where on the vast border between psychiatry and medicine a patient's pathologic condition is located is the psychiatric consultant's fundamental task. As for any physician, his or her chief responsibility is diagnosis. The C-L psychiatrist (i.e., practitioner of psychosomatic medicine) is aided in this enterprise, by appreciation of four key differences between general hospital psychiatry and practice in other venues: clinical approach, environment, style of interaction, and use of language.

Clinical Approach

The late senior psychiatrist at the Massachusetts General Hospital (MGH) and founding director of its Psychosomatic Medicine–Consultation Psychiatry Fellowship Program, Dr. George Murray, advised his trainees to think in three ways when consulting on patients: physiologically, existentially, and "dirty." Each element of this tripartite conceptualization is no more or less important than the other, and the most accurate formulation of a patient's problem will prove elusive without attention to all three.

First, psychiatrists are physicians and, as such, subscribe to the medical model: altered bodily structures and functions lead to disease; their correction through physical means leads to restoration of health. Although allegiance to this model may be impolitic in this era of biopsychosocial holism, the degree of morbidity in general hospitals is ever more acute and the technology brought to bear against it increasingly more sophisticated.[3] Consultation psychiatrists who fail to keep pace with their medical and surgical colleagues jeopardize their usefulness to physicians and patients alike.

Alongside the physiologic frame of mind, consultation psychiatrists must think existentially; that is, they must nurture a healthy curiosity about the meaning of illness to their patients at this particular moment in their patients' lives and the circumstances in which their patients find themselves at particular moments in the course of illness.

For example, what does it mean to the patient in Case 3 that both of her two pregnancies have been complicated by pre-eclampsia? How might this meaning relate to her unshakeable fear that she will become dangerously hypertensive at home? How does this fear impact her ability to care for her children and how does it impact her husband? To be curious about such matters, the consulting psychiatrist must first *know* the details of the patient's situation, largely achieved by a careful reading of the chart, and then *ask* the patient about it.

Consultation psychiatrists are wise to maintain a measured skepticism toward patients' and others' statements, motivations, and desires. In other words, they should consider the possibility that the patient (or another informant) is somehow distorting information to serve his or her own agenda. Providers of history can distort the truth in myriad ways, ranging from innocuous exaggeration of the truth to outright lies; their aims are equally legion: money, revenge, convenience, and cover-up of peccadilloes, infidelities, or crimes. For example, the beleaguered mother of a young woman with borderline personality disorder embellished her daughter's suicidal comments in an effort to secure involuntary commitment for her daughter and respite for herself. By paying attention to his or her own countertransference—his or her personal reading of the limbic music[4] emanating from the mother–daughter dyad—the psychiatric consultant called in to assess the patient's suicidal thoughts ably detected the mother's self-serving distortion and thus avoided unwitting collusion with it. This special case of distortion to remove a relative to a mental or other hospital has been termed the *gaslight phenomenon*.[5–7] Although thinking "dirty" is merely a realization that people refract reality through the lens of their own personal experience, other health professionals—even some psychiatrists—bristle at even a consideration, let alone a suggestion, that patients and their families harbor unseemly ulterior motives. Consequently, this perspective does not make the consultation psychiatrist many friends; his or her thinking "dirty" may even earn him or her an unsavory reputation. However, neither an ever-widening social circle nor victory in popularity contests is the C-L psychiatrist's *raison d'être*—competent doctoring is.

Environment

The successful psychiatric consultant must be prepared to work in an atmosphere less formal, rigid, and predictable than one typically found in an office or a clinic; flexibility and adaptability are crucial. Patients are often seen in two-bedded rooms with nothing but a thin curtain providing only the appearance of privacy; roommates—as well as nurses, aides, dietary personnel, and other physicians—are frequent interlocutors.[8] Cramped quarters are the rule, with IV poles, tray tables, and one or two chairs, leaving little room for much else. When family members and other visitors are present, the physician may ask them to leave the room; alternatively, he or she may invite them to stay to "biopsy" the interpersonal dynamics among the family and friends, as was done in the case of the borderline patient described previously. The various alarms and warning signals of medical equipment (e.g., IV pumps, cardiac monitors, ventilators) and assorted catheters and tubes traveling into and out of the patient's body add to the unique ambiance of the bedside experience that distinguishes it from the quiet comfort afforded by a private office. Perhaps off-putting at first, for the psychiatrist who, as Lewis Glickman in his book on consultation put it (as cited in Cassem[1]), loves medicine and is fascinated with medical illness, the exigencies of life and work in a modern hospital quickly become compelling.

Style of Interaction

The adaptability required by these environmental circumstances allows the psychiatric consultant to be more flexible in his or her relations with the patient. For example, psychiatric consultants should permit themselves to crouch at the bedside; lowering themselves to the recumbent patient's level can diminish apprehension and minimize the inherent power differential between doctor and patient. Shaking hands or otherwise laying on hands may achieve the same end. Performance of a physical examination provides an excellent opportunity to allay anxiety and dramatically distinguishes consultation work from office-based psychiatry, where any touching of a patient—let alone physical examination—is considered taboo (rightly or wrongly). An offer to make the person more comfortable by adjusting the bed or getting the patient something to drink before beginning the interview goes a long way in building rapport. When the patient is unable to do even these simple things unaided, it is simply a kind, human gesture. When the patient tends toward the cantankerous and irascible, concern for the patient's comfort may prevent the patient from expelling the consultant from the room. Finally, as a simple matter of respect, one should make every effort to leave the room as one found it (e.g., if towels and sheets are removed from a chair before sitting on it, they should be replaced upon getting up).

Use of Language

Allowance for flexibility also extends to psychiatrists' use of language; they can feel freer than they might in other practice settings to use humor, slang expressions, and perhaps even foul language.[9] All of these varieties of verbal expression create a temporarily jarring juxtaposition between the stereotypical image of the staid physician and the present one; defenses may be briefly disabled just long enough to connect with the truth and allow connection with the patient. For example, in a technique taught by Murray, the psychiatrist raised a clenched fist in front of an angry but

CASE 7

A 30-year-old man with leukemia refractory to bone-marrow transplantation was admitted with graft-versus-host disease. His mother and sister kept a near-constant vigil at his bedside. When he refused to eat and to talk to his family and the nurses, the psychiatrist was summoned. Quickly sizing up the situation, the consultant said to the young man, "It must be a pain to have your mother constantly hovering over you." The patient grinned slightly and answered in the affirmative.

anger-phobic patient and asked him, "If you had one shot, where would you put it?" In this case, the sight and sound of a "healer" in boxer's pose inquiring about placement of a "shot" creates a curious, even humorous, incongruity that disarms the patient's defenses and allows an otherwise intolerable emotion (anger) to emerge (if it is there in the first place). A variant of this maneuver, substitution of a verbal expression of anger for the physical one, is also possible.

Lack of the formal arrangements of office-based psychiatric practice makes such techniques permissible in the general hospital, often to the delight of residents, who sometimes feel unnecessarily constrained in their interpersonal comportment and in whom even a little training unfortunately does much to limit their natural spontaneity.

THE PROCESS OF PSYCHIATRIC CONSULTATION IN THE GENERAL HOSPITAL

With this general overview of the art of consultation, we next outline the step-by-step approach to the actual performance of a psychiatric consultation. Table 2-1 summarizes the key points elaborated in the following text.

Speak Directly With the Referring Clinician

The consultative process begins with the receipt of the referral. With experience, the sensitive consultant begins to formulate preliminary hypotheses even at this early stage. For example, the consultant recognizes a particular unit within the hospital or an individual physician and recollects previous consultations that originated from these sources. In addition, he or she may discern a difference in the way this consultation request was communicated compared with the form of previous requests. In a form of parallel process, this alteration in the usual routine—even if subtle and only in retrospect—often reflects something about the patient. Throughout the consultative process, these crude preliminary hypotheses thus formed are refined and ultimately either accepted or rejected. The continual revision of previous theories as additional data become available is a fundamental process in C-L psychiatry as it is in the whole of medicine.

The reason for the consultation stated in the request might differ from the real reason for the consultation. The team might accurately sense a problem with the patient but not capture it precisely. In some cases, they may be quite far afield, usually when the real reason for the consultation is difficulty in the management of a difficult patient.[10] It is up to the consultant to identify the core issue and ultimately address it in the consultation. Practically speaking, a special effort to contact the consultee is not usually required, because, in general, in the course of reading the chart or reviewing laboratory data, one encounters a member of the team and can inquire then about the consultation request.

TABLE 2-1 Procedural Approach to Psychiatric Consultation
Speak directly with the referring clinician.
Review the current and pertinent past records.
Review the patient's medications.
Gather collateral data.
Interview and examine the patient.
Formulate a diagnosis and management plan.
Write a note.
Speak directly again with the referring clinician.
Provide periodic follow-up.

Review the Current and Pertinent Past Records

A careful review of the current medical record is indispensable to a thorough and comprehensive evaluation of the patient. Perhaps no other element of the consultative process requires as much discipline as this one. The seasoned consultant is able to accomplish this task quite efficiently, knowing fruitful areas of the chart to mine. For example, nursing notes often contain behavioral data often lacking from other disciplines' notes; a well-written consultation provided by another service can provide a general orientation to a case. However, in the current era of widespread use of electronic medical records, when copying and pasting parts of previous notes often substitutes for crafting new ones, the consultant must take care not to propagate error by failing to check primary data personally. Other bountiful areas of the chart include notes written by medical students (who tend to be the most thorough of all), physical and occupational therapists (for functional data), and speech pathologists (for cognitive data). In reading the chart, the focus of the psychiatric consultant's attention varies according to the nature of the case and the reason for the consultation. In cases in which sensorium is altered, for example, careful note of changes in level of awareness, behavior, and cognition should be made, especially as they relate to changes in the medical condition and treatment.

Review the Patient's Medications

Regardless of the particulars of a case, detailed evaluation of medications, paying special attention to those recently initiated or discontinued, is always in order. For example, in Case 2, knowledge that the HIV-positive man had recently initiated treatment with efavirenz was key to diagnosing the cause of his nightmares. Important medications the patient might have taken before admission, including those on which he may be physiologically dependent (e.g., benzodiazepines, narcotic analgesics), might inadvertently have been excluded from his current regimen. Patients who have been transferred among various units in the hospital may be at particular risk of such inadvertent omissions. In cases in which mental status changes resulting from withdrawal phenomena top the differential diagnosis, careful construction of a timeline of the patient's receipt of psychoactive agents is often the only way to identify the problem. In much the same way as infectious-disease specialists chart the administration of antibiotics in relation to culture results, and dermatologists plot newly prescribed medications against the appearance of rashes, the psychiatric consultant tabulates mental status changes, vital signs, and dosages of psychoactive medications to clarify the diagnostic picture. Such a procedure exemplifies the industry and discipline required of the competent consultant.

Gather Collateral Data

The gathering of collateral information from family, friends, and outpatient treaters is no less important in consultation work than in other psychiatric settings. For several reasons (e.g., altered mental status, denial, memory impairment, malingering), patients' accounts of their history and current symptoms are often vague, spotty, and unreliable. Although data from other sources is therefore vital, the astute psychiatrist recognizes that their information, too, may be distorted by the same factors and by selfish interests, as already described. Consultation psychiatrists must guard against accepting any one party's version of events as the truth, and must maintain an open mind in constructing a history informed by multiple sources.

Interview and Examine the Patient

Next follows the interview of the patient and performance of a mental status examination, in addition to relevant portions of the physical and neurologic examinations.

A detailed assessment of cognitive function is not necessary in all patients. If there is no evidence that a patient has a cognitive problem, a simple statement to the effect that no gross cognitive problem is apparent, is sufficient. However, even a slight hint that a cognitive disturbance is present should trigger performance of a more formal screen. We recommend the Folstein Mini-Mental State Examination (MMSE)[11] and the Montreal Cognitive Assessment[12] for this purpose and supplement this test with others that specifically target frontal executive functions (e.g., clock drawing, Luria maneuvers, and cognitive estimations). Any abnormalities that arise on these bedside tests should be comprehensively evaluated by formal neuropsychological testing. It is convenient if a psychologist—especially one trained specifically in neuropsychology—is affiliated with the consultation service. Conversely, if a patient is obviously inattentive, we would argue that performance of the MMSE (or similar tests) is not indicated, because one can predict *a priori* poor performance resulting from the subject's general inattention to the required tasks.

The consultant should, at the very least, review the physical examinations performed by other physicians. This does not, however, preclude doing his or her own examination of relevant systems, including the CNS, which, unless the patient is on the neurology service or is known to have a motor or a sensory problem, has likely been left unexamined. A number of physical findings can be discerned simply by observation: pupillary size (noteworthy with opioid withdrawal or intoxication); diaphoresis, either present (from fever, or from alcohol or benzodiazepine withdrawal) or absent (associated with anticholinergic intoxication); and adventitious motor activity (e.g., tremors, tremulousness, or agitation). Vital signs are especially relevant in cases of substance withdrawal, delirium, and other causes of agitation. Primitive reflexes (e.g., snout, glabellar, grasp), deep-tendon reflexes, extraocular movements, pupillary reaction to light, and muscle tone are among the key elements of the neurologic examination that the psychiatrist often checks.

Formulate a Diagnosis and Management Plan

Any physician's tasks are two-fold: diagnosis and treatment. This dictum is no different for the psychiatrist, whether in the general hospital or elsewhere. To arrive at a diagnosis, laboratory testing comes after the history and examination. By the time a psychiatric consultation is requested, most hospitalized patients have already undergone extensive laboratory testing, including comprehensive metabolic panels and complete blood cell counts; these should be reviewed. In constructing the initial parts of a management plan, the psychiatric consultant should attend to diagnostics and specifically consider each of the tests listed in Table 2-2.

Toxicology screens of both serum and urine are required any time a substance-use disorder is suspected and in cases of altered sensorium, intoxication, or withdrawal.

Well known by every student of psychiatry, syphilis, thyroid dysfunction, and deficiencies of vitamin B_{12} and folic acid are always included in an exhaustive differential diagnosis of virtually every neuropsychiatric disturbance. Although it is certainly possible that these conditions can *cause* any manner of psychiatric perturbation (e.g., dementia, depression, mania), more commonly these ailments co-exist with other conditions, which together *contribute* to psychiatric disturbances. Although blood tests and treatments for these diseases are relatively easily accomplished, these tests should not be recommended reflexively in every case but only when a specific reason dictates (e.g., vitamin testing for anemia).

For purposes other than evaluation of acute intracranial hemorrhage, cerebral magnetic resonance imaging (MRI) is preferred to computed tomography (CT). MRI provides higher resolution and greater detail, particularly of subcortical structures of interest to the psychiatrist. A thorough consultation is incomplete without a reading of the actual radiology report of the study; merely reviewing the telegraphic summary in a house officer's progress note is insufficient, because important findings are often omitted. For example, an MRI scan that shows no abnormalities other than periventricular white matter changes is invariably recorded as "normal" or as showing "no acute change." Although periventricular white matter changes are not acute, they are certainly not normal and they should be documented

TABLE 2-2 Laboratory Tests in Psychiatric Consultation

Toxicology
• Serum
• Urine
Serology
• Rapid plasma reagin
• VDRL test
Thyroid stimulating hormone
Vitamin B_{12} (cyanocobalamin)
Folic acid (folate)
Electroencephalography
Cerebrospinal fluid analysis
Neuroimaging
• Head computed tomography
• Brain magnetic resonance imaging

VDRL, Venereal Disease Research Laboratory.

in a careful psychiatric consultation note. They may be evidence of insults that form a substrate for depression or dementia and may be a predictive sign of sensitivity to usual dosages of psychotropic medications.

Electroencephalography (EEG) can be particularly helpful to document the presence of generalized slowing in patients thought by their primary physicians to have a functional problem. Such indisputable evidence of electric dysrhythmia often puts a sudden end to the primary team's skepticism. In cases of suspected complex partial seizures, depriving the patient of sleep the night before the EEG increases the test's sensitivity. Continuous EEG and video monitoring or ambulatory EEG monitoring may be necessary to catch aberrant electric activity. As with neuroimaging reports, the consultant psychiatrist must read the EEG report himself or herself; non-psychiatrists commonly equate the absence of "organized electrographic seizure activity" with normality, even though focal slowing may be evidence of seizure activity.

CSF analysis is often overlooked by psychiatrists and other physicians. However, it should be considered in cases of altered mental status with fever, leukocytosis, or meningismus and when causes of be-clouded consciousness are not obvious. In some cases (e.g., in the vignette of the man with HSV presented previously), some conditions initially considered causative are not, and the true culprit is identified only after a lumbar puncture is performed.

Any suspicion of a somatic symptom disorder (especially conversion disorder) should trigger referral for psychological testing with the Minnesota Multiphasic Personality Inventory (MMPI) or the shorter Personality Assessment Inventory. For example, MMPI results of the young female graduate student in Case 4 may demonstrate the conversion (or psychosomatic) V pattern of marked elevations on the hypochondriasis and hysteria scales and a normal or slightly elevated result on the depression scale. These pencil-and-paper tests can also be useful in assessments of psychological contributions to pain. Projective testing (e.g., Rorschach inkblots) is more common in outpatient venues.

Write a Note

The psychiatric consultation note should be a model of clear, concise writing with careful attention to specific, practical diagnostic and therapeutic recommendations. Several reviews of this topic are available.[13,14] If the stated reason for the consultation differs from the consultee's more fundamental concern, both should be addressed in the note. If the referring physician adopts the consultant's recommendations, he or she should be able to transcribe them directly into computerized order-entry systems. "Note wars," criticism of the consultee, accusations of shoddy work, pejorative labels, and jargon should be avoided. If the consultee chooses a diagnostic or therapeutic course equally appropriate to the consultant's suggested choice, an indication of agreement is more prudent than rigid insistence on the psychiatrist's preference. The consultant should avoid prognostication (e.g., "This patient will probably have decision-making capacity after his infection has resolved" or "This patient will likely need psychiatric hospitalization after he recovers from tricyclic antidepressant [TCA] toxicity"). Such forecasts do not engender confidence in the consultant's skill if they prove inaccurate; may be invoked by the consultee even when they no longer apply; and are unnecessary if routine follow-up is provided.

Speak Directly Again With the Referring Clinician

The consultative process is not complete without further contact, either by phone or in person, with the referring physician or other member of the patient's team, especially if the diagnosis or recommended intervention warrants immediate attention.

Provide Periodic Follow-up

The committed consultant sees the patient as often as is necessary to treat him or her competently, and the consultant holds himself or herself accountable for tracking the patient's clinical progress, following up on laboratory tests, refining earlier diagnostic impressions, and modifying diagnostic and treatment recommendations. The consultation comes to an end only when the problem for which the consultant was called resolves, any other concerns identified by the consultant are fully addressed, or the patient is discharged or dies. Rarely do any of these outcomes occur after a single visit, making repeated visits the rule and availability, even at inopportune times, crucial. However, the consultant is not obligated to continue consulting on a case when his or her recommendations are clearly being ignored.[15] In these cases, it is appropriate to sign off. In some settings, psychiatric consultants may be expected to secure insurance coverage for psychiatric admissions and locate available psychiatric beds.

PRINCIPLES OF PSYCHIATRIC TREATMENT IN THE GENERAL HOSPITAL

As in other practice settings, in the general hospital, psychiatric treatment proceeds on biological, psychological, and social fronts.

Biological Management

When prescribing psychopharmaceuticals for medically ill patients taking other medications, the consultant must be aware of pharmacokinetic profiles, drug–drug interactions, and adverse effects. These topics are considered in depth in Chapter 38.

Pharmacokinetic Profiles

Pharmacokinetics refers to a drug's absorption, distribution, metabolism, and excretion. Because an acutely medically ill patient might not be able to take medications orally, absorption is a primary concern in the general hospital setting. Often in such situations (e.g., in an intubated patient), a nasogastric tube is in place and medications can be crushed and administered through the nasogastric tube. However, if one is not in place, the psychiatric consultant is obliged to consider medications that can be given intramuscularly, intravenously, or in suppository form. In addition, orally disintegrating formulations may be available (e.g., mirtazapine, olanzapine, risperidone); these formulations still work enterally.

Many psychotropic medications are metabolized in the liver and excreted through the kidneys. Thus, impaired hepatic and renal function can lead to increased concentrations of parent compounds and pharmacologically active metabolites. This problem is readily overcome by using lower initial doses and increasing them slowly. However, concern for metabolic alterations in medically ill patients should not justify use of homeopathic doses for indeterminate durations, because most patients ultimately tolerate and require standard regimens.

Drug–Drug Interactions

Many psychopharmaceuticals are metabolized by the cytochrome P450 isoenzyme system; many also inhibit various isoforms in this extensive family of hepatic enzymes, and the metabolism of many is, in turn, inhibited by other classes of medication, thus creating fertile ground for drug–drug interactions in patients taking several medications. This topic is reviewed extensively in Chapter 38. Psychiatric consultants should also be aware that cigarette smoking induces the metabolism of many drugs. When patients are hospitalized and thus stop or curtail smoking, serum concentrations of these drugs (e.g., clozapine) increase, and the propensity for adverse effects thus also increases.

TABLE 2-3 Personality Assessment and Management in the General Hospital

PERSONALITY TYPE	MAJOR TRAITS	REACTION TO ILLNESS	RECOMMENDED STRATEGIES
Dependent	Craves special attention Expects services on demand Requires constant reassurance	Perceived abandonment generates feeling of helplessness Increased anxiety prompts more demands	Express desire to provide comprehensive care Make minor concessions if possible
Obsessive	Values detail and order Becomes anxious with uncertain outcomes Well defended against fear and pain	Illness represents threat to self-control Need for certainty and control prevents questioning of staff, thus increasing anxiety	Provide ample information, using and defining medical terms Ally with patient's desire for mastery Allow patient to participate in medical decisions
Histrionic	Prematurely trusts others Uses repression, denial, and avoidance Dramatizes feelings	Illness represents threat to masculinity or femininity	Recognize patient's grace under pressure Omit details in reassuring patient
Masochistic	Plays the martyr role Seems to enjoy suffering Feels unappreciated	Illness represents deserved punishment Illness is welcomed as a form of suffering Lack of recognition of martyr status risks non-compliance	Appreciate patient's suffering Recommend treatment as an additional burden that will aid others
Paranoid	Is suspicious, wary, and guarded Readily feels slighted Bickers when feeling persecuted	Illness represents an external assault Medical interventions generate suspicions and fear of harm	Inform patient completely about tests and treatments Acknowledge difficulty of illness
Narcissistic	Requests and receives help with difficulty Strives to appear smart, strong, and superior Fears dependence	Illness challenges self-esteem and superior stance Efforts to appear effectual and strong are redoubled	Recognize patient's strengths and knowledge Allow patient to participate in medical decisions Expect gaps in history, because more illness connotes weakness
Schizoid	Is aloof, uninvolved, and detached Prefers solitary occupations	Illness requires contact with caregivers Rejection risk spurs greater withdrawal	Recognize preference for isolation Minimize intrusions Assure patient of interest and concern

Adapted from Shuster JL, Stern TA: Intensive care units. In Wise MG, Rundell JR, editors: *The American Psychiatric Publishing textbook of consultation–liaison psychiatry: psychiatry in the medically ill*, ed 2, Washington, 2002, American Psychiatric Publishing, pp 753–770; Kahana RJ, Bibring GL: Personality types in medical management. In Zinberg NE, editor: *Psychiatry and medical practice in a general hospital*, New York, 1965, International Universities Press, pp 108–123; and Wool C, Geringer ES, Stern TA: The management of behavioral problems in the ICU. In Rippe JM, Irwin RS, Alpert JS et al, editors: *Intensive care medicine*, ed 2, Boston, 1991, Little, Brown, pp 1906–1916.

Adverse Effects

Depending on the practice venue, the profile of adverse effects of concern to the psychiatrist varies. For example, the likelihood that TCAs will cause dry mouth and sedation may be of more concern in the outpatient setting than in the general hospital, where concern about the cardiac-conduction and gut-slowing effects will likely be of greater importance in patients recovering from myocardial infarction (MI) or bowel surgery. Traditional neuroleptics—often relegated to second-line in otherwise healthy patients with psychosis—may be preferable to the atypical agents in general medical settings, where patients with obesity, diabetes mellitus, and dyslipidemia may be seen for the complications of these conditions (e.g., MI, stroke, diabetic ketoacidosis).

Psychological Management

Psychological management of the hospitalized medically ill patient begins—as does all competent treatment—with diagnosis. That is, the psychiatric consultant first appraises the patient's psychological strengths and vulnerabilities. Armed with this psychological balance sheet, the psychiatrist then uses this information therapeutically in how he or she phrases questions and comments to the patient and describes the patient to the medical and nursing staff. Several schemas have been developed to aid in such a personality assessment.[10,16,17] Groves' formulation is reviewed in Chapters 36 and 43; Table 2-3 summarizes Kahana and Bibring's approach.[16]

The consultant must realize that the patient may find the psychiatrist the only outlet available to vent his or her feelings about treatment in the hospital. This is an appropriate function of the consultant—and, in fact, may be the tacit reason for the consultation. Relieved of his or her feelings, often hostile and at odds with the team's treatment efforts, the patient is thus better able to work with the team.

Social Management

Psychiatric consultants may be called on to help make decisions about end-of-life care (e.g., do-not-resuscitate and do-not-intubate orders), disposition to an appropriate living situation (e.g., home with services, assisted-living residence, skilled nursing facility, or nursing home), short-term disability, probate guardianship for a patient deemed clinically unable to make medical decisions for himself or herself, and involuntary psychiatric commitment. For patients who are agitated and thereby place themselves and others in harm's way, the consultant may recommend the use of various restraints (e.g., Posey vests, mitts [to prevent removing IV and other catheters], soft wrist restraints, and leather wrist and ankle restraints) and constant observation.

SUMMARY

Regardless of the practice setting, the basics of competent psychiatric care remain the diagnosis of affective, behavioral, and cognitive disturbances and their treatment by pharmacologic, psychological, and social interventions. The psychiatrist in the general hospital applies these fundamentals while remaining *accessible* to the consultee and to the patient, *adaptable* to the exigencies of the hospital environment, and *flexible* in clinical approach and interpersonal style. The consultation psychiatrist adheres to the tenets of competent doctoring: accountability, commitment, industry, and discipline.

REFERENCES

Access the reference list online at https://expertconsult.inkling.com/.

The Doctor–Patient Relationship

3

Christopher Gordon, M.D.
Gene V. Beresin, M.D., M.A.

OVERVIEW

The doctor–patient relationship—despite all the pressures of accountable care, complex and demanding electronic health records, and other systemic complications—remains one of the most profound partnerships in the human experience; in it, one person reveals to another his or her innermost concerns, in hope of healing.[1,2] In this deeply intimate relationship, when we earn our patients' trust, we are privileged to learn about fears and worries that our patients may not have shared—or ever will share—with another living soul; patients literally put their lives and well-being in our hands. For our part, we hope to bring to this relationship technical mastery of our craft, wisdom, experience, and humility as well as our physicianly commitment to stand by and with our patient—that is, not to be driven away by any degree of pain, suffering, ugliness, or even death itself. We foreswear our own gratification, beyond our professional satisfaction and reward, to place our patients' interests above our own. We hope to co-create a healing relationship, which Ventres and Frankel have elegantly termed "shared presence"[3] in which our patients can come to understand with us the sources of suffering and the options for care and healing, and to partner with us in the construction of a path toward recovery.

In clinical medicine, the relationship between doctor and patient is not merely a vehicle through which to deliver care. Rather, it is one of the most important aspects of care itself. Excellent clinical outcomes—in which patients report high degrees of satisfaction, work effectively with their physicians, adhere to treatment regimens, experience improvements in the conditions of concern to them, and proactively manage their lives to promote health and wellness—are far more likely to arise from relationships with doctors that are collaborative and in which patients feel heard, understood, respected, and included in treatment planning.[4–7] On the other hand, poor outcomes—including non-compliance with treatment plans, complaints to oversight boards, and malpractice actions—tend to arise when patients feel unheard, disrespected, or otherwise out of partnership with their doctors.[8–10] Collaborative care not only leads to better outcomes but also is more efficient than non-collaborative care in achieving good outcomes.[11,12] The relationship matters.

An effective doctor–patient relationship may be even more critical to successful outcomes in psychiatry than it is in other medical specialties. In psychiatry, more than in most branches of medicine, there is a sense that when the patient is ill, there is something wrong with the person as a whole, rather than that the person has, or suffers from, a discrete condition. Our language aggravates this sense of personal defectiveness or deficiency in psychiatric illness. We tend to speak of "being depressed" or "being bipolar" as if these are qualities of the whole person rather than a condition to be dealt with. Even more hurtfully, we sometimes speak of people as "borderlines" or "schizophrenics," as if these labels sum up the person as a whole. This language, together with the persistent stigma attached to mental illness in our culture, amplifies the shame and humiliation that patients may experience in any doctor–patient interaction[13] and makes it even more imperative that the physician works to create a safe relationship.

Moreover, if we seek to co-create a healing environment in which the patient feels understood, psychiatry more than any other branch of medicine requires us to attend thoughtfully to the whole person, even to parts of the person's life that may seem remote from the person's primary concern. This is especially salient in the general hospital, where a patient's medical problem may cause clinicians to overlook critically important aspects of the person's current relationships and social environment, from long-standing psychological issues, and from the person's spiritual orientation. Often, these psychological, social, or spiritual aspects shed light on the person's distress (Figure 3-1). There must be time and space in the doctor–patient relationship to know the person from several perspectives:[14] in the context of the person's biological ailments and vulnerabilities; in the setting of the person's current social connections, supports, and stressors; in the context of the person's earlier psychological issues; and in the face of the person's spirituality.[15]

UNIQUE ASPECTS OF THE DOCTOR–PATIENT RELATIONSHIP IN THE GENERAL HOSPITAL

In the general hospital, the doctor–patient relationship has several unique features. To begin with, a medical problem is usually the cornerstone of doctor–patient encounters. This simple fact has several key consequences.

First, the relationship occurs in the context of a complex interplay of psychiatric and medical symptoms and illnesses (see Figure 2-1) that may each stem from a variety of etiologies; the doctor–patient relationship must assess and attempt to address each of these domains.

Second, the dynamics of power and trust in the doctor–patient relationship may be different from those in outpatient

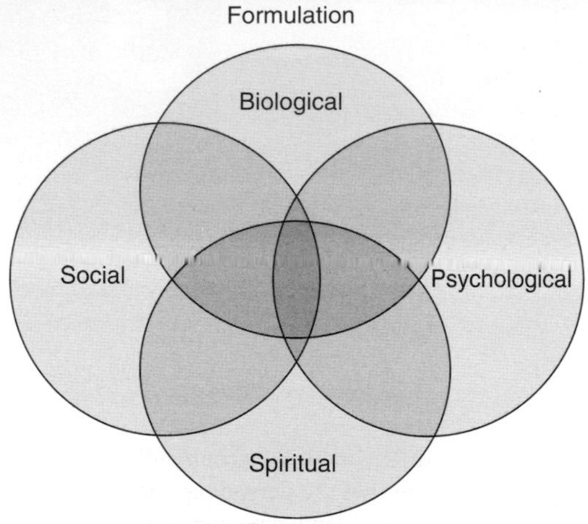

Figure 3-1. Graphic representation of frameworks that facilitate an understanding of the patient.

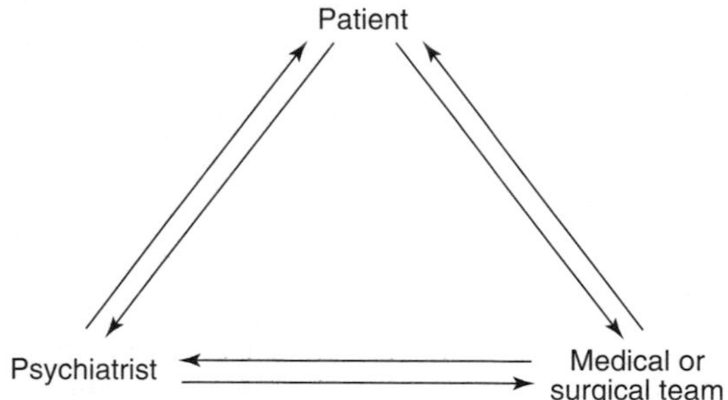

Figure 3-2. Patient–doctor relationships in the general hospital.

settings. In the hospital, patients usually have not asked for a meeting with a psychiatrist, and may not welcome such a meeting. For instance, a psychiatrist may be called to evaluate a patient who is refusing treatment or who has developed hallucinations after a cholecystectomy. The context of care affects the patient's willingness and ability to engage in a relationship with a psychiatric physician. Doctors must be mindful of patient autonomy—which is typically strained by illness—and strive to maintain a patient-centered approach.

Third, the presence of a primary medical or surgical team changes a dyadic relationship into a complex doctor–patient–doctor triad. Both sets of physicians and the patient can feel pulled in different directions when there is disagreement about treatment. Physicians and patients alike tend to categorize illness and treatments as "medical" and "psychiatric."[16] Successful doctor–patient relationships collaborate in the service of patient care (Figure 3-2).

Fourth, the hospital environment challenges privacy, space, and time and hinders the clinical encounter. For example, assessing whether a patient who is losing weight after a stroke is depressed may be especially difficult because of barriers to communication. The hospital roommate may have visitors who interrupt or inhibit the patient,[17] or the patient may have intrinsic barriers to communication (e.g., an aphasia or intubation). Chapter 2 reviews some differences in approach, language, and style that may be applicable to care in the general hospital. Ultimately, regardless of setting, the doctor–patient relationship is at the core of the clinical encounter. The following sections will explore the provision of patient-centered care, conduct of the clinical interview, and creation of a clinical formulation and treatment plan; all of these are facilitated by a therapeutic doctor–patient relationship.

THE OPTIMAL HEALING ENVIRONMENT: PATIENT-CENTERED CARE

Although cultural factors limit the validity of this generalization, patients generally prefer care that centers on their own concerns; addresses their perspective on these concerns; uses language that is straightforward, is inclusive, and promotes collaboration; and respects the patient as a fully empowered partner in decision-making.[18–20] This model of care may be denoted by the term *patient-centered care*[11,21,22] or, even better, *relationship-centered care*. In *Crossing the Quality Chasm*, the Institute of Medicine identified person-centered practices as key to achieving high-quality care that focuses on the unique perspective, needs, values, and preferences of the individual patient.[23] Person-centered care involves a collaborative relationship in which two experts—the practitioner and the patient—attempt to blend the practitioner's knowledge and experience with the patient's unique perspective, needs, and assessment of outcome.[20,22,24,25]

In relationship-centered practice, the physician does not cede decision-making authority or responsibility to the patient and family but rather enters into a dialogue about what the physician thinks is best. Most patients and families seek a valued doctor's answer to the question (stated or not), "What would you do if this were your family member?" This transparent and candid collaboration conveys respect and concern. Enhanced autonomy involves a commitment to know the patient deeply, to respect the patient's wishes, to share information openly and honestly (as the patient desires), to involve others at the patient's discretion, and to treat the patient as a partner (to the greatest extent possible).

In patient-centered care, there is active management of communication to avoid inadvertently hurting, shaming, or humiliating the patient through careless use of language or other slights. When such hurt or other error occurs, the practitioner apologizes clearly and in a heartfelt way to restore the relationship.[26]

The role of the physician in patient-centered care is one of an expert who seeks to help a patient co-manage his or her health to whatever extent is most comfortable for that particular person. The role is not to cede all important decisions to the patient.[23,27]

The patient-centered physician attempts to accomplish six goals (Table 3-1).[28] First, the physician endeavors to create conditions of welcome, respect, and safety so that the patient can reveal his or her concerns and perspective. Second, the physician endeavors to understand the patient as a whole person, listening to both the "lyrics" and the "music" of what is communicated. Third, the physician confirms and demonstrates his or her understanding through direct, non-jargonistic language to the patient. Fourth, if the physician successfully establishes common ground on

TABLE 3-1 Six Goals of Patient-Centered Care[28]

- Create conditions of safety, respect, and welcome.
- Seek to understand the patient's perspective.
- Confirm an understanding of the problem(s) via direct communication.
- Synthesize information into diagnoses and problem lists.
- Formulate and share thoughts about the illness.
- Negotiate a plan of action with the patient.

the nature of the problem as the patient perceives it, an attempt is made to synthesize these problems into workable diagnoses and problem lists. Fifth, through the use of technical mastery and experience, a path is envisioned toward healing, and it is shared with the patient. Finally, together, the physician and patient can then negotiate the path that makes the most sense for this particular patient.

Through all of this work, the physician models and cultivates a relationship that values candor, collaboration, and authenticity; it should be able to withstand and even welcome conflict, as a healthy part of human relationships.[27] In so doing, the physician–patient partnership forges a relationship that can withstand the vicissitudes of the patient's illness, its treatment, and conflict in the relationship itself. In this way, the health of the physician–patient relationship takes its place as an important element on every problem list, to be actively monitored and nurtured as time passes.

Physician Practice in Patient-Centered Care

Physicians' qualities have an impact on the doctor–patient relationship. These qualities support and enhance—but are not a substitute for—technical competence and cognitive mastery. Perhaps most important is a quality of mindfulness,[29] as described by Messner,[30] acquired through a process of constant autognosis, or self-awareness. Mindfulness appreciates that a person's emotional life (i.e., of both the physician and the patient) has meaning and importance and deserves our respect and attention. Mindfulness involves acceptance of feelings in both parties without judgment and with the knowledge that feelings are separate from acts. It also enhances an awareness of our ideals, values, biases, strengths, and limitations—again, in both the patient and doctor.

Mindfulness, which springs from Buddhist roots,[31] has offered wisdom to the practice of psychotherapy (e.g., helping patients tolerate unbearable emotions without action and helping clinicians tolerate the sometimes hideous histories their patients share with them).[32] It helps physicians find a calm place from which to build patient relationships.[33] Mindfulness also counsels us to be compassionate, without a compulsion to act on feelings. This quality is an invaluable asset to consultation psychiatrists in the general hospital, particularly with difficult patients who evoke strong emotions in medical and surgical teams. Thus, the physician can be informed by the wealth of his or her inner emotional life, without being driven to act on these emotions; this can serve as a model for the relationship with the patient.

Empathy (the ability to imagine a patient's perspective, express genuine care and compassion, and communicate understanding back to the patient) is another important quality for physicians.[34] Stated differently, empathy involves "identifying a patient's emotional state accurately, naming it, and responding to it appropriately."[35] Studies have shown that physician empathy promotes more complete history-taking, enhances patient satisfaction, and improves adherence to treatment.[34,36] Conversely, simple reassurance without empathic exploration of the patient's concerns has been linked to increased visits and cost.[37] Empathy may even decrease medical–legal risk;[38] one study by Ambady and colleagues suggested that surgeons' tone of voice corresponded to malpractice rates.[39]

Communication of empathy can be achieved by both verbal and non-verbal means. Listening, establishing eye contact, expressing emotion (e.g., through facial expressions and body language, such as leaning forward, and modulating the tone of voice) are several components of empathy. Other personal qualities in the physician that promote healthy and vibrant relationships with patients include humility, genuineness, optimism, good humor, candor, a belief in the value of living a full life, and transparency in communication.[40]

Important communication skills include the ability to elicit the patient's perspective, help the patient feel understood, explain conditions and options using clear and non-technical language, generate input and consensus about paths forward in care, acknowledge difficulty in the relationship without aggravating it, welcome input and even conflict, and work through difficulty.[41–43]

One of the most important ingredients of successful doctor–patient relationships (and one that is in very short supply) is time.[44] There is simply no substitute for, or quick alternative to, sitting with a person and taking the time to get to know that person in depth, in a private setting free from intrusions and interruptions. In the general hospital, where there are frequent interruptions, this scenario may seem impossible. However, most physicians know that patients want our full and undivided attention.

COLLABORATION AROUND HISTORY-TAKING

One major goal of an initial interview is to generate a database that will support a comprehensive differential diagnosis. However, there are other over-arching goals, including demystifying and explaining the process of collaboration, finding out what is troubling and challenging to the patient, co-creating a treatment path to address these problems, understanding the person as a whole, encouraging the patient's participation, welcoming feedback, and modeling a mindful appreciation of the complexity of human beings (including our inner emotional life).[45,46] At the end of the history-taking—or to use more collaborative language, after building a history with the patient[47]—a conversation should be feasible about paths toward healing and the patient's and doctor's mutual roles in that process (in which the patient feels heard, understood, confident in the outcome, and committed to the partnership).

Effective Clinical Interviewing

Effective skills and traits for clinical interviewing include friendliness, warmth, a capacity to help patients feel at ease in telling their stories, and an ability to engage the person in a mutual exploration of what is troubling him or her. Demystification of the clinical encounter, by explaining what we are doing before we do it and by making our thinking as transparent and collaborative as possible, promotes good interviews.[48] Similarly, pausing often to ask the patient if we understand clearly or seeking the patient's input and questions promotes bidirectional conversations (rather than one-sided interrogation) and can yield deeper information.[49]

One useful technique involves offering to tell the patient what we already know about him or her. For example, "I wonder if it would be helpful if I told you what Dr. Smith mentioned to me when she called to refer you to me? That way, if I have any information wrong, you could straighten it out at the outset." In the emergency department, in which we usually have a chart full of information, or when doing consultations on medical–surgical patients, this technique allows us to "show our cards" before we ask the patient to reveal information about himself or herself. Moreover, by inviting correction, we demonstrate at the outset that we value the person's input. This technique also allows us to put the person's story in neighborly, non-pathological language, setting the stage for the interview to follow. For example, if the chart reveals that the person has been drinking excessively and may be depressed, we can say, "It looks like you have been having a hard time recently," leaving the patient with the opportunity to fill in the details.[50]

Having opened the interview, the doctor remains quiet to make room for the person to tell his or her story, encouraging (with body language, open-ended questions, and other encouragement) the person to say more. The temptation to jump too early to closed-ended symptom checklists should be eschewed. One study of 73 recorded doctor–patient encounters revealed that doctors interrupted patients after an average of 18 seconds and did not allow them to complete their opening statement in 69% of cases.[51] We should venture to listen deeply, to both the words and the music.

After a reasonable amount of time, it is often helpful for the physician to summarize what he or she has heard and to establish whether he or she understands accurately what the patient is trying to say. Saying, "Let me see if I understand what you are saying so far" is a good way of moving to this part of the interview. In reflecting back to the patient our summary of what we have heard, careful use of language is important. Whenever possible, use of inflammatory or otherwise inadvertently hurtful language should be avoided (e.g. "So it sounds like you were hallucinating and perhaps having other psychotic symptoms"), in favor of neighborly, neutral language ("Sounds like things were difficult—did I understand you to say you were hearing things that troubled you?"). Whenever possible, it is preferable to use the exact words that the patient has used to describe his or her emotional state. For example, if the person says, "I have been feeling so tired, just so very, very tired—I feel like I have nothing left," and we say, "It sounds as if you have been exhausted," we may or may not convey to the person that we have understood them; however, if we say, "You have been just so terribly tired," it is more likely that the person will feel understood.

One measure of rapport comes from getting the "nod"—that is, simply noticing if in the early stages of the interview, the patient is nodding at us in agreement and otherwise giving signs of understanding and of feeling understood.[48] If the nod is absent, it is a signal that something is amiss—either we have missed something important, have inadvertently offended the person, have failed to explain our process, or have otherwise derailed the relationship. A clinical interview without the nod is an interview in peril. Often a simple apology if a person has been kept waiting or an acknowledgment of something in common ("Interesting—I grew up in Maryland, too!") can go a long, long way toward creating connection and rapport.

Having established a tone of collaboration, identified the problem, and perceived the nod, the next area of focus is the history of the present illness. Letting the person tell his or her story is important when eliciting the history of the present illness. For many people, it is a deeply healing experience merely to be listened to in an empathic and attuned way.[50] It is best to listen actively (by not interrupting and by not focusing solely on establishing the right diagnosis) and to make sure to "get it right" from the patient's point of view. When the physician hypothesizes that the patient's problem may be more likely to be in the psychological or interpersonal realm, it is especially important to give the patient a chance to share what is troubling him or her in an atmosphere of acceptance and empathy.

In taking the history of the present illness, under the pressure of time, the physician may erroneously rely too heavily on symptom checklists or ask a series of closed-ended questions to rule in or rule out a particular diagnosis (e.g., major depression). Doing this increases the risk of prematurely closing off important information that the patient might otherwise impart about the social or psychological aspects of the situation.

Having sketched in the main parameters of the person's history of the current issue, it may be wise to inquire about the last time the patient felt well with respect to this problem: the earliest symptoms recollected; associated stresses, illnesses, and changes in medications; attempts to solve the problem and their effects; and how the person elected to get help for the problem at the present time. This may be a time to summarize, review, and request clarification.

As the interviewer moves to different sections of the history, he or she may want to consider explaining what he or she is doing and why: "I'd like now to ask some questions about your psychiatric history, if any, to see if anything like this has happened before." This guided interviewing tends to demystify what the interviewer is doing and to elicit collaboration.[48,52] Chapter 4 discusses each component of the psychiatric interview in more detail.

The social and developmental history offers a rich opportunity for data-gathering in the social and psychological realms. Where the person grew up; what family life was like; what culture the person identifies with; how far the person advanced in school; what subjects the person preferred; and what hobbies and interests the person has, are all fertile lines of pursuit. Marital and relationship history, whether the person has been in love, who the person admires most, and who has been most important in the person's life are even deeper probes into this aspect of the person's experience. A deep and rapid probe into a person's history can often be achieved by the simple question, "What was it like for you growing up in your family?"[53] Spiritual orientation and practice (e.g., whether the person ever had a spiritual practice and, if so, what happened to change it) fit well into this section of the history.[54]

The formal mental status examination continues the line of inquiry that was begun in the history of present illness (i.e., the symptom checklists to rule in or rule out diagnostic possibilities and to ask more about detailed signs and symptoms to establish pertinent positives and negatives in the differential diagnosis).

An extremely important area, and one all too frequently given short shrift in diagnostic evaluations, is the area of the person's strengths and capabilities. As physicians, we are trained in the vast nosology of disease and pathology, and we admire the most learned physician as one who can detect the most subtle or obscure malady; indeed, these are important physicianly strengths, to be sure. But there is regrettably no comparable nosology of strengths and capabilities. Yet, in the long road to recovery it is almost always the person's strengths on which the physician relies to make a partnership toward healing. It is vitally important that the physician notes these strengths and lets the person know that the physician sees and appreciates them.[47]

Sometimes strengths are obvious (e.g., high intelligence in a young person with a first-break psychosis or a committed and supportive family surrounding a person with recurrent depression). At other times, strengths are more subtle or even counterintuitive—for example, seeing that a woman who cuts herself repeatedly to distract herself from the agony of remembering past abuse has found a way to live with the unbearable; this is a strength. Notable, too, may be her strength to survive, her faith to carry on, and other aspects of her life (e.g., a history of playing a musical instrument, a loving concern for children, a righteous rage that galvanizes her to make justice in the world). Whatever the person's strengths, we must note them, acknowledge them, and remember them. An inability to find strengths and capacities to admire in a patient (alongside other attributes that may be a great deal less admirable) is almost always a sign of countertransference malice and bears careful thought and analysis.

Finally, a clinical diagnostic interview should always include an opportunity for the patient to offer areas for discussion: "Are there areas of your life that we have not discussed that you think would be good for me to know about?" or "Are there things we have mentioned that you'd like to say more about?" or "Is there anything I haven't asked you about that I should have?"

PLANNING THE PATH FORWARD: CREATING A CLINICAL FORMULATION

Having heard the patient's story, the physician next formulates an understanding of the person that can lead to a mutually developed treatment path. The formulation contextualizes and complements the diagnosis. A diagnosis describes a condition that can be reasonably delineated and described to the person and that implies a relatively foreseeable clinical course; usually it implies options of courses of treatment. As important as a diagnosis is in clinical medicine, a diagnosis alone is insufficient for effective treatment planning and is an inadequate basis for work by the doctor–patient dyad.

In psychiatry, one method for creating a formulation is to consider each patient from a bio-socio-psycho-spiritual perspective, thinking about each patient from each of these four perspectives.[15]

The first of these is biological: Could the person's suffering be due, entirely or in part, to a biological condition of some sort (either from an acquired condition [such as hypothyroidism] or a genetic "chemical imbalance" [such as some forms of depression and bipolar disorder])? The second model is social: Is there something going on in the person's life that is contributing to his or her suffering, such as an abusive relationship, a stressful job, a sick child, or financial trouble? The third model is psychological: Although this model is more subtle, most patients will acknowledge that practically everyone has baggage from the past, and sometimes this baggage contributes to a person's difficulties in the present. The fourth model is spiritual: Although this model is not relevant for all people, sometimes it is very important. For people who at one point had faith but lost it, or for whom life feels empty and meaningless, conversation about the spiritual aspects of their suffering sometimes taps into important sources of difficulty and sometimes into resources for healing.[54]

These four models—biological "chemical imbalances," current social stressors, psychological baggage, and spiritual issues—taken together provide an excellent framework for understanding most people (see Figure 3-1). One of the beauties of this method is that these models are not particularly pathologizing or shame-inducing. On the contrary, they are normalizing and emphasize that all of us are subject to these same challenges. This opens the way to collaboration.

Whereas the biological, social, and spiritual models are fairly easy to conceptualize, the formulation of psychological issues can seem particularly daunting to physicians and patients alike, given that every person is dizzyingly complex. It can seem almost impossible to formulate a psychological perspective of a person's life that is neither simplistic and jargon-ridden nor uselessly complex (and often jargon-ridden). A useful method for making sense of the psychological aspects of the person's life is to consider whether there are recurrent patterns of difficulty, particularly in important relationships as the person looks back on his or her life.[15] The most useful information when assessing this model is information about the most important relationships in this person's life (in plain, non-technical terms—not only current important relationships, for which we need to assess current social function, but also past important relationships). In this way, for example, it may become clear that the person experienced his relationship with his father as abusive and hurtful and has not had a relationship with any other person in authority since then that has felt truly helpful and supportive. This information in turn may shed light on the person's current work problems and illuminate some of the person's feelings of depression.

Underlying our inquiry regarding whether there may be significant recurrent patterns in the person's life that shed light on his or her current situation is the critical notion that these patterns almost always began as attempts to cope and represent creative adaptations or even strengths. Often, these patterns—even when they involve self-injury or other clearly self-destructive behaviors—begin as creative solutions to apparently insoluble problems. For example, self-injury may have represented a way of mastering unbearable feelings and may have felt like a way of being in control while remaining alive under unbearable circumstances. It is important that the doctor appreciates that most of the time these self-defeating behaviors began as solutions and often continue to have adaptive value in the person's life. If we fail to appreciate the creative, adaptive side of the behavior, the person is likely to feel misunderstood, judged harshly, and possibly shamed.

Practically everyone finds the four models understandable and meaningful. Moreover, and importantly, these four models avoid language that overly pathologizes the person, and they use language that tends to universalize the patient's experience. This initial formulation can be a good platform for a more in-depth discussion of diagnostic possibilities. With this framework, the differential diagnosis can be addressed from a biological perspective, and acute social stressors can be acknowledged. The diagnosis and treatment can be framed in a manner consistent with the person's spiritual orientation. Fleshing out the psychological aspects can be more challenging, but this framework creates a way of addressing psychological patterns in a person's life and his or her interest in addressing them and the ability to do so.

TREATMENT PLANNING

Having a good formulation as a frame for a comprehensive differential diagnosis permits the doctor and the patient to look at treatment options (including different modalities or even alternative therapies or solutions not based in traditional medicine), and to engage in person-centered shared decision-making.[55] It is possible from this vantage point to look together at the risks and benefits of various approaches, as well as the demands of different approaches (the time and money invested in psychotherapy, for example, or the side effects from many medication trials). The sequence of treatments, the location, the cost, and other parameters of care can all be made explicit and weighed together.

This approach also is effective in dealing with situations in which the physician's formulation and that of the patient differ, so that consultation and possibly mediation can be explored.[15] For example, the physician's formulation and differential diagnosis for a person might be that the person's heavy drinking constitutes alcohol abuse or possibly dependence and that cessation from drinking and the active pursuit of sobriety is a necessary part of the solution to the patient's chronic severe anxiety and depression. The patient, on the other hand, may feel that if the doctor would offer more effective treatment for his anxiety and depression, he would then be able to stop drinking. An explicit formulation enables the patient and the doctor to see where and how they disagree and to explore alternatives. For example, in Case 1, the physician could offer to meet with family members with the patient, so both could get family input into the preferred solution; alternatively, the physician could offer the patient a referral for expert psychopharmacologic consultation to test the patient's hypothesis.

CASE 1

Mrs. A, a 41-year-old executive and mother of three daughters (aged 12, 10, and 6 years) was admitted to the hospital for intractable depression. Three years earlier, her husband, also an executive, had suffered a severe anoxic brain injury that left him in a coma for several weeks. When he awoke, he had severe anterograde amnesia, and was unable to hold new information in his memory for more than a minute. Although he was grossly impaired by this deficit, and had some other sequelae of his anoxia (e.g., incontinence) he appeared entirely well. He had returned home, where Mrs. A was now his principal caregiver, in addition to her working full-time and caring for their three children.

Mrs. A's depression had responded poorly to vigorous treatment with antidepressants, supportive psychotherapy, and social work input to optimize supports. She had had a course of electroconvulsive therapy, which had only a short-lived benefit. She yearned for death as the only way out of the nightmare her life had become. A devout Catholic however, for Mrs. A, suicide was not an option, though it beckoned her, and took all of her will to resist.

As she and her doctor struggled to find a way to help her, her doctor shared what he thought about using a bio-socio-psycho-spiritual formulation, both as a way of understanding the person, and as a way of finding paths toward healing. Mrs. A's family history was positive for depression, so she was vulnerable biologically. Her social situation was catastrophically difficult. She also acknowledged that in her family, she had always been a caregiver and that it seemed to be her lot in life to bear whatever came her way, much as her mother had done before her (perhaps a psychological contribution to her difficulty). Her doctor also wondered about spiritual aspects.

Mrs. A shared that when her husband had lain in his coma, she'd prayed fervently for his recovery. A devout person, it was her practice to pray several times each day. When her husband awakened, but as a living ghost, it seemed as though it was a cruel joke. "God and I," she said, "are not speaking."

This understanding deepened the connection between the doctor and Mrs. A. She felt that she had a safe place in her relationship with her doctor in which she was deeply understood. Over many months, her despair lessened and she found a way back into her life, including an active practice of her faith.

In either case, however, the use of an explicit formulation in this way can identify problems and challenges early in the evaluation phase and can help the physician avoid getting involved in a treatment under conditions that make it likely to fail. Mutual expectations can be made clear (e.g., the patient must engage in a 12-step program, get a sponsor, and practice sobriety for the duration of the treatment together), and the disagreement can be used to forge a strong working relationship, or the physician and patient may agree not to work together.

The formulation and differential diagnosis are of course always in flux, as more information becomes available and the doctor and patient come to know each other more deeply.

TABLE 3-2 Strategies to Build the Doctor–Patient Relationship

- Encourage the patient to tell his or her story.
- Explain the process of the clinical encounter at the outset.
- Use open-ended questions early in the interview.
- Elicit the patient's understanding of the problems.
- Summarize information and encourage the patient to correct any misinformation.
- Look for the "nod" as an indication of collaboration.
- Provide transitional statements when moving to new sections of the history.
- End the interview with an opportunity for the patient to add or correct information.
- Formulate according to the bio-socio-psycho-spiritual model.
- Share your formulation with the patient and negotiate a plan for treatment.

Part of the doctor's role is to welcome and nurture, to change, and to promote growth, allowing the relationship to grow as part of the process (Table 3-2).[15]

OBSTACLES AND DIFFICULTIES IN THE DOCTOR–PATIENT RELATIONSHIP

Lazare and colleagues[25] pioneered the patient's perspective as a customer of the healthcare system. Lazare[13] subsequently addressed the profound importance of acknowledging the potential for shame and humiliation in the doctor–patient encounter and most recently has written a treatise on the nature and power of true, heartfelt apology.[26] Throughout his work, Lazare addressed the inevitable occurrence of conflict in the doctor–patient relationship (as in all important human relationships) and offered wise counsel for negotiating with the patient as a true partner to find creative solutions.[56]

Conflict and difficulty may arise from the very nature of the physician's training, language, or office environment. Physicians who use overly technical, arcane, or obtuse language distance themselves and make communication difficult. Physicians may lose sight of how intimidating, arcane, and forbidding medical practice—perhaps especially psychiatry—can appear to the uninitiated, unless proactive steps toward demystification occur. Complex and demanding electronic health records can draw the physician's focus and attention, possibly to the detriment of the doctor–patient relationship.[57] Similarly, overreliance on so-called objective measures, such as symptom checklists, questionnaires, tests, and other measurements, may speed diagnosis but alienate patients from effective collaboration. More insidious may be assumptions regarding the supposed incapacity of psychiatric patients to be full partners in their own care. Hurtful, dismissive language, or a lack of appreciation for the likelihood that a patient has previously experienced hurtful care, may damage the relationship.[16,18] Overly brief, symptom-focused interviews that fail to address the whole person, as well as his or her preferences, questions, and concerns, are inadequate foundations for an effective relationship.

Conflict may also arise from the nature of the problem to be addressed. In general, patients are interested in their illness—how they experience their symptoms, how their health can be restored, how to ameliorate their suffering—whereas physicians are often primarily concerned with making an accurate diagnosis of an underlying disease.[58] Moreover, physicians may erroneously believe that the patient's chief complaint is the one that the patient gives voice to first, whereas patients often approach their doctors warily, not leading with their main concern, which they may not voice at all unless conditions of safety and trust are established.[59] Any inadvertent shaming of the patient makes the emergence of the real concern all the less likely.[13]

Physicians may misunderstand a patient's readiness to change and assume that once a diagnosis or problem is identified, the patient is prepared to work to change it. In actuality, a patient may be unable or unwilling to acknowledge the problem that is obvious to the physician or, even if able to acknowledge it, may not be prepared to take serious action to change it. Clarity about where the patient is in the cycle of change[60,61] can clarify such misunderstanding and help the physician direct his or her efforts at helping the patient become more ready to change, rather than fruitlessly urging change to which the patient is not committed. Similarly, physicians may underestimate social, psychological, or spiritual aspects of a person's suffering that complicate the person's willingness or ability to partner with the physician toward change. A deeply depressed patient, for example, whose sense of shame and worthlessness is so profound that the person feels that he or she does not deserve to recover, may be uncooperative with a treatment regimen until these ideas are examined in an accepting and supportive relationship.

Conflict may arise, too, over the goals of the work. Increasingly, mental health advocates and patients promote recovery as a desired outcome of treatment, even for severe psychiatric illness. Working toward recovery in schizophrenia or bipolar disorder, which most psychiatrists regard as life-long conditions that require ongoing management, may seem unrealistic or even dishonest.[62]

It may be useful for physicians to be aware that the term *recovery* is often used in the mental health community to signify a state analogous to recovery from alcoholism or other substance abuse.[63] In this context, one is never construed to be a recovered alcoholic but rather a recovering alcoholic—someone whose sobriety is solid; who understands his or her condition and vulnerabilities well; who takes good care of himself or herself; and who is ever alert to risks of relapse, to which the person is vulnerable for his or her entire life.

In a mental health context, *recovery* similarly connotes a process of reclaiming one's life, taking charge of one's options, and stepping out of the position of passivity and victimization that major mental illness often entails, particularly if it involves involuntary treatment, stigmatization, or downright oppression. From this perspective, recovery means moving beyond symptomatic control of the disease to having a full life of one's own design (including work, friends, sexual relationships, recreation, political engagement, spiritual involvement, and other aspects of a full and challenging life).

Other sources of conflict in the doctor–patient relationship may include conflict over methods of treatment (a psychiatrist, perhaps, who emphasizes medication to treat depression to the exclusion of other areas of the patient's life, such as a troubled and depressing marriage), over the conditions of treatment (e.g., the frequency of interactions or access to the physician after hours), or over the effectiveness of treatment (e.g., the psychiatrist believes that antipsychotic medications restore a patient's function, whereas the patient believes the same medications create a sense of being drugged and "not being myself").[20]

In these examples, as in so many challenges on the journey of rendering care, an answer may lie not solely in the doctor's offered treatment, nor in the patient's resistance to change, but in the vitality, authenticity, and effectiveness of the doctor–patient relationship.

CONCLUSION

The doctor–patient relationship is a key driver of clinical outcomes—both in promoting desired results and in preventing adverse outcomes. An effective doctor–patient relationship involves both parties in co-creating a working relationship that is reliable, effective, and durable. The doctor–patient relationship in the general hospital has several unique features, including limited privacy, the interplay of medical and psychiatric illness, and the interplay of relationships among the psychiatrist, the patient, and the medical or surgical team. The relationship promotes good outcomes by creating an empowered, engaged, and active partnership with patients who feel heard and accurately understood by their physicians. Successful relationships require physicians to practice a welcoming stance, participatory decision-making, and mindfulness about both the patient's and the physician's inner lives. Especially in psychiatry, the physician must understand and relate to the patient as a whole person, which requires both accurate diagnosis and formulation, blending biological, social, psychological, and spiritual perspectives. Conflict is an inevitable aspect of all important relationships and, properly managed, can deepen and strengthen them. In the doctor–patient relationship, conflict can arise from many sources and can either derail the relationship or provide an opportunity to improve communication, alliance, and commitment.

REFERENCES

Access the reference list online at https://expertconsult.inkling.com/.

The Psychiatric Interview

4

Gene V. Beresin, M.D., M.A.
Christopher Gordon, M.D.

OVERVIEW

The purpose of the initial psychiatric interview is to build a relationship and a therapeutic alliance with an individual or a family, and to collect, organize, and synthesize information about present and past thoughts, feelings, and behaviors. The relevant data derive from several sources: observing the patient's behavior with the examiner and with others present (including medical staff); attending to the emotional responses of the examiner; obtaining pertinent medical, psychiatric, developmental, educational, occupational, social, cultural, and spiritual history (using collateral resources if possible); and performing a mental status examination. The initial evaluation should enable the practitioner to develop a clinical formulation that integrates biological, social, and psychological dimensions of a patient's life and establish provisional clinical hypotheses and questions—the differential diagnosis—that need to be tested empirically in future clinical work.[1]

A collaborative review of the formulation and differential diagnosis can provide a platform for developing (with the patient) options and recommendations for treatment, taking into account the patient's amenability for therapeutic intervention.[2] Finally, the interview must generate a relationship both with the patient and with the primary medical or surgical team as the basis of future collaboration for treatment.

Few medical encounters are more intimate and potentially frightening and shameful than the psychiatric examination.[3] As such, it is critical that the examiner create a safe space for the kind of deeply personal self-revelation required.

Several methods of the psychiatric interview are examined in this chapter. These methods include the following: promoting a healthy and secure attachment between doctor and patient that promotes self-disclosure and reflection and lends itself to the creation of a coherent narrative of the patient's life; appreciating the context of the interview that influences the interviewer's clinical technique; establishing an alliance around the task at hand and fostering effective communication; considering awareness of one's personal implicit biases that may influence history gathering, establishing a relationship, and offering options for treatment;[4] collecting data necessary for creating a formulation of the patient's strengths and weaknesses, a differential diagnosis, and recommendations for treatment, if necessary; educating the patient about the nature of emotional, behavioral, and interpersonal problems, and psychiatric illnesses (while preparing the patient for a psychiatric intervention, if indicated and agreed upon, and setting up arrangements for follow-up); using special techniques with children, adolescents, and families; understanding difficulties and errors in the psychiatric interview; and documenting the clinical findings for the medical record and communicating with other clinicians involved in the patient's care.

CASE 1

Mr. C, a 96-year-old man presented to the emergency department (ED) the day after he fell the previous night in his assisted-living facility; while on the way to the bathroom he tripped and fell. There was no pain, no head injury, and no loss of consciousness. He had called his 65-year-old son (a physician) and they agreed that Mr. C could probably return to bed and that they would talk the next day.

The day after the fall, Mr. C called his primary care provider (PCP) and reported that he had not urinated that day. He was told to go to the ED. His son, who was notified, met him at the hospital. His medications included a diuretic for hypertension, metoprolol for an arrhythmia, and escitalopram for anxiety. He had been treated for prostate cancer 6 years earlier, with excellent results.

In the ED he was alert and articulate, and able to describe his medical, social, and psychiatric history. His son corroborated the history. The consultant frequently turned to the son to obtain parts of the history. Mr. C also had a 60-year-old daughter. His wife had died 10 years previously from cancer. He said that he was dizzy and short of breath. His work-up revealed that his hematocrit had dropped from a baseline of 35.3 to 29, and he had a large hematoma in his left chest, with six fractured ribs. There was no pneumothorax. Mr. C received a blood transfusion.

In the ED, he became disoriented and agitated, and began talking to his wife. His son informed the nurse and a psychiatric consultation was ordered. About 2 hours later, the psychiatric consultant arrived and noted that Mr. C was oriented (times three), that his recent and remote memory was intact, and his speech was normal in flow and form. His mood and affect were normal and he did not recall having spoken with his deceased wife. He denied hallucinations, paranoia, or suicidal ideation. The psychiatrist's interview included a lengthy discussion of his passion for fishing, boating, and gourmet cooking. They talked about his life-long work as an entrepreneur, and the loving relationship he had with his late wife. They also talked about their mutual love for sushi. He made frequent jokes about the long wait for a bed, and the frantic pace in the ED. Given Mr. C's long wait in the ED, he thought it might be a good idea for the hospital to have room service and this might help in the financial problems in the healthcare system, and he suggested that the hospital leadership might consult him for advice. He noted that serving fish would be wonderful for raising everyone's omega-3 fatty acids.

After Mr. C was admitted to the medical floor, he again became disoriented, agitated, and needed restraint (as he was attempting to pull out his intravenous lines and to leave his bed). The psychiatrist returned to his bedside, noted the changes in his mental status, and suggested low-dose haloperidol and lorazepam for what appeared to be an episode of delirium.

Later that evening, the consultant returned to find the man much improved. Upon greeting him, the psychiatrist was asked how he was doing with establishing room service, particularly now that he was in his room. They talked about the terrible quality of the hospital food, and the need for changes to the healthcare system, as well as a sushi bar in the hospital.

Unfortunately, delirium recurred despite moderately increased doses of haloperidol. The consultant discussed the case with the psychiatric resident covering the consultation service. The resident asked the attending consultant if the recurrent delirium might be complicated by alcohol withdrawal. The resident, who spent considerable time alone with Mr. C inquired about his daily use of alcohol and noted that he tended to drink up to a fifth of vodka nightly to aid a chronic sleep problem. The senior consultant realized that his history was deficient, largely because he did not ask about alcohol or substance use, and reflected that his history was influenced by the presence of the patient's son, who was a physician. He appreciated that he inadvertently omitted sensitive but essential parts of the interview in an effort to avoid shaming the patient and his son. This appreciation resulted in ordering lorazepam and having a more detailed discussion of substance use and his sleep disturbance.

LESSONS FROM ATTACHMENT THEORY, NARRATIVE MEDICINE, AND MINDFUL PRACTICE

I'm the spirit's janitor. All I do is wipe the windows a little bit so you can see for yourself.

— Godfrey Chips, Lakota Medicine Man[5]

Healthy interactions with "attachment figures" in early life (e.g., parents) promote robust biological, emotional, and social development in childhood and throughout the life cycle.[6] The foundations for attachment theory are based on research findings in cognitive neuroscience, genetics, and brain development, and they indicate an ongoing and life-long dance between an individual's neural circuitry, genetic predisposition, brain plasticity, and environmental influences.[7] Secure attachments in childhood foster emotional resilience[8] and generate skills and habits of seeking out selected attachment figures for comfort, protection, advice, and strength. Relationships based on secure attachments lead to effective use of cognitive functions, emotional flexibility, enhancement of security, assignment of meaning to experiences, and effective self-regulation.[7] In emotional relationships of many sorts, including the student–teacher and doctor–patient relationships, there may be many features of attachment present (such as seeking proximity, or using an individual as a "safe haven" for soothing and as a secure base).[9]

What promotes secure attachment in early childhood, and how may we draw from this in understanding a therapeutic doctor–patient relationship and an effective psychiatric interview? The foundations for secure attachment for children (according to Siegel) include several attributes ascribed to parents[7] (Table 4-1).

We must always be mindful not to patronize our patients and to steer clear of the paternalistic power dynamics that could be implied in analogizing the doctor–patient relationship to one between parent and child; nonetheless, if we substitute "doctor" for "parent" and similarly substitute "patient" for "child," we can immediately see the relevance

TABLE 4-1 Elements That Contribute to Secure Attachments

- Communication that is collaborative, resonant, mutual, and attuned to the cognitive and emotional state of the child.
- Dialogue that is reflective and responsive to the state of the child. This creates a sense that subjective experience can be shared, and allows for the child "being seen." It requires use of empathy, "mindsight," and an ability to "see," or be in touch with, the child's state of mind.
- Identification and repair of miscommunications and misunderstandings. When the parent corrects problems in communication, the child can make sense of painful disconnections. Repair of communication failures requires consistent, predictable, reflective, intentional, and mindful caregiving. The emphasis here is on mindfulness and reflection. Mindfulness in this instance is an example of a parent's ability for self-awareness, particularly of his or her emotional reactions to the child and the impact of his or her words and actions on the child.
- Emotional communication that involves sharing feelings that amplify the positive and mitigate the negative.
- Assistance in the child's development of coherent narratives that connect experiences in the past and present, creating an autobiographical sense of self-awareness (using language to weave together thoughts, feelings, sensations, and actions as a means of organizing and making sense of internal and external worlds).

to clinical practice. We can see how important each of these elements is in fostering a doctor–patient relationship that is open, honest, mutual, collaborative, respectful, trustworthy, and secure. Appreciating the dynamics of secure attachment also deepens the meaning of "patient-centered" care. The medical literature clearly indicates that good outcomes and patient satisfaction involve physician relationship techniques that center on reflection, empathy, understanding, legitimization, and support.[10,11] Patients reveal more about themselves when they trust their doctors, and trust has been found to relate primarily to behavior during clinical interviews[11] rather than to any preconceived notion of competence of the doctor or behavior outside the office.

Particularly important in the psychiatric interview is the facilitation of a patient's narrative. The practice of narrative medicine involves an ability to acknowledge, absorb, interpret, and act on the stories and struggles of others.[12] Charon[12] describes the process of listening to patients' stories as a process of following the biological, familial, cultural, and existential thread of the situation. It encompasses recognizing the multiple meanings and contradictions in words and events; attending to the silences, pauses, gestures, and non-verbal cues; and entering the world of the patient, while simultaneously arousing the doctor's own memories, associations, creativity, and emotional responses—all of which are seen in some way by the patient.[12] Narratives, as with all stories, are co-created by the teller and the listener. Storytelling is an age-old part of social discourse that involves sustained attention, memory, emotional responsiveness, non-verbal responses and cues, collaborative meaning-making, and attunement to the listener's expectations. It is a vehicle for explaining behavior. Stories and storytelling are pervasive in society as a means of conveying symbolic activity, history, communication, and teaching.[7] If a physician can assist the patient in telling his or her story effectively, reliable and valid data will be collected and the relationship solidified. Narratives are facilitated by authentic, compassionate, and genuine engagement.

A differential diagnosis detached from the patient's narrative is arid; even if it is accurate it may not lead to an effective and mutually designed treatment path. By contrast, an accurate and comprehensive differential diagnosis that is supported by an appreciation of the patient's narrative is experienced by both patient and physician as more three-dimensional, more real, and more likely to lead to a mutually created and achievable plan, with which the patient is much more likely to "comply."

Creating the optimal conditions for a secure attachment and the elaboration of a coherent narrative requires mindful practice. Just as the parent must be careful to differentiate his or her emotional state and needs from the child's and be aware of conflicts and communication failures, so too must the mindful practitioner. Epstein[13] noted that mindful practitioners attend in a non-judgmental way to their own physical and mental states during the interview. Their critical self-reflection allows them to listen carefully to a patient's distress, to recognize their own errors, to make evidence-based decisions, and to stay attuned to their own values so that they may act with compassion, technical competence, and insight.

Self-reflection is critical in psychiatric interviewing. Reflective practice entails observing ourselves (including our emotional reactions to patients, colleagues, and illness); our deficits in knowledge and skill; our personal styles of communicating; our responses to personal vulnerability and failure; our willingness or resistance to acknowledge error, to apologize, and to ask for forgiveness; and our reactions to stress. Self-awareness allows us to be aware of our own thinking, feelings, and action, while we are in the process of practicing. It is important in the elaboration of a patient's narrative to separate it from one's own. We all have life experiences that may house unconscious associations and biases that may inadvertently color or influence our perception of the stories related by our patients. For example, our attitudes toward gender, sexual orientation, race, ethnicity and culture, are often colored by implicit bias, and these may become barriers to an empathic psychiatric interview. The more we are able and willing to confront our hidden judgmental attitudes, the better we are able to foster truly collaborative relationships, gather history impartially, and engage in patient-centered care.[4] By working in this manner, a clinician enhances his or her confidence, competence, sensitivity, openness, and lack of defensiveness—all of which assist in fostering secure attachments with patients, and help them share their innermost fears, concerns, and problems.

THE CONTEXT OF THE INTERVIEW: FACTORS INFLUENCING THE FORM AND CONTENT OF THE INTERVIEW

All interviews occur in a context. Awareness of the context may require modification of clinical interviewing techniques. There are four elements to consider: the setting, the situation, the subject, and the significance.[14]

The Setting

Patients are exquisitely sensitive to the environment in which they are evaluated. There is a vast difference between being seen in an emergency department (ED), on a medical floor, on an inpatient or partial hospital unit, in a psychiatric outpatient clinic, in a private doctor's office, in a school, or in a court clinic. In the ED or on a medical or surgical floor, space for private, undisturbed interviews is usually inadequate. Such settings are filled with action, drama, and hospital personnel who race around. ED visits may require long waits and contribute to impersonal approaches to patients and negative attitudes towards psychiatric patients. For a patient with borderline traits who is in crisis, this can only create extreme frustration and exacerbate chronic fears of deprivation, betrayal, abandonment, aloneness, and regression.[15] For these and for higher functioning patients, the public nature of the environment and the frantic pace of the emergency service may make it difficult for the patient to present personal, private material calmly. It is always advisable to ask the patient directly how comfortable he or she feels in the examining room, and to try to ensure privacy and a quiet environment with minimal distractions.

The setting must be comfortable for the patient and the physician. If the patient is agitated, aggressive, or threatening, it is important to calmly assert that the examination must require that everyone is safe and that we will only use words and not actions during the interview. Hostile patients should be interviewed in a setting in which the doctor is protected. In some instances, local security may need to be called to ensure safety.

The Situation

Many individuals seek psychiatric help because they are aware that they have a problem. Given the limitations placed on psychiatrists by some managed care panels, access to care may be severely limited. It is not unusual for a patient to present to an ED in crisis after having called multiple psychiatrists, only to find that their practices are all filled. The frustrating process of finding a psychiatrist sets the stage for some patients to either disparage the field and the healthcare system, or to idealize the psychiatrist who has made the time for the patient. In either case, much goes on before the first visit that may significantly affect the initial interview. To complicate matters, the evaluator needs to understand previous experience with psychiatrists and psychiatric treatment. Sometimes a patient has had a negative experience with another psychiatrist—perhaps the result of a mismatch of personalities, a style that was ineffective, a treatment that did not work, or other problems. Many will wonder about a repeat performance. In all cases, in the history and relationship-building, it is propitious to ask about previous treatments (e.g., what worked and what did not, and particularly how the patient felt about the psychiatrist). There should be reassurance that this information is held in confidence, though in a hospital setting, the clinician should discuss that information may be shared with the medical or surgical team.

Other patients may come in reluctantly or even with great resistance. Many arrive in the ED at the request or demand of a loved one, friend, colleague, or employer because of behaviors deemed troublesome. The patient may deny any problem or simply be too terrified to confront a condition that is bizarre, unexplainable, or "mental." Some conditions are ego-syntonic, such as anorexia nervosa. A patient with this eating disorder typically sees the psychiatrist as the enemy—as a doctor who wants to make her "get fat." For resistant patients, it is often very useful to address the issue at the outset. With an anorexic patient referred by her internist and brought in by family, one could begin by saying, "Hi, Ms. Jones. I know you really don't want to be here. I understand that your doctor and family are concerned about your weight. I assure you that my job is first and foremost to understand your point of view. Can you tell me why you think they wanted you to see me?" Another common situation with extreme resistance is the individual with alcohol abuse who is brought in by a spouse or friend (and clearly not ready to stop drinking). In this case you might say, "Good morning, Mr. Jones. I heard from your wife that she is really concerned about your drinking, and your safety, especially when driving. First, let me tell you that neither I nor anyone else can stop you from drinking. That is not my mission today. I do want to know what your drinking pattern is, but more than that, I want to get the picture of your entire life to understand your current situation." Extremely resistant patients may be brought involuntarily to an emergency service, often in restraints, by police or ambulance, because they are considered dangerous to themselves or others. It is typically terrifying, insulting, and humiliating to be physically restrained. Regardless of the reasons for admission, unknown to the psychiatrist, it is often wise to begin the interview as follows: "Hi, Ms. Carter, my name is Dr. Beresin. I am terribly sorry you are strapped down, but the police and your family were very upset when you locked yourself in the car and turned on the ignition. They found a suicide note on the kitchen table. Everyone was really concerned about your safety. I would like to discuss what is going on, and see what we can do together to figure things out."

In the general hospital, a physician is commonly asked to perform a psychiatric evaluation on a patient who is hospitalized on a medical or surgical service with symptoms arising during medical or surgical treatment. These patients may be delirious and have no idea that they are going to be seen by a psychiatrist. This was never part of their agreement when they came into the hospital for surgery, and no one may have explained the risk of delirium. Some may be resistant, others confused. Other delirious patients are quite cognizant of their altered mental status and are extremely frightened. They may wonder whether the condition is going to continue forever. For example, if we know a patient has undergone abdominal surgery for colon cancer, and has been agitated, sleepless, hallucinating, and delusional, a psychiatric consultant might begin, "Good morning, Mr. Harris. My name is Dr. Beresin. I heard about your surgery from Dr. Rand and understand you have been having some experiences that may seem kind of strange or frightening to you. Sometimes after surgery, people have a reaction to the procedure or the medications used that causes difficulties with sleep, agitation, and mental confusion. This is not unusual, and it is generally temporary. I would like to help you and your team figure out what is going on and what we can do about this." Other requests for psychiatric evaluation may require entirely different skills, such as when the medical team or emergency service seeks help for a family who lost a loved one.

In each of these situations, the psychiatrist needs to understand the nature of the situation and to take this into account when planning the evaluation. In the aforementioned examples, only the introduction was addressed. However, when we see the details (discussed next) about building a relationship and modifying communication styles and questions to meet the needs of each situation, other techniques might have to be employed to make a therapeutic alliance. It is always helpful to find out as much ancillary information as possible before the interview. This may be done by talking with the medical team and primary care physicians, by looking in an electronic medical record or patient chart, and by talking with family, friends, or professionals (such as police or emergency medical technicians).

The Subject

Naturally, the clinical interview needs to take into account features of the subject (including age, developmental level, gender, and cultural background, among others). Moreover, one needs to determine "who" the patient is. In families, there may be an identified patient (e.g., a conduct-disordered child or a child with chronic abdominal pain). However, the examiner must keep in mind that psychiatric and medical syndromes do not occur in a vacuum. Although the family has determined an "identified patient," the examiner should consider that, when evaluating the child, all members of the environment need to be part of the evaluation. A similar situation occurs when an adult child brings in an elderly demented parent for an evaluation. It is incumbent on the evaluator to consider the home environment and caretaking, in addition to simply evaluating the geriatric patient. In couples, one or both may identify the "other" as the "problem." An astute clinician remains neutral (i.e., does not "take sides") and allows each person's perspective to be clarified.

Children and adolescents require special consideration. Though they may, indeed, be the "identified patient," they are embedded in a home life that requires evaluation; the parent(s) or guardian(s) must help administer any prescribed treatment (e.g., psychotropic or behavioral). Furthermore, the developmental level of the child needs to be considered in the examination. Young children may not be able to articulate what they are experiencing. For example, an 8-year-old boy who has panic attacks may simply throw temper tantrums and display oppositional behavior when asked to go to a restaurant. Although he may be phobic about malls and restaurants, his parents simply see his behavior as defiance. When asked what he is experiencing, he may not be able to describe palpitations, shortness of breath, fears of impending doom, or tremulousness. However, if he is asked to draw a picture of himself at the restaurant, he may draw himself with a scared look on his face and with jagged lines all around his body. Then when specific questions are asked, he is able to acknowledge many classic symptoms of panic disorder.

Evaluation of adolescents raises additional issues. While some may come willingly, others are dragged in against their will. In this instance, it is very important to identify and to empathize with the teenager: "Hi, Tony. I can see this is the last place you want to be. But now that you've been hauled in here by your folks, we should make the best of it. Look, I have no clue what is going on, and don't even know if you are the problem! Why don't you tell me your story?" Teenagers may indeed feel like hostages. They may have *bona fide* psychiatric disorders or may be stuck in a terrible home situation. The most important thing the examiner must convey is that the teenager's perspective is important, and that this will be looked at, as well as the parent's point of view. It is also critical to let adolescents, as all patients, know about the rules and limits of confidentiality. Many children think that whatever they say will be directly transmitted to their parents. Surely this is their experience in school. However, there are clear guidelines about adolescent confidentiality, and these should be delineated at the beginning of the clinical encounter. Confidentiality is a core part of the evaluation, and it will be honored for the adolescent; it is essential that this be communicated to them so they may feel safe in divulging very sensitive and private information without fear of repercussion. Issues such as sexuality, sexually transmitted diseases, substance abuse, and mental health are protected by state and federal statutes. There are, however, exceptions; one major exception is that if the patient or another is in danger by virtue of an adolescent's behavior, confidentiality is waived.[16]

The Significance

Psychiatric disorders are commonly stigmatized and subsequently are often accompanied by profound shame, anxiety, denial, fear, and uncertainty. Patients generally have a poor understanding of psychiatric disorders, either from lack of information, myth, or misinformation from the media (e.g., TV, radio, and the internet).[17] Many patients have preconceived notions of what to expect (bad or good), based on the experience of friends or family. Some patients, having talked with others or having searched online, may be certain or very worried that they suffer from a particular condition, and this may color the information presented to an examiner. A specific syndrome or symptom may have idiosyncratic significance to a patient, perhaps because a relative with a mood disorder was hospitalized for life, before the deinstitutionalization of people with mental disorders. Hence, he or she may be extremely wary of divulging any indication of severe symptoms lest life-long hospitalization results. Obsessions or compulsions may be seen as clear evidence of losing one's mind, having a brain tumor, or "becoming like Aunt Jessie with a chronic psychosis."[14] Some patients (based on cognitive limitations) may not understand their symptoms. These may be normal, such as the developmental stage in a school-age child, whereas others may be a function of mental retardation, autistic spectrum disorder, or cerebral lacunae secondary to multiple infarcts following embolic strokes.

Finally, there are significant cultural differences in the way mental health and mental illness are viewed. Culture may influence health-seeking and mental health-seeking behavior, the understanding of psychiatric symptoms, the course of psychiatric disorders, the efficacy of various treatments, or the kinds of treatments accepted.[18] Psychosis, for example, may be viewed as possession by spirits. Some cultural groups have much higher completion rates for suicide, and thus previous attempts in some individuals should be taken more seriously. Understanding the family structure may be critical to the negotiation of treatment; approval by a family elder could be crucial in the acceptance of professional help.

ESTABLISHING AN ALLIANCE AND FOSTERING EFFECTIVE COMMUNICATION

Studies of physician–patient communication have demonstrated that good outcomes flow from effective communication; developing a good patient-centered relationship is characterized by friendliness, courtesy, empathy, and partnership building, and by the provision of information. Positive outcomes have included benefits to emotional health, symptom resolution, and physiologic measures (e.g., blood pressure, blood glucose level, and pain control).[19–22]

In 1999, leaders and representatives of major medical schools and professional organizations convened at the Fetzer Institute in Kalamazoo, Michigan, to propose a model for doctor–patient communication that would lend itself to the creation of curricula for medical and graduate medical education, and for the development of standards for the profession. The goals of the Kalamazoo Consensus Statement[23] were to foster a sound doctor–patient relationship

TABLE 4-2 Building a Relationship: the Fundamental Tasks of Communication

- Elicit the patient's story while guiding the interview by diagnostic reasoning.
- Maintain an awareness that feelings, ideas, and values of both the patient and the doctor influence the relationship.
- Develop a partnership with the patient and form an alliance in which the patient participates in decision-making.
- Work with patients' families and support networks.

Open the Discussion

- Allow the patient to express his or her opening statement without interruption.
- Encourage the patient to describe a full set of concerns.
- Maintain a personal connection during the interview.

Gather Information

- Use both open- and closed-ended questions.
- Provide structure, clarification, and a summary of the information collected.
- Listen actively, using verbal and non-verbal methods (e.g., eye contact).

Understand the Patient's Perspective

- Explore contextual issues (e.g., familial, cultural, spiritual, age, gender, and socioeconomic status).
- Elicit beliefs, concerns, and expectations about health and illness.
- Validate and respond appropriately to the patient's ideas, feelings, and values.

Share Information

- Avoid technical language and medical jargon.
- Determine if the patient understands your explanations.
- Encourage questions.

Reach Agreement on Problems and Plans

- Welcome participation in decision-making.
- Determine the patient's amenability to following a plan.
- Identify and enlist resources and supports.

Provide Closure

- Ask if the patient has questions or other concerns.
- Summarize and solidify the agreement with a plan of action.
- Review the follow-up plans.

and to provide a model for the clinical interview. The key elements of this statement are summarized in Table 4-2, and are applicable to the psychiatric interview.

BUILDING THE RELATIONSHIP AND THERAPEUTIC ALLIANCE

All psychiatric interviews must begin with a personal introduction and establish the purpose of the interview; this helps create an alliance around the initial examination. The interviewer should attempt to greet the person warmly and use words that demonstrate care, attention, and concern. Note-taking and use of computers should be minimized and, if used, should not interfere with ongoing eye contact. The interviewer should indicate that this interaction is collaborative, and that any misunderstandings on the part of patient or physician should be immediately clarified. In addition, the patient should be instructed to ask questions, interrupt, and provide corrections or additions at any time. The time frame for the interview should be announced. In general, the interviewer should acknowledge that some of the issues and questions raised will be highly personal, and that if there are issues that the patient has real trouble with, he or she should let the examiner know. Confidentiality should be assured at the outset of the interview. If the psychiatrist is meeting a hospitalized patient at the request of the primary medical or surgical team, this should be stated at the outset.

These initial guidelines set the tone, quality, and style of the clinical interview. An example of a beginning is, "Hi, Mr. Smith. My name is Dr. Beresin. It is nice to meet you. Your surgeon, Dr. Jones, asked me to meet with you because he is concerned that you haven't eaten or taken any of your medications since you've been in the hospital. I would like to discuss some of the issues or problems you are dealing with so that we can both understand them better, and figure out what kind of assistance may be available. I will need to ask you a number of questions about your life, both your past and present, and if I need some clarification about your descriptions I will ask for your help to be sure I 'get it.' If you think I have missed the boat, please chime in and correct my misunderstanding. Some of the topics may be highly personal, and I hope that you will let me know if things get a bit too much. We will have about an hour to go through this, and then we'll try to come up with a reasonable plan together. I do want you to know that everything we say is confidential. Do you have any questions about our job today?" This should be followed with an open-ended question about the reasons for the interview.

One of the most important aspects of building a therapeutic alliance is helping the patient feel safe. Demonstrating warmth and respect is essential. In addition, the psychiatrist should display genuine interest and curiosity in working with a new patient. Preconceived notions about the patient should be eschewed. If there are questions about the patient's cultural background or spiritual beliefs that may have an impact on the information provided, on the emotional response to symptoms, or on the acceptance of a treatment plan, the physician should note at the outset that if any of these areas are of central importance to the patient, he or she should feel free to speak about such beliefs or values. The patient should have the sense that both doctor and patient are exploring the history, life experience, and current symptoms together.

For many patients, the psychiatric interview is probably one of the most confusing examinations in medicine. The psychiatric interview is at once professional and profoundly intimate. We are asking patients to reveal parts of their life they may only have shared with extremely close friends, a spouse, clergy, or family, if anyone. And they are coming into a setting in which they are supposed to do this with a total stranger. Being a doctor may not be sufficient to allay the apprehension that surrounds this situation; being a trustworthy, caring human being may help a great deal. It is vital to make the interview highly personal and to use techniques that come naturally. Beyond affirming and validating the patient's story with extreme sensitivity, some clinicians may use humor and judicious self-revelation. These elements are characteristics of healers.[24]

An example should serve to demonstrate some of these principles. A 65-year-old deeply religious woman was seen to evaluate delirium following cardiac bypass surgery. She told the psychiatric examiner in her opening discussion that she wanted to switch from her primary care physician, whom she had seen for more than 30 years. As part of her postoperative delirium, she developed the delusion that he may have raped her during one of his visits with her. She felt that she could not possibly face him, her priest, or her family, and she was stricken with deep despair. Although the examiner may have recognized this as a biological consequence of her surgery and postoperative course, the patient's personal experience spoke differently. She would not immediately accept an early interpretation or explanation that her brain was not functioning correctly. In such a situation, the examiner must verbally acknowledge her perspective, seeing the problem through her eyes, and helping her see that he or she "gets it." For the patient, this was a horrible nightmare. The interviewer might have said, "Mrs. Jones, I understand how awful you must feel. Can you tell me how this could have happened, given your long-standing and trusting relationship with your doctor?" She answered that she did not know, but that she was really confused and upset. When the examiner established a trusting relationship, completed the examination, determined delirium was present, and explained the nature of this problem, they agreed on using haloperidol to improve sleep and "nerves." Additional clarifications could be made in a subsequent session after the delirium cleared.

As noted earlier, reliable mirroring of the patient's cognitive and emotional state and self-reflection of one's affective response to patients are part and parcel of establishing secure attachments. Actively practicing self-reflection and clarifying one's understanding helps to model behavior for the patient, as the doctor and patient co-create the narrative.

Giving frequent summaries to "check in" on what the physician has heard may be very valuable, particularly early on in the interview, when the opening discussion or chief complaints are elicited. For example, consultation was requested after a 22-year-old woman who was hospitalized for emergency surgery refused to go to a rehabilitation facility. During the course of the psychiatric interview, the physician elicited a history of obsessive–compulsive symptoms during the past 2 years that led her to be housebound. The interviewer said, "So, Ms. Thompson, let's see if I get it. You have been stuck at home and cannot get out of the house because you have to walk up and down the stairs for a number of hours. If you did not 'get it right,' something terrible would happen to one of your family members. You also noted that you were found walking the stairs in public places, and that even your friends did not understand this behavior, and they made fun of you. You mentioned that you had to 'check' on the stove and other appliances being turned off, and could not leave your car, because you were afraid it would not turn off, or that the brake was not fully on, and again, something terrible would happen to someone. And you said to me that you were really upset because you knew this behavior was 'crazy.' How awful this must be for you! Did I get it right?" The examiner should be sure to see both verbally and non-verbally that this captured the patient's problem. If positive feedback did not occur, the examiner should attempt to see if there was a misinterpretation, or if the interviewer came across as judgmental or critical. One could "normalize" the situation and reassure the patient to further solidify the alliance by saying, "Ms. Thompson, your tendency to stay home, stuck, in the effort to avoid hurting anyone is totally natural given your perception and concern for others close to you. I do agree, it does not make sense, and appreciate that it feels bizarre and unusual. I can see why it would be upsetting to have to wait any longer to return home. I think we can better understand this behavior, and later I can suggest ways of coping and maybe even overcoming this situation through treatments that have been quite successful with others. However, I do need to get some additional information. Is that OK?" In this way, the clinician helps the patient feel understood—that anyone in that situation would feel the same way, and that there is hope. But more information is needed. This strategy demonstrates respect and understanding and provides support and comfort, while building the alliance.

DATA COLLECTION: BEHAVIORAL OBSERVATION, THE MEDICAL AND PSYCHIATRIC HISTORY, AND MENTAL STATUS EXAMINATION

Behavioral Observation

There is a lot to be learned about patients by observing them before, during, and after the psychiatric interview. It is useful to see how the patient interacts with support staff as well as with family, friends, or others who accompany him or her to the appointment. In the interview, one should take note of grooming, the style and state of repair of clothes, mannerisms, normal and abnormal movements, posture and gait, physical features (such as natural deformities, birth marks, cutting marks, scratches, tattoos, or piercings), skin quality (e.g., color, texture, and hue), language (including English proficiency, the style of words used, grammar, vocabulary, and syntax), and non-verbal cues (such as eye contact and facial expressions). All these factors contribute to a clinical formulation.

The Medical and Psychiatric History

Table 4-3 provides an overview of the key components of the psychiatric history.

Presenting Problems

The interviewer should begin with the presenting problem using open-ended questions. The patient should be encouraged to tell his or her story without interruptions. Many times the patient will turn to the doctor for elaboration, but it is best to let the patient know that he or she is the true expert and that only he or she has experienced this situation directly. It is best to use clarifying questions throughout the interview. For example, "I was really upset and worked up" may mean one thing to the patient and something else to an examiner. It could mean frustrated,

TABLE 4-3 The Psychiatric History

Identifying Information
Name, address, phone number, and e-mail address
Insurance
Age, gender, marital status, occupation, children, ethnicity, and religion
For children and adolescents: primary custodians, school, and grade
Primary care physician
Psychiatrist, allied mental health providers
Referral source
Sources of information
Reliability

Chief Complaint/Presenting Problem(s)

History of Present Illness
Onset
Perceived precipitants
Signs and symptoms
Course and duration
Treatments: professional and personal
Effects on personal, social, and occupational or academic function
Co-morbid psychiatric or medical disorders
Psychosocial stressors: personal (psychological, medical), family, friends, work/school, legal, housing, and financial
Safety assessment: presence of suicidal or homicidal ideation, plan, intent, past attempts, access to weapons
Assessment of pain

Past Psychiatric History

Previous Episodes of the Problem(s)
Symptoms, course, duration, and treatment (inpatient or outpatient)
Suicide attempts or self-injurious behavior (dates, methods, consequences)

Psychiatric Disorders
Symptoms, course, duration, and treatment (inpatient or outpatient)

Past Medical History
Medical problems: past and current
Surgical problems: past and current
Accidents
Allergies
Immunizations
Current medications: prescribed and over-the-counter medications
Other treatments: acupuncture, chiropractic, homeopathic, yoga, and meditation
Tobacco: present and past use
Substance use: present and past use
Pregnancy history: births, miscarriages, and abortions
Sexual history: birth control, safe sex practices, and history of, and screening for, sexually transmitted diseases

Review of Systems

Family History
Family psychiatric history
Family medical history

Personal History: Developmental and Social History

Early Childhood
Developmental milestones
Family relationships
Family culture and languages

Middle Childhood
School performance
Learning or attention problems
Family relationships
Friends
Hobbies
Abuse

Adolescence
School performance (include learning and attention problems)
Friends and peer relationships
Family relationships
Psychosexual history
Dating and sexual history
Work history
Substance use
Problems with the law

Early Adulthood
Education
Friends and peer relationships
Hobbies and interests
Marital and other romantic partners
Occupational history
Military experiences
Problems with the law
Domestic violence (including emotional, physical, sexual abuse)

Midlife and Older Adulthood
Career development
Marital and other romantic partners
Changes in the family
Losses
Aging process: psychological and physical

Adapted from Beresin EV: *The psychiatric interview*. In: Stern TA, editor: *The ten-minute guide to psychiatric diagnosis and treatment*. New York, 2005, Professional Publishing Group.

anxious, agitated, violent, or depressed. Such a statement requires clarification. So, too, does a comment, such as "I was really depressed." Depression to a psychiatrist may be very different for a patient. To some patients, depression means aggravated, angry, or sad. It might be a momentary agitated state or a chronic state. Asking more detailed questions not only clarifies the affective state of the patient, but also transmits the message that he or she knows best and that a real collaboration and dialogue is the only way we will figure out the problem. In addition, once the patient's words are clarified, it is very useful to use the patient's own words throughout the interview to verify that you are listening.[25]

When taking the history, it is vital to remember that the patient's primary concerns may not be the same as the physician's. For example, although the examiner may be concerned about escalating mania due to high-dose steroids, the patient may be more concerned about her husband's unemployment and how this is making her agitated and sleepless. The psychiatrist may be called to consult on managing the steroid-induced mania, whereas the patient may be focused on how the psychiatrist may help her and her husband cope with family finances. In this case, her concerns should be validated. Additionally, the consultant should gently re-direct her attention to her hospitalization and indicate that he is concerned about her inability to sleep and level of emotional intensity. If the patient feels the clinician and she are on the same page, this will facilitate the interview and enable the clinician to get a more detailed history and establish a diagnosis of mania. It is always useful to ask, "What are you most worried about?" and "What would you hope I could do to help?"

In discussing the presenting problems, it is best to avoid a set of checklist questions, but one should cover the bases to create a differential diagnosis based on the *Diagnostic and Statistical Manual* (5th edition; DSM-5). It is best to focus largely on the chief complaint and presenting problems and to incorporate other parts of the history around this. The presenting problem is the reason for a referral and is probably most important to the patient, even though additional questions about current function and the past medical or past psychiatric history may be more critical to the examiner. A good clinician, having established a trusting relationship, can always re-direct a patient to ascertain additional information (such as symptoms not mentioned by the patient, and the duration, frequency, and intensity of symptoms). Also, it is important to ask how the patient has coped with the problem and what is being done personally or professionally to help it. One should ask if there are other problems or stressors, medical problems, work, or family issues that exacerbate the current complaint. This is particularly relevant for patients who are hospitalized, because the period of hospitalization can have profound repercussions on a patient's emotional stability, family, finances, and future. After a period of open-ended questions about the current problem, the interviewer should ask questions about mood, anxiety, and other behavioral problems and how they affect the presenting problem.

A key part of the assessment of the presenting problem should be a determination of safety. Questions about suicide, homicide, domestic violence, and abuse must be included in the review of the current situation. Additionally, one must assess the patient's level of comfort and degree of physical and emotional pain. Finally, one should ascertain how motivated the patient is for getting help and how the patient is faring in personal, family, social, and professional life. Without knowing more, since this is early in the interview, the examiner should avoid offering premature reassurance, but provide support and encouragement for therapeutic assistance that will be offered in the latter part of the interview.

Past Psychiatric History

After the initial phases of the interview, open-ended questions may shift to more focused questions. In the past psychiatric history, the interviewer should inquire about previous DSM-5 diagnoses (including the symptoms of each, partial syndromes, how they were managed, and how they affected the patient's life). A full range of treatments, including outpatient, inpatient, and partial hospital care, should be considered. One should assess whether the patient has ever considered or attempted suicide. If so, ask what prompted the attempt, when it occurred, what means were used, and what the consequences were. In addition, one should also assess self-harm behaviors (such as cutting, burning, or intentional recklessness). It is most useful to ask what treatments, if any, were successful, and if so, in what ways. By the same token, the examiner should ask about treatment failures. This, of course, will contribute to the treatment recommendations provided at the close of the interview. This may be a good time in the interview to get a sense of how the patient copes under stress. What psychological, behavioral, and social means are employed in the service of maintaining equilibrium in the face of hardship? It is also wise to focus not just on coping skills, defenses, and adaptive techniques in the face of the psychiatric disorder, but also on psychosocial stressors in general (e.g., births, deaths, loss of jobs, problems in relationships, and problems with children). Discerning a patient's coping style may be highly informative and contribute to the psychiatric formulation. Does the patient rely on venting emotions, on shutting affect off and wielding cognitive controls, on using social supports, on displacing anger onto others, or on finding productive distractions (e.g., plunging into work)? Further, does the patient have a common strategy for dealing with stress, such as using meditation, prayer, exercise, or use of alcohol or other substances? Again, knowing something about a person's style of dealing with adversity uncovers defense mechanisms, and use of healthy or unhealthy behaviors, reveals something about personality, and aids in the consideration of treatment options. For example, a person who avoids emotion, uses reason, and sets about to increase tasks in hard times may be an excellent candidate for a cognitive-behavioral approach to a problem. An individual who relies on venting emotions, turning to others for support, and working to understand the historical origins of his or her problems may be a good candidate for psychodynamic psychotherapy, either individual or group.

Past Medical History

A number of psychiatric symptoms and behavioral problems are secondary to medical conditions, to the side effects of medications, and to drug–drug interactions (including those related to over-the-counter medications). The past medical history needs to be thorough and must include: past and current medical and surgical conditions; past and current use of medications (including vitamins, herbs, and non-traditional remedies); use of substances (e.g., tobacco, alcohol, and other drugs—past and present); an immunization and travel history; pregnancies; menstrual history; a history of hospitalizations and day surgeries; accidents (including sequelae, if any); and sexual history (including use of contraception, abortions, history of sexually transmitted diseases, and testing for the latter). For hospitalized patients, assessment should include a thorough review of the patient's current hospital course, relevant laboratory test results and imaging studies, medication changes, and history from nurses, doctors, and social workers.

Review of Systems

By the time the examiner inquires about past medical history and review of systems, a checklist type of questioning is adopted in lieu of the previous format of interviewing. It is useful to elicit a complete review of systems following the medical history. A number of undiagnosed medical disorders may be picked up in the course of the psychiatric interview. For instance, night sweats, weight loss, and easy bruising in an elderly man with apathy, may signify a malignancy that could be mistaken for depression. Many patients do not routinely see their primary care physician, and psychiatrists have a unique opportunity to consider medical conditions and their evaluation in the examination. Although not a formal part of the interview, laboratory testing is a core part of the psychiatric examination. Though this chapter refers to the interview, the review of systems may alert the clinician to order additional laboratory tests and consult the primary care physician about medical investigations.

Family History

The fact that many illnesses run in families requires an examiner to ask about the family history of medical, surgical, and psychiatric illnesses, along with their treatments.

Social and Developmental History

The developmental history is important for all psychiatric patients, but especially for children and adolescents, because prevention and early detection of problems may lead to interventions that can correct deviations in development. The developmental history for early and middle childhood and adolescence should include questions about: developmental milestones (e.g., motor function, speech, growth, and social and moral achievements); family relationships in the past and present; school history (including grade levels reached and any history of attention or learning disabilities); friends; hobbies; jobs; interests; athletics; substance use; and any legal problems. Questions about adult development should focus on: the nature and quality of intimate relationships; friendships; relationships with children (e.g., natural, adopted, products of assisted reproductive technology, and stepchildren); military history; work history; hobbies and interests; legal issues; and financial problems. Questions should always be asked about domestic violence (including a history of physical or sexual abuse in the past and present).

The social history should include questions about a patient's cultural background, including the nature of this heritage, how it affects family structure and function, belief systems, values, and spiritual practices. Culture can inform a patient's explanatory model of an illness for which he or she is hospitalized, and may affect his or her interactions with medical staff. Questions should be asked about the safety of the community and the quality of the social supports in the neighborhood, the place of worship, or other loci in the community.

Assessing social factors (such as the availability of housing and primary supports) is of vital importance for hospitalized patients. For instance, knowing that a depressed patient is in danger of being evicted from her apartment while in the hospital is critical in performing an adequate safety assessment.

Use of Collateral Information

In addition to the patient interview, it is quite useful to obtain collateral information. Patients may have impaired insight into their behavior, so talking to other important people in the patient's life (such as a spouse or partner, siblings, children, parents, friends, and clergy) can yield important clinical information. For example, a patient who appears paranoid and mildly psychotic may deny such symptoms or not see them as problems. To understand the nature of the problem, its duration and intensity, and its impact on function, others may need to be contacted (with informed consent, of course). This applies to many other conditions, particularly substance use disorders, in which the patient may deny the quantity used and the frequency of effects of substances on everyday life.

In the general hospital, several factors (e.g., delirium, confusion, dementia, pain, or sedation) can limit the patient's ability to give a full history. Collateral information is especially important in these cases. With the patient's permission, one should perform a thorough review of the medical chart. Medical personnel (including nurses, social workers, physical therapists, and primary care physicians) can provide data about the patient's symptoms and course. Moreover, they may know the patient over several years and have a useful perspective of the patient's attitudes toward illness and coping style.

Obtaining consent to contact others in a patient's life is useful not only for information gathering, but for the involvement of others in the treatment process, if needed. For children and adolescents, this is absolutely essential, as is obtaining information from teachers or other school personnel.

The Mental Status Examination

The mental status examination is part and parcel of any medical and psychiatric interview. Its traditional components are indicated in Table 4-4. Most of the data needed in this model can be ascertained by asking the patient about elements of the current problems. Specific questions may be needed for the evaluation of perception, thought, and cognition. Most of the information in the mental status examination is obtained by simply taking the psychiatric history and by observing the patient's behavior, affect, speech, mood, thought, and cognition.

TABLE 4-4 The Mental Status Examination

General appearance and behavior: grooming, posture, movements, mannerisms, and eye contact
Speech: rate, flow, latency, coherence, logic, and prosody
Affect: range, intensity, lability
Mood: euthymic, elevated, depressed, irritable, anxious
Perception: illusions and hallucinations
Thought (coherence and lucidity): form and content (illusions, hallucinations, and delusions)
Safety: suicidal, homicidal, self-injurious ideas, impulses, and plans
Cognition:

- Level of consciousness
- Orientation
- Attention and concentration
- Memory (registration, recent and remote)
- Calculation
- Abstraction
- Judgment
- Insight

Perceptual disorders include abnormalities in sensory stimuli. There may be misperceptions of sensory stimuli, known as *illusions*, for example, micropsia or macropsia (objects that appear smaller or larger, respectively, than they are). Phenomena such as this include distortions of external stimuli (affecting the size, shape, intensity, or sound of stimuli). Distortions of stimuli that are internally created are hallucinations and may occur in one or more of the following modalities: auditory, visual, olfactory, gustatory, or kinesthetic.

Thought disorders may manifest with difficulties in the form or content of thought. Formal thought disorders involve the way ideas are connected. Abnormalities in form may involve the logic and coherence of thinking. Such disorders may herald neurologic disorders, severe mood disorders (e.g., psychotic depression or mania), schizophreniform psychosis, delirium, or other disorders that impair reality testing. Examples of formal thought disorders are listed in Table 4-5.[26,27]

Disorders of the content of thought pertain to the specific ideas themselves. The examiner should always inquire about paranoid, suicidal, and homicidal thinking. Other indications of disorder of thought content include delusions, obsessions, and ideas of reference (Table 4-6).[27]

The cognitive examination includes an assessment of higher processes of thinking. This part of the examination is critical for a clinical assessment of neurologic function, and is useful for differentiating focal and global disorders, delirium, and dementia. The traditional model assesses a variety of dimensions (Table 4-7).[28]

Alternatively, the Mini-Mental State Examination[29] may be administered. This instrument is commonly used to assess dementia. One large study revealed a sensitivity of 87% and specificity of 82% of diagnosing dementia with a cut-off score of 24 out of 30 points. Use of this instrument cannot make the diagnosis of a mild dementia or focal neurologic deficits. Its value may also be limited by the patient's educational level and primary language. Finally, the instrument is often invalid in the presence of delirium or other processes that impair attention and concentration.[30]

TABLE 4-5 Examples of Formal Thought Disorders

Circumstantiality: a disorder of association with the inclusion of unnecessary details until one arrives at the goal of the thought
Tangentiality: use of oblique, irrelevant, and digressive thoughts that do not convey the central idea to be communicated
Loose associations: jumping from one unconnected topic to another
Clang associations: an association of speech without logical connection dictated by the sound of the words rather than by their meaning; it frequently involves using rhyming or punning
Perseveration: repeating the same response to stimuli (such as the same verbal response to different questions) with an inability to change the responses
Neologism: made-up words; often a condensation of different words; unintelligible to the listener
Echolalia: persistent repetition of words or phrases of another person
Thought-blocking: an abrupt interruption in the flow of thought, in which one cannot recover what was just said

TABLE 4-6 Disorders of Thought Content

Delusions: fixed, false, unshakable beliefs
Obsessions: persistent thoughts that cannot be extruded by logic or reasoning
Idea of reference: misinterpretation of incidents in the external world as having special and direct personal reference to the self

SHARING INFORMATION AND PREPARING THE PATIENT FOR TREATMENT

The conclusion of the psychiatric interview requires summarizing the symptoms and history and organizing them into a coherent narrative that can be reviewed and agreed on by the patient and the clinician. This involves recapitulating the most important findings and explaining the meaning of them to the patient. It is crucial to obtain an agreement on the clinical material and the way the story holds together for the patient. If the patient does not concur with the summary, the psychiatrist should return to the relevant portions of the interview in question and revisit the topics that are in disagreement.

This part of the interview should involve explaining one or more diagnoses to the patient (their biological, psychological, and environmental etiologies), as well as a formulation of the patient's strengths, weaknesses, and style of managing stress. The latter part of the summary is intended to help ensure that the patient feels understood. The next step is to delineate the kinds of approaches that the current standards of care would indicate are appropriate for treatment. If the diagnosis is uncertain, further evaluation should

TABLE 4-7 Categories of the Mental Status Examination

Orientation: for example, to time, place, person, and situation
Attention and concentration: for example, remembering three objects immediately, and in 1 and 3 minutes; spelling "world" backwards; performing digit span; and serially subtracting 7 from 100
Memory: registration, both recent and remote
- Registration is typically a function of attention and concentration
- Recent and remote memory are evaluated by recalling events in the short and long term

Calculations
Abstraction: assessed by the patient's ability to interpret proverbs or other complex ideas
Judgment: evaluated by seeing if the patient demonstrates an awareness of personal issues or problems, and provides appropriate ways of solving them
Insight: an assessment of self-reflection and an understanding of one's condition or the situation of others

be recommended to elucidate the problem or co-morbid problems. This might require one or more of the following: further laboratory evaluation; medical, neurologic, or pediatric referral; psychological or neuropsychological testing; use of standardized rating scales; or consultation with a specialist (e.g., a psychopharmacologist or a sleep disorders or substance abuse specialist).

Education about treatment should include reviewing the pros and cons of various options. This is a good time to dispel myths about psychiatric treatments, either pharmacotherapy or psychotherapy. Both of these domains have significant stigma associated with them. For patients who are prone to shun pharmacotherapy (not wanting any "mind-altering" medications), it may be useful to "medicalize" the psychiatric disorder and note that common medical conditions involve attention to biopsychosocial treatment.[14] For example, few people would refuse medications for treatment of hypertension, even though it may be clear that the condition is exacerbated by stress and lifestyle. The same may be said for the treatment of asthma, migraines, diabetes, and peptic ulcers. In this light, the clinician can refer to psychiatric conditions as problems of "chemical imbalances"—a neutral term—or as problems with the brain, an organ people often forget when talking about "mental" conditions. A candid dialogue in this way, perhaps describing how depression or panic disorder involves abnormalities in brain function, may help. It should be noted that this kind of discussion should in no way be construed or interpreted as pressure—rather as an educational experience. Letting the patient know that treatment decisions are collaborative and patient-centered is absolutely essential in a discussion of this order.

A similar educational conversation should relate to the use of psychotherapies. Some patients disparage psychotherapies as "mumbo jumbo," lacking scientific evidence. In this instance, discussion can center around the fact that scientific research indicates that experience and the environment can affect biological function. An example of this involves talking about how early trauma affects child development, or how coming through an experience in war can produce post-traumatic stress disorder, a significant dysfunction of the brain. Many parents will immediately appreciate how the experiences in childhood affect a child's mood, anxiety, and behavior, though they will also point out that children are born with certain personalities and traits. This observation is wonderful because it opens a door for a discussion of the complex and ongoing interaction among brain, environment, and behavior.

THE EVALUATION OF CHILDREN AND ADOLESCENTS

Psychiatric disorders in children and adolescents will be discussed elsewhere in this book. In general, children and adolescents pose certain unique issues for the psychiatric interviewer. First, a complete developmental history is required. For younger children, most of the history is taken from the parents. Rarely are young children seen initially away from their parents. Observation of the child is critical. The examiner should notice how the child relates to the parents or caregivers. Conversely, it is important to note whether the adult's management of the child is appropriate. Does the child seem age-appropriate in terms of motor function and growth? Are there any observable neurologic impairments? The evaluator should determine whether speech, language, cognition, and social function are age-appropriate. If possible, the examiner should provide toys for the evaluation in the ED or hospital floor. Collateral information from the pediatrician and schoolteachers is critical to verify or amplify parental and child-reported data.

Adolescents produce their own set of issues and problems for the interviewer.[31] A teenager may or may not be accompanied by a parent. However, given the developmental processes that surround the quests for identity and separation, the interviewer must treat the teen with the same kind of respect and collaboration as with an adult. The issue and importance of ensuring confidentiality have been mentioned previously. The adolescent also needs to hear at the outset that the interviewer needs to obtain permission to speak with parents or guardians, and that any information received from them would be faithfully transmitted to the patient.

Although all the principles of attempting to establish a secure attachment noted previously apply to the adolescent, the interview of the adolescent is quite different from that of an adult. Developmentally, teenagers are capable of abstract thinking and are becoming increasingly autonomous. At the same time, they are struggling with grandiosity that alternates with extreme vulnerability and self-consciousness and managing body image, sexuality and aggression, mood lability, and occasional regression to dependency—all of which makes an interview and relationship difficult. The interviewer must constantly consider what counts as normal adolescent behavior and what risk-taking behaviors, mood swings, and impulsivity are pathological. This is not easy, and typically teenagers need a few initial meetings for the clinician to feel capable of co-creating a narrative—albeit a narrative in progress. The stance of the clinician in working with adolescents requires moving in a facile fashion between an often-needed professional authority figure and a big brother or sister, camp counselor, and friend. The examiner must be able to know something about the particular adolescent's culture, to use humor and exaggeration, to be flexible, and to be empathic in the interview, yet not attempt to be "one of them." It is essential to validate strengths and weaknesses and to inspire self-reflection and some philosophical thinking—all attendant with the new cognitive developments since earlier childhood. References to individuals, situations, and problems in pop culture, such as YouTube videos, reality television shows, films, or young adult novels, may identify instances with which the teenager identifies. Discussing these examples may help understand the youth during the interview and further solidify a therapeutic alliance.

DIFFICULTIES AND ERRORS IN THE PSYCHIATRIC INTERVIEW

Dealing With Sensitive Subjects

A number of subjects are particularly shameful for patients. Such topics include sexual problems, excessive substance use and other addictions, financial matters, impulsive behavior, bizarre experiences (such as obsessions and compulsions), domestic violence, histories of abuse, and symptoms of psychosis. Some patients will either deny or avoid discussing these topics. In this situation, non-threatening, gentle encouragement, and acknowledgment of how difficult these matters are, may help. If the issue is not potentially dangerous or life-threatening to the patient or to others, the clinician may omit some questions known to be important in the diagnosis or formulation. If it is not essential to obtain this information in the initial interview, it may be best for the alliance to let it go, knowing the examiner or another clinician may return to it as the therapeutic relationship grows.

In other situations that are dangerous (such as occurs with suicidal, homicidal, manic, or psychotic patients), in which pertinent symptoms must be ascertained, questioning is crucial, no matter how distressed the patient may become. In some instances when danger seems highly likely, transfer to a psychiatric hospital may be necessary for observation and further exploration of a serious disorder. Similarly, an agitated patient who needs to be assessed for safety may need sedation, restraints, or eventual transfer to a psychiatric hospital, to complete a comprehensive evaluation, particularly if the cause of agitation is not known and the patient is not collaborating with the evaluative process.

Disagreements About Assessment and Treatment

There are times when a patient disagrees with a clinician's formulation, diagnosis, and treatment recommendations. Or the disagreement may be between the patient and the medical staff, with the psychiatrist in the challenging position of the intermediary. In either case, it is wise to listen to the patient and hear where there is conflict. This can serve to re-establish the alliance. It also may diffuse the patient's need to defend himself or herself against what he or she may perceive as doctors "ganging up" on him or her. Then, the evaluator should systematically review what was said and how he or she interpreted the clinical findings. The patient should be encouraged to correct misrepresentations. Sometimes clarification will help the clinician and patient come to an agreement. At other times, the patient may deny or minimize a problem. In this case, additional interviews may be necessary. It is sometimes useful to involve a close relative or friend, if the patient allows this. If the patient is a danger to self or others, however, protective measures will be needed, short of any agreement. If there is no imminent danger, explaining one's clinical opinion and respecting the right of the patient to choose treatment must be observed. It may also be necessary to work with the medical team to reach a compromise that takes into consideration the patient's goals and wishes when they differ from that of the medical team.

Errors in Psychiatric Interviewing

Common mistakes made in the psychiatric interview are provided in Table 4-8.

TABLE 4-8 Common Errors in the Psychiatric Interview

- Premature closure and false assumptions about symptoms.
- False reassurance about the patient's condition or prognosis.
- Defensiveness around psychiatric diagnoses and treatment, with arrogant responses to myths and complaints about psychiatry.
- Omission of significant parts of the interview, due to theoretical bias of the interview (e.g., mind–body splitting).
- Recommendations for treatment when diagnostic formulation is incomplete.
- Inadequate explanation of psychiatric disorders and their treatment, particularly not giving the patient multiple options for treatment.
- Minimization or denial of the severity of symptoms, due to overidentification with the patient; countertransference phenomenon (e.g., as occurs with treatment of a "very important person," VIP, in a manner inconsistent with ordinary best practice, with a resultant failure to protect the patient or others).
- Failure to establish a genuine, empathic rapport (e.g., by using brusque language, tone, or body posture).
- Use of an angry or dismissive style in response to a patient who is guarded or hostile.
- Inadvertently shaming or embarrassing a patient, and not offering an apology.

CONCLUSION

The purpose of the psychiatric interview is to establish a therapeutic relationship with the patient to collect, organize, and synthesize data that can become the basis for a formulation, differential diagnosis, and treatment plan. A fundamental part of establishing this relationship is fostering a secure attachment between doctor and patient, in order to facilitate mutual and open communication, to correct misunderstandings, and to help the patient create a cohesive narrative of his or her past and present situation. Interviews in the general hospital require modification in techniques in order to take into account four elements of the context: the setting, the situation, the subject, and the significance. Data collection should include behavioral observation, medical and psychiatric history, and a mental status examination.

The clinician should conclude the interview by summarizing the findings and the formulation, seeking agreement with the patient, and negotiating appropriate follow-up arrangements. All clinicians should be aware of difficulties in the psychiatric interview (such as shameful topics and disagreements about assessment or treatment). Common errors in an interview include premature closure and false assumptions about symptoms, false reassurance about a patient's condition, defensiveness around psychiatric diagnosis and treatment, maintenance of a theoretical bias about mental health and illness, inadequate explanations about psychiatric disorders and their treatment, minimization of the severity of symptoms, and inadvertent shaming of a patient without offering an apology.

REFERENCES

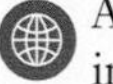
Access the reference list online at https://expertconsult.inkling.com/.

Functional Neuroanatomy and the Neurologic Examination

5

Joel Salinas, M.D., M.B.A., M.Sc.
Joan A. Camprodon, M.D., M.P.H., Ph.D.

For the psychiatric consultant, the neurologic examination is an important component of every patient evaluation. By reviewing the main components of the standard examination and attempting to relate them to anatomic constructs, the consulting psychiatrist may gain a theoretical and pragmatic framework for the neurologic examination that can facilitate case formulation, differential diagnosis, and treatment planning.

FUNCTIONAL NEUROANATOMY

At its most basic level, the nervous system allows us to interact with external stimuli, serving as a bridge between the environment and our internal mental and physical worlds. In humans, there is a large evaluation step between stimulus and response, which allows for a carefully chosen (or programmed) response that is additionally influenced by an actual or perceived situational context. Using an information-processing model, we can map these concepts in three distinct steps: *input* of sensory information through perceptual modules, the internal integration and *evaluation* of this information, and the production of a *response*. These steps are carried out by four main anatomic systems in the brain: the *thalamus*, the *cortex*, the *medial temporal lobe*, and the *basal ganglia* (Figure 5-1).

Sensory organs provide information about physical attributes of incoming information. Details of physical attributes (e.g., temperature, sound frequency, color) are conveyed through multiple segregated channels in each perceptual module. Information then passes through the thalamus, which serves as the gateway to cortical processing for all sensory data with the exception of olfaction. Specifically, it is the relay nuclei (ventral posterior lateral, medial geniculate, and lateral geniculate) that convey sensory information from the sensory organs to the appropriate area of primary sensory cortex (i.e., S1, A1, or V1) (Figure 5-2).

The first step in the integration and evaluation of incoming stimuli occurs in unimodal association areas of the cortex, where physical attributes of one sensory domain are linked together. A second level of integration is reached in multimodal association areas, including regions in the parietal lobe and prefrontal cortex, which link together the physical attributes from different sensory domains. A third level of integration is provided by input from limbic and paralimbic regions of the brain, including the cingulate cortex and regions of the medial temporal lobe (hippocampus and amygdala). At this level of integration, the brain creates a representation of experience that has the spatiotemporal resolution and full complexity of the outside world, imbued with emotion and viewed in the context of prior experience. Evaluation and interpretation involve the comparison of new information with previously stored information and current expectations or desires, which allows the brain to classify information as new or old, or as threatening or non-threatening.

Based on the result of evaluation and interpretation, the brain then creates a response. The regions involved in generating, for example, motor responses, include the motor cortex, the basal ganglia, the motor nuclei of the thalamus, and the cerebellum. The basal ganglia, which include the striatum (made up of the caudate and the putamen) and the globus pallidus, are charged with integrating and coordinating this motor output. The striatum receives input from the motor cortex, projecting to the globus pallidus. The globus pallidus in turn relays the neostriatal input to the thalamus. The thalamus then projects back to the cortical areas that gave rise to the corticostriatal projections, thereby closing the cortico-striato-pallido-thalamo-cortical (CSPTC) loop. This loop is thought to be the means by which motor control is enacted; damage to regions in this loop leads to disorders, such as Parkinson's disease and Huntington's disease. In addition to motor responses, the brain generates other types of outputs, such as cognitive decision-making, emotional reactions, or socially meaningful behavioral responses. These outputs also rely on similar frontal CSPTC loops, which start in non-motor parts of the frontal cortex, such as the dorsolateral prefrontal, the medial prefrontal, or the orbitofrontal cortices. Structural or physiologic lesions to these systems lead to the cognitive, affective, or behavioral signs and symptoms that constitute neuropsychiatric syndromes.

CASE 1

Mr. H, a 43-year-old man, was brought to the Emergency Department (ED) after he was found wandering barefoot on the street; he was belligerent and disheveled. On presentation, his vital signs and a basic screening evaluation for intoxication or acute medical illness were normal. Psychiatry was consulted to assess his capacity to leave the hospital against medical advice. On interview, Mr. H was alert but disoriented; his mood was elevated and he had grandiose, paranoid, and persecutory delusions. He was irritable, easily distracted, and angrily insisted that his health was "100% perfect."

On neurologic examination, his visual fields were full to confrontation, his extraocular movements were intact in all directions with smooth pursuit, his face was symmetric, and his speech was slightly dysarthric. There was no evidence of myoclonus or asterixis, but perioral and bilateral upper extremity tremors were present with posture. Muscle bulk, tone, and strength were normal and symmetric. Deep tendon reflexes were brisk and symmetric. There was no evidence of primitive reflexes; he had normal plantar responses. There was symmetric withdrawal of all four extremities to painful stimuli. There were no gross ataxic movements in the extremities or trunk. Gait had normal posture, stride, arm swing, and turns, though widened stance and he fell with tandem gait. Romberg's sign was present. These findings prompted an MRI of the brain with and without gadolinium, which revealed left greater than right mesial temporal and basal ganglionic inflammation. Additional serum studies, including HIV, syphilis rapid plasma reagin (RPR), fluorescent treponemal antibody absorption test (FTA-ABS), and serum paraneoplastic antibodies, were negative. Lumbar puncture revealed a normal opening pressure. CSF analysis revealed a normal glucose, no leukocytosis, and an elevated total protein. CSF viral studies were negative, but the Venereal Disease Research Laboratory (VDRL) test was highly elevated. Treatment was initiated for diagnosis of neurosyphilis with intravenous penicillin for 2 weeks. Mr. H had a gradual improvement in his mental status and was discharged to a physical rehabilitation hospital.

THE NEUROLOGIC EXAMINATION

The neurologic examination is a set of steps designed to probe the input, integration/evaluation, and output domains of information processing. Here, we provide an overview of the examination, using this framework. For complete details, see standard texts of neurology.

Input

Sensory information enters the central nervous system (CNS) by two routes: spinal nerves and cranial nerves. The former

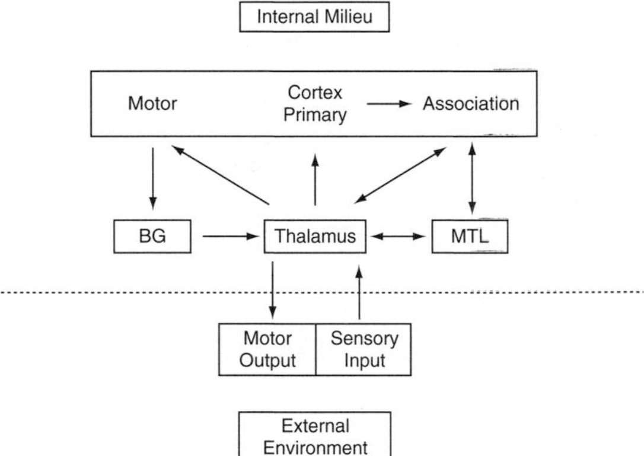

Figure 5-1 Basic circuitry of information processing. BG, basal ganglia; MTL, medial temporal lobe.

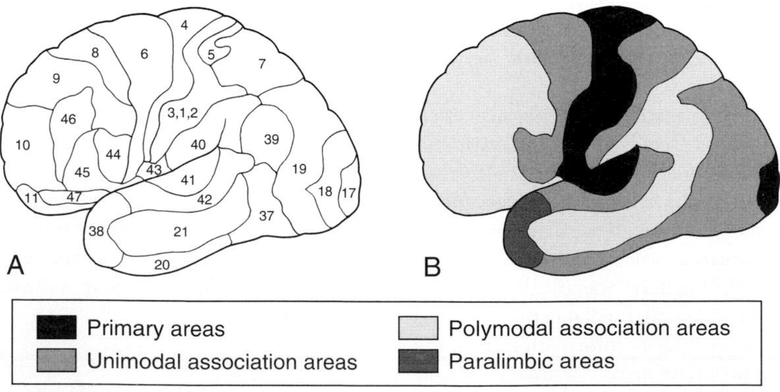

Figure 5-2 Functional role of areas in the human cerebral cortex. (A) Map of cytoarchitectonic areas according to Brodmann. The parcellation of the cortical mantle into distinct areas is based on the microscopic analysis of neurons in the six layers of the cortex. (B) Map of functional areas according to Mesulam. The primary sensory areas (visual = area 17; auditory = areas 41, 43; somatosensory = areas 3, 1, 2) and the primary motor area 4 are indicated in *black*. The association areas, dedicated to one stream of information processing (visual = areas 18, 19, 20, 37; auditory = area 42; somatosensory = areas 5, 7, 40; motor = areas 6, 44), are indicated in *dark gray*. The polymodal association areas, where all sensory modalities converge, are indicated in *light gray*. The temporal pole is part of the paralimbic areas, which occupy large regions on the medial surface of the brain (i.e., cingulate cortex and parahippocampal cortex). *((A) from Brodmann K:* Vergleichende lokalisationslehre der grosshirnrinde in ihren prinzipien dargestellt auf grund des zellenbaues, *Leipzig, Germany, 1909, JA Barth; (B) from Mesulam M-M:* Principles of behavioral neurology, *Philadelphia, 1985, FA Davis.)*

handle somatosensory information presented to the body, and the latter handle somatosensory information presented to the face and each of the remaining special senses (vision, hearing, smell, and taste).

Peripheral Sensory Examination

Peripheral sensation allows tactile exploration of our environment. The most thorough examiner could not test every square inch of the body for intact sensation, though it would not be necessary. Knowledge of the full sensory examination is important for the patient with a focal sensory complaint (see other texts for detailed information on peripheral nerve examination[1–9]). The main sensory modalities include the following:

Pain: Tested by pinprick (using disposable sterile pins)

Temperature: Tested by touching the skin with a cold metal object (e.g., a tuning fork);

Light touch: Tested by simply brushing the patient's skin with your hand or a moving wisp of cotton;

Vibration sense: Tested by applying a "buzzing" tuning fork to osseous prominences of the distal lower extremities;

Proprioception: Efficiently tested by Romberg's maneuver. One can ask the patient to stand with the feet as close together as possible while still maintaining stability. Then ask the patient to close their eyes, ensuring the patient that you will not let him or her fall. The patient with poor proprioception will begin to sway and lose balance after closing their eyes. Falling during the maneuver indicates the presence of Romberg's sign, a manifestation of severe proprioceptive sensory loss.

In Addition, Complex Associative Sensory Modalities of Clinical Relevance Include

Stereognosis: The ability to recognize objects using touch, which can be tested by placing common objects (e.g., a coin) in the patient's hand and asking the patient to name the items, with the eyes closed.

Graphesthesia: The ability to recognize numbers or letters traced on the skin, most often using the palm, with the patient's eyes closed. As with stereognosis, primary sensory modalities must be intact for this test to have meaning.

Sensory (I, II, VIII) and Sensorimotor (V, VII, IX, X) Cranial Nerves

Seven cranial nerves serve an input function and are known as sensory (I, II, VIII) or sensorimotor (V, VII, IX, X) cranial nerves to distinguish them from those that exclusively play a motor/output role (Table 5-1).

Olfactory Nerve (Cranial Nerve I)

The first cranial nerve runs along the orbital surface of the frontal lobe, an area that is otherwise clinically silent. Lesions (e.g., a frontal lobe meningioma) in this area may produce behavioral dysregulation, such as impulsivity, with or without unilateral anosmia. In addition, anosmia can be an early sign of neurodegenerative conditions before the onset of cognitive or motor symptoms. Routine testing of smell is therefore important. A small vial of coffee provides a simple and convenient method for testing smell, but olfaction can also be tested with an inexpensive smell identification test booklet. The nostrils should be tested separately.

Optic Nerve (Cranial Nerve II)

The optic nerve and its posterior radiations run the entire length of the brain and produce different patterns of symptoms and signs depending on where they are compromised; therefore, a thorough evaluation can be quite informative. There are five components to the visual examination:

Funduscopy: Because the optic nerve is the only nerve that can be visualized directly with an ophthalmoscope, the funduscopic examination reveals much about its integrity, the systemic vascular system, and the presence of increased intracranial pressure.

TABLE 5-1 The Cranial Nerves

NUMBER	NAME	SENSORY (INPUT), MOTOR (OUTPUT), OR BOTH?	FUNCTION
I	Olfactory	Sensory	Olfaction
II	Optic	Sensory	Vision
III	Oculomotor	Motor	Innervation of extraocular musculature
IV	Trochlear	Motor	Innervation of extraocular musculature
V	Trigeminal	Both	Facial sensation + innervation of muscles of mastication
VI	Abducens	Motor	Innervation of extraocular musculature
VII	Facial	Both	Taste + innervation of muscles of facial expression
VIII	Vestibulocochlear	Sensory	Hearing + balance
IX	Glossopharyngeal	Both	Taste + innervation of stylopharyngeus muscle
X	Vagus	Both	Parasympathetic innervation + innervation to muscles of larynx and pharynx
XI	Spinal accessory	Motor	Innervation of the sternocleidomastoid and trapezius muscles
XII	Hypoglossal	Motor	Innervation of tongue

Visual acuity: Poor vision can profoundly impair a person's ability to function or orient himself and is often reversible with corrective lenses or surgery. Acuity is easily assessed in each eye while the patient is wearing current corrective lenses.

Pupillary measurement: Pupillary size represents the delicate balance between sympathetic and parasympathetic input to the ciliary muscles of the eye. The presence of abnormally large or small pupils reflects an imbalance and may be an important sign of disease or toxicity. Similarly, an inequality in pupillary size (anisocoria) can be an important hallmark of a severe intracranial pathologic condition. Each pupil is measured in millimeters with measurements clearly documented for future reference, including whether measurement was performed in a light or dark room.

Pupillary reaction: The direct and consensual pupillary reaction to light, and the near reaction (accommodation), assess any damage in the afferent and efferent pathways that compose the pupillary response. A penlight and close observation are all that are necessary.

Confrontational visual fields: Because the visual system runs from the retina to the occipital cortex, involving a substantial area of the CNS, lesions anywhere along this pathway lead to visual field deficits. Importantly, the patient is almost never aware of this abnormality of vision. Careful testing is therefore required. One can sit directly in front of the patient, and have him or her look at a single point between your eyes. The eyes should be tested separately by bringing an object (e.g., a pin or a wiggling finger) into each visual quadrant. For the patient who is unable to cooperate in this fashion, having them count fingers displayed in each quadrant is another option. Assessing for blink to visual threat in each quadrant may be viable in more inattentive patients.

Trigeminal Nerve (Cranial Nerve V)

The sensory component of the trigeminal nerve captures somatosensory information from the face via the ophthalmic (V1), maxillary (V2), and mandibular (V3) branches. Testing light touch (by stroking the face with your fingers) or temperature sensitivity (using a cold metal tuning fork) is usually adequate. Simply asking, "Does this feel normal on both sides?" will detect any major abnormalities worth further investigation.

Facial Nerve (Cranial Nerve VII)

The sensory component of the facial nerve (chorda tympani) transmits taste from the anterior two-thirds of the tongue. Testing this aspect of the facial nerve involves the application of a sweet, sour, or salty solution (via a cotton-tipped swab) to the outstretched tongue. The yield of this component of the examination without specific gustatory complaints is minimal.

Acoustic Nerve (Cranial Nerve VIII)

In addition to its role in the maintenance of equilibrium (via the vestibular branch), the VIIIth cranial nerve is the primary input channel for auditory information. Rubbing fingers together near the ear may bring out high-pitched hearing deficits, a finding typically associated with presbycusis that can exacerbate confusional states.

Glossopharyngeal and Vagus Nerves (Cranial Nerves IX and X)

These two nerves innervate the palate, pharynx, and larynx and are important for speech and swallowing. The IXth cranial nerve also conducts taste and touch sensation for the posterior third of the tongue. Lesions of these two nerves are clinically meaningful as they cause dysarthric, or aphonic speech, dysphagia, and drooling (see later for more details).

Integration and Evaluation

Several automatic or reflexive responses (e.g., pupillary light reflex and corneal reflex in the sensory evaluation) can be tested, including three sets of reflexes (proprioceptive, nociceptive, and primitive) commonly probed in a standard neurologic examination.

In addition, higher-level information processing also occurs in the brain. This is not a pre-programmed reflex but a flexible and adaptive output that is generally dependent on the environment (external and internal) leading to a wide range of cognitive, behavioral, and affective responses.[6] The mental status examination is the clinical tool to evaluate these functions.

Reflexes

Proprioceptive reflexes: Proprioceptive reflexes, also known as deep tendon reflexes (DTRs), are based on the simple reflex arcs that are activated by stretching or tapping. Because they are influenced by the descending corticospinal tracts, DTRs can provide important information on the integrity of this pathway at several levels. The reader is probably familiar with the methods used to elicit the five major DTRs: biceps, triceps, brachioradialis, quadriceps (knee), and Achilles (ankle). The grading of each reflex is on a 4-point scale with a score of 2 (2+) designated as normal, though special attention is placed on asymmetry in reflex strength (e.g., difference between upper versus lower extremities or left versus right extremities).

Nociceptive reflexes: Nociceptive reflexes are based on reflex arcs located in the skin (rather than muscle tendons) and are therefore elicited by scratching or stroking. These include the abdominal, cremasteric, and anocutaneous reflexes, none of which is extensively used clinically. The major nociceptive reflex of clinical value is the plantar reflex. Stroking the sole of the foot should elicit plantar flexion of the toes. Babinski's sign, marked by an extensor response (i.e., dorsiflexion) of the toes, often with fanning of the toes and flexion of the ankle, is seen in pyramidal tract disease.

Primitive reflexes (release reflexes): Primitive reflexes are present at birth but disappear in early infancy. Their reappearance later in life is abnormal and reflects cortical disease, often attributed but not exclusive to the frontal lobes. They include the grasp reflex (stroking the patient's palm leads to an automatic clutching of your finger between his or her thumb and index finger); the glabellar reflex (cessation of the natural blink response in response to repetitive tapping on the forehead, also known as Meyerson's sign); and the snout reflex (gentle tapping over the patient's upper lip causes a puckering of the lips). Note that this may also elicit a suck response, or a turning of the head toward the stroking stimulus (rooting reflex).

The Mental Status Examination

The brains of higher mammals, particularly the human, have the added capacity to integrate sensory information across domains, to evaluate this information, and to react in a manner consistent with past experience, current context, or future expectations. The ability to use these higher-level faculties is often considered part of the mental status examination. For routine purposes, the following four components compose an adequate examination. These components, unlike other features of the neurologic examination, are best done in sequence because the preceding basic functions must be intact to perform more complex tasks.

Executive Function and Attention

Executive function is a term that encompasses the different cognitive capacities responsible for organizing behavior: e.g., attention/concentration, working memory, cognitive control/inhibition, planning, and multi-tasking. Historically, the psychiatric literature has used the term "attention" and "consciousness" interchangeably when discussing the mental status exam, particularly when it relates to conditions, such as delirium. Consciousness lies on a continuum from full alertness to coma and although the two extremes are generally obvious, the middle ground can be subtle and is generally characterized by attentional deficits. Because inattention leads to indirect disruption of all other cognitive functions, attention should be tested in all patients. Some common tests of attention include "*serial 7s*" (asking the patient to subtract 7 from 100 and to then continue to serially subtract 7 from the remainder) and *digit span* (having the patient repeat a randomly presented list of digits; a normal capacity is between five and seven digits, or having the patient spell a five-letter word backwards, such as *world*).

Language

Language is the means by which we present our thoughts to each other. As with other cognitive functions, language can be extraordinarily complex, with entire texts on aphasiology dedicated to its study. In general, the following simple three questions allow the examiner to draw valid conclusions about language in the individual patient:

Is the language *fluent* or *non-fluent?* Independent of the actual words, does the speech sound like a language? Loss of the normal inflection and spacing of normal speech leads to non-fluent language production.

Is *comprehension* normal or abnormal? Does the patient seem to understand what you are saying? A request to complete a one-step to three-step command is an adequate assessment, although complex commands may test more than just receptive language function. Asking simple yes/no questions (e.g., "Were you born in Mexico?" or "Are we in the kitchen?") is another common method.

Is *repetition* normal or abnormal? One can have a patient repeat a phrase such as "no ifs, ands, or buts." This particular phrase is quite sensitive given the difficulty of repeating conjunctions.

Because language is a multimodal function, core language deficits should be observed in both spoken and written forms.

Memory

Memory function is generally divided into the following three components:

Immediate recall is the ability to hold information for instant use (e.g., remembering a phone number given by the operator long enough so it may be dialed). Immediate recall is heavily dependent on attention and therefore considered a form of executive function. It can be tested by both digit span and phrase repetition. Asking the patient to repeat three named items (e.g., piano, monkey, and blue) is another commonly used method.

Short-term memory involves the ability to store information for later use. Asking the patient to reproduce the three previously named items after a span of 2 to 5 minutes is a common test of episodic memory.

Long-term memory involves the recall of past events. This is nearly impossible to test accurately at the bedside without a close friend or relative of the patient because the examiner is rarely privy to details of remote events from the patient's life. Asking about well-known national events or people (e.g., "How did JFK die?") depends on the age and educational background of the patient. Accurate assessment often requires a standardized battery of questions available in full neuropsychological testing.

Visual–Spatial Skills

Clock-drawing: Have the patient fill in a large circle with numbers in the form of a clock. When completed, ask the patient to set the hands at "10 past 11" or "10 to 2." This test captures different aspects of cognition, including executive function and visual–spatial skills. Abnormalities can occur in planning (e.g., manifested by poor spacing between numbers) or in positioning of the hands (with a style that reflects being stimulus-bound) that may belie a lesion involving executive control networks. Complete absence of detail on one side of the clock (usually the left side) may represent a hemi-neglect syndrome associated with a right parietal lobe lesion.

Output

Although there are many potential responses to environmental stimuli, including subtle changes in the internal hormonal or neurochemical milieu, the response often involves some type of motor output. The examination of this output can be divided into a motor (or muscular) component and a coordination component.

Motor (III, IV, VI, XI, XII) and Sensorimotor (V, VII, IX, X) Cranial Nerves

These cranial nerves are responsible for motor function in the head and neck and are tested by examining the functionality of the muscles they subserve. For example, cranial nerves III, IV, and VI innervate the extraocular muscles that allow the eye to scan its environment. They are therefore tested in examining the range of eye movements in all directions by having the patient track one's finger or a salient object. Cranial nerve V can be assessed with opposing force to the muscles of mastication, though of greater importance is the assessment of cranial nerve VII, which innervates the facial muscles and can be tested by observing the face at rest (e.g., noting facial new-onset asymmetry, such as nasolabial fold flattening, or significant ptosis) or with action (i.e., asking the patient to raise their forehead, close their eyes tightly against opposition, smile, or puff their cheeks). Weakness of cranial nerve IX can be noted by listening for dysarthria in speech or dysphasia, which can be assessed by asking the patient to voluntarily cough, clear their throat, swallow, and, if safe, to drink a sip of water while noting if there is a change in the quality of speech after swallowing. Cranial nerve XI can be tested by observation and confrontation with shoulder shrugging and horizontal head rotation. Cranial nerve XII can be assessed by asking the patient to protrude their tongue and push against the inside of their mouth while applying opposing external force.

Motor Examination

There are four aspects evaluated in the motor examination: abnormal movements, muscle tone, bulk, and strength. The four aspects may be affected separately.

Abnormal movements can be broadly classified as syndromes of movements that are decreased (e.g., akinesia or bradykinesia) or increased (e.g., tremors, tremulousness, fasciculation, myokymia, dyskinesia, dystonia, athetosis, chorea, asterixis, myoclonus, stereotypies, or simple and complex tics). Each movement is assessed first with passive observation followed by changes in posture and action, such as arms and hands outstretched, or during ambulation. A clear narrative description is most valuable. More structured elements to note for each movement include occurrence (e.g., at rest, with action, or with specific tasks or postures); character/phenotype (e.g., simple, complex, or patterned; rhythmic or irregular; tonic or clonic; high or low amplitude); rate (e.g., fast or slow frequency); and location (e.g., focal or diffuse; specific body parts involved; symmetry or laterality; synchronous or asynchronous).

Muscle tone refers to the resistance of a limb to passive movement through its normal range of motion. To examine for tone, one can have the patient fully relax the arms and legs to allow the physician to determine the degree of stiffness during passive motion. An increased level of tone, noted by rigidity or spasticity as can be seen in Parkinsonism, is an important finding that may underlie an upper motor neuron or extrapyramidal lesion.

Assessment of *muscle bulk* can be extraordinarily challenging because of natural variation in body habitus and the role of weightlifting or exercise (i.e., "bulking up"), but remains important as muscle atrophy can be an important lower motor neuron sign of neurodegenerative disease, such as amyotrophic lateral sclerosis. Muscles that are unaffected by weightlifting or exercise (e.g., the facial muscles or the intrinsic muscles of the hand) may therefore provide the best estimate of overall muscle bulk.

In testing *muscle strength*, it is impractical (and unnecessary) to test each of the several hundred muscles in the human body. If the patient has a focal motor complaint, knowledge of major muscle groups in the proximal and distal limbs becomes important. Muscle strength is graded from 0 (no motion) to 5 (normal strength).

Observation of gait is an excellent screening test for the patient without focal weakness. If the patient is able to rise briskly and independently from a seated position and walk independently, gross motor deficits can be confidently ruled out. The ability to walk on one's heels and toes further ensures distal lower-extremity strength. Gait must be tested in all patients, particularly in older adults, for whom a fall can be a life-threatening event.

Coordination

Coordination reflects the ability to orchestrate and control movement, and it is crucial in the translation of movement into productive activity. Although the cerebellum plays a lead role in motor coordination, several other structures (e.g., the basal ganglia and red nucleus) are involved.

The complexity of walking makes it an ideal screening test for coordination ability. Humans have a particularly narrow base when standing upright; with any degree of incoordination (ataxia), the patient needs to widen the base to remain upright. Balance becomes even more difficult when other sensory information is removed, forming the basis for Romberg's maneuver where the patient is asked to stand with their feet together and eyes closed. Romberg's sign is present if the patient begins to fall and is absent if the patient only has mild postural instability. The sensitivity of screening is further increased by having the patient walk heel-to-toe (as on a tightrope). The ability to do this smoothly and quickly makes major impairment in coordination unlikely.

Diadochokinesia refers to the alternating movements made possible by the paired nature of agonist and antagonist muscle activity in coordinated limb movement. Abnormalities of this function are detected by several simple maneuvers, including rapid alternating movements (quick pronation or supination of the forearm, or finger/foot tapping). In tapping a rhythm with cerebellar damage, the rhythm is poorly timed with incorrect emphases.

REFERENCES

Access the reference list online at https://expertconsult.inkling.com/.

Limbic Music: The Band Plays On

6

Nicholas Kontos, M.D.
Anna R. Weissman, M.D.
John B. Taylor, M.D., M.B.A.

When you talk with the patient, you should listen, first, for what he wants to tell, secondly for what he does not want to tell, thirdly for what he cannot tell.

— L.J. Henderson 1935[1]

I have to say that as a psychiatric interviewer I learned as much from a 3-year residency with monkeys as I did in a 3-year residency with humans.

— G.B. Murray 1987[2]

INTRODUCTION

First appearing in 1987 in an internally published collection of essays celebrating the 50th anniversary of the Massachusetts General Hospital Department of Psychiatry,[2] George Murray's "Limbic Music" is a rare example of the medical literature producing actual *literature*. Its synthesis of neuroscience, philosophy, clinical wisdom, and engaging writing was, like Dr. Murray himself, unique. Subsequent versions of that essay in the journal *Psychosomatics*,[3] and in every edition of this *Handbook*, inspired many psychiatrists' career paths and practice patterns.

Dr. Murray retired a year after the last edition of this book was published, and he died 2 years later. Those of us left with the daunting task of carrying on his tradition of "Limbic Music" urge (or even toothlessly command) the reader to track down and read one of its past incarnations. What follows here is less an update, sequel, or remix of the preceding "Music" than a song heavily inspired by earlier work. One does not discard a Miles Davis record when another trumpeter tests out his chops on a new album. The former makes the latter possible and perhaps even part of something bigger than it otherwise would or could be on its own. As justification for his 1990 publication of "Limbic Music" in *Psychosomatics*, Dr. Murray reproduced a letter of encouragement from his mentor, Dr. Thomas Hackett. We, in turn, offer up Figure 6-1 as proof of permission and pedigree for this effort.

This chapter inherits a few core iterative themes from that pedigree. First, the limbic system concept is advanced here in a way that bucks against an intellectual bias that privileges "higher" (read: "cortical") cognitive functions over "lower" (read: "primitive") emotional, conditioned, and instinctive functions in routine and aspirational human life. Second, important parts of our individual and shared existences go on outside of conscious awareness; it is important for psychiatrists to understand some of the anatomic, philosophical, and psychological ideas that expand this truth beyond more prosaic teaching about the "unconscious." Third, to the alert, this knowledge presents opportunities to access the limbic domain, and an imperative to respect it.

WHY LIMBIC MUSIC?

Why introduce, let alone carry forward, "Limbic Music" in this text? One cannot justify attention to the limbic system with a trite, "because it's there," since for more than four decades there has been debate over whether or not it is[4]—but more on that to come. Instead, the limbic system and the Limbic Music concept provide a site where philosophy, psychology, and biology can co-mingle in ways that are clinically practical. Make no mistake, though; while the limbic system is fertile scientific ground, its clinical usage in this chapter does not always reflect 100% established brain–behavior relationships.

Dr. Murray made no bones about his paper being "primarily heuristic."[5] Some aspects of Limbic Music stray into the realm of metapsychology. Describing an emotionally detached, hyper-rationalized person as an "overgrown neocort" or a mercurial, shallow thinker as a "thin-layer neocort"[2] exemplifies the descriptive utility of indulging in neuroanatomic metaphor. However, couching metapsychology in the jargon of neuroscience does not make it *ipso facto* real. It is easy to find "skeptics and enthusiasts in neuropsychiatry."[6] Hyman notes the prematurity of claims sometimes staked by those willing to extrapolate from current neuroscience a complete lack of free will in those who suffer from addictions,[7] and Uttal[8] arguably puts the lie to a neuroscience of "love" being ready for pedagogic prime time in psychiatry training.[9] On the other hand, skepticism is mobilized by some in the ironic service of defending their own non-biologically referent meta-psychologies (e.g., psychodynamics).[10,11]

Limbic Music favors neuroanatomically referenced explanations, does not shy away from potential accusations of "dualism," but also recognizes that brain-based explanations are meaningless unless attached to the outside world as understood through psychology and philosophy. Stretching the music metaphor, Limbic Music treats these sometimes adversarial ways-of-understanding like the treble and bass clefs. A holist might see them (correctly) as artificially

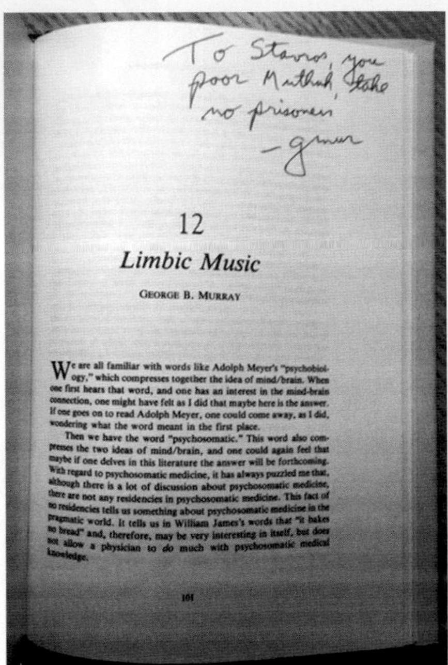

To Stavros, you
no prisoners

12

Limbic Music

George B. Murray

We are all familiar with words like Adolph Meyer's "psychobiology," which compresses together the idea of mind/brain. When one first hears that word, and one has an interest in the mind-brain connection, one might have felt as I did that maybe here is the answer. If one goes on to read Adolph Meyer, one could come away, as I did, wondering what the word meant in the first place.

Then we have the word "psychosomatic." This word also compresses the two ideas of mind/brain, and one could again feel that maybe if one delves in this literature the answer will be forthcoming. With regard to psychosomatic medicine, it has always puzzled me that, although there is a lot of discussion about psychosomatic medicine, there are not any residencies in psychosomatic medicine. This fact of no residencies tells us something about psychosomatic medicine in the pragmatic world. It tells us in William James's words that "it bakes no bread" and, therefore, may be very interesting in itself, but does not allow a physician to *do* much with psychosomatic medical knowledge.

101

Figure 6-1. A blessing, of sorts, to the lead author (*aka*, "Stavros").

dividing up the unity of musical notes. But it does not take a dualist to see that some instruments, not to mention our bodies, are constructed such that composition, performance, and appreciation demand that the clefs sometimes be cleft. The same goes for mind–body, bio-psycho-social, and other ways of thinking about, interacting with, and treating our patients.[12]

So why privilege the brain, let alone the limbic system? Because it is the target organ of our specialty, because the explanation of disease through biological theory is the distinguishing trait of the Western medical tradition of which psychiatry is part,[13] and because cognitive neuroscience is marching inexorably toward validating a materialist, brain-based understanding of psychological phenomena.[14] Some would argue that, for clinicians, this understanding can be achieved without using the brain as an intermediary. Those arguing otherwise need to be wary of pushing their luck further than contemporary neuroscience can support.[15] However, even (misguidedly) putting aside the neglected need for greater neuropsychiatric competency among psychiatrists, an everyday, pragmatic biological model of unconscious processes, which is the essence of Limbic Music, does not get much air time.

Most other models of mind that incorporate unconscious elements (e.g., ego psychology, object relations theory, self-psychology) are taught with reference to their respective psychotherapies. Infrequent exceptions do exist, and, interestingly, tend to appear in the psychosomatic literature.[16,17] Limbic Music fills a void that even these approaches to personality/coping categorization and life narratives cannot. That is, Limbic Music, like any music, need not serve a preconceived function. It may, as with other approaches, lead to a formulation or an intervention, but it is playing, and can be played, from the very start of a clinical interaction. Dr. Murray enjoyed using "limbic probes" (Table 6-1),[18,19] which can be used to elicit "squelched" affect, test hunches, convey understanding, hold an emotional mirror up to the patient, demonstrate what cannot be tolerated if spoken aloud, comfort, or even strategically antagonize a patient. Mental health professionals often speak of using themselves as instruments; Limbic Music augments this idea by making the model itself an instrument. Not just that, it embraces the uncertainty principle by which that instrument simultaneously takes the measure of and influences (or, some would say, manipulates) the patient.

WHAT IS LIMBIC MUSIC?

As we will later see about the limbic system itself, Dr. Murray's definition of limbic music was simultaneously fuzzy edged and potent. "*Limbic music* is a term that denotes the existential, clinical raw feel emanating from the patient. It is a truer rendering of the patient's clinical state than is articulate speech."[5] It arises from processes that subserve, among other things, survival-related functions, and exert their effects via neuroanatomic structures and pathways that bypass downstream association cortex. This definition partially recalls Paul MacLean's initial proposals of the "visceral brain," for which he later coined the term, "limbic system" (note: earlier usage of the term "limbic," by Willis and Broca referred to the "border," or limbus, formed by the cingulate and parahippocampal gyri around the corpus callosum and rostral brainstem). MacLean entertained the possibility that the limbic system is "not at all unconscious … but rather eludes the grasp of the intellect because its animalistic and primitive structure makes it impossible to communicate in verbal terms." He connected the intellect with "the word brain."[20]

While agreeing in principle about a language-limbic disconnect, Dr. Murray bristled (or worse) at the depiction of the limbic system as "animalistic and primitive." He had disdain for an "Olympian"[5] view of humans as ideally and uniquely rational creatures who are at their best when suppressing their limbic urges. The lofty viewpoint finds some loose correspondence between MacLean's "triune brain," with its reptilian complex, paleomammalian complex (corresponding to his concept of the limbic system), and neomammalian complex,[21] and Plato's tripartite soul with its appetitive, spirited, and rational parts[22] (and perhaps even Freud's id, ego, and superego).

Evolution and Western philosophy thus seem to grade our humanity and morality based on our respective rational:emotive ratios. However, this view comes under fire not only from 30 years of "Limbic Music," but also from figures in contemporary philosophy, psychology, and neuroscience. Plato himself saw his tripartite soul as optimally operating in harmony with itself, not necessarily as a constant top-down hierarchy. Lakoff and Johnson,[23] in their book, *Philosophy in the Flesh*, make a compelling case against a Western philosophical tradition that views conscious reason as the defining feature of humanity and the measuring stick of virtue. They note that "abstract reason builds on and makes use of forms of perceptual and motor inference present in 'lower' animals." Meanwhile, "we think of our 'higher' (moral and rational) selfstruggling to get control over our 'lower' (irrational and amoral) self." Yet these ideas, and that of "thought-as-language" are really metaphors for a

TABLE 6-1 "Limbic Probe" Examples

Probe	Content	Goal
"The Frank Jones Story"	"I'm gonna tell you a story. Tell me what you think of it. I have a friend named Frank Jones. His feet are so big he has to put his pants on over his head" (said without humor). Patient responds. "Can he do it?"	Type 1 Response: Laugh. "No." Type 2: Laugh. "Yes" + implausible reason. Type 3: No laugh. "Yes" ± reason. Initially thought to discriminate between delirium and dementia based on relative intactness of limbic system vs cortex. Does not do this, but is a gross (and fun) brief screen for cognitive dysfunction.[18]
"The Cup Push"	"How do you feel about that (cup)?" Patient looks and responds quizzically. Move cup a bit towards edge of table. "How about it now?" Patient less quizzical; more amused vs annoyed vs indifferent. Repeat until stopped or theatrically balance cup half off edge.	Screen for obsessive character. Tolerance for loss of control proportional to distance cup can be moved before annoyance (if any) occurs. Best response ever: Examiner moved cup 1 inch. Patient instantly pushed it back where it was, stating "I liked it THERE!" But then was able to talk about why being in the hospital is so hard.
"The Fist"	"What's this?" (putting up clenched fist and waving it about—not at patient—with pseudo-aggressive expression) Patient (eventually) gets your drift. "If you had one pop with this, where would you put it?"	Screen for direction and tolerance of suspected rage. "Oh my, no one. Never," in sad tone. – "Ineluctable bepissment." "Myself," often in sad tone – Depression. "God," often with guilty tone – Demoralization. "That bastard, ____," with laughter and mock guilt – OK. "That bastard, ____," with glee – Watch out. "No one," sincerely – a saint.
Profanity	Casually, but strategically use profanity as punctuation. First time is the telling time. Must come naturally to you. Authenticity is important. If necessary, might ask first if patient is offended by profanity.	Catch an honest affective response in a "squelched" patient. Amygdala responsiveness greater to unexpected stimuli.[19]

brain that is largely operating outside of our own awareness.[23]

The "psychological unconscious" as a major influencer of human behavior takes several forms, many, if not most, of which are subsumed under the functions of the limbic system. Khilstrom[24] identifies many of these, bringing to light that the psychological unconscious can even include some highly complex cognitive processes. These bleed into the realm of emotion in cases of prosopagnosia, where patients with downstream visual association cortex lesions or disconnection syndromes can still feel affective responses to faces they do not consciously recognize, likely due to preserved connections between (relatively) upstream visual association cortex and limbic and paralimbic areas. In "desynchrony," behavioral or physiological correlates of emotion are expressed without the agent being consciously aware of what is occurring.[24]

Moving from psychology to metapsychology, the prosopagnosia situation described above is not too far afield from transference reactions. We can easily view the latter as "limbic" responses, through one or more of the consciousness-bypassing routes cited below, to incomplete information with enough valence to activate the bypass connections. Desynchrony is seen every day in what is often casually brushed aside by psychiatrists and patients as a "nervous laugh" (both parties conveniently not registering that these quick chuckles sometimes sound more sadistic than nervous). Most often bubbling up from the limbic depths when the conversation edges towards anger or fear (begging for speculation on the role of the amygdala), these laughs demand that the interviewer make quick decisions about whether or not to bring them to light and/or continue the line of inquiry that elicited them. "Higher"-level cortex may be your friend or enemy here, playing dumb or clamping down on a limbic system that has shown too much of its hand (a state, when persistent, referred to by Dr. Murray as "ineluctable bepissment" and signaling a smoldering, long-suffering state), surrendering to the gratification and peril of opening the floodgates of rage, or being guided to a state of Platonic harmony where true feelings and "cortical squelch" can co-exist in a state of well-modulated honesty.

Habib Davanloo's Intensive Short Term Dynamic Psychotherapy indirectly exemplifies many of the points just raised.[25] Davanloo's approach touches upon neurophysiology, including involuntary motor responses and autonomic nervous system activity, in listening for Limbic Music (though he does not use the term), and making decisions about what to do with it.[25] In his "central dynamic sequence," the patient's laughter might be met with light pressure ("You just laughed while telling me how difficult your husband is. Did you notice that?") that is incrementally increased ("You just did it again. Do you always laugh when you are starting to talk about something uncomfortable?" "And there it is again. Why are you putting up this wall?"), or decreased depending on responses that range from modulated but honest emotion, to hyper-rationalization, to autonomic dyscontrol (e.g., how many times have you had an emotionally intense consultation interrupted by borborygmi and the patient's departure to the bathroom?). In Davanloo's work, we see a model that, removed from its formal psychotherapeutic context and translated via the concept of Limbic Music, can be used in a multitude of ways in the interactions and assessments of routine consultation psychiatry. The same could be done with many other psychotherapeutic approaches.

WHERE DOES LIMBIC MUSIC COME FROM AND WHAT DOES IT WANT?

Limbic Music emanates from the limbic system and conveys emotion. If only it were that easy. Table 6-2 is an oversimplified representation of the expansion of the limbic system from its humble beginnings as a grossly, then architectonically, defined "border zone" with mainly olfactory functions, to its current status as a functionally and connectivity defined "system" or assembly of sub-systems with a range of functions.[26–28]

The argument that there is no limbic system was already mentioned. Generally credited as starting with Brodal[4] in 1969, this argument hinges on the idea that the limbic system was even then incorporating and connecting to so much of the brain that its boundaries and status as a system

TABLE 6-2 Anatomic Expansion of the Limbic System[26–28]

Investigator	*Circa*	Corticoid areas and subcortical nuclei	Allocortical and mesocortical areas	Neocortical areas	Brainstem/ cerebellum
Willis	1664		Cingulate, parahippocampal gyrus		
Broca	1878		Same as Willis; expands concept		
Papez	1937	Hypothalamus, mammillary bodies, anterior thalamus, fornix	Hippocampus	Precuneus	
Yakovlev	1950	Amygdala	Medial orbitofrontal, olfactory cortex incl. part of insula, temporal pole		
MacLean	1955+	Septum			Midbrain central gray, reticular activating system
Nauta	1958+	"Limbic forebrain"		Frontal neocortical connections	Raphe nuclei, ventral tegmental area
Heimer	1970+	Ventral striatum, ventral pallidum, extended amygdala, septal nuclei	Entire hippocampal/ parahippocampal complex, insula (greater portion)	Medial frontal, retrosplenial	
Nieuwenhuys	1996				Vagal-solitary complex, parabrachial nucleus, tegmental nuclei
Schmahmann	1997+				Medial cerebellum
Connectivists (e.g., Sporns)	2010+			"Default Mode Network" incl.: Medial prefrontal, posterior cingulate, lateral prefrontal, retrosplenial, cortical midline (some mesocortical overlap)	

would reach a point of meaninglessness. Note that the limbic system described in Table 6-2 is cumulative, with few, if any, structures eliminated over time.

Recently, Heimer et al.[26] suggested that "the limbic system is a concept in perpetual search for a definition," and that the "anatomical characterization of such a comprehensive functional system ... may be impossible without enlisting practically the entire brain".[26] These same authors, however, ultimately find utility and reality in the limbic system based on the robustness of its connections to the hypothalamus, neuromodulatory nuclei in the brainstem, and the cortical regions most affiliated with emotional functions. Simultaneously acknowledging and embracing the expansiveness of their "greater limbic lobe," they remark that "when the amygdala speaks, the entire brain listens."

Other neuroscientists who embrace a larger limbic system do so by dividing it into parts. Rolls,[27] for example, in a recent review, concludes that there are two limbic systems that are connected but double dissociated. One is organized around the orbitofrontal cortex and amygdala, involving (non-exclusively) anterior cingulate and parietal cortex, as well as ventral striatum, hypothalamus, and brainstem nuclei.[28] This limbic system, which loosely corresponds to Mesulam's olfactocentric paralimbic belt,[29] is thought to subserve emotion, reward valuation/learning, and reward-related decision-making. Rolls' second limbic system is organized around the hippocampus, involving (non-exclusively) the entorhinal, parahippocampal, perirhinal, and posterior cingulate cortices, as well as the connected fornix–mammillary bodies–anterior thalamus. This limbic system, which loosely corresponds to Mesulam's hippocampocentric paralimbic belt[29] and the well-known Papez circuit,[30] is thought to subserve episodic memory. It is affected by emotional states, but is not dependent on or generative of them.

In another multiple-limbic-systems scheme, Catoni et al.[28] add a third system corresponding to the default mode network. This system is believed to involve (non-exclusively) anterior cingulate, other medial prefrontal, posterior cingulate, and retrosplenial cortices, as well as the precuneus. Active mainly, but not only, in the resting state, the default mode network operates in a "mode of cognition that is directed internally rather than being externally driven and that is concerned with self and social context,"[31] thus subserving functions, such as introspection, theory of mind, and working memory.

These models of the limbic system(s) reiterate Dr. Murray's focus on the hippocampus and amygdala in "Limbic Music." They also illustrate the proliferation of brain areas thought to participate in limbic functions, which, in turn, have proliferated to include not just emotion, but forms of learning, reward valuation, episodic memory, introspection, empathy, and even some aspects of working memory. Neuroscience has clearly widened its scope to include more than even Dr. Murray's re-formulation, by way of Lazarus,[32] of the limbic "4-Fs" as pertaining to "gender role, territoriality, and bonding."[5] It has also forced the question of what the boundary is between emotion and cognition, or whether there even is one. Heimer et al.[26] acknowledge as much, pointing out that the basal forebrain/ventral striatum funnel of their greater limbic lobe mirrors the subcortical paths of other cortical and cerebellar regions. Uttal[8] very matter-of-factly refers frequently to "emotions and other cognitive functions," only stopping briefly to say it is "incontestable that emotional responses ... are at least a useful adjunct to higher level cognitive processes *if not another one of them*" [italics added].[8]

So where does this leave Limbic Music? Initially put forth by Dr. Murray as an expression of the limbic system as a mind–brain mediator, it now additionally emerges as a means of considering the mysteries of consciousness itself. Of course, this being a "handbook of general hospital psychiatry," we should avoid getting (further) bogged down in philosophy and neuroscience. Suffice it to say that the human brain, and its limbic system(s) in particular, is set up such that much or most of its processing goes on outside of our awareness. This "non-conscious" (a term perhaps preferable to "unconscious" due to the baggage the latter carries) processing may occur through LeDoux's[33] "low road" cortical bypass, routing incompletely processed, high-priority, sensory information via the thalamus directly to the amygdala; through connections between limbic structures and upstream sensory cortex that "flavor" the way situational perception occurs using prior learning that may, in turn, have been acquired limbically;[26] through unimodal association to paralimbic/limbic cortical connections;[29] through "bottom-up" interoceptive mechanisms kicked off by pre-conscious autonomic activation;[34,35] or through any of the many mechanisms of the aforementioned "psychological unconscious."

All of these non-conscious goings-on influence behavior in ways that are similarly non-conscious (until we and/or helpful others attend to them). At the same time, they express our authentic selves as much or more than our deliberate choices and actions. Limbic Music is playing constantly, but infrequently given a close listen. We now examine a few selected examples of the concept being tested out.

THE POLYVAGAL THEORY

There has been disagreement in the field of cognitive psychology about the impact of the limbic system. Some say emotion is partially independent of cognition; others say that emotions are products of cognition; and still others, as noted above, say that emotions *are* cognition. These ideas are not mutually exclusive, though limbic music focuses on emotions arising on their own without prior conscious cognitive processes. This position is supported by Porges' polyvagal theory and the concept of neuroception.[36]

Polyvagal theory postulates that social behavior is dependent on autonomic reactivity. Porges bases his theory on the evolution of the autonomic nervous system (ANS), pointing to three phylogenetic stages.[36] He relates these three stages to distinct sub-systems of the ANS: the ventral vagal complex, the sympathetic nervous system, and the dorsal vagal complex. These response systems are responsible for social engagement, mobilization, and immobilization, respectively. Porges[36] also suggests that the ANS risk response apparatus follows a phylogenetic hierarchy, starting with the newest, social engagement system (ventral vagal complex) and, when all else fails, reverting to the most primitive, immobilization system (the dorsal vagal complex).

Through these vagal circuits, the nervous system continuously evaluates risk by processing sensory information. Key to the polyvagal theory is the notion that the neural evaluation of risk does not require conscious awareness. This process, termed "neuroception," is distinct from perception and is capable of distinguishing environmental and visceral features that are safe, dangerous, or life-threatening.[37] Limbic activation and neuroception of bodily states, or interoception, actually can precede and influence eventual conscious responses and experiences. Besides providing another reason to be impressed with William James by seeming to validate the James-Lange theory of emotion,[38] the polyvagal theory adds to our list of non-conscious drivers of expression/behavior.

MICROEXPRESSIONS

In prior versions of "Limbic Music," Dr. Murray states that,

> *... dogs have a visible 'limbicometer,' their tails. Whether a dog's tail wags or not, with what frequency, and with what vigor all tell us about the dog's feelings. Probably the closest thing to a limbicometer in humans is the smile. In this context, a smile is the limbic recognition of reality before it is fully understood by the intellect (neocortex).*[5]

This insight might be expanded to include the entire human face. Two-thirds of communication is non-verbal. Facial expressions of emotion are universal and provide a critical source of Limbic Music. Fortunately, our ability to recognize facial expressions is innate, cross-cultural, and evolutionarily preserved.[39]

Unlike a dog's tail, however, the human face can lie. As much as "Limbic Music" emphasizes non-conscious emotional behavior, facial expressions can, of course, be voluntarily modulated by varying the number of areas involved, the duration of the expression, or the excursion of the facial muscles. They can be falsified entirely, through simulation, neutralization, and masking. Humans are naturally poor lie detectors, and mental health clinicians are no exceptions.[40] Hundreds of studies have shown the rate of detection of deception to be just over 50%—about as accurate as a coin toss.[41]

Deception giveaways can, however, be spotted in facial morphology, the timing of an expression, the location of an expression in a conversation, and through "microexpressions," facial movements lasting less than half a second. Though the term was introduced by psychologist Paul Ekman, the phenomenon was first described by psychoanalytic researchers Haggard and Issacs.[42] After watching hours of psychotherapy films frame-by-frame at one-sixth the normal speed, they noted "micromomentary facial expressions ... that are so short-lived they seem to be quicker than the eye."[42] Haggard and Issacs[42] initially believed these expressions were signs of repressed emotion; however, Ekman later determined that they can also reveal emotions that have been deliberately concealed.

As such, increased accuracy at lie detection is a skill that can be learned. Just a few hours of formal training in laypeople can improve the ability to read microexpressions. This ability is retained a few weeks after initial training and is also associated with higher third-party ratings of sociocommunicative skills.[43] For people with schizophrenia who have emotional recognition impairment, microexpression training can close the gap to the point that they cannot be distinguished in this area from untrained controls.[44]

Microexpression research teaches us that limbic music has a volume knob and a tuner that, for good or for ill, humans can learn to manipulate. It does not, however, have an off-button.

IMPLICIT BIAS

Each day consists of an endless number of decisions, from the mundane (lunch: sandwich or salad?) to the critical (career: law school or medical school?). Every decision is informed by the innumerable decisions made before it and the resulting life experiences. It is therefore important to realize that it is nearly impossible to encounter a novel situation and arrive at an unbiased decision. Implicit bias, or unconscious bias, is the idea that prior decisions and experiences unconsciously influence future decisions. Because this information is not consciously recalled, there is a lack of awareness of the baggage of life experiences carried around. These biases may lead to behavior that differs from those beliefs that are consciously voiced.[45] Online tests, such as the Implicit Association Tests (http://implicit.harvard.edu/implicit) measure implicit biases in a variety of demographic domains.

Prejudice and stereotyping involve different, but interacting, neuroanatomic structures. Prejudice "reflects an evaluative or emotional component of social bias" while stereotypes "represent the cognitive component—the conceptual attributes linked to a particular group as defined by a culture or society."[46] The amygdala, evaluating threat and reward, interacts with the insula (visceral subjective emotion), striatum (instrumental approach response), ventral medial prefrontal cortex (empathy and mentalizing), and orbitofrontal cortex (affective judgment), functioning to support the development and voicing of prejudice; in contrast, the anterior temporal lobe, representing stereotype-related knowledge, interacts with the inferior frontal gyrus (stereotype activation), lateral temporal lobe (semantic and episodic memory), and dorsal medial prefrontal cortex (impression formation), result in stereotyping and resultant actions.[46] Those actions may be prodded along in opposition to our conscious self-images. For example, Phelps et al.[47] found amygdala activation in white subjects exposed to unfamiliar black faces (but not unfamiliar white faces), independent of their consciously held race attitudes. The amygdala activation correlated with indirect measures of physiologic states of alarm.[47] The limbic system can sometimes play ugly music while the "high-minded" neocortex blithely turns a deaf ear to it.

Prejudice, with its reliance on the amygdala, is rapid and instinctual, while stereotypes involve the recruitment of memory. Both work in concert, but with the allowance of time, a more nuanced response can be achieved that merges the recognition of these more immediate processes with cortical involvement. Studies have shown that implicit bias toward demographic groups such as gender, race, and class is widespread throughout society.[48,49] Recognizing this universal truth is the first step toward mitigating its influence on clinical decision-making, which has been shown to be affected by unconscious bias.[50]

Yet implicit bias, if acknowledged, can be a useful clinical tool. Much has been made of the challenges of unconscious bias and its presumed negative effects on clinical decision-making.[51] However, the seed of countertransference is, essentially, prejudice; psychiatrists use this internally generated information to guide their interview trajectory, modulate their own affect, inform their diagnoses, and make inferences about their patients' interactions in the world. Allowing implicit bias to evolve into a fully formed thought both allows for the generation of a useful hypothesis (provided the psychiatrist is attuned to his or her own experiences and biases) and allows for mitigation of a potentially harmful instinctive response. Implicit bias develops into heuristics that allow the seasoned psychiatrist to draw upon prior clinical encounters to inform current clinical encounters. Of course, allowing unconscious bias to assist, rather than dictate, decision-making requires a tricky balancing act of consciously acknowledging bias without allowing it to overwhelm.

CLINICAL EXAMPLES

CASE 1

A 72-year-old, independently living woman, is admitted for work-up of a lung mass. She is noted by staff to be "forgetful," during education and consent discussions. Psychiatry is consulted to assess dementia. She performs poorly on the Montreal Cognitive Assessment when administered by the resident. She seems withdrawn and disinterested during subsequent interviewing by the attending psychiatrist, who suggests that "seeing me is not your number one priority, is it?" and requests "just one test and then I'll leave you alone." A $1, $10, and $20 bill are each "hidden" in locations initially shown to the patient. Some jokes are made about her possibly "pretending to forget where my money is ... don't let me leave without it." After 10 minutes of surprisingly permitted further interaction during which she acknowledged and discussed her fear about cancer, the patient is asked to "tell me where my money is." She readily recalls the denominations and their respective locations – six out of six items spanning verbal and visuo-spatial recent recall.

This woman does not care about remembering random memory items on a cognitive screen. It is not hard to use one's own limbic system to hypothesize about what is really distracting her. Some humor and empathy, along with the use of a limbically activating array of memory items (residents may need to borrow money to perform this "test"), led to a more genuine display of feelings and cognitive ability than were initially evident.

CASE 2

A 50-year-old man with a "diagnosis" of "mood disorder NOS" and an electronic medical record history of over a dozen psychiatric hospitalizations for self-presentations with suicidal ideation never succeeded by follow-through with outpatient care, presents with suicidal ideation and chest pain. A cardiac origin is excluded that day. During psychiatric consultation for "placement," the patient is spontaneously effusive and detailed about his suicidal thinking but will not describe other psychological experiences. He mentions having been recently assaulted by a man who is going to be tried for battery. The patient knows and intensely dislikes this man, briefly smiling and becoming animated about the subject when it initially came up. The interviewing psychiatrist returns to the topic later, asking the patient if he expects his assailant to "get what's coming to him" in court. Big smile and a nod; "he's on probation." The trial is revealed to be a week away. Asked if he plans to be there to be a witness or to "just see him suffer," the patient replies in the emphatic affirmative. He is discharged despite a now-tepid reassertion of suicidal ideation, and after his refusal to discuss what his actual needs might be and how they might be better addressed.

While perhaps manipulative, the psychiatrist in this case noted incongruities between this patient's "word brain" and Limbic Music. Through his own choice of words, the psychiatrist attempted to communicate with the patient's limbic system and obtained consistent and specific future orientation that belied the patient's assertions of suicidality. The patient's survival was confirmed by an almost identical presentation not long afterward.

CONCLUSION

Originally introduced by Dr. George Murray in 1987, "Limbic Music" is a concept with neuroanatomic, psychological, and philosophical aspects. It is sometimes discussed in a factual way, and sometimes metaphorically. In both instances, it utilizes a neuroscientific frame of reference, in the form of the limbic system. This framework is felt to not only make the Limbic Music concept informative, but also more versatile in some situations than are theories of emotion bound to therapeutic interventions. The limbic system that "plays" Limbic Music, and the functions attributed to it, have expanded and become controversial over time. But so long as Limbic Music is rooted in the brain structures, emotions, and non-conscious forces that govern human lives, it will play tunes that psychiatrists would be well advised to listen to—in their patients, and in themselves.

REFERENCES

Access the reference list online at https://expertconsult.inkling.com/.

Psychological and Neuropsychological Assessment

7

Mary K. Colvin, Ph.D., A.B.P.P.
Mark A. Blais, Psy.D.
Sheila M. O'Keefe, Ed.D.
Dennis K. Norman, Ed.D., A.B.P.P.
Janet Sherman, Ph.D.

OVERVIEW

Psychological and neuropsychological assessments can be invaluable in cases where there is a question regarding differential diagnosis, a change in functioning from a premorbid baseline, or when a baseline is needed to assess the efficacy of planned treatments. Clinical psychologists who have doctoral and postdoctoral training in assessment perform these types of evaluations, generally working in a consultative role. Psychological evaluations focus on distinguishing between different types of psychopathology and broadly characterize cognitive and emotional functioning. Neuropsychological evaluations focus on relating an observed pattern of performances on cognitive tests to brain function and are often most helpful when there are complex differential diagnostic questions at the interface of psychiatry and neurology. Both types of evaluations involve clinical interviews, review of available records, and the administration of standardized tests that are designed to tap specific functions. Test data are interpreted using normative data for each measure that allows for comparison of an individual to the general population as well as a characterization of the individual's pattern of strengths and weaknesses. A written report is provided to the referring provider and the psychologist may also meet with the patient to review the findings and recommendations. This chapter describes both types of evaluations, using cases to illustrate the types of measures and findings.

PSYCHOLOGICAL ASSESSMENT

Psychological assessments are most commonly requested when there is a question regarding psychiatric diagnosis. For example, psychological evaluations are often requested when there are questions regarding the nature of a mood or anxiety disorder, personality features, or how an individual's overall level of cognitive functioning may interact with emotional functioning and treatment. Evaluations are performed in outpatient and inpatient settings, and are often more comprehensive in the outpatient setting. The request for psychological testing might be framed as portrayed in Case 1.

CASE 1

Please conduct a psychological assessment on Ms. B, a 28-year-old, right-handed, single attorney to help determine if her presentation represents depression with suicidality and/or atypical personality functioning.

Ms. B initially presented to the Emergency Department with complaints of extreme back pain. The physician noted mild confusion and disorientation and Ms. B was admitted to the medical service for further evaluation. By the next morning, her mental status had improved. However, she continued to complain of extreme back pain and made vague suicidal statements. A pain work-up and psychiatric consultation were both ordered.

A review of the medical chart revealed that she had graduated from a prestigious university and law school and was employed at a large legal firm. She had developed severe back pain secondary to multiple equestrian injuries that occurred while riding competitively in college. She had received various diagnoses for her pain and there had been multiple unsuccessful interventions, including medication trials, surgery, and limited progress as a patient on an inpatient pain rehabilitation unit. Ms. B's current prescribed medications included diazepam (5 mg BID), amitriptyline (100 mg QHS), and oxycodone–acetaminophen (Percocet; one tablet QHS). The pain service consultant was unsure about the diagnosis. The psychiatric consultant found her to be guarded (with regard to her mood and the level of her suicidal ideation). She reported no history of depression or suicide attempts. She got into frequent struggles with the nursing staff over the hospital's smoking rules.

Later that same day, Ms. B completed a brief, but fairly comprehensive psychological assessment. The test battery included: the Wechsler Abbreviated Scale of Intelligence (2nd edition; WASI-II);[1] the Rorschach inkblot test;[2] four Thematic Apperception Test (TAT) cards;[3] and the Personality Assessment Inventory (PAI).[4] The WASI-II was selected for its brief administration time (20 to 30 minutes) and its ability to provide an estimate of the patient's overall level of intellectual functioning, including verbal and non-verbal abilities. The Rorschach, a performance measure of personality functioning, was selected given her guardedness and unwillingness to openly discuss her emotional functioning. The PAI, a self-report measure of psychopathology was also selected because it has embedded validity indices to determine whether a respondent has completed the task with sufficient attention and willingness to disclose personal experiences. Compared with other self-report inventories, the PAI is relatively short (344 items), and contains a number of treatment-planning scales that can provide important information.

Ms. B's assessment was conducted in her semi-private room. Although this was not an ideal situation, hospital evaluations are commonly performed in this fashion. Ms. B completed all of the testing without complaint. The WASI-II data indicated that her overall level of intellectual functioning generally falls well above the average range, though there was a notable discrepancy between her verbal and non-verbal abilities with superior range Verbal Comprehension Index (Standard Score = 120; 91st percentile) and low average range Perceptual Reasoning Index (Standard Score = 87; 19th percentile).

With regard to Ms. B's implicit psychological function, the Rorschach depression index was positive and suggested either current depression or a propensity to depressive experiences. The suicide constellation was negative. Although her adaptive psychological resources were adequate, situational stress was overwhelming her ability to cope. Her affective experience was dominated by helplessness, painful internalized affect, and unmet dependency–nurturance needs. Together these findings suggested possible depression resulting from situational factors. She was not psychotic, but her thinking was over personalized and idiosyncratic. The experience of anger also decreased her reasoning and judgment. She had a self-centered and narcissistic character style. She did not process her feelings but instead tried to minimize them through intellectualization or externalization (projection).

The PAI was considered to provide a picture of her explicated psychological world. The PAI profile was valid. She reported minimal psychopathology. Her mean elevation on the 10 clinical scales was well within the range of non-patients (average T-score = 53), suggesting either that she was experiencing little overt distress or that she was reluctant to express emotional pain. Either way, she did not appear to others, including her caregivers, to be psychologically impaired. She reported mild clinical depression (T-score = 71) and excessive concern about her physical function (T-score = 85). On further clinical interview, her excessive physical complaints and concerns overshadowed her depressive symptoms. A grandiose sense of self, consistent with the pronounced signs of a narcissistic character style on the Rorschach, was also indicated by one of the PAI subscales. On the treatment consideration scales, she indicated minimal interest in psychologically oriented treatments, high levels of social stress, and minimal suicidal ideation (T-score = 54).

Impressions and Recommendations

Overall, the assessment strongly suggested the presence of a clinical depression. Depression was likely masked to some extent by both the patient's focus on her physical function (back pain) and her inability or unwillingness to express her emotional pain. As a result, her depression was likely more significant and disruptive to her functioning than she reported, particularly given her personality functioning, which is likely to include an immature, self-centered view of the world and narcissistic traits. She did not appear to be actively suicidal either on the self-report or performance tests. However, given her emotionally overwhelmed and depressed state of being and her reduced coping ability. Ms. B should be considered at an increased risk (over and above being depressed) for impulsive self-harm. Her safety should be monitored closely.

The significant discrepancy between her verbal and non-verbal abilities on intellectual testing raised several questions for further exploration, including whether there is a longstanding developmental condition (e.g., a non-verbal learning disability) or whether there has been a change in cognitive functioning (i.e., an acquired condition) secondary to medical (neurological, pain, medication effects, etc.) and/or psychiatric factors (e.g., depression). Such findings should prompt further medical evaluation, specifically a neurological exam to rule out right hemisphere dysfunction. A neuropsychological evaluation following stabilization of her emotional functioning would also be appropriate to help hone in on the factors contributing to her uneven cognitive abilities. Regardless of etiology, this profile is sometimes associated with a tendency to be detail-oriented at the expense of "seeing the big picture" and others may overestimate her level of function because of her strong verbal communication skills.

Psychotherapy will be challenging given her personality style, but is nonetheless recommended. The primary focus should be practical efforts to improve her coping skills and function. Once her functioning stabilizes, the focus of therapy might be expanded to include her interpersonal style. If her cognitive profile reflects an idiopathic developmental condition (e.g., a non-verbal learning disability), she may also have difficulties with social communication that further limit her everyday functioning and this could be targeted in individual psychotherapy.

Assessment of Intellectual Functioning

The conceptualization and assessment of intelligence have evolved over time. Current models emphasize a dimensional approach in which an estimate of current intellectual functioning is derived from performances on a number of subtests that assess different types of cognitive skills.[5] A full discussion of the theories of intelligence is beyond the scope of this chapter, but generally speaking, IQ scores are meant to capture the patient's current ability to perform and adapt in the everyday setting.

The Wechsler intelligence tests are very commonly used to assess intellectual functioning and allow for assessment across the life span. The series includes the Wechsler Preschool and Primary Scale of Intelligence-IV (for ages 2–7 years);[6] the Wechsler Intelligence Scale for Children-V (for ages 6–16 years);[7] and the Wechsler Adult Intelligence Scale-IV (for ages 16–89 years).[8] An abbreviated version of the Wechsler IQ test for ages 6–90 (Wechsler Abbreviated Scale of Intelligence, 2nd edition; WASI-II).[1] All the

Wechsler scales provide a Full Scale IQ score as well as clinical index scores that group similar cognitive abilities, including verbal and non-verbal abilities. With the exception of the WASI-II, the Wechsler scales also provide composite indices for working memory and processing speed. The Full Scale IQ and index scores have a mean of 100 and standard deviation (SD) of 15. The normative data allow the examiner to determine whether certain index scores are statistically higher than others. When there is significant variability among the index scores, the overall estimate of Full Scale IQ should be interpreted with some degree of caution, as the patient's performances may vary depending on task demands.

Tests of Personality, Psychopathology, and Psychological Function

Objective psychological tests, also called *self-report tests*, are designed to clarify and quantify a patient's personality function and psychopathology. Objective tests use a patient's response to a series of true/false or multiple-choice questions to broadly assess psychological function. These tests are called *objective* because their scoring involves standardized procedures and the application of normative data. Objective tests provide excellent insight into how patients see themselves and want others to see and treat them. Self-report tests allow the patient to communicate their psychological difficulties to their caregivers directly.

The Minnesota Multiphasic Personality Inventory–2 (MMPI-2) is a 567-item true/false, self-report test of psychological function.[9] It was designed to provide an objective measure of abnormal behavior, basically to separate subjects into two groups (normal and abnormal) and to further categorize the abnormal group into specific classes. The MMPI-2 contains 10 clinical scales that assess major categories of psychopathology and three validity scales designed to assess test-taking attitudes. MMPI-2 validity scales are (L) lie, (F) infrequency, and (K) correction. The MMPI-2 clinical scales include (1) Hs, hypochondriasis; (2) D, depression; (3) Hy, conversion hysteria; (4) Pd, psychopathic deviate; (5) Mf, masculinity–femininity; (6) Pa, paranoia; (7) Pt, psychasthenia; (8) Sc, schizophrenia; (9) Ma, hypomania; and (10) Si, social introversion. More than 300 new or experiential scales have also been developed for the MMPI-2. The MMPI-2 is interpreted by determining the highest two or three scales, called a *code type*. For example, a 2–4–7 code type indicates the presence of depression (scale 2), impulsivity (scale 4), and anxiety (scale 7), along with the likelihood of a personality disorder.[9]

The Millon Clinical Multiaxial Inventory-III (MCMI-III) is a 175-item true/false, self-report questionnaire designed to identify both symptom disorders and personality disorders.[10] The MCMI-III is composed of 3 modifier indices (validity scales); 10 basic personality scales; 3 severe personality scales; 6 clinical syndrome scales; and 3 severe clinical syndrome scales. One of the unique features of the MCMI-III is that it attempts to assess a wide variety of psychopathology simultaneously. Given its relatively short length (175 items vs 567 for the MMPI-2), the MCMI-III has an advantage in the assessment of patients who are agitated, whose stamina is significantly impaired, or who are suboptimally motivated.

The PAI[4] is one of the newest objective psychological tests. The PAI includes 344 items and a 4-point response format (false, slightly true, mainly true, and very true) to make 22 non-overlapping scales. These 22 scales include: 4 validity scales, 11 clinical scales, 5 treatment scales, and 2 interpersonal scales. The PAI covers a wide range of psychopathology and other variables related to interpersonal function and treatment planning (including suicidal ideation, resistance to treatment, and aggression). The PAI possesses outstanding psychometric features and is an ideal test for broadly assessing multiple domains of relevant psychological function.

A patient's response style can have an impact on the accuracy of his or her self-report. Validity scales are incorporated into all major objective tests to assess the degree to which a response style may have distorted the findings. The three main response styles are careless or random responding (which may indicate that someone is not reading or cannot understand the test), attempting to "look good" by denying pathology, and attempting to "look bad" by over-reporting pathology (a cry for help or malingering).

Performance tests (formerly known as projective tests) of psychological function differ from objective tests, in that they are less structured and require more effort on the part of the patient to make sense of, and to respond to, the test stimuli. As a result, the patient has a greater degree of freedom to demonstrate his or her own unique personality characteristics. Performance tests are more like problem-solving tasks, and they provide insights into a patient's style of perceiving, organizing, and responding to external and internal stimuli. When data from objective and performance tests are combined, they can provide a fairly complete picture or description of a patient's range of psychological function.

The Rorschach inkblot test consists of 10 cards that contain inkblots (five are black and white; two are black, red, and white; and three are various pastels), and the patient is asked to say what the inkblot might be. The test is administered in two phases. First, the patient is presented with the 10 inkblots one at a time and asked, "What might this be?" The patient's responses are recorded verbatim. In the second phase, the examiner reviews the patient's responses and inquires where on the card the response was seen (known as *location* in Rorschach language) and what about the blot made it look that way (known as the *determinants*).[11] For example, a patient responds to Card V with "A flying bat." The practitioner asks, "Can you show me where you saw that?" The patient answers, "Here. I used the whole card." The practitioner asks, "What made it look like a bat?" The patient answers, "The color, the black made it look like a bat to me."

The examining psychologist reviews these codes rather than the verbal responses to interpret the patient's performance. Rorschach "scoring" has been criticized for being subjective. However, over the last 40 years, Exner and colleagues have developed a Rorschach scoring system (called the *Comprehensive System*) that has demonstrated acceptable levels of reliability.[11] Using the scoring system, high interrater reliability coefficients can be obtained (e.g., kappa >0.80) and are required for all Rorschach variables reported in research studies. Rorschach data are particularly valuable for quantifying a patient's contact with reality and the quality of his or her thinking.

The Thematic Apperception Test (TAT) is helpful in revealing a patient's dominant motivations, emotions, and core personality conflicts.[3] The TAT consists of a series of 20 cards in which drawings depict people in various interpersonal interactions. The cards were intentionally drawn to be ambiguous. The TAT is administered by presenting 8 to 10 of these cards, one at a time, with the following instructions: "Make up a story about this picture. Like all good stories, it should have a beginning, middle, and an ending. Tell me how the people feel and what they are thinking." Although there is no standard scoring method for the TAT (making it more of a clinical technique than a psychological test proper), when a sufficient number of cards are presented, meaningful information can be obtained. Psychologists typically assess TAT stories for emotional themes, level of emotional and cognitive integration, interpersonal relational style, and view of the world (e.g., whether it is seen as a helpful or hurtful place). This type of data can be particularly useful in predicting a patient's response to psychotherapy. Recent research has shown that TAT narratives can be reliably scored to reveal level of personality organization, emotional regulation, identity integration and social understanding.[12]

Psychologists sometimes use performance drawings (freehand drawings of human figures, families, houses, and trees) as a supplemental assessment procedure. These are clinical techniques rather than tests because there are no formal scoring methods. Despite their lack of psychometric grounding, drawings can sometimes be very revealing. For example, psychotic subjects may produce a human figure drawing that is transparent and shows internal organs. Still, it is important to remember that drawings are less reliable and less valid than other tests reviewed in this chapter.[13]

NEUROPSYCHOLOGICAL ASSESSMENT

Neuropsychological assessment is a specialty within clinical psychology that focuses on understanding brain–behavior relationships using standardized psychological measures. The main goal of a neuropsychological evaluation is to relate a patient's test performance to both the status of his or her central nervous system and real-world functional capacity. In addition to assessing intellectual and general psychological functioning, a complete neuropsychological assessment evaluates abilities within six major cognitive domains: attention, executive functions, language (expressive and receptive), memory (immediate and delayed recall in verbal and visual modalities), and visual–spatial functions. Higher-order motor functions may also be assessed. While the domains focused on in this evaluation are similar to those within a mental status examination used by neurologists, it provides a deeper, more comprehensive, and better-quantified assessment. The application of a battery of tests covering these major cognitive areas allows for a broad assessment of the patient's strengths and areas of weakness or impairment and provides some indication as to how these may impact real-world adaptation. The request for neuropsychological testing might be framed as portrayed in Case 2.

CASE 2

Mr. A is a 20-year-old, right-handed male with a childhood history of attention-deficit hyperactivity disorder (ADHD) and a seizure disorder. He developed psychotic symptoms approximately 4 years ago and these prompted a recent psychiatric hospitalization for stabilization. A neuropsychological evaluation was requested to assess his current cognitive function, establish a baseline to monitor his future course, aid in differential diagnosis, and guide treatment. Assistance in determining the degree to which his presentation may reflect focal neurologic dysfunction was requested.

Mr. A was recently discharged from a psychiatric unit, where he was being treated for symptoms of schizophrenia that included hallucinations (in multiple perceptual systems) and dysregulated behavior. Despite a long history of emotional and behavioral concerns (including a diagnosis of ADHD at the age of 9, seizures that were clinically diagnosed at age 12, and visual hallucinations that first developed at the age of 16), there was no history of significant developmental delays or learning difficulties. He has completed some college courses. Since his diagnosis with a seizure disorder, he has been treated with antiepileptic medication, and a variety of antidepressants and anti-anxiety agents were attempted in his mid to late teens. Antipsychotics were started in the past year. He denied use of substances within the past 4 months, but has a past history of regular marijuana use and had taken hallucinogenic mushrooms, and used inhalants.

Mr. A's evaluation included a review of medical records, an interview with him and his mother, and a discussion with his outpatient treaters. The following tests were administered: Test of Premorbid Functioning (TOPF);[14] Wechsler Adult Intelligence Scale (4th edition; WAIS-IV);[8] Wechsler Memory Scale-IV (WMS-IV)[15] Logical Memory, WMS-IV Visual Reproduction, Trail Making Test;[16] Stroop Color Word Test;[17] Controlled Oral Word Association Test (COWA);[18] Conners' Continuous Performance Test (CPT), 3rd edition;[19] Boston Naming Test;[20] Hooper Visual Organization Test;[21] Rey-Osterrieth Complex Figure;[22] Grooved Pegboard Test;[23] and PAI.[4] Mr. A cooperated fully with the evaluation. Overall, his performance was believed to be a valid reflection of his current behavior and level of function. Performances on embedded measures of performance and symptom validity were within normal limits (i.e., all the psychological tests were valid and interpretively useful).

Intellectual Functioning

Based on his performance on a test of word reading, premorbid intellectual functioning is estimated to fall in the average range for age (TOPF, 40th percentile). Consistent with this estimate, his performance on the WAIS-IV indicated that his current level of intellectual functioning falls in the average range for age (Full Scale IQ Standard Score = 91, 27th percentile). However, his performance on measures of verbal abilities (Verbal Comprehension Index, Standard Score = 98, 45th percentile) was significantly higher than on measures of non-verbal abilities (Perceptual Reasoning Index, Standard Score = 90, 25th percentile). Working memory (Working Memory Index, Standard Score = 86, 18th percentile), and processing speed (Processing Speed Index, Standard Score = 89, 23rd percentile) fell in the low average range for age. The magnitude of the discrepancy between his verbal and non-verbal abilities was statistically significant, raising the possibility of relative right hemisphere inefficiency.

Memory

Performances on measures of verbal memory were also stronger than on measures of visual memory, again pointing to possible greater right-hemisphere dysfunction. Immediate recall of narrative passages (WMS-IV Logical Memory) was average (37th percentile). After a delay period, free recall fell to the low average range (16th percentile). Qualitatively, Mr. A's recall of the two stories was disjointed, and some facts were misrepresented which raises some concerns about his functional verbal memory. However, delayed recognition of the material was grossly accurate, indicating that he is able to retain information that he learns. In contrast to verbal memory, immediate visual memory (ability to recall designs) fell in the borderline to low average range (9th percentile). After a delay, free recall fell in the low average range (16th percentile) and delayed recognition was intact. Thus, there was no evidence of loss of visual information over time.

Language

He was able to comprehend complex instructions, suggesting that his receptive language skills were intact. On the Boston Naming Test, he was able to correctly name 52 items (out of 60) spontaneously (16th percentile), which is below aptitude-based expectations. When provided with phonemic cues, his score improved to 58 (out of 60). This degree of improvement suggested some mild word retrieval problems. Consistent with this, verbal fluency was reduced. Phonemic fluency fell in the borderline range (FAS = 20 words, 3rd percentile). Semantic fluency was slightly stronger and fell in the low average range for age (animals = 16 words, 18th percentile). His ability to define the meaning of words and to describe similarities between words was average (WAIS-IV Vocabulary, 37th percentile, WAIS-IV Similarities, 37th percentile).

Visual–Spatial

Mr. A had some difficulty on measures assessing visuo–spatial functions. Construction of block designs was low average (WAIS-IV Block Design, 16th percentile), and he frequently broke the gestalt of the design he was trying to copy. Similarly, while his copy of the Rey Complex Figure was basically accurate, it was notable for a piecemeal approach that did not indicate an appreciation of the overall gestalt. On the Hooper Visual Organization Test, where he was asked to identify pictured objects presented in cut-up pieces, his performance was on the border of normal and impaired. His ability to quickly identify which "puzzle pieces" might be combined to make a pattern fell in the lower end of the average range (WAIS-IV Visual Puzzles, 25th percentile).

Attention and Executive Function

There were difficulties with aspects of attention and executive function. His passive span of auditory attention was intact (WAIS-IV Digit Span Forward) but performances on measures of auditory working memory were slightly reduced (WAIS-IV Digit Span Backward, 16th percentile; WAIS-IV Digit Span Sequencing, 9th percentile). His performance on a measure of sustained attention was notable for impulsivity and poor vigilance (Conners CPT). Processing speed fell in the low average to average range and he was slower as task demands increased (WAIS-IV Coding, 16th percentile; WAIS-IV Symbol Search, 37th percentile). Consistent with this, his performance on a straightforward visuomotor sequencing task and rapid naming task were low average to average (Trail Making Test Part A, 30th percentile; Stroop Rapid Naming, 21st percentile). When a set-shifting component was added to the sequencing task, he made three impulsive errors suggesting problems with inhibition of his behavior (Trail Making Test Part B). Sustained inhibition was low average (Stroop Color Word Interference, 9th percentile).

Motor Function

Mr. A is right-handed. His performance on a measure of fine motor coordination and speed (Grooved Pegboard Task) indicated an expected right-hand advantage but it is notable that dexterity with his left hand was borderline to low average (14th percentile) and weaker than his average dexterity with his right hand (50th percentile).

Emotional Function

The patient's PAI profile revealed elevations on the depression and schizophrenia scales. All three of the depression subscales (cognitive, affective, and physiological) were elevated (indicating a strong likelihood of major depression), as were all three schizophrenia subscales (psychotic experiences, social isolation, and thought disorder). Mr. A also reported having a stimulus-seeking personality style and little motivation for psychological treatment. Both of these features will complicate his treatment.

Impressions

The neuropsychological evaluation revealed three principal findings: (1) given his reported developmental history, Mr. A's premorbid and current intellectual functioning likely falls in the average range for age. (2) His profile is lateralizing with test findings indicating that left hemisphere functions are stronger than right hemisphere functions. (3) There are significant difficulties with aspects of attention and executive functions that contribute to weaknesses in cognitive efficiency, including his ability to learn and recall new information, and implicate dysfunction within networks involving the frontal lobes. With regard to etiology, the degree of difficulty with attention and executive function is consistent with his psychiatric history, including ADHD, depression, and possibly an emerging schizophrenia-spectrum illness. The weaknesses in skills related to right hemisphere function are less likely to be fully accounted for by his current psychiatric symptoms. This may be related to developmental factors, including his seizure disorder. Given this, follow-up with neurology would be appropriate.

An Overview of Neuropsychological Assessment Methods

Many neuropsychologists use a composite and flexible battery of tests. Tests are standardized, meaning that there are specific task instructions and administration methods and that there is normative data available for a specific population that allows for statistical comparison between an individual patient's performance and the normative group. A composite battery is usually comprised of measures of intellectual and cognitive function that cover the major domains of cognitive functioning and allow for depth of exploration within specific areas relevant to the referral question.[24] Here we review some of the more common neuropsychological tests that might be used to compose a battery or to assess specific cognitive functions. For a more comprehensive description of these tests and normative data, the reader is referred to Spreen and Strauss or Lezak.[25,26]

Attention and Executive Functions

These skills are generally related to the function of networks involving the frontal lobes of the brain. Attention and concentration are central to most complex cognitive processes. While a number of subcortical brain networks are involved in basic orienting, networks involving the frontal and parietal cortices are critically involved in the guidance of attention.[27] "Executive function" refers to a collection of higher-order cognitive processes that allow an individual to access and apply knowledge and these critically depend on functioning of the frontal cortices.

Focal attention is generally assessed by measuring the amount of information that can be held in mind for short periods of time and is closely related to working memory, which captures the patient's ability to mentally manipulate information in mind. In the auditory domain, this is commonly assessed by asking patients to repeat, reverse, and order sequences of digits (e.g., WAIS-IV Digit Span).[8] In addition to working memory, commonly assessed basic executive function skills include processing speed (i.e., how quickly an individual can integrate and act upon new information), set-shifting, self-monitoring, and inhibitory control. Processing speed is often assessed using timed graphomotor (pencil-and-paper) tests (WAIS-IV Coding, WAIS-IV Symbol Search, Trail Making Test).[8,15] Set-shifting or multitasking is often assessed by asking a patient to alternate between two different tasks (e.g., Trail Making Test Part B).[15] Self-monitoring can be evaluated across the entire neuropsychological battery through rates of intrusion and perseverative errors but also on formal measures requiring the manipulation of well-learned sequences (e.g., WMS-III Mental Control).[28] Inhibitory control is often assessed by asking a patient to keep from performing a prepotent action (e.g., Stroop Color Word Interference Test).[16,29]

Higher-order executive functions include judgment, planning, logical reasoning, and the modification of behavior on the basis of external feedback. All of these functions are extremely important for effective real-world function. Abstract reasoning and judgment are typically assessed using verbal and visual material (e.g., WAIS-IV Similarities; WAIS-IV Matrix Reasoning).[8] Planning may be assessed by observing a patient's approach to a complex self-directed task (e.g., Rey-Osterrieth Complex Figure, Tower of London).[22,30] Concept formation and mental flexibility are commonly assessed using the Wisconsin Card Sorting Test (WCST), which requires the patient to determine how to sort cards by integrating response feedback and shifting to occasional changes in the sorting criteria.[31]

Language

Brain networks subserving language function are widespread, with the majority of functions critically depending on the left hemisphere. Specifically, comprehension (receptive language) and expression are generally dependent on the left hemisphere, with comprehension relying on temporal networks surrounding Wernicke's area and expression relying on frontal networks including Broca's area. Skills related to reading and writing often involve areas at the junction of the parietal and temporal cortices. While the majority of language-based skills are typically left lateralized, there is evidence that language processes related to social communication (e.g., interpretation of tone of voice or facial affect) may involve the right hemisphere. Thus, comprehensive assessment of language function includes measures of expressive and receptive (comprehension) language, across a variety of stimulus modalities (oral, auditory, and written). In addition to language knowledge, neuropsychological evaluation should include some assessment of functional communication, including the quality of spoken language and social communication.

For receptive language, patients are often asked to match pictures to spoken words (e.g., Peabody Picture Vocabulary Test, 4th edition),[32] or to follow a series of commands (e.g., Mini-Mental Status Exam [MMSE],[33] Addenbrooke's Cognitive Estimation [revised; ACE-R],[34] observation of response to instructions). For expressive language, patients may be asked to spell words or generate simple sentences (e.g., MMSE, ACE-R) or to name pictured objects (Boston Naming Test, Expressive Vocabulary Test, 2nd edition).[20,35] Verbal fluency, including phonemic and semantic fluency, is also critical in determining the efficiency of word retrieval networks. Formal assessment of social communication is relatively recent and measures include those from the Clinical Evaluation of Language Functions (5th edition; CELF-5) or the Wechsler Advanced Clinical Solutions (ACS).[36,37]

Higher-Order Visual Functions

While both brain hemispheres are involved in basic perceptual processing, higher-order skills, including spatial and constructional skills, are typically lateralized to the right hemisphere. Assessment may include tasks that require pattern analysis and completion (e.g., WAIS-IV Matrix Reasoning), spatial reasoning or mental rotation (e.g., WAIS-IV Visual Puzzles, Hooper Visual Organization Test).[8,21] Constructional tasks commonly include copying shapes or designs (e.g., Rey-Osterrieth Complex Figure) or manipulating blocks to match a pictured design (WAIS-IV Block Design).[8,22]

Learning and Memory

Learning and memory are complex processes that involve multiple brain networks. Broadly speaking the processing of learning and memory can be broken into three phases: (1) learning or acquisition; (2) storage or consolidation; and (3) retrieval. The learning and retrieval phases are closely aligned with attention and executive functions, as strategic encoding and efficient retrieval may depend upon processing speed, set-shifting, planning, and organization. Thus, these aspects of memory are generally dependent upon networks involving the frontal lobes. In contrast, the memory storage phase is critically dependent upon the medial temporal lobes, including the hippocampi. Furthermore, depending on the type of material (verbal or visual), the two brain hemispheres may be differentially involved.

Thus, an evaluation of memory should include both verbal and visual memory systems, measure immediate and delayed recall, assess the pattern and rate of new learning, and explore for differences between recognition (memory with a retrieval cue) and unaided recall. The Wechsler Memory Scale (4th edition; WMS-IV) is a commonly used memory inventory.[15] Its statistical properties allow for a detailed evaluation of memory function and is jointly normed with the Wechsler Adult Intelligence Scale (4th edition; WAIS-IV), allowing for more meaningful comparisons between IQ and memory.[8] Other measures include list-learning tasks (e.g., California Verbal Learning Test [2nd edition; CVLT-II] or Hopkins Verbal Learning Task–Revised; HVLT-R) or design-learning tasks (e.g., Brief Visuospatial Memory Test – Revised; BVMT-R).[38–40]

Higher-Order Sensory and Motor Functions

A neuropsychological evaluation often also includes measures of sensory and motor function that typically depend on networks involving the frontal and parietal cortices and may help to determine whether there is a hemispheric asymmetry. Tests of motor function include the Finger-Tapping Test (the average number of taps per 10 seconds with the index finger of each hand),[25] grip strength (using the hand dynamometer), dexterity (e.g., Grooved Pegboard Task),[23] and praxis (e.g., imitative tool use). Sensory tests include Finger Localization Tests (naming and localizing fingers on the subject's and examiner's hand) and Two-Point Discrimination and Simultaneous Extinction Test (measuring two-point discrimination threshold and the extinction or suppression of sensory information by simultaneous bilateral activation).[25]

Statistical Analysis and Interpretation

Raw scores on test measures are converted to standard scores based on normative data for each test. These standard scores correspond to percentiles based on demographic factors (age, education, and sometimes gender) and allow for comparison across tests. Interpretation of neuropsychological test findings involves comparing patients' performances to an estimated baseline and determining whether the test data reveal a pattern of strengths and weaknesses that may imply compromised neurological functioning. The neuropsychologist also relates this pattern to known patterns of cognitive dysfunction in developmental and acquired syndromes to determine whether the patterns of strengths and weaknesses are consistent with a particular etiology. The precise scores obtained from a neuropsychological evaluation also allow for monitoring of a patient's functioning, with re-evaluations (typically a year or more after an initial evaluation to avoid 'practice effects'), very helpful in determining progression of disease or response to treatment.

Neuropsychological Screening Instruments

A number of brief neuropsychological assessment tools are used in clinical practice. Brief assessment tools are not a substitute for a comprehensive neuropsychological assessment, but they can be useful as screening instruments for time-limited evaluations or when patients cannot tolerate a comprehensive test battery (e.g., on an inpatient psychiatry or medical service). These screening tools generally include tasks that assess the major areas of cognitive function (attention, executive functions, learning and memory, language, and visuospatial functions). Two commonly employed screening measures are the Repeatable Battery for the Assessment of Neuropsychological Status (RBANS) which can be employed across the life span and the Mattis Dementia Rating Scale (2nd edition; DRS-2) for older adults suspected of having cognitive impairment.[41,42]

Integration With Psychological Assessment Tools

Neuropsychologists screen for current symptoms of major mental illness through the clinical interview and through the use of standardized checklists. Neuropsychological assessment can include more detailed assessment of personality and emotional functioning, including some of the more extensive measures detailed earlier in the chapter (e.g., Personality Assessment Inventory[4]). The extent of psychological testing typically varies depending on the skills of the neuropsychologist as well as the referral question. Thus, if the referring psychiatrist would like for this to be addressed, it should be discussed at the time of the referral. Results of psychological testing can be integrated with neuropsychological testing to understand how the patient responds to emotional stimuli and interacts with his or her environment.

Common Neuropsychological Assessment Referral Questions for Psychiatrists

Neuropsychological evaluations are clearly warranted when there is a question of an acute or subacute change in cognitive, emotional, or social functioning related to neurological function. For these cases, the precipitant may be known (e.g., traumatic brain injury, brain tumor, seizure) or suspected (e.g., a neurodegenerative disease). Many chronic medical conditions are also associated with psychiatric symptoms and cognitive dysfunction, including autoimmune disorders (e.g., multiple sclerosis). The course of symptoms may be static, progressive, or waxing and waning, and the degree to which this can be characterized will assist the neuropsychologist in differential diagnosis.

Neuropsychological evaluations are also helpful when there is concern about whether cognitive, emotional, and social functioning is atypical. In childhood and adolescence, neuropsychological testing can track the development of certain skills and can help with differential diagnosis. For example, a psychiatrist treating a child for emotional and behavioral dysregulation may seek a neuropsychological evaluation to help determine whether the child has attention deficit hyperactivity disorder (ADHD) or another neurodevelopmental condition, such as an autism spectrum disorder (ASD) or learning disability. Once a diagnosis is determined, a neuropsychological evaluation can make recommendations as to the most appropriate interventions and treatment and can also quantify the impact of interventions on behavior. The psychiatrist may also wish to refer for a neuropsychological re-evaluation once the child has been treated with medication and psychotherapy for ADHD to determine the effectiveness of those interventions and whether there are residual symptoms that are interfering with cognitive functioning and need management (e.g., anxiety).

At the other end of the life span, neuropsychological assessment is helpful in distinguishing between cognitive difficulties caused by psychiatric disorders and difficulties caused by neurological disorders. One of the most common referral questions is whether an older patient's memory problems are due to depression or an incipient neurodegenerative process. By evaluating the profile of deficits obtained across a battery of tests, a neuropsychologist can help distinguish between these two disorders. For example, depressed patients tend to have problems with attention, concentration, and memory (new learning and retrieval), whereas patients with early dementia of the Alzheimer's type have problems with delayed recall (retention) and word-finding or naming problems, with relative preservation of attention.

Neuropsychological assessments can often aid in treatment planning for patients with moderate to severe psychiatric illness. Neuropsychological assessment informs treatment planning by providing objective data (a test profile) regarding the patient's cognitive skills (deficits and strengths). The availability of such data can help clinicians and family members develop more realistic expectations about the patient's functional capacity.[43] This can be particularly helpful for patients suffering from severe disorders, such as schizophrenia. The current literature indicates that neuropsychological deficits are more predictive of long-term outcome in schizophrenic patients than are either positive or negative symptoms.[44]

Whether a patient is capable of living independently is a complex and often emotionally charged question. Neuropsychological test data can provide one piece of the information needed to make a reasonable medical decision in this area. In particular, neuropsychological test data regarding memory function (both new learning rate and delayed recall) and executive function (judgment and planning) have been shown to predict failure and success in independent living. However, any neuropsychological test data should be thoughtfully combined with information from an occupational therapy evaluation, assessment of the patient's psychiatric status, and input from the family (when available) before rendering any judgment about a patient's capacity for independent living.

OBTAINING AND UNDERSTANDING TEST REPORTS

Referring a patient for an assessment should be like referring a patient to any professional colleague. Psychological and neuropsychological testing cannot be done "blind." The psychologist will want to hear relevant information about the case and may ask the referring practitioner for specific questions that need to be answered (this is called the referral question). On the basis of this case discussion and referral question, the psychologist will select an appropriate battery of tests designed to obtain the desired information. It is helpful if the referrer prepares the patient for the testing by reviewing why the consultation is desired and that neuropsychological evaluations often take 3 or more hours to complete. The referrer should expect the psychologist to evaluate the patient in a timely manner and provide verbal feedback, a "wet read," quickly. The written report should follow shortly thereafter (inpatient reports are typically produced within 48 hours and outpatient reports are generally available within 2 weeks, although this may vary depending on the setting).

The psychological assessment report is the written statement of the psychologist's findings. It should be understandable and should be stated plainly and answer the referral question(s). The report should contain relevant background information, a list of the tests used in the consultation, a statement about the validity of the results and the confidence the psychologist has in the findings, a detailed integrated description of the patient, and clear recommendations. It should contain test data (e.g., IQ scores) as appropriate to allow for meaningful follow-up testing. To a considerable degree, the quality of a report (and the assessment consultation) can be judged from the recommendations provided. A good assessment report should contain a number of useful recommendations. The referrer should never read just the summary of a test report; this leads to the loss of important information, because the whole report is really a summary of a very complex consultation process.

In contrast to the written report from a personality assessment, the written neuropsychological testing report tends to be less integrated. The test findings are provided and reviewed for each major area of cognitive function (intelligence, attention, memory, language, reasoning, and construction). These reports typically contain substantial amounts of data to allow for meaningful retesting comparison. The neuropsychological assessment report should provide a brief summary that reviews and integrates the major findings and also contains useful and meaningful recommendations. As with all professional consultations, the examining psychologist should be willing to meet with the referrer and/or the patient to review the findings. This is especially important as the information that is provided by psychological and neuropsychological evaluations can help with diagnostic questions, with questions regarding further investigations that may be helpful, and with recommendations regarding how to best move forward in terms of clinical management to enhance a patient's functioning.

REFERENCES

Access the reference list online at https://expertconsult.inkling.com/.

Diagnostic Rating Scales and Laboratory Tests

8

Joshua L. Roffman, M.D., M.M.sc.
David Mischoulon, M.D., Ph.D.
Theodore A. Stern, M.D.

Although the interview and the mental status examination compose the primary diagnostic tools in psychiatry, the use of standardized rating scales and laboratory tests provides important adjunctive data. In addition to ruling out medical and neurologic explanations for psychiatric symptoms, the quantitative instruments described in this chapter play important clinical roles in clarifying disease severity, identifying patients who meet sub-syndromal criteria within a particular diagnosis, assessing response to treatment, and monitoring for treatment-related side effects. Rating scales are similarly applied in research studies to enroll patients and are often developed initially for this purpose.

DIAGNOSTIC RATING SCALES

Diagnostic rating scales (or rating instruments) translate clinical observations or patient self-assessments into objective measures. Clinically, rating scales can screen for individuals who need treatment, evaluate the accuracy of a diagnosis, determine the severity of symptoms, or gauge the effectiveness of a given intervention. In clinical research, rating scales ensure the diagnostic homogeneity of subject populations, essentially helping to define phenotypic categories, and assess outcomes of study interventions. Ideal rating instruments in both settings should demonstrate good reliability (i.e., the ability to relate consistent and reproducible information) and validity (i.e., the ability to measure what they intend to measure). Although clinician-administered instruments are generally more reliable and valid, self-completed patient instruments are less time-consuming and more readily utilized. In either case, careful consideration should be given to the clinical meanings and consequences of their results, as well as to cultural factors that could affect performance. The following sections summarize commonly used rating scales for general psychiatric diagnosis as well as specific disorders and treatment-related conditions.

GENERAL PSYCHIATRIC DIAGNOSTIC INSTRUMENTS

The Structured Clinical Interview for the *Diagnostic and Statistical Manual of Mental Disorders*, 5th edition (DSM-5), (SCID-5)[1–3] is the most commonly used clinician-administered diagnostic instrument in psychiatry. An introductory segment relies on open-ended questions to elucidate demographic, medical, and psychiatric histories, as well as medication use. The remainder is organized into modules that cover most major Axis I disorders (Mood [Depressive] Disorders, Psychotic Disorders, Bipolar Disorder, Substance Use Disorders, Anxiety Disorders, Obsessive-Compulsive Disorder [OCD], Sleep-Wake Disorders, Eating Disorders, Somatic Symptom Disorders, Externalizing Disorders, Trauma Disorders, and Adjustment Disorders). The SCID-5 lists some Axis I disorders as "optional" and these do not need to be assessed unless necessary for a particular study (e.g., Separation Anxiety Disorder, Hoarding Disorder, Trichotillomania, and Intermittent Explosive Disorder). Other DSM-5 changes reflected in the SCID-5 include the elimination of the bereavement exclusion for a major depressive episode, and the re-categorization of OCD, Post-Traumatic Stress Disorder (PTSD), and Acute Stress Disorder as independent from Anxiety Disorders. Based on patient responses, the rater determines the likelihood that criteria for a DSM-5 diagnosis will be met. The SCID is reliable but time-consuming; for this reason, it is used primarily in research. The derivative SCID-clinical version (SCID-CV) provides a simplified format more suitable for clinical use. A similar, but more compact and easily administered, structured diagnostic interview is the Mini International Neuropsychiatric Interview (MINI).[4] Also administered by the clinician, the MINI uses "yes/no" questions that cover the major Axis I disorders, as well as antisocial personality disorder and suicide risk. Following administration of a diagnostic instrument, the 7-point Clinical Global Improvement (CGI) scale may be used to determine both severity of illness (CGI-severity [S]) and degree of improvement following treatment (CGI-improvement [I]).[5] On the CGI-S, a score of 1 indicates normal, whereas a score of 7 indicates severe illness; a 1 on the CGI-I corresponds to a high degree of improvement, whereas a 7 means the patient is doing much worse.

Mood Disorders

Considered the "gold standard" for evaluating the severity of depression in clinical studies, the Hamilton Rating Scale for Depression (HAM-D)[6] may be used to monitor the patient's progress during treatment, after the diagnosis of major depression has been established. This clinician-administered scale exists in several versions, ranging from 6 to 31 items; answers by patients are scored from 0 to 2 or 0 to 4 and tallied to obtain an overall score. Standard scoring for the 17-item HAM-D-17 instrument, frequently used in research studies, is listed in Table 8-1. A decrease of 50% or more in the HAM-D score is often considered to indicate a positive treatment response, whereas a score of 7 or less is considered equivalent to a remission. The longer versions of the HAM-D include questions about atypical depression symptoms (such as overeating and oversleeping), seasonal depression, psychotic symptoms, psychosomatic symptoms, and symptoms associated with OCD.

The Montgomery–Asberg Depression Rating Scale (MADRS) is a 10-item clinician-administered scale, designed to be particularly sensitive to antidepressant treatment effects in patients with major depression.[7] The HAM-D and the MADRS are well correlated with each other, with the MADRS sampling a smaller symptom set, but including anhedonia and concentration difficulties not collected in the HAM-D. The MADRS provides a short but reliable scale, optimized for rapid clinical use. There is a 15-item version of the MADRS that covers atypical depressive symptoms, such as overeating and oversleeping.

The Beck Depression Inventory (BDI)[8] is a widely used 21-item patient self-rating scale that can be completed in a few minutes. Scores on the BDI can be used both as a diagnostic screen and as a measure of improvement over time. For each item, patients choose from among four answers, each corresponding to a severity rating from 0 to 3. The correlation between total scores and the severity of depression is provided in Table 8-2. Although easy to administer and to score, the BDI also excludes atypical neurovegetative symptoms.

Fewer rating scales have been designed to assess mania. Two instruments for assessing manic symptoms, the Manic State Rating Scale (MSRS)[9] and Young Mania Rating Scale (Y-MRS)[10] have been designed for use on inpatient units; they demonstrate high reliability and validity. Whereas the 26-item MSRS gives extra weight to grandiosity and to paranoid–destructive symptoms, the Y-MRS examines primarily symptoms related to irritability, speech, thought content, and aggressive behavior. Neither scale has been as extensively evaluated for reliability and validity as have its counterparts geared toward depression. Newer scales, such as the Bipolar Depression Rating Scale (BDRS), have been designed to capture episodes of bipolar depression, focusing more on mixed symptoms than the above-noted studies designed for unipolar depression.[11]

TABLE 8-1 Scoring the HAM-D

SCORE	INTERPRETATION
0–7	Not depressed
8–15	Mildly depressed
16–25	Moderately depressed
>25	Severely depressed

HAM-D, Hamilton Rating Scale for Depression.

TABLE 8-2 Scoring the BDI

SCORE	INTERPRETATION
0–7	Normal
8–15	Mild depression
16–25	Moderate depression
>25	Severe depression

BDI, Beck Depression Inventory.

Psychotic Disorders and Related Symptoms

Instruments for assessing psychotic symptoms are nearly always administered by clinicians. Two of the broader and more frequently used instruments are the Brief Psychiatric Rating Scale (BPRS)[12] and the Positive and Negative Syndrome Scale (PANSS).[13] The BPRS was designed to address symptoms common to schizophrenia and other psychotic disorders, as well as severe mood disorders with psychotic features. Items assessed include hallucinations, delusions, and disorganization, as well as hostility, anxiety, and depression. The test is relatively easy to administer and takes about 20 to 30 minutes. The total score, often used to gauge the efficacy of treatment, provides a global assessment and therefore lacks the ability to track sub-syndromal items (e.g., positive vs negative symptoms). Alternatively, the PANSS includes separate scales for positive and negative symptoms, as well as a scale for general psychopathology. The PANSS requires more time to administer (30 to 40 minutes); related versions for children and adolescents are available.

More focused attention to positive and negative symptoms characterize the Scale for the Assessment of Positive Symptoms (SAPS)[14] and the Scale for the Assessment of Negative Symptoms (SANS),[15] respectively. The 30-item SAPS is organized into domains that include hallucinations, delusions, bizarre behavior, and formal thought disorder; the 20-item SANS covers affective flattening and blunting, alogia, avolition-apathy, anhedonia-antisociality, and attentional impairment. The scales are particularly useful to document specific target symptoms and measure their response to treatment, but their proper administration requires more training than do the global scales.

The proclivity of neuroleptics to induce motoric side effects has driven the creation of standardized rating scales to assess these treatment-related conditions. The Abnormal Involuntary Movement Scale (AIMS)[16] is the most widely used scale to rate tardive dyskinesia. Ten items evaluate orofacial movements, limb–truncal dyskinesias, and global severity on a 5-point scale; the remaining two items rule out contributions of dental problems or dentures. The Barnes Akathisia Rating Scale[17] evaluates both objective measures of akathisia, as well as subjective distress related to restlessness. Both scales are administered easily and rapidly and may be used serially to document the effects of chronic neuroleptic use or changes in treatment.

Anxiety Disorders

A variety of rating scales are available to assess anxiety symptoms as well as specific anxiety disorders (e.g., panic disorder, social phobia, OCD, PTSD, and generalized anxiety disorder; GAD). Two of the more frequently used scales, both clinically and for research purposes, are described here: the Hamilton Anxiety Rating Scale (HAM-A)[18] and the Yale–Brown Obsessive Compulsive Scale (Y-BOCS).[19,20] The HAM-A provides an overall measure of anxiety, with particular focus on somatic and cognitive symptoms; worry, which is a hallmark of GAD, receives less attention. The clinician-administered scale consists of 14 items and, when scored, does not distinguish specific symptoms of a specific anxiety disorder. A briefer six-item version, the Clinical Anxiety Scale, is also available. The most widely used scale for assessing severity of OCD symptoms, the Y-BOCS, is also clinician-administered and yields global as well as obsessive and compulsive subscale scores. Newer self-report and computer-administered versions have compared favorably to the clinician-based gold standard. The Y-BOCS has proven useful both in initial assessments and as a longitudinal measure.

Attention Disorders

Rating scales for attention disorders in children are numerous and include clinician-administered instruments, along with self-reports and scales completed by teachers, parents, and other caregivers.[21] Current diagnostic criteria for attention-deficit/hyperactivity disorder (ADHD) in children and adolescents require impairment across multiple settings, necessitating a multi-informant assessment. The Conners Rating Scales are the most popular and well-researched rating scales and exist in several versions, including parent and teacher questionnaires, an adolescent self-report scale, and both full and abbreviated length scales.[22] The full scale is limited in use by its length (20–30 minutes to administer), but it provides a large normative base and well-tested reliability. Completed by parents or teachers, the ADHD Rating Scale-IV (ADHD RS-IV) derives directly from DSM symptom criteria and provides a faster (5–10 minutes), reliable screening that can help to identify children in need of additional evaluation and monitor treatment effects in children treated for ADHD.[23] The Adult ADHD Self-Report Scale (ASRS) is an 18-item self-rating scale that focuses on difficulties with concentration, organization, and psychomotor restlessness.[24] The checklist takes about 5 minutes to complete and can alert the treating clinician to the need for a more in-depth interview and assessment. A 6-item screening tool, taken out of the full ASRS, provides a rapid (less than 2 minutes) method for screening general clinic populations.

Substance Abuse Disorders

The CAGE Questionnaire (Table 8-3)[25] is a brief, clinician-administered tool used to screen for alcohol problems in many clinical settings. CAGE is an acronym for the four "yes/no" items in the test, which requires less than 1 minute to administer. "Yes" answers to two or more questions indicate a clinically significant alcohol problem (sensitivity has been measured at 0.78 to 0.81, specificity at 0.76 to 0.96), and positive screening suggests the need for further evaluation. The Alcohol Use Disorders Identification Test (AUDIT) is a 10-item questionnaire designed to detect problem drinkers at the less severe end of the spectrum, prior to the development of alcohol dependence and associated medical illnesses and major life problems from drinking.[26] The AUDIT can quickly screen for hazardous alcohol consumption (sensitivity 0.92 and specificity 0.94) in outpatient settings and permit early intervention and treatment for alcohol-related problems, often before the brief CAGE questions would be positive. A widely used scale to assess past or present clinically significant drug-related diagnoses, the Drug Abuse Screening Test (DAST)[27] is a 28- or 20-item self-administered instrument that takes several minutes to complete. If the subject answers "yes" to five or more questions, a drug abuse disorder is likely. The instrument includes consequences related to drug abuse (without being specific about the drug); it is most useful in settings where drug-related problems are not the patient's chief complaint.

TABLE 8-3 The CAGE Questionnaire

C	Have you ever felt you should **C**ut down on your drinking?
A	Have people **A**nnoyed you by criticizing your drinking?
G	Have you ever felt bad or **G**uilty about your drinking?
E	Have you ever had a drink first thing in the morning to steady your nerves or get rid of a hangover (**E**ye opener)?

Cognitive Disorders

Cognitive scales are useful for screening out organic causes for psychopathologic conditions and can help the clinician determine whether more formal neuropsychological, laboratory, or neuroimaging work-ups are warranted. It is important to consider the patient's intelligence, level of education, and literacy before interpreting results. The Folstein Mini-Mental State Examination (MMSE)[28] is used ubiquitously in diagnostic interviews as well as to follow cognitive decline over time in neurodegenerative disorders. The MMSE is administered by the clinician. It includes items that test orientation to place (state, county, town, hospital, and floor) and time (year, season, month, day, and date); registration and recall of three words; attention and concentration (serial 7s or spelling the word *world* backward); language (naming two items, repeating a phrase, understanding a sentence, following a three-step command); and visual construction (copying a design). The total score ranges from 0 to 30, with a score of 24 or lower indicating possible dementia. Although highly reliable and valid, the MMSE demonstrates less sensitivity early in the course of Alzheimer's disease and other dementing disorders, and pays little attention to executive function. In clinical practice, the MMSE is often supplemented by clock drawing and Luria maneuvers to more fully assess frontal function.

The clock drawing test is a simple, bedside assessment of general cognitive dysfunction.[29] When asked to draw a clock face with the hands set to a specified time (e.g., 10 minutes to 2), the patient must demonstrate several cognitive processes, including auditory comprehension of the instructions, assessment of the semantic representation of a clock, planning ability, and visual–spatial and visual–motor skills, to successfully complete the task. Although performance can be assessed informally, several structured scoring measures have been described in the literature.[29–31]

Earlier detection of neurodegenerative disorders can be achieved with the Mattis Dementia Rating Scale (DRS).[32] Administered by a trained clinician, the DRS consists of questions in five domains: attention, initiation and perseveration, construction, conceptualization, and memory. Subscale items are presented hierarchically, with the most difficult items presented first; if the subject can perform these correctly, many of the remaining items in the section are skipped and scored as correct. The total score ranges from 0 to 144 points. In addition to early detection, the DRS can be used in some cases to differentiate dementia that results from different neuropathological conditions, including Alzheimer's disease, Huntington's disease, Parkinson's disease, and progressive supranuclear palsy. We refer the reader to Chapter 11 in this text for additional details on the work-up, assessment, and quantification of dementia.

LABORATORY TESTS

Although primary diagnoses in psychiatry are based on clinical phenomenology, physical examination and laboratory studies are often essential to rule out organic causes in the differential diagnosis for psychiatric symptoms.[33,34] Consideration should be given to dysfunction in multiple organ systems, toxins, malnutrition, infections, vascular abnormalities, neoplasm, and other intracranial problems (Table 8-4 organizes many of these using the mnemonic VICTIMS DIE). Certain presentations are especially suggestive of an organic cause, including onset after the age of 40 years, history of chronic medical illness, or a precipitous course. Laboratory tests are also important for following serum levels of certain psychiatric medications and for surveillance for treatment-related side effects. The following sections describe routine screening tests as well as specific serum, urine, cerebrospinal fluid (CSF), and other studies that are considered in the determination of the differential diagnosis and in treatment monitoring. The use of electroencephalography and neuroimaging studies is also described later in this chapter vis-à-vis diagnosis of neuropsychiatric conditions.

Routine Screening

The decision to order a screening test should take into account its ease of administration, the likelihood of an abnormal result, and the clinical implications of abnormal results (including management). Although no clear consensus exists about which tests to order in a routine screening battery for new-onset psychiatric symptoms, in practice routine screening tests include the complete blood cell (CBC) count; serum chemistries including electrolytes, glucose, calcium, magnesium, phosphate, and tests of renal function; erythrocyte sedimentation rate; and levels of vitamin B_{12}, folate, thyroid-stimulating hormone, and rapid plasma reagin (RPR). Often urine and serum toxicology screens, liver function tests (LFTs), and urinalysis are added as well.

Psychosis and Delirium

Evaluation of new-onset psychosis or delirium must include a full medical and neurologic work-up; potential causes for mental status changes include central nervous system (CNS)

TABLE 8-4 Organic Causes for Psychiatric Symptoms, Recalled by the Mnemonic "VICTIMS DIE"

Vascular	Multi-infarct dementia Other stroke syndromes Hypertensive encephalopathy Vasculitis
Infectious	Urinary tract infection and urosepsis Acquired immunodeficiency syndrome Brain abscess Meningitis Encephalitis Neurosyphilis Tuberculosis Prion disease
Cancer	Central nervous system tumors (primary or metastatic) Endocrine tumors Pancreatic cancer Paraneoplastic syndromes
Trauma	Intracranial hemorrhage Traumatic brain injury
Intoxication/withdrawal	Alcohol or other drugs Environmental toxins Psychiatric or other medications (side effects or toxic levels)
Metabolic/nutritional	Hypoxemia Hyper/hyponatremia Hypoglycemia Ketoacidosis Uremic encephalopathy Hyper/hypothyroidism Parathyroid dysfunction Adrenal hypoplasia (Cushing's syndrome) Hepatic failure Wilson's disease Acute intermittent porphyria Pheochromocytoma Vitamin B_{12} deficiency Thiamine deficiency (Wernicke–Korsakoff syndrome) Niacin deficiency (pellagra)
Structural	Normal pressure hydrocephalus
Degenerative	Alzheimer's disease Parkinson's disease Huntington's disease Pick's disease
Immune (autoimmune)	Systemic lupus erythematosus Rheumatoid arthritis Sjögren's syndrome
Epilepsy	Partial complex seizures/temporal lobe epilepsy Postictal or intraictal states

TABLE 8-5 Life-Threatening Causes of Delirium, Recalled by the Mnemonic "WWHHHHIMPS"

Wernicke's encephalopathy
Withdrawal
Hypertensive crisis
Hypoperfusion/hypoxia of the brain
Hypoglycemia
Hyper/hypothermia
Intracranial process/infection
Metabolic/meningitis
Poisons
Status epilepticus

lesions, infections, intoxication, medication effects, metabolic abnormalities, and alcohol or benzodiazepine withdrawal (Table 8-5 organizes the life-threatening causes of delirium, using the mnemonic WWHHHHIMPS).[35] If an organic causal agent is not clearly established by virtue of the history, physical examination, and the screening studies listed previously, additional testing should include an electroencephalogram (EEG) and neuroimaging. Blood or urine cultures should be sent if there is suspicion for a systemic infectious process. Lumbar puncture is indicated (once an intracranial lesion and elevated intracranial pressure have been ruled out) if patients present with fever, headache, photophobia, or meningeal symptoms; in addition to sending routine CSF studies (e.g., opening pressure, appearance, Gram stain, culture, cell counts, and levels of protein and glucose), depending on the clinical circumstances, consideration should also be given to specialized markers (e.g., antigens for *Cryptococcus*, herpes simplex virus, Lyme disease, and other rare forms of encephalitis, including paraneoplastic syndromes, autoimmune encephalitides, and prion diseases; acid-fast staining; and cytological examination for leptomeningeal metastases). With appropriate clinical suspicion, other tests to consider include serum heavy metals (e.g., lead, mercury, aluminum, arsenic, copper), ceruloplasmin (which is decreased in Wilson's disease), and bromides.

Patients receiving certain antipsychotic medications (e.g., thioridazine, droperidol, pimozide, ziprasidone—as well as haloperidol when high-dose intravenous administration is required for the treatment of agitated delirious patients) should have a baseline electrocardiogram (ECG) as well as periodic follow-ups to monitor for QTc prolongation. Serum levels of antipsychotics can be useful both as a measure of compliance and to monitor for drug interactions (e.g., carbamazepine can decrease haloperidol levels).[36] The atypical antipsychotic clozapine causes agranulocytosis in 1% to 2% of patients taking the medication, necessitating weekly CBC testing for the first 6 months. At the initiation of treatment, a patient must have a white blood cell (WBC) count of >3500 cells/mm^3 and an absolute neutrophil count (ANC) >2000 cells/mm^3. If treatment proceeds without interruption (i.e., with laboratory values remaining above these thresholds), CBC testing can be spaced to biweekly testing after 6 months and to monthly after 1 year of treatment. If the WBC or ANC drops significantly (by more than 3000 or 1500 cells/mm^3, respectively), or in the case of mild leukopenia (WBC 3000 to 3500 cells/mm^3) or granulocytopenia (ANC 1500 to 2000 cells/mm^3), the patient should be monitored closely and have biweekly CBCs checked. In the case of moderate leukopenia (WBC 2000 to 3000 cells/mm^3) or granulocytopenia (ANC 1000 to 1500 cells/mm^3), treatment should be interrupted, CBCs checked daily until abnormalities resolve, and the patient may be re-challenged with clozapine in the future. If the WBC drops below 2000 cells/mm^3 or the ANC drops below 1000 cells/mm^3, clozapine should be permanently discontinued (i.e., patients should not be challenged in the future). In this case, the patient may need inpatient medical hospitalization with daily CBCs. Physicians and pharmacists who dispense clozapine must report laboratory values through national registries. As an aside, if a patient on clozapine develops signs of myocarditis, treaters should immediately check the WBC, troponin, and an ECG; interrupt treatment with clozapine; and refer the patient for medical evaluation.

Other adverse neuropsychiatric side effects of antipsychotic medications include the risk of seizure, changes in prolactin levels, and the onset of neuroleptic malignant syndrome (NMS). A baseline EEG can be helpful in patients taking more than 600 mg/day of clozapine because of an increased incidence of seizures at higher doses. Patients taking typical antipsychotics and risperidone should have prolactin levels checked if they manifest galactorrhea, menstrual irregularities, or sexual dysfunction. NMS should be suspected in patients who develop high fever, delirium, muscle rigidity, and elevated serum creatine phosphokinase levels while taking antipsychotic medications.

Finally, it is becoming increasingly clear that antipsychotic medications, particularly second-generation antipsychotics, are associated with weight gain and the development of metabolic syndrome. This is particularly concerning in patients with schizophrenia, who are more likely to be overweight or obese than those in the general population. Consensus guidelines recommend baseline and routine monitoring of weight, body mass index, waist circumference, blood pressure, and fasting glucose and lipid profiles.[37,38]

Mood Disorders and Affective Symptoms

Although depressive symptoms often reflect a primary mood disorder, they may also be associated with a number of medical conditions, including thyroid dysfunction, folate deficiency, Addison's disease, rheumatoid arthritis, systemic lupus erythematosus, pancreatic cancer, Parkinson's disease, and other neurodegenerative disorders. Clinical suspicion for any of these disorders should drive further laboratory testing, in addition to the routine screening battery listed previously. First-break manic symptoms warrant especially careful medical and neurologic evaluation, and patients who present with these symptoms often receive a laboratory work-up analogous to that described previously for a new-onset psychosis.

Patients who receive pharmacotherapy for mood disorders often require serum levels of the drug being prescribed (and its metabolite) to be checked periodically, as well as baseline and follow-up screening for treatment-induced organ damage. Tricyclic antidepressants (TCAs) can cause cardiac conduction abnormalities, including prolongation of the PR, QRS, or QT intervals; patients taking TCAs should have a baseline ECG to assess for conduction delays, especially if they have a history of pathologic cardiac conditions. TCA levels are useful in several clinical situations, including when the patient reports side effects at low doses, in geriatric or medically ill patients, when there is a question of compliance, or in an urgent clinical situation that requires rapid achievement of therapeutic levels (e.g., in a severely suicidal patient). Steady state levels are usually not achieved for 5 days after starting the medication or changing the dose; TCA trough levels should be obtained 9 to 12 hours after the last dose. No guidelines support routine checking of blood levels once a stable maintenance dose has been achieved, except in the noted circumstances or with changes in the clinical picture.

The selective serotonin re-uptake inhibitors (SSRIs), while considered very safe, require precautions in the cases of citalopram and escitalopram, since doses higher than 40 mg of citalopram and 20 mg of escitalopram have been associated with QT prolongation.[39] Patients who require high doses of these agents should have a baseline ECG and periodic monitoring to ensure no QT interval prolongation.

Lithium, a remarkably effective drug for bipolar disorder, has a bevy of adverse effects spanning numerous organ systems. Lithium can induce adverse effects on the thyroid gland, the kidney, and the heart, as well as cause a benign elevation of the WBC count; accordingly, baseline and follow-up measures of the CBC count with a differential, serum electrolytes, blood urea nitrogen (BUN), creatinine, thyroid function tests (TFTs), urinalysis, and ECG should be obtained. Pregnancy tests should also be obtained in women of childbearing years given the risk of teratogenic effects (e.g., Ebstein's anomaly) that are associated with use in the first trimester. There is general consensus that therapeutic lithium levels range from 0.4 to 1.2 mEq/L, although certain patients may have idiosyncratic responses outside of this range. Elderly patients with slower rates of drug metabolism and lower volumes of distribution, for example, may experience side effects within this typical range and may require maintenance at lower serum levels with a narrower therapeutic window. Steady state levels can be checked after 4 to 5 days. Lithium levels can change dramatically during or immediately after pregnancy or if patients are taking thiazide diuretics, non-steroidal antiinflammatory drugs, angiotensin-converting enzyme inhibitors, angiotensin receptor blockers, or in those who have deteriorating renal function or are dehydrated. Patients on a stable maintenance dose of lithium should have levels checked no less than once every 6 months, along with routine renal and thyroid function testing.

Patients taking carbamazepine or valproic acid for bipolar disorder should have baseline and follow-up CBCs, electrolytes, and LFTs, in addition to routine level monitoring, typically every 6 months. In the case of carbamazepine, which can cause agranulocytosis, the CBC should be checked every 2 weeks for the first 2 months of treatment, and then at least once every 3 months thereafter. Pregnancy tests should be considered for women of childbearing age.

Anxiety

The medical differential for new-onset anxiety is broad; it includes drug effects, thyroid or parathyroid dysfunction, hypoglycemia, cardiac disease (including myocardial infarction and mitral valve prolapse), respiratory compromise (including asthma, chronic obstructive pulmonary disease, and pulmonary embolism), and alcohol or benzodiazepine withdrawal. Rare causes, such as pheochromocytoma, porphyria, and seizure disorder, should be investigated if suggested by other associated clinical features. Based on this broad differential diagnosis, laboratory work-up may include TFTs, serum glucose or glucose tolerance testing, chest x-ray examination, pulmonary function tests, cardiac work-up, urine vanillylmandelic acid or porphyrins, and an EEG.

Care of the Geriatric Population

Given the increased likelihood of medical conditions that cause psychiatric symptoms in older adults, special attention should be given to organic causal agents. Especially common are mental status changes resulting from urinary tract infections, anemia, thyroid disease, dementia, and iatrogenic effects from medications. Kolman[40] described five particularly useful tests for older adults: clean-catch urinalysis and culture, a chest x-ray examination, a serum B_{12} level, an ECG, and a BUN. Although the National Institutes of Health Consensus Development Conference identified the history and physical examination as the most important diagnostic tests in older adult psychiatric patients, they also specifically recommended checking a CBC, serum chemistries, TFTs, RPR, B_{12}, and folate levels. If clinically indicated, additional testing should include neuroimaging, an EEG, and a lumbar puncture. With suspected early dementia, in addition to the DRS (see Rating Scales, discussed earlier), positron emission tomography (PET) may be useful diagnostically.[41]

Substance Abuse

Substance abuse and withdrawal should always be considered in patients with mental status changes. Substances available for testing in serum and urine are summarized in Table 8-6. Alcohol levels can be quickly assessed using breath analysis (breathalyzer). It is important to remember that serum levels of alcohol do not necessarily correlate with the timing of withdrawal symptoms, especially in patients with chronically high alcohol levels (e.g., withdrawal starts well before the serum alcohol level reaches zero). Patients who present with a history of alcohol abuse should have LFTs and a CBC count checked; if macrocytic anemia is present, B_{12} and folate levels should also be assessed. Chronic liver damage can lead to coagulopathy (as manifested by an elevated prothrombin time or international normalized ratio; INR) and other manifestations of synthetic failure (e.g., low albumin level). In the case of cocaine abuse, there should be a low threshold for obtaining an ECG with any cardiac symptom.

Eating Disorders

As part of their medical evaluation, patients who present with severe eating disorders should have routine laboratory studies to evaluate electrolyte status and nutritional measures (e.g., albumin level). Patients who are actively purging can present with metabolic alkalosis (manifested by an elevated bicarbonate level), hypochloremia, and hypokalemia. Serum aldolase levels can be increased in those who abuse ipecac; chronic emesis can also lead to elevated levels of amylase. Cholecystokinin levels can be blunted in bulimic patients, relative to controls, following ingestion of a meal. Finally, patients who abuse laxatives chronically may present with hypocalcemia.

TABLE 8-6 Serum and Urine Toxicology Screens

SUBSTANCE	SERUM DETECTION	URINE DETECTION
Alcohol	1–2 days	1 day
Amphetamine	Variable	1–2 days
Barbiturates	Variable	3 days to 3 weeks
Benzodiazepines	Variable	2–3 days
Cocaine	Hours to 1 day	2–3 days
Codeine, morphine, heroin	Variable	1–2 days
Delta-9-THC	N/A	~30 days, longer if chronic use
Methadone	15–29 hours	2–3 days
Phencyclidine	N/A	8 days
Propoxyphene	8–34 hours	1–2 days

N/A, not applicable.

Pharmacogenomic Testing

In recent years, research has greatly expanded knowledge of individual genetic variability, particularly as it applies to the metabolism of and response to psychotropic medications. A major focus has been on the cytochrome P450 (CYP) system, responsible for metabolism of many psychotropic agents (summarized in Table 8-7). Commercially available tests, including one FDA-approved test, permit examination of an individual's CYP polymorphisms through gene chip technology, suggesting patients who may be slow or rapid metabolizers of the substrate drugs.[42]

The advent of Deplin (5-methyltetrahydrofolate; 5-MTHF), a prescription form of folate, has stimulated interest in testing for a methylene tetrahydrofolate reductase (MTHFR) polymorphism found in about 10% to 12% of the population. Individuals with the C–>T MTHFR polymorphism, particularly in the homozygotic form, cannot convert folic acid normally and may develop deficiencies that could contribute to depression.[43] Because 5-MTHF can cross the blood–brain barrier directly without undergoing the various chemical conversions of the folic acid pathway, individuals with the MTHFR polymorphism could benefit from addition of 5-MTHF to their medication regimen, both from the standpoint of general health as well as alleviation of depression.[44]

In theory, knowledge gained from these kinds of tests might help clinicians make dosing decisions for particular patients, potentially facilitating treatment with certain

TABLE 8-7 Cytochrome P450 Isoenzymes Active in Metabolizing Commonly Prescribed Psychotropic Medications

CYP1A2	CYP2C9	CYP2C19	CYP2D6	CYP3A3/4/5
Amitriptyline	Fluoxetine	Amitriptyline	Amitriptyline	Alprazolam
Clomipramine	Moclobemide	Citalopram	Amphetamines	Amitriptyline
Clozapine	Ramelteon	Clomipramine	Aripiprazole	Aripiprazole
Duloxetine	THC	Clozapine	Atomoxetine	Buspirone
Fluvoxamine		Diazepam	Clozapine	Carbamazepine
Haloperidol		Imipramine	Codeine	Clozapine
Imipramine		Moclobemide	Desipramine	Haloperidol
Methadone		Ramelteon	Dextromethorphan	Imipramine
Mirtazapine		Sertraline	Duloxetine	Lamotrigine
Olanzapine			Fluoxetine	Methadone
Ramelteon			Haloperidol	Midazolam
Tacrine			Hydrocodone	Nefazodone
			Methadone	Oxcarbazepine
			m-CPP	Pimozide
			Mianserin	Quetiapine
			Nortriptyline	Risperidone
			Olanzapine	Trazodone
			Oxycodone	Triazolam
			Paliperidone	Zaleplon
			Paroxetine	Zolpidem
			Phenothiazines	Ziprasidone
			Risperidone	
			Sertraline	
			Thioridazine	
			Tricyclics (TCAs)	
			Venlafaxine	

medications with narrow therapeutic windows. Recent guidelines, however, have not supported the clinical use of such tests in treating non-psychotic major depression with SSRIs, for example, because of the relatively high cost and lack of available evidence for clinical benefit.[45] Other pharmacogenomic tests work to predict the clinical response to clozapine, development of agranulocytosis from clozapine, and development of antipsychotic-induced metabolic syndrome, though none are in routine clinical use at this time. Genotype testing for serotonin receptor and transporter variations are available but not yet clinically proven. Current research focuses heavily on the pharmacogenetics of antidepressants, and the use of peripheral blood-based biomarkers as predictors of clinical response,[46] but no tests for clinical response are yet available outside of the research setting. The concept of personalized prescriptions, or tailoring drugs to an individual's genetic makeup, remains a future goal and research interest for psychiatry, but pharmacogenomic tests have not yet reached routine clinical practice.

CASE 1

Mr. B, a 30-year-old molecular biologist was diagnosed with major depression 2 years earlier. He had tried several antidepressants, with only a partial response at best. He was currently taking paroxetine (40 mg daily) when he presented to his psychiatrist's office for a regular follow-up visit. At the time, Mr. B was endorsing mildly depressed mood, anhedonia, mild fatigue, diminished concentration, and poor appetite. He was reluctant to have his paroxetine dose increased, because he felt it was already contributing to his daytime tiredness.

During the visit, Mr. B reported that he had recently gone to a commercial lab where they tested people for various enzymatic polymorphisms. Mr. B's profile, which he gave to the psychiatrist, showed that he had a heterozygous C-to-T mutation in the gene for methylene tetrahydrofolate reductase (MTHFR), an enzyme involved in the interconversion of folate. Mr. B wondered whether he might be deficient in folate and if this could be contributing to his depression.

The psychiatrist ordered a test for folate levels, and instructed the patient to return in 2 weeks. The test results showed folate levels in the low–normal range, which is often seen in individuals with this polymorphism. Because folate metabolism is important to many vital cellular functions, the psychiatrist prescribed Deplin (5-MTHF) 15 mg/day as an adjunct to the paroxetine, since a study had shown the benefit of 5-MTHF augmentation in depressed individuals. One month later, Mr. B reported that his depression was considerably improved with the addition of 5-MTHF.

THE ELECTROENCEPHALOGRAM

The EEG employs surface (and sometimes nasopharyngeal) electrodes to measure the low-voltage electric activity of the brain. Used primarily in the evaluation of epilepsy and other neurologic disorders, the EEG is often useful in evaluating organic causes of psychiatric symptoms.

Electroencephalogram signals are presumed to reflect primarily cortical activity, especially from neurons in the most superficial cortical cell layers. The frequencies of electric activity have been divided into four bands: delta (0 to 4 Hz), theta (4 to 8 Hz), alpha (8 to 12 Hz), and beta (>12 Hz). The awake state is characterized by an alpha predominance. Beta waves emerge during stage 1 sleep (drowsiness); during stage 2, vertex sharp theta and delta waves are observed. Delta waves are seen in stages 3 and 4 sleep. During rapid eye movement sleep, the EEG will record low-voltage fast waves with ocular movement artifacts. Sleep deprivation, hyperventilation, and photic stimulation can sometimes activate seizure foci. For patients with non-epileptiform EEGs but a residual high suspicion for seizure activity, serial studies, sleep-deprived studies, or long-term monitoring can produce a higher yield. Video long-term monitoring can help link often infrequent clinical events with the associated electrical patterns.

Electroencephalogram patterns associated with neuropsychiatric conditions are summarized in Table 8-8. EEG findings in generalized, absence, and partial complex seizure disorders are well characterized and are diagnostic. When

TABLE 8-8 EEG Findings Associated With Neuropsychiatric Conditions

Condition	EEG Finding
Seizure	
• Generalized	• Bilateral, symmetric, synchronous, paroxysmal spikes; sharp waves followed by slow waves
• Absence	• 3-Hz spike–wave complexes
• Complex partial	• Temporal lobe spikes, polyspikes, and waves
Pseudoseizure	Normal EEG
Delirium	• Generalized theta and delta activity
• Hepatic or uremic encephalopathy	• Triphasic waves
Dementia	
• Alzheimer's and vascular	• Alpha slowing of the background
• Subacute sclerosing panencephalitis and Creutzfeldt–Jakob disease	• Periodic complexes accompanying myoclonic jerks
Locked-in syndrome	• Normal EEG
Persistent vegetative state	• Slow and disorganized EEG
Death	• Electrocerebral silence
Medications	
• Benzodiazepines and barbiturates	• Beta activity
• Neuroleptics and antidepressants	• Non-specific changes
Focal lesion	• Focal delta slowing
Increased intracranial pressure	• FIRDA

EEG, electroencephalogram; FIRDA, frontal, intermittent, rhythmic delta activity.

interpreted within the context of the clinical presentation, abnormal EEG data can help support several other broad diagnostic categories, including delirium, dementia, medication-induced mental status changes, and focal lesions. Normal data can provide support for diagnoses of pseudo-seizures and locked-in syndrome, but they are not able to rule out a variety of ictal states because of limitations on the placement of surface electrodes. Although an increased number of EEG abnormalities have been described in a variety of primary psychiatric disorders, at present the EEG is not clinically useful to definitively rule in any primary psychiatric diagnosis.

NEUROIMAGING

Neuroimaging has emerged as a powerful tool in both neuropsychiatric research and in the clinical investigation of organic causal agents for psychiatric presentations; however, rarely do neuroimaging studies establish a primary psychiatric diagnosis. Although less invasive than other diagnostic tests, imaging studies come with their own risks to the patient, and they remain costly.[47] Following a thorough initial evaluation, the decision to use neuroimaging needs to be made on a case-by-case basis; at present, the major objective of neuroimaging studies in patients with psychiatric symptoms is to prevent missing a treatable brain lesion. A suggested list of indications for brain imaging in psychiatric patients is given in Table 8-9. The following sections describe the major neuroimaging techniques currently available, as well as their clinical utility.

Computed Tomography

Computed tomography (CT) scans use multiple x-rays to provide cross-sectional images of the brain. On CT films, areas of increased beam attenuation (e.g., of the skull) appear white, whereas those of low attenuation (e.g., gas) appear black, and those of intermediate attenuation (e.g., soft tissues) appear in shades of gray. Contrast material may be used to visualize areas where the blood–brain barrier has been compromised, for example, by tumors, bleeding, inflammation, and abscesses; however, up to 5% of patients can develop idiosyncratic reactions to contrast media, manifested by hypotension, nausea, flushing, urticaria, and anaphylaxis. CT scans can be obtained rapidly and are the imaging modality of choice in identifying acute hemorrhage and trauma, as well as in situations in which magnetic resonance imaging (MRI) is contraindicated. CT scans are generally better tolerated by patients with anxiety or claustrophobia. Although useful in examining gross pathological conditions, CT lacks the resolution to detect subtle white matter lesions or changes in smaller structures, such as the hippocampi and basal ganglia. Because CT scans use ionizing radiation, they are contraindicated in pregnancy.

Although CT scans have a well-established role in the identification of structural abnormalities responsible for psychiatric symptoms in patients with organic lesions, they cannot be used to diagnose primary psychiatric illness. However, there are non-specific structural changes visible on CT that have been consistently identified in the brains of psychiatric patients. Since Weinberger and co-workers[48] first described increased ventricular-to-brain ratios in patients with schizophrenia, several investigators have observed enlarged ventricles in those with eating disorders, alcoholism, bipolar disorder, dementia, and depression.

TABLE 8-9 Indications for Neuroimaging in Patients With Psychiatric Symptoms

New-onset psychosis[a]
New-onset delirium[a]
New-onset dementia
Onset of any psychiatric problem in a patient >50 years old[a]
An abnormal neurologic examination
A history of head trauma
During an initial work-up for ECT

[a]When initial history, physical examination, and laboratory studies are not definitive.

ECT, electroconvulsive therapy.

Magnetic Resonance Imaging

Magnetic resonance imaging (MRI), which provides detailed images of the brain in axial, sagittal, and coronal planes, takes advantage of the interaction between protons and an external magnetic field. In the magnetic field of the MRI scanner, hydrogen protons in the water molecules of the brain become aligned as dipoles with, or against, the field. A radiofrequency pulse is applied, shifting the spin on the protons to a higher energy level; when the signal is turned off, spin returns to the ground state and the proton releases energy. The frequency of energy release (or relaxation) depends on the chemical environment surrounding the proton. A coil that detects the energy emission generates signals that are processed by the scanner to create images. Adjusting the relaxation time parameters (known as T1 and T2) can result in images that are "weighted" differently; whereas T1-weighted images provide anatomic detail and gray–white matter differentiation, T2-weighted images highlight areas of pathologic conditions.

Magnetic resonance imaging is considered superior to CT for differentiation of white and gray matter, identification of white matter lesions (e.g., in multiple sclerosis, vasculitis, and leukoencephalitis), and visualization of the posterior fossa. As with CT, contrast medium may be used to identify lesions where the blood–brain barrier has been compromised. MRI is contraindicated in patients with metallic implants (including pacemakers) and is often less tolerable to patients because of the longer length of the study, the enclosed space, and the noise.

MRI may be used clinically to rule out structural brain lesions in patients with psychiatric symptoms, including acute psychosis or delirium, severe mood disorder, and abrupt personality changes. In addition to the structural changes that CT scans are capable of detecting, MRI appears to be more sensitive at detecting atrophic changes in dementia, inflammation-induced edema, and white matter lesions. Compared with CT, MRI is capable of detecting acute strokes earlier, using a method called diffusion-weighted imaging.

Functional MRI (fMRI), which is primarily a research tool at present, uses a process of acquisition sequences to approximate cerebral blood flow; accordingly, one can infer regions of brain activation and deactivation at rest, as well as during execution of sensory, motor, or cognitive tasks. Certain patterns of activation have emerged consistently in dementia, major depression, schizophrenia, and OCD. Although fMRI is not currently considered a diagnostic or clinical tool, it is starting to provide enhanced knowledge about psychiatric illnesses and psychotropic medications, which will likely help guide research, drug development, and clinical practice in the future.

A related imaging modality, magnetic resonance spectroscopy (MRS), permits *in vivo* measurements of certain markers of brain tissue metabolism and biochemistry. For example, using proton-based MRS, one can measure local concentrations of *N*-acetyl aspartate (a putative marker of neuronal integrity), choline (a marker of membrane turnover), creatine (a marker of intracellular energy metabolism), glutamine, glutamate, and gamma-aminobutyric acid. Localized reductions in *N*-acetyl aspartate have been implicated in multiple neuropsychiatric disorders, including schizophrenia, temporal lobe epilepsy, Alzheimer's disease, acquired immune deficiency syndrome dementia, and Huntington's disease. In the near future, the combined use of fMRI and MRS holds great promise for delineating abnormal structure–function relationships underlying psychopathologic conditions.[49]

Positron Emission Tomography/Single Photon Emission Computed Tomography

Positron emission tomography (PET) employs radioactive markers to visualize directly cortical and subcortical brain functioning. Some examples of these markers include F-18 fluorodeoxyglucose (which provides a picture of brain glucose metabolism), oxygen-15 (a surrogate for regional cerebral blood flow), and receptor-specific radioligands (which indicate activity at neurotransmitter receptors). Studies can be performed only where an on-site cyclotron is present to prepare the emitter tracers. Single photon emission computed tomography (SPECT) uses photon-emitting nucleotides measured by gamma detectors to localize brain activation or pharmacologic activity; commonly used tracers include xenon-133 and technetium Tc-99m hexamethylpropyleneamine (which measure cerebral blood flow) and, as in PET, radioligands with specific receptor activity. Although PET scans provide greater spatial and temporal resolution, signal-to-noise ratio, and variety of ligands, SPECT is more readily available, better tolerated, and less expensive.

Although both PET and SPECT are primarily used as research tools in delineating pathophysiology and rational drug designs, clinical use of these techniques is becoming increasingly common. PET and SPECT may be used in concert with the EEG to determine seizure foci, especially in patients with partial complex seizures; during a seizure, scans can demonstrate areas of increased metabolism, whereas interictally the focus will be hypometabolic and hypoperfused. Moreover, in both Alzheimer's disease and multi-infarct dementia, abnormal patterns of cortical metabolism and receptor function as evidenced on PET and SPECT appear to predate structural changes visible on MRI.[50,51] With the continued development of receptor-specific ligands and other functional markers, these imaging modalities may continue to find a more prominent role in clinical diagnosis and management.

CONCLUSION

Although diagnosis in psychiatry continues to rely primarily on the interview and other clinical phenomenology, diagnostic rating scales and laboratory testing serve important roles in eliminating organic causal agents from the differential diagnoses, monitoring the effects of treatment, and guiding further management decisions. Neuroimaging has provided a non-invasive means to detect subtle neurophysiological dysfunction in psychiatric patients and has begun to find meaningful clinical as well as research applications. It is clear that these quantitative measures will assume increasing prominence and importance in 21st century psychiatry.

REFERENCES

Access the reference list online at https://expertconsult.inkling.com/.

Depressed Patients

9

Benjamin G. Shapero, Ph.D.
Paolo Cassano, M.D., Ph.D.
George I. Papakostas, M.D.
Maurizio Fava, M.D.
Theodore A. Stern, M.D.

OVERVIEW

A major depressive disorder (MDD) serious enough to warrant professional care affects approximately 16% of the general population during their life-time.[1] Both the Epidemiological Catchment Area (ECA) study and the National Comorbidity Survey study have found that MDD is prevalent, with cross-sectional rates of up to 6.6%.[1] Although this condition ranks first among reasons for psychiatric hospitalization (23.3% of total hospitalizations), it has been estimated that 80% of all persons suffering from it are either treated by non-psychiatric personnel or are not treated at all.[2]

Depression is second only to hypertension as the most common chronic condition encountered in general medical practice.[3] Depression is estimated to rival virtually every other known medical illness with regard to its burden of disease morbidity early in this millennium.[4] With respect to physical function, depressed patients score, on average, 77.6% of normal function, with advanced coronary artery disease (CAD) and angina being 65.8% and 71.6%, respectively, and back problems, arthritis, diabetes, and hypertension ranging from 79% to 88.1%.[5] MDD has also been characterized by increased mortality.[6–8] In the general population, suicide accounts for about 0.9% of all deaths. Depression is the most important risk factor for suicide, with about 21% and 18% of the patients with recurrent depressive disorders and dysthymic disorder, respectively, attempting suicide.

Depressed patients often have co-morbid medical illnesses (e.g., arthritis, hypertension, backache, diabetes mellitus [DM], and heart problems). Similarly, the presence of one or more chronic medical conditions raises the recent (6-month) and life-time prevalence of mood disorders. Patients affected by chronic and disabling physical illnesses are at higher risk of depressive disorders, with rates being typically >20%. Among patients hospitalized for CAD, 30% present with at least some degree of depression.[9] Patients with DM also have a two-fold increased prevalence of depression, with 20% and 32% rates in uncontrolled and controlled studies, respectively, conducted with depression symptom scales.[10,11] Depression is also more common in obese persons than it is in the general population.[12] At the Massachusetts General Hospital (MGH), the psychiatric consultant called to see a medical patient makes a diagnosis of MDD in approximately 20% of cases, making MDD among the most common problems seen for diagnostic evaluation and treatment. The prevalence of chronic medical conditions in depressed patients is higher regardless of the medical context of recruitment, with an overall rate ranging from 65% to 71% of patients.[13] Several studies indicate that depression significantly influences the course of concomitant medical diseases. In general, the more severe the illness, the more likely depression is to complicate it.[14] Some degree of depression in patients hospitalized for CAD is associated with an increased risk of mortality, and also with continuing depression for at least the first year after hospitalization.[9] Proceeding to cardiac surgery while suffering from MDD, for example, is known to increase the chance of a fatal outcome.[15] Depression in the first 24 hours after myocardial infarction (MI) was associated with a significantly increased risk of early death, re-infarction, or cardiac arrest.[16] Even in depressed outpatients, the risk of mortality, chiefly as a result of cardiovascular disease, is more than doubled.[17] The increased risk of cardiac mortality has also been confirmed in a large community cohort of individuals with cardiac disease who presented with either MDD or minor depression.[18] Those subjects without cardiac disease but with depression also had a higher risk (from 1.5- to 3.9-fold) of cardiac mortality.[18]

In patients with type 1 or 2 diabetes, depression was associated with a significantly higher risk of DM-specific complications (e.g., retinopathy, nephropathy, neuropathy, macrovascular complications, and sexual dysfunction).[19] Data from the Hispanic Established Population for the Epidemiologic Study of the Elderly indicated that death rates in this population were substantially higher when a high level of depressive symptoms was co-morbid with DM (odds ratio, OR 3.84).[20] Depression symptom severity is also associated with poor diet and with poor medication adherence, functional impairment, and higher healthcare costs in primary care patients with DM.[21]

In acutely ill hospitalized older persons, the health status of patients with more symptoms of depression is more likely to deteriorate and less likely to improve during and after hospitalization.[22] Under-recognition and under-treatment of depression in the elderly have been associated in primary care with increased medical utilization.[23] Among the elderly (age ≥65 years), a significant correlation exists between depression and the risk of recurrent falls, with an OR of 3.9 when four or more depressive symptoms are present. These data are of particular importance because falls in the elderly are a well-recognized public health problem.[24]

Patients with cancer and co-morbid depression are at higher risk for mortality[25] and for longer hospital stays. Unfortunately, despite the impact of depression on overall morbidity, functional impairment, and mortality, a significant proportion of those with depression (43%) fail to seek treatment for their depressive symptoms.[26]

Failure to treat depression leaves the patient at risk for further complications and death. There is a clinical sense, moreover, that any seriously ill person who has neurovegetative symptoms, and who has given up and wishes that he or she were dead, is going to do worse than if he or she had hope and motivation. MDD, even if the patient is healthy in every other way, requires treatment. When a seriously ill person becomes depressed, the failure to recognize and to treat the disorder is even more unfortunate.

Prompt and effective treatment of medical co-morbidity is equally important for the outcome of depression. In a study of patients with DM, the severity of depression during follow-up was related to the presence of neuropathy at study entry, and to incomplete remission during the initial treatment trial.[27] By the 10th year of insulin-dependent DM, roughly 48% of a sample of young diabetics developed at least one psychiatric disorder, with MDD being the most prevalent (28%).[28] In addition to DM, other medical and neurologic conditions have been associated with an increased risk for MDD. For example, Fava and colleagues'[29] review showed that MDD is a life-threatening complication of Cushing's syndrome, Addison's disease, hyperthyroidism, hypothyroidism, and hyperprolactinemic amenorrhea, and that treatment that primarily addresses the physical condition may be more effective than antidepressant drugs for such organic affective syndromes. A study of computerized record systems of a large staff-model health maintenance organization showed that patients diagnosed as being depressed had significantly higher annual health care costs and higher costs for every category of care (e.g., primary care, medical specialty care, medical inpatient care, and pharmacy and laboratory costs) than patients without depression.[30] Depressive disorders are likely to cause more disability than are most other chronic diseases (e.g., osteoarthritis, DM), with a possible exception being MI.[31]

MAKING THE DIAGNOSIS OF DEPRESSION

The criteria for MDD according to the *Diagnostic and Statistical Manual of Mental Disorders*, 5th edition (DSM-5)[32] should be applied to the patient with medical illness in the same way as to a patient without medical illness. The DSM-5 has a category for mood disorders "due to" another medical condition. A stroke in the left hemisphere, for example, is commonly followed by a syndrome clinically indistinguishable from MDD. It can now be referred to as a "major depression-like" condition when full criteria are met. Our recommendation is to diagnose a mood disorder using the DSM-5 criteria. A depressive disorder that does not meet full-threshold due to its duration or to the number of symptoms that cause clinically significant distress or impairment can now be diagnosed as an "Other Specified Depressive Disorder" in the DSM-5, which is often referred to as minor depression—a distinction that is important in the medically ill.

The DSM-5 classification of MDD involves clear-cut changes in affect, cognition, and neurovegetative functions. The common feature of MDD is the presence of depressed mood and/or a loss of interest/pleasure, which is accompanied by somatic and cognitive changes that significantly affect the individual's ability to function.

Diagnosis is crucial to treatment. Three questions face the consultant at the outset: (1) Does the patient manifest depression? (2) If so, is there an organic cause, such as use of a medication that can be eliminated, treated, or reversed? (3) Does it arise from the medical condition (e.g., Cushing's disease), and treatment of that condition will alleviate it, or must it be treated itself (e.g., post-stroke depression; PSD)?

Major Depression

Depression is a term used by most to describe even minor and transient mood fluctuations. It is seen everywhere and is often thought to be normal; therefore, it is likely to be dismissed even when it is serious. This applies all the more to a patient with serious medical illness: If a man has terminal cancer and meets the full criteria for MDD, this mood state is regarded by some as "appropriate." Depression is used here to denote the disorder of MDD—a seriously disabling condition for the patient, capable of endangering the patient's life; it is not just an emotional reaction of sadness or despondency. If, while recovering from an acute stroke, a patient has a severe exacerbation of psoriasis, no one says that the cutaneous eruption is appropriate, even though the stress associated with the stroke has almost certainly caused it. Moreover, caregivers are swift to treat the exacerbation. When a patient with a history of MDD lapses into severe depression 1 month after beginning radiation therapy for an inoperable lung cancer, some may see a connection to the prior depressive illness and hasten to treat it. Far more common is the conclusion that anyone with that condition would be depressed. The majority of terminally ill cancer patients do not develop MDD no matter how despondent they feel. If a patient is hemorrhaging from a ruptured spleen, has lost a great deal of blood, becomes hypotensive, and goes into shock, no one calls this appropriate. Like shock, depression is a dread complication of medical illness that requires swift diagnosis and treatment.

Two assumptions are made here: (1) A depressive syndrome in a medically ill patient shares the pathophysiology of a (primary) major affective disorder, and (2) proper diagnosis is made by applying the same criteria. Patients who suffer from unipolar depressive disorders typically present with a constellation of psychological and cognitive (Table 9-1), behavioral (Table 9-2), and physical and somatic (Table 9-3) symptoms. Because far less epidemiologic information is available on depression in the medically ill, the requirement that the dysphoria be present for 2 weeks or longer should be regarded as only a rough approximation in the medically ill. According to the DSM-5,[32] at least five of the following nine symptoms should be present most of the day, nearly every day, and should include either depressed mood or loss of interest or pleasure:

1. Depressed mood, subjective or observed
2. Markedly diminished interest or pleasure in all, or almost all activities
3. Significant (more than 5% of body weight per month) weight loss or gain

TABLE 9-1 Unipolar Depressive Disorders: Common Psychological and Cognitive Symptoms

Depressed mood
Lack of interest or motivation
Inability to enjoy things
Lack of pleasure (anhedonia)
Apathy
Irritability
Anxiety or nervousness
Excessive worrying
Reduced concentration or attention
Memory difficulties
Indecisiveness
Reduced libido
Hypersensitivity to rejection or criticism
Reward dependency
Perfectionism
Obsessiveness
Ruminations
Excessive guilt
Pessimism
Hopelessness
Feelings of helplessness
Cognitive distortions (e.g., "I am unlovable")
Preoccupation with oneself
Hypochondriacal concerns
Low or reduced self-esteem
Feelings of worthlessness
Thoughts of death or suicide
Thoughts of hurting other people

TABLE 9-2 Unipolar Depressive Disorders: Common Behavioral Symptoms

Crying spells
Interpersonal friction or confrontation
Anger attacks or outbursts
Avoidance of anxiety-provoking situations
Social withdrawal
Avoidance of emotional and sexual intimacy
Reduced leisure-time activities
Development of rituals or compulsions
Compulsive eating
Compulsive use of the internet or video games
Workaholic behaviors
Substance use or abuse
Intensification of personality traits or pathologic behaviors
Excessive reliance or dependence on others
Excessive self-sacrifice or victimization
Reduced productivity
Self-cutting or mutilation
Suicide attempts or gestures
Violent or assaultive behaviors

4. Insomnia or hypersomnia
5. Psychomotor agitation or retardation that is observable by others
6. Fatigue or loss of energy
7. Feelings of worthlessness or excessive or inappropriate guilt (which may be delusional), not merely about being sick

TABLE 9-3 Unipolar Depressive Disorders: Common Physical and Somatic Symptoms

Fatigue
Leaden feelings in arms or legs
Difficulty falling asleep (early insomnia)
Difficulty staying asleep (middle insomnia)
Waking up early in the morning (late insomnia)
Sleeping too much (hypersomnia)
Frequent naps
Decreased appetite
Weight loss
Increased appetite
Weight gain
Sexual arousal difficulties
Erectile dysfunction
Delayed orgasm or inability to achieve orgasm
Pains and aches
Back pain
Musculoskeletal complaints
Chest pain
Headaches
Muscle tension
Gastrointestinal upset
Heart palpitations
Burning or tingling sensations
Paresthesias

8. Diminished ability to think or concentrate, or indecisiveness
9. Recurrent thoughts of death (not just a fear of dying), recurrent suicidal ideation without a plan, or a suicide attempt or a specific plan for committing suicide.

Two questions (does the patient suffer from depressed mood? is there diminished interest or pleasure?) have a high sensitivity (about 95%), but unfortunately a low specificity (57%), for diagnosing MDD. Consequently, posing these two questions can be useful as a first approach to the patient who presents with risk factors for depression. However, further inquiry is required to establish the diagnosis. Although depressive disorders are frequently associated with medical illnesses, the DSM-5 considers that potential medical illnesses underlying depressive symptoms should be excluded before making the diagnosis of MDD. This hierarchical approach is typically ignored by clinicians, who tend to make the diagnosis of MDD even in the presence of comorbid medical conditions that may be etiologically related to the condition itself. Nevertheless, the issue of differential diagnosis with medical diseases still exists, as patients may present with transient demoralization as a result of their physical illness or of fatigue or other cognitive and neurovegetative symptoms (but not fulfilling the criteria for MDD or even minor depression). For instance, weight loss and fatigue may also be associated with a variety of disorders (e.g., DM, cancer, thyroid disease). The medical and psychiatric history, together with the physical examination, should guide any further diagnostic work-up.

The aforementioned DSM-5 symptoms may at first seem invalid in the medically ill. If the patient has advanced cancer, how can one attribute anorexia or fatigue to something other than the malignant disease itself? Four of the nine diagnostic symptoms could be viewed as impossible to ascribe exclusively to depression in a medically ill patient: sleep difficulty, anorexia, fatigue or energy loss, and difficulty concentrating. Endicott[33] developed a list of symptoms that the clinician can substitute for, and count in place of, these four: fearful or depressed appearance; social withdrawal or decreased talkativeness; brooding, self-pity, or pessimism; and mood that is not reactive (i.e., the patient cannot be cheered up, does not smile, or does not react positively to good news). Although this method is effective, Chochinov and colleagues[34] compared diagnostic outcomes using both the regular (Research Diagnostic Criteria) and the substituted criteria in a group of medically ill patients. If one held the first two symptoms to the strict levels—that is, depressed mood must be present most of the day, nearly every day, and loss of interest applies to almost everything—the outcome for both diagnostic methods yielded exactly the same number of patients with the diagnosis of MDD.

The first help comes from discovery of symptoms that are more clearly the result of MDD, such as the presence of self-reproach ("I feel worthless"), the wish to be dead, or psychomotor retardation (few medical illnesses in and of themselves produce psychomotor retardation; hypothyroidism and Parkinson's disease are two of them). Insomnia or hypersomnia can also be helpful in the diagnosis, although the patient may have so much pain, dyspnea, or frequent clinical crises that sleep is impaired by these events. The ability to think or concentrate, as with the other symptoms, needs to be specifically asked about in every case.

CASE 1

Mr. H, a 24-year-old graduate student without a psychiatric history reported some unusual aches during his annual physical. After a full work-up, it was determined that his A_{1C} was high, and upon fasting blood work, his blood sugar level was above diabetic levels (126 mg/dL) and he was thought to have type 2 diabetes (DM). His physician provided him with instructions to manage his newly diagnosed condition, including eating healthy, exercising, and monitoring serum glucose, and requested that he return to the office in 3 months.

Upon his return, Mr. H reported being unable to follow the doctor's instructions, and indeed his blood sugar levels remained above the targeted threshold. Mr. H also described being shocked by the news and feeling as though there was no hope. He also reported feeling tired all the time, sleeping poorly, and that he was concentrating poorly in classes. Due to these new symptoms, his physician requested a consultation to determine whether Mr. H was also struggling with depression, which might have been impacting his adherence to her instructions.

The consultant interviewed Mr. H and reviewed his medical records and medications. He was able to rule-out that his mood change was due to medication. Although the consultant was aware of normative reactions to a new diagnosis, he considered whether Mr. H's presenting concerns were a result of DM or co-occurring MDD. Mr. H already presented with sleep, concentration, and energy difficulties. Upon further questioning, Mr. H also reported considerable guilt over his present condition, stating "this is my fault" and described feelings of hopelessness and pessimism. He also described spending more time watching television alone and socializing less; he also found that the exercise and diet plan that his doctor suggested was too hard.

The consultant determined that Mr. H met criteria for MDD. His decision was based on the criteria of having five of nine MDD symptoms that were present most of the day, nearly every day. These also represented a change after his diagnosis and significant functional impairment. Of note, although some symptoms may be ascribed to DM, these symptoms would have also presented prior to his diagnosis. In addition, the presence of low self-esteem, guilt, hopelessness and apathy were more clearly a result of MDD. He conveyed these results to Mr. H's primary care physician and recommended starting adjunctive treatment for MDD.

Unfortunately, to some, a request for psychiatric consultation is tantamount to saying that physical symptoms are only "in your head" or are the result of malingering. Instead, depression is as much a somatic as a psychic disorder. The somatic manifestations of depression (e.g., insomnia, restlessness, anhedonia) may even be construed as proof to a patient that they have no "psychic" illness. "No, doctor, no way am I depressed; if I could just get rid of this pain, everything would be fine." Persistence and aggressive questioning are required to elicit the presence or absence of the nine symptoms.

If the history establishes six of nine symptoms, the consultant may not be certain that three of them have anything to do with depression but may just as likely stem from a co-morbid medical illness. If the patient was found to be hypothyroid, the treatment of choice would not be antidepressants but judicious thyroid replacement. Usually, however, everything is being done for the patient to alleviate the symptoms of the primary illness. If this appears to be the case, our recommendation is to make the diagnosis of MDD and proceed with treatment.

States Commonly Mislabeled as Depression

Up to one-third of patients referred for depression have, on clinical examination, neither MDD nor minor depression. By far the most common diagnosis found among these mislabeled referrals at the MGH has been an organic mental syndrome. A quietly confused patient may look depressed. The patient with dementia or with a frontal lobe syndrome caused by brain injury can lack spontaneity and appear depressed. Fortunately, the physical and mental status examinations frequently reveal the tell-tale abnormalities. Another unrecognized state, sometimes called "depression" by the consultee and easier for the psychiatrist to recognize, is anger. The patient's physician, realizing that the patient has been through a long and difficult illness, may perceive reduction in speech, smiling, and small talk on the patient's part as depression. The patient may thoroughly resent the illness, be irritated by therapeutic routines, and be fed up with the hospital environment but, despite interior smoldering rage, may remain reluctant to discharge wrath in the direction of the physician or nurses.

Excluding Organic Causes of Depression

When clinical findings confirm that the patient's symptoms are fully consistent with MDD, the consultant must still create a differential diagnosis of this syndrome. Could the same constellation of symptoms be caused by a medical illness or its treatment? Should the patient's symptoms be caused by an as yet undiagnosed illness, the last physician with the chance of detecting it is the consultant. Differential diagnosis in this situation is qualitatively the same as that described for considering causes of delirium (see Chapter 10). With depression, although the same process should be completed, certain conditions more commonly produce depressive syndromes and are worthy of comment.

Review of the medications that the patient is taking generally tells the consultant whether the patient is receiving something that might alter mood. Ordinarily, one would like to establish a relationship between the onset of depressive symptoms and either the start of, or a change in, a medication. If such a connection can be established, the simplest course is to stop the agent and monitor the patient for improvement. When the patient requires continued treatment, as for hypertension, the presumed offending agent can be changed, with the hope that the change to another antihypertensive will be followed by resolution of depressive symptoms. When this fails or when clinical judgment warrants no change in medication, it may be necessary to start an antidepressant along with the antihypertensive drug. The literature linking drugs to depression is inconclusive at best. Clinicians have seen depression following use of reserpine and steroids[35] and from withdrawal from cocaine, amphetamine, and alcohol. Despite anecdotal reports, β-blockers do not appear to cause depression. It has been suggested that depression in some cases appears as a reaction to subclinical cardiovascular symptoms,[36] so the differential diagnosis should also take into account medical conditions. The most common central nervous system (CNS) side effect of a drug is confusion or delirium, and this is commonly mislabeled as depression because a mental status examination has not been conducted.

Abnormal laboratory values should not be overlooked, because they may provide the clues to an undiagnosed abnormality responsible for the depressive symptoms. Laboratory values necessary for the routine differential diagnosis in psychiatric consultation should be reviewed. A work-up is not complete if the evaluation of thyroid and parathyroid function is not included. MDD is never "appropriate" (e.g., "This man has inoperable lung cancer metastatic to his brain and is depressed, which is appropriate"). MDD is a common and dread complication of many medical illnesses as they become more severe. To call it anything else is to endanger the patient and neglect one of the worst forms of human suffering. The disability associated with depressive illness is seldom recognized, yet it and mental illness in general show a stronger association with disability than with severe physical diseases.[37] In general, the more serious the illness, the more likely the patient is to succumb to a depressive episode. Careful studies have found a high incidence of MDD in hospitalized medical patients.[14] For more than 50 years, carcinoma of the pancreas has been associated with psychiatric symptoms, especially depression, which in some cases seems to be the first manifestation of the disease.[38] Two carefully controlled studies have shown these patients to have significantly more psychiatric symptoms and major depression than patients with other malignancies of gastrointestinal origin, leading some to suspect that depression in this case is a manifestation of a paraneoplastic syndrome.[38,39]

Stroke

Direct injury to the brain can produce changes of affect that progress to a full syndrome of MDD. Morris and co-workers[40] have intensively studied mood disorders that result from strokes. Left-hemisphere lesions involving the prefrontal cortex or basal ganglia are the most likely to be associated with post-stroke depression (PSD) and to meet criteria for MDD or dysthymia.[40] Depressive symptoms appear in the immediate post-stroke period in about two-thirds of patients, with the rest manifesting depression by the 6th month. Additional risk factors for developing MDD were a prior stroke, pre-existing subcortical atrophy, and a family or personal history of an affective disorder. Aphasia did not appear to cause depression, but non-fluent aphasia was associated with depression; both seemed to result from lesions of the left frontal lobe. Although the severity of functional impairment at the time of acute injury did not correlate with the severity of depression, depression appeared to retard recovery. Among patients with left-hemispheric damage, those who were depressed showed significantly worse cognitive performance, which was seen in tasks that assessed temporal orientation, frontal lobe function, and executive motor function. Successful treatment of PSD has been demonstrated by double-blinded studies with nortriptyline[41] and trazodone[42] and been reported with electroconvulsive therapy (ECT)[43] and use of psychostimulants.[44] In fact, one study has shown that nortriptyline was more effective than fluoxetine in treating depressive symptoms in patients with PSD.[45] Early and aggressive treatment of PSD is required to minimize the cognitive and performance deficits that this mood disorder inflicts on patients during the recovery period.

Right-hemisphere lesions deserve special attention. When the lesion was in the right anterior location, the mood disorder tended to be an apathetic, indifferent, state associated with "inappropriate cheerfulness." However, such patients seldom look cheerful and may have complaints of loss of interest, or even worrying. This disorder was found in 6 of 20 patients with solitary right-hemisphere strokes (and in none of 28 patients with single left-hemisphere lesions).

Prosody is also a problem for those with a right hemisphere injury. Ross and Rush[46] focused on the presentation of aprosodia (lack of prosody or inflection, rhythm, and intensity of expression) when the right hemisphere is damaged. A patient with such a lesion could appear quite depressed and be labeled as having depression by staff and family but simply lacks the neuronal capacity to express or recognize emotion. If one stations oneself out of the patient's view, selects a neutral sentence (e.g., "The book is red"), asks the patient to identify the mood as mad, sad, frightened, or elated, and then declaims the sentence with the emotion to be tested, one should be able to identify those patients with a receptive aprosodia. Next, the patient is asked to deliver the same sentence with a series of different emotional tones to test for the presence of an expressive aprosodia. Stroke patients can suffer from both aprosodia and depression, but separate diagnostic criteria and clinical examinations exist for each one.

Dementia

Primary dementia, even of the Alzheimer's type, increases the vulnerability of the patients to suffering MDD, even though the incidence is not as high as it is in multi-infarct or vascular dementia. The careful post-mortem studies of Zubenko and colleagues[47] supported the hypothesis that the pathophysiology of secondary depression is consistent with theories of those for primary depression. Compared with demented patients without depression, demented patients with MDD showed a 10- to 20-fold reduction in cortical norepinephrine levels.

Multi-infarct or vascular dementia so commonly includes depression as a symptom that Hachinski and associates[48] included it in the Ischemia Scale. Cummings and co-workers[49] compared 15 patients with multi-infarct dementia with 30 patients with Alzheimer's disease and found that depressive symptoms (60% vs 17%) and episodes of MDD (4/15 vs 0/30) were more frequent in patients with the former.

Subcortical Dementias

Patients with Parkinson's disease and Huntington's disease commonly manifest MDD. In fact, Huntington's disease may present as MDD before the onset of either chorea or dementia.[50] The diagnosis is made clinically. Some have noted that as depression in the Parkinson's patient is treated, parkinsonian symptoms also improve, even before the depressive symptoms have subsided. This is especially striking when ECT is used,[51] although the same improvement has been reported after use of tricyclic antidepressants (TCAs). Treatment of MDD in either disease may increase the comfort of the patient and is always worth a try. Because Huntington's patients may be sensitive to the anticholinergic side effects of TCAs, anticholinergic agents should be tried first.

Because HIV-1 is neurotropic, even asymptomatic HIV-seropositive individuals, when compared with seronegative controls, demonstrate a high incidence of electroencephalographic abnormalities (67% vs 10%) and more abnormalities on neuropsychological testing.[52] The unusually high life-time and current rates of mood disorders in HIV-seronegative individuals at risk for AIDS[53] demands an exceedingly high vigilance for their appearance in HIV-positive persons. Depression, mania, or psychosis can appear with AIDS encephalopathy, but the early, subtler signs (e.g., impaired concentration, complaints of poor memory, blunting of interests, lethargy) may respond dramatically to antidepressants, such as psychostimulants.[54] The selective serotonin re-uptake inhibitors (SSRIs) (such as sertraline, fluoxetine, and paroxetine) have also been effective in the treatment of depression in HIV-positive patients.[55] A small open trial also supports the use of bupropion in these patients.[56]

We recommend that pharmacologic treatment be considered seriously whenever a patient meets criteria for either minor depression or MDD.

CHOICE OF AN APPROPRIATE ANTIDEPRESSANT TREATMENT

The properties, side effects, dosages, and drug interactions of antidepressant medications are discussed elsewhere in this volume. Whenever MDD is diagnosed, the effort to alleviate symptoms almost always includes somatic treatments. The consultant who understands the interactions among antidepressants, illnesses, and non-psychotropic drugs is best prepared to prescribe these agents effectively. ECT remains the single most effective somatic treatment of depression. A nationwide review has only sustained its merit.

Prescribing Antidepressants for the Medically Ill

Ever since sudden death in cardiac patients was first associated with amitriptyline,[57,58] physicians have tended to fear the use of TCAs when cardiac disease is present. However, depression itself is a life-threatening disease, and it should be treated. Choice of an agent often begins with the knowledge that a patient is especially troubled by insomnia; however, in patients with certain medical illnesses, the decision must be made on a case-by-case basis, taking into consideration the side effect profile (risk), the anticipated benefits, and potential drug–drug interactions. In obese diabetic patients, fluoxetine has ameliorated mean blood glucose levels, daily insulin requirements, and glycohemoglobin levels,[59] perhaps by improving insulin sensitivity.[60] In contrast, TCAs, such as nortriptyline, may actually worsen glycemic control.[61] However, TCAs have been found to be superior to fluoxetine in decreasing pain secondary to diabetic neuropathy.[62]

One could also make a similar argument for patients with hypercholesterolemia, because the SSRI fluvoxamine has decreased serum cholesterol levels,[63] whereas TCAs appear to increase cholesterol levels.[64]

With respect to making a decision based on insomnia, the sedative potency of the available antidepressants can generally be predicted by their *in vitro* affinity for the histamine H_1 receptor. Table 9-4 shows these values.[65] The antihistaminic property of these drugs gives a reasonably good estimate of their sedative properties. Trazodone, which has low affinity for the H_1 receptor, is, however, a sedating agent.

This same property can also be used to predict how much weight gain may be associated with use of the antidepressant. Patients troubled by obesity may be placed at additional risk if treated with those agents higher on the list. For the most part, the SSRIs, bupropion, nefazodone, trazodone, and venlafaxine have negligible antihistaminic potency. The monoamine oxidase inhibitors (MAOIs) generally have low sedative potency, although phenelzine sulfate can produce complaints of drowsiness. Mirtazapine,[66] a powerful antagonist of the H_1 receptor, is quite sedating and can be associated with significant weight gain.

All antidepressants in the cyclic, SSRI, and MAOI categories usually correct sleep disturbances (insomnia or hypersomnia) when these are symptoms of depression, a therapeutic effect not thought to be related to their effects on brain histamine. Therefore, this discussion highlights a

TABLE 9-4 Relationship of Antidepressants to Neurotransmitter Receptors

ANTIDEPRESSANT	EFFECT ON BIOGENIC AMINE UPTAKE: POTENCY[a]		SELECTIVITY FOR BLOCKING UPTAKE OF 5-HT OVER NE	AFFINITIES[b] FOR NEUROTRANSMITTER RECEPTORS							
				HISTAMINE		*ADRENERGIC*		*SEROTONIN*		*MUSCARINIC*	*DOPAMINE*
	5-HT	*NE*		H_1	H_2	α_1	α_2	S_1	S_2	*ACh*	D_2
Doxepin	0.36	5.3	0.068	420	0.6	4.2	0.091	0.34	4.0	1.2	0.042
Amitriptyline	1.5	4.2	0.36	91	2.2	3.7	0.11	0.53	3.4	5.5	0.10
Imipramine	2.4	7.7	0.31	9.1	0.4	1.1	0.031	0.011	1.2	1.1	0.050
Clomipramine	18	3.6	5.2	3.2	–	2.6	0.031	0.014	3.7	2.7	0.53
Trimipramine	0.040	0.20	0.2	370	33.3	4.2	0.15	0.012	3.1	1.7	0.56
Protriptyline	0.36	100	0.0035	4	0.05	0.77	0.015	0.011	1.5	4.0	0.043
Nortriptyline	0.38	25	0.015	10	0.12	1.7	0.040	0.32	2.3	0.67	0.083
Desipramine	0.29	110	0.0026	0.91	0.08	0.77	0.014	0.010	0.36	0.50	0.030
Amoxapine	0.21	23	0.0094	4	–	2	0.038	0.46	170.0	0.10	0.62
Maprotiline	0.030	14	0.0022	50	–	1.1	0.011	0.0083	0.83	0.18	0.29
Trazodone	0.53	0.020	26	0.29	–	2.8	0.20	1.7	13.0	0.00031	0.026
Fluoxetine	8.3	0.36	23.0	0.016	–	0.017	0.008	0.0042	0.48	0.050	–
Bupropion	0.0064	0.043	0.15	0.015	–	0.022	0.0012	0.0059	0.0011	0.0021	0.00048
Sertraline	29	0.45	64.0	0.0041	–	0.27	–	–	–	0.16	0.0093
Paroxetine	136.0	3	45.0	0.0045	–	0.029	–	–	–	0.93	0.0031
Fluvoxamine	14.0	0.2	71.0	–	–	–	–	–	–	–	–
Venlafaxine	2.6	0.48	5.4	0	–	0	–	–	–	0	0
Nefazodone	0.73	0.18	4.2	–	–	–	–	–	–	–	–
Mirtazapine	–	–	–	200.00	–	0.2	5	–	0.2	0.040	–
(Dextroamphetamine)[c]	2	–	–	–	–	–	–	–	–	–	–
(Diphenhydramine)[c]	–	–	–	7.1	–	–	–	–	–	–	–
(Phentolamine)[c]	–	–	–	–	–	6.7	–	–	–	–	–
(Yohimbine)[c]	–	–	–	–	–	–	62	–	–	–	–
(Methysergide)[c]	–	–	–	–	–	–	–	–	7.8	–	–
(Atropine)[c]	–	–	–	–	–	–	–	–	–	42	–
(Haloperidol)[c]	–	–	–	–	–	–	–	–	–	–	23

[a] $10^7 \times I/K_i$, where K_i = inhibitor constant in molarity.

[b] $10^7 \times I/K_d$, where K_d = equilibrium dissociation constant in molarity.

[c] Drugs in parentheses are not antidepressants.

ACh, acetylcholine; 5-HT, serotonin; NE, norepinephrine.

Adapted from Richelson E: Pharmacology of antidepressants—characteristics of the ideal drug, *Mayo Clin Proc* 69: 1069–1081, 1994.

sedative effect of the drugs that occurs in addition to, and independent of, these agents' ability to correct the specific sleep disturbances of MDD (e.g., to lengthen rapid-eye-movement sleep latency).

Occasionally, the consultant may encounter a patient in whom antihistamines have been tried and have failed to achieve a therapeutic effect, such as in the treatment of an urticarial rash or the itching associated with uremia. Doxepin hydrochloride, possibly the most potent antihistamine in clinical medicine, has demonstrated superiority with a 10-mg dose when compared with 25 mg of diphenhydramine hydrochloride.[67]

Threatening the successful use of antidepressants is the presence of unwanted side effects. The three groups of side effects that are particularly relevant for the treatment of depression in the acute medical setting are orthostatic hypotension (OH), anticholinergic effects, and cardiac conduction effects. The clinical ratings for these three side-effect groups with current antidepressants are presented in Table 9-5. We will discuss side effects specific to each antidepressant class, and side effects associated with abrupt discontinuation of antidepressant treatment. When these side effects are understood, safe clinical prescription of antidepressant drugs is far more likely.

Orthostatic Hypotension

Orthostatic hypotension (OH) is not directly related to each drug's *in vitro* affinity for the α_1-noradrenergic receptor. Table 9-5 presents the drugs with a clinical rating of their likelihood of causing an orthostatic drop in blood pressure (BP). In general, among the TCAs, tertiary amine agents are more likely to cause an orthostatic fall in BP than are secondary amines. For reasons that are not clearly understood, imipramine, amitriptyline, and desipramine are the TCAs most commonly associated with clinical mishaps, such as falls and fractures. The orthostatic effect appears earlier than the therapeutic effect for imipramine and is objectively verifiable at less than half the therapeutic plasma level. Hence, the drug may have to be discontinued long before a therapeutic plasma level is reached. Once postural symptoms develop, increasing the dosage of the antidepressant may not make the symptoms worse.

Paradoxically, a pre-treatment fall of more than 10 mmHg in orthostatic BP actually predicts a good response to antidepressant medication in older adult depressed patients.[68,69] Naturally, younger patients may tolerate a fall in BP more easily than older patients, so an orthostatic fall in BP may not produce symptoms serious enough to require discontinuation of the drug. The presence of cardiovascular disease increases the likelihood of OH. When patients with no cardiac disease take imipramine, the incidence of significant OH is 7%. With conduction disease, such as a bundle-branch block (BBB), the incidence rises to 33%, and with congestive heart failure (CHF), it reaches 50%.[70] Of the traditional TCAs, nortriptyline has been shown to be the least likely to cause OH, an extremely valuable factor when depression in cardiac or older adult patients requires treatment.[71] MAOIs cause significant OH with about the same frequency as imipramine (i.e., often). Moreover, the patient starting on an MAOI usually does not experience OH until the medication is having a significant therapeutic effect, roughly 2 to 4 weeks later.

Among other agents, trazodone is associated with OH moderately often, as is mirtazapine. Fluoxetine, sertraline, paroxetine, citalopram, fluvoxamine, bupropion, venlafaxine, and psychostimulants are essentially free of this side effect. Bupropion, psychostimulants, and venlafaxine may raise systolic BP slightly in some patients. Some have noted that even though the objective fall in standing BP continues for several months, some patients with initial symptoms accommodate subjectively and no longer complain of the side effect.

Anticholinergic Effects

The anticholinergic effects of TCAs are a nuisance for many patients. Urinary retention, constipation, dry mouth, confusional states, and tachycardia are the most common. The increase in heart rate is usually manifested as a sinus tachycardia that results from muscarinic blockade of vagal tone on the heart. As many as 30% of normal individuals respond to amitriptyline with tachycardia.[72] This side effect correlates nicely with the *in vitro* affinity of each drug for the acetylcholine muscarinic receptor (see Table 9-4). As seen in the table, amitriptyline is the most anticholinergic of the antidepressants, with protriptyline a close second. These two agents regularly cause tachycardia in the medically ill, and one should monitor the heart rate as the dosage is increased. If significant tachycardia results, another agent may have to be used. Many hospitalized patients, particularly those with ischemic heart disease, are already being treated with β-blockers, such as propranolol. When this is the case, the β-blocker usually protects the patient from developing a significant tachycardia.

All of the cyclic agents except trazodone are anticholinergic. If one switches from, for example, imipramine to desipramine because the patient developed urinary retention, the patient is quite likely to develop urinary retention again on desipramine. Amoxapine and maprotiline are not significantly less anticholinergic than desipramine. Trazodone is almost devoid of activity at the muscarinic receptor, and it is a reasonable choice when another agent has caused unwanted anticholinergic side effects.

Fluoxetine, bupropion, venlafaxine, and the MAOIs exert minimal activity at the acetylcholine muscarinic receptor; hence, they can also be useful alternatives when these side effects impair a patient's access to an antidepressant. There is laboratory evidence (see Table 9-4) with anecdotal clinical support that paroxetine is more anticholinergic, close in *in vitro* potency to imipramine. Similarly, in Richelson's[65] laboratory, sertraline and maprotiline appear to have quite similar anticholinergic effects. For maprotiline, this effect is clinically noticeable (e.g., dry mouth) but usually mild. Similar mild effects seem to accompany the use of mirtazapine. Effects of fluvoxamine and nefazodone are generally mild.

Cardiac Conduction Effects

All TCAs appear to prolong ventricular depolarization. This tends to produce a lengthening of the P-R and QRS intervals as well as of the Q-T interval corrected for heart rate (QTc) on the electrocardiogram (ECG). When the main effect of these agents is measured by His-bundle electrocardiography, the His-ventricular portion of the recording is preferentially prolonged. That is, these drugs, which are sodium-channel blockers, tend to slow the electric impulse as it passes through the specialized conduction tissue known as the His-Purkinje

TABLE 9-5 Characteristics of Antidepressant Drugs

	ELIMINATION HALF-LIFE (h)	SEDATIVE POTENCY	ANTICHOLINERGIC POTENCY	ORTHOSTATIC HYPOTENSION	CARDIAC ARRHYTHMIA POTENTIAL	TARGET DOSAGE (mg/day)	DOSAGE RANGE (mg/day)
Tricyclics							
Doxepin	17	High	Moderate	High	Yes	200	75–400
Amitriptyline	21	High	Highest	High	Yes	150	75–300
Imipramine	28	Moderate	Moderate	High	Yes	200	75–400
Trimipramine	13	High	Moderate	High	Yes	150	75–300
Clomipramine	23	High	High	High	Yes	150	75–300
Protriptyline	78	Low	High	Moderate	Yes	30	15–60
Nortriptyline	36	Moderate	Moderate	Moderate	Yes	100	40–150
Desipramine	21	Low	Moderate	Moderate	Yes	150	75–300
Others							
Citalopram	33	Low	Low	Low	Low	20	20–80
Escitalopram	22	Low	Low	Low	Low	10	10–20
Maprotiline	43	High	Moderate	Moderate	Yes	150	75–300
Trazodone	3.5	High	Lowest	Moderate	Yes	150	50–600
Fluoxetine	87	Low	Low	Lowest	Low	20	40–80
Sertraline	26	Low	Low	Lowest	Low	50	50–200
Paroxetine	21	Low	Low–moderate	Lowest	Low	20	20–60
Fluvoxamine	19	Low	Low	Low	Low	200	50–300
Bupropion	15	Low	Low	Lowest	Low	200	75–300
Venlafaxine	3.6	Low	Low	Low	Low	300	75–375
Desvenlafaxine	10	Low	Low	Low	Low	50	50–400
Duloxetine	12	Low	Low	Low	Low	40	40–120
Nefazodone	3	Moderate	Low	Low	Low	300	300–600
Mirtazapine	30	High	Low	Low	Low	15	15–45
Selegiline (transdermal)	18	Low	Low	Moderate	Low	6	6–12
Monoamine oxidase inhibitors	–	Low	Low	High	Low	–	–

system. This makes them resemble in action the class IA arrhythmic drugs, such as quinidine and procainamide hydrochloride. In practical terms, this means that depressed cardiac patients with ventricular premature contractions, when started on an antidepressant, such as imipramine, are likely to experience improvement or resolution of their ventricular irritability, even if the abnormality is as serious as inducible ventricular tachycardia. Both imipramine and nortriptyline have proved efficacy as antiarrhythmics and share the advantage of a half-life long enough to permit twice-daily doses.[73–75]

Ordinarily, this property does not pose a problem for the cardiac patient who does not already have disease in the conduction system. The patient who already has conduction system disease is the focus of concern. First-degree heart block is the mildest pathologic form and probably should not pose a problem for antidepressant treatment. When the patient's abnormality exceeds this (e.g., right BBB, left BBB, bifascicular block, BBB with a prolonged P-R interval, alternating BBB, or second- or third-degree atrioventricular, AV, block), extreme caution is necessary in treating the depression. Cardiology consultation is almost always already present for the patient. Electrolyte abnormalities, particularly hypokalemia or hypomagnesemia, increase the danger to these patients, and they require careful monitoring.

Occasionally, the question arises clinically whether one of the cyclic agents is less likely than another to cause a quinidine-like prolongation in conduction, particularly when the patient already shows some intraventricular conduction delay. Maprotiline should be regarded as similar to the TCAs in its effects on cardiac conduction. Amoxapine has been touted to have fewer cardiac side effects, based on patients who had taken overdoses. Although these patients were noted to have suffered seizures, coma, and acute renal failure, the authors thought it worth noting that less cardiac toxicity resulted,[76,77] but atrial flutter and fibrillation have been reported in patients taking amoxapine.[78,79] Trazodone does not prolong conduction in the His-Purkinje system, but aggravation of the pre-existing ventricular irritability has been reported.[80] Hence, clinical caution cannot be abandoned.

MAOIs are remarkably free of arrhythmogenic effects, although there are several case reports of atrial flutter or fibrillation, or both, with tranylcypromine. Consultees tend to dread them, fearing drug and food interactions.

How, then, should the consultant approach the depressed patient with conduction disease? Depression can itself be life-threatening and more damaging to cardiac function than a drug. Therefore, it must be treated. In the case of a depressed patient with cardiac conduction problems, one can begin with an SSRI, bupropion, venlafaxine, nefazodone, or mirtazapine. Should the depression not remit completely, reasonable options include augmentation with a psychostimulant or switching to a psychostimulant. Should the patient improve, the stimulant can be continued as long as it is helpful. By starting with a low dosage (2.5 mg of either dextroamphetamine or methylphenidate), one is reasonably assured that toxicity will not result. The fragile patient can have heart rate and BP monitored hourly for 4 hours after receiving the drug. If no beneficial response is noted, the next day the dosage should be raised to 5 mg (our usual starting dosage), then to 10, 15, and 20 mg on successive days, if necessary. Some response to the stimulant should be seen, even a negative one (e.g., feeling tenser, "wired," or agitated). Of course, an elevation of heart rate or BP may be a reason to stop the trial. The degree of clinical vigilance must match the clinical precariousness of the patient. Discussion of the type and intensity of monitoring takes place with the consultee.

The role of the psychiatric consultant is to recommend aggressive treatment for depression, with the consultee helping to decide what means is appropriate and to detect possible side effects. If the patient's depression fails to remit despite a number of adequate antidepressant trials, an MAOI is reasonable even with an unstable cardiac condition, provided that the patient can tolerate the OH that may result. The adage, "start low, go slow," which is so appropriate in the treatment of older adult patients, is also a good rule for medically unstable patients.

If the depression has left the patient dangerously ill, suicidal, or catatonic, ECT is the treatment of choice. When an antidepressant can be used, monitoring must take into account both the development of a steady state (which typically takes about five half-lives of the drug) and the rate at which the dosage is being increased. When the patient requires a daily dosage increase, a daily rhythm strip may be necessary as well as another one, five half-lives after reaching the level thought to represent the therapeutic dosage. Plasma levels are especially useful when a 4- to 8-week drug trial is judged worthwhile. Reliable levels have been established only for nortriptyline hydrochloride (50 to 150 ng/mL), desipramine hydrochloride (> 125 ng/mL), and imipramine hydrochloride (>200 ng/mL).

Myocardial Depression

Antidepressants have not been shown to impair left ventricular function significantly in depressed or non-depressed patients with either normal or impaired myocardial contractility.[81–84] Even with TCA overdose, impairment of left ventricular function is generally mild.[85] Hence, CHF is not an absolute contraindication to antidepressant therapy.[83–85] The patient with heart failure is far more vulnerable to OH; hence the SSRIs, bupropion, venlafaxine, and nortriptyline, are the preferred agents.

A severely depressed patient could suffer an acute MI. Both conditions are a threat to survival, and the MI is no contraindication to antidepressant treatment. ECT or drugs may be mandatory. Using the previously mentioned principles, psychiatrists and cardiologists must combine their efforts to restore the patient's health.

Other Side Effects (Specific to Each Antidepressant Class)

Other common side effects of bupropion include anxiety and nervousness, agitation, insomnia, headache, nausea, constipation, and tremor. Bupropion is contraindicated in the treatment of patients with a seizure disorder or bulimia, because the incidence of seizures is approximately 0.4% at dosages up to 450 mg/day, and increases almost 10-fold at higher dosages.

Common side effects of venlafaxine include nausea, lack of appetite, weight loss, excessive sweating, nervousness, insomnia, sexual dysfunction, sedation, fatigue, headache, and dizziness.

Mirtazapine's side effects include dry mouth, constipation, weight gain, and dizziness. The relative lack of significant drug–drug interactions with other antidepressants makes mirtazapine a good candidate for combination strategies (i.e., combining two antidepressants together at full dosages).

Trazodone's most common side effects are drowsiness, dizziness, headache, and nausea, with priapism being an extremely rare but potentially serious side effect in men.

Antidepressant Discontinuation Syndrome

Several reports have described discontinuation-emergent adverse events with abrupt cessation of SSRIs and venlafaxine,[86,87] including dizziness, insomnia, nervousness, nausea, and agitation. The likelihood of developing these symptoms may be inversely related to the half-life of the SSRI used, because these symptoms are more likely to develop after abrupt discontinuation of paroxetine and to a lesser degree with sertraline, with few symptoms seen with fluoxetine discontinuation.

Hepatic Metabolism

Essentially all antidepressants are metabolized by the hepatic P450 microsomal enzyme system. The interactions produced by the competition of multiple drugs for these metabolic pathways are complex. For example, mirtazapine is a substrate for, but not an inhibitor of, the 2D6, 1A2, and 3A4 isoenzymes.

How long antidepressants need to be maintained in patients with MDD associated with medical illness is not known. Even though patients with primary affective disorder should be maintained on their antidepressant for more than 6 months, the same requirement is not clear for patients with MDD in the medical setting. In patients with PSD, and possibly in other instances in which primary brain disease or injury appears to cause depression, antidepressants should be continued for 6 months or longer.

Thioridazine

A final caution about cardiovascular toxicity should include discussion of thioridazine. Notorious among neuroleptics for its potential cardiac side effects, this drug should not be used in combination with TCAs unless there is a special need. It, too, possesses quinidine-like properties, has been associated with reports of sudden death that antedate similar reports with TCAs,[88] and has been implicated in the causation of ventricular tachycardia alone[89] and in combination with desipramine.[90] Thioridazine's anticholinergic potency is high (roughly equivalent *in vitro* to that of desipramine), which can be troublesome. This property, however, might make it particularly useful to treat the delirium of a patient with Parkinson's disease. As little as 5 to 10 mg can be helpful in such a patient. Again, it is important to avoid hypokalemia and hypomagnesemia, which predispose patients to cardiac rhythm disturbances.

OTHER DSM-5 DIAGNOSES OF DEPRESSION

Persistent Depressive Disorder (Formerly Dysthymic Disorder)

The DSM-5 consolidated chronic MDD and dysthymic disorder into persistent depressive disorder. For the diagnosis of persistent depressive disorder (diagnosis code 300.40), DSM-5 specifies a chronic state of depression for more than 2 years. To qualify, the patient must have depressed mood for most of the day, on more days than not, and have two or more of the following six symptoms: (1) poor appetite or overeating; (2) insomnia or hypersomnia; (3) low energy or fatigue; (4) low self-esteem; (5) poor concentration or difficulty making decisions; and, (6) feelings of hopelessness.

Adjustment Disorder With Depressed Mood

Adjustment disorder with depressed mood (code 309.00) is probably the most over-used diagnosis by consultation psychiatrists. It should not be given to a medical patient unless the depressive reaction is maladaptive, either in intensity of feeling (an over-reaction) or in function (e.g., when a despondent patient interacts minimally with caregivers and family).

Bereavement

Bereavement (code V62.82) refers to the death of a loved one. In the case of the medical patient, it is the self that is mourned after a narcissistic injury (e.g., an MI). DSM-5 cautions clinicians to consider carefully the normative response to loss versus a depressive episode. They note that a distinguishing feature of grief is the predominant effect of feelings of emptiness and loss, whereas in a major depressive episode (MDE), it is feelings of a persistent depressed mood and the inability to anticipate happiness or pleasure.[32] In acute grief, MDD can be a difficult diagnosis, but, when it is present, it requires treatment (perhaps even more than when it is present without acute grief). Clues helpful to determine the presence of MDD include: (1) guilt beyond that about actions taken around the time of the death of the loved one; (2) thoughts of death (other than wanting to be with the lost person) or feeling one would be better off dead—suicidal ideation should count in favor of MDD; (3) morbid preoccupation with worthlessness; (4) marked psychomotor retardation; (5) prolonged and marked functional impairment; and, (6) hallucinations other than seeing, hearing, or being touched by the deceased person. The symptoms that are the principal components of the complicated grief factor are yearning for, and preoccupation with, thoughts of the deceased, crying, searching for the deceased, disbelief about the death, being stunned by the death, and inability to accept the death.

DESPONDENCY CONSEQUENT TO SERIOUS ILLNESS

Despondency in serious illness appears to be a natural response and is here regarded as the psychic damage done by the disease to the patient's self-esteem. Bibring's[91] definition of depression is "response to narcissistic injury." The response is here called *despondency* and not *depression* because depression is reserved for those conditions that meet the research criteria for primary or secondary affective disorder. In any serious illness, the mind sustains an injury of its own, as though the illness, for example, MI, produces an ego infarction. Even when recovery of the diseased organ is complete, recovery of self-esteem appears to take somewhat longer. In patients who had an MI, for example, although the myocardial scar has fully formed in 5 to 6 weeks, recovery of the sense of psychological well-being seems to require 2 to 3 months.

Management of the Acute Phase of Despondency

A mixture of dread, bitterness, and despair, despondency presents the self as broken, scarred, and ruined. Work and relationships seem jeopardized. Now it seems to the patient too late to realize career or personal aspirations. Disappointment with both what has and what has not been accomplished haunts the individual, who may now feel old and like a failure. Concerns of this kind become conscious early in acute illness, and their expression may prompt consultation requests as early as the second or third day of hospitalization.[92]

Management of these illness-induced despondencies is divided into acute and long-term phases. In the acute phase, the patient is encouraged but never forced to express such concerns. The extent and detail are determined by the individual's need to recount them. Many patients are upset to find such depressive concerns in consciousness and even worry that this signals a "nervous breakdown." It is therefore essential to let patients know that such concerns are the normal emotional counterpart of being sick and that even though there will be ups and downs in their intensity, these concerns will probably disappear gradually as health returns. It is also helpful for the consultant to be familiar with the rehabilitation plans common to various illnesses, so that patients can also be reminded, while still in the acute phase of recovery, that plans for restoring function are being activated.

Self-esteem often falters in seriously ill persons even though they have good recovery potential. Hence, efforts to learn what the sick person is like can help the consultant alleviate the acute distress of a damaged self-image. The consultant should learn any "defining" traits, interests, and accomplishments of the patient so that the nurses and physicians can be informed of them. For example, after learning that a woman patient had been a star sprinter on the national Polish track team preparing for the 1940 Olympics, the consultant relayed this both in the consultation note and by word of mouth to her caregivers. "What's this I hear about your having been a champion sprinter?" became a common question that made her feel not only unique but appreciated. The objective is to restore to life the real person within the patient who has serious organic injuries or impairment.

Few things are more discouraging for the patient, staff, or consultant than no noticeable sign of improvement. Psychological interventions, however, can be helpful. For example, getting a patient with severe CHF out of bed and into a reclining chair (known for 25 years to produce even less cardiovascular strain than the supine position)[93] can provide reassurance and boost confidence. For some patients with severe ventilatory impairments and difficulty weaning from the respirator, a wall chart depicting graphically the time spent off the ventilator each day (one gold star for each 5-minute period) is encouraging. Even if the patient's progress is slow, the chart documents and dramatizes each progressive step. Of course, personal investment in very ill persons may be far more therapeutic in itself than any gimmick, but such simple interventions have a way of focusing new effort and enthusiasm on each improvement.

Management of Post-Acute Despondencies: Planning for Discharge and After

Even when the patients are confident their illness is not fatal, they usually become concerned that it will cripple them. Such psychological "crippling" is a normal hazard of organic injury. Whether the patient had an uncomplicated MI and is still employable, or has chronic emphysema with a carbon dioxide tension of 60 mmHg, only restoration of self-esteem can protect him or her from emotional incapacitation. Even when the body has no room for improvement, the mind can usually be rehabilitated. Arrival home from the hospital often proves to be a vast disappointment. The damage caused by illness has been done, acute treatment is completed, and health professionals are far away. Weak, anxious, and demoralized, the patient experiences a "homecoming depression."[94] Weakness is a universal problem for any individual whose hospitalization required extensive bed rest; in fact, it was the symptom most complained of by one group of post-MI patients visited in their homes.[94] Invariably the individuals attribute this weakness to the damage caused by the disease (e.g., to the heart, lungs, and liver). A large part of this weakness, however, is the result of muscle atrophy and the systemic effects of immobilization.

Fear can be omnipresent after discharge from the hospital. The least bodily sensation, particularly in the location of the affected organ, looms as an ominous sign of the worst recurrence (e.g., MI, malignancy, gastrointestinal bleeding, or perforation), metastatic spread, (another) infection, or some new disaster that will cripple the individual even further. Most of the alarming symptoms felt in the early post-hospital days are so trivial that they would never have been noticed before, but the threshold is far lower now, and patients may find any unusual sensation a threat. When the alarm has passed, they may feel foolish or even disgusted with themselves for being hypochondriacal. It helps to know in advance that such hypersensitivity to bodily sensations commonly occurs, that it is normal, and that it will be time-limited. Although there are wide ranges in the time it takes for this problem to disappear, a well-adjusted patient who had an uncomplicated MI requires from 2 to 6 months for these fears to resolve (far more time than the recovery of the myocardium). With specific measures, this time may be shortened.

Whether the person can improve a physical function such as oxygen consumption (e.g., as after an MI or gastrointestinal bleeding) or cannot do so at all (e.g., after chronic obstructive pulmonary disease), the mental state is basically the same—a sense of imprisonment in a damaged body that is unable to sustain the everyday activities of a reasonable life. The illness has mentally crippled the individual. Horizons have shrunk drastically, so that the person may feel literally unable or afraid to leave the house, to walk across a room, or to stray far from the phone. Moreover, such people are likely to regard routine activities like walking, riding a bike, or raking leaves as too exhausting or dangerous. For some individuals, life comes to a near standstill.

The best therapy for such psychological constriction is a program that emphasizes early and progressive mobilization in the hospital and exercise after discharge. A physician might naturally be wary of prescribing this for a person with severe chronic obstructive pulmonary disease who is dyspneic while walking at an ordinary pace. For some significantly impaired chronic pulmonary patients,[95] however, objective exercise tolerance can be increased as much as 1000-fold. The improvement is the result of better limb muscle conditioning. The patient does not have to change pulmonary function at all to experience significantly greater endurance.[96] Several self-imposed restrictions (e.g., never being far from an oxygen tank) are dramatically relieved. The psychiatric consultant should be aware that patients with chronic pulmonary disease that is considered to be irreversible can be significantly helped by a specific rehabilitation program.[97] Just as the original illness or injury can be demoralizing, so can the seeming snail's pace of recovery. This normal despondency can further retard rehabilitation. Few things heal self-esteem as effectively as regaining the sense of a sound body. The consultant who helps the patient grieve for those losses beyond restoration, while correcting misconceptions about inactivity and encouraging the patient to shoulder the work of recovery, shortens the convalescence of both body and mind.

REFERENCES

Access the reference list online at https://expertconsult.inkling.com/.

Delirious Patients

10

Jason P. Caplan, M.D.

Delirium has probably replaced syphilis as "the great imitator" because its varied presentations have led to misdiagnoses among almost every major category of mental illness. Delirium is a syndrome caused by an underlying physiologic disturbance and marked by a fluctuating course of impairments in consciousness, attention, and perception. Thus, delirium is often mistaken for: depression, when the patient has a withdrawn or flat affect; mania, when the patient has agitation and confusion; psychosis, when the patient has hallucinations and paranoia; anxiety, when the patient has restlessness and hypervigilance; dementia, when the patient has cognitive impairments; and for substance abuse, when the patient has impairment in consciousness. With so diverse an array of symptoms, delirium assumes a position of diagnostic privilege in the *Diagnostic and Statistical Manual of Mental Disorders*, 5th edition (DSM-5),[1] in that almost no other diagnosis can be made in its presence.

Sometimes, delirium is referred to as an acute confusional state, a toxic-metabolic encephalopathy, or acute brain failure; unquestionably, it is the most common cause of agitation and one of the most common triggers for psychiatric consultation in the general hospital. Even more noteworthy, delirium is a signifier of, often serious, somatic illness.[2] Delirium has been associated with increased length of stay in hospitals,[3] with an increased cost of care,[4,5] and an increased risk of mortality even after correction for other covariates.[6] Among intensive care unit (ICU) patients, prospective studies have noted that delirium occurs in 31% of admissions;[7] when intubation and mechanical ventilation are required, the incidence soars to 81.7%.[6] Placed in this context, the consequences of misdiagnosis of delirium can be severe; prompt and accurate recognition of this syndrome is paramount for all clinicians.

CASE 1

Mr. J, a 67-year-old man, was admitted to the hospital for elective lumbar spine surgery in the context of chronic back pain. His medical history was significant only for hypertension and hypercholesterolemia that was treated with losartan and simvastatin, respectively. He had no history of psychiatric illness. His hospital course was complicated by a dehiscence of his surgical wound that required a protracted hospitalization and total bedrest.

Psychiatry was consulted on hospital day 15 to assess for depression. In speaking with the nurse practitioner from the neurosurgery service, the consultant learned that over the prior several days Mr. J had stopped speaking with staff and family, was not allowing his vital signs to be checked, and was now refusing oral medications. The consultant spoke with the bedside nurse who confirmed these behaviors and further noted "he's just given up!"

The consultant introduced himself to Mr. J whose response was to raise an eyebrow and turn his head away. The consultant then further explained the purpose of his visit, noting that staff and family were concerned that he may be depressed. Mr. J remained non-verbal. The consultant stated that "sometimes I speak to folks who have had the sort of surgery you have had and are on all the medications you're on and they tell me that sometimes they worry that they see things or hear things that other people don't seem to see or hear. Has anything like that happened to you?" Mr. J then turned his head back to the consultant and nodded his head in the affirmative. The consultant went on to discuss the phenomenon of delirium; that it is due to a medical illness, is not representative of primary psychiatric illness, and the symptoms can be effectively managed. Mr. J then engaged in the interview, revealing that he had been seeing animals running through his hospital room and was worried that he was "losing my marbles." Cognitive exam revealed prominent deficits of attention and short-term memory.

A battery of laboratory studies revealed a previously undiagnosed urinary tract infection and antibiotic treatment was initiated. After reviewing an EKG to check Mr. J's QTc, haloperidol 1 mg IV every 6 hours was initiated with resultant resolution of Mr. J's hallucinations and improvements in attention and memory. This regimen was tapered over the subsequent several days without re-emergence of symptoms of delirium.

DIAGNOSIS

The essential features of delirium, according to the DSM-5, are a disturbance of attention and awareness accompanied by cognitive deficits that develop over a short period of time and tend to wax and wane over the course of the day in the setting of evidence that these deficits are the direct physiologic consequences of a physiologic condition (including medical illness, substance intoxication or withdrawal, and toxin exposure). Disturbance of the sleep–wake cycle is also common, sometimes with nocturnal worsening (sundowning) or even by a complete reversal of the night–day cycle, though, despite previous postulation and ongoing hospital folklore, sleep disturbance alone does not cause delirium.[8] Similarly, the term *ICU psychosis* persists in the medical lexicon; this is an unfortunate and lazy misnomer because it assigns the environment of the ICU as the cause of delirium, effectively allowing the clinician to shrug off any burden of having to explore this syndrome further, and it inaccurately limits the symptomatology of delirium to psychosis.[8] Despite wide variation in the presentation of the delirious patient, the hallmarks of delirium, although perhaps less immediately apparent, remain quite consistent from case to case.

Impaired attention has long been regarded as the main deficit of delirium.[9,10] This inattention (along with an acute onset, waxing and waning course, and overall disturbance of consciousness) forms the core features of delirium, whereas other related symptoms, such as withdrawn affect, agitation, hallucinations, and paranoia, serve as a frame that can sometimes be so prominent as to distract from the picture itself.

Psychotic symptoms (such as visual or auditory hallucinations and delusions) are common among patients with delirium.[11] Sometimes the psychiatric symptoms are so bizarre or so offensive (e.g., an enraged and paranoid patient shouts that pornographic movies are being made in the ICU) that diagnostic efforts are distracted. The delirium-inducing hypoglycemia of a man with diabetes can be missed in the Emergency Department (ED) if the accompanying behavior is threatening, uncooperative, and resembling that of an intoxicated person.

Although agitation can distract clinicians from making an accurate diagnosis of delirium, disruptive behavior alone will almost certainly garner some attention. The hypoactive presentation of delirium is more insidious, because the patient is often thought to be depressed or anxious because of the medical illness. Studies of quietly delirious patients show the experience to be as disturbing as the agitated variant;[12] quiet delirium is still a harbinger of serious medical pathology.[13,14]

The core similarities found in cases of delirium have led to postulation of a final common neurologic pathway for its symptoms. Current understanding of the neurotransmitter imbalance involved in delirium is one of hyperdopaminergia and hypocholinergia.[15] The ascending reticular activating system (RAS) and its bilateral thalamic projections regulate alertness, with neocortical and limbic inputs to this system controlling attention. Because acetylcholine is the primary neurotransmitter of the RAS, medications with anticholinergic activity can interfere with its function, resulting in the deficits in alertness and attention that are the heralds of delirium. Similarly, it is thought that loss of cholinergic neuronal activity in the elderly (e.g., resulting from microvascular disease or atrophy) is the basis for their heightened risk of delirium. Release of endogenous dopamine due to oxidative stress is thought to be responsible for the perceptual disturbances and paranoia that so often lead to mislabeling the delirious patient "psychotic." As discussed later, cholinergic agents (e.g., physostigmine) and dopamine blockers (e.g., haloperidol) have proved efficacious in managing delirium.

Early detection of changes in cognition can be key to timely identification and treatment of delirium (and perhaps of a heretofore undiagnosed somatic illness responsible for the delirium). Unfortunately, studies have revealed that non-psychiatrist physicians are quite unreliable in their ability to identify delirium accurately, and most patients referred to psychiatric consultation services with purported depression are ultimately found to have delirium.[16] Because consultation psychiatrists cannot perform repeated examinations on all patients admitted to the general hospital (even on those at high risk for delirium), a number of screening protocols designed to be administered serially by nursing staff have been developed and validated for use. Some of the most commonly used of these scales are summarized in Table 10-1.[17–23]

DIFFERENTIAL DIAGNOSIS

As useful as screening protocols may be, treatment relies on a careful diagnostic evaluation; there is no substitute for a systematic search for the specific cause of delirium. The temporal relationship to clinical events often gives the best clues to potential causes. For example, a patient who extubated himself was almost certainly in trouble before self-extubation. When did his mental state actually change? Nursing notes should be studied to help discern the first indication of an abnormality (e.g., restlessness, mild confusion, anxiety). If a time of onset can be established as a marker, other events can be examined for a possible causal relationship to the change in mental state. Vital signs can reveal periods of hypotension or fever. The highest temperature recorded will also be key. Operative procedures and the use of anesthetics can also induce a sustained period of hypotension or reveal unusually large blood loss that requires replacement. Laboratory values should be scanned for abnormalities that could be related to an encephalopathic state. Initiation or discontinuation of a drug, the onset of fever or hypotension, or the acute worsening of renal function, if in proximity to the time of mental status changes, become likely culprits.

Without a convincing temporal connection, causes of delirium should be investigated based on their likelihood in the unique clinical situation of the patient. In critical care settings, there are several (life-threatening) states that the clinician can consider routinely. These are states in which intervention needs to be especially prompt because failure to make the diagnosis may result in permanent central nervous system (CNS) damage. These conditions are Wernicke's disease, hypoxia, hypoglycemia, hypertensive encephalopathy, hyper- or hypothermia, intracerebral hemorrhage, meningitis or encephalitis, poisoning (exogenous or iatrogenic), and status epilepticus. These conditions are usefully recalled by the mnemonic device "WHHHHIMPS" (Table 10-2). Other less urgent but still acute conditions that require intervention include intracranial bleeds, sepsis, hepatic or renal failure, thyrotoxicosis or myxedema, delirium tremens, and complex partial seizures. If these conditions are not already ruled out, they are easy to verify. A broad review of conditions commonly associated with delirium is provided by the mnemonic "I WATCH DEATH" (Table 10-3).

Bacteremia commonly clouds a patient's mental state. In prospectively studied seriously ill hospitalized patients, delirium was commonly correlated with bacteremia.[24] In that study, the mortality of septic patients with delirium

TABLE 10-1 Delirium Assessment Tools

TOOL	STRUCTURE	NOTES
Confusion Assessment Method (CAM)[17]	Full scale of 11 items Abbreviated algorithm targeting four cardinal symptoms	Intended for use by non-psychiatric clinicians
Confusion Assessment Method for the Intensive Care Unit (CAM-ICU)[18]	Algorithm targeting four cardinal symptoms	Designed for use by nursing staff in the ICU
Intensive Care Delirium Screening Checklist (ICDSC)[19]	8-item screening checklist	Bedside screening tool for use by non-psychiatric physicians or nurses in the ICU
Delirium Rating Scale (DRS)[20]	Full scale of 10 items Abbreviated 7- or 8-item subscales for repeated administration	Provides data for confirmation of diagnosis and measurement of severity
Delirium Rating Scale—Revised–98 (DRS-R-98)[21]	16-item scale that can be divided into a 3-item diagnostic subscale and a 13-item severity subscale	Revision of DRS is better suited to repeat administration
Memorial Delirium Assessment Scale (MDAS)[22]	10-item severity rating scale	Grades severity of delirium once diagnosis has been made
Neecham Confusion Scale[23]	10-item rating scale	Designed for use by nursing staff and primarily validated for use in elderly populations in acute medical or nursing home setting

ICU, intensive care unit.

TABLE 10-2 Life-Threatening Causes of Delirium: "WHHHHIMPS"

Wernicke's disease
Hypoxia
Hypoglycemia
Hypertensive encephalopathy
Hyperthermia or hypothermia
Intracerebral hemorrhage
Meningitis or encephalitis
Poisoning (exogenous or iatrogenic)
Status epilepticus

TABLE 10-3 Conditions Commonly Associated With Delirium: "I WATCH DEATH"

CATEGORY	CONDITIONS
Infectious	Encephalitis, meningitis, syphilis, pneumonia, urinary tract infection
Withdrawal	From alcohol or sedative–hypnotics
Acute metabolic	Acidosis, alkalosis, electrolyte disturbances, liver or kidney failure
Trauma	Heat stroke, burns, following surgery
CNS pathology	Abscesses, hemorrhage, seizure, stroke, tumor, vasculitis, or normal pressure hydrocephalus
Hypoxia	Anemia, carbon monoxide poisoning, hypotension, pulmonary embolus, lung or heart failure
Deficiencies	Of vitamin B_{12}, niacin, or thiamine
Endocrinopathies	Hyper- or hypoglycemia, hyper- or hypoadrenocorticism, hyper- or hypothyroidism, hyper- or hypoparathyroidism
Acute vascular	Hypertensive encephalopathy or shock
Toxins or drugs	Medications, pesticides, or solvents
Heavy metals	Lead, manganese, or mercury

was higher than that in septic patients with a normal mental status. In the elderly, regardless of the setting, the onset of confusion should trigger concern about infection. Urinary tract infections (UTIs) and pneumonias are among the most common infections in older patients, and when bacteremia is associated with a UTI, confusion is the presenting feature nearly one-third (30%) of the time.[25] Once a consultant has eliminated these common conditions as possible causes of a patient's disturbed brain function, there is time enough for a more systematic approach to the differential diagnosis. While an old medical adage tells us to think of horses when we hear hoofbeats, it behooves the psychiatric consultant to maintain an awareness of the zebras and unicorns that might have evaded detection. A comprehensive differential diagnosis, similar to the one compiled by Ludwig[26] (expanded in Table 10-4) is recommended. A quick review of this list is warranted even when the consultant is relatively sure of the diagnosis.

Prior medical records, no matter how lengthy, cannot be overlooked without risk. Some patients have had psychiatric consultations for similar difficulties on prior admissions. Others, in the absence of psychiatric consultations, have caused considerable trouble for their caregivers. Similar to a patient's psychiatric history, the family psychiatric history can help make a diagnosis, especially if a major mood or anxiety disorder, alcoholism, schizophrenia, or epilepsy is present.

Examination of current and past medications is essential because pharmacologic agents (in therapeutic doses, in overdose, or with withdrawal) can produce psychiatric

TABLE 10-4 Differential Diagnosis of Delirium

GENERAL CAUSE	SPECIFIC CAUSE
Vascular	Hypertensive encephalopathy Cerebral arteriosclerosis Intracranial hemorrhage or thrombosis Emboli from atrial fibrillation, patent foramen ovale, or endocarditic valve Circulatory collapse (shock) Systemic lupus erythematosus Polyarteritis nodosa Thrombotic thrombocytopenic purpura Hyperviscosity syndrome Sarcoid Posterior reversible encephalopathy syndrome (PRES) Cerebral aneurysm
Infectious	Encephalitis Bacterial or viral meningitis, fungal meningitis (*cryptococcal, coccidioidal, Histoplasma*) Sepsis General paresis Brain, epidural, or subdural abscess Malaria Human immunodeficiency virus Lyme disease Typhoid fever Parasitic (*toxoplasma, trichinosis, cysticercosis, echinococcosis*) Behçet's syndrome Mumps
Neoplastic	Space-occupying lesions, such as gliomas, meningiomas, abscesses Paraneoplastic syndromes Carcinomatous meningitis
Degenerative	Dementias Huntington's disease Creutzfeldt–Jakob disease Wilson's disease
Intoxication	Chronic intoxication or withdrawal effect of drugs, including sedative-hypnotics, opiates, tranquilizers, anticholinergics, dissociative anesthetics, anticonvulsants
Neurophysiologic	Epilepsy Postictal states Complex partial status epilepticus
Traumatic	Intracranial bleeds Postoperative trauma Heat stroke Fat emboli syndrome
Intraventricular	Normal-pressure hydrocephalus
Vitamin deficiency	Thiamine (Wernicke–Korsakoff syndrome) Niacin (pellagra) B_{12} (pernicious anemia)
Endocrine/metabolic	Diabetic coma and shock Uremia Myxedema Hyperthyroidism Parathyroid dysfunction Hypoglycemia Hepatic or renal failure Porphyria Severe electrolyte or acid/base disturbances Cushing's or Addison's syndrome Sleep apnea Carcinoid Whipple's disease
Autoimmune	Autoimmune encephalitides Steroid-responsive encephalopathy associated with thyroiditis (SREAT)/Hashimoto's encephalopathy Systemic lupus erythematosus Multiple sclerosis
Poisoning	Heavy metals (lead, manganese, mercury) Carbon monoxide Anticholinergics Other toxins
Anoxia	Hypoxia and anoxia secondary to pulmonary or cardiac failure, anesthesia, anemia
Psychiatric	Depressive pseudodementia, catatonia, Bell's mania

symptoms. These medications must be routinely reviewed, especially in patients whose drugs have been stopped because of surgery or hospitalization or whose drug orders have not been reconciled during transfer between services or institutions. Of all causes of an altered mental status, use of and withdrawal from drugs are probably the most common. Some, such as lidocaine, are quite predictable in their ability to cause encephalopathy; the frequency and severity of symptoms are dose-related. Other agents usually cause delirium only in someone whose brain is already vulnerable, as in a patient with a dementia. Table 10-5 lists some drugs used in clinical practice that have been associated with delirium.

The number of drugs that can be involved either directly or indirectly (e.g., because of drug interactions) is numerous. Fortunately, there are an array of resources (including websites and smartphone applications) that easily allow for identification of these issues.[27] Once identified, the usual treatment is to stop the offending drug or to reduce the dosage; however, at times this is not possible. Elderly patients, those with impairments of metabolism (e.g., hepatic or renal failure), and those with neurodevelopmental disorders or a history of significant head injury are more susceptible to the toxic actions of many of these drugs.

Psychiatric symptoms in medical illness can have other causes. Besides the abnormalities that can arise from the

TABLE 10-5 Drugs Commonly Used in Clinical Practice That Have Been Associated With Delirium

Antiarrhythmics	**Tricyclic Antidepressants**	**Dopamine Agonists (Central)**	**Monoamine Oxidase Inhibitors**
Disopyramide	Amitriptyline	Amantadine	Tranylcypromine
Lidocaine	Clomipramine	Bromocriptine	Phenelzine
Mexiletine	Desipramine	Levodopa	Procarbazine
Procainamide	Imipramine	Selegiline	**Narcotic Analgesics**
Propafenone	Nortriptyline	**Ergotamine**	Meperidine (normeperidine)
Quinidine	Protriptyline	**GABA Agonists**	Pentazocine
Tocainide	Trimipramine	Baclofen	Podophyllin (topical)
Antibiotics	**Anticonvulsants**	Benzodiazepines	**Non-Steroidal Antiinflammatory Drugs**
Aminoglycosides	Phenytoin	Eszopiclone	Ibuprofen
Amodiaquine	Levetiracetam	Zaleplon	Indometacin
Amphotericin	**Antihypertensives**	Zolpidem	Naproxen
Cephalosporins	Captopril	**Immunosuppressives**	Sulindac
Chloramphenicol	Clonidine	Aminoglutethimide	**Other Medications**
Gentamicin	Methyldopa	Azacitidine	Clozaril
Isoniazid	Reserpine	Chlorambucil	Cyclobenzaprine
Metronidazole	**Antiviral agents**	Cytosine arabinoside (high dose)	Lithium
Rifampin	Acyclovir	Dacarbazine	Ketamine
Sulfonamides	Interferon	FK-506	Sildenafil
Tetracyclines	Ganciclovir	5-Fluorouracil	Trazodone
Ticarcillin	Nevirapine	Hexamethylmelamine	Mefloquine
Vancomycin	**Barbiturates**	Ifosfamide	**Sympathomimetics**
Anticholinergics	**β-Blockers**	Interleukin-2 (high dose)	Aminophylline
Atropine	Propranolol	L-Asparaginase	Amphetamine
Benztropine	Timolol	Methotrexate (high dose)	Cocaine
Diphenhydramine	**Cimetidine, Ranitidine**	Procarbazine	Ephedrine
Eye and nose drops	***Digitalis* Preparations**	Tamoxifen	Phenylephrine
Scopolamine	**Disulfiram**	Vinblastine	Phenylpropanolamine
Thioridazine	**Diuretics**	Vincristine	Theophylline
Trihexyphenidyl	Acetazolamide		**Steroids, ACTH**

Adapted from Cassem NH, Lake CR, Boyer WF: Psychopharmacology in the ICU. In Chernow B, editor: *The pharmacologic approach to the critically ill patient*, Baltimore, 1995, Williams & Wilkins, pp 651–665; and Drugs that may cause psychiatric symptoms, *Med Letter Drugs Ther* 2002; 44:59–62.
ACTH, adrenocorticotropic hormone; GABA, gamma aminobutyric acid.

effect of the patient's medical illness (or its treatment) on the CNS (e.g., the abnormalities produced by systemic lupus erythematosus or high-dose steroids), the disturbance may be the effect of the medical illness on the patient's mind (the subjective CNS), as in the patient who thinks he or she is "done for" after a myocardial infarction, quits, and withdraws into hopelessness. The disturbance can also arise from the mind, as a conversion symptom or as malingering about pain to get more narcotics. Finally, the abnormality may be the result of interactions between the sick patient and his or her environment or family (e.g., the patient who is without complaint until the family arrives, at which time the patient promptly looks acutely distressed and begins to whimper continuously). Nurses are commonly aware of these sorts of abnormalities, although they may refrain from documenting them in the medical record.

THE EXAMINATION OF THE PATIENT

Appearance, level of consciousness, thought, speech, orientation, memory, mood, judgment, and behavior should all be assessed. In the formal mental status examination (MSE), one begins with the examination of consciousness. If the patient does not speak, a handy common-sense test is to ask oneself, "Do the eyes look back at me?" One could formally rate consciousness by using the Glasgow Coma Scale (Table 10-6), a measure that is readily understood by consultees in other specialties.[28]

Delirious patients are occasionally unwilling to participate in a psychiatric examination, often because they fear that they are "going crazy" and the presence of a psychiatric consultant at the bedside magnifies these concerns. Indeed, patients may be reluctant to report subjective experiences, such as hallucinations or paranoia, because they do not want hospital staff or family to think that they have "lost it." Leading the interview with an explanation that such symptoms are relatively normal in the setting of illness, do not represent a primary psychiatric illness, and can be effectively managed may serve to establish rapport with these reluctant interviewees. If the patient cooperates with an examination, attention should be examined first because if this is disturbed, other parts of the examination may be invalid. One can ask the patient to repeat the letters of the alphabet that rhyme with "tree." (If the patient is intubated, ask that a hand or finger be raised whenever the letter of the recited alphabet rhymes with "tree.") Then the rest of the MSE can be performed. The Folstein Mini-Mental State Examination (MMSE),[29] which is presented in Table 4-8, is usually included. Specific defects are more important than is the total score. Other functions, such as writing, are often abnormal in delirium.[9] Perhaps the most dramatic (though difficult to score objectively) test of cognition is the clock drawing test, which can provide a broad survey of the patient's cognitive state (Figure 10-1).[30] A more recently developed and validated bedside test, the Montreal Cognitive Assessment (MoCA),[31] usefully incorporates some aspects of the MMSE (i.e., tests of memory, attention, and orientation) with tests of more complex visuospatial and executive function (including clock drawing and an adaptation of the Trail Making B task). Although not specifically validated for detecting delirium, the MoCA (available at www.mocatest.org, in a variety of languages) has been consistently shown to have greater sensitivity than the MMSE for mild cognitive impairment in a variety of conditions and typically requires less than 10 minutes to administer.

TABLE 10-6 Glasgow Coma Scale

CRITERION	SCORE
Eye Opening (E)	
Spontaneous	4
To verbal command	3
To pain	2
No response	1
Motor (M)	
Obeys verbal command	6
Localizes pain	5
Flexion withdrawal	4
Abnormal flexion (decortication)	3
Extension (decerebration)	2
No response	1
Verbal (V)	
Oriented and converses	5
Disoriented and converses	4
Inappropriate words	3
Incomprehensible sound	2
No response	1
Coma Score = (E + M + V)	Range 3 to 15

The patient's problem can involve serious neurologic syndromes as well; however, the clinical presentation of the patient should direct the examination. In general, the less responsive and more impaired the patient is, the more one should look for *hard signs*. A directed search for an abnormality of the eyes and pupils, rigidity (nuchal or otherwise), hyperreflexia, hung-up reflexes, one-sided weakness or asymmetry, gait, Babinski's reflexes, *gegenhalten*, *mitgehen*, absent vibratory and position senses, hyperventilation, or other specific clues can help verify or reject hypotheses about causality that are stimulated by the abnormalities in the examination.

Frontal lobe function deserves specific attention. Grasp, snout, palmomental, suck, and glabellar responses are helpful when present. Hand movements thought to be related to the premotor area (Brodmann's area 8) can identify subtle deficiencies. The patient is asked to imitate, with each hand separately, specific movements. The hand is held upright, a circle formed by thumb and first finger ("okay" sign), then the fist is closed and lowered to the surface on which the elbow rests. In the Luria sequence, one hand is brought down on a surface (a table or one's own leg) in three successive positions: extended with all five digits parallel ("cut"), then as a fist, and then flat on the surface ("slap"). Finally, both hands are placed on a flat surface in front of the patient, one flat on the surface, the other resting as a fist. Then the positions are alternated between right and left hands, and the patient is instructed to do the same.

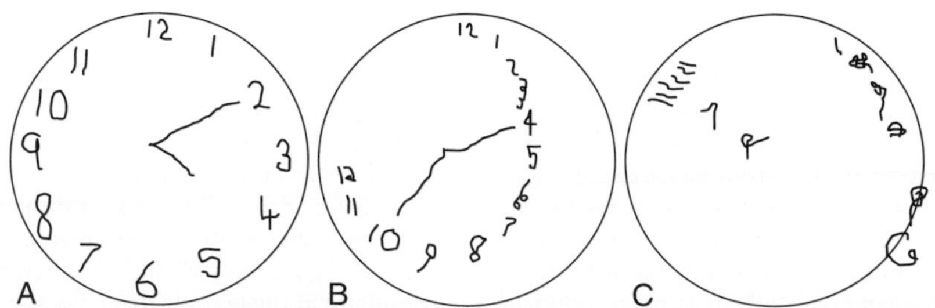

Figure 10-1. The clock drawing test. The patient is provided with a circular outline and asked to draw the numbers as they appear on the face of a clock. Once the numbering is complete, the patient is asked to set the hands to a particular time (often "ten past" the hour to test if the patient can suppress the impulse to include the number *10*). (A) This drawing demonstrates good planning and use of space. (B) This drawing features some impulsiveness because the numbers are drawn out without regard for actual location, and the time "ten past four" is represented by hands pointing to the digits *10* and *4*. Note the perseveration indicated by the extra loops on the digits *3* and *6*. Impulsiveness and perseveration indicate frontal lobe dysfunction. (C) This drawing demonstrates gross disorganization, although the patient took several minutes to draw the clock and believed it to be a good representation.

For verbally responsive patients, their response to the "Frank Jones story" can be gauged ("I have a friend, Frank Jones, whose feet are so big he has to put his pants on over his head. How does that strike you?"). Three general responses are given. Type 1 is normal: The patient sees the incongruity and smiles (a limbic response) and can explain (a neocortical function) why it cannot be done. Type 2 is abnormal: The patient smiles at the incongruity (a limbic connection), but cannot explain why it cannot be done. Type 3 is abnormal: The patient neither gets the incongruity nor can explain its impossibility. Even in patients unable to respond verbally, attempts to elicit a limbic response through humor or absurd incongruity can help gauge their level of impairment.

Laboratory studies should be carefully reviewed, with special attention paid to indicators of infection or metabolic disturbance. Toxicology screens are also helpful in allowing the inclusion or exclusion of substance intoxication or withdrawal from the differential diagnosis. Neuroimaging can prove useful in detection of intracranial processes that can result in altered mental status. Of all the diagnostic studies available, the electroencephalogram (EEG) may be the most useful tool in the diagnosis of delirium. Engel and Romano[32] reported in 1959 their (now classic) findings on the EEG in delirium, namely, generalized slowing to the theta-delta range in the delirious patient, the consistency of this finding despite wide-ranging underlying conditions, and resolution of this slowing with effective treatment of the delirium. EEG findings might even clarify the etiology of a delirium, because delirium tremens is associated with low-voltage fast activity superimposed on slow waves, sedative–hypnotic toxicity produces fast beta activity (>12 Hz), and hepatic encephalopathy is classically associated with triphasic waves.[33] When faced with a consultee who insists that a patient's delirium is actually a primary psychiatric illness requiring admission to a psychiatric unit (i.e., transfer off their service), an abnormal EEG can provide incontrovertible evidence to the contrary.

SPECIFIC MANAGEMENT STRATEGIES FOR DELIRIUM

The antiepileptic medication levetiracetam has been associated with a number of neuropsychiatric adverse effects, including delirium.[34] In these cases, the medication can usually be switched to an alternate antiepileptic but problems are seldom so simple. Often the drugs (such as corticosteroids), that cause delirium cannot be changed without causing harm to the patient. Alternatively, pain can cause agitation in a delirious patient. Morphine sulfate can relieve pain but can unfortunately lead to decreases in blood pressure and respiratory rate.

Psychosocial or environmental measures are rarely effective in the treatment of a *bona fide* delirium of uncertain or unknown cause. Nevertheless, it is commendable to have hospital rooms with windows, calendars, clocks, and a few mementos from home on the walls;[35] soft and low lighting at night; and, when available, a loving family in attendance to reassure and reorient the patient. Indeed, these measures have been codified into a number of delirium-prevention protocols. A meta-analysis of these protocols has demonstrated efficacy in reducing the incidence of delirium and it is likely that simply paying attention to the specter of delirium is useful in forestalling it, regardless of which specific protocol is used.[36] However, once the proverbial genie is out of the bottle, it is unlikely that these environmental factors will be sufficient to manage it. The psychiatric consultant is often summoned because psychosocial measures have failed to prevent or to treat the patient's delirium. Mechanical restraints are available and quite useful to protect patients from inflicting harm on themselves or staff. One or several of these is often in place when the consultant arrives. One hoped-for outcome of the consultation is that the use of these devices can be reduced or eliminated.

When the cause of the delirium seems straightforward, the treatment revolves around resolution or reversal of the underlying cause. A discovered deficiency can be replaced (e.g., of blood, oxygen, thiamine, vitamin B_{12}, levothyroxine, or glucose). Pathologic conditions can be treated (e.g., volume replacement for hypotension, diuretics for pulmonary edema, antibiotics for infection, calcium for hypocalcemia, or dialysis for acute lithium toxicity). Implicated drugs can be stopped or reduced.

Specific antidotes can reverse the delirium caused by some drugs. Flumazenil and naloxone reverse the effects of benzodiazepines and opioid analgesics, respectively. However, caution is required because flumazenil can precipitate seizures in a benzodiazepine-dependent patient, and naloxone can also precipitate opioid withdrawal in an opioid-dependent patient.

Anticholinergic delirium can be reversed by intravenous (IV) physostigmine in doses starting at 0.5 to 2 mg. Caution is essential with use of this agent because the autonomic nervous system of the medically ill is generally less stable than it is in a healthy patient who has developed an anticholinergic delirium as a result of a voluntary or accidental overdose. Moreover, if there is a reasonably high amount of an anticholinergic drug on board that is clearing from the system slowly, the therapeutic effect of physostigmine, although sometimes quite dramatic, is usually short lived. The cholinergic reaction to intravenously administered physostigmine can cause profound bradycardia and hypotension, thereby multiplying the complications.[37,38] A continuous IV infusion of physostigmine has been successfully used to manage a case of anticholinergic poisoning.[39] Because of the diagnostic value of physostigmine, one might wish to use it even though its effects will be short-lived. If one uses an IV injection of 1 mg of physostigmine, protection against excessive cholinergic reaction can be provided by preceding this injection with an IV injection of 0.2 mg of glycopyrrolate. This anticholinergic agent does not cross the blood–brain barrier and should protect the patient from the peripheral cholinergic actions of physostigmine.

DRUG MANAGEMENT

Definitive treatment of delirium requires identification and treatment of the underlying somatic etiology, but all too often, the cause of delirium is not readily identified or treated. Even when the cause has been identified, effective treatment can still take considerable time. These situations call for management of the symptoms of delirium.

Benzodiazepines (e.g., lorazepam) are often effective in mild agitation in the setting of withdrawal from drugs that work at the chloride channel (including alcohol, benzodiazepines, and barbiturates). Morphine is also often used because it calms agitation and is easily reversed if hypotension or respiratory depression ensues. These agents should be used with caution since they themselves can cause or exacerbate confusion. This occurs much less often with neuroleptics.

Neuroleptics are the agent of choice for delirium. Haloperidol is probably the agent most commonly used to treat agitated delirium in the critical care setting; its effects on blood pressure, pulmonary artery pressure, heart rate, and respiration are milder than those of the benzodiazepines, making it an excellent agent for delirious patients with impaired cardiorespiratory status.[40]

Although haloperidol can be administered orally, acute delirium with extreme agitation typically requires use of parenteral medication. IV administration is preferable to intramuscular (IM) administration for a number of reasons. First, because drug absorption may be poor in distal muscles if delirium is associated with circulatory compromise or shock. The deltoid is probably a better IM injection site than the gluteus muscle, but neither is as reliable as the IV route. Second, because the agitated patient is commonly paranoid, repeated painful IM injections can increase the patient's sense of being attacked or harmed. Third, IM injections can complicate interpretations of muscle enzyme studies if enzyme fractionation is not readily available. Fourth, and most importantly, haloperidol is less likely to produce extrapyramidal symptoms (EPS) when given IV than when given IM or by mouth (PO), at least for patients without a prior serious psychiatric disorder.[41]

In contrast to the immediately observable sedation produced by IV benzodiazepines, IV haloperidol has a mean distribution time of 11 minutes in normal volunteers;[42] this may be even longer in critically ill patients. The mean half-life of IV haloperidol's subsequent, slower phase is 14 hours. This is still a more rapid metabolic rate than the overall mean half-lives of 21 and 24 hours for IM and PO doses. The PO dose has about half the potency of the parenteral dose, so 10 mg of PO haloperidol corresponds to 5 mg given IV or IM.

Haloperidol has not been approved by the Food and Drug Administration (FDA) for IV administration, and since it has been off-patent since the 1980s, there is no pharmaceutical company that will fund the studies required to gain such approval. IV haloperidol is, however, the standard of care for the management of delirium in hospitals around the world.

Over decades of clinical use in medically ill patients, IV haloperidol has been associated with few side effects on blood pressure, heart rate, respiratory rate, or urinary output and has been linked with few EPS. The reason for the latter is not known. Studies of the use of IV haloperidol in psychiatric patients have not shown that these side effects were fewer, perhaps because patients with psychiatric disorders are more susceptible to EPS.[41]

Before administering IV haloperidol, the IV line should be flushed with 2 mL of normal saline. Occasionally, haloperidol precipitates with heparin, and because many lines in critical care units are heparinized, the 2-mL flush is advised. Phenytoin precipitates with haloperidol, and mixing the two in the same line must be avoided. The initial bolus dose of haloperidol usually varies from 0.5 to 20 mg; usually 0.5 mg (for an elderly person) to 2 mg is used for mild agitation, 5 mg is used for moderate agitation, and 10 mg for severe agitation. A higher initial dose should be used only when the patient has already been unsuccessfully treated with reasonable doses of haloperidol. To adjust for haloperidol's lag time, doses are usually staggered by at least a 30-minute interval. If one dose (e.g., a 5-mg dose) fails to calm an agitated patient after 30 minutes, the next higher dose, 10 mg, should be administered. Calm is the desired outcome. Partial control of agitation is usually inadequate, and settling for this only prolongs the delirium or guarantees that excessively high doses of haloperidol will be used after the delirium is controlled.

Haloperidol can be combined every 30 minutes with simultaneous parenteral lorazepam doses (starting with 1 to 2 mg). Because the effects of lorazepam are noticeable within 5 to 10 minutes, each dose can precede the haloperidol dose, be observed for its impact on agitation, and be increased if it is more effective. Some believe that the combination leads to a lower overall dose of each drug.[43]

After calm is achieved, agitation should be the sign for a repeat dose. Ideally the total dose of haloperidol on the second day should be a fraction of that used on day 1. After complete lucidity has been achieved, the patient needs to be protected from delirium only at night, by small doses of haloperidol (1 to 3 mg), which can be given orally. As in the treatment of delirium tremens, the consultant is advised to stop the agitation quickly and completely at the outset rather than barely keep up with it over several days. The maximum total dose of IV haloperidol to be used as an upper limit has not been established, although IV administration of single bolus doses of 200 mg has been used,[44] and more than 2000 mg has been used in a 24-hour period. The highest requirements have been seen with delirious patients on the intra-aortic balloon pump.[45] A continuous infusion of haloperidol has also been used to treat severe, refractory delirium.[46] It has previously been argued that (despite strong empirical clinical evidence) high-dose haloperidol made little pharmacologic sense, given the high rates of dopamine receptor blockade at relatively low doses. *In vitro* and animal model research has revealed that the butyrophenone class of neuroleptics (haloperidol and droperidol) protect neurons from oxidative stress via their effects at the sigma receptor.[47,48] This mechanism of action may provide the physiologic basis for the clinical benefits of high-dose haloperidol.[49]

When delirium does not respond and agitation is unabated, one might wonder if the neuroleptic (e.g., haloperidol) is producing akathisia. The best indication as to whether the treatment is causing agitation is the patient's description of an irresistible urge to move—usually the limbs, lower more often than upper. If dialogue is possible, even nodding yes or no (provided that the patient understands the question) can confirm or exclude this symptom. If the patient cannot communicate, limited options remain: to decrease the dose or to increase it and judge by the response. In our experience, it is far more common for the patient to receive more haloperidol and to improve.

Hypotensive episodes following the administration of IV haloperidol are rare and almost invariably result from hypovolemia. Local caustic effects on veins do not arise. IV haloperidol is generally safe for epileptic patients and for patients with head trauma, unless psychotropic drugs are contraindicated because the patient needs careful neurologic monitoring. Although IV haloperidol may be used without mishap in patients receiving epinephrine drips, after large doses of haloperidol a pressor other than epinephrine (e.g., norepinephrine) should be used to avoid unopposed β-adrenergic activity. IV haloperidol does not block a dopamine-mediated increase in renal blood flow. It also appears to be the safest agent for patients with chronic obstructive pulmonary disease.

As with all neuroleptic agents, IV haloperidol has been associated with the development of torsades de pointes (TDP).[50–54] Particular caution is urged when levels of potassium and magnesium are low (because these deficiencies independently predict TDP), when a baseline prolonged QT interval is noted, when hepatic compromise is present, or when a specific cardiac abnormality (e.g., mitral valve prolapse or a dilated ventricle) exists. Progressive QT widening after administration of haloperidol should alert one to the danger, however infrequent it may be in practice (4 of 1100 cases in one report).[51] Delirious patients who are candidates for IV haloperidol require careful screening. Serum potassium and magnesium should be within the normal range, and a baseline electrocardiogram (ECG) should be checked for the pre-treatment QT interval corrected for heart rate (QTc). If necessary, potassium and magnesium should be repleted and the QTc and levels of potassium and magnesium should be monitored regularly for the duration of neuroleptic treatment. QT interval prolongation occurs in some patients with alcoholic liver disease; this finding is associated with adverse outcomes (e.g., sudden cardiac death).[55] A multitude of other commonly used medications also carry the potential for QTc prolongation (some of the usual offenders are summarized in Table 10-7). Medication lists should be reviewed closely for other agents that could be discontinued or therapeutically exchanged if QTc prolongation becomes a concern. Administration of haloperidol is based (as are all decisions in medicine) on a risk:benefit calculus. Thus, there may be circumstances where administration of haloperidol is reasonable even in the face of a prolonged QTc.

Other available parenteral first-generation neuroleptics for treatment of agitation are perphenazine, thiothixene, trifluoperazine, fluphenazine, and chlorpromazine. Perphenazine is approved for IV use as an antiemetic. Chlorpromazine is extremely effective, but its potent α-blocking properties can be dangerous for critically ill patients. When administered IV or IM, it can abruptly decrease total peripheral resistance and cause a precipitous fall in cardiac output. Nevertheless, used IV in small doses (10 mg) it can be safe and effective in the treatment of delirium.

The commonplace use of second-generation neuroleptics in general psychiatric practice and the availability of injectable formulations of olanzapine and ziprasidone has prompted investigation of these agents in managing delirium.[56] Risperidone has the most data available supporting its use, and multiple studies show it to be efficacious and safe for treating delirium;[57–59] one small randomized double-blind comparative study found no significant difference in efficacy compared with oral haloperidol.[60] Randomized controlled trials of olanzapine and quetiapine have shown some benefit in terms of ameliorating the severity of delirium.[61–65] Studies that have attempted to compare second-generation neuroleptics with haloperidol have, to date, been limited by two key confounders. First, they employ the oral formulation of haloperidol in order to allow for successful blinding (since none of the second-generation drugs is available intravenously). Second, IV haloperidol is often used as the "bailout" medication for episodes of uncontrolled agitation in the study subjects–thus, subjects in the second-generation arms of these studies still receive IV haloperidol (sometimes more frequently than those receiving oral haloperidol). All drugs in this class feature an FDA black box warning indicating an increased risk of death when used to treat behavioral problems in elderly patients with dementia. Similar warnings regarding a potential increased risk of cerebrovascular events are reported for risperidone, olanzapine, and aripiprazole. One study examining the mean prolongation of the QTc for various neuroleptic agents on a per-dose-equivalent basis revealed that haloperidol was associated with the lowest increase of all the drugs tested.[66] With decades of clinical experience in the use of haloperidol, and a relative dearth of available data on these newer agents, haloperidol remains the agent of choice for treating delirium.

TABLE 10-7 Non-Neuroleptic Medications Associated With Prolongation of the QT Interval

ANTIARRHYTHMICS	ANTI-INFECTIOUS	OTHER
Amiodarone	Atazanavir	Alfuzosin
Disopyramide	Azithromycin	Amantadine
Dofetilide	Chloroquine	Arsenic trioxide
Flecainide	Ciprofloxacin	Bepridil
Ibutilide	Clarithromycin	Chloral hydrate
Procainamide	Erythromycin	Cisapride
Quinidine	Foscarnet	Citalopram
Sotalol	Gatifloxacin	Dolasetron
	Gemifloxacin	Escitalopram
	Halofantrine	Felbamate
	Levofloxacin	Granisetron
	Moxifloxacin	Indapamide
	Ofloxacin	Isradipine
	Pentamidine	Lapatinib
	Sparfloxacin	Levomethadyl
	Telithromycin	Lithium carbonate
	Voriconazole	Methadone
		Nicardipine
		Octreotide
		Ondansetron
		Oxytocin
		Probucol
		Ranolazine
		Sunitinib
		Tacrolimus
		Tizanidine
		Vardenafil
		Venlafaxine

Randomized controlled trials of medications for delirium prevention have shown that perioperative administration of olanzapine, risperidone, and IV (but not oral) haloperidol may reduce the incidence of delirium.[67–70] A meta-analysis of five such trials supported the prophylactic use of neuroleptics to ward off delirium.[71] Additional randomized controlled trials have demonstrated that regularly scheduled doses of ramelteon and ondansetron can also reduce the incidence of delirium.[72,73] There is some limited evidence suggesting that the pro-cholinergic action of cholinesterase inhibitors provides some protection against the development of delirium,[74,75] though multiple trials have failed to demonstrate any efficacy of these agents in the treatment of active delirium. For patients undergoing surgery, one study has demonstrated a 20% to 30% reduction in use of intraoperative anesthetic agents and a 35% decrease in postoperative delirium when operative anesthesia is measured by bispectral index (BIS) monitoring as compared with treatment as usual.[76]

DELIRIUM IN SPECIFIC DISEASES

Critically ill patients with human immunodeficiency virus (HIV) infection may be more susceptible to the EPS of haloperidol and to neuroleptic malignant syndrome (NMS),[77–80] leading an experienced group to recommend use of molindone.[80] Molindone is associated with fewer such effects; it is available only as an oral agent, and it can be prescribed from 5 to 25 mg at appropriate intervals or, in a more acute situation, 25 mg every hour until calm is achieved. Risperidone (0.5 to 1 mg per dose) is another recommended oral agent. If parenteral medication is required, 10 mg of chlorpromazine has been effective. Perphenazine is readily available for parenteral use as well, and 2-mg doses can be used effectively.

Delirious patients with Parkinson's disease pose a particular problem because dopamine blockade aggravates their condition. If oral treatment of delirium or psychosis is possible, clozapine, starting with a small dose of 6.25 or 12.5 mg, is probably the most effective agent available that does not exacerbate the disease. With the risk of agranulocytosis attendant to the use of clozapine, quetiapine can play a valuable role in this population because its very low affinity for dopamine receptors is less likely to exacerbate this disorder.[81]

Adding medications to the regimen of a patient with hepatic compromise is always fraught with risk of toxicity from that agent or from extant drugs whose metabolism is upset by the disturbance of an already over-burdened cytochrome system. In this population, paliperidone is a useful option since it does not require significant hepatic metabolism.[82]

Benzodiazepines (particularly diazepam, chlordiazepoxide, and lorazepam) are routinely used to treat agitated states, particularly delirium tremens, and alcohol withdrawal.[83] Neuroleptics have also been used as adjunctive agents successfully, and both have been combined with clonidine. Trials of barbiturates may be successful as well. When all else fails, IV alcohol is also extremely effective in treating alcohol withdrawal states. The inherent disadvantage is that alcohol is toxic to liver and brain, although its use can be quite safe if these organs do not show already extensive damage, and it is sometimes quite safe even when they do. Nonetheless, use of IV alcohol should be reserved for extreme cases of alcohol withdrawal when other, less-toxic measures have failed. A 5% solution of alcohol mixed with 5% dextrose in water run at 1 mL per minute often achieves calm quickly. Treatment pathways have been developed to provide nonpsychiatric clinicians with guidance on the management of alcohol withdrawal,[84] though care must always be taken to ensure that benzodiazepines are not inappropriately administered because they almost certainly exacerbate a delirium that results from any other cause.[85]

Propofol is commonly used to sedate critically ill patients and can also be extremely effective in managing agitation. It has moderate respiratory depressant and vasodilator effects, although hypotension can be minimized by avoiding boluses of the drug. Impaired hepatic function does not slow metabolic clearance, but clearance does decline with age, and its half-life is significantly longer in the elderly. This drug's rapid onset and short duration make it especially useful for treating short periods of stress. When rapid return to alertness from sedation for an uncompromised neurologic examination is indicated, propofol is a nearly ideal agent;[86] however, its use in treating a prolonged delirious state has specific disadvantages.[87] Delivered as a fat emulsion containing 0.1 g of fat per milliliter, propofol requires a dedicated IV line, and drug accumulation can lead to a fat-overload syndrome that has been associated with overfeeding and with significant CO_2 production, hypertriglyceridemia, ketoacidosis, seizure activity 6 days after discontinuation, and even fatal respiratory failure.[88,89] Obese patients provide a high volume of distribution, and their doses should be calculated using estimated lean, rather than actual, body mass. If the patient is receiving fat by parenteral feeding, this must be accounted for or eliminated and adequate glucose infusion must be provided to prevent ketoacidosis. Although no clear association has been demonstrated with addiction, tolerance, or withdrawal, doses seem to require escalation after 4 to 7 days' infusion. Seizures seen after withdrawal or muscular rigidity during administration are poorly understood. The drug is costly, especially when used for prolonged infusions.

Dexmedetomidine is a selective α_2-adrenergic agonist used for sedation and analgesia in the ICU setting. Its action on receptors in the locus ceruleus results in anxiolysis and sedation, and agonism of spinal cord receptors provides analgesia. This unique mechanism of action allows effective management in agitation without the risks of respiratory depression, dependence, and deliriogenesis associated with the benzodiazepines traditionally employed in the ICU.[90] Its relative lack of amnestic effect might further limit its use as monotherapy in the treatment of the delirious patient owing to an increased likelihood of distressing recollections persisting from the period of sedation.[91] In current practice, dexmedetomidine can serve as a useful (but costly) adjunct agent to quell agitation when more traditional approaches have met with limited success.

CONCLUSION

Of all psychiatric diagnoses, delirium demands the most immediate attention because delay in identifying and treating this syndrome might allow the progression of serious and irreversible pathophysiologic changes. Unfortunately, delirium is all too often under-emphasized, misdiagnosed, or altogether missed in the general hospital setting.[92–94] Indeed, it was not until their most recent editions that major medical and surgical texts corrected chapters indicating that delirium was the result of anxiety, depression, or the hospital milieu, rather than an underlying somatic cause that required prompt investigation. In the face of this tradition of misinformation, it often falls to the psychiatric consultant to identify and manage delirium while alerting and educating others to its significance.

REFERENCES

Access the reference list online at https://expertconsult.inkling.com/.

Patients With Neurocognitive Disorders

11

Franklin King IV, M.D.
Ilse R. Wiechers, M.D., M.P.P., M.H.S.

As life expectancy extends and the baby boomer generation begins to reach geriatric age, we will confront an epidemic of neurocognitive disorders (NCDs) in general hospitals. The number of cases of Alzheimer's disease (AD), the most common cause of NCD, is expected to quadruple in the coming decades.[1] Unfortunately, most NCDs (used interchangeably in this chapter with the term "dementia"), including AD, are incurable, but progression can be slowed if the condition is identified and managed appropriately; only a few neurocognitive illnesses are reversible. Given that a major task for consultation psychiatrists is to assist in the diagnosis and treatment of NCDs, this chapter provides an overview of these disorders and an approach to their identification and management.

Often, the request to see an inpatient on a medical or surgical floor is for a behavioral disturbance associated with delirium, not for cognitive difficulties alone. Nonetheless, the risk of developing delirium is between two to five times higher in patients with a NCD, and an episode of delirium may unmask a previously undiagnosed NCD. Conversely, delirium itself is also a risk factor for later development of a NCD.[2] Thus, the presence of delirium in an elderly patient should lead the consultant to conduct a thorough evaluation in search of a potentially coexisting NCD.

Another common request is for the evaluation of depressive symptoms associated with a NCD. It may be challenging to determine whether the mood symptoms are causing, coexisting with, or resulting from neurocognitive difficulties.[3] Determining the sometimes subtle differences in the history and presentation of delirium, depression, and AD, can be helpful in the diagnosis of these disorders (Table 11-1).

Other presenting problems should alert the physician to an underlying NCD. These include poor medication adherence and injuries that could be accounted for by memory impairment. For example, many elderly patients experience burns as a result of dangerous cooking methods. Another reason for referral may be the patient's difficulty in coping with the inpatient setting itself. Despite a gradual cognitive decline, the patient may have functioned adequately in his or her familiar home setting. In the alien environment of the hospital, however, unfamiliar people provide care on an unusual schedule. As a result, trusted coping mechanisms may fail; anxiety, dysphoria, agitation, or paranoia can develop.

CASE 1

Mr. G, a 74-year-old retired chef without a known psychiatric history and a medical history significant for hypertension, was admitted for treatment of gout after 2 days of worsening foot and knee pain. Colchicine therapy was initiated. His first 24 hours passed uneventfully but on his second night, he abruptly yelled at his nurse and showed "aggressive posturing" while she was attempting to take his evening vital signs. Psychiatry was consulted for evaluation and management of this behavior.

On interview, Mr. G was alert and agitated; however, he was oriented only to name and "a hospital" and could not state why he had been admitted. He told the consultant, "the nurses stole my clothes and my wallet! I'm going home! Where's my wife?" The consultant calmly heard Mr. G's concerns and offered reassurance that his belongings had been stored for safekeeping while he was in the hospital. Mr. G remained suspicious, but calmed somewhat after the consultant requested that staff retrieve his belongings and bring them to the patient.

When Mr. G's wife arrived for evening visitation hours, the consultant was able to organize a discussion with her, the nurse, and the night-float resident, whereby the reason for hospitalization was revisited with Mr. G. An interview conducted with Mr. G's wife alone revealed that he had got lost several times recently, and that she had taken over paying bills due to errors he had made over the past year. He had also become "confused" during a family trip the previous summer.

For the duration of his stay, Mr. G's personal effects were placed around him to create an atmosphere of familiarity, and the entire team worked to ensure that he was frequently re-oriented to date, location, and the purpose of admission. He was discharged without further incident, and an outpatient neuropsychology appointment was arranged.

EPIDEMIOLOGY

Improvements in public health, nutrition, and medical care for the elderly have led to a dramatic increase in the US population over the age of 65. Furthermore, those who live beyond the age of 90, the so-called oldest old, are the

TABLE 11-1 Clinical Features of Delirium, Depression, and Alzheimer's Disease

	DELIRIUM	DEPRESSION	ALZHEIMER'S DISEASE
Onset of initial symptoms	Abrupt Difficulty with attention and disturbed consciousness	Relatively discrete Dysphoric mood or lack of pleasure	Insidious Memory deficits—verbal and/or spatial
Course	Fluctuating—over days to weeks	Persistent—usually lasting months if untreated	Gradually progressive, over years
Family history	Not contributory	May be positive for depression	May be positive for AD
Memory	Poor registration	Patchy/inconsistent	Recent > remote
Memory complaints	Absent	Present	Variable—usually absent
Language deficits	Dysgraphia	Increased speech latency	Confrontation naming difficulties
Affect	Labile	Depressed/irritable	Variable—may be neutral

fastest-growing segment of the US population.[4] The significance of the aging population lies in the fact that age is a risk factor for dementia. Although the results of epidemiologic studies vary depending on the subjects sampled and the method employed, dementia occurs in approximately 14% of all individuals over the age of 71, rising to 37% in those over the age of 90 and 50% in older non-agenarians.[5,6] The global prevalence of dementia was estimated at over 35.6 million people in 2010; the number of people affected will double every 20 years, reaching over 115 million by 2050.[7]

The most common type of dementia (accounting for 50% to 70% of cases) is AD. Vascular dementia (which can have a number of different etiologies) is the second most common type of dementia and can exist independently, but frequently co-occurs with other dementias, especially AD. Dementia with Lewy bodies (DLB) is the next most common, followed by the less common forms of dementia, such as frontotemporal dementia (FTD), dementias associated with Parkinson's disease, and Creutzfeldt–Jakob disease (CJD).

DIAGNOSIS

In an effort to define disorders characterized by cognitive dysfunction, the *Diagnostic and Statistical Manual of Mental Disorders*, 5th edition (DSM-5) has replaced the term "dementia" with "major neurocognitive disorder".[8] The diagnosis of major NCD has also changed; memory impairment is no longer necessary but instead there must be a significant decline from previous level of functioning in at least one cognitive domain (e.g., memory, executive function, language, or social cognition).

Features of various NCDs may include aphasia (a difficulty with any aspect of language), apraxia (the impaired ability to perform motor tasks despite intact motor function), agnosia (an impairment in object recognition despite intact sensory function), or a disturbance of executive function (including the ability to think abstractly, as well as to plan, initiate, sequence, monitor, and stop complex behavior). Associated features include impaired judgment, poor insight, personality change, and psychiatric symptoms (e.g., persecutory delusions and hallucinations, particularly visual). Motor disturbances (falls, ataxia, parkinsonism, and extrapyramidal signs) and dysarthria (slurred speech) may be associated with certain NCDs.

Additional essential elements for a diagnosis of a major NCD include a significant impact on independent functioning and the occurrence of impairment outside the exclusive context of a delirium. These final criteria are necessary to rule out age-associated memory impairment, congenital mental retardation, and life-threatening acute confusional disorders.

Scores of specific disorders can cause cognitive impairment (Table 11-2). The consultant cannot have in-depth knowledge of all of them but can identify common or typical and rare or unusual presentations. In addition, certain associated physical findings can direct the consultant to particular diagnoses (Figure 11-1).

Many elderly individuals complain of memory difficulties, often involving learning new information or names or finding the right words. In most circumstances, such lapses are normal. The term *mild cognitive impairment (MCI)* was coined to label an intermediate category between the normal cognitive losses that are associated with aging and those linked with dementia, and correspond in the *DSM-5* to the diagnosis of mild NCD. MCI is characterized by a notable decline in memory or other cognitive functions compared with age-matched controls, without significant impairment in independent functioning. MCI is common among the elderly, although estimates vary widely depending on the diagnostic criteria and assessment methods employed; some, but not all, individuals with MCI progress to dementia. The identification of those at risk for progression of cognitive impairment is an active area of research.[9]

Neurocognitive Disorder Due to Alzheimer's Disease

Alzheimer's disease (AD) is a progressive, irreversible, and fatal brain disease that affects memory, thinking, and behavior. The classic brain lesions of AD are known as neurofibrillary tangles (composed of hyperphosphorylated tau protein) and neuritic plaques (composed of amyloid β peptides). Although a definitive diagnosis of AD relies upon postmortem findings of these lesions, detailed clinical assessments (by psychiatrists, neurologists, and neuropsychologists), in combination with use of structural and functional neuroimaging and certain biomarkers, have a high concordance rate with autopsy-proven disease.[10]

TABLE 11-2 Causes of Cognitive Impairment: Diagnoses by Categories With Representative Examples

Degenerative	HIV dementia
Alzheimer's disease	HIV-associated infection
Frontotemporal dementias	Syphilis
Dementia with Lewy bodies	Lyme encephalopathy
Corticobasal degeneration	Subacute sclerosing panencephalitis
Huntington's disease	Creutzfeldt–Jakob disease
Wilson's disease	Progressive multifocal leukoencephalopathy
Parkinson's disease	Parenchymal sarcoidosis
Multiple system atrophy	Chronic systemic infection
Progressive supranuclear palsy	**Demyelinating**
Psychiatric	Multiple sclerosis
Depression	Adrenoleukodystrophy
Schizophrenia	Metachromatic leukodystrophy
Vascular	**Autoimmune**
Vascular dementia	Systemic lupus erythematosus
Binswanger's encephalopathy	Polyarteritis nodosa
Amyloid dementia	**Drugs/Toxins**
Diffuse hypoxic/ischemic injury	*Medications*
Obstructive	Anticholinergics
Normal-pressure hydrocephalus	Antihistamines
Obstructive hydrocephalus	Anticonvulsants
Traumatic	β-blockers
Chronic subdural hematoma	Sedative–hypnotics
Chronic traumatic encephalopathy	*Substance Abuse*
Post-concussion syndrome	Alcohol
Neoplastic	Inhalants
Tumor—Malignant—primary and secondary	PCP
Tumor—Benign (e.g., frontal meningioma)	*Toxins*
Paraneoplastic limbic encephalitis	Arsenic
Infections	Bromide
Chronic meningitis	Carbon monoxide
Post-herpes encephalitis	Lead
Focal cerebritis/abscesses	Mercury
	Organophosphates

Progressive memory loss is the hallmark of AD. Other common cognitive clinical features include impairment of language, visual–spatial ability, and executive function. Patients may be unaware of their cognitive deficits, but this is not uniformly the case. There may be evidence of forgetting conversations, having difficulty with household finances, being disoriented to time and place, and misplacing items regularly. At least two domains of cognitive impairment, including progressive memory decline (that affects functional ability), are required to make a clinical diagnosis of AD.[11] In addition to its cognitive features, AD is associated with a number of neuropsychiatric symptoms, even in its mildest phases. In particular, irritability, apathy, and depression are common early in the course of the disease, whereas psychosis (including delusions and hallucinations) tends to occur later.[12]

Vascular Neurocognitive Disorder

Vascular neurocognitive disorder, commonly called vascular dementia, refers to a variety of vascular-related causes of dementia, including multi-infarct dementia and small-vessel disease. The pathophysiology of vascular dementia can be related to recurrent or localized embolic strokes, smaller subcortical strokes (e.g., lacunar infarcts), or cerebral hemorrhages. It is important to keep in mind that cerebral hemorrhages (resulting from hypertension or amyloid angiopathy) require a different type of clinical management than does typical vascular occlusive disease, and that dementia develops in 15% to 30% of patients after a stroke.[13]

The clinical features of vascular dementia depend on the localization of the lesions; both the type of cognitive deficits and the time course of the cognitive changes vary. Embolic or large-vessel stroke-related dementia often progresses in a step-wise pattern, with intervening periods of stability punctuated by abrupt declines in cognitive function. Although this might be considered the classic presentation, it is not the most common.[14] Presentations that involve relatively isolated psychotic symptoms in the setting of preserved memory should also raise the possibility of vascular dementia. Similarly, apathy, executive dysfunction, and a relatively intact memory are suggestive of a small-vessel ischemic process.

The main difficulty that arises in the diagnosis of vascular dementia is distinguishing it from AD. Classically, vascular dementia was distinguished from AD on the basis of an abrupt onset and a step-wise course, although with small-vessel, subcortical disease, acute changes may not be

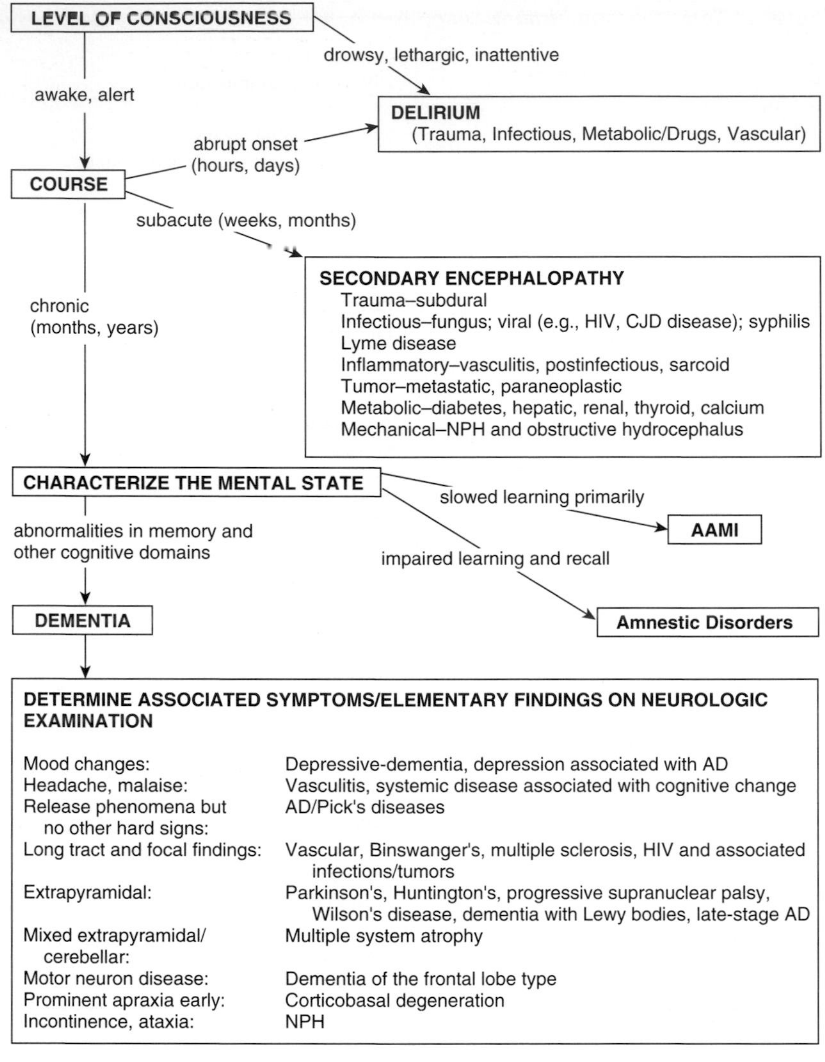

Figure 11-1. An algorithm for dementia diagnosis. AAMI, Age-associated memory impairment; CJD, Creutzfeldt–Jakob disease; AD, Alzheimer's disease; HIV, human immunodeficiency virus; NPH, normal-pressure hydrocephalus. *(Schmahmann JD: Neurobehavioral manifestations of focal cerebral lesions. In: Geriatric Psychiatry. Harvard Medical School and Massachusetts General Hospital Continuing Medical Education Course Syllabus. Boston, MA. 1995.)*

appreciated. In addition, prominent executive dysfunction and preserved recognition memory are also suggestive of vascular dementia. However, the symptoms of vascular dementia frequently overlap with those of AD; in fact, evidence of both is often found at autopsy.

Neurocognitive Disorder With Lewy Bodies

Neurocognitive disorder with Lewy bodies, or dementia with Lewy bodies (DLB), share clinical features of both AD and idiopathic Parkinson's disease (IPD); this makes accurate diagnosis a challenge. The main pathologic features of DLB are protein deposits called *Lewy bodies*, composed of α-synuclein in the cortex and brainstem.[15] Features that suggest DLB include parkinsonism, visual hallucinations (which occur early, in contrast to the pattern seen in AD), a fluctuating course, an extreme sensitivity to neuroleptic medications, autonomic dysfunction (with falls), and executive and visual–spatial dysfunction (with relatively spared language and memory function). Rapid eye movement (REM) sleep–behavior disorder may precede the onset of other symptoms by several years. As in IPD, depression is common. DLB differs from IPD in that in the former, motor symptoms occur within 1 year of the onset of cognitive problems; in contrast, motor symptoms in IPD typically precede cognitive problems by several years. Although these clinical features are helpful in the identification of the disease, clinical–pathologic concordance remains poor, and postmortem pathologic findings of Lewy bodies in the cerebral cortex, amygdala, and brainstem are necessary to confirm the diagnosis.[16]

Frontotemporal Neurocognitive Disorder

Frontotemporal neurocognitive disorder, or frontotemporal dementias (FTDs), are a heterogeneous group of disorders that involve degeneration of different regions of the frontal and temporal lobes, resulting in a variety of clinical presentations. Currently included under the category of FTDs are three clinical variants: behavioral-variant frontotemporal dementia (BV-FTD, accounting for 50% to 70% of FTD in the United States), and primary progressive aphasias, which are subdivided into a semantic variant PPA and a non-fluent variant PPA.[17] FTDs tend to manifest at younger ages than typical AD, with the majority of cases occurring in people younger than 65 years of age.

The classic hallmarks of FTD, particularly BV-FTD, are behavioral features, usually out of proportion to, or preceding, cognitive impairment. In general, there is a subtle onset and a progression of symptoms (with loss of judgment, disinhibition, impulsivity, loss of empathy and social tact, and interpersonal withdrawal). Other common symptoms are stereotypies, excessive oral–manual exploration, selective eating habits, wanderlust, excessive joviality, displays of sexually provocative behaviors, and use of inappropriate words or actions. In later stages, parkinsonism is common. Clinical presentations of FTD vary depending on the relative involvement of the hemisphere (right or left) or lobe (frontal or temporal) affected.[18] Patients may initially have more involvement of the right temporal lobe than the left and exhibit primarily a behavioral syndrome with emotional distance, irritability, and disruption of sleep, appetite, and libido. With greater initial left than right temporal lobe involvement, patients tend to exhibit more language-related problems, including anomia, word-finding difficulties, repetitive speech, and loss of semantic information (i.e., semantic variant PPA).[19] In some cases of FTD, the frontal lobes may be involved more than the temporal lobes. In these instances, patients exhibit symptoms of elation, disinhibition, apathy, or aberrant motor behavior.

Neurocognitive Disorder Due to Another Medical Condition

NCDs caused by other medical conditions include a broad range of disorders that are causally associated with cognitive impairment: structural lesions; trauma; infections; endocrine, nutritional, and metabolic disorders; and autoimmune diseases. Two notable examples include NCDs caused by normal-pressure hydrocephalus (NPH) and CJD.

NPH is recognized by the classic clinical features of gait disturbance, frontal systems dysfunction, and urinary incontinence.[20] Intermittent pressure increases are thought to cause ventricular expansion over time, with damage to the adjacent white matter tracts that connect the frontal lobes. Evaluation usually includes structural brain imaging (magnetic resonance imaging, MRI; or computed tomography, CT) that demonstrates ventricular enlargement that is out of proportion to the atrophy present.

CJD is a rare disorder that causes a characteristic triad of dementia, myoclonus, and distinctive periodic electroencephalographic (EEG) complexes. CJD is caused by prions, novel proteinaceous infective agents that induce changes in the cerebral cortex and lead to the distinctive microscopic, vacuolar appearance of spongiform encephalopathy. The cerebrospinal fluid in almost 90% of CJD cases contains traces of prion proteins detected by a routine lumbar puncture. Treatment of afflicted individuals is supportive, insofar as the condition follows a characteristic course, with death arriving after an average of 6 months.[21]

Substance/Medication-Induced Neurocognitive Disorder

To establish the diagnosis of substance/medication-induced NCD, there must be evidence from the history, physical examination, or laboratory data that cognitive deficits consistent with dementia are probably caused by exposure to a substance or medication. The diagnosis cannot be made during a period of acute intoxication or during drug withdrawal. The most common cause of this type of disorder is chronic alcohol use,[22] but toxins, poisons, inhalants, sedative–hypnotics, and other medications are also causes.

Neurocognitive Disorders Due to Multiple Etiologies

In the diagnostic section of the DSM-5, the phrase "neurocognitive disorder due to multiple etiologies" serves to emphasize that a patient can have more than one cause for cognitive decline. Although many combinations can occur, perhaps the most common is the co-existence of AD and vascular disease. Some authorities refute this assertion, suggesting that diffuse DLB is the second most common primary neurocognitive disorder and that its combination with AD is not sufficiently recognized.[23] AD can also co-exist with reversible causes of dementia (e.g., vitamin B_{12} deficiency, hypothyroidism), further emphasizing the importance of a thorough medical and neurologic work-up.

EVALUATION OF NEUROCOGNITIVE DISORDERS

Brain failure deserves at least as careful an assessment as the failure of any other organ. Only through thoughtful evaluation can remediation of the cognitive decline be possible. Although in most cases the goal of treatment is not a cure, there is still much that can be done to help afflicted patients and their families. The evaluation requires a reliable history (cognitive, psychiatric, medical, and family), complete medical and neurologic examinations, appropriate laboratory testing, and assessments of the mental status and cognitive function.

History

A meticulous cognitive history is an extremely sensitive diagnostic tool. Onset, course, and associated symptoms must be elicited carefully because these details of history often provide critical diagnostic clues. Because of time constraints, consultants may be inclined to limit their history-taking to the patient alone. Although some mildly impaired patients may have sufficient capacity to provide an accurate account of their deficits, many (owing to their amnesia, agnosia, or failure of insight) do not. To rely solely on the patient's report is unwise; it may be inaccurate, and it will be incomplete. Additional history is best obtained from people who frequently spend time with the patient, such as family members or close friends. It is important to interview informants away from the patient because informants are often uncomfortable discussing evidence of cognitive decline in the presence of the patient. Even a phone call to a family member or a friend can be helpful, as can a review of old medical records, when available.

A good cognitive history must establish the time at which cognitive changes first became apparent. This information provides important clues regarding the nature of the disorder because some diseases (e.g., CJD) are well known for causing a rapid rate of decline. If the time of onset of the disorder is known, the rate of decline can be estimated by seeing how long it has taken the patient to reach the current level of dysfunction. The rate of progression can only be approximated; however, it is helpful for family members to have such estimations so that plans for the future can be facilitated.

Next, it is important to determine the nature of the behavioral changes that were evident when the disease began. This information can also be helpful in the diagnostic process. For example, an early symptom of FTD is personality change, as manifested by inappropriate behavior, whereas the early symptoms of AD may involve increased passivity or apathy and a gradual, progressive decline in the ability to learn new information. Several years after the onset of the disease, when most patients are actually diagnosed, the cognitive symptoms of the two disorders may be quite similar, so information about the initial symptoms may be critical.

It is also important to determine whether the initial symptoms developed gradually or suddenly. If the onset of illness was insidious, as in AD, the family may realize only in retrospect that a decline has occurred. In contrast, a series of small strokes may produce symptoms of sudden onset, even if lesions were not evident on a CT scan or MRI of the head. Delirium generally has an acute onset as well. However, if it results from a condition such as a gradually developing drug toxicity, its onset may be subacute or insidious.

The manner in which symptoms have progressed also provides important diagnostic information. Stepwise deterioration characterized by sudden exacerbation of symptoms is typical of vascular dementia. A physical illness (e.g., pneumonia, a hip fracture) in a patient with AD, however, can also cause a sudden decline in cognitive function. Thus, careful questioning is necessary to determine the underlying cause of a step-wise decline in function.

Accurate histories of cognitive function are difficult to obtain because most patients and family members are not attuned to subtle behavioral changes. Important aspects of the medical history may not be recognized. For example, the family may state that the first symptoms of the disease were the patient's anxiety and depression about work. Only after further inquiry will family members remember several episodes that preceded the onset of work-related anxiety in which the patient could not remember how to deal with a complex situation or learn how to use new equipment.

Family members may also have difficulty understanding why certain subtle distinctions are important for diagnosis. For example, they may report that the patient's first symptom was forgetfulness, but when asked to provide instances of this forgetfulness, they may explain that the patient had difficulty installing a new knob in the kitchen or had trouble finding a familiar location. Both features would suggest spatial difficulty more than memory difficulty. In addition, an unwillingness to admit that certain impairments exist may prevent family members from providing accurate information.

Finally, family members may even misinterpret direct questions. Although a history of a gradual, progressive decline is essential to the diagnosis of AD, informants frequently state that the disorder came on suddenly because they suddenly became aware that something was wrong. This realization by the family often coincides with external events (e.g., a trip to an unfamiliar place prevented the patient from employing over-learned habits and routines and thus exposed the cognitive decline). The hospital is obviously one such setting; it is not uncommon for family members to state, "He was fine until he got here!" When this appears, it is necessary to determine when subtle symptoms of cognitive change first occurred. Usually, family members can recall episodes that they had previously ignored that suggest an earlier change in cognitive function. Annual family gatherings or holiday events are useful occasions about which to inquire.

It is also important to determine the patient's current functional status. This information is best obtained in an informal manner by asking about the patient's typical day. Alternatively, scales, such as the activities of daily living (ADL) and the instrumental activities of daily living (IADL) scales (Table 11-3), have been developed for this purpose. The ADL scale surveys six basic areas of function and determines whether the individual can perform these tasks independently or with assistance.[24] The IADL scale provides a sense of a patient's executive functions.[25] A substantial discrepancy between the functional and cognitive status of the patient generally suggests the presence of a psychiatric illness. For purposes of comfort, safety, rehabilitation, and determination of appropriate level of care, ADL and IADL results should be evaluated carefully.

The psychiatric history, with particular attention paid to reports of past mood or psychotic disorders, may assist in the differentiation of cognitive changes observed in depression from those of a primary NCD. Although cognitive changes can be seen in depression, the history and mental status examination usually allow the physician to separate

TABLE 11-3 Assessment of Functional Status

ACTIVITIES OF DAILY LIVING (ADL)	INSTRUMENTAL ACTIVITIES OF DAILY LIVING (IADL)
Bathing	Ability to use telephone
Dressing	Shopping
Toileting	Food preparation
Transferring	Housekeeping
Continence	Laundry
Feeding	Mode of transportation
	Responsibility for own medications
	Ability to handle finances

Adapted from Katz S, Downs TD, Cash HR et al: Progress in the development of the index of ADL, Gerontologist 10:20–30, 1970; and Lawton MP, Brody EM: Assessment of older people: self-maintaining and instrumental activities of daily living, Gerontologist 9: 179–186, 1969.

depression from a NCD or suggest that both are present. Neurovegetative symptoms of depression may be difficult to link specifically to mood or cognitive disorders because anergia, sleep disturbance, and appetite changes can be seen in both depression and NCDs. Thus, it is important to modify the questions asked to encompass the possibility of cognitive impairment. For example, if the tasks are simplified and within the capabilities of a non-depressed, demented patient, the patient is typically able to carry them out. Similarly, if food is presented in a manner that the patient can manage, such as meat cut into bite-size pieces, the patient may show a newfound gusto in his or her appetite (see Table 11-1).

In reviewing the medical history, the physician should consider whether surgical procedures (e.g., gastrectomy predisposing to vitamin B_{12} deficiency) or medical illnesses (e.g., hypertension, systemic lupus erythematosus) contribute to the symptoms of cognitive dysfunction. It is crucial to determine whether the patient was exposed to toxins (e.g., lead or other heavy metals, carbon monoxide), or has a history of head trauma. Careful questioning should cover alcohol and drug usage (not just current patterns), including a past history of abuse or overuse. Many non-psychotropic agents, including those sold over-the-counter, can have negative effects on cognition. For example, antihistamines and antispasmodic drugs can cause cognitive difficulties. Valuable historical data include information regarding impairments in hearing or vision, incontinence, falls, and gait disturbances.

The family history is also helpful. Certain NCDs (e.g., Huntington's disease) have definite genetic modes of transmission (e.g., autosomal dominant), whereas for others (e.g., certain vascular dementias) the specific mode of transmission may be unclear, but their prevalence is much higher in affected families than in the population at large. Several familial subtypes of AD with genetic loci have been identified. An estimated 7% of cases with an onset before the age of 60 are familial, with an autosomal dominant inheritance. Several genes, including beta-amyloid precursor protein and presenilin 1 and 2, have been associated with early-onset AD.[26] For the majority of patients with AD, there appears to be a complex interaction among genetic and other factors.[27,28] Variations in the gene for apolipoprotein E (APOE) may increase the risk of developing AD or predispose to earlier onset,[27] and APOE remains the only documented late-onset AD gene.[28]

Medical and Neurologic Examination

The consultant should review recent examinations in the medical record to assess their adequacy and accuracy. The cognitive portion of prior examinations may note only that the patient was alert and oriented. Additionally, if notes report "disorientation," it is often unclear from the chart whether the patient could not remember the day of the week or whether he or she was confused or psychotic. Consequently, the psychiatric consultant should look for medical and neurologic findings that are associated with NCDs. For example, focal areas of muscle weakness and pyramidal signs may suggest vascular dementia. The presence of extrapyramidal movements may point to one of the NCDs that principally affects subcortical motor areas. Mild to moderate AD, however, may also be associated with extrapyramidal symptoms (EPS) and other neurologic signs.[29] A comprehensive neurologic examination should include careful assessment of ocular function, gait, and praxis, as well as the presence of any frontal release signs.

Laboratory Examination

Table 11-4 lists laboratory and other tests that are typically ordered as part of a dementia evaluation. Whenever possible and appropriate, results of prior testing in other settings should be obtained. For example, a chest x-ray examination or CT scan should not be re-ordered if one was recently done unless an acute change has occurred. Additional tests (e.g., serum copper and ceruloplasmin for Wilson's disease or serum and urine porphyrins for acute intermittent porphyria) should be requested when the history and examination suggest a particular disorder.

Mental Status Examination

The bedside psychiatric examination covers considerable territory, but it focuses on assessments of affective and psychotic signs and symptoms. The physician should probe

TABLE 11-4 Recommended Laboratory Studies in a Dementia Work-Up
Blood Studies
Complete blood cell count
Vitamin B_{12}
Folate
Sedimentation rate
Glucose
Calcium
Phosphorus
Magnesium
Electrolytes
Liver function tests
Thyroid-stimulating hormone
Creatinine, blood urea nitrogen
Cholesterol (high-density lipoprotein/low-density lipoprotein)
Triglycerides
Syphilis serology
HIV testing
Other Studies
Urinalysis
Electrocardiogram
CT or MRI
Representative Additional Studies Based on History and Physical Findings
Chest x-ray examination
Electroencephalogram
Non-invasive carotid studies
Rheumatoid factor, antinuclear antibody, and other autoimmune disorder screens
Lumbar puncture
Drug levels
Heavy metal screening

CT, computed tomography; HIV, human immunodeficiency virus; MRI, magnetic resonance imaging.

for mood symptoms, irritability or tearfulness, and nihilistic or suicidal thinking. Depressed elderly patients may, among their somatic complaints, describe decrements in memory. Depressed patients, as opposed to patients with AD, however, may perform better on more difficult memory tasks than on simple ones. Depressed patients are also more likely to show poor effort on testing (e.g., "I don't know" answers) compared with patients with AD, who are more likely to confabulate when they don't know an answer.

Positive psychotic symptoms can be present in primary psychiatric disorders, such as psychotic depression or schizophrenia, but they can also be suggestive of delirium or dementia. The prevalence of psychosis in moderate to severe AD is estimated at approximately 40%, with delusions predominating over hallucinations.[30] Usually, delusions in patients with AD are of a paranoid nature, often involving the mistaken belief that misplaced items have been stolen. With progression of the disease, so-called *delusional misidentification syndromes* develop, with the patient believing that loved ones are actually imposters (i.e., Capgras syndrome).[31] Illusions and hallucinations, usually of a visual nature, tend to occur with advanced AD. For example, some patients describe seeing "little people" entering their homes. Despite their unusual nature, not all hallucinations or delusions are troublesome to the patient. Mood and psychotic symptoms can occur as part of the clinical picture of many NCDs. Generally, they are non-specific. However, taken together with other elements of the assessment, such symptoms can provide clues as to whether a psychiatric disorder or a NCD is present.

Bedside Neurocognitive Assessment

Domains of cognitive function that require rapid and accurate bedside assessment can be remembered with the mnemonic "A CALM VISAGE" (the face the consultant would put forward when confronted with a patient who is difficult to diagnose). These domains include the following: Attention, Conceptualization, Appearance/behavior, Language, Memory, VISual–spatial, Agnosia and apraxia, General intelligence, and Executive function.

Attention is important to consider because simple attentional abilities must be preserved if any other cognitive task is to be performed adequately. If the patient has difficulty concentrating on a task for even a few minutes at a time, assessment of other domains will likely be inaccurate. For this reason, attention is evaluated first. Auditory and visual attention can be assessed easily by means of digit span and letter cancellation tests. For the digit span test, the patient is asked to repeat a series of numbers spaced 1 second apart. The examiner provides gradually increasing spans; unimpaired individuals are able to repeat five to seven numbers. For the letter cancellation test, the patient is asked to cross off a particular letter each time he or she observes it in any series of letters. A gross assessment can be inferred from how well the patient responds to questions during an interview. The physician should note whether the level of arousal appears to fluctuate or the patient seems easily distracted during the interview.

Tasks that examine conceptualization include tests of concept formation, abstraction, set-shifting, and set-maintenance. Similarities and proverbs are useful in this regard.

Observation of appearance and behavior is helpful in determining whether patients are able to care adequately for themselves. Detecting that a patient's buttons are misaligned, for example, may suggest that he or she has spatial difficulties or an apraxia.

Language testing for aphasia should include evaluation of comprehension, repetition, reading, writing, and naming. If aphasia has been ruled out or is not suspected, confrontation naming (e.g., of objects and their parts, such as jacket and lapel or watch and strap) should be included in an assessment of the older individual because impairments in naming ability (anomia) occur with age but are prominent in a number of disorders, including AD. In addition, alterations in verbal fluency (tested by having the patient name as many animals or words beginning with a certain letter as possible in a minute) are seen in many neurocognitive diseases.[32]

The presence of memory dysfunction, despite no longer being essential in the *DSM*, remains highly common and important in the diagnosis of a NCD. The nature and severity of the memory impairment can serve as a guide to diagnosis, but the assessment of memory is complicated by the fact that changes in memory capacity normally occur with aging. Normal elders may require more time to retain new information. Therefore careful testing is important to differentiate normal from pathologic memory performance. Testing should include not only short-term memory but also memory of personal events (e.g., details of marriage, names of children) and significant historical dates (e.g., John F. Kennedy's assassination, September 11).

Assessment of visual–spatial abilities may be more difficult in older than in younger individuals because of the frequency of visual–sensory deficits in the elderly. It is difficult to enlarge certain test stimuli to evaluate this domain; therefore figure copying (e.g., of intersecting pentagons or a cube) is the most useful method of assessment.

When agnosia or apraxia is evident, the patient's disease is usually quite advanced. *Agnosia* is diagnosed when a patient fails to recognize a familiar object, despite intact sensory function. With *apraxia*, the patient's ability to carry out motor tasks is impaired, despite intact motor systems and an understanding of the tasks. For example, the patient is unable to mimic the use of common objects (e.g., use of a toothbrush) or to carry out well-learned motor behaviors (e.g., pretending to blow out a candle). A subtle finding is "organification of praxis" in which the subject, for example, uses a finger as the toothbrush.

In addition to the areas of assessment previously mentioned, the examiners should estimate general intelligence to determine whether the patient has access to previously acquired knowledge. A rough approximation can be inferred from the patient's highest level of education. Alternatively, the vocabulary subtest of *The Wechsler Adult Intelligence Scale–Revised* can be used to estimate level of intelligence.[33]

A simple, yet often revealing measure of executive functioning is the clock-drawing test, where the patient is asked to draw a clock face with the hands set at a non-simple time, such as "ten past eleven" or "ten to two."

Standardized Cognitive Testing

Non-standard testing developed by the clinician can be used to evaluate the cognitive domains noted previously, but a variety of standardized, brief mental status tests can be useful as well. However, although screening tests may identify cognitive difficulties, they are not sufficient to establish a diagnosis of dementia.

Commonly used screening tests are the Mini-Mental State Examination (MMSE)[32] and the Blessed Dementia Scale.[34] Both have high test–retest reliability, and are relatively brief, taking 5 to 15 minutes to administer. Historically, the MMSE has been the most often used in clinical settings because it assesses a broad range of cognitive abilities (i.e., attention, concentration, memory, language, spatial ability, and set-shifting) in a simple, straightforward manner. Scores on the MMSE range from 0 to 30, with scores above 26 generally indicating normal cognitive function. Mildly impaired patients typically obtain MMSE scores of 20 to 26; moderate impairment is reflected in scores of 11 to 20; and severe impairment is indicated by scores of 10 or lower. A cut-off score of 23 is generally recommended as suggestive of cognitive dysfunction; however, the application of this cut-off score must be modified in light of the patient's education level. For example, an extremely bright, well-educated patient may score 29 or 30, despite having significant impairment.

The MMSE is a useful screening tool in the assessment of demented patients with mild to moderate cognitive impairments, but it is less helpful in the evaluation of severely impaired patients. The quantification of cognitive abilities in severely impaired patients can serve a variety of needs, including the ability to follow patients throughout an intervention trial, the assessment of spared abilities (which health care professionals can use in the development of management strategies), and the examination of the relationship among post-mortem neurochemical and neuropathologic findings and cognitive status shortly before death. The Test for Severe Impairment (TSI) is a useful scale for severely impaired patients that can contribute to improved patient management.[35] It minimizes the need for the patient to use language skills because severely impaired patients often have minimal intact verbal skills. Nonetheless, the TSI can evaluate motor performance, language comprehension, language production, immediate and delayed memory, general knowledge, and conceptualization.

Patients with MCI/mild NCD often score within the normal range on the dementia screening tools discussed previously. The Montreal Cognitive Assessment (MoCA) was created as a 10-minute screening tool to assist in the detection of MCI.[36] It assesses many cognitive domains, and although somewhat more challenging than the MMSE, it assesses executive and abstract functions in a superior manner. Components of the visual–spatial and executive function testing include a brief "Trails B," copying a cube, and drawing a clock. The MoCA is available free of charge for non-commercial clinical use and available online (www.mocatest.org) in a multitude of languages (Figure 11-2). As the MoCA covers additional cognitive domains, and may be more sensitive than the MMSE in detecting MCI, it is increasingly used as the initial measurement of choice at some institutions.[37]

With all structured tests, the examiner must not simply look at the total score but rather assess the qualitative areas of low and high function. The pattern of deficits may confirm a diagnostic opinion. Conversely, determining that areas of function have been preserved assists the clinician in making recommendations to the patient and the family for adaptive coping with the dementia.

TREATMENT CONSIDERATIONS

The approach to treatment of an NCD depends on the specific diagnosis established as well as on the troublesome symptoms and signs that must be managed. Treatment is divided into three broad categories: medical and surgical interventions, behavioral interventions, and pharmacotherapy. Pharmacotherapy can be divided further into treatments for cognitive symptoms and neuropsychiatric symptoms of dementia.

Medical and Surgical Interventions

Some NCDs can be helped dramatically by surgical interventions. For example, the treatment for NPH is removal of cerebrospinal fluid by way of a lumbar puncture or ventriculoperitoneal shunting. It is important to perform cognitive and motor testing before and after the removal of a large volume of cerebrospinal fluid.[38] Similarly, draining of frontal subdural hematomas can improve patients' cognition and behavior.

Other reversible medical disorders that cause dementia should be corrected. For example, thyroid repletion in the myxedematous patient improves cognitive function. In many conditions, however, damage has already been done, and repletion may provide only marginal improvement. For example, a patient who had deteriorated over several years was found to have an extremely low vitamin B_{12} level. Her dementia was profound, and it did not respond to intramuscular injections of vitamin B_{12}. Further deterioration of her cognition and other nervous system functions, however, may have been prevented by the treatment.

Sometimes the reduction or elimination of drugs can be helpful. For example, elimination of highly anticholinergic (e.g. diphenhydramine, oxybutynin) or sedative-hypnotic medications (e.g., diazepam) can lead to improvement in drug-induced memory impairment. Care must be taken, however, to avoid a withdrawal syndrome caused by too abrupt a discontinuation, especially with benzodiazepines and barbiturates.

Searching for treatable contributors to cognitive decline is important, even when the principal diagnosis is AD. Identification of co-existing medical conditions that have a deleterious effect on the patient's cognition is critical. For example, the aggressive treatment of a urinary tract infection improves not only physical comfort but also intellectual function (because infection in the setting of AD usually causes delirium). Pain, too, may have a negative effect on cognition and is often overlooked in patients with dementia admitted to the general hospital.[39] A patient whose AD was manageable at home became severely aggressive and more confused owing to the discomfort of an impacted bowel. Another patient with presumed vascular dementia showed

MONTREAL COGNITIVE ASSESSMENT (MoCA)

NAME :
Education :
Sex :
Date of birth :
DATE :

VISUOSPATIAL / EXECUTIVE

[ ]

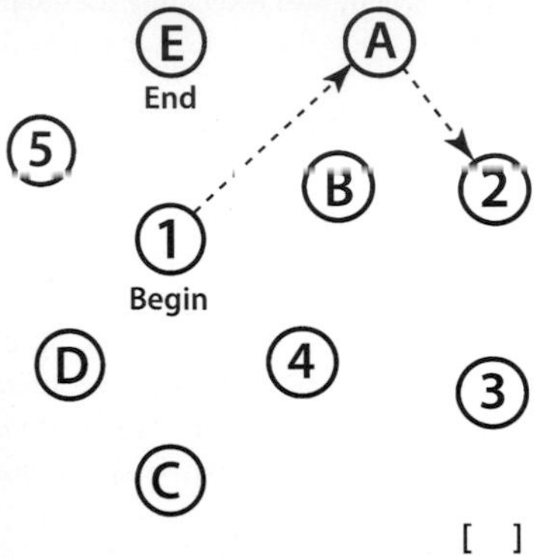

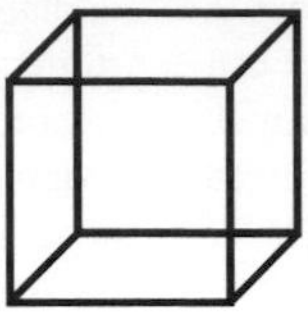

Copy cube [ ]

Draw CLOCK (Ten past eleven) (3 points)

[ ] Contour [ ] Numbers [ ] Hands

POINTS ___/5

NAMING

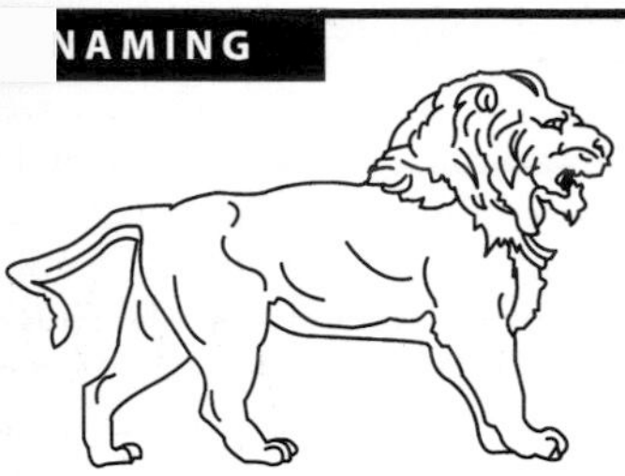

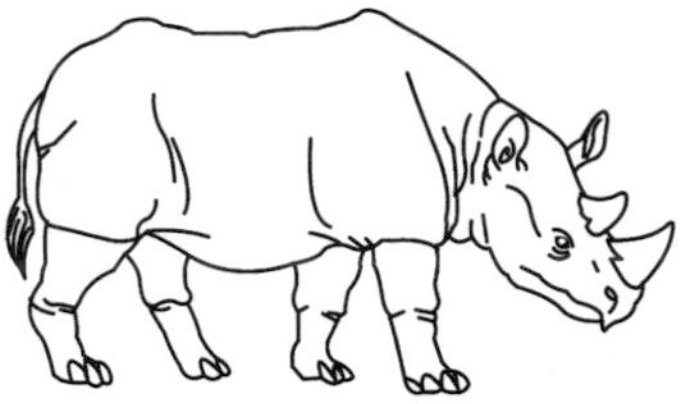

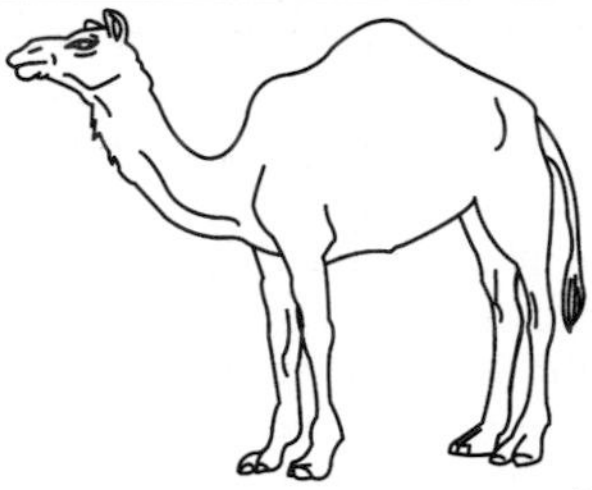

[ ] [ ] [ ] ___/3

MEMORY Read list of words, subject must repeat them. Do 2 trials, even if 1st trial is successful. Do a recall after 5 minutes.

	FACE	VELVET	CHURCH	DAISY	RED
1st trial					
2nd trial					

No points

ATTENTION Read list of digits (1 digit/ sec.). Subject has to repeat them in the forward order [ ] 2 1 8 5 4
Subject has to repeat them in the backward order [ ] 7 4 2 ___/2

Read list of letters. The subject must tap with his hand at each letter A. No points if ≥ 2 errors
[ ] F B A C M N A A J K L B A F A K D E A A A J A M O F A A B ___/1

Serial 7 subtraction starting at 100 [ ] 93 [ ] 86 [ ] 79 [ ] 72 [ ] 65
4 or 5 correct subtractions: **3 pts**, 2 or 3 correct: **2 pts**, 1 correct: **1 pt**, 0 correct: **0 pt** ___/3

LANGUAGE Repeat : I only know that John is the one to help today. [ ]
The cat always hid under the couch when dogs were in the room. [ ] ___/2

Fluency / Name maximum number of words in one minute that begin with the letter F [ ] _____ (N ≥ 11 words) ___/1

ABSTRACTION Similarity between e.g. banana - orange = fruit [ ] train – bicycle [ ] watch - ruler ___/2

DELAYED RECALL	Has to recall words **WITH NO CUE**	FACE [ ]	VELVET [ ]	CHURCH [ ]	DAISY [ ]	RED [ ]	Points for UNCUED recall only	___/5
Optional	Category cue							
	Multiple choice cue							

ORIENTATION [ ] Date [ ] Month [ ] Year [ ] Day [ ] Place [ ] City ___/6

© Z.Nasreddine MD Version 7.1 **www.mocatest.org** Normal ≥26 / 30 TOTAL ___/30
Administered by: ____________ Add 1 point if ≤ 12 yr edu

Figure 11-2. The Montreal Cognitive Assessment (MoCA). *(Copyright Z. Nasreddine M.D. Reproduced with permission. The test and instructions may be accessed at* www.mocatest.org.*)*

some improvement in cognition after treatment for congestive heart failure.

Behavioral Interventions

Once drug effects and contributing medical conditions are identified and managed, acute behavioral symptoms associated with dementia may subside. The environmental strangeness of the hospital, however, may be enough to trigger new psychiatric and behavioral problems, such as paranoid ideation and agitation.

Often, behavioral management alone reduces certain symptoms. Non-pharmacologic interventions are considered first-line treatment because there is evidence to support efficacy and minimal potential for adverse events; therefore, they should be used in every case.[40,41] The basic approaches are well known but bear repeating (Table 11-5). When considering behavioral interventions, always remember the ABCs of behavioral analysis: antecedent, behavior, and consequences. For example, a patient is easily upset and confused when she cannot remember her nurse; as a result, she yells and sometimes throws things at the nurse when she comes into the room, putting both the patient and nurse in danger (e.g., from inadvertent removal of intravenous lines or being struck by thrown objects). When tailoring behavioral interventions, the physician should consider each aspect of the behavioral analysis. Possible solutions to the aforementioned case include posting the names of providers in the patient's room, removing potentially dangerous objects from within reach of the patient's bed, and reassuring the patient.

The manner in which staff members communicate with the patient is also important. Speaking loudly enough (but not too loudly) is a critical first step. Decreased hearing acuity affects all elders, but this does not mean that shouting is necessary. The content of what is said should be simple and to the point. If the patient has considerable expressive language difficulties, questions should be framed so that a yes-or-no response is adequate. Reassurance and distraction are preferred responses to patients who are paranoid or easily distressed.[42]

TABLE 11-5 Examples of Behavioral Management for Dementia Patients

Re-orient to the environment (e.g., clock, calendar); post names of care providers
Simplify communication (e.g., yes/no questions)
Reassure, distract, and re-direct (e.g., familiar pictures from home)
Use eyeglasses and hearing aids appropriately
Encourage activity and exercise
Offer soothing therapies (e.g., music therapy or aromatherapy)
Provide one-on-one supervision

Pharmacotherapy

Cognitive Symptoms

Pharmacotherapies in dementia target both cognitive decline and the neuropsychiatric symptoms of dementia. Because AD is associated with cholinergic dysfunction, cholinesterase inhibitors (ChE-Is) have been developed and are now widely used in treatment (Table 11-6). The commonly used ChE-Is in the United States include donepezil, rivastigmine, and galantamine. A fourth agent, tacrine, was discontinued in 2013 because of its association with hepatotoxicity. The ChE-Is differ in their pharmacologic properties, administration regimens, drug interactions, and effect on hepatic enzymes. The most common side effects include nausea, vomiting and diarrhea; other bothersome adverse effects include insomnia or vivid dreams, fatigue, muscle cramps, incontinence, bradycardia, and syncope. As a result, these drugs may be contraindicated in the setting of bradycardia or sick sinus syndrome; severe asthma and peptic ulcer disease may also be relative contraindications. A patch form is now available for rivastigmine, which appears to decrease its gastrointestinal side effects.

In patients with AD, all the ChE-Is have been shown to slow progression of cognitive and functional decline, as well as to potentially improve neuropsychiatric symptoms (see below).[43,44] Treatment with these agents should begin as early as possible in patients with AD.[45] Evidence suggests use of ChE-Is is also warranted in dementia related to vascular disease[46] and a recent meta-analysis supported the use of ChE-Is in Parkinson's disease dementia, though efficacy in DLB was unclear.[47]

Goals of therapy with ChE-Is include a delay in cognitive decline, a delay of functional decline, and treatment or prevention (or both) of the development of behavioral symptoms. It is important to note that the downhill slope of the illness will continue. ChE-Is also have a small beneficial effect on burden and active time use among caregivers of persons with AD.[48]

Memantine, an N-methyl-D-aspartate antagonist, is approved by the Food and Drug Administration for treatment

TABLE 11-6 Characteristics of Cholinesterase Inhibitors

DRUG	CHEMICAL CLASS	TOTAL DAILY DOSE	REGIMEN	ADVERSE EVENTS
Donepezil	Piperidine	5–10 mg	Daily	GI, headaches, weakness
Rivastigmine	Carbamate	6–12 mg (oral), 4.6–9.5 mg (transdermal)	Twice daily (oral) or daily (transdermal)	GI, headaches, dizziness
Galantamine	Tertiary alkaloid	16–24 mg	Once daily (extended release) or twice daily (immediate release)	GI, insomnia

Adapted from Daly EJ, Falk WE, Brown, P: Cholinesterase inhibitors for behavioral disturbance in dementia, *Curr Psychiatry Rep* 2001; 3:251–258.
GI, gastrointestinal.

of moderate to severe AD. Memantine normalizes levels of glutamate, a neurotransmitter involved in learning and memory, and which in excessive quantities is thought to contribute to neurodegeneration. Common side effects include dizziness, agitation, headache, and confusion. Evidence indicates that adding memantine to the regimen of patients with moderate to severe AD (who were already receiving stable doses of donepezil) results in better outcomes on measures of cognition, ADL, and behavior.[49,50]

Initiating pharmacotherapy for cognitive symptoms is not usually in the domain of the psychiatric consultant in the general hospital; this is typically the work of outpatient treaters. However, one reason to consider starting these medications in an inpatient medical setting might be to monitor for side effects and tolerability in patients with significant co-morbid medical illnesses. Initiation of ChE-Is may also be considered in this setting for treatment of neuropsychiatric symptoms, as described later. The consultant may be asked to consider reasons to stop ChE-Is, such as side effects, new medical contraindications, poor compliance, or rapid decline in the patient's illness. Any benefits of treatment are rapidly lost upon discontinuation.

Neuropsychiatric Symptoms

Behavioral interventions remain the first-line treatment for managing the neuropsychiatric symptoms of NCDs.[51] However, particularly in the acute hospital setting, pharmacotherapy may also be useful, although certain symptoms are poorly responsive to drug therapies. For example, the motor restlessness and wandering behavior seen in patients with AD are typically non-responsive to medications; in addition, some treatments (e.g., neuroleptics that cause akathisia) may actually aggravate the problem.[52] When other symptoms, such as visual hallucinations or delusions, cause no distress to the patient and are not dangerous, medication is not required. When treatment is necessary, the golden rule of geriatric pharmacotherapy is, "Start low and go slowly." This maxim applies whether target symptoms relate to apathy, depression, psychosis, agitation, or some combination of these domains.

Apathy is the most common behavioral change in AD.[53] It is defined as a lack of motivation relative to the prior level of function, with a decrease in goal-directed behaviors, goal-directed cognition, and emotional responsiveness.[54] The lack of motivation must not be attributable to intellectual impairment, emotional distress, or a diminished level of consciousness. It is important to distinguish apathy from depression in patients with dementia because the treatments are different (Table 11-7). Treatments for apathy include use of psychostimulants,[55] dopamine agonists (e.g., bupropion, amantadine),[56] and ChE-Is.[57]

The depressive component of any dementia should be assessed and treated aggressively. If the degree to which affective symptoms are contributing to cognitive dysfunction is unclear, a therapeutic trial of an antidepressant should be employed. Choice of an agent is based principally on the side effects it produces; other considerations include drug–drug interactions and cost. The selective serotonin reuptake inhibitors (SSRIs, e.g., citalopram, sertraline), as well as bupropion and mirtazapine have favorable side effect profiles and should be considered. However, there is a paucity of literature to support their use in depression associated with dementia, given somewhat mixed findings on efficacy in recent meta-analyses.[58,59] Additionally, a large, multicenter trial developed by a consensus panel assembled by the National Institute of Mental Health found no difference between administration of 100 mg of sertraline to the placebo-treated group.[60] Care should be taken to avoid those drugs with greater anticholinergic side effects (e.g., paroxetine). Nortriptyline has been used effectively in depression following strokes and is generally well-tolerated. Tertiary amine tricyclic antidepressants (TCAs) that are highly anticholinergic (e.g., amitriptyline, imipramine) should be avoided.

Hallucinations (particularly visual), delusions (e.g., paranoid, persecutory, somatic), and agitation (which can take the form of motor restlessness, verbal outbursts, or physical aggression) are common in patients with dementia.[61] Before any medication is instituted, reversible causes (e.g., infection, pain, drug effects) should be investigated. If the symptoms are causing significant distress and placing the patient or caregiver at risk, and if non-pharmacologic interventions have failed, the first-line treatment is an antipsychotic medication.

First-generation or typical antipsychotics (e.g., haloperidol, trifluoperazine, perphenazine, thiothixene) have been well studied and show modest improvement in target symptoms.[62] However, elderly patients may be particularly sensitive to the side effects of these agents (e.g., sedation, postural hypotension, EPS), and are at particularly increased risk for developing tardive dyskinesia.[63] Second-generation or atypical antipsychotics (e.g., risperidone) have also been well studied in patients with dementia, however, direct comparison of atypical antipsychotics in the CATIE-AD trial (which randomized patients to olanzapine, quetiapine, risperidone, or placebo) found no differences among treatments in the main outcome, time to all-cause discontinuation.[64] Meta-analyses of randomized controlled trials of atypical antipsychotics have found small but statistically significant improvements in neuropsychiatric symptoms of dementia;[65] however, in other studies, trials were limited by high drop-out rates, side effects, and worsening of cognition.[66]

Further complicating the picture is the evidence showing an increased risk of cerebrovascular adverse events in patients with dementia taking atypical antipsychotics.[67] The risk of death in patients taking typical antipsychotics is comparable with or higher than the rates in patients taking atypical antipsychotics.[68–70] More recent data have found that the use of both typical and atypical antipsychotic drugs carries a similar, dose-related increased risk of sudden cardiac death.[71]

TABLE 11-7 Apathy Versus Depression in Alzheimer's Disease

	APATHY	DEPRESSION
Mood	Blunted	Dysphoric
Attitude	Indifferent	Pessimistic, hopeless
Self-concept	Bland	Self-critical
Thoughts/actions	Decreased initiative and persistence	Guilty, suicidal

Thus, the clinician facing the challenge of treating a dementia patient with psychosis or agitation must carefully weigh the risk of not treating neuropsychiatric symptoms against the risks of the treatment previously discussed. This requires consideration of the evidence supporting efficacy of a given agent, the morbidity and risk associated with the target symptoms, the patient's medical conditions, and the risks and benefits of the proposed antipsychotic being considered. It is essential that the clinician obtain informed consent from the patient's healthcare decision-maker before starting any antipsychotic medications. In general, dosing of atypical antipsychotics is lower in elderly patients than other populations. In addition to oral forms, some agents may be administered intramuscularly when required.[72] Usage should be reassessed periodically, particularly because target symptoms may subside with disease progression, and adverse events, such as tardive movement disorders, occur frequently in this population and typically do not resolve spontaneously.[73]

Treatment of psychosis and agitation associated with Parkinson's disease requires special mention. High-potency neuroleptics may aggravate tremor and bradykinesia and should be avoided. Clozapine has been found to be useful in controlling psychotic symptoms in patients with Parkinson's disease and DLB;[74,75] however, careful consideration of risk is necessary, given a recent study found use of antipsychotics is associated with an increased mortality risk in patients with Parkinson's disease.[76] In 2016, the US Food and Drug Administration approved pimavanserin, the first drug to be given an indication for treatment of hallucinations and delusions specifically associated with Parkinson's disease.

Several additional medications can be used in addition to antipsychotics in patients with agitation. The short-acting lorazepam (in an oral dosage of 0.25 to 1 mg) may be helpful when administered before an uncomfortable or potentially frightening procedure, such as a lumbar puncture or MRI scan. However, due to the many risks associated with use of benzodiazepines in the elderly (e.g. falls, hip fractures, sedation, worsening cognition), protracted use of benzodiazepines, especially long-acting agents or those with active metabolites (e.g. diazepam, clonazepam), is discouraged.[77–79] The use of buspirone for treatment of agitation has been reported, but at least a few weeks are necessary to achieve a modest benefit with this agent.[80]

Among the antidepressants, a Cochrane review found sertraline and citalopram to be beneficial in reducing agitation, and SSRIs and trazodone were generally well tolerated when compared to antipsychotics.[81] More recently, a randomized control trial showed citalopram to be beneficial in reducing agitation in patients with AD, although patients in the citalopram arm experienced worsening of cognition and QTc interval prolongation.[82] Trazodone has been the subject of many case reports demonstrating behavioral improvement in agitated, demented patients,[83] and has been found effective at decreasing irritability, agitation, depressive symptoms and eating disorders in a small, randomized controlled trial in patients with FTD.[84]

Trazodone has also been found effective for treatment of sleep disturbances in patients with AD, with sedative effects usually rapidly achieved at a dose of 50 mg.[85] Although generally well-tolerated, trazodone may induce postural hypotension and priapism. Evidence also supports use of melatonin to treat sleep disturbance in dementia, showing improvement in sleep efficacy and total sleep time, with no reports of severe adverse events.[86]

Mood stabilizers and other anticonvulsants have been used to treat agitation associated with dementia. While valproic acid has shown some promise in case reports and open label studies, results of meta-analyses of fully blinded, randomized controlled trials have not supported its routine use for treating agitation in demented patients.[87,88] Pooled data for carbamazepine have been mixed, although two randomized trials found efficacy supporting its use.[88] In these studies, both valproate and carbamazepine were better tolerated than atypical antipsychotics and efficacy was achieved in many cases at subtherapeutic dose ranges. However, drug–drug interactions need to be closely monitored when using these agents. The use of gabapentin and lamotrigine have been shown to be modestly effective in case series, although no randomized studies have been published.[89] Of note, gabapentin may worsen neuropsychiatric symptoms in DLB.[90] Lithium is not routinely used unless there is a pre-existing history of bipolar disorder, while oxcarbazepine has not been found to be helpful.[91]

There is also growing evidence that ChE-Is and memantine have modest benefit for neuropsychiatric symptoms in AD and possibly other related dementias with cholinergic deficits.[43,49,92] Evidence suggests that apathy, depression, or aberrant motor behavior are most likely to improve with use of ChE-Is; however, they have not been found effective in the treatment of either agitation or aggression.[93] Mood symptoms and apathy have most commonly responded to ChE-Is, whereas memantine has been associated with a reduction in irritability and agitation.[57] However, a recent randomized control trial specifically examining the efficacy of memantine in agitation in dementia found no benefit over placebo.[94] Thus, using ChE-Is or memantine for neuropsychiatric symptoms offers another alternative to antipsychotic medications in patients with dementia, though the effects of these drugs appear modest and often provide only temporary improvement.

CONCLUSION

As the population ages, the number of people with NCDs is increasing dramatically; most have AD or vascular dementia. The role of the psychiatric consultant in the diagnosis and treatment of NCDs is important, particularly in the identification of treatable psychiatric and behavioral symptoms.

Family members are the hidden victims of progressive dementia. They typically appreciate the consultant's communication about the diagnosis and the expected course of the disorder. They can benefit from advice about how best to relate to the patient, how to restructure the home environment, and how to seek out legal and financial guidance if appropriate. Family members also should be made aware of the assistance available to them through such organizations as the Alzheimer's Association.

REFERENCES

Access the reference list online at https://expertconsult.inkling.com/.

Psychotic Patients

Oliver Freudenreich, M.D.
Daphne J. Holt, M.D., Ph.D.
Donald C. Goff, M.D.

12

Psychosis, broadly defined, is a gross impairment of reality testing. Psychosis can result from a wide range of psychiatric and medical disturbances and may take several forms. The elderly woman, who lies quietly in bed listening to Satan whisper, bears little resemblance to the wildly agitated young man who accuses the nursing staff of trying to poison him. Hallucinations and delusions are the two classic psychiatric symptoms whose presence would indicate that the patient has lost touch with reality (i.e., suffers from psychosis). Hallucinations, which are sensory perceptions in the absence of an external source, can occur in any sensory modality and may take the form of voices, visions, odors, or even complex tactile perceptions (such as electric shocks, or the sensation that one is being fondled). Delusions are firmly held beliefs that other members of the patient's societal group would judge to be false. Delusions range from beliefs that are plausible, albeit unlikely (such as being monitored by the National Security Agency), to bizarre convictions (e.g., that one's internal organs have been replaced with empty beer cans). Delusional individuals cling to their beliefs with unfaltering conviction even in the face of overwhelming evidence to the contrary. Another category of psychotic symptoms comes under the rubric of a formal thought disorder, which refers to a disruption in the form, or organization, of thinking. Patients with a formal thought disorder may be incoherent to the point of producing word salad; they may not be able to make sense of reality or to communicate their thoughts to others.

When called to see a patient with psychosis, the psychiatric consultant can be of immediate help by ensuring that the patient and staff are safe; moreover, he or she can demystify this often-frightening condition. Psychosis can best be approached by proceeding with a well-ordered differential diagnosis, which transforms the patient's condition in the eyes of medical staff from insanity, with all its disturbing connotations, to a more comprehensible disorder of brain function.

CASE 1

Mr. A, a 45-year-old man who lived in a group home for patients with serious mental illness, had been going to a community mental health center for his psychiatric care. He had long-standing schizophrenia that had been treated with clozapine for 10 years. Mr. A was brought to the Emergency Department for abdominal pain. He was admitted to the surgical service for an acute abdomen and found to have a toxic megacolon that required a hemicolectomy.

Psychiatry was consulted to help manage Mr. A's medications and perioperative agitation. Clozapine was held and haloperidol was used to manage agitation. Even though his prior treatment with clozapine contributed to the development of toxic megacolon (because of clozapine's anticholinergic properties), the patient and his family considered clozapine an essential medication, as it had stabilized his illness course after a decade of failed treatments with other antipsychotics. Clozapine was therefore re-started at a low dose and carefully titrated to his previous dose during the hospitalization.

The hospitalization was also used to address two other concerns: Mr. A's basic medical care and his nicotine use. Mr. A had not seen his primary care doctor in many years, and he had been smoking cigarettes since high school, currently smoking two packs per day. Thus, the psychiatric consultant requested basic screening laboratory tests (i.e., hemoglobin A_{1c} and lipid profile) to assess for metabolic side effects that can emerge from long-term treatment with clozapine. His hemoglobin A_{1c} was found to be elevated but pre-diabetic. In addition, Mr. A received nicotine patches during the hospitalization to manage nicotine withdrawal and the psychiatric consultant used motivational interviewing to engage Mr. A around smoking cessation as a critical health goal to reduce his cardiovascular mortality risk. Follow-up with a primary care doctor to address diabetes prevention was arranged as part of his hospital discharge plan. Mr. A also agreed to start a smoking cessation group at his community mental health center and discuss pharmacotherapy for smoking cessation (e.g., varenicline) with his outpatient psychiatrist. Last, the group home received a note from the psychiatry consultation-liaison service about the prevention of constipation in clozapine patients. As a result of this hospital admission, Mr. A became more engaged in managing his own medical health and better linked to healthcare services.

DIAGNOSTIC EVALUATION

It cannot be stressed enough that the presence of psychotic symptoms does not always mean that a primary psychiatric disorder like schizophrenia is present. Therefore, the diagnostic assessment of a psychotic patient begins with a thorough consideration of toxic or medical conditions that can present with psychosis (Table 12-1).[1,2] A medical history, review of systems, family history, and physical examination are crucial elements of this process because most organic causes can be identified on this basis. A bedside examination of cognitive function should be performed. The Mini-Mental State Examination supplemented by the clock-drawing test will usually suffice as an initial cognitive screen. Serious deficits in attention, orientation, and memory suggest delirium or dementia rather than a primary psychotic illness. However, only more comprehensive neurocognitive testing will establish the more subtle yet functionally relevant cognitive difficulties with processing speed, working memory, verbal memory, and executive function that almost all patients with schizophrenia, including first-episode patients, experience to some degree.[3,4] Careful delineation of the temporal course of psychotic symptoms is of particular diagnostic importance. History from family about the patient is often the most critical aspect for piecing together how the illness unfolded over time. One should consider whether the disorder is chronic, episodic, or of recent onset. A typical prodromal period of unspecific anxiety and depression for several months followed by attenuated psychotic symptoms and increasing role failure that eventually gives rise to psychosis at the syndromal level is a typical time course for beginning schizophrenia.[5,6] The temporal relationship of psychotic symptoms to mood episodes, substance use, medication use, and medical or neurologic illness should be carefully reviewed. Substance misuse, such as intoxication with stimulants[7] or synthetic cannabinoids, is potentially reversible and in the latter case an increasingly common cause of psychosis that leads to emergency room visits.[8] Many other illegal drugs and legal medications have the potential to cause psychosis; unfortunately, causality is often difficult to prove (Table 12-2). Such substance-induced psychoses should be considered if the psychosis is of new onset, if there is no personal history of psychosis, or if the psychosis starts in the hospital, particularly if a delirium is present. A urine toxicologic screening test might identify unsuspected drug use, but it would not rule out drug-induced

TABLE 12-1 Selected Medical Conditions Associated With Psychosis

- Epilepsy
- Head trauma (history of)
- Dementias
  - Alzheimer's disease
  - Pick's disease
  - Lewy body disease
- Stroke
- Space-occupying lesions and structural brain abnormalities
  - Primary brain tumors
  - Secondary brain metastases
  - Brain abscesses and cysts
  - Tuberous sclerosis
  - Midline abnormalities (e.g., corpus callosum agenesis, cavum septi pellucidi)
  - Cerebrovascular malformations (e.g., involving the temporal lobe)
- Hydrocephalus
- Demyelinating diseases
  - Multiple sclerosis
  - Leukodystrophies (metachromatic leukodystrophy, X-linked adrenoleukodystrophy, Marchiafava–Bignami disease)
  - Schilder's disease
- Neuropsychiatric disorders
  - Huntington's disease
  - Wilson's disease
  - Parkinson's disease
  - Friedreich's ataxia
- Autoimmune disorders
  - Systemic lupus erythematosus
  - Rheumatic fever (history of)
  - Paraneoplastic syndromes
  - Myasthenia gravis
  - NMDA receptor encephalitis
- Infections
  - Viral encephalitis (e.g., herpes simplex, measles including SSPE, cytomegalovirus, rubella, Epstein–Barr, varicella)
  - Neurosyphilis
  - Neuroborreliosis (Lyme disease)
  - HIV infection
  - CNS-invasive parasitic infections (e.g., cerebral malaria, toxoplasmosis, neurocysticercosis)
  - Tuberculosis
  - Sarcoidosis
  - *Cryptococcus* infection
  - Prion diseases (e.g., Creutzfeldt–Jakob disease)
- Endocrinopathies
  - Hypoglycemia
  - Addison's disease
  - Cushing's syndrome
  - Hyperthyroidism and hypothyroidism
  - Hyperparathyroidism and hypoparathyroidism
  - Hypopituitarism
- Narcolepsy
- Nutritional deficiencies
  - Magnesium deficiency
  - Vitamin A deficiency
  - Vitamin D deficiency
  - Zinc deficiency
  - Niacin deficiency (pellagra)
  - Vitamin B_{12} deficiency (pernicious anemia)
- Metabolic disorders
  - Amino acid metabolism (Hartnup disease, homocystinuria, phenylketonuria)
  - Porphyrias (acute intermittent porphyria, porphyria variegata, hereditary coproporphyria)
  - GM_2 gangliosidosis
  - Fabry's disease
  - Niemann–Pick type C disease
  - Gaucher's disease, adult type
- Chromosomal abnormalities
  - Sex chromosomes (Klinefelter's syndrome, XXX syndrome)
  - Fragile X syndrome
  - VCFS

CNS, central nervous system; HIV, human immunodeficiency virus; SSPE, subacute sclerosing panencephalitis; VCFS, velo-cardio-facial syndrome.

TABLE 12-2 Substances Associated With Psychosis

Drugs of Abuse
Associated With Intoxication
Alcohol
Amphetamine
Anabolic steroids
Cannabis including synthetic cannabinoids
Cocaine
Designer drugs (wide variety of chemical classes)
Hallucinogens: LSD, MDMA
Inhalants: glues and solvents
Opioids (meperidine)
Phencyclidine (PCP), ketamine
Sedative–hypnotics (including withdrawal): barbiturates and benzodiazepines
Associated With Withdrawal
Alcohol
Sedative–hypnotics
Medications (Broad Classes With Selected Medications)
Anesthetics and analgesics (including NSAIDs)
Anticholinergic agents and antihistamines
Antiepileptics (with high doses)
Antihypertensive and cardiovascular medications (e.g., digoxin)
Anti-infectious medications (antibiotics, e.g., fluoroquinolones, TMP/SMX; antivirals, e.g., nevirapine; tuberculostatics, e.g., INH; antiparasitics, e.g., metronidazole, mefloquine)
Antiparkinsonian medications (e.g., amantadine, levodopa)
Chemotherapeutic agents (e.g., vincristine)
Corticosteroids (e.g., prednisone, ACTH)
Interferon
Muscle relaxants (e.g., cyclobenzaprine)
Over-the-counter medications (e.g., pseudoephedrine, caffeine in excessive doses)
Toxins
Carbon monoxide
Heavy metals: arsenic, manganese, mercury, thallium
Organophosphates
Key Diagnostic Questions to Determine Causality Between a Substance and Psychosis
Does the patient have a history of psychosis?
Does the patient have a history of illicit drug use?
Did the psychosis start after a medication was started? After the patient came to the hospital?
Is there evidence of delirium?

ACTH, adrenocorticotropic hormone; INH, isoniazid; LSD, D-lysergic acid diethylamide; MDMA, methylenedioxymethamphetamine; NSAID, non-steroidal antiinflammatory drug; TMP/SMX, trimethoprim/sulfamethoxazole.

psychosis if it were negative, nor would a positive toxicologic screening test necessarily establish a cause for the psychosis, because co-morbid substance use and abuse is common in psychotic disorders. Many designer drugs that are freely available over the Internet require specialized and dedicated testing that is usually not available.[9] Routine laboratory testing includes determination of a sedimentation rate, a complete blood cell count, serum electrolytes, urinalysis, and levels of calcium, glucose, creatinine, and blood urea nitrogen. In addition, liver function tests, thyroid function tests, and syphilis serology (specific, such as the fluorescent treponemal antibody absorption test), are appropriate. Human immunodeficiency virus (HIV) testing should be recommended. Extended work-ups may include karyotyping for chromosomal abnormalities or urine testing for metabolic disorders.[10] The diagnostic yield from neuroimaging of the brain (magnetic resonance imaging, MRI; or computed tomography, CT) is low in the absence of localizing neurologic findings.[11] Neuroimaging should be obtained, however, in cases with atypical or unresponsive psychotic symptoms when psychotic symptoms first appear and should be considered even in cases with typical psychotic features, because the long-term costs and morbidity of this disorder are potentially quite high in relation to the expense of diagnostic procedures. The electroencephalogram (EEG) can be useful when evaluating a confused patient where a delirium is suspected or when a history of serious head trauma or symptoms suggestive of a seizure disorder are present.[12–14] An EEG is rarely helpful if it is employed as a routine screening procedure. Similarly, a lumbar puncture is not necessary for a routine work-up, but it can be lifesaving if a treatable central nervous system (CNS) infection is suspected. NMDA receptor encephalitis is a newly delineated autoimmune disorder of particular concern to psychiatrists since patients might initially present with only psychiatric symptoms.[15] Making this diagnosis quickly is critical to initiate immunotherapy and requires a lumbar puncture to detect NMDA receptor antibodies.[16]

Several neuropsychiatric disorders in particular should be considered during the diagnostic work-up of a patient with psychosis.[17] Huntington's disease is suggested by family history of Huntington's disease, dementia, and choreiform movements; psychotic symptoms may occur before motor and cognitive symptoms become prominent.[18] Parkinson's disease also may present with psychosis, along with bradykinesia, tremor, rigidity, and a festinating gait. With disease progression, psychosis is common and can be the result of illness and not just of medications.[19] The diagnosis of Parkinson's disease can be complicated by exposure to neuroleptics—review of the time course of neurologic symptoms in relation to the use of antipsychotics should clarify this diagnostic possibility. Wilson's disease may also present with psychotic symptoms, tremor, dysarthria, rigidity, and a gait disturbance.[20] Kayser–Fleischer rings, which are golden-brown copper deposits that encircle the cornea, are pathognomonic for this disease. However, a slit-lamp exam is needed to detect them early on. The diagnosis can be confirmed by measuring concentrations of ceruloplasmin in the urine and serum. Finally, acute intermittent porphyria is characterized by acute episodes of abdominal pain, weakness, and peripheral neuropathy; this condition may be associated with psychosis.[21] Because this is a hereditary (autosomal dominant) illness, a family history often points to this diagnosis. During acute attacks, levels of δ-aminolevulinic acid and porphobilinogen are elevated in the urine.

It is impractical and ill-advised to attempt to rule out all conceivable diseases that could cause psychosis. The more tests are ordered without clinical concern for a particular disease, the more false-positive test results will occur.[22] Thankfully, a thoughtful approach that combines clinical history and a physical examination (including a neurologic examination) with selected laboratory tests will usually suffice to exclude treatable medical illnesses and provide a medical baseline for future reference. Table 12-3 suggests one screening battery that accomplishes these important initial diagnostic goals.

After an organic cause has been ruled out, the psychiatric differential diagnosis of psychosis flows from the diagnostic criteria contained in the "Psychotic Disorders" section of the *Diagnostic and Statistical Manual of Mental Disorders*, 5th edition (DSM-5).[13] It should be emphasized, however, that these criteria are guidelines for diagnosis and a tool for a common language; they are to be used only in conjunction with a full understanding of the descriptions of the syndrome as described in textbooks (Table 12-4). A clear, longitudinal view of the illness is necessary to identify affective episodes and to determine whether the patient's level of function has declined. In addition, the range and severity of psychotic and negative symptoms as well as the neurocognitive impairment must be determined. Psychotic patients are often unable to provide an accurate history; therefore information must be collected from as many sources as possible. In one study, information necessary for diagnosis, such as the presence of persecutory delusions, was missed more than 30% of the time when the assessment was based on the interview only.[24] Concurrent substance abuse is also frequently missed in patients with schizophrenia if toxicologic screening is not performed.[25]

If major depression and mania are not present and have not played a prominent role in the past, the diagnosis is likely to be schizophrenia, delusional disorder, or schizotypal personality disorder (depending on the severity of the illness). To meet criteria for schizophrenia according to DSM-5, the patient must have demonstrated a decline in function and displayed, for at least 4 weeks, symptoms of the active phase, which can consist of delusions, hallucinations, or disorganized speech. So-called "Schneiderian first-rank symptoms" (e.g., voices conversing or keeping up a running commentary) are characteristic for schizophrenia, albeit neither pathognomonic nor obligatory.[26] Other active-phase symptoms include grossly disorganized behavior and catatonia as well as negative symptoms. Negative symptoms of schizophrenia fall into two main clusters: a cluster of reduced affective experience or expression (i.e., affective blunting and alogia) and an amotivation cluster (i.e., avolition, anhedonia, and asociality).[27] The diagnosis of schizophrenia

TABLE 12-3 Medical Work-Up for First-Episode Psychosis

Physical exam with emphasis on neurologic exam
Vital signs
Weight and height (BMI), waist circumference[a]
Electrocardiogram (ECG)[a]
Laboratory Tests
Broad Screening and Medical Baseline:
Complete blood count (CBC)
Electrolytes including calcium
Renal function tests (BUN/creatinine)
Liver function tests
Erythrocyte sedimentation rate (ESR)
Antinuclear antibody (ANA)
Fasting glucose
Fasting lipid profile[a]
Hemoglobin A_{1c}[a]
Consider prolactin level[a]
Hepatitis C (if risk factors are present)[a]
Pregnancy test (in women of childbearing age)
Urine drug screen
Exclude Specific Treatable Disorders:
Thyroid stimulating hormone (TSH)
Fluorescent treponemal antibody absorbed (FTA-ABS)
HIV test
Ceruloplasmin
Vitamin B_{12}
Neuroimaging
MRI (preferred over CT)
Ancillary Tests
Expand etiological search if indicated, taking into account epidemiology: e.g., chest x-ray, electroencephalogram (EEG), lumbar puncture, karyotype, heavy metal testing, Lyme antibodies, NMDA receptor autoantibodies, and other autoantibodies
Expand medical monitoring if indicated: e.g., eye exam (if risk factors for cataracts are present)

[a]Not for diagnostic purposes but to establish baseline for longitudinal medical monitoring.

Modified from Freudenreich O, Schulz SC, Goff DC: Initial medical work-up of first-episode psychosis: a conceptual review, *Early Interv Psychiatry* 3:10–18, 2009.

TABLE 12-4 Psychiatric Disorders That May Present With Psychosis

Continuous Psychosis
Schizophrenia
Schizoaffective disorder, bipolar type (with prominent episodes of mania)
Schizoaffective disorder, depressed type (with prominent depressive episodes)
Delusional disorder (plausible, circumscribed delusions)
Shared psychotic disorder (in which delusions are induced by another person)
Episodic Psychosis
Depression with psychotic features
Bipolar disorder (manic or depressed)
Schizophreniform disorder (<6 months' duration)
Brief psychotic disorder (<1 month duration)
Key Diagnostic Questions
Has a reversible, organic cause been ruled out?
Are cognitive deficits prominent (delirium or dementia)?
Is the psychotic illness continuous or episodic?
Have psychotic symptoms (active phase) been present for at least 4 weeks?
Has evidence of the illness been present for at least 6 months?
Is there evidence of a decline in level of functioning?
Are negative symptoms present?
Are mood episodes prominent?
Have there been episodes of major depression or mania?
Do psychotic features occur only during affective episodes?

is made only after evidence of the illness has been present for at least 6 months—if symptoms have been present for less than 6 months, the provisional diagnosis of schizophreniform disorder is used. Patients whose psychotic symptoms remit within 4 weeks of their onset are diagnosed as having a brief psychotic disorder if no organic cause is identified.

If the patient's condition does not meet the criteria for schizophrenia or schizophreniform disorder, but one or more delusions are present, the diagnosis of delusional disorder is made, provided that the patient does not exhibit severe deterioration in function outside of the circumscribed delusional system. Typical delusions are often quite plausible and include the belief that one has a physical defect or medical condition or that one is being followed, poisoned, infected, loved by a famous person, or cheated on by a spouse. Patients who do not meet the active phase criteria for schizophrenia but who present with chronic, bizarre, or idiosyncratic thoughts or behaviors are classified as having schizotypal personality, which probably is a less severe form of schizophrenia.

If the patient meets criteria for major depression and has exhibited psychotic symptoms only during episodes of depression, the diagnosis is major depression with psychotic features. If psychotic features characteristic of schizophrenia have also occurred for a substantial amount of time during periods when the patient was euthymic, the illness is classified as schizoaffective disorder, depressed type if depressions have been prominent throughout the course of the illness, or schizophrenia with superimposed depression if bouts of depression have been infrequent. Patients who have experienced manic episodes and who have been psychotic only during affective episodes are diagnosed as having bipolar disorder. If psychosis has been present between manic and depressive states, the diagnosis is schizoaffective disorder, bipolar type, or schizophrenia with superimposed mood disorder; again, the diagnosis depends on how prominent a role affective episodes have played in the overall course of the illness. The proper psychiatric diagnosis of a patient who is psychotic on a cross-sectional examination requires an intimate knowledge of the patient's longitudinal course, something that is often unavailable during an inpatient admission. As a result, initial diagnostic impressions need to be revised as more longitudinal history becomes available.

CLINICAL PICTURES AND CORRESPONDING PROBLEMS ON THE MEDICAL WARD

It is often surprising to see that psychotic patients do perfectly well when admitted to a medical or surgical service; they tend to require little in the way of special treatment. One survey found that only half of patients with schizophrenia admitted to a general hospital required psychiatric consultation.[28] Interestingly, the most common reason for a psychiatric consultation in patients with schizophrenia admitted to the medical service of the Massachusetts General Hospital was "schizophrenia" (30%); there was no specific question.[29] This may reflect a concern that is evoked by managing a patient with schizophrenia. Other referrals revolve around depression (16%), capacity assessment (14%), and help with prescription of psychotropic medications (10%). For patients with psychotic disorders, the role of the consultation psychiatrist in the general hospital can be seen as three-fold: conducting conventional consultations with an emphasis on making a correct diagnosis and instituting proper treatment, educating staff about the nature of schizophrenia, and serving as an advocate for the chronically mentally ill so that they can receive standard and comprehensive medical care.[30,31] In one chart review study, patients with schizophrenia who needed a medical or surgical admission had higher rates of complications in the form of infections and postoperative complications compared to patients who did not carry a schizophrenia diagnosis.[32] Effective consultation and advocacy could thus have real-life implications for some patients with schizophrenia.[33]

The specific form of illness that a patient with schizophrenia manifests determines the nature of the staff's concerns as well as the staff's level of comfort. Studies have demonstrated that the symptoms of schizophrenia tend to cluster into at least three groups: reality distortion (e.g., delusions, hallucinations), disorganization (e.g., formal thought disorder, inappropriate affect), and negative symptoms (e.g., apathy, anhedonia, social withdrawal, alogia, flat affect).[34,35] A fourth symptom domain, cognitive deficits, has been re-discovered.[36] Schizophrenia was once known as dementia praecox because of its prominent cognitive problems. The majority of patients with schizophrenia display a varying admixture of symptoms from all four symptom domains that leads to significant variability among patients. Some patients, however, exhibit prominent symptoms from only one category, and the difficulties they encounter in the general hospital are determined by which cluster of symptoms predominates.

In all cases, a question can arise as to whether the patient is competent to make treatment decisions. Some patients may already have a guardian who must be involved in treatment decisions; if not, assessment for competency and initiation of appropriate legal steps may be necessary to ensure proper medical treatment. It is crucial to assess to what degree, if at all, delusions affect the patient's decision-making. The consultant should make it clear that patients with psychosis may have the capacity to make certain decisions, such as weighing risks and benefits of proceeding with or refusing medical treatment, even when their judgment is impaired in other realms. The idiosyncratic speech manifest by some patients may give an exaggerated impression of cognitive impairment, whereas their capacity to understand aspects of their medical condition may be adequate. With patience and explanations that account for cognitive limitations, many patients with schizophrenia are able to participate meaningfully in their medical care, despite some cognitive impairment.[37] Put differently: a diagnosis of schizophrenia *per se* is not an indication of lack of capacity.

The Paranoid or Delusional Patient

Patients with schizophrenia whose symptoms are restricted to complex delusional systems and hallucinations used to be called "paranoid." In the absence of overt disorganization and negative symptoms, individuals with paranoid schizophrenia may go unnoticed by hospital staff. These patients often conceal all psychiatric symptoms and fail to exhibit the bizarre appearance and speech that attract attention in others with schizophrenia. Patients with paranoid schizophrenia may antagonize nursing staff because of their anger, argumentativeness, or patronizing manner. Nursing staff often appreciate learning that these annoying characteristics are actually common features of the illness. Despite complex and bizarre delusional beliefs, these individuals may elude detection and complete a medical or surgical hospitalization without incident. Difficulties arise when circumstances in the hospital collide with an individual's delusions. The patient who believes that the Mafia is attempting to kill him may refuse all hospital food for fear of being poisoned. Others become convinced that their physicians are members of the conspiracy that is plotting against them or that the surgeons have implanted a microchip intended to control or monitor their thoughts. To assess safety and to anticipate potential problems with compliance, the psychiatric consultant must understand the full scope of the person's delusional system and the nature of any hallucinatory experiences.

Because paranoid patients usually are reluctant to reveal their delusional beliefs, the consultant must proceed carefully and deliberately. A direct, interrogatory approach often convinces the patient that conspirators sent the interviewer. Because delusional individuals are preoccupied and distressed by their delusional beliefs, it is usually sufficient to engage them in a neutral, non-threatening discussion about their current interests and activities. Comments that seem out of place or inappropriate to the content may provide clues as to the subject of the delusional system, and these should be explored. Questions should never imply a judgment about psychopathology, but rather they should demonstrate the interviewer's interest and concern. Examples of such questions include, "Are you safe? Have you noticed any strange coincidences? Are you aware of anyone trying to play with your mind? How do you understand what is happening to you? What is it that you overhear from others about this?" The interviewer should neither agree with the delusion nor attempt to reality-test—impartial interest and concern are usually a welcome relief to a delusional patient. This technique is sometimes called *partial joining of perspectives*.[38] Ideally, the consultant can serve as an intermediary, listening to the concerns of both the patient and the hospital staff; as a consequence he or she can mediate misunderstandings.

In addition to persecutory delusions, somatic delusions may also pose unique problems for the patient with schizophrenia admitted to a medical service. In a retrospective chart survey, McGilchrist and Cutting[39] found that more than half of patients with schizophrenia described somatic delusions. These delusions were typically bizarre (such as the belief that a third arm is growing out of one's chest) and could usually be immediately recognized as delusional. Having heard a patient's somatic delusions, however, medical staff tend to discount other somatic complaints. The consultant may be needed to help sort out which physical complaints merit further investigation by hospital staff and which delusional concerns are best ignored.

The Disorganized Patient

The disorganized patient can be problematic on a medical service. Disordered speech may make communication about medical symptoms difficult and may interfere with discussions about treatment options. If disorganization is subtle, the patient may merely appear stubborn or oppositional, and make routine nursing tasks difficult. One major area of concern for disorganized patients is their lack of judgment and behavioral control. These patients may engage in inappropriate behaviors (such as masturbating or disrobing in public, stealing food, and smoking in restricted areas). Of even greater concern is the occasional violent or self-injurious behavior of an agitated, disorganized patient. These patients typically require aggressive pharmacotherapy and may require physical restraints or round-the-clock attendants. A review of past behavioral problems, which can be provided by outpatient caregivers or family, can help the consultant anticipate behavioral problems that are likely to arise during a medical or surgical hospitalization.

The Patient With Negative Symptoms or Neurocognitive Deficits

Individuals with schizophrenia who display prominent negative symptoms may encounter unique difficulties when admitted to medical or surgical services. Moreover, negative symptoms are often compounded by cognitive deficits, particularly in the realms of sustained attention, memory, and executive function. Patients may seem indifferent to their medical problems and unappreciative of their care. Nursing staff can easily be put off by the poor hygiene and soiled clothing. Sustaining empathy and enthusiasm for the care of a withdrawn, unmotivated patient can require unusual efforts by nursing staff. This process may be facilitated by the psychiatric consultant, who can explain that poor hygiene, apathy, and deficits in interpersonal skills are symptoms of illness that require management and that should not be interpreted as willful or as a weakness of character. Often, if the consultant can provide a description of the patient as a vibrant, healthy young adult before onset of the illness, nursing staff can find it easier to empathize. When ongoing treatment or rehabilitation is required after discharge, a comprehensive plan should be developed to provide supervision for avolitional patients, who otherwise would be unlikely to follow through with treatment. If little history about the patient's baseline level of function is available, it is important to rule out other causes of negative symptoms, such as a hypoactive delirium or a seizure disorder.[40]

The Manic Patient

Although psychotic features in patients with schizophrenia are often bizarre and idiosyncratic, patients who are manic are much more likely to present with grandiose delusions that typically impair judgment and self-esteem. These patients may be difficult to manage because of their boundless energy and their grandiose misinterpretation of their situation. Staff may at first mistake mania for unusually high energy, talkativeness, and positive self-esteem; eventually they turn to the psychiatric consultant when the patient refuses to stop pacing or to stop talking to other patients late at night, or when he or she is belligerent or insists that he or she is free of any medical problems. Patients with irritable or dysphoric mania may present with persecutory delusions and can be superficially indistinguishable from a patient with paranoid schizophrenia. Management of the manic patient should begin with containment and isolation from distracting stimuli and behavioral temptations. Short-term behavioral control can be achieved with use of antipsychotics in combination with benzodiazepines,[41] whereas the ultimate goal of sustained remission with the prevention of relapse requires a therapeutic blood level of lithium carbonate, valproic acid, or another mood stabilizer.

The Psychotic Depressed Patient

The delusions of the psychotically depressed patient usually reflect ruminative concerns about guilt, worthlessness, or physical decrepitude. These patients may puzzle their medical or surgical caregivers with exaggerated bodily concerns and illogical descriptions of organ dysfunction. Their overwhelming sense of hopelessness and sense of being responsible for their plight may also interfere with attempts to involve them in treatment decisions—they may seem more interested in euthanasia than care and cure. Some psychotically depressed patients withdraw and may become mute and catatonic. Persecutory delusions also occur in psychotic depression, but these beliefs tend to be less bizarre than those encountered in patients with schizophrenia. In fact, it may be quite difficult to discern whether strangers are actually attempting to break into the patient's house or whether family members are stealing the elderly aunt's savings. Treatment of psychotic depression typically requires either a course of electroconvulsive therapy or the use of an antipsychotic agent, plus an adequate dose of an antidepressant.[42]

The Elderly Psychotic Patient

Psychotic symptoms are relatively common among the medically ill or disabled elderly. One survey found that 21% of newly admitted nursing home patients were delusional, and approximately 4% of elderly individuals in the community suffer from persecutory delusions.[43] Isolation and sensory impairment probably contribute to the higher incidence of paranoia and agitation in the elderly. *Late paraphrenia* is an older term still used to describe such patients.[44] In addition, older individuals are at particular risk for a host of organic causes of psychosis, importantly dementia and delirium. Psychosis is present in 50% of deliria that are easily missed if psychosis overshadows the core features of a delirium.[45] Polypharmacy is a risk factor for delirium in the elderly. Late-onset schizophrenia, which occurs after the age of 45 and may first present in old age, usually occurs in women and appears as a paranoid psychosis.[46] Psychotic symptoms are quite common in patients with Alzheimer's disease; approximately one-third of patients with Alzheimer's disease develop paranoid delusions, and 7% develop auditory hallucinations.[47] Management of psychosis in the elderly involves, first and foremost, a comprehensive screening for organic causes, plus supportive measures and the judicious use of antipsychotics. Supportive measures should be individualized but include reassurance, visits from family to alleviate isolation, strategies to maintain the sleep–wake cycle, and measures to compensate for sensory or cognitive deficits, such as providing clear and repeated instructions, to counteract misinterpretations of reality. If antipsychotics are used to treat the psychosis of Alzheimer's disease, clinicians face two problems. For one, antipsychotics must be used with great care, because they may increase the risk of death in the dementia population.[48] Moreover, antipsychotics have limited efficacy for the neuropsychiatric complications of Alzheimer's disease including psychosis.[49] Unfortunately, safer or more effective options may not always be available, although citalopram can help reduce agitation.[50] If antipsychotics are used as part of a comprehensive treatment plan to manage agitation or psychosis in a patient with dementia, the response to treatment should be monitored with a rating scale and periodic attempts be made to remove the antipsychotic.[51]

MANAGEMENT OF PSYCHOTIC PATIENTS

General Considerations

As has been emphasized, the first step in approaching the treatment of a psychotic patient is to clarify the diagnosis, along with any prior psychotropic medication use. Delirium, which is characterized by fluctuations in mental status and by confusion, must be recognized and the underlying cause addressed. The pharmacologic management of delirium is described in Chapter 10. Specific information about individual antipsychotic agents and drug–drug interactions is provided in Chapter 38.

Target symptoms for antipsychotics fall into three categories: (1) psychotic symptoms (e.g., hallucinations, delusions, disorganization); (2) agitation (e.g., distractibility, affective lability, tension, increased motor activity); and (3) negative symptoms (e.g., apathy, flat affect, social isolation, poverty of speech). The last category responds to an antipsychotic best if symptoms are the result of active psychosis (e.g., a patient is withdrawn because of psychotic preoccupation). The pharmacologic treatment of psychotic symptoms is similar in many ways to the treatment of infection with antibiotics—the clinician needs to choose the proper medication at a sufficient dose and then await therapeutic results while monitoring side effects. Contrary to common wisdom, a response to antipsychotics can often be seen after a few days or even after a single dose, particularly for agitation.[52]

Psychotic symptoms and agitation usually improve with antipsychotics, regardless of cause. Most causes of organic psychosis, such as stimulant intoxication (e.g., amphetamines, cocaine), also respond readily to antipsychotics. The decision whether to use an antipsychotic in cases of organic psychosis should be informed by a weighing of the anticipated duration and severity of the psychosis and the potential side effects of the drug. When time-limited psychoses, such as those produced by psychoactive substances or psychosis accompanying a delirium, are treated with an antipsychotic, care should be taken that this medication not be inadvertently continued indefinitely after the patient is discharged from the hospital, particularly if a first-generation antipsychotic is used; the risk of irreversible tardive dyskinesia (TD) must be considered.

Drug Selection

Selection of an antipsychotic agent is usually guided by efficacy considerations, side effect profiles, and available formulations (i.e., tablet, rapidly dissolving wafer, liquid, IM, IV, or depot preparations). First-generation antipsychotics, which act by blocking dopamine D_2 receptors, are of similar efficacy and differ primarily in their potency (i.e., the dose required for their clinical effect) and in their side effects.[53] Second-generation antipsychotics were developed based on the observation that clozapine, though an effective antipsychotic, did not cause extrapyramidal symptoms (EPS).[54] However, several seminal large randomized treatment trials known by their acronyms, CATIE, CUtLASS, and EUFEST, have been unable to clearly establish superior efficacy of second-generation antipsychotics as a class.[55–57] It has, however, also become clear that not all second-generation including the newest antipsychotics are alike; each drug needs to be considered individually. Clozapine remains the "gold standard" with regard to efficacy, and it is preferred for patients who are exquisitely sensitive to dopamine blockade like patients with Parkinson's disease; of the other second-generation agents, evidence suggestive of enhanced efficacy is strongest for olanzapine.[58]

High-potency, first-generation agents continue to have their strongest support in the short-term treatment of medically compromised agitated patients; they have been relatively free of serious medical side effects. In the outpatient setting, adherence to antipsychotics is a major treatment goal to reduce relapse.[59] As many as 70% of patients with schizophrenia do not take their medications as prescribed, in part because of ongoing substance use, medication side effects, and lack of insight, but also because of a poor response to treatment. Several first- and second-generation long-acting injectable antipsychotics (LAIs) are available to assist in improving adherence. LAIs play no role in the short-term management of patients. Patients who are managed with LAIs as outpatients can usually be simply continued as per their injection schedule if they are admitted medically. It is important to remember that it takes several months for LAIs to be fully eliminated from the body after stopping them, which can obviously be problematic for patients who develop neuroleptic malignant syndrome.

If a patient has been taking an antipsychotic with good results, it is often best not to make changes in the regimen unless medical problems or potential drug interactions necessitate a switch, as switches in stabilized patients can be detrimental.[60] Exacerbations in otherwise stable patients, particularly if related to stress and accompanied by depressive symptoms, usually improve without altering the medication or raising the dosage. Benzodiazepines can be used temporarily, if needed, to manage symptom exacerbations.[61]

First-generation Antipsychotics

Low-potency first-generation antipsychotic agents, such as chlorpromazine (CPZ), should be prescribed in dosages of 300 to 600 CPZ mg-equivalents/day; they are associated with orthostatic hypotension, anticholinergic side effects, sedation, and weight gain, and they are less readily or safely administered in a parenteral fashion.[53] High-potency agents, such as haloperidol, are more likely to produce EPS, such as acute dystonia, parkinsonism, and akathisia (see later). Haloperidol is available for parenteral (including IV) administration. In the setting of serious medical illness, particularly if other medications with anticholinergic or hypotensive side effects are being administered, haloperidol is typically the antipsychotic of choice. It is important to minimize the small risk of torsades de pointes from parenteral haloperidol by reducing risk factors for it (e.g., hypokalemia, hypomagnesemia) and by tracking the QTc. Although considerable inter-individual variability exists, daily oral doses of haloperidol between 5 and 15 mg are adequate for the vast majority of patients; increasing the dose beyond this dose range may only aggravate side effects without improving antipsychotic efficacy. IM and IV administration tend to require roughly half that dose. In the elderly, 0.5 mg to 2 mg of haloperidol at bedtime may be sufficient. If a patient has not previously received an antipsychotic, it is best to start with a low dose (e.g., haloperidol 2 to 5 mg orally) before increasing it to a standard therapeutic dose.

Extrapyramidal Side Effects and Tardive Dyskinesia

Younger patients (i.e., those younger than 40 years of age) started on high-potency first-generation antipsychotics are especially vulnerable to developing an acute dystonic reaction during the first week of treatment.[62] Dystonia, the sudden constriction of muscles, is a frightening and uncomfortable experience; when manifested as a laryngeal spasm, it can be life-threatening. The occurrence of dystonia early in treatment jeopardizes future compliance with antipsychotics; therefore it is important to anticipate and treat this side effect aggressively. Prophylaxis with an anticholinergic agent, such as benztropine 1 to 2 mg twice daily, substantially reduces the likelihood of a dystonic reaction even in a high-risk patient.[63] Dystonia is less common with the use of second-generation agents than with first-generation high-potency agents; moreover, it probably does not occur with either quetiapine or clozapine.

Akathisia is an extremely unpleasant sensation of motor restlessness that is primarily experienced in the lower extremities in patients who receive an antipsychotic medication. For the psychotic patient hospitalized on a medical service, akathisia can make bedrest unbearable. Akathisia substantially increases the risk that a patient will leave the hospital against medical advice, and it has been associated with self-injurious behaviors as well as with a worsening of psychosis. Untrained staff frequently mistake akathisia for psychotic agitation, which leads to unfortunate escalations of antipsychotic doses. For patients in acute distress, diazepam 10 mg can provide immediate relief. For the long-term management, dose reduction may improve akathisia; if relief is not obtained, propranolol (10 to 20 mg two to four times daily) is often helpful. Even more effective is a switch to a second-generation antipsychotic, which usually resolves the problem. Akathisia may occur with the dopamine D_2 partial agonists (e.g., aripiprazole, brexpiprazole) and may resolve spontaneously over several weeks.

Antipsychotic-induced parkinsonism can easily be mistaken for depression or for the negative symptoms of schizophrenia.[64] The presence of tremor and rigidity distinguishes this side effect in more severe cases; subtle cases can easily be missed. Parkinsonian side effects commonly improve with a reduction of the neuroleptic dosage or with addition of an antiparkinsonian agent (e.g., benztropine 1 to 2 mg twice daily or amantadine 100 mg two or three times daily). Because anticholinergic agents impair attention and memory and can produce a vast array of troublesome side effects in the elderly, long-term use of these agents should be avoided.[65] A newer medication, pimavanserin, a selective serotonin 5-HT_{2A} inverse agonist, can be effective for psychosis in Parkinson's disease;[66] if unsuccessful, either clozapine or quetiapine are essentially free of EPS but may be associated with other side effects in the elderly.

Tardive dyskinesia rarely appears after less than 6 months of treatment with an antipsychotic; once present, TD may be irreversible.[67] TD usually takes the form of involuntary, choreiform movements of the mouth, tongue, or upper extremities, although a dystonic form has also been described.[68] Studies suggest that the risk for developing TD with first-generation agents is approximately 5% per year of exposure, with a life-time risk possibly as high as 50% to 60%.[69] The incidence of TD is much higher in the elderly, although a substantial proportion of these cases may represent spontaneously occurring dyskinesias.[70] As part of informed consent, patients requiring prolonged antipsychotic treatment with first-generation agents should be educated about the risk of developing TD after their acute psychosis has been treated and before 6 months has elapsed. Preliminary evidence that indicated α-tocopherol (vitamin E), at dosages of 400 to 1200 IU daily, improved symptoms of TD was not supported by a much larger controlled trial; thus the best treatment for TD is prevention.[71] Clozapine has not been linked to TD; switching a patient from a conventional agent to clozapine increases the likelihood of improvement in TD.[72] Lowering the dose of a conventional antipsychotic or switching to an atypical agent can occasionally produce a "withdrawal dyskinesia," which either resolves within 6 weeks, or unmasks an underlying dyskinesia that was previously suppressed by the antipsychotic.[73] Tetrabenazine, which is approved to treat the chorea of Huntington's disease, is often used to treat serious TD.[74] Valbenazine, a derivative of tetrabenazine, is under clinical development.[75] (See also Chapter 21 for more information about antipsychotic-induced movement disorders.)

Second-generation Antipsychotics

Second-generation antipsychotics (including the dopamine partial agonists, aripiprazole, brexpiprazole, and cariprazine) as a class, produce fewer neurologic side effects (e.g., dystonia, akathisia, parkinsonism) than first-generation agents;[76] they are also associated with less TD (about 0.8% per year).[77] In this class, risperidone is most likely to induce EPS, particularly at dosages higher than 6 mg/day. It is important to appreciate that second-generation antipsychotics differ substantially with regard to other side effects. Risperidone and its active and marketed metabolite, 9-hydroxyrisperidone (paliperidone), are unique among the second-generation agents because of their propensity to produce hyperprolactinemia. Aripiprazole by contrast can lower prolactin levels.[78] Clozapine, olanzapine, and iloperidone have been associated with substantial weight gain that can be a major obstacle to adherence. Risperidone and quetiapine are associated with intermediate weight gain, and ziprasidone and lurasidone appear to produce little or no weight gain.[79,80] Considerable research over the past decade has focused on the effects of second-generation antipsychotics on glucose metabolism and lipids. The observed insulin-resistance and dyslipidemia are only in part explained by weight gain, and some antipsychotics seem to directly affect metabolism.[81] Despite differences in the propensity to cause metabolic side effects, it is recommended that all patients who receive second-generation antipsychotics be carefully monitored, with particularly close monitoring of patients at higher risk (e.g., with a family history of diabetes; a history of clozapine or olanzapine treatment).[82]

Lurasidone and aripiprazole have the smallest effect among the second-generation antipsychotics on cardiac conduction. Clozapine, risperidone, quetiapine, iloperidone, and ziprasidone have alpha-adrenergic effects that necessitate dose titration to avoid orthostatic hypotension; paliperidone can be given without titration. Of those, clozapine produces the most hypotension and tachycardia. Ziprasidone and iloperidone appear to prolong the QT interval more than other atypical agents, but less than thioridazine.[83] Serious cardiac events have been rare in patients treated with ziprasidone (not differing from placebo in registration trials), and reported cases of overdose have been benign. The large observational ZODIAC study of ziprasidone patients found no increase in mortality when compared with olanzapine-treated patients.[84] However, ziprasidone's effect on cardiac repolarization may be problematic in the presence of underlying heart disease or when it is added to other agents with similar effects. Potential cardiac toxicity remains a clinical concern with all antipsychotics. A large retrospective cohort study did not find a difference between first- and second-generation antipsychotics in associated risk for sudden death.[85] Instead, both classes produced a dose-related increase in risk for sudden death.

For patients who have difficulty swallowing, rapidly dissolvable formulations are available for several antipsychotics, including asenapine, aripiprazole, clozapine, olanzapine, and risperidone.

Clozapine, although clearly possessing unique antipsychotic efficacy, can produce many bothersome and even potentially lethal side effects, including agranulocytosis (in approximately 1% of patients), sialorrhea, weight gain, hypotension, tachycardia, seizures, impairment of esophageal and bowel motility, and urinary incontinence. Clozapine has also been linked to cardiomyopathy, pericarditis, and pulmonary embolism. Despite the list of potentially serious medical complications, clozapine was found to decrease mortality more than other antipsychotic agents;[86] this net positive effect on mortality rates probably reflects the magnitude of its protective effect against suicide in contrast to its relatively low frequency of serious adverse effects. However, any potential protection from death due to suicide has to be weighed against the possibility of a premature death from cardiovascular disease for the individual patient.[87]

If a patient is to be started or re-started on clozapine, a colleague with experience in the use of this agent should be consulted to determine how frequently to monitor neutrophil counts and to outline strategies for the initiation and optimization of the dosage of this unique agent. Clozapine treatment should not be unnecessarily interrupted when patients are admitted to a medical or surgical service, because abrupt discontinuation has been associated with acute worsening of psychosis and with cholinergic rebound. If clozapine has been discontinued for more than 2 days, clozapine should be re-introduced at a low dose and titrated upward toward the patient's previous optimal dose. A cautious approach is necessary to avoid hypotension, bradycardia, or syncope. It is ill-advised to start clozapine *de novo* in a patient during a complicated medical admission.

Treating Agitation

Usual therapeutic doses of antipsychotics do not always treat agitation associated with psychosis successfully. Benzodiazepines can effectively enhance the tranquilizing effect of antipsychotics or be used alone for the treatment of agitation.[41] Lorazepam can be combined (in the same syringe) with haloperidol for acute behavioral control—usually 1 mg of lorazepam is given with 5 mg of haloperidol intramuscularly. An inhaled version of the mid-potency antipsychotic loxapine is also available to treat agitation associated with bipolar disorder or schizophrenia in emergency situations.[88] Once agitation is controlled, the patient can be started on a usually therapeutic dose of an antipsychotic, with a benzodiazepine (e.g., lorazepam 1 to 2 mg) given as needed or as a standing order two to three times daily for as long as is needed. Typically, as the psychotic symptoms improve with use of an antipsychotic, use of a benzodiazepine often becomes unnecessary. Alternatively, several second-generation antipsychotics (i.e., aripiprazole, olanzapine, and ziprasidone) are available for IM use for the control of agitation.

Neuroleptic Malignant Syndrome

Neuroleptic malignant syndrome (NMS) is a rare, potentially lethal complication of neuroleptic treatment characterized by hyperthermia, rigidity, confusion, diaphoresis, autonomic instability, elevated creatine phosphokinase (CPK), and leukocytosis.[89] Although the first symptoms of NMS may involve mental status changes, the syndrome may evolve gradually and culminate in fever and an elevated CPK. NMS probably occurs in fewer than 1% of patients who receive first-generation antipsychotics, although sub-syndromal cases may be much more common.[90] Parallels have been drawn between NMS and malignant hyperthermia (which results from general anesthesia), largely on the basis of common clinical characteristics. Patients with a history of either NMS or malignant hyperthermia, however, do not appear to be at increased risk for developing the other syndrome, and analysis of muscle biopsy specimens has not consistently demonstrated physiological overlap between the two conditions. Most cases of malignant hyperthermia are due to a genetic mutation in the ryanodine receptor that regulates calcium movement in muscle tissue.[91] Lethal catatonia is a spontaneously occurring syndrome that may be indistinguishable from NMS that reportedly can occur in the absence of neuroleptic treatment.[92] In addition, antipsychotic agents may impair temperature regulation, and thus may produce low-grade fever in the absence of other symptoms of NMS.[93] The clinician's immediate response to NMS should be to discontinue antipsychotic medications and hospitalize the patient to allow for IV fluids and cooling. Whether bromocriptine or dantrolene facilitates recovery remains the subject of debate. It is important that re-institution of antipsychotics is delayed until at least 2 weeks after the episode of NMS has resolved.[94] NMS has been associated with all antipsychotics, including clozapine and other second-generation antipsychotics.[95] It has been suggested that a variant of NMS without rigidity may result from use of second-generation antipsychotics; if such a syndrome occurs, it is probably quite rare, and typical presentations (i.e., with muscular rigidity) are to be expected.

Drug Interactions With Antipsychotic Agents

Antipsychotic drugs interact with other medications as a result of alterations of hepatic metabolism and combined use of drugs with additive side effects (such as anticholinergic effects or impairments of cardiac conduction). Most first-generation antipsychotics are extensively metabolized by the 2D6 isoenzyme of the hepatic P450 enzyme system, whereas second-generation agents generally have more variable hepatic metabolism, typically involving isoenzymes 3A4, 1A2, and 2D6.[53] Fortunately, the therapeutic index (safety/risk ratio) of antipsychotic drugs is quite large, and interactions with agents that inhibit hepatic metabolism are unlikely to be life-threatening, but may increase side effects. Clozapine produces the most serious adverse effects when blood levels are dramatically elevated; obtundation and cardiovascular effects have been associated with inhibition of clozapine metabolism by fluvoxamine or erythromycin. Fluvoxamine, a selective serotonin re-uptake inhibitor (SSRI), has been shown to quadruple clozapine plasma concentrations.[96] Some patients experience a doubling of clozapine blood levels when they quit smoking, along with sedation and worsening of other side effects. Addition of 2D6 inhibitors (e.g., SSRIs) to first-generation antipsychotics would be expected to increase EPS, but in one placebo-controlled trial this was not clinically significant, despite substantial increases in blood levels of haloperidol and fluphenazine.[97] Drugs that pan-induce hepatic metabolism, such as certain anticonvulsants (e.g., carbamazepine, phenobarbital, phenytoin), may lower blood concentrations of most antipsychotics substantially and cause loss of therapeutic efficacy.

Considerable inter-individual variability exists for the metabolism of antipsychotic drugs, even without the complication of drug interactions. Therapeutic plasma concentrations have been best established for haloperidol because it is the antipsychotic least complicated by active metabolites. Plasma concentrations between 5 and 15 ng/mL have been associated with an optimal therapeutic response.[98] Clozapine has been found to be effective at serum concentrations of between 200 and 300 ng/mL, although some patients might benefit from levels above 350 ng/mL.[99] The risk of toxicity, particularly seizures, is generally believed to be significant at levels above 1000 ng/mL although individual vulnerability (brain damage, alcoholism) plays a role.

Great care must be taken if low-potency agents (such as chlorpromazine or clozapine) are combined with other highly anticholinergic drugs, because the additive anticholinergic activity may produce confusion, urinary retention, and constipation. In addition, low-potency antipsychotics can depress cardiac function and can significantly impair cardiac conduction when added to class I antiarrhythmic agents (such as quinidine and procainamide). Ziprasidone and iloperidone also significantly affect cardiac conduction and should not be combined with low-potency phenothiazines or with antiarrhythmic agents.

WORKING WITH THE PATIENT AND THE FAMILY

Patients with schizophrenia may be unable to directly express their fears or concerns; instead, they may exhibit anxiety or insomnia and may become increasingly delusional in the face of stress. Efforts to anticipate and answer a patient's unspoken fears about his or her medical status can greatly alleviate other symptoms, although this process may need to be repeated daily. Patients with schizophrenia may also lack the capacity to "filter out" extraneous stimuli in their environment and so may become easily overwhelmed or overly stimulated in a busy, chaotic environment. Placing a patient with schizophrenia in as quiet and orderly a room as possible can help the patient retain a sense of control and foster reality testing. The patient's need for privacy should be respected, and nursing staff should be advised that some patients with schizophrenia do not respond to overly nurturing or seemingly intrusive attention.

Families of patients with schizophrenia can be an invaluable source of information in any setting; they can help establish the diagnosis and identify potential behavioral problems. Family members might have a clear idea if poor adherence or illicit drug use contribute to psychiatric problems. Patients are poor judges of cognitive problems and functional limitations, whereas family members can often provide a more accurate picture of these domains. Working with families is always important; it is arguably most important when the patient experiences or is recovering from his or her first psychotic episode. Education about the illness, a discussion about the use of medication, and identification of the early signs of relapse after remission can start in the hospital and help with the transition to outpatient care. Families need to know about the risk for suicide in schizophrenia because they could be the first ones to recognize that a patient is becoming hopeless or disillusioned after discharge. It has been well demonstrated that educating families about the illness and helping them develop reasonable expectations for their loved one with schizophrenia significantly improves the course of the illness and is time well spent.[100]

MORE PROBLEMS IN THE CARE OF PSYCHOTIC PATIENTS

Assessment of Dangerousness

The public has long associated mental illness with violence. However, any such link is complex, and having a mental illness *per se* does not predict violence.[101] Instead, clinicians need to assess well-established predictors of violence, particularly substance use and past violence, preferably not only by self-report which is unreliable. An important component cause of violence that should not be overlooked is sociopathy.[102] Obviously, unmitigated psychosis or manic irritability can potentially result in acts of violence.[103] Although assaultive behavior is probably more likely in disorganized patients as a result of impaired control of aggression, violent acts such as homicide, which involve planning or complex behaviors, are much more likely in patients with persecutory or religious delusions (when they are convinced that they have no alternative but to act violently—either to defend themselves or family or to obey God's command). Negative symptoms reduce the risk for violence because afflicted patients are less likely to initiate activity. Command hallucinations appear to increase the risk of violence only when the individual interprets the voices within a delusional system in such a way that the voices cannot be disobeyed.[104] For example, a patient may believe that it is God's voice giving orders to attack someone believed to be possessed by Satan. Although the potential for violence from disorganized or delusional patients is a cause for concern, homicide is committed by fewer than 1% of patients with schizophrenia. Psychiatric treatment of psychosis is a critical violence prevention task for psychiatrists.

Suicide is a main cause of premature death in patients with schizophrenia; 5% of patients with schizophrenia commit suicide and as many as 50% make an attempt.[105] In addition to delusions and hallucinations, depression and substance abuse are important risk factors for suicide. The consultant must explore carefully these risk factors as well as any history of violent or self-injurious behaviors. In patients at high risk for violence or suicide, the antipsychotic clozapine should be considered. Studies have shown a specific protective effect of clozapine on violence[106] and suicide that may not be shared by other antipsychotics.[107]

Even in patients with schizophrenia with a history of violence, unusual diagnoses of concurrent illnesses such as encephalitis need to be ruled out.[108] Regardless of its cause, in cases in which risk of violence or self-harm is ongoing in the hospital, patients must be monitored continuously. If safe, a sitter is preferred over use of restraints, but some situations require restraints for the safety of the patient, other hospital patients, and staff. However, the indication for restraint must be clear, and restraint has to be part of an overall treatment plan. Inappropriate use of restraint is not only unjust, but any restraint carries risks, such as deep vein thrombosis and death from pulmonary embolism.[109]

Pain Threshold in Schizophrenia

A large literature suggests that patients with schizophrenia may have dramatically elevated pain thresholds, which can obscure serious medical problems.[110,111] In one study, 21% of schizophrenic patients did not describe pain associated with a perforated peptic ulcer, and 37% felt no pain during acute appendicitis. It has been estimated that more than 95% of the general public would experience excruciating pain with either condition. The mechanism underlying this often-dramatic analgesic effect remains unclear, but it does not appear to be the result of medication. It is important for the psychiatric consultant to make medical colleagues aware of this characteristic of patients with schizophrenia, so that the existence of serious pathologic processes is not dismissed because of an absence of typical manifestations of pain.[112]

Psychogenic Polydipsia (Water Intoxication)

Psychogenic polydipsia is defined as chronic or intermittent ingestion of large volumes of water; it is reported in 6% to 17% of chronically ill patients with serious mental illness. Polydipsia is most frequently observed in patients with schizophrenia, in whom it generally appears 5 to 15 years after the onset of illness.[113] While historically associated with institutionalized patients, 15% of outpatients show excessive water intake.[114] Polydipsia may lead to several complications, including bladder dilatation, enuresis, incontinence, hydronephrosis, renal failure, and congestive heart failure. Approximately 25% to 50% of patients with polydipsia develop hyponatremia within the first 10 years of this condition. Often referred to as *water intoxication*, symptoms of polydipsia with hyponatremia include nausea, vomiting, blurred vision, tremors, cramps, ataxia, confusion, lethargy, seizures, coma, and death. Polydipsia with hyponatremia should be considered a serious complication of psychotic illness that requires careful evaluation and management. Acute care includes supportive treatment, fluid restriction, normal saline, and, in severe cases, use of hypertonic saline. Fluid restriction can be difficult to implement in patients who have no clear understanding of their contribution to the problem. Rapid correction of an abnormal serum sodium level is unwise, however, because it can lead to congestive heart failure and central pontine myelinolysis. A medical admission is often necessary until the serum sodium normalizes. Long-term management includes frequent monitoring of serum sodium concentrations and restriction of fluid intake when possible. *Vaptans* are a new class of medicines to manage hyponatremia. While clinicians might try them to treat hyponatremia due to psychogenic polydipsia, they are probably prohibitively expensive in most settings, particularly for chronic use.[115] Switching from conventional neuroleptics to clozapine may significantly improve polydipsia and hyponatremia in some patients.[116]

Medical Co-morbidities

As a group, patients with schizophrenia carry a high burden of medical illnesses, including, among others, obesity, diabetes, cardiovascular disease, HIV infection, and hepatitis.[117] Cardiovascular disease is the primary contributor to an average reduction in life expectancy of two decades or more, a gap that seems to be worsening.[118] Cancer (particularly lung cancer) is, after cardiovascular disease, the second most frequent medical cause of death in patients with schizophrenia.[119] Unfortunately, part of the excess mortality related to these medical illnesses is iatrogenic, because antipsychotics, regardless of class, can potentially contribute to cardiac deaths directly (i.e., from sudden death), and more indirectly via the development of cardiac disease (due to weight gain, diabetes, and dyslipidemia). Appropriate attention to the medical care of patients with psychotic illnesses has emerged as an important mandate for psychiatrists.[120] A medical hospital admission provides an excellent opportunity to review the adequacy of medical treatment for these patients, with emphasis on the highly prevalent metabolic syndrome (about 40% in the CATIE sample mentioned earlier[121]), cardiovascular risk factors, and antipsychotic-related problems. Patients who do not have a primary care doctor can be identified and linked with community providers. In selected patients, screening for the metabolic syndrome, hepatitis C, and HIV infection can be accomplished during a hospitalization, particularly if it is unlikely to occur otherwise.[33]

Cigarette Smoking

Several decades ago, smoking cigarettes was almost ubiquitous in patients with a serious mental illness: approximately 85% of patients with schizophrenia smoked, usually quite heavily.[122] While progress has been made, the rate of everyday smokers among patients with mental illness is still higher than the general population.[123] It is especially concerning that 50% of young patients with schizophrenia smoke, which is a much higher rate than their peers.[124] For those patients who still smoke, quitting should be one of the most important health goals, particularly in the light of the aforementioned burden of cardiovascular disease in this population. Most patients with schizophrenia want to and with the right supports can quit smoking.[125] A hospital admission might provide a window of opportunity to motivate the patient for a quit attempt, particularly if the admission was related in some way to smoking. During an admission, nicotine dermal patches can provide some protection against nicotine withdrawal. Smoking reduces the drug levels of most antipsychotic drugs, particularly drugs that are metabolized by the 1A2 P450 enzyme system (e.g., olanzapine, clozapine). During lengthier hospital stays, the possible effects (e.g., an increase in EPS) of forced abstinence on drug metabolism should be considered; this effect is not mediated by nicotine, but by tar products, and hence not reversed by nicotine patches.[126] Smoking cessation treatment needs to be comprehensive and combine pharmacotherapy with behavioral treatment. While bupropion and nicotine replacement therapy alone or in combination are good medication choices to help some patients with schizophrenia quit smoking, varenicline is the most effective medication to help patients quit and importantly remain abstinent.[127] Compared with other populations, where short-term pharmacotherapy is sufficient to assist in quitting but not needed for long-term abstinence, many patients with schizophrenia benefit from maintenance treatment to prevent relapse.[128] Varenicline has been studied in many patients with psychiatric illnesses, including psychosis and has in general been found to be safe, with neuropsychiatric side effect rates being similar between placebo-treated and varenicline-treated patients.[129]

CONCLUSION

Medication Adherence and Insight Into Illness

One hallmark of schizophrenia is an often striking lack of insight into their mental illness: its symptoms, consequences, and need for treatment.[130] A psychotic patient who has just been involuntarily committed to a psychiatric hospital after fighting with police might report that the reason for the admission was that he came for coffee. Thankfully, this is an extreme example, and many patients have at least some understanding of the role of psychiatric treatment and can participate meaningfully in decisions regarding use of antipsychotics. Clinicians need to determine the specific reason for poor antipsychotic adherence so that specific remedies can be sought.[131] In some patients, supervision is all that is required, whereas in others, one of the assisted treatment options (such as assertive community treatment, ACT) will be required. There is little doubt that for the great majority of patients, maintenance antipsychotics must play a pivotal role in preventing psychotic relapse. This is true for patients who have been ill for many years, and for patients who are recovering from their first psychotic episode. In one study of first-episode psychosis patients who discontinued maintenance antipsychotics, 78% and 96% of patients experienced another psychotic episode within 1 and 2 years, respectively.[132] The prevention of further psychotic episodes is paramount because psychotic episodes come at a high cost to the patient: professional lives are interrupted; there is stigma and embarrassment associated with a psychiatric hospitalization; and there is always the danger of violence, accidental injury, and death. On the other hand, medical hospital staff can be reassured that antipsychotics can usually be held for a brief medical hospital stay or procedure *if necessary* because relapse is typically measured in weeks or months, not days, for remitted patients. For most patients with stable schizophrenia who require a medical admission these long-term adherence issues are not usually relevant, and house staff can simply continue the psychiatric outpatient regimen.

REFERENCES

Access the reference list online at https://expertconsult.inkling.com/.

13 Anxious Patients

Sean P. Glass, M.D.
Mark H. Pollack, M.D.
Michael W. Otto, Ph.D.
Curtis W. Wittmann, M.D.
Jerrold F. Rosenbaum, M.D.

OVERVIEW

Clinical challenges in the diagnosis and treatment of anxiety are abundant in the general hospital setting: discerning normal from pathologic anxiety, differentiating medical from psychiatric causes, and choosing effective therapeutic approaches. In addition to a knowledge of medical and psychiatric differential diagnoses, the clinician may rely on a variety of strategies and interventions that involve pharmacologic, cognitive-behavioral, interpersonal, and psychodynamic skills. The ubiquity of anxiety and the non-specific nature of anxiety symptoms can confound the care of the patient. Pathologic anxiety symptoms and behavior may be attributed to other physical causes or, when viewed as "only anxiety," may be prematurely dismissed as insignificant.

Anxiety refers to a state of anticipation of alarming future events, whereas fear is a result of perceived imminent threat.[1] The former is the same distressing experience of dread and foreboding as the latter, except that it derives from an unknown internal stimulus or is inappropriate to the reality of the current situation. Anxiety is manifested in the physical, affective, cognitive, and behavioral domains. The possible physical symptoms of anxiety reflect autonomic arousal and include an array of bodily perturbations (Table 13-1). The anxious state ranges from edginess and unease to terror and panic. Cognitively, the experience is one of worry, apprehension, and thoughts concerned with emotional or bodily danger. Behaviorally, anxiety triggers a multitude of responses concerned with diminishing or avoiding the distress.

The importance of recognizing and attending to the suffering of the anxious patient is not always readily apparent, given the universality of the experience of anxiety. Anxiety is expected and normal as a transient response to stress and may be a necessary cue for adaptation and coping. Excessive or pathologic anxiety, however, is no more a normal state than is the production of excess thyroid hormone.

Pathologic anxiety is distinguished from a normal emotional response by four criteria: autonomy, intensity, duration, and behavior. *Autonomy* refers to suffering that, to some extent, has a life of its own, with a minimal basis in recognizable environmental stimuli. *Intensity* refers to the level of distress; the severity of symptoms is such that the patient's level of anguish moves the physician to offer relief. The *duration* of suffering also can define anxiety as pathologic. Symptoms that are persistent rather than transient, possibly adaptive, indicate a disorder and they are a call to evaluation and treatment. Finally, *behavior* is a critical criterion; if anxiety impairs coping, if normal function is disrupted, or if behavior such as avoidance or withdrawal results, the anxiety is of a pathologic nature.

Stereotyped syndromes of pathologic anxiety are described in the American Psychiatric Association's *Diagnostic and Statistical Manual of Mental Disorders* (DSM).[2] Changes in the DSM-5 diagnostic criteria for anxiety disorders include the re-categorization of obsessive–compulsive disorder (OCD), post-traumatic stress disorder (PTSD), and acute stress disorder. These syndromes will all be included in this chapter given the pervasiveness of anxiety and fear that is common to all of these disorders. In epidemiologic studies, anxiety disorders have been found to be among the most common psychiatric disorders in the general population.[3] This observation predicts that a significant percentage of the general hospital population would also suffer from anxiety symptoms. Some patients suffer from an anxiety disorder before admission to the hospital for medical care, but medical and surgical settings are also associated with the onset of anxiety symptoms as a consequence of hospitalization, medical illness, or treatment (e.g., adjustment disorder with anxious mood and organic anxiety disorder).[4]

THE NATURE AND ORIGIN OF ANXIETY

Despite the protean physiologic manifestations of anxiety, the experience of anxiety can be divided into two broad categories: (1) an acute, severe, and brief wave of intense anxiety with impressive cognitive, physiologic, and behavioral components, and (2) a lower-grade persistent distress, quantitatively distinct and also with some qualitative differences. Pharmacologic and epidemiologic observations suggest a clinically relevant distinction between these two states.

In light of phenomenologic similarities, fear and anxiety most likely reflect a common underlying neurophysiology. The first category of anxiety resembles acute fear or alarm in response to life-threatening danger: a cognitive state of terror, helplessness, or sense of impending disaster or doom, with autonomic but primarily sympathetic activation, and an urgency to flee or seek safety. The second type of anxiety corresponds to a state of alertness with a heightened sense of vigilance to possible threats and with less intense levels of inhibition, physical distress, and behavioral impairment.

TABLE 13-1 Physical Signs and Symptoms of Anxiety

Anorexia	Muscle tension
"Butterflies" in stomach	Nausea
Chest pain or tightness	Pallor
Diaphoresis	Palpitations
Diarrhea	Paresthesias
Dizziness	Sexual dysfunction
Dry mouth	Shortness of breath
Dyspnea	Stomach pain
Faintness	Tachycardia
Flushing	Tremulousness
Headache	Urinary frequency
Hyperventilation	Vomiting
Light-headedness	

The two fear states resemble the clinical syndromes of panic attacks and generalized or anticipatory anxiety. As innate responses for protecting the organism and enhancing survival, panic and vigilance are normal when faced with threatening stimuli. As anxiety or psychopathologic symptoms, other factors besides actual physical threat must be implicated as triggers or causes. Of several explanatory models proposed, the biological model places emphasis on the nervous system, the psychodynamic on meanings and memories, and the behavioral on learning.

Animal and neuronal receptor studies suggest that a number of central systems are involved in fear and pathologic anxiety.[5,6] The alarm or panic mechanism is likely to have a critical component involving central noradrenergic mechanisms, with particular importance placed on a small retropontine nucleus, the primary source of the brain's norepinephrine, the locus ceruleus (LC). When this key to sympathetic activation is stimulated in monkeys, for example, an acute fear response can be elicited with distress vocalizations, fear behaviors, and flight. Furthermore, destruction of the LC leads to abnormal complacency in the face of threat.[7] Biochemical perturbations that increase LC firing similarly elicit anxious responses in animals and humans that are blocked by agents that decrease LC firing, some of which are in clinical practice as anti-panic agents (e.g., antidepressants, alprazolam).[8]

Another critical system involves limbic system structures, including the amygdala and septohippocampal areas. An important role of the limbic system is to scan the environment for life-supporting and life-threatening cues, as well as to monitor internal or bodily sensations, and to integrate these with memory and cognitive inputs in assessing the degree of threat and need for action to maintain safety.[9]

Vigilance, or its psychopathologic equivalent, generalized anxiety, most probably involves limbic system activity: limbic alert. Benzodiazepine receptors in high concentrations in relevant limbic system structures may play a role in modulating limbic alert, arousal, and behavioral inhibition[10] by increased binding of the inhibitory neurotransmitter gamma-aminobutyric acid (GABA).[11] As one might expect, there are neuronal connections between the LC and the limbic system. An increased firing rate of LC neurons may serve as a rheostat to generate levels of arousal from vigilance to alarm.

A number of neurotransmitters are implicated as modulators of both the limbic alert and the central alarm systems. For example, LC firing is regulated by the α_2-noradrenergic autoreceptors as well as by 5-hydroxytryptamine (5-HT), serotonin receptors, GABA-benzodiazepine receptors, and opioid and other receptors. The limbic system also has important GABA-benzodiazepine receptor and serotonergic modulations. Peptides, such as cholecystokinin,[12] have also been implicated as potential activators of the alarm system, and an accruing body of work points to abnormalities in corticotropin-releasing factor and hypothalamic–pituitary axis function as critical in the genesis and maintenance of pathologic affective states.[13] As a critical function, the central security system is endowed with redundancy of regulation.

When inappropriately activated, vigilance and alarm (the stereotyped functions of the security system) are manifested as psychopathology: anxiety states. The more sustained, variably intense, but distressing arousal state of vigilance (i.e., preparation for threat) becomes generalized anxiety. The sudden, stereotyped, and intense (but false) alarm response is a panic attack.

Cognitive-behavioral formulations of anxiety disorders, although attending to possible differences in biological reactivity, focus primary attention on the information processing and behavioral reactions that characterize an individual's anxiety experience. Although anxiety patterns may stem from a variety of experiences, including (mis)information, observational learning, and direct conditioning events with real or perceived trauma, the enduring consequences of such learning can be found in current patterns of behavior. In cognitive-behavioral formulations, emphasis is placed on the role of thoughts and beliefs (cognitions) in activating anxiety, as well as on the role of avoidance or other escape responses in maintaining both fear and faulty thinking patterns. Faulty cognitions are frequently marked by the over-prediction of the likelihood or degree of catastrophe of negative events and may focus on external experiences (e.g., "my colleagues will laugh at me if I ask this question") or internal experiences (e.g., "I am going to lose control if this anxiety gets worse"). Intolerance and catastrophic misinterpretations of the anxiety experience itself play a role in a variety of anxiety conditions and can help propel mild anxiety into a full, intense panic attack. Attempts to neutralize anxious feelings, with avoidance or compulsive behavior, can serve to lock in anxiety reactions and help to develop the chronic arousal and anticipatory anxiety that marks many anxiety disorders.

Recent evidence has offered a bridge between neurobiological and cognitive-behavioral understandings of anxiety. Increased attention has been paid to the consolidation of memories after traumatic experiences and potential therapeutic interventions (e.g., blocking of the noradrenergic or glucocorticoid systems to decrease the potential for developing PTSD after trauma). Knowledge of the *N*-methyl-D-aspartate (NMDA) system's involvement in the extinction of learned behaviors has offered the possibility of pharmacologic enhancement of cognitive-behavioral therapy (CBT) techniques. D-cycloserine, a partial NMDA agonist, has facilitated treatment of specific phobias, obsessive–compulsive disorder (OCD), panic disorder, and social anxiety disorders when combined with CBT.[14]

Developmental experiences receive particular emphasis in psychodynamic approaches to anxiety. Although Freud's early writing implied a more physiologic basis for anxiety attacks in terms of undischarged libido, later emphasis was on anxiety as a signal of threat to the ego, signals elicited because of events and situations with similarities (symbolic or actual) to early developmental experiences that were threatening to the vulnerable child (traumatic anxiety), such as separations, losses, certain constellations of relationships, and symbolic objects or events (e.g., snakes, successes). More recently, psychodynamic thinking has emphasized object relations and the use of internalized objects to maintain affective stability under stress.

Phobic disorders, associated with the experience of panic, anticipatory anxiety, or no anxiety symptoms at all (depending on the success of avoidance behavior), serve to illustrate the different models of understanding anxiety. The biological view recognizes the stereotyped nature of phobias. Most of the objects and situations in everyday life that truly threaten us are rarely selected as phobic stimuli; children, who proceed normally through a variety of developmental phobias (e.g., strangers, separation, darkness), rarely become phobic of objects and situations that parents attempt to associate with danger (e.g., electric outlets and roads), and most phobic stimuli have meaning in the context of biological preparedness and were presumably selected through evolution.[15] Most human phobias are of objects and situations that make sense in the context of enhancing survival before the dawn of civilization: places of restricted escape, groups of strangers, heights, and snakes, for example. Social phobias—for example, fear of scrutiny by others—resemble the intense discomfort elicited in primates introduced into a new colony or in any animal simply being stared at. A glare is a threat. When panic attacks and anticipatory anxiety heighten the general sense of danger and insecurity, a variety of phobias may be manifested as part of the patient's increased concern with security and safety.

The principal explanatory models in psychiatry of how a normal protective system might become the source of distress and dysfunction include the biological (with its emphasis on constitutional vulnerability), the cognitive-behavioral (with its emphasis on self-perpetuating patterns of cognitions and behaviors), and the psychodynamic (with its emphasis on meanings, memories, and internal representations derived from developmental experience). The pragmatic and pluralistic modern clinician should not regard these models as mutually exclusive. Potential biological vulnerabilities, for example, may never become manifest without specific developmental experiences, sustained adversity, or trauma. Accumulating evidence indicates that for anxiety disorders, as with affective and psychotic disorders, biological systems are responsive to, and perturbable by, environmental influences. Potentially dysregulated (i.e., anxiety-prone) neurobiological systems may remain homeostatic until developmental experience, life events, or other stressors disturb them. An integrated model predicts risk for manifested anxiety disorders as a consequence of constitutional vulnerability shaped by developmental experience (whether harmful or protective) and, in later (adult) life, either activated or influenced by environmental factors and maintained by ongoing chains of maladaptive cognitions and avoidance responses.

ANXIETY IN THE MEDICAL SETTING

Although some distress from anxiety is expected as a routine consequence of hospitalization, anxiety may also be a significant clinical issue in the treatment of patients in a medical setting. The hospitalized patient encounters a world of both internal and external dangers: assaults on bodily integrity in the form of uncomfortable procedures and forced intimacy with strangers; the atmosphere of illness, pain, and death; and separation from loved ones and familiar surroundings. The patient typically experiences uncertainty about his or her illness and its implications for the patient's capacity to work and maintain social and family relationships. Just as depression has been described as a "psychobiological final common pathway" of a number of interacting determinants,[16] it is likely that anxiety too represents a multiple-determined expression of the variety of psychological, biological, and social factors having impact on the patient.

The anxious patient can be a diagnostic challenge. The presence of anxiety may represent the patient's reaction to the meaning and implications of medical illness or to the medical setting, a manifestation of the physical disorder itself, or the expression of an underlying psychiatric disorder. The distinction between anxiety as a symptom and anxiety as a syndrome, may be difficult to make in the medical setting, where there may be an overlap between normal situational anxiety or fear, anxiety-like symptoms resulting from a variety of organic disease states and their treatments, and the characteristic presentation of anxiety disorders.

Methodological obstacles surface in attempts to identify the nature and prevalence of anxiety in medical patients.[17] Studies of anxiety in the medical setting are often difficult to interpret because of a lack of clarity of case definition and assessment measures, heterogeneity of the study populations, absence of appropriate control groups, and the non-specific and often transitory nature of the anxiety symptoms themselves.

Approximately 60% of patients with psychiatric conditions are treated by primary care practitioners; the most common disorders are depression and anxiety.[18,19] In a study of patients who presented to a group of primary care physicians, anxiety was the fifth most common diagnosis overall; others suggest this may be an underestimate.[20,21] Anxiety is the chief complaint of 11% of patients presenting in primary care settings.[22] This prevalence is mirrored by the high rate of prescribing benzodiazepines by primary care physicians.[23] Panic disorder has a reported prevalence of 1% to 2% in the general population,[24] as compared with 6% to 10% of patients in a primary care setting[25] and 10% to 14% of patients in a cardiology practice.[26] Patients with anxiety disorders, furthermore, are but a subgroup of those for whom anxiety is a complicating factor in their diagnosis and treatment in the hospital.

In view of the likely frequency of normal anxiety in this setting, there must be special circumstances surrounding those patients identified by primary caregivers as deserving psychiatric attention. Although some overly anxious patients go unrecognized, those who generate concern have impressed their caregivers in some way by the autonomy, intensity, duration, or behavior associated with their distress. Several typical scenarios of anxiety in the general hospital can be recognized.

Anxiety From Failure to Cope

For most patients, potentially overwhelming stressors of hospitalization are mitigated by a variety of coping mechanisms. The sources of threat and the flood of perceptions signaling potential danger are managed by common strategies: rationalization and self-reassurance ("I've come this far," "the doctors know what they're doing," "safest place in the world"); denial and minimization ("the chest pain is just heartburn," "these machines will protect me"); religious faith; support from family and friends; and other strategies determined by the patient's personality style.

Even for those without a pre-illness anxiety disorder, coping strategies may fail and yield to a sense of fear and vulnerability. A host of factors may be implicated in this failure: personality features with brittleness or a tendency to regress in the face of threat (or paradoxically in a setting that evokes passivity and offers access to nurturance), the suddenness of the onset of threat (acute, life-threatening medical or surgical disease), unavailability of familial or other social support, feelings of aloneness or abandonment, or the unconscious meaning of the particular illness or injury. The patient becomes frightened, trembles, cannot sleep, repeatedly seeks attention and reassurance, registers excessive pain complaints and other physical symptoms, and becomes disruptive and unable to manage the fear. For many, especially the young or those with organic brain syndromes (e.g., mental retardation or dementia), catastrophic emotional responses are more readily triggered.

CASE 1

A psychiatric consultation request was received for a 17-year-old high school junior following an above-the-knee amputation for osteogenic sarcoma without evidence of metastasis at the time of surgery. He had returned to school with a prosthesis and had done well. Some months later, a pulmonary metastasis was discovered, and he was re-hospitalized for surgery and chemotherapy. Although anticipating a favorable outcome at this point, his behavior was unlike that of his prior hospitalization. He raged at caregivers, acted panicky, and withdrew from contact. Consultation was sought for treatment of his anxiety.

He was a tall, handsome, athletic young man admired by his peers, a leader who managed his life with braggadocio and pseudo-independence. For the first time in his illness, he was overwhelmed and frightened. Two critical issues emerged from the interview. First, in the past, he had had a great deal of support from his peers, but lately he had refused their visits. He was embarrassed by hair loss from chemotherapy. Second, during this hospitalization, his father, feeling overwhelmed by this turn of events, had decreased the frequency of visits to his son, claiming increased work demands.

Two interventions calmed the acute anxiety. First, an effort was made to find a well-suited wig; second, a psychotherapeutic contact with the father helped him to manage his grief adequately to increase the frequency of visits, and thereby relieve his son's separation anxiety.

Although the oncologist's request was for an anxiolytic prescription, recognition of the failure of coping ability yielded the appropriate therapy for the acute anxiety.

This case serves to underscore two points: previously well-adapted individuals can become anxious in the face of serious or life-threatening illness; and, despite the appropriateness of anxiety in the face of serious illness, other factors, potentially remediable, may be involved in triggering anxious symptoms or behavior. In this case, troublesome behavior was evident; for others, only more subtle physical symptoms may have occurred.

PTSD Resulting From Traumatic Procedures

In recent years, increasing attention has been paid to the role of serious medical illness and invasive procedures in producing reactions that approach or meet criteria for PTSD. For example, symptoms of PTSD have been documented in patients after myocardial infarction (MI), coronary artery bypass graft surgery,[27] and treatment for breast cancer,[28] traumatic brain injury,[29] and in those who require intensive care (a setting associated with increased morbidity and mortality).[30] Estimates of rates of PTSD in these samples of patients range from 5% to 10%,[28] with rates of PTSD in patients hospitalized after traumatic physical injuries as high as 30% to 40%.[31] The emergence of PTSD is considered most likely when a traumatic event is perceived as both uncontrollable and life-threatening[32] as such, any attempts to help patients regain or maintain a sense of control over their experiences may prevent or reduce emergent distress.

CASE 2

Ms. B, a 52-year-old woman with a history of depression, anxiety, chronic back pain, and severe peripheral vascular disease, was admitted to the hospital as preparation for a femoral artery–popliteal artery bypass. Consultation was requested for management of anxiety because surgery had previously been attempted but was aborted when the patient became acutely anxious when the staff began to disrobe her.

During the course of the consultation, Ms. B revealed that she had been the victim of a sexual assault at age 24. In the past, she had not needed treatment for symptoms related to this event. However, during the preparation for surgery, she began to re-experience her trauma while she was being disrobed.

Education was provided to Ms. B regarding the sequence of events that would take place leading up to and during the operation. The surgical staff was educated about the effects of past trauma and the need for special consideration regarding this patient. An agreement was made to allow the patient to disrobe herself prior to the initiation of the surgery. This increased her sense of control and she was able to tolerate the surgery, which went well.

This case demonstrates the importance of the events that take place during a hospitalization, but also a patient's prior experiences with trauma. By talking with Ms. B and identifying the historical factors as well as the present conditions that made this experience difficult for her, a plan was devised to alleviate as much of her anxiety as possible. Under these conditions, she was able to take a more active role and complete the necessary medical procedure.

Memory of events during anesthesia has been documented in controlled trials,[33,34] leading to recommendations that the surgical staff provide reassurance to patients during surgery and monitor their own verbalizations in the presence of anesthetized patients. Intraoperative awareness occurs in 1–2 of every thousand cases and may occur with general anesthesia as well as with sedation/regional anesthesia.[35] Risk factors for intraoperative awareness include use of light anesthesia (that is often used in conjunction with cardiac surgery, surgery following an acute trauma, and cesarean deliveries), and a history of intraoperative awareness.[35] The modified Bruce interview is commonly used as a screening tool for the detection of intraoperative awareness.[36] Intraoperative methods to reduce awareness of events include the use of monitoring end-tidal anesthetic concentration and the use of EEG-derived bispectral index to monitor levels of sedation.[35] Both of these methods have proven effective at reducing rates of intraoperative awareness.[37] Bispectral index is recommended when intravenous (IV) sedative–hypnotics or heterogeneous anesthetic agents are used primarily for sedation. End-tidal anesthetic gas concentration can be used if inhaled agents are utilized.

Reactions to awareness during surgery include generalized anxiety and irritability, repetitive nightmares, and preoccupation with death, as well as reluctance to discuss the memory or associated symptoms.[38] More severe reactions have also been documented, including the full emergence of PTSD after experiences of awareness during surgery. Rates of PTSD after intraoperative awareness have been reported to be as high as 70%.[39] Patients who are aware during surgery may face the terrifying experience of pain occurring in conjunction with anesthesia-induced paralysis (ensuring that no overt coping or escape responses are available), and fear of death. As memories of the trauma emerge, patients may face the full spectrum of PTSD symptoms, including: re-experiencing symptoms (intrusive memories, nightmares, and over-responsivity to cues of the surgery); avoidance of reminders of the experience (e.g., avoidance of strong emotions, prone bodily positions or sleep, medical television shows, colors similar to those of surgical scrub suits); and symptoms of pervasive autonomic arousal (e.g., exaggerated startle, sleep difficulties, hypervigilance, and irritability). Timely identification of this syndrome can aid in rapid referral for full psychiatric evaluation and treatment, which may include both cognitive-behavioral and pharmacologic interventions.

Anxiety That Interferes With Evaluation or Treatment

A request for consultation may be a consequence of anxiety that interferes with a patient's evaluation or treatment: refusal of work-up or treatment because of fear of pain or discomfort, catastrophic interpretation of physical symptoms or of the planned work-up ("they're looking for cancer") with an excessively fearful response, or the need to minimize or deny a potentially serious condition and its implications, limiting cooperation with evaluation.

CASE 3

Examination of Mrs. C, a 38-year-old woman, revealed a large breast lump. Although initially reluctant, she eventually agreed to a mammogram. In the waiting room, she became increasingly anxious and, when her name was called, refused to come in for the test. A psychiatric consultation was called to provide management of the patient's anxiety to permit the mammogram.

An attractive woman, she had stopped working as a teacher 12 years earlier after marrying a successful business executive and having the first of her two children. On interviewing, she spoke of a favorite aunt who had died of breast cancer after disfiguring surgeries, and of her own fear of a similar lesion. She was plagued by the thought that the loss of a breast would cause her husband to lose interest and abandon her. She had not informed her husband of her current medical situation.

Meeting subsequently with both husband and wife, the psychiatrist gave explicit information about the possibility of malignancy and treatment options. The husband's manifest interest, support, and affection were reassuring; after the mammogram, a benign lump was removed.

Discovery of the meaning to the patient of the illness and the procedure permitted an intervention that sufficiently reduced her anxiety to allow evaluation and treatment. As with any situational anxiety, the fear of serious or fatal illness can be managed with education, support, cognitive and behavioral strategies, and at times, the short-term use of benzodiazepines.

Review of a patient's conceptualization of his or her medical condition, the procedures the patient faces, and the patient's interpretation of symptoms offers the physician the opportunity to correct cognitive distortions that may needlessly engender anxiety. Care should be taken in discussing symptoms and procedures, with sensitivity to an individual's coping style. The clinician should elicit the patient's conceptualization of his or her condition (or upcoming procedure) and provide corrective information when distortions are encountered.

Additional strategies may be helpful when phobias about select medical procedures are encountered. For example, the enclosed chamber of the magnetic resonance imaging (MRI) scanner presents a phobic challenge to some individuals, engendering fears of overwhelming anxiety because of the inability to "escape" the MRI scanner quickly. For individuals with a history of claustrophobia, panic disorder, or PTSD, pre-treatment with medications (e.g., benzodiazepines) or CBT may be required. In less severe cases, anxiety may be managed with simple procedures designed to maximize the patient's sense of safety and control. For example, compliance and comfort during the MRI scan may be aided by explaining to the patient the periods when he or she can shift positions or rub his or her hands together, the patient's ability to communicate with the nurse or technician, the patient's understanding of sounds and sensations to be experienced during the procedure, and the patient's ability to terminate the procedure, if need be. Initial practice of being moved into and out of the scanning chamber before the actual experience, as well as discussion of normal sensations of heat and anxiety experienced by patients while being scanned, can help normalize the experience and prevent catastrophic interpretations. There is evidence from analogue studies that information about the somatic sensations to be experienced during a procedure can help reduce anxiety and panic reactions.[40] Instruction in comforting imagining may also aid the patient in tolerating the procedure.

Anxiety that occurs in patients with a known and potentially fatal illness is more accurately termed *fear* because there is a known danger. Such fear, however, can adversely affect the course of illness and treatment. A study of survivors of MI, for example, indicated that 95% had increased tension and anxiety, and of one group of post-MI patients discharged from the hospital, 40% did not return to work; in 80%, psychological impairment, including anxiety, was the cause.[41]

Worry that activity will cause further heart damage or death interferes with rehabilitation and the return to autonomous function. The most effective therapeutic approaches for these patients center on education, group discussion, and support and stress management techniques.[42] Anxious patients with a diagnosed serious or fatal illness require treatment that includes education in addition to the possible use of supportive, cognitive-behavioral, or insight-oriented psychotherapy and anxiolytic or antidepressant medications.

Among patients with medical disorders, such as gastrointestinal (GI) disorders or allergies, the course and symptoms of the illness may be exacerbated by anxiety.[42,43] Anxiety, as with other emotional responses, may adversely affect normal physiologic function; asthma symptoms are exacerbated by emotional arousal or stress, and the increased symptoms generate further anxiety.[44] Psychological and emotional responses and behavior possibly affect the survival of patients with cancer through effects on the immune system.[45]

Medical Illnesses That Mimic Anxiety Disorder

Anxiety symptoms may be the principal manifestation of an underlying medical illness.[46] Of patients referred for psychiatric treatment, 5% to 42% have been reported as having an underlying medical illness responsible for their distress, with depression and anxiety as frequent complaints.[47,48] Of reported cases of medical illnesses causing anxiety symptoms, 25% have been secondary to neurologic problems; 25% to endocrinologic causes; 12% to circulatory, rheumatoid, or collagen vascular disorders and chronic infection; and 14% to miscellaneous other illnesses.[46] A most common cause of anxiety may be alcohol and drug use; the anxiety results from either intoxication or, more typically, withdrawal states.[49]

The clinical presentation of anxiety in the medical setting takes many forms. The bewildering array and variable nature of the physical and psychic symptoms reported by anxious patients may lead the physician to overlook symptoms related to another disorder.[4] The relative contribution of situational, psychiatric, and physiologic factors to the presentation of anxiety-like symptoms in a medical patient is often murky. The number of medical illnesses, furthermore, that may generate or exacerbate anxiety symptoms (Table 13-2) clearly renders an exhaustive evaluation for each of them impractical. A thorough yet efficient evaluation of the differential diagnostic possibilities, however, includes the following considerations:[46,50]

1. In a patient with a known medical illness, the condition and its associated complications and treatment may be the cause of anxiety. For example, in the asthmatic patient, hypoxia, respiratory distress, and sympathomimetic bronchodilators may all contribute to the experience of anxiety. In some patients, risk factors or predisposition, such as a family history of medical illness capable of causing anxiety-like symptoms (e.g., thyroid disease), may be clues to diagnosis.
2. In medical illnesses considered mimics of anxiety, the quality of anxiety symptoms when closely examined may be different from that seen in primary anxiety disorders. For example, Starkman and associates[51] studied 17 patients with pheochromocytoma and compared their anxiety symptoms with those of a group of 52 patients with anxiety and related disorders. Most patients with pheochromocytoma did not meet the criteria for panic disorder or generalized anxiety disorder (GAD); none developed agoraphobic symptoms, and their overall severity of symptoms was lower. There was a significant lack of psychological as opposed to physical symptoms of anxiety in most of these patients.
3. Similarly, patients with primary anxiety disorders are more likely to have emotional trauma related to the onset of anxiety, daily symptoms, neurotic features, and gradual resolution of symptoms after an attack and are less likely to have a loss of speech or consciousness during an episode of anxiety than are patients with anxiety associated with temporal lobe epilepsy.[52] Thus, the lack of a significant emotional experience of anxiety or the occurrence of anxiety only coincidental with particular physical events (e.g., a run of ventricular tachycardia on a cardiac monitor or spike activity on an electroencephalogram) may suggest the presence of an organic anxiety syndrome. Evaluation directed toward the somatic system (e.g., GI or cardiac) most prominently affected by anxiety symptoms may provide the greatest yield from further diagnostic investigations.
4. In patients with an onset of anxiety symptoms after the age of 35 years, a lack of personal or family history of anxiety disorders, a negative childhood history of anxiety symptoms, an absence of significant life events heralding or exacerbating anxiety symptoms, a lack of avoidance behavior, and a poor response to standard anti-anxiety agents, the presence of an organically based anxiety syndrome should be considered.
5. Even for the apparently healthy patient, particular scrutiny should be directed at more common conditions associated with anxiety: arrhythmias, thyroid abnormalities, excessive caffeine intake, and other drug use. Anxiety-like symptoms may be the first clue to a withdrawal syndrome in a patient with unreported regular sedative–hypnotic (e.g., ethchlorvynol, glutethimide, or a benzodiazepine) or alcohol use before admission to the hospital. Intoxication or withdrawal from prescription or over-the-counter medication or substances of abuse should also be suspected. Up to 3% of individuals have been reported to develop psychiatric symptoms after using prescribed or over-the-counter medication.[53]

TABLE 13-2 Selected Medical Causes of Anxiety

Endocrine
Adrenal cortical hyperplasia (Cushing's disease)
Adrenal cortical insufficiency (Addison's disease)
Adrenal tumors
Carcinoid syndrome
Cushing's syndrome
Diabetes mellitus
Hyperparathyroidism
Hyperthyroidism
Hypoglycemia
Hypothyroidism
Insulinoma
Menopause
Ovarian dysfunction
Pancreatic carcinoma
Pheochromocytoma
Pituitary disorders
Premenstrual syndrome
Testicular deficiency

Drug-Related
Intoxication
Analgesics
Antibiotics
Anticholinergics
Anticonvulsants
Antidepressants
Antihistamines
Antihypertensives
Antiinflammatory agents
Antiparkinsonian agents
Aspirin
Caffeine
Chemotherapy agents
Cocaine
Digitalis
Hallucinogens
Neuroleptics
Steroids
Sympathomimetics
Thyroid supplements
Tobacco
Withdrawal
Ethanol
Narcotics
Sedative–hypnotics

Cardiovascular and Circulatory
Anemia
Cerebral anoxia
Cerebral insufficiency
Congestive heart failure
Coronary insufficiency
Dysrhythmias
Hyperdynamic β-adrenergic state
Hypovolemia
Mitral valve prolapse
Myocardial infarction
Type A behavior

Respiratory
Asthma
Hyperventilation
Hypoxia
Pneumonia
Pneumothorax
Pulmonary edema
Pulmonary embolus

Immunologic-Collagen Vascular
Anaphylaxis
Polyarteritis nodosa
Rheumatoid arthritis
Systemic lupus erythematosus
Temporal arteritis

Metabolic
Acidosis
Acute intermittent porphyria
Electrolyte abnormalities
Hyperthermia
Pernicious anemia
Wilson's disease

Neurologic
Brain tumors (especially in the third ventricle)
Cerebral syphilis
Cerebrovascular disorders
Combined systemic disease
Encephalopathies (toxic, metabolic, infectious)
Epilepsy (especially temporal lobe epilepsy)
Essential tremor
Huntington's disease
Intracranial mass lesion
Migraine headaches
Multiple sclerosis
Myasthenia gravis
Organic brain syndrome
Pain
Polyneuritis
Post-concussive syndrome
Post-encephalitic disorders
Posterolateral sclerosis
Vertigo (including Ménière's disease and other vestibular dysfunction)

Gastrointestinal
Colitis
Esophageal dysmotility
Peptic ulcer

Infectious Disease
Acquired immunodeficiency syndrome
Atypical viral pneumonia
Brucellosis
Malaria
Mononucleosis
Tuberculosis
Viral hepatitis

Miscellaneous
Nephritis
Nutritional disorders
Other malignancies (e.g., oat cell carcinoma)

CASE 4

A psychiatric consultation was requested from the medical service for Ms. D, a 31-year-old secretary, who developed anxiety attacks shortly after learning that she had contracted syphilis from her boyfriend. She had previously experienced spontaneous anxiety attacks in her mid-20s that had remitted early in a 6-month course of the TCA imipramine, and she had been symptom free since. During the interview with the psychiatrist, Ms. D manifested anger and sadness about her boyfriend's infidelity and her own victimization, as well as anxiety about the future of their relationship. Her anxiety attacks, however, were different from those she had previously experienced. They consisted of blurred vision; dull bi-parietal headaches, primarily left-sided; numbness in her extremities; and feelings of dizziness. She reported feeling anxious after the onset of these symptoms. On further questioning, Ms. D described a history of menstrual irregularities over the past 2 to 3 years, and galactorrhea. Her prolactin level was found to be elevated, and a computed tomography scan revealed a pituitary adenoma. Surgical resection of the adenoma resulted in resolution of her anxiety attacks, although she elected to pursue psychotherapy to consider issues raised by the difficulties in her relationship.

This case serves to illustrate the following points. The presence of a history of an anxiety disorder or a recent stressor does not eliminate the need to consider medical illness in the differential diagnosis of a new or different presentation of anxiety. Ms. D's experience of anxiety attacks was primarily somatic, and it was fortuitous that she had a history of more typical anxiety attacks for comparison; the nature of her symptoms led to a careful exploration for neurologic disease and allowed an appropriate and timely intervention.

Anxiety That Mimics Medical Illness

The autonomic arousal associated with anxiety states allows anxiety to present as a great imitator of medical illness. Patients with anxiety disorders repeatedly visit their primary care physicians or make the rounds of a variety of medical practitioners to seek a medical diagnosis to explain their symptoms. Along the way, they may be considered hypochondriacs, deceptive, or just nervous, and they may receive benzodiazepines or reassurance but fail to be offered adequate or definitive treatment. Patients with untreated panic disorder, for example, have increased rates of alcoholism and sedative–hypnotic abuse, presumably in an attempt to self-medicate.[21,54] Sheehan and associates[55] noted that 70% of patients with panic disorder in their series had been to at least 10 medical practitioners without receiving a diagnosis or adequate treatment. They had high somatization scores on the Symptom Checklist-90, which decreased with the treatment of the panic disorder. The majority of these patients met the criteria for somatization disorder and tended to focus on the somatic symptoms of the untreated panic disorder. The nature of a patient's complaints may contribute to missed diagnosis and misdiagnosis. More than 90% of patients with panic present primarily with somatic complaints.[21] Although 95% of patients with mood or anxiety disorders are correctly diagnosed if the affective symptoms are their presenting complaint, only 48% are accurately assessed if they present with somatic complaints.[56] Individuals with somatization disorder are nearly 100 times more likely than those in the general population to suffer from a co-morbid panic disorder.[57] Of 55 patients with panic disorder referred by primary care physicians in one study, 49 (89%) initially presented with one or two somatic complaints and were misdiagnosed for months to years.[21] The three most common somatic loci of symptoms were cardiac, GI, and neurologic, with 45 (81%) of the 55 patients presenting with a pain complaint. These patients may focus on specific physical symptoms, such as chest pain or diarrhea, thereby obscuring other anxiety symptoms, or they may deny affective or cognitive responses to avoid the stigmatization of psychiatric illness. As noted, anxiety may also exacerbate pre-existing physical conditions, such as asthma, which then become the focus of the attention of both the patient and the physician.

The cost of unrecognized and untreated anxiety disorders in patients is high in terms of continued suffering, inefficient use of medical personnel, and costly repetitive diagnostic procedures. In one study of "high utilizers" of medical services, 58% had a mood or anxiety disorder, including 22% with panic disorder.[58] Clancy and Noyes[59] have documented the high rate of medical specialty consultations and procedures (most commonly cardiologic, neurologic, and GI) requested by patients with panic disorder. In one series of patients with chest pain who were undergoing coronary arteriography, Bass and co-workers[60] noted that 61% of the patients with insignificant coronary disease had psychiatric morbidity on a standardized interview, as opposed to only 23% of those with significant coronary disease. In those with normal coronary arteries, the most common psychiatric diagnosis was an anxiety disorder. Recognition and treatment of the anxiety disorder, in some cases, may have eliminated the necessity for arteriograms. In another study, 30% of patients admitted to a cardiac care unit were determined to have no coronary disease but were subsequently diagnosed with panic disorder.[61] Wulsin and colleagues[62] noted that 43% of patients who presented to the Emergency Department (ED) with chest pain had panic attacks, and 16% had panic disorder; patients with panic disorder who presented to the ED with chest pain made more subsequent medical and ED visits than those without panic disorder.[63] Richter and associates[64] estimated that the average patient with non-cardiac chest pain spends US$3500 per year on ED, physician, hospital visits, and medications. In one series,[22] panic disorder exacerbated the symptoms of patients with pre-existing medical disease and led to multiple hospitalizations—a trend that was reversed with treatment of the panic disorder. Dirks and associates[65] reported that patients with chronic asthma and high levels of anxiety had more hospitalizations than asthmatic patients with physiologic illness of comparable severity but normal degrees of anxiety.

Anxiety may play an especially important role in the intensification of hypochondriacal concerns. Once a fear of disease is activated, that fear provides a context for organizing subsequent experiences, including the experience of anxiety symptoms. The fear of disease helps direct attention to somatic symptoms, including anxiety-related symptoms, and can help engender a self-perpetuating cycle of vigilance, worry, and disease concern.[66,67]

Although consideration of the medical differential diagnosis for anxiety is crucial, recognition and treatment of anxiety disorders is essential in preventing inefficient use of medical resources and patient exposure to costly and occasionally dangerous diagnostic and therapeutic procedures. Failure to make the pertinent psychiatric diagnosis may result in a patient continuing to "doctor shop" in the search to discover "what's really wrong with me," with repeated diagnostic procedures resonating with the patient's hypochondriacal concerns. Untreated anxiety can exacerbate symptoms of existing medical pathologic conditions and drive a cycle of escalating help-seeking behavior and hospitalization.

CASE 5

An ED psychiatric consultation was requested for Mr. E, a 35-year-old man, seen acutely by cardiology staff six times in the past month for chest pain and tachycardia. He had been admitted to the cardiac care unit twice, where MIs were ruled out. An extensive negative work-up at another hospital had included a cardiac angiogram. After being told "there's nothing wrong with your heart, you're just nervous" and being given a prescription for diazepam, he sought emergency treatment at our institution in the hope that "they'll find out what's wrong." He had refused previous consultations with psychiatry in the fear that he would be dismissed as "a head case," but he finally agreed to evaluation at the insistence of the medical team.

He was an athletic-looking salesman in his 30s, a self-described "take-charge kind of guy" without any previous psychiatric or medical history. He had a family history of hypertension and was concerned about potential "inherited heart problems." His electrocardiogram recorded a sinus tachycardia of 120 beats/minute and ST-T wave changes deemed secondary to the elevated rate. The episodic periods of anxiety, chest pain, tachycardia, diaphoresis, and hyperventilation had begun approximately a year earlier without clear precipitants during highway driving and had caused him to pull off the road and to seek emergency medical treatment. He reported anticipating long trips with trepidation lest the episodes of chest pain be repeated.

His diagnosis was panic disorder with mild agoraphobia, and treatment was initiated with alprazolam. He felt reassured that he was not crazy and had a definable condition for which treatment was available. The panic attacks remitted shortly thereafter, as did the patient's use of emergency medical services.

Treatment with a number of agents can dramatically relieve the spells and secondary complications of panic disorders, thus underscoring the importance of early diagnosis. Furthermore, because of the physical nature of the symptoms, general medical and ED evaluators need to be alert to the clinical phenomena of a panic attack. Patients who describe their symptoms as anxiety or who evolve a major depression may be more likely to be identified as having a psychiatric disorder. Given the dramatic physical complaints in a variety of bodily systems, however, as with depression, in which somatic symptoms may dominate the presentation and mask diagnosis, an analogy may be made with missed or masked panic disorder.

The absent report of the affective, behavioral, or cognitive components of a panic attack can obscure the diagnosis in the face of paroxysmal physical symptoms. One case report[68] described a patient with a symptom picture that suggested a panic attack but the patient failed to describe the emotional experience of anxiety or panic; alexithymia, or the inability to describe one's emotions, was offered as a possible mechanism for the clinical picture. The predominance of physical symptoms or the absence of cognitive or behavioral responses, however, may not reflect alexithymia or a cognitive impairment, but rather variability in symptom expression. Some patients suffer panic attacks without experiencing a need to flee; others experience panic attacks without a sense of terror or dread, but do not necessarily lack the ability to describe their own emotions.

Most patients with clinically significant panic attacks also suffer limited-symptom attacks that feature only one or two physical symptoms. These may be interspersed with major attacks and may be either situational or unexpected, consisting, for example, of runs of tachycardia or bouts of flushing, hyperventilation, or dizziness. Panic disorder, in its early stages, may be manifested exclusively by such minor attacks. Similarly, as anti-panic therapy is effective, both unexpected and situational limited-symptom attacks may be the last vestige of the disorder or continue to represent a residual disorder.

As stated, patients vary in the primary somatic locus of anxiety distress.[50] For example, predominant panic attack symptoms may appear as cardiovascular symptoms (tachycardia or palpitations), neurologic symptoms (dizziness or paresthesias), respiratory symptoms (dyspnea), GI symptoms (diarrhea), and so forth. Recurrent limited-symptom attacks may therefore be initially indistinguishable from symptoms of a number of disorders in these systems (see Table 13-2). Limited-symptom attacks also may be a harbinger of progression to the full syndrome, but in some cases they may also be disabling themselves and progress to such panic disorder complications as persistent anxiety, phobic avoidance, and depression.

CASE 6

Mr. F, a 32-year-old married factory supervisor, had been out of work for 2 years because of stomach pain, nausea, and vomiting. He described his discomfort as "gnawing pains" that would occur paroxysmally, followed by vomiting with little warning. In the previous 5 years, he had had extensive GI work-ups and medical management, vagotomy and pyloroplasty, and ultimately hemigastrectomy without relief of symptoms. He was totally disabled and was referred for psychiatric evaluation. The following features were noted: (1) His severe pain was paroxysmal with lower-grade persistent symptoms; (2) diazepam helped diminish, but did not eradicate, his symptoms; (3) he was homebound and described attacks of stomach pain and vomiting only when he left his apartment, e.g., to go shopping; (4) the onset had followed the break-up of a relationship; (5) a major depression had evolved.

On treatment with sertraline (co-administered with diazepam), he experienced complete symptomatic relief in 6 weeks and with maintenance treatment, remained symptom free for 5 years. He sought and found a new job after treatment and has been continuously employed for the past 5 years. He recalled frequently needing to leave school as a child because of a nervous stomach.

This case reflects a missed or masked diagnosis of panic disorder because of the predominance of a limited-symptom attack resembling a GI syndrome. Clues to a diagnosis of panic disorder were evident, and appropriate treatment led to dramatic improvement in this disabled patient. Features reminiscent of more typical patients with panic disorder were identified before definitive treatment, including severe paroxysmal and lower-grade persistent symptoms, onset with a major life event, agoraphobic features, a childhood history suggesting separation anxiety, partial relief with benzodiazepines, and secondary depression. No family history of panic attacks or agoraphobia was reported in this case.

Panic Disorder Associated With Medical Illness

An association between panic disorder and other medical illnesses has been described. More than one-third of patients with chronic obstructive pulmonary disease have an anxiety disorder, including 8% to 25% with panic disorder.[69–71] Pollack and associates[72] found an elevated prevalence of panic disorder (11%) among patients referred to a general hospital for pulmonary function testing, including two-thirds of those with chronic obstructive pulmonary disease. Almost half of all patients evaluated reported substantial symptoms of anxiety.

Katon[21] and Noyes and co-workers[73] reported an increased incidence of peptic ulcers and hypertension in patients with panic disorder. Close to a third of patients with irritable bowel syndrome have panic disorder, and 44% of panic patients have irritable bowel syndrome; symptoms of both conditions improve with treatment of the panic disorder.[74]

Retrospective studies by Coryell and colleagues[75] suggest an increased risk of premature mortality from cardiac disease in men with panic disorder. Patients with mitral valve prolapse (MVP) have been diagnosed much more frequently (30% to 50%) with panic disorder.[76,77] Studies have indicated that the relationship is coincidental and there are no associations between MVP, panic disorder, social anxiety disorder, or other anxiety disorders.[78]

PRIMARY ANXIETY DISORDERS

Patients with a number of primary psychiatric disorders may present with anxiety in the medical setting. A history of psychiatric illness may precede the patient's entry into the medical setting and then be exacerbated by the medical condition. For some, however, the onset of symptoms associated with a psychiatric disorder is provoked by the stress of medical illness.

Panic Disorder

A panic attack usually lasts minutes with fairly stereotypical physical, cognitive, and behavioral components. Patients with panic disorder may experience these attacks intermittently over time or in clusters and, as stated, may develop a number of complications, including persistent anxiety, phobic avoidance, depression, alcoholism, or other drug overuse.

Physical symptoms (e.g., cardiac, respiratory, neurologic, and GI symptoms) are experienced as if there is a sudden surge of autonomic, primarily sympathetic, arousal. Cognitively, the patient feels a sense of terror or fear of losing control, dying, or going crazy and behaviorally often feels driven to flee from the setting in which the attack is experienced to a safe, secure, or familiar place or person.

The initial attack that appears to "turn on" the disorder, the herald attack, is particularly well remembered by the patient. Subsequent attacks may be a mixture of spontaneous, unexpected attacks and those preceded by a buildup of anticipatory anxiety; the latter, called situational attacks, occur in settings in which the patient might sense being at risk for panic, such as crowded places. Attacks may be major, with four or more symptoms, or limited-symptom attacks with fewer symptoms.

Panic disorder has its typical onset in early adult life and afflicts women two to three times as commonly as men. More than half of patients with panic disorder have a history of anxiety disorders beginning in childhood.[79] The disorder is familial and very likely has a genetic basis, given a higher concordance in monozygotic as compared with dizygotic twins,[80] but it is not clear whether a genetic influence is specific to panic disorder or whether it represents a general anxiety-proneness that may be expressed variably as any of a number of anxiety disorders.

The onset of the disorder in a clinical population typically follows either a major life event, such as a loss, threat of loss, other upheavals in work or home situations, or some physiologic event, such as medical illness (e.g., hyperthyroidism, vertigo) or drug use (marijuana, cocaine). For example, some patients whose first or herald attack appears to be triggered by a physiologic perturbation, such as following marijuana use, may continue thereafter with persistent or recurrent symptoms without further drug use.

A panic attack, like an endogenous false alarm, appears to turn on a state of vigilance or post-panic anxiety that resembles GAD. Between attacks, patients may remain symptomatic with low-level constant anxiousness and anticipatory anxiety that may crescendo into panic in certain situations or be punctuated by panic unexpectedly.

In this state of vigilance, phobic avoidance may occur as a complication. The patient may develop mild or extensive phobic avoidance, usually of travel or places of restricted escape, immediately after the onset of attacks, after a number of attacks, or never at all. In some cases, the phobic avoidance evolves as a progressive constriction with the cumulative avoidance of settings where attacks have occurred.

Major depressive episodes may also complicate the course of the patient with panic disorder and occur in up to two-thirds of cases.[81] For some, the demoralization attending the sustained distress and progressive disability of panic disorder extends to a typical depression with characteristic signs and symptoms. As noted, the relationship between panic and depression is a complicated one, however. Some patients manifest no depressive symptoms; for others, it is unclear which disorder is primary because symptoms arise concurrently. Alcohol use can temporarily tame the distress of panic disorder but soon yields to rebound symptoms, thereby setting the stage for alcohol overuse.

Generalized Anxiety Disorder

Patients with GAD suffer from chronic worry about a number of life circumstances (e.g., finances or danger to loved ones) that is difficult to control and is present on more days than not, for longer than 6 months.[2] These patients are often called "nervous" or "worriers" by family or friends. Their anxiety is accompanied by a number of somatic and cognitive symptoms associated with motor tension and autonomic hyperactivity (e.g., muscle tension, restlessness, difficulties concentrating, and sleep disturbances). Although the disorder may be differentiated from panic disorder by the persistent rather than episodic nature of the symptoms, careful questioning often reveals that patients with GAD may experience panic attacks as well.[82,83] Many patients with GAD in the medical setting manifest anxiety in addition to the symptoms of other psychiatric disorders (e.g., panic disorder, depression, or alcohol abuse).[84]

Specific Phobias

Patients with specific phobias are afraid of circumscribed situations or objects (e.g., heights, closed spaces, animals, or the sight of blood).[2] Exposure to the feared stimulus results in intense anxiety and avoidance that interferes with the patient's life. Some patients are so afraid of needles or blood, that compliance with procedures in the medical setting is nearly impossible. Acute treatment with benzodiazepines may decrease the patient's anxiety to the point where he or she agrees to treatment. The only consistently effective treatment for specific phobias, however, is behavioral therapy, a technique that involves exposure and desensitization to the feared object or situation.[85]

Social Phobia (Social Anxiety Disorder)

Social phobia, also referred to as social anxiety disorder, is diagnosed when the patient perceives that he or she will be the object of public scrutiny and fears that he or she will behave in a way that will be humiliating or embarrassing.[2] This perception leads to persistent fear and avoidance, or to endurance with intense distress. Circumscribed situations may be feared (e.g., speaking before a group, performance anxiety, writing or eating in the presence of others, or urinating in public lavatories); many patients experience more global difficulties in which most social interactions are difficult. Again, depression and alcoholism can frequently occur with social phobia.[86,87] Patients with a social phobia may have intense anxiety in the hospital because they are under intense scrutiny by others. Long-term treatments include antidepressants with selective serotonin re-uptake inhibitors (SSRIs) (fluoxetine, sertraline, paroxetine, fluvoxamine, citalopram, escitalopram), serotonin–norepinephrine re-uptake inhibitors (SNRIs) (venlafaxine), and monoamine oxidase inhibitors (MAOIs) (phenelzine, tranylcypromine) generally being more effective than TCAs (e.g., imipramine, desipramine, nortriptyline), β-blockers (for performance anxiety rather than generalized social phobia), or CBT. Some reports support the clinical efficacy of high-potency benzodiazepines (HPBs) (e.g., clonazepam,[88] alprazolam[89]) for the treatment of social phobia; when immediate intervention is necessary, the use of these agents is appropriate.

Post-traumatic Stress Disorder

Patients with PTSD have experienced or witnessed a traumatic event involving death or serious injury to themselves or others and responded with feelings of intense fear, horror, or helplessness.[2] Afflicted patients frequently re-experience the traumatic event. They have recurrent dreams or suddenly act or feel as though the event is recurring (i.e., a flashback). Individuals with PTSD frequently avoid situations that remind them of the event and may become numb, irritable, or hypervigilant and experience difficulty with sleep or concentration. Although much attention has been directed toward PTSD in combat veterans, PTSD can occur in civilians who suffer life-threatening accidents or assaults or who have survived natural disasters. PTSD is unfortunately common and often unrecognized in the medical setting, with reported rates of PTSD in over one-third of patients hospitalized after traumatic injury, such as occurring in motor vehicle accidents, assaults, or fires.[31,90] Injured patients who develop PTSD have increased functional impairment and problem-drinking when followed up a year after surgery.[91]

Acute stress disorder involves the development of dissociation and re-experiencing symptoms along with avoidance, anxiety, increased arousal, and significant distress or impairment lasting up to 4 weeks after a trauma.[2] The presence of acute stress disorder is associated with the development of PTSD.[92]

There is growing interest in whether early intervention for trauma victims can prevent the development of PTSD. There are scarce data on the effectiveness of primary PTSD prevention.[93] Despite being a widely used intervention after trauma, data show that single-session debriefing after a traumatic event has no benefit in preventing PTSD.[93,94] In contrast, more extensive, multiple-session cognitive-behavioral interventions incorporating information, cognitive re-structuring, and exposure elements, appear effective.[93,95] Pharmacologic interventions have also demonstrated potential benefit in reducing the morbid sequelae of trauma. Glucocorticoid administration is currently the most effective pharmacologic intervention in preventing PTSD.[93,95] Studies consistently show a reduced incidence of PTSD after administration of high doses of hydrocortisone after different types of traumatic events in both critically ill as well as healthy cohorts. SSRIs are considered first-line for the treatment of chronic PTSD,[96] however early use aimed at preventing PTSD[15] is equivocal, with one small RCT showing no benefits versus placebo with escitalopram and another small RCT demonstrating lower PTSD rates with sertraline versus placebo.[93] It should be noted that the study samples were small, the ages of participants varied greatly, as did the nature of traumatic events in each study.

Propranolol has been investigated in numerous studies as a PTSD prevention strategy. While there have been mixed results, the majority of studies including large RCTs have not shown that propranolol is effective in PTSD prevention.[93] Benzodiazepines have been consistently shown to have no effect on preventing PTSD when given after a traumatic experience.[93] Furthermore, they may have "PTSD-enhancing" effects by interfering with extinction learning.[95] Morphine has been shown to be associated with lower rates of developing PTSD when given after traumatic events, however, these have been small observational studies and no RCTs are currently available to confirm its benefits.[93,95] Ketamine, a dissociative NMDA-receptor antagonist, has been studied as a potential strategy to prevent PTSD in surgical patients with mixed results; further study is warranted.[93]

Though early treatment strategies aimed at preventing PTSD are scarce and understudied, it is well established that both CBT[97] and SSRI pharmacotherapy are effective first-line interventions for the treatment of established or chronic PTSD.[98] They are frequently co-administered to improve outcome.

Obsessive–Compulsive Disorder

Patients with OCD suffer from recurrent, intrusive, unwanted thoughts (i.e., obsessions, such as the fear of hurting a loved one or the fear of contamination) or compulsive behaviors or rituals (such as repetitive hand-washing or checking a door multiple times to make sure it is locked).[2] The obsessions and compulsions are distressing and time consuming (i.e., they may take more than 1 hour/day) and interfere with the patient's normal function. In the medical setting, the patient with OCD may suffer a marked increase in anxiety if physical disability or hospital routine makes it impossible for him or her to perform compulsive rituals. CBT aimed at reducing the patient's obsessive thoughts and compulsive behavior has demonstrated clear efficacy for OCD. Benzodiazepine therapy may be necessary to control overwhelming anxiety, particularly in acute treatment. Effective long-term treatments include use of serotonergic antidepressants (e.g., SSRIs, clomipramine) as well as behavioral therapy.

Other Psychiatric Disorders

Anxiety symptoms may be associated with a number of psychiatric disorders (such as schizophrenia, depression, and bipolar disorder) other than primary anxiety disorders. Vague uneasiness extending to severe anxiety may either precede or accompany the symptoms of schizophrenia. Patients with significant degrees of anxiety may have a reduced level of function and manifest withdrawal that superficially resembles schizophrenia. The presence of hallucinations, delusions, and bizarre and disordered thinking, a marked degree of social withdrawal, and a characteristic pre-morbid personal and family history usually allows an uncomplicated differentiation of schizophrenia from anxiety disorders.

The relationship between anxiety and depression is complex. Weissman and co-workers[99] reported an increased prevalence of both panic disorder and depression in the families of probands with both disorders. One estimate holds that one-third of patients with panic disorder, with or without agoraphobia, develop a secondary major depression, and 22% have had a major depressive disorder before developing panic disorder.[100] The incidence of a major depressive episode in patients with panic disorder has been reported as ranging between 28% and 90%, depending on the diagnostic criteria used.[101] Leckman and associates[102] found that 58% of a group of depressed patients had anxiety symptoms meeting criteria for agoraphobia, panic disorder, or GAD.

Although this overlap between syndromes can make the distinction between anxiety and depression difficult, a number of clinical considerations may be useful. Psychomotor retardation, persistent dysphoria, early morning awakening, diurnal variation, a sense of hopelessness, and suicidal thoughts are more indicative of depression. Patients with an anxiety disorder have often not lost interest in their usual activities but rather have lost the ability to negotiate them comfortably. They are more likely to report autonomic hyperactivity, derealization, perceptual distortions, and anxious impatience than hopelessness.[49] Advances in neurobiology at this time offer few diagnostic markers for differentiating anxiety and depressive disorders. The sleep of patients with panic disorders differs from the sleep of depressives during all-night polysomnograms.[103] There are also differences in physiologic parameters and platelet receptor-binding patterns between anxious and depressed patients.[104,105]

The principal concern in differentiating depression from anxiety is to not overlook treatment with an antidepressant and, in particular, to avoid the common scenario of prescribing only a benzodiazepine for the anxiety component of a depression, thereby leaving the depression untreated. Fortunately, the frequent overlap in clinical presentations between primary depressive and primary anxiety disorders is mirrored by an overlap in therapeutic considerations. One important consideration, however, is the possibility that depressed symptoms may reflect an underlying bipolar (manic-depressive) disorder. Anxiety disorders are a common co-morbidity among bipolar individuals.[106] However, the use of antidepressants in bipolar patients may precipitate mania and provoke greater mood cycling. Bipolar disorder should be considered in the differential diagnosis of depression, particularly in those patients with a history of marked mood instability or a family history of manic-depressive illness, as well as in individuals who become more agitated or dysphoric after antidepressant administration. For bipolar patients, use of an anticonvulsant may treat both the mood and the anxiety disorder, with use of benzodiazepines, in preference to antidepressants, considered for persistent anxiety in individuals without a substance abuse diathesis. Although cognitive-behavioral interventions for anxiety and depression differ in both their focus and procedures, it is not unusual for treatment of one condition to extend benefit to the associated disorder. For example, the CBT of panic disorder is associated with improvement in co-morbid depression. Nonetheless, co-morbidity generally serves as a predictor of worse overall treatment response to CBT, just as it does for pharmacologic approaches.[107]

TREATMENT

The nature of the medical setting favors expedient interventions, such as drug treatment to ease acute distress, because of the time-limited nature of medical and surgical stays (Table 13-3). Nonetheless, as illustrated by the case examples, comprehensive assessments, including systematic scrutiny of cognitive and psychosocial factors, may lead to practical interventions short of formal psychotherapy, including CBT. In addition, disrupted relations with family members may be provocative, and family interventions may prove therapeutically expedient.

Pharmacologic Treatment of Panic Disorder

The drug treatment of anxiety essentially involves selecting agents for panic, GAD, or both. As with recognizing the primacy of depression in some anxious patients, if the presence of panic attacks is overlooked, treatment for generalized anxiety alone is likely to be inadequate, and patient suffering will continue. Familiarity with panic disorder, its complications, and its treatments is a necessary resource in evaluating and caring for anxious patients.

Although early intervention offers the likelihood of preventing complications, many patients come for treatment after years of symptoms and disability. Even in the face of chronicity, however, most patients achieve substantial if not dramatic benefit with available treatments, which include anti-panic pharmacotherapy and CBT. Given the apparent primacy of the panic attack in the distress and evolution of complications of the disorder, our usual approach is to initiate anti-panic medications for patients who continue to experience panic attacks, with the expectation of regression and remission of complications once the attacks have ceased. For patients with residual phobic avoidance despite the prevention of panic attacks, behavioral and cognitive strategies are employed. For some patients, behavioral and cognitive strategies are employed initially, especially when the frequency and intensity of unexpected panic are minimal, with pharmacotherapy subsequently applied if emergence or exacerbation of panic attends the behavioral program.

Antidepressants

The SSRIs (including fluoxetine, sertraline, paroxetine, citalopram, escitalopram, and fluvoxamine) have become first-line agents for the treatment of panic disorder as well as other anxiety disorders[108,109] because of their broad spectrum of efficacy, favorable side effect profile, and lack of cardiotoxicity. Although effective, these agents may worsen anxiety for some patients at the initiation of treatment. Thus, treatment of panic patients or the anxious depressed should be initiated at half or less of the usual starting dosage

TABLE 13-3 Selected Pharmacologic Treatments for Anxiety Disorders

AGENT	USUAL INITIAL DOSAGE (mg)	DOSAGE RANGE (mg)	CHIEF DOSAGE LIMITATIONS	DISORDERS
Tricyclic Antidepressants (TCAs)				
Imipramine	10–25	150–300	Jitteriness, TCA side effects	PD, AG, GAD, PTSD, OCD
Clomipramine	25	25–250	Sedation, weight gain, TCA side effects	PD, AG, GAD, PTSD
Monoamine Oxidase Inhibitors (MAOIs)				
Phenelzine	15–30	45–90	Diet, MAOI side effects	PD, AG, SP, ?GAD, OCD, PTSD
Selective Serotonin Re-Uptake Inhibitors (SSRIs)				
Fluoxetine	10	10–80	SSRI side effects	PD, AG, SP, OCD, PTSD
Sertraline	25	25–200	SSRI side effects	PD, AG, SP, OCD, PTSD
Paroxetine	10	10–50	SSRI side effects	PD, AG, SP, OCD, PTSD
Paroxetine-CR	12.5	12.5–62.5	SSRI side effects	PD, AG, SP, OCD, PTSD
Fluvoxamine	50	50–300	SSRI side effects	PD, AG, SP OCD, PTSD
Citalopram	10	20–60	SSRI side effects	PD, AG, SP, OCD, PTSD
Escitalopram	5	10–20	SSRI side effects	PD, AG, SP, OCD, PTSD
Serotonin–Norepinephrine Re-Uptake Inhibitor (SNRI)				
Venlafaxine	37.5	75–225	SSRI side effects, hypertension	PD, AG, SP, OCD, PTSD
Benzodiazepines				
Alprazolam	0.25 QID	2–10/day	Sedation, discontinuation syndrome	PD, AG, GAD, SP, ?SpP
Clonazepam	0.25 QHS	1–5/day	Abuse, psychomotor and memory impairment	PD, AG, GAD, SP, ?SpP
Diazepam	2.5	5–30/day	–	GAD, SpP, PD, SP
Other Anxiolytics				
Buspirone	5 TID	15–60/day	Dysphoria	GAD
Propranolol	10–20	10–160/day (maintenance use)	Depression	SP, ?PD, ?GAD

AG, agoraphobia; GAD, generalized anxiety disorder; OCD, obsessive–compulsive disorder; PD, panic disorder; PTSD, post-traumatic stress disorder; SP, social phobia; SpP, specific phobia.

(e.g., fluoxetine 5–10 mg/day, sertraline 25 mg/day, paroxetine 10 mg/day—or 12.5 mg/day of the controlled-release formulation—citalopram 10 mg/day, escitalopram 5 mg/day, and fluvoxamine 50 mg/day) to minimize the early anxiogenic effect. Dosages can usually be raised, after about 1 week of acclimation, to typical therapeutic levels. Typical target dosages for this indication are fluoxetine 20–40 mg/day, paroxetine 20–60 mg/day (25–72.5 mg/day of the controlled-release formulation), sertraline 100–150 mg/day, citalopram 20–60 mg/day, escitalopram 10–20 mg/day, and fluvoxamine 150–250 mg/day, although some patients may respond at lower levels. Patients with OCD and PTSD may require higher dosages (e.g., fluoxetine 60–80 mg/day) to receive maximal benefit.

Onset of benefit with the SSRIs and other antidepressants usually occurs after 2 to 3 weeks of treatment. Although generally better tolerated for acute and long-term treatment than older available classes of antidepressants, SSRIs may be associated with transient or persistent adverse effects, including nausea and other GI symptoms, headaches, sexual dysfunction, and apathy. Despite their reputation as stimulating agents, sleep disturbance is generally not a persistent or significant problem during SSRI therapy. The SSRIs are usually administered in the morning; emergent sleep disruption can usually be managed by the addition of hypnotic agents.

The extended-release SNRI venlafaxine has also demonstrated efficacy for the treatment of panic disorder and the other anxiety disorders. As with other antidepressants, it may cause uncomfortable stimulation early in the treatment of anxious patients, so dosing should be initiated with low dosages (i.e., venlafaxine 37.5 mg/day). Other antidepressants, such as mirtazapine, are also probably effective for the treatment of anxiety disorders, but the systematic data supporting their use for these indications are limited. Trazodone appears to be less effective for panic disorder than other agents; studies assessing the effectiveness of bupropion for panic disorder are small and have shown mixed results.

The TCA imipramine hydrochloride has well-established efficacy in panic disorder.[110] Although other TCAs are probably also effective (e.g., desipramine is frequently employed because of its lower anticholinergic burden), this class of agents has several drawbacks, including a delayed onset of benefit and treatment-emergent adverse effects. In addition to the usual TCA side effects (such as dry mouth, constipation, and orthostatic hypotension), panic patients are particularly prone to a sudden worsening of their disorder with the first doses. To minimize the effect of this adverse response, treatment can be initiated with small test doses (e.g., 10 mg of imipramine hydrochloride). If this is well tolerated, standard antidepressant dosing can be pursued; for others, the adverse response typically fades over a few days, thus allowing an upward titration of dosage. For a small percentage of patients, this apparent worsening of the disorder does not subside. Mavissakalian and Perel[111] reported that a reasonable target dosage of imipramine for treatment of panic disorder and agoraphobia in most patients is approximately 2.25 mg/kg per day (usually between 100 and 200 mg/day for most patients), with a total plasma level of 75 to 150 ng/mL for imipramine and its metabolite, desipramine.

The MAOI phenelzine has stood up well in clinical use and controlled trials,[110] and many clinicians believe that MAOIs may be the most comprehensively effective agents for treating panic disorder, blocking panic attacks, relieving depression, and offering a confidence-enhancing effect of considerable value to the patient needing to recover from vigilance and phobic avoidance. Except for postural hypotension, MAOIs are free of most of the early TCA and SSRI side effects, including the anxiogenic response. Unfortunately, as treatment proceeds, a variety of challenging problems emerge, including insomnia, weight gain, edema, sexual dysfunction, nocturnal myoclonus, and other unusual symptoms. Further, many anxious patients are most circumspect about the dietary precautions and instructions about hypertensive crises. Because the SSRIs and the MAOIs offer similar spectra of efficacy in terms of treating panic disorder, social phobia, and atypical depressive symptoms, along with a superior safety and side-effect profile, they are generally used first in most patients. MAOIs, however, may be effective in patients failing to respond to other interventions; thus, although this has not been systematically studied, many clinicians believe that no patient should be considered truly treatment refractory to pharmacotherapy until the patient has had an MAOI trial.

Benzodiazepines

When treatment refusal, treatment discomfort from side effects, and treatment failure are considered, the need for a better-tolerated and effective anti-panic treatment is apparent. In some respects, benzodiazepines, such as alprazolam and clonazepam, fit this need. They have demonstrated anti-panic efficacy as well as patient acceptability and a reasonable record of safety. In addition, they provide the speed of action that is desirable in a medical setting. Although it was once believed that higher-potency agents, such as alprazolam and clonazepam, were more effective than lower-potency agents, such as diazepam, for the treatment of panic, it appears that all benzodiazepines may be effective at equivalent dosages (i.e., 4 mg/day of alprazolam and 40 mg/day of diazepam).[112]

The usual dosage range for most panic disorder patients receiving alprazolam is 2 to 8 mg/day, with most achieving a benefit from around 4 to 6 mg/day. Clinical response is evident early, but lower dosages are necessary to initiate treatment so that the patient can accommodate to sedation. Most patients adapt within a few days to the sedating effects, and this allows a stepwise increase in panic-blocking doses. Adaptation to sedation usually occurs without a loss of therapeutic benefit, but some upward adjustment may be required after the first 2 weeks. A small percentage of patients appear particularly sensitive to the drug and experience persisting sedation despite time and careful titration. Alprazolam must be given in divided doses, usually three to four times a day, because of its relatively short duration of action; a recently introduced extended-release formulation permits once-a-day dosing. It does not change the elimination half-life or need for a gradual taper with discontinuation.

Despite the ease of administration of alprazolam and frequently dramatic results even in the first days of treatment, clinical drawbacks include concerns about abuse and dependency, rebound symptoms between doses, withdrawal, and early relapse. The abuse potential of alprazolam, like that of other benzodiazepines, varies widely among clinical populations; patients with a history of alcohol or other substance abuse are most at risk for abusing benzodiazepines. Numerous studies are reassuring that panic patients treated with benzodiazepines do not experience therapeutic tolerance or dosage escalation; in fact, dosages of benzodiazepines generally decrease over the maintenance period, often despite the presence or persistence of untreated anxiety symptoms.[113] Most well-informed panic and phobic patients who have endured severe distress over time treat their medication with respect and understand the wisdom of maintaining the lowest effective dose; thus, unless there is evidence that a particular patient is at risk, the use of this agent appears generally safe for the disorder under consideration. As with any benzodiazepine, without controlled prescribing for targeted symptoms, inappropriate use may occur. As seen with a benzodiazepine with a relatively short half-life, the discontinuation of alprazolam therapy, especially after long-term treatment, without a gradual taper tailored to the individual patient's sensitivity to decreasing dosages, may be followed by rebound symptoms (worsened anxiety) or a withdrawal syndrome.

With the pharmacokinetic drawbacks associated with a short half-life agent in mind, the longer-acting high-potency benzodiazepine (HPB) clonazepam, has been effective for those patients who require an HPB. Because of its long half-life (15 to 50 hours), clonazepam is generally administered on a twice-a-day dosage schedule, with patients less likely to experience interdose rebound and withdrawal symptoms than on shorter-acting agents.

With a milligram-for-milligram potency approximately twice that of alprazolam, clonazepam's effective dosage range for panic patients is between 1 and 5 mg/day when given in morning and bedtime doses. Sedation is the limiting factor in dosage titration and is managed by initiating treatment with a low bedtime dosage and titrating upward if symptoms persist and sedation resolves. An initial dosage as low as 0.25 mg may be used in drug-naive patients or those particularly sensitive to benzodiazepines. Greater dosages may be given at bedtime than in the morning if the patient is not readily accommodating to sedation, but many patients function without sedation on equal morning and bedtime dosages, as with alprazolam.

The effect of a daily dose on panic attacks and generalized anxiety is apparent within a few days. Some patients, for unclear reasons, develop depressive symptoms as a treatment-emergent adverse effect when taking alprazolam or clonazepam. Resolution of depressive symptoms typically occurs with the introduction of an antidepressant; benzodiazepine treatment can then be withheld with the expectation of a comprehensive response to the antidepressant. Combined treatment can again be used if anxiety symptoms break through the antidepressant treatment.

Some clinicians initiate combined treatment with an antidepressant and an HPB to obtain the rapid anxiolysis associated with HPB treatment, decrease the activation associated with initiation of antidepressant therapy, and provide antidepressant coverage of co-morbid or benzodiazepine-induced depression. For many patients, the HPB can be tapered after a few weeks when the antidepressant begins to exert therapeutic effects; however, some patients remain on combined treatment with benefit and without adverse consequences.

Pharmacologic Treatment of Generalized Anxiety

As noted previously, the SSRIs and the SNRIs have become first-line pharmacologic agents for the treatment of anxiety disorders, including GAD. They are better tolerated than the older classes of antidepressants and have a broad spectrum of efficacy, which is a critical clinical concern given the high rates of co-morbidity, particularly depression affecting the generally anxious individual. In addition, SSRIs and SNRIs do not have significant abuse potential, which is an important consideration for generally anxious individuals with a predisposition to substance abuse. However, use of these agents may be associated with side effects, including sexual dysfunction and GI distress, that may adversely affect compliance. The delay in the onset of therapeutic benefit is a relative disadvantage for antidepressants as well as for buspirone; the call to intervene with medication for the anxious patient in the hospital typically requires a response with a more immediate-acting agent. Thus, benzodiazepines are usually used for acute management of anxiety, with antidepressant addition or substitution considered in patients requiring maintenance pharmacotherapy, particularly those with a depressive or substance abuse diathesis.

Benzodiazepines, by dint of their efficacy, tolerability, and rapid onset of effect, have long been the mainstay of anxiolytic pharmacotherapy, although the clinical decision to prescribe these agents for symptom relief is a difficult one. The attitudes of individual physicians toward prescribing may be characterized as falling along a spectrum between pharmacologic Calvinism and psychotropic hedonism, reflecting a personal and moral stance toward prescribing medication for the relief of psychic distress. The abundant literature on anti-anxiety agents falls short of providing reliable measures for diagnosis and prescribing. Given the ubiquity of anxiety in hospital settings, the physician must frequently confront the question of whether to prescribe. The use of a benzodiazepine for the distressed, anxious patient is often a therapeutic act analogous to the provision of pain relief.

When compared with barbiturates and non-barbiturate sedative and hypnotic agents (meprobamate, ethchlorvynol, glutethimide, methaqualone, and others), the benzodiazepines are more selectively anxiolytic, with less sedation and less morbidity and mortality in overdose and acute withdrawal. Because using a benzodiazepine represents a clinical decision to offer symptomatic relief, the critical clinical assessment is to evaluate the patient's response. The patient's coping should be enhanced in addition to, and as a consequence of, relief from suffering.

Choice of Benzodiazepine

All available benzodiazepines are effective in treating generalized anxiety. Drug selection is based on pharmacokinetic properties, which determine the rapidity of onset of effect, the degree of accumulation with multi-dosing, the rapidity of offset of clinical effect, and the risk of drug discontinuation syndrome.

For single or acute dosing, the onset of effect is determined by the rate of absorption from the stomach, and the offset by distribution from plasma into lipid stores. The half-life of a drug predicts the amount of accumulation of drug in plasma with multi-dosing and the speed of washout on drug discontinuation (and thus the quickness of return of symptoms or the risk of rebound and withdrawal). For example, a rapidly absorbed, lipophilic agent, such as diazepam, given acutely, has a rapid but relatively short-lived effect; with repeated dosing, however, plasma levels are higher than for a short half-life drug at steady state. The long half-life offers some tapering effect to help protect against rebound or withdrawal on discontinuation.

The clinician can choose a drug to have a fast onset for greater clinical effect, a slow onset to minimize sedation or confusion, short action to allow rapid clearing, or long action to minimize inter-dose or post-treatment rebound symptoms (Table 13-4). Treatment begins with low doses (e.g., diazepam 5 to 10 mg/day or its equivalent) and upward titration. Dosages vary, but for usual situational anxiety, 30 to 40 mg of diazepam a day or its equivalent are not usually exceeded.

Patients in whom benzodiazepine therapy is being prescribed to manage acute situational reactions should expect that treatment will be of limited duration. For specific phobic anxiety (e.g., fear of flying), occasional use is indicated. For generalized anxiety, using anxiolytics for periods of exacerbation may be effective, although increasing recognition of the distress and chronicity associated with persistent anxiety has underscored the observation that many patients often report sustained improvement and improved quality of life with maintenance treatment.

Precautions in Prescribing

A withdrawal syndrome, usually mild but potentially severe depending on the dose and the duration of treatment, may follow abrupt cessation of therapy. For patients receiving usual doses for less than 3 to 4 weeks—during hospitalization, for example—without prior use of sedatives, the risk of an abstinence syndrome is less. In general, however, treatment is discontinued by tapering doses, gradually adjusting decrements according to patient response.

Over-use of medication and drug-seeking from multiple sources is a concern for outpatient prescribing, but with the controlled use of drugs in the hospital, particular vigilance is appropriate primarily for the patient with a history of drug or alcohol abuse.

The sedative effects of benzodiazepines are additive with those of other CNS depressants, and plasma levels are higher with the use of certain drugs, such as cimetidine. A few patients, particularly with use of HPBs, are prone to increased hostility, aggression, and rage eruptions.

Pharmacologic Alternatives to Benzodiazepines

Anticonvulsants (including valproate, gabapentin, topiramate, and lamotrigine) are increasingly being studied and used for a range of anxiety disorders, with some (e.g., gabapentin) administered as an alternative to benzodiazepines because of their sedating properties and tolerability.[114] Although typical neuroleptics (e.g., trifluoperazine) have long been used in clinical practice for the treatment of anxiety, concerns about extrapyramidal effects and tardive dyskinesia have limited this practice. Based on accruing open-label reports and controlled studies, the atypical neuroleptics also appear to have anxiolytic effects across a variety of conditions.[115]

However, although less likely to be associated with neurologic side effects (e.g., extrapyramidal symptoms, tardive dyskinesia) than older-generation agents,[116] the severity of potential metabolic consequences (e.g., weight gain, diabetes, increased triglycerides) associated with these agents suggests that caution must be taken when prescribing them.

β-Blocking drugs, such as propranolol hydrochloride, have proved useful in alleviating some of the peripheral autonomic symptoms of anxiety (such as tremor and tachycardia). Although of second-line or third-line importance in treating panic attacks or more cognitively experienced symptoms (e.g., worry), β-blockers are often impressively useful in the performance-anxiety subtype of social phobia and when persistent peripheral symptoms (somatic anxiety) predominate. Agents, such as atenolol, that are less able to cross the blood–brain barrier than propranolol may have advantages for patients who experience fatigue or dysphoria when taking propranolol. Effective doses vary, and treatment requires upward titration from low initial doses.

Buspirone is a non-benzodiazepine anxiolytic without sedative and anticonvulsant properties or abuse potential.

TABLE 13-4 Characteristics of Commonly Used Benzodiazepines

DRUG	HALF-LIFE (h)	DOSAGE EQUIVALENT (mg)	ONSET	SIGNIFICANT METABOLITES	TYPICAL ROUTE OF ADMINISTRATION
Midazolam (Versed)	1–12	2.0	Fast	No	IV, IM
Oxazepam (Serax)	5–15	15	Slow	No	PO
Lorazepam (Ativan)	10–20	1.0	Intermediate	No	IV, IM, PO
Alprazolam (Xanax)[a]	12–15	0.5	Intermediate-fast	No	PO
Chlordiazepoxide (Librium)	5–30	10	Intermediate	Yes	PO, IV
Clonazepam (Klonopin)[a]	15–50	0.25	Intermediate	No	PO
Diazepam (Valium)	20–100	5.0	Fast	Yes	PO, IV
Flurazepam (Dalmane)	40	15.0	Fast	Yes	PO
Clorazepate (Tranxene)	30–200	7.5	Fast	Yes	PO

[a]Commonly used to treat panic disorder.

It interacts with postsynaptic 5-HT (serotonin) receptors as a partial agonist and with dopamine receptors but apparently not with the benzodiazepine-GABA receptor.[116] Buspirone is ineffective in panic disorder, and although clinical trials suggest that it is effective for the treatment of GAD, many clinicians and patients have found it disappointing for this indication as well. For some patients, this may in part result from a latency of therapeutic response of weeks, similar to the antidepressants, and the presence of a critical beneficial dose threshold. The dosage range is 5 to 20 mg three times a day.

Cognitive-behavioral Therapy

For patients with persisting anxiety symptoms, cognitive-behavioral strategies similar to those used for ambulatory patients with anxiety disorders may be adapted to the hospitalized medical patient. CBT for anxiety disorders brings to bear an array of cognitive re-structuring, exposure, and symptom management techniques that target the core fears and behavioral pattern characterizing each anxiety disorder. Cognitive interventions include a variety of procedures to challenge and re-structure the inaccurate and maladaptive cognitions that increase anxiety and help maintain anxiety disorders. Procedures range from informational discussions, self-monitoring, and Socratic questioning to the construction of behavioral experiments in which patients can directly examine the veracity of anxiogenic expectations. A reliance on corrective experiences also lies at the heart of exposure interventions that provide patients with opportunities to extinguish learned fears, by directly confronting (in a hierarchical fashion) feared events and sensations. Symptom management techniques typically include relaxation and breathing re-training procedures to help eliminate anxiogenic bodily reactions. In addition, training in problem-solving or social skills may be necessary to eliminate behavioral deficits hat help maintain anxiety disorders. Similarly, couples sessions may be required to change family patterns that help maintain avoidant or other anxiety-related behaviors.

CBT centers on the elimination of core features of each disorder, with treatment for panic disorder targeting fears of arousal, anxiety, and panic symptoms; treatment for social phobia targeting fears of negative evaluations by others; and treatment for PTSD targeting fears of cues of the traumatic event, including fears of the memory and anxiety symptoms accompanying the memory of the trauma. Treatment for GAD focuses on the aberrant worry process itself but also includes symptom management procedures, and treatment for OCD focuses on breaking the link between intrusive thoughts, anxiety, and compulsive behaviors using exposure techniques combined with compulsion-response prevention.

The success of these strategies has made them among the most promising in the treatment literature, with the efficacy of CBT equaling or surpassing that of alternative treatments.[97,117–121] Nonetheless, referral for CBT may be limited by the availability of clinicians specializing in these methods. In addition, the hospital setting may not allow timely initiation of treatment or the completion of basic treatment packages. Basic treatment interventions are commonly delivered in a series of 12 to 16 sessions, although patients may respond much earlier. For patients unresponsive, uninterested, or unwilling to make the initial time investment required for CBT, pharmacotherapy offers the most efficacious alternative.

REFERENCES

Access the reference list online at https://expertconsult.inkling.com/.

Patients With Alcohol Use Disorder

14

Mladen Nisavic, M.D.
Shamim H. Nejad, M.D.

OVERVIEW

Alcohol remains one of the most prevalent and clinically relevant drugs of abuse, with an estimated 75 million people worldwide meeting criteria for an alcohol use disorder (AUD) in 2004.[1] In the United States, two-thirds of all adults consume alcoholic beverages; an estimated 8 million Americans meet criteria for a severe AUD. Furthermore, approximately 500,000 individuals each year experience acute alcohol withdrawal severe enough to require pharmacologic management.[2] The annual healthcare cost related to alcohol use exceeds US$250 billion, and an estimated 85,000 deaths a year in the United States alone can be attributed to alcohol use.[3,4] Alcohol accounts for roughly one-tenth of all deaths among working-age US adults.[5] Thus, it is no surprise that alcohol is responsible for more psychiatric and neuropsychiatric problems in general hospitals than from all other substances combined. Studies estimate that 25% to 50% of all patients hospitalized for injuries are intoxicated at the time of their trauma and that the prevalence of alcohol-related problems in medical inpatients ranges from 12.5% to 30%.[5,6]

Given the prevalence of alcohol use in our society and the potential for significant medical, psychiatric, and psychosocial complications associated with chronic use and alcohol withdrawal, all psychiatrists who work in general hospitals should be skilled in the recognition and treatment of AUD. In fact, failure to diagnose and effectively treat alcohol use in hospitalized patients is exceedingly costly (in terms of morbidity and expense); a retrospective study at a major teaching hospital estimated that $4.3 million of charges were sustained by 160 patients with a substance use disorder (SUD) over a 23-day period and these could be attributed directly to the patients' SUD.[7] Prompt identification of patients with AUD in particular, and initiation of acute inpatient treatment (including acute withdrawal management, engagement with an addiction consultation service and identification of suitable aftercare resources), has been associated with improved outcomes (e.g., abstinence, longer time since the last drink, job performance, and personal happiness).[8,9]

CASE 1

Mr. T, a 55-year-old unkempt homeless man was admitted to the hospital after sustaining 30% total body surface area burns to his face, chest, and upper extremities. His examinations fluctuated between profound sedation and assaultive behavior, when attempts were made to arouse him. Examiners also commented on the "smell of alcohol" on his breath. Review of prior notes indicated an extensive history of visits for alcohol intoxication, albeit without concerns for self-harm. EMT notes indicated that Mr. T's injuries were not self-inflicted, and instead resulted from an altercation. There was no clear history of alcohol and substance use (beyond presumed daily drinking), and no history of complicated withdrawal. His medical record was replete with requests to leave the hospital against advice after acute intoxication resolved.

Mr. T was admitted to the burn service with a plan for urgent wound exploration and management. Psychiatry consult was requested "STAT" for assistance with agitation, as well as for prophylaxis and management of alcohol withdrawal.

His initial examination was notable for tachycardia (with a heart rate of 120 beats/minute), systolic hypertension (with a blood pressure, BP, of 165/80 mmHg), and an oxygen level of 96% on 3L nasal cannula. Laboratory tests were notable for a blood alcohol level (BAL) of 3,600 mg/mL, as well as for cannabis detected on the urine toxicology screen. Otherwise, labs indicated elevated transaminases (ALT 120 U/L, AST 235 U/L), but a normal MCV (95) and a normal PTT/INR.

Mr. T received a total of 10 mg of intravenous (IV) lorazepam while in the Emergency Department (ED), and he was deeply sedated. His neurologic exam did not reflect any signs, including tremor, suggestive of imminent alcohol withdrawal, but did reveal mild horizontal nystagmus. The mental status exam remained consistent with encephalopathy, but was without paranoid ideation or hallucinations. When he awoke, Mr. T stated that he "drinks a lot, 100 beers a day," and then he fell asleep.

Following surgery, Mr. T was started on a phenobarbital taper (based on his ideal body weight, his expected high risk for withdrawal, and his high risk of associated complications). He tolerated the treatment well. His mental status remained "pleasantly confused" and his vital signs showed persistent low-grade tachycardia, although both improved with wound debridement and treatment of his infectious contributors. As his mental status continued to improve further, Mr. T also agreed to meet with clinicians from the addiction consultation team to manage his alcohol use disorder (AUD). After 3 weeks on the inpatient burn surgical service, Mr. T was transferred to an inpatient medical rehabilitation program with a plan to transition him to an outpatient addiction treatment program after discharge.

SCREENING FOR ALCOHOL USE DISORDER

Alcohol use is widespread; roughly 50% of the adult US population reports using alcohol within the past 30 days, although there is considerable variation in the pattern and severity of use. The National Institute on Alcohol Abuse and Alcoholism (NIAAA) defines two categories of problematic drinking:

- Use of more than 14 drinks per week or more than 4 drinks on any day, for men under the age of 65 years
- Use of more than 7 drinks per week or more than 3 drinks on any day for women and/or any adult 65 years and older.[10]

Nearly 30% of all US adults who use alcohol do so in a potentially unhealthy manner, including 15% who exceed the recommended daily limit, 10% who exceed both daily and weekly limits, and 2% who exceed the weekly limit alone.[10] The highest rates of risky alcohol use occur in younger adults (18–29 years old), males, and Native Americans.[11]

Many tools are available to providers to help identify risky alcohol use. These include a variety of questionnaires that can be administered to inpatients or outpatients. Laboratory testing can be useful (especially if there is a concern for minimization of reported use), although such tests are not routinely recommended for screening purposes. The most commonly encountered screening tools are outlined in Tables 14-1 and 14-2, and include the AUDIT-C screening test (Table 14-1) and the CAGE questionnaire (Table 14-2). The AUDIT-C asks three questions and is considered positive when scores are >4 in men or are >3 in women, with a 90% sensitivity, and an 80% specificity rate. The CAGE asks four questions; >2 positive responses carries 77% sensitivity and 79% specificity for the detection of an AUD.[12] If the CAGE is used for screening, even a single response should be considered as screening positive.

TABLE 14-1 AUDIT-C Questionnaire for Alcohol Problems Screening[a]

1. How often did you have a drink containing alcohol in the past year?
   - Never (0 points)
   - Monthly or less (1 point)
   - 2–4 times per month (2 points)
   - 2–3 times per week (3 points)
   - >4 times per week (4 points)
2. In the past year, how many drinks did you have on a typical day when you were drinking?
   - 1–2 (0 points)
   - 3–4 (1 point)
   - 5–6 (2 points)
   - 7–9 (3 points)
   - >10 (4 points)
3. How often did you have six or more drinks on one occasion in the past year?
   - Never (0 points)
   - Less than monthly (1 point)
   - Monthly (2 points)
   - Weekly (3 points)
   - More than once a week, or daily (4 points)

[a]AUDIT-C is scored 0–12, with score >4 (men) and >3 (women) considered positive for problematic drinking.

ACUTE INTOXICATION AND THE PSYCHIATRIC SEQUELAE OF ALCOHOL USE

Ethanol, the primary active component of alcoholic beverages, is a water-soluble alcohol compound primarily absorbed via the gastrointestinal (GI) mucosa of the duodenum and small intestine (80%) and the stomach (20%).[13] The compound undergoes hepatic metabolism via alcohol dehydrogenase; in fact, a smaller distribution volume and reduced expression of this enzyme in women is believed to account for their increased susceptibility to alcohol intoxication. In most individuals, peak serum alcohol levels are reached 30–90 minutes following ingestion. Resolution of the acute toxidrome follows steady-state kinetics, so that a 70-kg male is expected to metabolize approximately 10 mL of absolute ethanol or 1.5 to 2 drink equivalents (1.5 oz whiskey = 5 oz wine = 12 oz beer) per hour.[14]

The effect of alcohol on the central nervous system (CNS) is surprisingly complex, and involves changes across multiple neurotransmitter systems. The primary mechanism of action is achieved through gamma amino butyric acid (GABA) agonism, which accounts for the CNS depressant effects of alcohol as well as for the behavioral disinhibition seen with use of the compound. With chronic exposure, further CNS changes occur, primarily in response to exogenously increased GABA tone, including a decrease in GABA receptors, decreased GABA production and decreased binding affinity to the receptor complex.[15] More importantly, these changes also lead to an increase in endogenous glutaminergic tone (an attempt to maintain homeostasis) and the development of complicated alcohol withdrawal symptoms.[16–18]

Signs and symptoms associated with acute alcohol intoxication are undoubtedly familiar to virtually all clinicians. Mild intoxication can present as impulsivity, elation, slight slurring of speech, and gait impairment. As the blood alcohol content increases, these findings become more pronounced, and include marked disinhibition, irritation, or even frankly aggressive behavior. The neurologic examination is notable for nystagmus, impaired coordination (ataxia), and unsteady gait. Attention and memory consolidation are commonly impaired, resulting in reduced recall of the intoxication, or even full "blackouts" in more severe cases. With severe

TABLE 14-2 CAGE Questionnaire for Alcohol Problems Screening[a]

C	Have you felt the need to **C**ut down on your drinking?
A	Have people **A**nnoyed you by criticizing your drinking?
G	Have you ever felt bad or **G**uilty about your drinking?
E	Have you had a drink first thing in the morning to steady your nerves or to get rid of a hangover (i.e., an "**E**ye opener")?

[a]A score of two positive items indicates the need for detailed assessment.

alcohol poisoning, CNS depression becomes prominent, leading to stupor and coma.

The clinical effect is dose-dependent, although much variability (based on the patient's gender, genetics, amount/rate of intake, co-ingestion of other drugs, and overall duration of alcohol use) exists. While the blood alcohol level (BAL) can reliably predict clinical effects in patients who only use alcohol socially, habituation and tolerance are common with chronic use, and in these individuals, little clinical evidence of intoxication may be seen despite an extremely elevated BAL.[19] In patients who use alcohol intermittently, a BAL <100 mg/dL, will produce euphoria, problems with coordination, and impaired attention. Higher levels (e.g., BAL 100–200 mg/dL) are associated with a worsening of motor deficits, impaired judgment, and an increased chance of assaultive/aggressive behavior. As BAL exceeds 300 mg/dL encephalopathy and CNS depression become prominent, and coma (and even death) can occur at BAL 400–500 mg/dL.

Initial work-up of acute alcohol intoxication should involve checking basic chemistry studies (as electrolyte imbalance is common with acute intoxication), a serum glucose, hepatic function, and a BAL. If co-ingestion is suspected, screening for other drugs of abuse is recommended, though it may not always be necessary with isolated alcohol intoxication. Treatment depends largely on the degree of intoxication observed:

- Mild to moderate intoxication can be managed supportively and patients may require little more than observation and serial assessments. IV fluids may be warranted if there is evidence (e.g., persistent tachycardia) of volume depletion. Agitation, if present, may respond to reduced stimulation/isolation, and in more severe cases, use of dopamine antagonists such as intravenous (IV) haloperidol (e.g., 2–5 mg), as it does not exacerbate sedation, and can be administered easily. In patients with a preference for the parenteral route, various atypical agents (e.g., olanzapine, quetiapine) should be considered. Benzodiazepines are also commonly used in this setting, although using them as sole agents for management of agitation may exacerbate acute intoxication and worsen agitation, over-sedation, and respiratory depression. Once an individual is no longer intoxicated, he or she can usually be discharged home, after screening for the severity/extent of use and discussing aftercare resources.
- Severe intoxication may require intensive supportive measures, including frequent assessment of physiologic parameters. With severe obtundation, patients may not be able to protect their airway and may require intubation. Hemodynamic changes may be seen, including tachycardia and hypotension, and patients may require IV hydration.

ALCOHOL WITHDRAWAL SYNDROME: IDENTIFICATION AND MANAGEMENT

Alcohol withdrawal can range from a state of mild discomfort that requires no medication to multi-organ failure that requires intensive care. In large part, this variability is a reflection of a series of changes in CNS receptor expression and function associated with chronic alcohol use (Figure 14-1). As previously discussed, alcohol enhances GABA activity and inhibits glutamate activity; this leads to a CNS depressant effect. In the setting of chronic alcohol use, the GABA system habituates, leading to a decrease in the number of GABA receptors, to changes in configuration of the receptor subunits, and to reduced rates of GABA synthesis. The result is one of decreased *endogenous* GABA tone. Similarly, chronic exposure to alcohol leads to changes in the glutamate neurotransmitter system, namely with an increase in the number of glutamate receptors. The overall effect is that of increased *endogenous* excitatory tone, representing an attempt to restore homeostasis and balance the increase in *exogenous* GABA tone caused by the use of alcohol. With abrupt cessation of alcohol use, this tenuous balance becomes disturbed quickly and a state marked by over-expression of excitatory neurotransmitters (glutamate, norepinephrine, dopamine) and reduced GABA tone develops. The specific types of neurotransmitters affected and the severity of aberration seen determine the clinical symptoms and the severity of the alcohol withdrawal syndrome observed.[16–18]

Table 14-3 summarizes three key clusters of symptoms observed in alcohol withdrawal. Type A symptoms are associated with minor (uncomplicated) withdrawal and reflect an overall decrease in GABA activity. The most common clinical findings with this type are anxiety, restlessness/irritability, insomnia, general malaise, and a *fine* tremor. Symptoms of types B and C are more prevalent in cases of severe (complicated) withdrawal and reflect an increase in noradrenergic and dopaminergic tone, respectively. Type B withdrawal symptoms include the hallmark increased

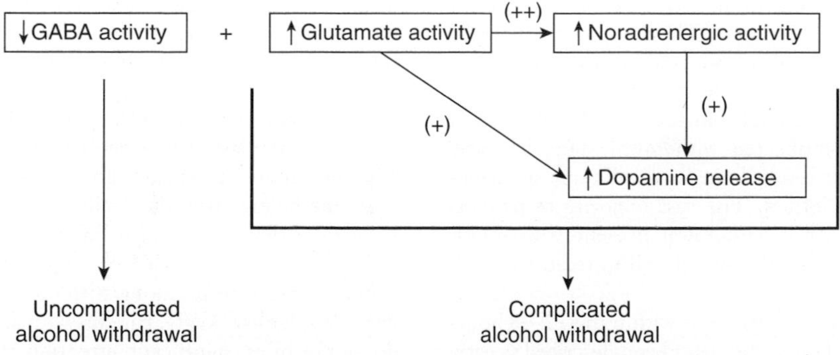

Figure 14-1 Neurotransmitters affected in alcohol withdrawal syndrome.

TABLE 14-3 Alcohol Withdrawal Syndrome Symptom Clusters, Receptors and Recommended Treatment Options

SYMPTOM CLUSTERS	COMMON SYMPTOMS	NEUROTRANSMITTERS AFFECTED	RECOMMENDED TREATMENT
A	Anxiety, restlessness, general malaise, nausea/emesis; *fine* tremor	Decreased GABA activity	GABA-agonists
B	*Coarse* tremor, hypertension, tachycardia, fever, diaphoresis	Increased glutamate and norepinephrine activity	Beta-blockers, alpha agonists
C	Confusion, encephalopathy, hallucinations, paranoid ideation, agitation	Increased glutamate and dopamine activity	Dopamine antagonists

sympathetic tone, with resultant *coarse* bilateral tremor, hypertension, tachycardia, fever, and diaphoresis. Since some patients attempt to fabricate type B findings (e.g., tremor), clinicians should examine patients for tongue fasciculations and monitor for the absence of tremor with distraction (e.g., observation from outside the room or providing a glass of water to consume while conducting the examination and observing for the presence of end-point tremor). Type C symptoms are marked by impairments of attention and by confusion, as well as by the symptoms of acute psychosis, including hallucinations (visual more often than auditory), paranoid ideation, and delusional thinking.

Given the range of neurotransmitters involved, treatment of alcohol withdrawal should be tailored to the specific symptom cluster observed, including use of benzodiazepines for type A symptoms, use of beta-blockers and alpha-adrenergic agents to treat refractory tachycardia/hypertension (type B symptoms), and use of dopamine antagonists for management of hallucinations, agitation, and paranoid delusions (type C symptoms). The clinician, however, should always ensure that one prioritizes type A > type B > type C unless there are type B or type C emergencies that need to be managed and treated acutely (e.g., concern for demand ischemia or hypertensive emergency).

Types of Alcohol Withdrawal Syndromes

Clinical hallmarks of the four major alcohol withdrawal syndromes are outlined below.

Early/uncomplicated withdrawal syndrome generally reflects CNS hyperactivity in the setting of alcohol discontinuation, and includes subjective sensations of anxiety and restlessness, as well as insomnia, fine tremor, changes in appetite/GI upset, diaphoresis, and headaches. These symptoms generally develop within the first 6–12 hours after cessation of use, and may even be observed in those with elevated BALs (a reflection of chronic use and habituation). Unless the patient progresses to a complicated withdrawal state, an early withdrawal syndrome is self-limited and will remit spontaneously within 24–48 hours. The vast majority of patients who experience alcohol withdrawal present with minor withdrawal symptoms, and respond well to treatment with benzodiazepines.

Alcohol withdrawal seizures occur within the 12–48 hours after the last drink, though they have been described as early as 1–2 hours after last use. Despite significant concerns in the hospital setting, alcohol withdrawal seizures are uncommon events seen in only 1% of unmedicated patients who undergo alcohol withdrawal. Moreover, the incidence of alcohol withdrawal seizures increases in patients with a pre-existing seizure disorder, prior head trauma, and a history of seizures related to alcohol discontinuation.[20] Classically, most alcohol withdrawal seizures fit the description of singular, self-limited, tonic-clonic convulsions and a report of multiple, prolonged seizures and/or progression to status epilepticus should raise concerns for alternative etiologies and prompt further diagnostic assessment. Although most patients do not require head imaging, CT and/or MRI scans can help exclude causes of ictal activity, and should be strongly considered in those who demonstrate focal neurologic findings, those with suspected head trauma, and those with an altered sensorium not due to acute intoxication. Multiple prior detoxifications predict withdrawal seizures more than the quantity or duration of a drinking history; this implies a kindling phenomenon with chronic alcohol use and detoxifications, similar to that observed in those patients with epilepsy. Most cases of alcohol withdrawal seizures are treated with benzodiazepines (e.g., IV/PO lorazepam) or longer-acting barbiturates (e.g., phenobarbital). There are limited data to support the use of other anti-epileptic drugs (AEDs) over benzodiazepines, unless the patient has a history of a seizure disorder, however care should be noted that no other AED, outside of phenobarbital, has been shown to be effective for moderate to severe alcohol withdrawal seizures in the acute setting. In other words, while they may reduce seizure activity from epilepsy, they do not influence seizure activity due to alcohol withdrawal seizures.

Alcoholic hallucinosis is a rare syndrome reflective of increased dopaminergic activity; it is commonly confounded by alcohol withdrawal delirium (AWD), which is often referred to as *delirium tremens*. The onset of symptoms is typically seen within 12–24 hours after the last drink. Without treatment, most symptoms will remit within 48 hours after the last drink (the earliest time point associated with delirium tremens).[18] The patients who experience alcoholic hallucinosis classically describe vivid visual hallucinations that may occur in an otherwise clear sensorium. Olfactory and tactile hallucinations are also noted with alcoholic hallucinosis, along with the presence of paranoid delusions. Unlike AWD, patients with alcoholic hallucinosis do not exhibit significant attention deficits, tremor, or autonomic dysregulation (the combination of these sets of symptoms essentially constitutes the diagnosis of alcohol withdrawal delirium). While alcoholic hallucinosis will invariably (and eventually) remit even without treatment, most patients will benefit from a brief course of dopamine antagonists, along with some GABA-agonists to provide a degree of anxiolysis. As with other types of acute psychosis, attention should be paid to patient safety and all patients with alcoholic hallucinosis should be assessed for self-harm and harm to others.

Alcohol withdrawal delirium (AWD), delirium tremens is a clinical syndrome characterized by autonomic hyperactivity (tachycardia, hypertension, hyperthermia), confusion/disorientation, hallucinations, and not uncommonly agitation. Visual hallucinations, including those of animals ("white mice" and "pink elephants"), are common, although hallucinations involving other sensory modalities have also been described. Delusional thinking and paranoia may exacerbate a patient's distress and lead to agitation or frank aggression. Most patients will develop AWD within 48–72 hours of discontinuing alcohol, although later onset has also been described. Untreated, the condition typically persists for 3–4 days, although it may persist longer and is associated with a significant risk for mortality and morbidity. While only 5% of all patients with AUD will develop AWD, the risk appears to be greater in the following populations:

- Patients with a history of AWD (strongest predictor)
- Patients with a history of chronic sustained daily drinking
- Older individuals (age >40)
- Patients with significant concurrent medical/surgical illnesses, including long bone fractures, burns, and head trauma
- Patients who develop withdrawal symptoms in the context of an elevated BAL
- Patients admitted >2 days since their last drink.[21–23]

While AWD was associated with a 37% mortality rate at the beginning of the last century, more recent estimates describe a mortality rate closer to 5%, undoubtedly a reflection of improved diagnosis, and management, particularly with advances in critical care. Most AWD-associated morbidity and mortality occurs in the setting of cardiopulmonary failure (e.g., arrhythmias, ischemic events, aspiration), infectious (e.g., aspiration pneumonia), metabolic derangements (e.g., acute hepatitis, pancreatitis, electrolyte abnormalities), and CNS injury.

Treatment of Alcohol Withdrawal

Uncomplicated alcohol withdrawal (accounting for the majority of patients) responds adequately to treatment with GABA-agonists, including various benzodiazepines or phenobarbital. Long-acting benzodiazepines (e.g., diazepam, chlordiazepoxide) have been preferred due to their longer half-life and associated self-tapering properties, which helps to create a smoother taper. One key exception is the populations with significant liver injury who require a taper with a short-acting agent (e.g., oxazepam, lorazepam) that does not undergo first pass hepatic metabolism; such agents are less likely to accumulate and to cause over-sedation. The duration of the taper, and overall dose required, will depend on a number of factors (e.g., the patient's pattern of alcohol use, genetics, hepatic metabolism, and the pharmacokinetics of the chosen drug). Thus, no single taper schedule may prove effective for all patients, and clinicians should expect considerable variation from patient-to-patient, particularly in those with co-morbid medical and surgical illness. In general, one should aim for light sedation as a target of treatment, to a degree that ensures patient comfort, and staff safety, and does not significantly obscure the neurologic examination.

Benzodiazepines can be administered either on a fixed schedule (i.e., a dose is given at fixed intervals even if symptoms of withdrawal are absent) or as symptom-triggered therapy. The latter method is most commonly utilized in detoxification centers and psychiatric units as it requires nursing staff with expertise in identification and treatment of alcohol withdrawal. In the general hospital setting, symptom-triggered therapy often proves to be challenging, as medical/surgical clinicians may lack familiarity with the CIWA scale, and its downstream consequences (e.g., a number of symptoms reported on the CIWA scale may be non-specific in the medically ill and may result in administration of sedatives due to other etiologies, leading to benzodiazepine excess and iatrogenic delirium). Fixed-dosing helps to avoid some of the unpredictability associated with symptom-triggered treatment, albeit at a risk of over-medicating and becoming benzodiazepine-intoxicated.

Regardless of the method used, management of withdrawal involves the use of increasingly large benzodiazepine doses until the patient appears comfortable and light sedation is attained. Subsequently, a benzodiazepine taper can be initiated and the dose is decreased by 25% to 30% per day until it has been discontinued.

One common clinical pitfall is using benzodiazepines for the management of symptoms associated with alcohol withdrawal, including type B and C symptoms. While benzodiazepines are excellent agents for managing symptoms related to decreased GABA tone, benzodiazepines have little impact on the management of refractory tachycardia and hypertension; these symptoms may be better addressed by hydration and by administration of beta-blockers, and/or alpha-adrenergic agents. Similarly, benzodiazepines should not be the sole agents for the management of alcohol withdrawal-related hallucinations or agitation; dopamine antagonists often offer better symptom control with less risk for over-sedation and intoxication.

Phenobarbital, the most commonly used AED in the world, presents an excellent alternative to benzodiazepines in general hospital settings. This medication demonstrates both GABA-agonism and glutamate-antagonism, and can thus directly address both major neurotransmitter-associated and acute withdrawal. Furthermore, it has reliable pharmacokinetics, and a long half-life, and it lacks a narrow therapeutic index; its only absolute contraindication is a history of Stevens–Johnson syndrome (SJS)/toxic epidermal necrolysis (TEN) or acute intermittent porphyria. Patients can be dosed based on their ideal body weight, with the target dose adjusted according to the patient's overall risk of withdrawal as well as the expected risk of complications. Initial loading doses are administered at 3-hour intervals as IM injections, while the subsequent taper can be administered orally. A serum level is obtained following the last IM dose and is used to monitor metabolic function, and to adjust subsequent dosing.[24–29]

Various AEDs (e.g., gabapentin, carbamazepine, valproate), have been proposed as agents for management of alcohol withdrawal, but none of these agents has appeared to confer the same degree of benefit as seen with benzodiazepines or phenobarbital.[30] Similarly, ethanol has been used, especially in patients who report their intention to resume drinking immediately on discharge.[31] Although the notion of administering ethanol in the hospital may appear novel and exciting, a number of practical complications arise that make other agents preferred alternatives in nearly all cases. Ethanol is difficult to titrate, has many adverse metabolic effects, and is overall unsafe in the general medical setting. Lastly, in the intensive care unit (ICU), dexmedetomidine and propofol have both been used as viable alternatives to benzodiazepines/phenobarbital for the treatment of alcohol withdrawal. Respiratory compromise and sedation with propofol, along with bradycardia and hypotension associated with dexmedetomidine, limits the use of these medications to the ICU setting.

In addition to the medications described, all patients treated for alcohol withdrawal should receive thiamine given their increased risk for Wernicke encephalopathy and Korsakoff psychosis. Doses of 200 mg daily are recommended for the prevention of the syndrome and carry no safety risk to the patient, while higher doses are recommended if an actual thiamine deficiency is suspected.

WERNICKE–KORSAKOFF SYNDROME

Victor and associates in their classic monograph *The Wernicke–Korsakoff syndrome* stated that "Wernicke's encephalopathy and Korsakoff's syndrome in the alcoholic, nutritionally deprived patient may be regarded as two facets of the same disease."[32] Although uncommon (by some estimates, <5% of all patients with chronic alcohol use) the diagnosis is often missed and should be considered in all patients who present with heavy alcohol use, especially if they may have other reasons for malnutrition (e.g., homelessness, head/neck cancer, cognitive impairment).

Wernicke's Encephalopathy

Wernicke's encephalopathy arises acutely and is classically characterized by a triad of ophthalmoplegia, ataxia, and mental status disturbance.[32] The ocular disturbance, which is necessary for the diagnosis, consists of paresis or paralysis of the lateral rectus muscles, nystagmus, and a disturbance in conjugate gaze. A global confusional state consists of disorientation, unresponsiveness, and derangement of perception and memory. Exhaustion, apathy, and profound lethargy are also part of the picture.

Once treatment with thiamine has been initiated for Wernicke's encephalopathy, improvement in the ocular findings is often evident within hours, while full recovery follows over days or weeks. Classically, it has been estimated that approximately one-third of patients recover from the state of global confusion within 6 days of treatment, another third recover within 1 month, and the remainder improve within 2 months. The global confusional state is almost always reversible, in marked contrast to the memory impairment of Korsakoff's psychosis.

Korsakoff's Psychosis

Korsakoff's psychosis, also referred to as *confabulatory psychosis* and *alcohol-induced persisting amnestic disorder*, is characterized by impaired memory in an otherwise alert and responsive person. Hallucinations and delusions are rarely encountered. Curiously, confabulation, long regarded as the hallmark of Korsakoff's psychosis, is not seen in the majority of cases and its absence should not preclude this diagnosis. The memory loss is generally bipartite. The retrograde component involves the inability to recall the past, and the anterograde component involves the lack of capacity for retention of new information. In the acute stage of Korsakoff's psychosis, the memory gap may be so blatant that the patient cannot recall simple items (such as the examiner's first name, the day, or the time) after a few minutes, even though the patient is provided with this information several times. As memory improves, usually within weeks to months, simple problems can be solved, limited always by the patient's span of recall.

The EEG may be unremarkable or might show diffuse slowing, while an MRI scan might demonstrate changes in the periaqueductal gray area, hippocampal formations, and the medial dorsal nucleus of the thalamus.[19]

Although often regarded as irreversible, a significant number of patients with Korsakoff's psychosis show some improvement over time. Classically, one expects 20% of the patients to recover more or less completely; however, 25% showed no recovery, and the rest recovered partially.

Treatment

Administration (IV or IM) of the B vitamin, thiamine, should be considered a routine component of early treatment for all intoxicated patients, preferably while still in the ED or immediately upon admission, whichever comes earlier.[33] Because subclinical cognitive impairment can occur even in apparently well-nourished patients, we recommend routine treatment with IV thiamine (as prophylaxis) for all intoxicated patients, as this prevents advancement of the disease and reverses at least a portion of the lesions affecting CNS territories.

For preventive measures, we often recommend using >100 mg of IV thiamine immediately, followed by 200 mg of thiamine (orally) while the patient remains in the hospital. If Wernicke/Korsakoff is suspected, treatment should consist of high-dose thiamine (500 mg IV three times per day for at least 3 days) followed by 500 mg IV/IM daily while symptoms persist. Because GI absorption of thiamine may be erratic, IV/IM formulations are much preferred to oral formulations. Lastly, thiamine should be administered before giving glucose, as the latter may precipitate or even exacerbate Wernicke's encephalopathy.[33,34]

PHARMACOTHERAPY FOR ALCOHOL USE DISORDER

Most of the treatment for AUD is centered on modifying the reinforcing effects that the compound has on the corticomesolimbic dopamine reward pathways. Thus, medications used for treatment of AUD will work on a variety of receptor systems (e.g., endogenous opioids, GABA, glutamate, and serotonin). Treatment should be initiated while the patient is hospitalized, and patients should remain on the medication for at least 6 months after attaining sobriety. Treatment courses longer than 6 months have not been well studied.

First-line treatment for AUD involves naltrexone and acamprosate. The two are briefly summarized below:

- Naltrexone, available in oral and IM depot form, exerts its pharmacologic effect through mu (μ)-opioid receptor blockade, which reduces the reinforcing effects of alcohol consumption. In animal studies, naltrexone has been found to reduce alcohol self-administration.[35] In humans, naltrexone has been found to reduce the rate and severity of alcohol consumption compared with placebo.[36,37] Oral naltrexone is commonly used at doses of 50 to 100 mg/day, while the IM formulation (Vivitrol) is used at doses of 380 mg every 4 weeks. Patients who require opioid agents (e.g., for pain management) should not be started on naltrexone; otherwise the drug is well tolerated with its most common side effects including nausea, fatigue, and low appetite. Rare cases of interstitial pneumonia and eosinophilic pneumonia have been reported with use of naltrexone.
- Acamprosate works through modulation of glutamate CNS transmission, and has been shown to reduce alcohol consumption rates compared to placebo in patients with severe AUD, as well as to increase the duration of abstinence by an average of 11%.[36,38] The drug is safe and is generally well tolerated, although dose adjustments may be needed in patients with renal failure (owing to primarily renal metabolism). The primary barrier to treatment may be reduced adherence in the setting of TID dosing.

In addition to these agents, a variety of other compounds have been use for pharmacologic management of AUD. Some of the most common are summarized below:

- Topiramate has been shown to reduce alcohol use in patients with severe AUD, but it does not carry FDA approval for this indication. It is believed to work through antagonizing kainate glutamate receptors and by interacting with GABA receptors.[39,40] Compared with other drugs listed here, topiramate initiation may require a gradual taper (to both initiate and discontinue the medication) and is associated with more frequent side effects, including cognitive dulling, weight loss, mood changes, and depression. As with many AEDs, topiramate should be avoided by pregnant women.
- Gabapentin, baclofen, SSRIs, and ondansetron have all been studied as potential options for treatment of AUD, although the data for most of these compounds have not been encouraging. A recent prospective placebo-controlled randomized trial of gabapentin in patients with AUD noted improvements with regard to rates of complete abstinence, reduction in heavy drinking, and improved mood/sleep and cravings in the treatment group. These results were more pronounced at higher doses of the medication (e.g., 1800 mg daily).[24]
- Disulfiram discourages drinking through negative reinforcement, as it precipitates an unpleasant physical reaction when an individual consumes alcohol while on this medication. The compound works by inhibiting aldehyde dehydrogenase, thus preventing the metabolism of acetaldehyde (the primary hepatic metabolite of alcohol breakdown). Accumulation of acetaldehyde leads to flushing, sweating, headache, palpitations, nausea, and vomiting. Efficacy of the compound is limited, and it often requires strong motivation or supervised conditions. With unsupervised treatment, disulfiram is less effective, as most patients will self-discontinue the medication before they resume drinking. Disulfiram should be avoided in patients with severe cardiovascular disease, pregnant women, and patients with psychosis. In general, the use of this medication has waned, given the alternatives.

PSYCHOSOCIAL TREATMENT OF ALCOHOL USE DISORDER

Brief substance use intervention in the general medical setting is well-developed and effective.[41] Even brief contact with an addiction consultant has led to improvement rates in 30% to 50% of patients several months after hospitalization. This effect is even more pronounced in those with no prior psychiatric illness and with good social function and resources.[42] Addiction consultation services to hospital physicians should assist with diagnosis, intervention, pharmacologic management, and post-acute care referral.

AUD causes diverse disruptions in people's self-awareness, communication skills, capacity for relationships, sense of purpose, and spirituality. Alcoholics Anonymous (AA), SMART recovery, and other peer-driven recovery services, have a record of success and benefit greatly from accessibility and low cost. If already established within AA, patients may benefit from visits from their sponsor or other group members while hospitalized. Alternatively, some hospitals have established AA meetings on-campus, and (if able and interested) patients should be encouraged to attend these while hospitalized. Recovery coaches offer an excellent alternative to the classic addiction clinician's approach and may be able to engage patients on a deeply personal level through shared experiences. Working with individuals in recovery may motivate the patient to engage with the team and be more trusting of the treatment options offered.

Key features of central intake include directly assisting patients with access to treatment, helping patients to call programs, subsidizing transportation to treatment program interviews, obtaining concrete services to diminish treatment obstacles (such as homelessness or lack of child care), and motivational interviewing. Motivational interviewing is a directed, patient-centered counseling for eliciting behavioral change by helping to explore and resolve ambivalence to change.[43] With this technique, the provider assesses the patient's losses and risks, helps the patient to recognize the underlying cause as substance abuse, and uncovers ambivalence about the potential value of treatment. By avoiding a threatening style of confrontation about denial, motivational interviewing has been found to enhance motivation for recovery.[43]

To be successful, any attempt at treating AUD in the inpatient setting should focus on much more than diagnosis of the disorder and management of the potential withdrawal syndrome. Patients should be assessed for their understanding of the problem and readiness to engage with addiction work. Pharmacologic treatments should be initiated while in the hospital, and patients should engage with substance use specialists to review outpatient resources and services to assist with recovery. Issues that may impede recovery, such as housing and legal issues, should be acknowledged and addressed whenever possible.

REFERENCES

Access the reference list online at https://expertconsult.inkling.com/.

Patients With Substance Use Disorders

15

Mladen Nisavic, M.D.
Shamim H. Nejad, M.D.

OVERVIEW

Without a doubt, substance use disorders (SUDs) present one of the gravest difficulties currently facing the United States healthcare system. Over the past two decades, the number of patients treated for substance use-related problems in the United States has grown steadily, and over the past 5 years it has reached epidemic proportions. Data from the Centers for Disease Control and Prevention (CDC) indicate that in the 10 years between 2004 and 2014, the mortality rates attributed to drug overdoses increased by 137%, including a staggering 200% increase in the rate of overdose deaths attributed to opioids. The increased mortality rates were independent of sex, age group, or ethnicity, and were evident across the country. In fact, the CDC estimates that nearly half a million persons in the United States died from drug overdoses between 2000 and 2014, and that drug-related fatalities were one and a half times higher than deaths from motor vehicle crashes in 2014.[1] Up to 80% of all drug-related fatalities appear to be unintentional, with 13% attributed to suicide, and the remainder classified as undetermined.

The increase in drug use has also led to increased utilization of healthcare services. The Drug Abuse Warning Network (DAWN) and the Substance Abuse and Mental Health Service Administration (SAMHSA) estimate that over 5 million Emergency Department (ED) visits in 2011 were related to drug use—a 100% increase over their 2004 data. Of these, nearly 2.5 million ED visits were attributed to medical emergencies related to drug abuse.

Clinical presentations in this domain are also becoming more complex. Of the 2.5 million ED visits identified by DAWN/SAMHSA in 2011, nearly one-half involved complications related to use of prescription medications, with the remainder being attributed to use of non-prescription illicit drugs. While the use of opioids, marijuana, and cocaine are seen most commonly, more than 50% of the patients present with co-ingestion of multiple substances, and there has been an increase in use of CNS stimulants, "club drugs," and hallucinogens.[2]

Successful treatment of this expanding group of patients requires that clinicians improve their management skills for SUDs and their sequelae. This involves timely and correct diagnosis of the substance use problem, recognition of key symptoms associated with intoxication or acute discontinuation/withdrawal, and appropriate initial management and treatment. It also involves meaningful engagement (including motivational enhancement techniques to assess readiness for recovery), identification of outpatient addiction resources, and use of medications to reduce craving and to maintain recovery. The chronic, relapsing, nature of substance use may inspire resignation and hopelessness in consulting clinicians, leading to a misperception that the consultation is unnecessary, or even futile. Because most clinicians fail to appreciate that the relapse rate for other common chronic medical disorders (e.g., diabetes, hypertension, asthma) exceeds that for SUDs, they do not treat substance abuse patients with comparable therapeutic diligence.[3] The Massachusetts General Hospital (MGH) has dedicated considerable effort and resources to adequately address the substance use epidemic within our local communities, starting with a hospital-wide effort to ensure that problems related to substance use are addressed with the same degree of compassion and persistence directed at other common relapsing medical disorders. Medical and surgical hospitalizations often provide extended periods during which patients are separated from their substance use, and thus hospitalization may present a unique opportunity to engage the patient in meaningful interventions.

CASE 1

Mr. B, a 36-year-old homeless man with a history of substance use and abuse (benzodiazepines, opiates, and stimulants), was admitted to the vascular surgery service with ischemia to his right hand and forearm. The injury was sustained when he relapsed on "heroin" (after 2 months of recovery), and became obtunded with a protracted period of immobility. An initial urine toxicology screen was positive for benzodiazepines and opioids, with further toxicology testing that confirmed the presence of clonazepam, methadone, and fentanyl. Psychiatric consultation was requested to assist with pain management and to provide assistance with addiction recovery treatment referral and resources.

On interview, Mr. B was alert, oriented, lucid, and forthcoming. He reported surprise, and then frank fear, that he "ended up this way—after all I only used once." He also appeared surprised that the toxicology screen revealed evidence of fentanyl and benzodiazepines, as he was "certain" he used heroin. He complained of pain, despite being on his methadone maintenance (75 mg/day), and expressed concern that his pain would be under-treated because of his history of substance use. His mood was appropriate to the clinical context: there was no evidence of depression.

Following initial stabilization, Mr. B underwent amputation of his right forearm and hand. During the perioperative period, he received a combination of long-acting opioids for basal analgesic control, as well as short-acting opioids for breakthrough pain. His methadone dose was increased to 90 mg/day, and was split into three-times-a-day dosing to optimize pain management. His short-acting opioids (intravenous [IV], then oral hydromorphone) were tapered gradually over 2 weeks while he remained in the inpatient setting.

With improved pain control, Mr. B more readily engaged in readiness work via motivational interviewing and he accepted addiction recovery services. He identified methadone maintenance as a key element to his recovery and noted no cravings on the higher dose of his medication. He found inspiration in his survival, and despite grieving the loss of his limb, expressed a strong readiness to maintain recovery. He worked closely with the consultation team to identify triggers for relapse and secured a safe disposition plan. By the end of his 2-week hospital stay, Mr. B held regular meetings with Narcotics Anonymous (NA) peers in the hospital. He maintained continuous contact with his methadone provider and allowed the consultation team to share their impressions with the clinic.

Mr. B was discharged to his parents' home, with a plan to follow-up with his methadone clinic and NA. He expressed (appropriate) anxiety on discharge, as he readily admitted that the road ahead of him would be challenging, but also noted hope and readiness to battle his addiction.

STIMULANTS

Cocaine

Cocaine is a tropane alkaloid naturally found in leaves of the *Erythroxylum coca* plant, a bush native to the Andes Mountains region of South America. To this day, leaves of the plant continue to be used by the indigenous people (typically chewed), for their anesthetic, stimulant, and hunger-suppressant effects. Over the past two centuries, the discovery of methods to reliably isolate the alkaloid combined with the ever-increasing demand for the compound, has led to cocaine becoming one of the most commonly abused drugs worldwide. An estimated 17 million people (about 0.4% of the world population) have used cocaine, a number only surpassed by cannabis and alcohol.[4] The widespread use of the drug, combined with potent stimulant effects has led to cocaine being one of the leading drugs of abuse (in terms of the frequency of ED contacts, general hospital admissions, violence, and other social problems). The DAWN ED data for 2011 reported 505,224 ED visits related to cocaine, compared with 455,668 ED visits for marijuana, and 258,482 ED visits related to heroin use—a staggering 40% of all ED visits related to illicit drug use.[2] Traditionally, the coca leaf is chewed to release the cocaine alkaloid, yet isolated cocaine is rarely ingested (commonly with a highly alkaline compound to prevent neutralization by the acidic milieu of the stomach). More commonly, cocaine is injected, insufflated or inhaled (as "crack") as the latter methods greatly increase the bioavailability of the drug.

Pharmacology and Mechanism of Action

Cocaine increases the monoamine neurotransmitter activity in the central nervous system (CNS) by blocking the pre-synaptic re-uptake transporters for dopamine, norepinephrine, and serotonin. Given the potent effects of cocaine on dopamine's availability within the CNS, much of the drug's stimulant and addictive effects have been ascribed to its effects on the corticomesolimbic dopamine reward circuits.[5,6] In addition to these effects, cocaine also acts by blocking voltage-gated sodium ion channels, an action that accounts for its effect as a local anesthetic and contributes to its cardiac toxicity.

The route of administration greatly influences the bioavailability of the drug, including its onset and duration of intoxication. Smoking (i.e., inhalation) and IV use generally lead to near instantaneous (seconds to minutes) effects, and most patients note that the drug's effects wear off within 30 minutes. Intranasal administration results in slower onset of symptoms (within 30 minutes) and the effects of the drug are similarly extended to up to 1 hour.

Cocaine is commonly co-administered with alcohol, which leads to the formation of cocaethylene, a compound with stimulant effects similar to that of cocaine, albeit with a longer half-life. This compound has also been noted to carry greater cardiac toxicity compared with cocaine alone.

Cocaine is extensively metabolized by the liver, and its metabolites are eliminated in the urine, most commonly as benzoylecgonine. This metabolite (rather than the parent compound) is detected by urine drug tests for cocaine; it can be detected as early as 4 hours after intake, and may remain detectable for up to 1 week after cocaine is used. There are no common false positives for urine cocaine screen.

Cocaine intoxication is associated with potent stimulant effects, including increased energy and alertness, bright (to frankly euphoric) affect, insomnia, as well as anorexia. Similar to other stimulants, cocaine is associated with an intensely pleasurable state and is commonly used to potentiate sexual activity. With higher doses, the unintended effects of cocaine may become apparent, including anxiety and panic attacks, restlessness, agitation, and violent behavior, as well as psychosis (manifesting as paranoid ideation, hallucinations, or delusional thinking). Signs of adrenergic hyperactivity (e.g., hyperreflexia, tachycardia, diaphoresis, mydriasis) may also be seen. More severe symptoms (e.g., hyperpyrexia, hypertension, cocaine-induced vasospastic events, such as stroke or myocardial infarction) are relatively rare among recreational users but are seen more commonly in patients who present to the ED for cocaine-related issues. Patients may manifest motor signs of CNS excitability, including tremor, myoclonus, and stereotyped movements of the mouth, face, or extremities (e.g., skin picking, "crack dancing," "boca torcida"). Infrequently, seizures may occur, even with first time use of the drug—most commonly these are manifest as generalized tonic-clinic seizures within the first 90 minutes after drug use.

Given its potent effects on the central and peripheral monoamine neurotransmitter systems, it is not surprising that cocaine has significant effects on most organ systems. In addition to stimulant and pro-ictal effects described previously, cocaine has been associated with increased rates of hemorrhagic and ischemic stroke, an effect postulated to be due to increased heart rate and blood pressure (due to sympathetic nervous system (SNS) activation), cerebral vasoconstriction, and vasospasm. Cocaine similarly increases risk for ischemic cardiac phenomena, and chest pain is one of the most frequent complaints in cocaine users who seek medical attention. Cocaine use has been associated with increased heart rate and blood pressure (via increased peripheral adrenergic activity), as well as vasoconstriction, both of which lead to reduced cardiac oxygen availability and increased risk for cardiac complications, including myocardial infarction. Furthermore, cocaine action as a sodium channel-blocker leads to an increased risk for cardiac arrhythmias, and even sudden death.

Intranasal cocaine use has been associated with rhinitis, sinusitis, and in severe cases, perforation of the nasal septum. Inhalation use leads to common respiratory symptoms, including shortness of breath, wheezing, and cough, but may also cause bronchitis, pulmonary edema, hemorrhage, and even a pneumothorax. While cocaine has not been shown to be a significant source of hepatotoxicity in humans, it can contribute to renal damage through direct (vasoconstriction of renal arteries) as well as indirect effects (through cocaine-induced rhabdomyolysis).

Cocaine discontinuation leads to an unpleasant, though rarely medically concerning, withdrawal syndrome. Nonetheless, DAWN data indicate that up to one-fourth of all drug-related detoxification-related ED visits were attributable to cocaine withdrawal. Patients commonly present with symptoms opposite to those seen with cocaine intoxication, including depression, fatigue, anhedonia, difficulties concentrating, as well as increased sleep and appetite. Patients may also exhibit drug cravings. In some cases, depression and psychomotor retardation observed with cocaine withdrawal may be so severe as to be accompanied by prominent hopelessness and suicidal ideation. In comparison with its behavioral effects, physical signs of cocaine withdrawal are usually mild and clinically unremarkable.

Psychiatric Sequelae of Cocaine Use

Cocaine use has been associated with the development of cocaine use disorder in up to one-sixth of all individuals exposed to the drug. Although euphoria is an intended effect of the drug, patients acutely intoxicated by cocaine may present with symptoms that resemble acute mania, a primary anxiety disorder, or a primary depressive disorder. The most serious psychiatric finding associated with cocaine intoxication is cocaine-induced psychosis, which frequently manifests as visual and auditory hallucinations, paranoid delusions, and (in severe cases) violent behavior. Some studies estimate its prevalence at 80% of all individuals with a cocaine use disorder. While these symptoms resemble those of a primary psychotic process, cocaine-induced psychosis may be differentiated by its transient nature, relative absence of negative symptoms, as well as more prominent visual and tactile hallucinations (e.g., "coke bugs").

Management

Cocaine intoxication can lead to significant medical as well as psychiatric consequences, and acute management should take both into consideration. As with all acute toxidromes, the ABC (airway, breathing, circulation) of stabilization are essential to initial patient management. Given the stimulant effects of cocaine outlined above, monitoring for tachycardia, hypertension, and associated end-organ damage (e.g., coronary ischemia, stroke) is essential with acute intoxication. Mild-to-moderate tachycardia and hypertension may respond to use of IV benzodiazepines. For refractory or severe hypertension, alpha-adrenergic agents (e.g., phentolamine) are commonly used. The use of beta-blockers in acute cocaine intoxication remains controversial, but this class of medications has been traditionally avoided for concerns of unopposed alpha-adrenergic stimulation and associated increased chances for vasospasm and cardiac ischemia.

Acute psychomotor agitation and anxiety can similarly be managed with benzodiazepines, while antipsychotics may be administered in cases of severe psychosis. In our experience, co-administration of IV lorazepam and IV haloperidol is often beneficial in these situations, with rapid resolution in agitation.

Sub-acute management of cocaine use may involve a brief course of benzodiazepines (for refractory anxiety and insomnia), as well as dopamine antagonists (for residual psychosis). The former should be used judiciously so as to avoid complications related to benzodiazepine misuse (e.g., dependence, diversion).

Longitudinally, cocaine use disorder is primarily managed through behavioral interventions, such as therapy and peer support groups. Most medications (including antidepressants, e.g., citalopram, dopamine antagonists; most anticonvulsants, e.g., carbamazepine, gabapentin; and certain dopamine agonists) have not shown consistent effectiveness in treating cocaine dependence. Disulfiram, varenicline, and naltrexone have also been used, again with mixed results. Agonist substitution therapy with long-acting oral stimulants (e.g., amphetamine) alone, or in combination with topiramate, has shown some promise; however, considerable risks regarding diversion and cardiac safety often present barriers to treatment.[7] A randomized clinical trial (RCT) of topiramate for the treatment of cocaine addiction showed evidence of greater efficacy than placebo at increasing the mean weekly proportion of cocaine non-use days and associated measures of clinical improvement among cocaine-dependent individuals.[8] Various therapeutic approaches have also been utilized to manage cocaine use disorder, including supportive, cognitive-behavioral, and motivational therapies, as well as peer support groups (such as Cocaine Anonymous), with mixed results. The behavioral intervention with the best evidence-based outcomes for the treatment of cocaine is the Matrix Model. This model provides a framework for engaging patients (as they learn about issues critical to addiction and relapse, receive direction and support from a trained therapist, and become familiar with self-help programs). Patients are also monitored closely for drug use through urine testing. Treatment includes elements of relapse prevention, family and group therapies, drug education, and self-help participation. Detailed treatment manuals contain worksheets for individual sessions; other components include family education groups, early recovery skills groups, relapse prevention groups, combined sessions, urine tests, 12-step programs, relapse analysis, and social support groups. A number of studies have demonstrated that participants treated using the Matrix Model show statistically significant reductions in drug and alcohol use, improvements in psychological indicators, and reduced high-risk behaviors associated with HIV transmission.[9]

Amphetamines and Other CNS Stimulants

Amphetamines include a diverse class of CNS stimulants that have been used since antiquity for medicinal, as well as recreational purposes. The practice of chewing Khat leaves in Ethiopia and Yemen, as well as use of the *Ephedra sinica* plant in ancient China offer some of the earliest examples of amphetamine use. Amphetamine was initially synthesized in 1887, but it was not until the 1930s that these drugs became widely used for treatment of colds and congestion and to promote alertness in battle-fatigued troops during the Second World War. In the 1950s, stimulants re-gained popularity as weight-loss aides, and soon thereafter became widely used as drugs of abuse. Despite increasing efforts to regulate the production and distribution of stimulants, the number of synthetic amphetamine compounds has risen in recent decades, and now includes not only the traditional amphetamines, but also methamphetamine (crystal meth), MDMA (ecstasy), and synthetic cathinones (bath salts).

Ongoing popularity of CNS stimulants as drugs of abuse is reflected in the epidemiologic data. According to data from DAWN, the number of ED visits related to non-medical use of CNS stimulants among adults aged 18 to 34 increased from 5605 in 2005 to 22,949 in 2011. As stimulants can mask the sedating effects of alcohol, the two compounds are commonly used in conjunction, and about 30% of all ED visits related to non-medical CNS stimulant use also involve alcohol.[2] Methamphetamine has been hailed as the fastest rising drug of abuse worldwide, and an estimated 4.7 million Americans are reported to have tried the drug. As the number of various amphetamines is considerable, and no toxicology tests will reliably screen for all compounds, it is essential that consulting physicians be familiar with the pharmacology of these drugs so as to be prepared to recognize the drug-related toxidrome and to provide appropriate management.

Pharmacology and Mechanism of Action

Similar to cocaine, most amphetamines exert their effect through stimulation of CNS alpha- and beta-adrenergic receptors, leading to a toxidrome marked by increased alertness, euphoria (or in severe cases anxiety and agitation), tachycardia, hypertension, and mydriasis. The specific mechanism of action is often drug-dependent, but most CNS stimulants propagate the release of amine neurotransmitters, including dopamine, serotonin and norepinephrine, although some may also act through re-uptake inhibition. The propensity of a specific amphetamine drug for a specific set of neurotransmitters may also differ, and this may in part be reflected by significant variability in clinical findings observed with these compounds. As an example, methamphetamine exerts its effect by increasing dopamine availability in the synaptic cleft through promoting the release of the neurotransmitter, blocking its re-uptake and degradation, and increasing the activity of enzymes necessary in dopamine synthesis.[10]

Acute intoxication on amphetamine compounds closely resembles that of cocaine, and is marked by central and peripheral hyperactivity, including physiologic changes (tachycardia, hypertension, hyperthermia, diaphoresis, and mydriasis) and mental status changes (euphoria, as the intended effect; anxiety, agitation, and violent behavior, as unintended effects). Cardiac problems, including chest pain, cardiac ischemia, and arrhythmias are rarely seen, but when present can lead to serious complications. Signs of CNS hyperexcitability, including seizures, tremors, and myoclonus, may occur with acute intoxication. Electrolyte abnormalities, related to dehydration due to reduced intake and insensible losses through hyperthermia, can lead to significant complications (including cardiac arrhythmias and renal failure). In particular, use of ecstasy (MDMA) has been linked with severe hyponatremia (in the setting of free-water losses) leading to obtundation and potentially fatal cerebral edema.

Psychiatric Sequelae of Amphetamine Use

Acute intoxication with amphetamines may present in a fashion similar to a number of primary psychiatric conditions, including panic attacks, mania (with decreased need for sleep, excitability, distractibility, euphoria, increased sexuality), or severe psychosis. Acute onset of symptoms without a prodrome characteristic for a primary psychiatric disorder, presence of visual and tactile hallucinations, a positive toxicology screen, and a history of drug use may all provide clues towards a secondary etiology of symptoms. Amphetamine-associated psychosis may persist considerably beyond the initial drug use, and may even recur during periods of abstinence from the drug. Physical examination may offer invaluable findings, including evidence of pupillary dilatation, poor dentition ("meth teeth" due to chronic dry mouth) and excoriations consistent with increased itching/skin picking. Furthermore, up to 30% to 40% of all patients who use amphetamines will have a co-morbid primary psychiatric disorder, including primary psychotic disorder (28.6%), primary mood disorder (32.3%), primary anxiety disorder (26.5%), or ADHD (30% to 40%).[11]

Depressive symptoms are commonly seen with discontinuation of the drug, and may be severe enough to meet the diagnostic criteria for major depressive disorder. While amphetamine discontinuation does not lead to a life-threatening withdrawal, it is important to assess the patient for presence of depression and even consider psychiatric hospitalization in severe cases.

Amphetamine use has been associated with deficits in episodic memory, executive functioning, language and motor skills, although the clinical relevance of these findings remains uncertain. Some of the changes are thought to be related to amphetamine-induced CNS toxicity. Animal research data have shown that methamphetamine use increases the permeability of blood–brain barrier (most importantly at the hippocampus), and may play a direct neurotoxic role through excitotoxic mechanisms (e.g., excessive glutamate release) and oxidative stress.[12]

Management

Acute amphetamine intoxication is managed in a manner similar to that of acute cocaine intoxication. IV benzodiazepines are commonly used as a first-line agent for both management of agitation/anxiety, and for centrally mediated hypertension and tachycardia. Alpha-blockers, such as phentolamine, have been preferred for severe hypertension refractory to benzodiazepine treatment, while beta-blockers have been avoided for fear of exacerbating cardiovascular toxicity.

No medications have shown consistent efficacy for long-term management of stimulant use disorder. This noted, both bupropion and mirtazapine have been studied in methamphetamine users, and show some promise, especially in milder cases, or if used in conjunction with therapy. In particular, the data (albeit limited) appear to favor mirtazapine—a 12-week trial of mirtazapine versus placebo in methamphetamine-dependent men-who-have-sex-with-men showed that the mirtazapine-treated group of patients was less likely to submit positive urine drug screens compared with the group receiving placebo.[13] The Matrix Model has shown some promise as a therapeutic approach to long-term behavioral management of patients with stimulant use disorders.

HALLUCINOGENS

Hallucinogens comprise a broad and diverse class of drugs of abuse, the unifying effect of which is their intended mode of action—to produce alteration in thinking, sensation, and reality perception. Widely used across many cultures, this group includes natural (e.g., hallucinogenic mushrooms, Peyote, *Salvia divinorum*) as well as synthetic compounds (e.g., lysergic acid diethylamine [LSD]). While these compounds have traditionally been used to heighten spiritual/religious experiences, most modern hallucinogen use is recreational, with the desired intent to produce perceptual alterations, including hallucinations or illusions, or to enhance emotional states. Commonly, the term "tripping" is used to describe acute intoxication with a hallucinogen, with the term "bad trip" used to describe acute intoxication marked by unintended sequelae (including anxiety, agitation, and paranoia).

LSD, synthesized in 1938 by Albert Hofmann, was the first synthetic hallucinogen and one of the best studied drugs in this class. Initially marketed as an anesthetic and adjunct for psychotherapy, the drug became popular as a psychedelic drug in the 1960s, and was listed as a drug of abuse, by 1966. Over the past two decades, use of LSD has diminished, as more users turn to alternative (and more readily available) compounds, including synthetic cannabinoids, phencyclidine (PCP), ketamine, and naturally occurring hallucinogen compounds.

Hallucinogen use is often sporadic, and relatively uncommon when compared with opioids and stimulants. Approximately 4.2 million individuals in the United States used hallucinogens in 2014, and these drugs account for only 7% of all United States ED visits related to illicit drugs.[2]

Pharmacology and Mechanism of Action

Given the sheer number and diversity of compounds characterized as hallucinogens, a detailed account of specific biochemical properties of each is beyond the scope of this chapter. Nonetheless, most of these compounds exert their effect through modulation of serotonin, dopamine, and glutamate—in particular through binding the 5-HT_{2A} receptors in the neocortical pyramidal cells.[14] Sympathomimetic effects, including pupillary constriction, tachycardia, hypertension, and hyperthermia are seen, though commonly they are not as severe as with stimulants and cocaine. A brief overview of the most-commonly used hallucinogenic compounds is presented below:

- *Lysergic acid diethylamine (LSD):* LSD is commonly used as a pill, or in liquid form (e.g., added to blotter paper). Its intended effect is to produce visual illusions, often characterized by intense colors and distortions, as well as emotional changes marked by euphoria and depersonalization. Time perception may also be distorted, with users often describing experience of reality as if in "slow motion." Most recreational users will maintain awareness that their experiences are drug-induced. Unintended effects are commonly seen with ingestion of higher doses of LSD and may include intense dysphoria, anxiety, or agitation. Panic, overwhelming fear, and even paranoia are classically described, and patients may lack the awareness that their bad trip is drug-induced. This, in turn, may cause impairment in judgment and lead to unintentional injury or even death.
- *Dextromethorphan (DXM):* DXM is easily available in various cough remedies, and is most commonly used in the adolescent population ("robo tripping"). The intended effect is to produce a trance-like dissociative state, though overdoses may also lead to paranoia, hallucinations, and in severe cases, coma. As DMX is commonly sold mixed with other compounds (including anticholinergic compounds and acetaminophen), all cases of suspected DMX intoxication should be monitored for potential additional toxicity related to these compounds.
- *Mescaline:* Mescaline is the active ingredient found in the peyote cactus (*Lophophora williamsii*), a plant native to the south-west United States. It is ingested as a tea prepared from the plant or as dried "buttons." Its effect is similar to that of LSD, though generally milder. While mescaline can be legally used by the members of Native American Church, reflecting its traditional use in religious ceremonies, all other use of the compound is considered illegal.
- *Psilocybin:* This hallucinogen compound is found in a number of mushroom species native to the Pacific Northwest and southern United States, commonly known by their street name of "magic mushrooms" or "shrooms." The mushrooms are commonly dried (to aid with storage/transport) and consumed with food. The intended effect is similar to LSD, though again milder, and may be preceded by significant gastrointestinal symptoms (nausea, vomiting) immediately upon consuming the compound. Accidental ingestion of otherwise toxic mushrooms can occur, as can unintended ingestion of other hallucinogens (e.g., lacing edible mushrooms with LSD).
- *Salvinorin A:* This compound is a kappa opioid agonist found in the leaves of the *Salvia divinorum* plant. It can be freely obtained through the Internet, and is not a federally controlled substance in the United States, further contributing to its rising popularity. Much like other hallucinogens, it can produce sensory distortions, although most users primarily reflect on emotional changes, including elevated mood, euphoria, as well as

introspection. It has a relatively short duration of action (generally 1–2 hours), especially when compared with other hallucinogenic compounds.

- *Phencyclidine (PCP, Angel dust):* PCP is a non-competitive antagonist of N-methyl-D-aspartate (NDMA) receptors, initially developed as an anesthetic agent. The drug can be insufflated, smoked, ingested, or used intravenously. At low doses, PCP produces a sense of detachment from one's surroundings and may lead to dissociation as well as amnesia. At higher doses, PCP intoxication may present with markedly bizarre (and often severely violent) behavior, hallucinations, and even catatonia. Physical examination may elicit nystagmus (vertical and horizontal), as well as signs of sympathomimetic toxicity (including mydriasis). Severe agitation is often a presenting problem for PCP-intoxicated patients, and appropriate measures to ensure the safety of healthcare staff must be considered when dealing with this toxidrome.
- *Ketamine (Special K):* Structurally similar to PCP, ketamine exerts its effect chiefly through NMDA receptor antagonism. Dependent on dosage, ketamine is capable of producing a wide variety of CNS effects, ranging from euphoria and dissociation to agitation, hallucinations, and coma. When used in the hospital setting, ketamine is a safe anesthetic, leading to conscious sedation and anesthesia. As a drug of abuse, ketamine is utilized to alter sensory perceptions, diminish alertness, and cause mild sedation. With overdose, patients may present with obtundation or even coma, while emergence from sedation may be marked by dissociation, confusion, and agitation. Respiratory and cardiovascular support is thus an essential component of acute management of ketamine intoxication. While ketamine overdose can be fatal, most complications have been described in patients co-ingesting drugs (e.g., stimulants or other sedatives). Physical exam may show nystagmus (though less common than with PCP), increased muscle tone, and pupillary dilatation. Chronic ketamine use can cause ketamine-induced ulcerative cystitis, which presents as incontinence, hematuria, and decreased bladder compliance/volume.

Psychiatric Sequelae and Management

Acute intoxication with hallucinogens may present in a fashion similar to mania (euphoria, overwhelming sense of well-being), as well as psychosis (given sensory misperceptions). Prominent visual phenomena, patient's awareness that the symptoms are drug-induced, dissociative experiences, and distorted sense of time may all point towards acute intoxication. The presence of severe vital sign changes is uncommon with these drugs, and if seen should raise concerns for co-ingestion. Containment and safety may be the only interventions warranted with milder cases of intoxication, though IV benzodiazepines co-administered with dopamine antagonists have been used to manage the agitated delirium observed in severe cases.

While hallucinogens are not known to induce primary psychosis, they may unmask latent psychotic illness, as well as lead to brief psychotic episodes (commonly lasting days to a week). Psychiatric containment may be warranted in these cases. Patients may also describe "flashback" experiences similar to those that develop with acute intoxication; it often arises weeks to months after the discontinuation of the drug.

Serotonin syndrome has been described with a number of hallucinogens, including LSD, and may occur in patients who take hallucinogens while also on other serotonergic agents, including SSRIs, MAOIs, or lithium.

CANNABIS AND SYNTHETIC CANNABINOIDS

Cannabis remains the most commonly used drug of abuse worldwide, with an estimated 2.5% of the world population (147 million people) having used the drug in 2014.[15] Cannabis use is particularly high in the adolescent and young adult populations across the United States. While cannabis remains illegal on the federal level, a growing number of states have passed legislation that legalizes possession and medical use of marijuana. Long-term effects of liberalization of marijuana use on the prevalence and severity of cannabis use disorder remain to be seen.

Besides cannabis, there has been a steady increase in the availability and use of synthetic cannabinoids over the last two decades. Commonly sold as "herbal remedies" and "natural products" these compounds go by a variety of street names, the most common of which are "K2" and "Spice." While synthetic cannabinoid intoxication resembles a marijuana "high," these drugs can be incrementally more potent and are often associated with pronounced psychiatric and neurologic pathology. As the number of synthetic cannabinoids available far exceeds the detection ability of most common drug assays, familiarity with this drug class and its effects remains essential.

Pharmacology and Mechanism of Action

Recreationally, cannabis is used in a variety of modes, including most commonly through inhalation and ingestion. The chemical exerts CNS effects primarily through the cannabinoid receptor (CB-1) found in the basal ganglia, substantia nigra, cerebellum, hippocampus, and cerebral cortex. CB-1 activation is associated with inhibition of release of several neurotransmitters including acetylcholine, glutamate, GABA, norepinephrine, and dopamine. Synthetic cannabinoids act on the same receptors as cannabis, but may differ in their potency (up to 800 times greater) and thus their clinical effects, because of differences in binding strength and affinity. Some of the synthetic cannabinoids have been shown to interact with other receptors, including NDMA and serotonin receptors.

Psychiatric Sequelae of Cannabis Use

Recreational cannabis use is seldom associated with medically significant side effects. Most cases of mild intoxication present with CNS depression (e.g., somnolence), while severe cases are often accompanied by unintended behavioral changes, including anxiety, dysphoria, or even agitation. Physical examination is classically notable for dry mouth, conjunctival injection, increased appetite ("munchies"), slurring of speech, and ataxia/nystagmus. Hyperemesis may be observed, often with chronic cannabis use, and may be indicative of cannabis hyperemesis syndrome. Classically, patients will report a pattern of chronic cannabis use, cyclical episodes of nausea/vomiting, and symptom relief with hot showers.

Synthetic cannabinoids may present with more pronounced symptoms compared with cannabis, including delirium, psychosis, severe psychomotor agitation, and (rarely) seizures. These drugs have also been associated with higher rates of cardiovascular and CNS toxicity.

Management

Most cases of marijuana intoxication are mild and generally self-limited. Most patients respond to supportive measures that target reduction of the level of stimulation and reassurance. Severe or persisting cases should raise concerns for exposure to synthetic cannabinoids or alternative psychoactive compounds. As with stimulants, use of short-acting benzodiazepines may reduce symptoms of anxiety that are often seen with the acute toxidrome. Synthetic cannabinoids may present with severe agitation, and thus may require considerably higher doses of benzodiazepines to achieve sedation. Monitoring and prompt management of medical sequelae is essential, including assessment of electrolyte abnormalities (related to insensible fluid losses and rhabdomyolysis), hyperthermia, and monitoring for seizures. In most severe cases, patients will warrant inpatient medical or psychiatric admission for assistance with symptom management.

HEROIN AND OTHER OPIOIDS

Opiates are some of the most important medicinal compounds, widely used for their ability to provide effective analgesia. They also constitute one of the most commonly encountered classes of drugs of abuse. With their use stretching back over millennia (opium was originally extracted from the poppy plant *P. somniferum*), opiates have played a significant role in religion, culture, and medicine. Over the last decade, recreational use of opioids has steadily risen across the United States, as have the associated unintended consequences (including overdoses and fatalities). Between 2004 and 2014, the number of heroin-related fatalities increased by a factor of five (3.3 deaths per 100,000 population), while fatalities involving all opioids increased to nine deaths per 100,000 population. In 2014, 61% of all drug overdose-related fatalities involved some type of opioid compound.[1,2] Natural and semi-synthetic opioids (e.g., oxycodone) account for the majority of all opioid-related unintended overdoses and fatalities, likely reflective of the widespread use of these drugs as pain-killers. Overdoses related to synthetic opioids (e.g., fentanyl) are becoming more prevalent, often as a result of clandestine drug manufacturing. Fueled by relatively low prices and widespread availability, rates of heroin use continue to increase, as do the numbers of overdoses/fatalities attributed to the drug.

Clinicians across all disciplines have considerable responsibility to prevent and reverse the epidemic of opioid-related morbidity and mortality. Judicious prescribing of opioids for pain relief remains an essential step in reducing availability of the drugs. Prompt recognition of the symptoms associated with opioid intoxication and withdrawal, including familiarity with medications used to manage sequelae of both, is an essential skill of acute inpatient management. Lastly, efforts should be made to ensure that all patients receive appropriate longitudinal assistance with their drug use, including maintenance opioid treatment strategies, medication-assisted strategies for abstinence, expanded access to naloxone, and behavioral treatment resources.

Pharmacology and Mechanism of Action

All opioid compounds exert their effect through interaction with one of three opioid receptor classes (mu, kappa, delta). Structurally, all opioid receptors are coupled to G proteins, which in turn activate second-messenger pathways in the target cell, including cAMP and calcium-mediated pathways. Although the opioid receptors are abundant throughout the central and peripheral nervous system, the distribution of specific receptor subtypes, the type of second-messenger pathway, and downstream effect on neurotransmitter release is markedly variable from site to site and accounts for the wide range of clinical effects observed with opiates. Activation of mu receptors in the CNS is associated with euphoria and reward pathway activation (via dopamine increase in the mesolimbic system), anxiolysis (via noradrenergic neurons in locus ceruleus), and analgesia (via inhibition of nociceptive information). Central mu receptor activation is also responsible for respiratory depression and sedation, while the stimulation of peripheral mu receptors results in cough suppression and gastrointestinal dysmotility. Mioisis, a classic sign of opioid intoxication, is mediated through kappa receptor activation.[16]

Management of Opioid Intoxication and Withdrawal

Acute intoxication with opioids presents with a clinical syndrome characterized by CNS depression (sedation), withdrawn to elated mood, and slurred speech. Physical examination is notable for mioisis, decreased bowel sounds, and may create cutaneous findings that confirm IV drug use (e.g., track-marks, fresh injection sites). Patients who inject a drug subcutaneously ("skin popping") may present with multiple soft tissue infections and abscesses at the injection sites. Vital signs are notable for reduced respiratory rate and normal-to-low heart rates. Hypothermia may be seen with severe overdose, as a result of prolonged environmental exposure versus impaired thermogenesis, while hyperthermia may alert to acute infection (e.g., aspiration pneumonia, bacteremia, or endocarditis).

Acute opioid overdose is a medical emergency and close attention should be paid to the patient's alertness and respiratory status. In severe cases, coma and respiratory arrest may ensue, requiring intensive care unit (ICU) level of care. Naloxone, a short-acting opioid antagonist, should be administered in all cases of suspected opioid overdose. It is available in a variety of formulations, including intravenous (IV), intramuscular (IM), and nasal, and it is a generally safe medication that lacks acute toxicity beyond the risk of precipitating acute withdrawal at higher doses. While initial doses of 0.05 mg can be used in patients with spontaneous ventilation, higher doses (0.2–1 mg) should be given to patients who are apneic or who present with cardiopulmonary arrest (2 mg). Naloxone should be administered to secure adequate ventilation rather than intact level of consciousness. With increasing presence of fentanyl as the adulterant in the heroin supply, patients may require multiple doses of naloxone (e.g., up to 8 doses) in the field and the ED. If withdrawal is accidentally precipitated, it should be managed through supportive measures; further opioid administration is not recommended. Once stabilized, the patient should be monitored for re-emergence of opioid toxicity and multiple administrations of naloxone may be required to maintain adequate respiration (due to naloxone's relatively short half-life).

Urine toxicology and urine opioid drug screening are not absolutely necessary for management of acute opioid toxidromes, but are recommended to differentiate various types of opioids ingested, and may alert the clinician to the presence of any co-ingested substances. Initial laboratory testing following acute overdose should also include serum glucose, serum electrolytes, and creatine kinase level (that may signal rhabdomyolysis). An ECG should be considered in cases where methadone overdose is suspected, so as to monitor for QTc prolongation. Chest imaging may be helpful to rule out aspiration. Once stabilized, patients may benefit from infectious disease screening (including HIV, hepatitis, syphilis) and liver function assessment (especially if maintenance treatment is considered).

The classic signs of opioid withdrawal are easily recognized and usually begin 8 to 12 hours after the last dose. The patient generally admits to the need for drugs and shows sweating, yawning, lacrimation, tremor, rhinorrhea, marked irritability, dilated pupils, and an increased respiratory rate. More severe signs of withdrawal (e.g., tachycardia, hypertension, nausea, vomiting, insomnia, abdominal cramps) occur 24 to 36 hours after the last dose. Untreated, the syndrome subsides in 5 to 10 days, and while uncomfortable, it is not life-threatening. Due to its longer half-life, patients withdrawing from methadone may not show symptoms until 24 to 30 hours after the last dose, and once present, the symptoms may persist for 2 to 4 weeks.

As data clearly show improved outcomes with opioid agonist therapy, acute detoxification is generally not recommended. However, in settings in which agonist therapy is not available or is potentially contraindicated, acute detoxification from opioids can be managed with a variety of methods, including supportive care and/or use of replacement therapy to taper the patient off opioids.

- *Supportive care:* Milder cases of opioid withdrawal can be managed by administering medications that counter some of the most challenging withdrawal symptoms. This includes acetaminophen for muscle aches, clonidine for autonomic symptoms, dicyclomine for GI cramps and diarrhea, and lorazepam for insomnia and anxiety. As this approach is generally less comfortable for the patient, it is associated with lower completion rates compared with withdrawal management through the use of opioid replacement therapy. Clonidine can be administered orally or as a transdermal patch, and patients should be monitored for hypotension and sedation.
- *Methadone:* Methadone is available in a variety of formulations (oral, IV, and IM), and its long half-life makes it particularly suitable for management of opioid withdrawal. Specific starting doses may be challenging to determine, and will depend on the patient's pattern of use; most patients note improvement of withdrawal symptoms, with doses between 10 and 30 mg/day. Methadone can be administered as a single daily dose, or divided into three doses. The latter approach is favored in the inpatient setting, as it minimizes the risk of over-sedation and allows for rapid dose titration, if needed. The QTc should be monitored, especially with dose escalation and initiation of treatment. Once the patient reaches a stable dose of methadone that leads to resolution of most withdrawal symptoms, the medication can be tapered by 10% to 25% per day until it has been discontinued. Patients with chronic methadone use may require a more protracted taper due to the long half-life of the drug.
- *Buprenorphine:* Buprenorphine is an efficacious alternative to methadone for short-term inpatient opioid detoxification. Patients are monitored for signs of opioid withdrawal and treated with sublingual doses of buprenorphine 2 to 4 mg. Once acute withdrawal symptoms have been stabilized, buprenorphine can be tapered over the course of 3 to 5 days. Patients typically report that a buprenorphine detoxification is more comfortable than is detoxification with either methadone or clonidine.

Although techniques that permit a safe, rapid, and medically effective detoxification from opiates seem highly attractive in an era of managed care, clinicians must understand that detoxification alone is rarely successful as a treatment for any addiction. Unless the patients are started on appropriate maintenance treatment (either with opioid agonists or naltrexone) and given access to appropriate long-term addiction resources, relapse rates following acute detoxification are extremely high. The resulting costs to the patient, to society, and to the healthcare system far outweigh any savings realized from a rapid and supposedly cost-effective detoxification protocol.

Pharmacotherapy for Maintenance of Opioid Use Disorder

Once sobriety has been achieved and the patient has completed detoxification, long-term abstinence from opiates should be pursued through maintenance pharmacotherapy and/or behavioral interventions. There are considerable data to support the pharmacologic approach to opioid maintenance treatment over non-pharmacologic options, and inpatient medical/surgical hospitalization may present an excellent opportunity to initiate treatment modalities and identify support resources for the patient following discharge.

Opioid Agonist Treatment

Opioid agonist treatment involves the use of either methadone or buprenorphine/naloxone to block the acute effects of other opiates, reduce drug cravings, and minimize behavioral consequences of chronic opioid use disorder. While the patient remains physiologically dependent on an opiate, maintenance therapy with either drug has not been associated with psychosocial problems associated with illicit drug use. Both methadone and buprenorphine/naloxone have been shown to reduce mortality related to opioid use disorder.[17]

Methadone is a long-acting opioid agonist and a Schedule II drug in the United States. As it carries a risk for diversion and abuse, methadone prescriptions are strictly regulated. Only licensed treatment programs can initiate methadone for opioid maintenance. In the general hospital setting, methadone cannot be initiated for these purposes, and the drug is commonly used in three specific situations—acute opioid withdrawal management, acute pain management, and continuing maintenance treatment in patients already on methadone therapy. To be eligible for methadone maintenance, the patient must present with documentation confirming at least 1 year of continuous use of opiates, with exceptions being patients who are pregnant, recently hospitalized, or incarcerated, and patients who have been on methadone maintenance within the past 2 years.

Methadone has been shown to be a safe and effective treatment choice for opioid maintenance treatment. Compared with placebo, methadone maintenance treatment has been associated with reduced rates of opioid-positive drug treatment, longer treatment duration, and greater retention rates. Methadone maintenance has also been associated with a reduced rate of HIV spread and with reduced mortality rates related to opioid use.[18]

Patients about to initiate long-term treatment with methadone should be informed about the risks associated with QTc prolongation, although in most cases, this risk is minimal compared with the risks presented by ongoing opioid use. Patients should also be counseled about the possibility of overdose. As a full opioid agonist, methadone has greater potential for overdose compared with buprenorphine, and these effects may be potentiated in patients still abusing opioids while on methadone maintenance.

Methadone is generally administered as a single daily dose, although split-dosing (e.g., three times a day) can be used in situations when methadone is prescribed for pain in addition to opioid maintenance. Most patients will initiate treatment at 30 mg on their first day, with an additional 10 mg given if the patient exhibits significant withdrawal symptoms 1 hour after the 30 mg dose. The dose is titrated in 5 to 10 mg increments every 3 to 5 days until a therapeutic dose is reached (generally 60 to 80 mg methadone/day). Some patients require doses greater than 100 mg/day, but close attention should be paid to sedation and respiratory compromise.

Buprenorphine is a partial μ-opioid agonist that has been shown to be a viable alternative to methadone in the management of opioid use disorder. When dispensed as a sublingual tablet in combination with naloxone, it has minimal potential for IV misuse and has demonstrated efficacy for maintenance treatment.[19] It has been approved for use in the office-based treatment of opiate dependence and provides an attractive alternative to methadone treatment for higher-functioning patients with moderate to severe opioid use disorders. Buprenorphine is classified as a Schedule III controlled substance, and can be dispensed only by specially trained and certified clinicians. As with methadone, buprenorphine maintenance treatment has been associated with fewer positive urines and greater treatment retention when compared with patients managed with non-pharmacologic measures alone.[20,21] Patients with untreated opioid use disorder started on buprenorphine maintenance during a medical hospitalization show increased drug sobriety and greater post-discharge follow-up with sobriety resources, compared with patients assigned to detoxification alone.[22]

Buprenorphine is relatively safe and appears to have a lower potential for lethal overdose compared with methadone. Most buprenorphine-related fatalities occur in patients who are abusing the drug intravenously, or with co-ingestion of other sedatives (e.g., benzodiazepines, alcohol).

Buprenorphine is typically administered in conjunction with naloxone as a sublingual tablet or strip. As naloxone has poor GI absorption, it is inactive when ingested and will not precipitate withdrawal. If the drug is crushed/dissolved and used intravenously, naloxone becomes active and will precipitate acute withdrawal—this effectively deters patients from abusing buprenorphine-naloxone. As buprenorphine is a partial opioid agonist, it can displace full agonist opioids from the receptor and precipitate withdrawal. When initiating the medication, it is thus essential that patients have been abstinent from other opioids and show symptoms consistent with moderate opioid withdrawal. Most patients in the outpatient setting are started on buprenorphine 4 mg and monitored for resolution of withdrawal symptoms. Additional 2 to 4 mg doses are administered if withdrawal symptoms persist 2 hours after the initial dose. On the following day, the patient is given a single dose consisting of the total doses received on the first day, and an additional 2 to 4 mg may be given for any residual withdrawal symptoms. In the inpatient hospital setting, buprenorphine/naloxone can be initiated faster, with patients receiving upwards of 8 to 12 mg over the first 24 hours in divided doses of 2 to 4 mg every 4 hours. Most patients will stabilize on doses of 8 to 16 mg/day, though some patients may require up to 32 mg/day. As with methadone, buprenorphine/naloxone can be used for analgesia in patients with chronic pain and opioid use. The patients commonly require split (e.g., TID) dosing of the drug, and should receive counseling that use of other opioid compounds for pain relief may precipitate acute withdrawal.

Opioid Antagonist Treatment

Opioid antagonists are used to prevent the user from experiencing opioid intoxication, and thus reinforce abstinence. This form of treatment is particularly effective in patients who are highly motivated or in patients who cannot be on opioid agonist treatment for personal/professional reasons. Naltrexone has been used as oral daily treatment (typically at doses of 50 mg/day), or as a long-acting injectable administered every 4 weeks (set dose of 380 mg per injection). The latter formulation appears to be overall more effective in treating opioid use disorder, as it requires less motivation from the patient. In comparison with placebo, long-acting IM naltrexone has been shown to reinforce abstinence and increase patient retention. It has also been shown to be effective in reinforcing abstinence in patients using more than one drug.

BENZODIAZEPINES AND OTHER SEDATIVE HYPNOTICS

Benzodiazepines

Benzodiazepines are a class of sedative–hypnotic agents with a wide variety of therapeutic roles, including management of anxiety disorders, seizures, insomnia, and GABA-mediated withdrawal states. Discovered accidentally in 1954 by Leo Sternbach, chlordiazepoxide (Librium) was the first benzodiazepine to be synthesized, followed by diazepam (Valium) in 1963, and some 50 other benzodiazepine compounds since. Nowadays, benzodiazepines are one of the staples of modern medicine and psychiatry—a versatile drug class commonly used in inpatient and outpatient settings, and readily prescribed by specialists (e.g., psychiatrists) as well as primary care physicians. While immensely useful in the appropriate clinical setting, benzodiazepines have a potential for abuse and dependence, and a withdrawal state produced by discontinuation of the drug may be life-threatening.

Pharmacology and Mechanism of Action

All benzodiazepines exert their effect via modulation of the gamma-aminobutyric $acid_A$ ($GABA_A$) receptor. Unlike many other drugs discussed in this chapter, benzodiazepines do not change the expression or synaptic availability of GABA, but act to increase the binding of the neurotransmitter to the $GABA_A$ receptor by modulating the receptor structure. The resulting effect is that of hyper-polarization of the target neuron and decreased ability to initiate an action potential. While different benzodiazepines generally share a similar molecular structure, the presence of various side-chains will account for the considerable variability observed in the metabolism pharmacodynamics and pharmacokinetics within the drug class.

It is clinically useful to categorize benzodiazepines based on their kinetics (e.g., onset of action, half-life), as well as the primary site of metabolism. These characteristics often determine how a particular drug is used clinically, and may also play an important role in its abuse potential. A detailed account of pharmacokinetics of common benzodiazepines is beyond the scope of this chapter. However, some of the key points are outlined below:

- *Onset of action:* Benzodiazepines with relatively quick onset of action (e.g., midazolam) have an important role in procedural sedation and management of acute anxiety states (e.g., clonazepam, alprazolam). Clinical experience suggests that the benzodiazepines with a faster onset of action (e.g., alprazolam, clonazepam) appear to be more likely sought after by patients abusing benzodiazepines as they produce an acute "high" sensation, unlike drugs with a slower onset of action (e.g., oxazepam).[23]
- *Half-life:* Benzodiazepines can be divided into three groups based on their half-life. Benzodiazepines with a short half-life (<12 hours) include oxazepam and midazolam. Generally, these drugs have few active metabolites, and are metabolized in a manner unaffected by liver disease. Midazolam is used as an anesthetic, given its rapid onset of action and quick clearance, while oxazepam is used for withdrawal management in patients with known hepatic disease. Intermediate-acting benzodiazepines include lorazepam and temazepam (half-life between 12 and 24 hours). Long-acting benzodiazepines (half-life >24 hours) include most other benzodiazepine compounds, including diazepam and chlordiazepoxide. Most of these drugs demonstrate significant hepatic metabolism, may have active metabolites, and tend to accumulate in tissues. Their long half-life makes these drugs a preferred choice for management of withdrawal states.[23]
- *Metabolism:* Most benzodiazepines are metabolized through the P450 system, namely the CYP3A4 and CYP2C19 enzymes. Drugs that inhibit the CYP3A4 enzyme (e.g., grapefruit juice, macrolide antibiotics, HIV protease inhibitors) may reduce benzodiazepine metabolism, and thus potentiate drug effect and potential toxicity. The inducers of CYP3A4 (e.g., phenobarbital, phenytoin, carbamazepine) will increase benzodiazepine metabolism and clearance. Lower benzodiazepine doses should be used in patients with known hepatic dysfunction. Lorazepam, oxazepam, and temazepam (easily remembered by the brief mnemonic "LOT") avoid first pass hepatic metabolism. These drugs are less susceptible to CYP interactions, and are considered to be safer in patients with known hepatic disease.[23]

Psychiatric Sequelae of Benzodiazepine Use

The intended effect of benzodiazepine use is to provide a reduction in anxiety, facilitate sleep, or induce sedation. When taken in excess, benzodiazepines may lead to overdose characterized by CNS depression similar to that seen with severe alcohol intoxication. Patients classically present with slurred speech, ataxia, confusion (which may lead to belligerence or agitation), and somnolence. Respiratory depression is uncommon with isolated benzodiazepine overdose, although the risk is increased with co-ingestion of other sedatives, including alcohol, and opioids. Severe intoxication may lead to stupor or coma and patients may require intubation for respiratory support. Commonly, patients will have benign vital signs, despite considerable sedation, which may help rule out other life-threatening causes of CNS depression. Toxicology screening will help differentiate between benzodiazepines and other sedatives, including alcohol, and may help identify potential co-ingestion.

Flumazenil, a specific benzodiazepine antagonist, reverses the life-threatening effects of a benzodiazepine overdose. An initial IV dose of 0.2 mg can be given over 30 seconds, followed by a second 0.2 mg IV dose if there is no response after 45 seconds. This procedure can be repeated at 1-minute intervals up to a cumulative dose of 5 mg. Although readily available, flumazenil is rarely used in clinical practice, as it may precipitate seizures in patients dependent on benzodiazepines, or in those taking tricyclic antidepressants. Most cases of benzodiazepine intoxication are thus managed through supportive care.

Benzodiazepine Withdrawal Management

Benzodiazepines can produce a state of physiologic dependence, especially when used in high doses for prolonged periods. Up to 45% of patients who receive stable, long-term doses show physiologic evidence of withdrawal with abrupt drug discontinuation. Withdrawal symptoms resemble those seen with alcohol and other sedative–hypnotics and include a state marked by subjective anxiety, irritability, and insomnia. Patients may show vital sign changes consistent with increased autonomic arousal (tachycardia, hypertension) and commonly present with a tremor ("shakes"). In severe cases, patients may develop delirium tremens or have one or more seizures—as both conditions are potentially life-threatening, prompt recognition and treatment of benzodiazepine withdrawal is a clinical priority.

The simplest approach to benzodiazepine detoxification in the outpatient setting is a gradual reduction in dose that may be extended over several weeks or months. This treatment approach is commonly reserved to highly motivated patients and patients without significant concern for misuse or diversion of the medication. When a more rapid inpatient detoxification is required, the use of phenobarbital, a longer-acting benzodiazepine, or controlled daily dosage reductions of the benzodiazepine at 15% to 25% daily may be considered. When phenobarbital is utilized, a target serum level of 15–30 μg/mL is utilized, with a controlled taper over the course, of at least 7 days.

An alternative approach may involve discontinuing the offending benzodiazepine altogether and starting the patient on a taper of a high-potency, longer-acting benzodiazepine (e.g., clonazepam or diazepam). This strategy is particularly useful for withdrawal from high-potency, intermediate-acting benzodiazepines (e.g., lorazepam). A clonazepam taper may mitigate acute withdrawal symptoms and also adequately manage the anxiety that most patients experience with rapid lorazepam discontinuation. Due to observed decreased sensitivity to other benzodiazepines, for alprazolam detoxification, we recommend either the use of a daily controlled taper of alprazolam at no more than 15% daily or detoxification with use of phenobarbital, as noted above.

Supplemental medication, such as the use of β-adrenergic blockers (propranolol), α-adrenergic agonists (clonidine), and dopamine antagonists, may offer some relief of subjective complaints, including anxiety and general malaise. These agents should never be utilized as monotherapy for the detoxification of patients from benzodiazepines.

SEDATIVE–HYPNOTICS

Use of CNS depressants accounts for a considerable portion of all ED visits related to suicide attempts and accidental overdoses (consequent to recreational use and self-medication). Although benzodiazepines are by far the most commonly abused sedative–hypnotic drug class in the United States, there are still areas where the non-medical use of barbiturates, such as butalbital (Fiorinal and Esgic) and carisoprodol (Soma), causes serious clinical problems.

Pharmacology and Mechanism of Action

A person intoxicated on a barbiturate typically presents with a clinical picture nearly identical to that seen with alcohol intoxication. Slurred speech, unsteady gait, and sustained vertical and/or horizontal nystagmus are commonly seen on the examination. Vital sign abnormalities may not be as pronounced as with alcohol intoxication, and patients may lack the odor of ethanol on their breath. Toxicology screening is essential to rule out co-ingestion, and also to differentiate benzodiazepine intoxication.

The behavioral effects of barbiturate intoxication can vary widely, even in the same person. With mild intoxication, patients may appear somnolent or display disinhibition (including excitement and loud behavior). More severe intoxication can present as aggressive behavior, or may lead to encephalopathy and coma. Bradycardia may be observed, but as with benzodiazepines, vital signs are generally unaffected in most patients. No specific antidotes are used for barbiturate poisoning, and most patients are managed supportively with a focus on airway management and prevention of secondary complications related to over-sedation (e.g., aspiration events).

Withdrawal Management

Sedative–hypnotic withdrawal syndromes resemble those seen with alcohol and benzodiazepines, and can present with a wide variety of symptoms already described in this chapter (e.g., anxiety, insomnia, hyperreflexia, diaphoresis, nausea, vomiting, and sometimes delirium and convulsions). Minor withdrawal symptoms begin 24 to 36 hours after the last dose—tachycardia, and in some cases tachypnea and fevers may also be seen. With more severe use, seizures and delirium tremens may occur. Grand mal seizures, if they occur, are seen between the 3rd and 7th days, although some cases occur as late as 14 days into a medically controlled detoxification.

Several techniques are available for managing barbiturate withdrawal. Patients may be gradually tapered off their drug of choice by a controlled taper of said agent. Alternatively, patients may be transitioned to a long-acting agent (e.g., phenobarbital) that can be given as needed based on the presence of withdrawal symptoms. As with other substances discussed in this chapter, following acute detoxification, most patients will benefit from referral to further addiction services, including formalized outpatient addiction treatment and peer support groups.

REFERENCES

Access the reference list online at https://expertconsult.inkling.com/.

Psychosomatic Conditions: Somatic Symptom and Related Disorders, Functional Somatic Syndromes, and Deception Syndromes

16

Nicholas Kontos, M.D.
Scott R. Beach, M.D., F.A.P.M.
Felicia Smith, M.D.
Donna B. Greenberg, M.D.

OVERVIEW

The 2003 approval by the American Board of Medical Specialties of "Psychosomatic Medicine" as a certified subspecialty of psychiatry evokes the obvious question of what this name means. Despite high-minded ideas about its referring to clinical and scientific attention to holistic approaches to health and disease, or to a bridge between psychiatry and the rest of medicine, for most medical professionals and many members of the lay public the term, "psychosomatic," brings to mind amplified, unfounded, or outright feigned medical concerns. Thus, our subspecialty's name, accurately or not, and for better or worse, implies foremost a focus on these sorts of patients and problems.

Psychosomatic is a blunt term and only one of many applied to somatic medical concerns that do not present "as advertised." Medically unexplained symptoms, symptoms of unknown origin, and somatoform disorders are just a few of the more professional (i.e., written) names applied to these problems. Crocks, invalids, and fakes are some of the less seemly (i.e., spoken) ones. This chapter will focus on three categories of "psychosomatic" presentations: the somatic symptom and related disorders; functional somatic syndromes; and deception syndromes. Borrowing and extending from Barsky,[1] *symptom amplification* will be used as an umbrella term for all three domains.

Before delving into the psychiatrically relevant ways in which somatic symptoms can present, it is worth noting that 60–80% of the American population experiences a somatic symptom in any given week.[2] Many of these people do not bring their complaints to the medical system, raising the issue that stoicism might represent the opposite end of a continuum from symptom amplification; one that might actually kill more people but which is not considered pathologic because the inconveniences of stoicism are not imposed on people who create diagnostic nomenclatures. That issue aside, sufferers who do present to doctors represent more than half of all ambulatory visits.[3] Only a small minority of them are found to have a clear "organic" etiology to their complaints.[4] Among the remaining majority, only a fraction prove to be diagnostically significant symptom amplifiers.[5] However, given the massive starting number, this fraction, accounting for 10% to 24% of outpatient visits, may represent the most frequent form of psychopathology seen by primary care providers.[6–8] Whether this large group is better accounted for by primary symptom amplification versus mood and anxiety disorders[9,10] or personality pathology[11,12] is a matter of debate.

The preceding epidemiology uses DSM-IV categories. Since the last edition of the MGH *Handbook of General Hospital Psychiatry*, the most significant update in the area of symptom amplification has been its diagnostic reconfiguration in DSM-5.[13] These changes were taken up for two main reasons. First, because the existing diagnoses contained redundancy and the prototypical disorder of the old category (somatization disorder) did not capture many of the patients of concern. Second, these being patients most often seen by non-psychiatrists, it was noted that these physicians did not use the existing DSM diagnoses.[14] There is hope (founded or not remains to be seen) that the new categorization will be both more useful and palatable to all doctors. In addition, there is some debate whether palatability to patients is a valid consideration here,[15,16] as clinical usefulness is balanced against the attempt to derive a scientifically derived classification system.

CASE 1

Ms. S, a 25-year-old woman, had a 5-year history of worsening lower back pain that initially occurred only when sitting at a work station for prolonged periods; it abruptly worsened 3 years ago after a seemingly minor fender bender. An MRI shortly afterwards revealed a herniated disc at L3–4. Ms. S has not worked since the accident. She moved back in with her parents shortly afterwards, and remains in litigation related to the accident, which she sees as being unfairly drawn out by the other driver's insurance company, especially given her financial situation. Attempts to treat her pain have been reported as ineffective, though she remains on chronic opioid therapy, as well as gabapentin and ibuprofen. She has consistently declined physical therapy referrals and recommendations of exercise, stating that she is too fatigued and in too much pain to tolerate either. Resistant to any inquiry about depressive symptoms, she at one point grudgingly accepted a trial of sertraline and reported severe nausea and diarrhea after two 25 mg doses. Further, the gastrointestinal symptoms did not resolve after she stopped the sertraline. Over the subsequent year, she was evaluated by two different gastroenterologists, the second of whom diagnosed her with irritable bowel syndrome. Despite reporting chronic diarrhea and an inability to keep food down, she had gained approximately 10 pounds a year since the automobile accident, perhaps relating to a life now dominated by allopathic and homeopathic medical visits, and devoid of any recreational activities of note, other than watching television from a chair bolstered by several memory foam back supports.

SOMATIC SYMPTOM AND RELATED DISORDERS

In the DSM-5, the term, "somatization," is no longer used diagnostically. This change represents almost a full circle change from the days of DSM-I and -II,[17,18] where "somatization" was similarly avoided. In those days, the meaning of somatization had expanded far beyond its original use by the psychoanalyst Wilhelm Stekel to indicate the defensive mechanism underlying conversion hysteria. Any expression of emotional or unconscious states was casually referred to as somatization. The early DSMs thus avoided the word somatization in favor of precision in etiologically distinguishing between "psychophysiologic disorders" (associated with the physiologic expressions of emotion) and "psychoneurotic reactions" (where loss of function was key and carried symbolic meaning).[19]

In today's purportedly "atheoretical" era of DSM, "somatization" finds itself discarded again; this time, not only because of its insinuations of psychodynamic causal factors, but also its connotation of absence of "real" somatic causes. The latter is a critical point in terms of understanding most of the disorders about to be described (including the functional somatic syndromes). A growing literature demonstrates that what is central in these disorders is not cryptogenesis of somatic symptoms. After all, many general medical problems (not to mention nearly all psychiatric ones) are poorly understood from an "organic" perspective. Instead, the crux of dysfunction here lies in *amplification* of the experience, import, or functional limitations caused by somatic symptoms.[20]

The remainder of this section is mainly descriptive, with passing mention of etiologic theories, which remain largely speculative and/or in scientific infancy. Treatment is discussed separately.

Somatic Symptom Disorder

Somatic symptom disorder (SSD) is the prototype diagnosis of the category bearing its name. In contrast to the smorgasbord approach that required a somewhat arbitrary and arcane multidomain symptom array in its predecessor, somatization disorder, SSD requires only that "one or more" symptoms form the focus of the patient's attention. Thus, in a rare display of "lumping" diagnoses, this change in DSM-5 obviates the need for the previous edition's pain and undifferentiated somatoform disorders. For a full "crosswalk" between DSM-IV Somatoform Disorders and DSM-5 Somatic Symptom and Related Disorders, see Figure 16-1.

The patient with SSD is characterized by preoccupation, anxiety, and "time and energy devoted" to their symptom(s) that are disproportionate to their severity, as determined by providers. This determination can be a very difficult task of cross-matching objective findings, clinical experience, and patient reports, as in the case of back pain and spinal imaging.[21] Still and unavoidably, the crux of this disorder is nonetheless "abnormal illness behavior"[22,23] or a mismanagement of the "sick role"[24] by the patient. While these characteristics are found to varying degrees in all of the SSD and related disorders, they are the crux of SSD. A major component of Parsons' sociologic conceptualization of the sick role is that the sick person justly acquires a degree of blamelessness for their symptoms, relief from duties incompatible with their malady, and an entitlement to care; these are balanced by an obligation to pursue health along with the help of one's providers. When one considers the plight of the guilt-ridden, overburdened, and unloved person, sickness can be "one-stop-shopping" from a primary gain point of view. From that same sociologic view, the pathology of SSD can be seen as a desperate clinging to the benefits of the sick role without fulfillment of the duty, that, along with sickness, purchases those benefits. This imbalance may be the cause of the variable consternation, and desperate indulgence that many providers and family members exhibit toward the SSD patient.[25–27]

Etiologic theories in SSD seem to exist in proportion to "schools" of psychiatry and cannot be given full justice here. Psychodynamic theories, originating in conversion hysteria as noted above, tend to hinge on defense mechanisms that "convert" unbearable or unacceptable feelings and impulses into bodily sensations. Originally coined by Nemiah,[28] alexithymia comes in and out of fashion as an explanation for why patients who are unable to recognize and describe their own emotions might instead experience them somatically. A cognitive model applied to somatization and hypochondriasis is presumed to still be applicable. Here, the symptom-amplifying patient is one who, already having a low threshold of detection for bodily sensations and variations, applies medical significance to those sensations, and behaves accordingly. This behavior often includes

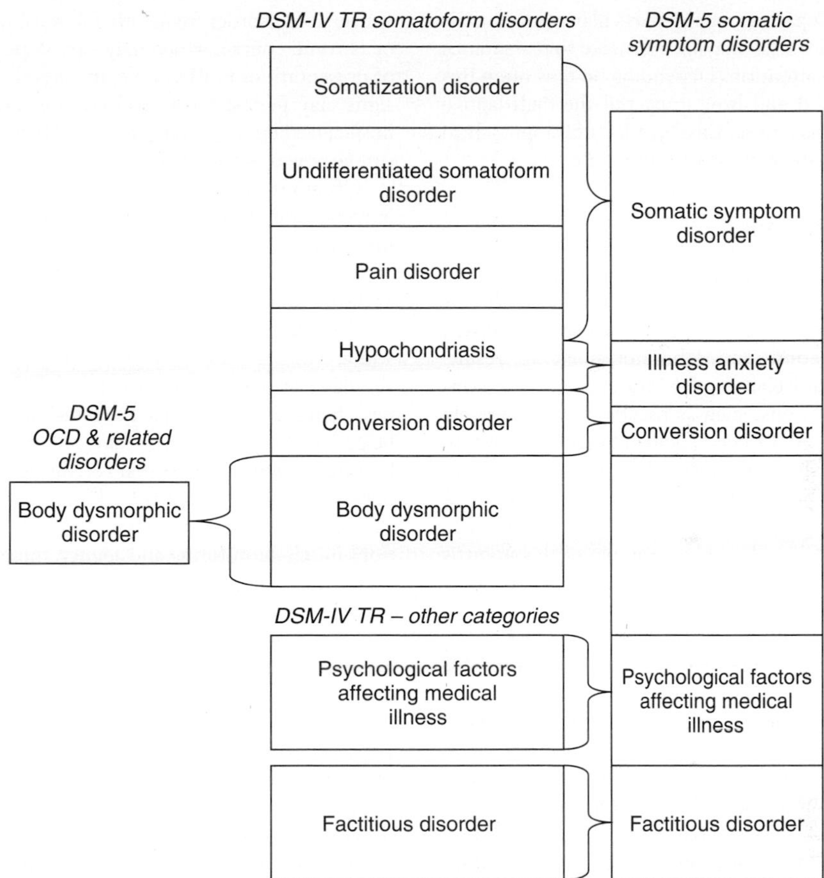

Figure 16-1. Transition of DSM-IV "Somatoform and Related Disorders" into DSM-V Classification.

limiting activities and seeming to relentlessly seek medical validation (and, usually unsuccessfully, functionally meaningful relief) of their suffering.[1] This mechanism is borne out by studies of the cognitive biases about health found in symptom-amplifying patients,[29] and overlaps with biological theories as represented in studies of the phenomenon of central sensitization.[30]

Epidemiology of SSD is yet to be determined. Extrapolating from prior conditions, SSD would be expected to be overrepresented among women, those with low education, low socioeconomic status, and a high rating in the personality trait of neuroticism. SSD must be present for 6 months to be diagnosed and is generally considered to be a chronic condition.

Illness Anxiety Disorder

Whereas the patient with SSD is preoccupied with symptoms, the patient with illness anxiety disorder (IAD) is preoccupied with the idea of having or contracting a major illness. He or she may not even have any active symptoms at a given point in time, and instead beset providers with requests for unwarranted screening tests such as "full body scans," or serially and progressively make restrictive lifestyle alterations based on the 11 o'clock news' "fear segments" or fringe health media. Alternatively, and as opposed to the above portrayal of stoicism, a person with IAD may avoid the healthcare system altogether, afraid of finding out something he does not wish to know. Thus, DSM-5 divides IAD into "care-seeking" and "care-avoidant" types.[13]

In the formative days of DSM-5, there was some debate as to whether IAD was better sorted among the anxiety or somatic symptom disorders, with arguments in favor of the latter coming out on top. It is felt to map best onto the DSM-IV diagnosis of hypochondriasis, though the DSM-5 committee predicts that it will capture only about 25% of these patients, leaving the rest to SSD.[13] Again, the presence or absence of somatic disease is immaterial to this diagnosis; the crux being the disproportionate nature of the patient's anxiety.

Extrapolating from studies of hypochondriasis, patients with IAD hold to a "restrictive concept of good health,"[31] as evidenced by their responses on scales such as the Health Norms Sorting Task, which asks if a person could be considered "healthy" while experiencing a variety of different somatic sensations.[32] A cognitive-behavioral model, much like that described above, minus the heightened symptom detection, is thought to hold sway over these patients and informs some promising psychotherapeutic approaches that may be adaptable to other SSDs.[33,34] As with any illness beliefs and behaviors, the patient's cultural and familial upbringing will have had a major influence, and (as with all SSDs) it is worth asking about family illness experiences/models, particularly in childhood.

Unlike the SSD patient, at any particular point in their illness, a patient with IAD may be amenable to reassurance and dutiful clinical attention. Depending on how often this attention is required and how impactful the maladaptive health beliefs are over time, this "patchwork" approach to the patient's problems may be of limited use.

Conversion Disorder

In a sense, psychiatry's original somatic symptom disorder, conversion disorder involves a loss or change in sensory or motor function that is suggestive of a neurological disorder, but lacks examination and laboratory/imaging results compatible with said change. DSM-5 accounts for non-neurologic presentations, such as pseudocyesis, separately under the heading of "Other Specified Somatic Symptom and Related Disorder." As with other somatic symptom disorders, incompatibility between signs and exam, laboratory, or radiologic findings does not necessarily mean complete absence of abnormality. The best example of this point is the oft-reported (though sometimes overblown) overrepresentation of conversion seizures (note: the standard term, "psychogenic nonepileptic seizures" [PNES], implies an unsubstantiated etiology) among patients with electrographic evidence of separate epileptic seizures.[35]

The possibility of psychiatric–neurologic co-existence can become a point of contention between psychiatrists and neurologists unless both are aware of it, and each has some basic knowledge of the others' work. On the subject of psychiatrists' attitudes towards conversion disorder work-ups, two other issues worth noting are that: (1) the idea that up to 30% of conversion disorders are later found to have neurologic disease has been debunked and the rate of false-positives for this diagnosis (about 5%) appears to be no higher than for other neurologic disorders;[36] (2) the idea of conversion disorder being a "diagnosis of exclusion" does not mean that psychiatrists should only be consulted at the end of a patient's work-up. For example, it has been convincingly argued[37] that psychiatric consultation should occur on the day of admission to an epilepsy monitoring unit (where rates of PNES are generally found to be 20% to 30%[38]), so as to normalize the possibility of conversion disorder early on.

DSM-5, in an effort to reduce the perceived underdiagnosis of conversion disorder, removed proof of unintentional sign production from the diagnostic criteria. The subsequent text addressing conversion disorder nonetheless clearly indicates that unintentional production is assumed, and that if feigning is suspected strongly enough, the differential shifts to factitious disorder or the non-disorder, malingering. Another important change in the DSM-5 criteria is the elimination of the need to identify a proximate psychological stressor presumably triggering conversion disorder. The previous requirement of this usually highly presumptive piece of detective work was not only an impediment to diagnosis, but also made an unsubstantiated psychodynamic etiologic assumption about all cases of conversion disorder.

The proximate-stressor requirement also runs counter to the longitudinal course of conversion disorder. More often than not, conversion disorder does *not* follow a stressor–conversion–relaxation–resolution pattern. Instead, conversion disorder frequently follows a relapsing–remitting or chronic course, which may vary depending on the type of presentation. For example, unilateral sensory and motor signs may persist for several years in the vast majority of hospitalized neurological patients. PNES frequency/presence similarly waxes and wanes in many patients.

Often referred to as "functional" deficits, the signs seen in conversion disorder ought to be looked at less as misleading than as misunderstood. The original historic meaning of "functional" in medicine, meant hidden or physiologic, as distinguished from visible, anatomic disease.[39] The physiologic underpinnings of conversion disorder remain "hidden," and are difficult to study given their protean nature (e.g., should conversion disorder patients with conversion blindness, hemiparesis, and "psychogenic" non-epileptic seizures be grouped together in the same study?). Still, an emerging literature suggests abnormal recruitment and connectivity between brain areas involved in arousal, planning, and execution of movements. Hypothesized to represent disruptions in self-monitoring and agency, these findings may also reflect the pathophysiologic underpinnings of the association between conversion disorder and trauma.[40]

Conversion disorder is seen more often in women. Age of onset is variable across most of the life span and across different manifestations of the illness. PNES may peak in the third decade and motor signs may peak in the fourth.[41] Treatment of conversion disorder is understudied. Suggestion of recovery is often employed, with hospitalized patients in particular often offered the prediction of a non-abrupt, progressive pattern of functional recovery. This technique likely has its heritage in psychoanalytically informed ideas about conversion "hysteria" and the theory/hope that a patient pathologically subject to suggestion will also be open to its therapeutic application. It is important that the psychiatric consultant emphasize the importance of physical therapy to patient and consultee alike, disconnecting this intervention from etiology and connecting it instead to deficit and recovery. Psychodynamic therapies are often recommended, and consultees often seem to assume this is a proven, effective, and standard treatment. Cognitive-behavioral therapies, including paradoxical approaches in which patients are coached through the precise, conscious simulation of their conversion signs, are under investigation.[42]

Psychological Factors Affecting Medical Illness

This diagnosis refers to abnormal illness behaviors that are adversely affecting the course or treatment of a conventionally defined and diagnosed medical condition. Psychological factors affecting medical illness exist on a range of severity from "mild" (i.e., increasing risk) to "extreme" (i.e., causing life-threatening risk), and encompassing just about any psychological state or personality trait (aside from those associated with a distinct psychiatric co-morbidity). It could be said that just about all of us have this condition, since just about none of us refrain from all behaviors detrimental to health, and that hypothetical person who unerringly behaves in a health-directed manner probably has illness anxiety disorder anyway. Perhaps conspicuously, this "diagnosis" does not end in the word "disorder."

Factitious Disorders

Factitious disorders are discussed later in this chapter, in the section on "Deception Syndromes." It is simply noted here that in previous iterations of the DSM, factitious disorders occupied a category of its own, "Factitious Disorders." Under this heading could be found factitious disorders with physical symptoms or psychological symptoms, and factitious disorder by proxy. Despite the preservation of its possible expression through psychological symptoms (e.g., lying about or simulating psychosis, reporting false suicidal ideation, or reporting non-lethally intended self-injury as a suicide attempt for "primary gain"), this diagnosis has been moved to the "Somatic Symptom and Related Disorders" category.

PSYCHIATRIC DIFFERENTIAL DIAGNOSIS

Depressive Disorders

The first consideration in patients with physical symptoms that seem out of proportion to objective findings is whether the patient is depressed. Major depressive disorder has a somatic dimension, and everything hurts more in the setting of depression.

Indeed, 75% of primary care patients with MDD or panic disorder seek treatment from their physicians for exclusively somatic symptoms.[6,43] The vegetative symptoms of MDD include insomnia, fatigue, anorexia, and weight loss; and depressed patients report more functional somatic symptoms (aches and pains, constipation, dizziness, etc.) than do other patients. Among primary care patients,[8] disabling chronic pain was present in 41% of those with MDD compared with 10% of those without MDD. Those patients with both chronic pain and MDD tended to have more severe affective symptoms and a higher prevalence of panic disorder. Even across cultures, the majority of patients with MDD spontaneously report only somatic symptoms; when pressed, however, 89% will also offer psychological symptoms.[44]

When MDD is diagnosed in the context of unexplained bodily complaints, depression should be treated promptly. Both affective and somatic symptoms may abate with systematic antidepressant treatment. Of course, MDD (as well as generalized anxiety disorder) is also a major comorbidity of somatic symptom disorders, seemingly present in a majority of these patients.[10] So, one must also be on guard against the false hope that, "if I just treat the depression, the 'somatizing' will disappear." Further, MDD itself can be difficult to diagnose in patients prone to amplified experiences and reporting of somatic symptoms. There is reason to believe they may also be prone to amplify certain psychological "symptoms" as well.[45] (For further coverage of affective disorders, see Chapter 9.)

Anxiety Disorders

Anxiety frequently co-occurs with functional somatic symptoms, distorting the cognitive appraisal of somatic symptoms and making even benign bodily sensations seem ominous and alarming. Anxious patients tend to catastrophize normal physiologic sensations and ailments. As noted in Chapter 13, many of the symptoms of panic disorder are somatic; they include dyspnea, palpitations, chest pain, choking, dizziness, paresthesias, hot and cold flashes, sweating, faintness, and trembling. As a result, patients in the midst of a panic attack may feel that they are unable to breathe or that they are dying. Patients with panic disorder may focus on the most prominent symptom and find the appropriate subspecialist; therefore, patients with medically unexplained symptoms and panic disorder present with chest pain in cardiology, nausea or diarrhea in gastroenterology, and dizziness in neurology.[46] Anxiety is also one of the most common features of MDD.[47]

When co-morbid with pain, anxiety can lower the pain threshold dramatically. In fact, some patients cannot distinguish anxiety from pain ("No, I am not frightened; I hurt!"). Pleas for pain relief may be related to anxiety rather than addiction or the neediness associated with personality disorder.

Substance Use Disorders

Physicians should always consider the diagnosis of alcohol abuse in a patient with multiple, vague somatic symptoms. Whether the patient consciously conceals alcohol dependency or fails to make the connection, the diagnosis may be elusive. Information from the patient's family may help ("What he calls headache and chest pains, Doctor, I call a hangover."). Because alcohol abuse systematically disrupts sleep, patients may begin using sedative–hypnotic substances as well. Insomnia, morning cough, pains in the extremities, dysesthesias, palpitations, headache, gastrointestinal (GI) symptoms, fatigue, bruises—none are strangers to the alcoholic. The effects of other addictive drugs may be similarly confounding. (See Chapters 14 and 15, for the diagnosis and treatment of substance abuse disorders.)

Psychotic Disorders

Sometimes a somatic complaint has the rigid, stereotyped character of a delusion and presents in a patient with a psychotic disorder. Here the key is to consider a psychotic disorder as a possibility from the perspective of a fuller mental status exam and a fuller past history. Patients with psychotic depression may have particularly negatively flavored somatic delusions (such as the conviction that one's abdominal organs are decomposing).

Delusional disorder of the somatic type presents a particular diagnostic challenge since the delusions of delusional disorder are, by definition, non-bizarre, at least insofar as they follow the laws of biology and physics. Patients with delusional disorder of the somatic type tend to be more circumscribed about the nature of their medical complaint in terms of its content, even as its consequences increasingly consume their lives. A (to some) controversial, yet prototypical example of this kind of somatic delusion is Morgellons disease which involves specific convictions about dermal infestation. Formerly known as Ekbom's syndrome,[48] Morgellons disease, as with other specific delusions and fringe beliefs, is increasingly difficult to pin down because of the spread of ideas and cohesion of sufferers through on-line resources.[49]

In contrast to delusional disorder, the somatic delusions of schizophrenia are generally so bizarre and idiosyncratic (e.g., that foreign bodies are inside an organ or orifice, that body parts are missing or deformed, or that a more mundane somatic issue is being caused by other parties at a distance) as to be easily recognized. But when a patient with schizophrenia complains of a symptom that is not bizarre (e.g., a headache or weakness), the rigid delusional dimension of psychosis may be missed. Making such a diagnosis with a thorough psychiatric history and examination is ordinarily no problem. Patients with schizophrenia can also have conversion symptoms (e.g., hemiparesis).

Nonetheless, physical symptoms in a patient with psychotic disorder must be taken seriously. The premature mortality in this seriously mentally ill population is significant. What component of this is due to symptoms being dismissed by providers distracted or biased by a psychotic disorder diagnosis is not entirely clear, but the fact that a schizophrenia diagnosis means a life foreshortened by an average of 15 years, is![50] It may be more common not to hear out a patient with schizophrenia and to miss a straightforward medical complaint.

Organic Mental Disorders

Somatizing cannot be localized to either a specific brain structure or a particular neurotransmitter system; however, patients with dementia or other organic brain disease can have functional somatic complaints, and the recognition of cognitive impairment may be the key to better care.

Personality Disorders

Although included in the differential diagnostic list of Table 16-1, personality disorders do not "cause" functional somatic symptoms. Rather, for the patient with these disturbances, the somatic symptom is a means to an end. For the individual with an antisocial personality, pain may be a means to get narcotics, to get out of work, or to escape trial. For the person with a dependent personality, functional weakness gains the attention and nurturance of others.[51] The borderline patient's somatic symptoms can become the focus for physicians and nurses, who may engage in a sadomasochistic struggle with the patient. The process begins with a helping relationship and ends with the rejection of a disappointed and outraged patient accused of wrongdoing. The "end" for this patient is the emotionally charged (usually hostile) relationship, and the failure to palliate the symptoms means to the patient that the physician simply does not care enough. Sometimes symptoms are reinforced by personality styles. Somatic symptoms are exaggerated by patients with a histrionic personality and may be the object of such intense fixations by those with compulsive, paranoid, schizotypal, and schizoid personalities, as to make these patients take on a hypochondriacal character.

TABLE 16-1 Differential Diagnosis of Functional Somatic Symptoms

Demonstrable Somatic Illness
With proportionate vs disproportionate illness behaviors
Psychiatric Differential Diagnosis
Depressive disorders
Anxiety disorders
Substance abuse disorders
Psychotic disorders
Organic mental disorders
Deception syndromes
Malingering
Factitious disorders
Somatoform disorders
Personality disorders

Functional Somatic Syndromes

Like somatoform disorders, functional somatic syndromes (FSS) are characterized by complaints that seem far out of proportion to any abnormalities found, and lack laboratory confirmation. These diagnoses depend on consensus criteria, description of symptoms, and a natural course of illness. The FSS vary from those with relatively more academic acceptance (e.g., irritable bowel syndrome, fibromyalgia) to those of more recent and lay prominence (e.g., chronic Lyme disease, electromagnetic hypersensitivity). Others straddle the line between the medical mainstream and the "fringe," partly depending on where and how they are discussed and managed (e.g., chronic fatigue syndrome, multiple chemical sensitivity).

The FSS are characterized by their respective cores of medically unexplained symptoms, with associated features, required to "rule in" those that have established diagnostic criteria.[52–55] Table 16-2 outlines salient features of four of the better characterized FSS (note: Table 16-2 uses chronic fatigue syndrome criteria rather than the systemic exertion intolerance criteria, as "proposed" by the Institute of Medicine, see below). There is an argument to be made that there are more commonalities than distinguishing features between them,[56] and there is substantial overlap in the phenomenology, epidemiology, and co-occurrence of these various syndromes. Depending on rigor of diagnosis, the FSS carry across-the-board co-morbidity with depressive and anxiety disorders;[57–60] a characteristic, of course, shared by the somatic symptom disorders. Patients with one FSS, when subjected to diagnostic investigation for another, are found generally to have both illnesses 30–70% of the time, with co-morbidities of >70% found in multiple studies.[61–63]

Those patients who seek medical care for FSS are more distressed, depressed, and under more life stress than community residents who have the same symptoms but who never seek out a physician. Indeed, all FSS could be said to have high rates of undiagnosed members of the general population who do not present themselves to the health care system or consider themselves markedly disabled, yet nonetheless "meet criteria" for these illnesses.[64–66] These findings reiterate the hypothesis that important features of FSS may have a low threshold of symptom detection and tendency to medically interpret somatic cues. Once the patient acquires a functional diagnosis (either by strict research criteria or by looser clinical criteria), that diagnosis is granted greater authority and legitimacy than a co-morbid psychiatric diagnosis. Physician and patient often collude to focus attention only on the somatic syndrome.

TABLE 16-2 Comparison of the Four Major Functional Somatic Syndromes

	CHRONIC FATIGUE SYNDROME[a]	IRRITABLE BOWEL SYNDROME[b]	FIBROMYALGIA[c]	MULTIPLE CHEMICAL SENSITIVITIES[d]
Exclusion of other somatic/ psychiatric cause	Required	Unnecessary	Unnecessary (specifically accommodates)	Unnecessary
Duration	≥6 months	≥6 months + 3 days/ month in last 3 months	≥3 months	"Chronic"
Severity criteria	Must be met	Unspecified "pain and discomfort"	Based on pain elicitation on exam	Nonspecific
Reproducibility/ relief of symptoms	Unnecessary	Relief with defecation	Based on pain elicitation on exam at 11/18 "tender point sites"	Reproducible with exposure, relief with removal of irritants
Ancillary symptoms	Four or more of: • Cognitive impairment • Sore throat • Tender lymph nodes • Muscle pain • Multi-joint pain • New headaches • Unrefreshing sleep • Post-exertion malaise	Onset associated with changes in frequency and form of stool	History of: • Bilateral pain • Pain above and below waist • Axial skeletal pain	• "Low levels" of irritant produce symptoms • Multiple irritants • Symptoms in multiple organ systems

Adapted from:
[a]Fukada K, Straus SE, Hickie I, et al: The chronic fatigue syndrome: A comprehensive approach to its definition and study. *Ann Intern Med* 121: 953–959, 1994.
[b]Longstreth GF, Thompson WG, Chey WD, et al: Functional bowel disorders. *Gastroenterology* 130: 1480–1491, 2006.
[c]Wolfe F, Smythe HA, Yunus MB, et al: The American College of Rheumatology 1990 criteria for the classification of fibromyalgia: Report of the multicenter committee. *Arthritis Rheum* 33: 160–172, 1990.
[d]Bartha RP, Baumzweiger W, Buscher DS, et al: Multiple chemical sensitivity: A 1999 consensus. *Arch Env Health* 54: 147–149, 1999.

The fact that the patient has been diagnosed with FSS should not limit aggressive treatment of co-morbid psychiatric diagnoses. The principles of care for somatoform disorders apply here as well. Rule out organic disease and diagnose and treat affective disorder, substance abuse, and the other psychiatric diagnoses. Knowing the patient, listening with respect for his or her suffering, setting limits, and keeping an ear for changes in medical complaints remain pivotal concepts. CBT is emerging from a number of rigorous intervention trials as an effective treatment for many of these syndromes.[67–69] The status of antidepressant pharmacotherapy for them has been systematically reviewed.[70]

Systemic Exertion Intolerance Disease

By consensus, systemic exertion intolerance disease (SEID), formerly known as myalgia encephalomyelitis/chronic fatigue syndrome (CFS), is defined by three core features: impaired day-to-day functioning because of fatigue persisting for 6 months and which is new, post-exertional malaise, and unrefreshing sleep.[71,72] Patients must also have either cognitive impairment or orthostatic intolerance.

The Institute of Medicine recommends thorough work-up for other possible medical or psychiatric causes of fatigue, though, unlike prior diagnostic criteria for CFS, no guidelines are given with regards to whether SEID can be diagnosed in the setting of other specific psychiatric disorders.

Though SEID was formerly associated with infection with Ebstein–Barr virus, no single virus has been shown to cause persistent, debilitating SEID. In the primary care setting, patients with postinfectious fatigue after 6 months are more likely to have had fatigue and psychological distress before the infection.[73] A history of dysthymia and more than eight medically unexplained symptoms not already listed in SEID criteria may predict prolonged disability in SEID patients.[74]

Suggested screening laboratory tests include a complete blood count, a sedimentation rate, liver and renal function tests, calcium, phosphate, glucose, thyroid-stimulating hormone (TSH), and urinalysis. Further tests, such as a magnetic resonance imaging (MRI) scan of the head to search for multiple sclerosis, should be guided by clinical findings.

There is no specific medical treatment for formal SEID. The choice of antidepressant for co-morbid mood disorder depends on its capacity to improve sleep but limit sedation. Graduated aerobic exercise programs have been shown in several studies to improve physical conditioning and reduce fatigue.[75] CBT programs increasingly appear to have established their effectiveness.[76,77] The goal is to help the patient achieve maximal function.

Fibromyalgia

Fibromyalgia is a syndrome of generalized muscle pain and tenderness at specific trigger points, detected by physical examination.[78] For diagnosis, pain must be present for 3 months at a similar level. Whereas the prior diagnosis relied on the number of trigger points, the 2011 modified criteria allow for significantly fewer trigger points in the presence of more and more disabling associated symptoms including fatigue, waking unrefreshed, cognitive symptoms, headaches, pain or cramps in lower abdomen, depression.[79] Affective disorders are common among FM patients who seek out rheumatologists.

For FM, amitriptyline (25 mg to 50 mg/day) and cyclobenzaprine (10 mg at bedtime) (both TCAs) to relieve pain and improve sleep seem to work at least briefly in some fraction of patients.[80,81] Pregabalin, duloxetine and milnacipran are all FDA-approved for the treatment of fibromyalgia.

Irritable Bowel Syndrome

Irritable bowel symptoms occur in 15% to 20% of the population, but people with the disorder who seek medical help compose a major component, 25% to 50%, of referrals to gastroenterologists.[82] The disorder affects females more than males and, although its causes are unknown, does appear to have a genetic component.[83,84]

The international criteria for IBS include continuous or recurrent symptoms (at least 3 days/month for at least 3 months) of abdominal pain or discomfort associated with two or more of the following: relief by defecation, onset associated with a change in stool frequency, or consistency.[85] The disorder is subtyped based on the predominant symptom into diarrhea, constipation, mixed and unsubtyped types.

Those who visit physicians have more severe symptoms and are more likely to have co-morbid psychiatric diagnoses than those who do not. Mood disorder, panic with agoraphobia (especially fear of leaving the house because of diarrhea), history of childhood abuse, and neuroticism are more prevalent among patients than among the general population.[86–89]

Again, diagnosis depends on criteria, natural history of illness, and absence of laboratory confirmation of another diagnosis. The clinical approach to IBS is similar to that for the somatoform disorders: rule out organic and psychiatric diagnoses. In the context of a relationship in which the physician continues to learn about the patient, the physician chooses somatic treatments that target the predominant symptom of pain, constipation, or diarrhea. A TCA has an analgesic effect at low doses but tends to cause constipation and be preferable for a patient with recurrent diarrhea. An SSRI seems the better choice for co-morbid panic disorder or OCD, particularly in patients with constipation.[90] Paroxetine is the most studied of the SSRIs for this use and results have been mixed.[91] If the patient tends to have diarrhea, loperamide, a constipating agent, may be useful. Fiber and dietary adjustments, including moving to a predominantly plant-based diet may relieve constipation. The principles of pain management in IBS parallel the principles of management in somatoform pain disorder.

Cognitive-behavioral therapy and interpersonal psychodynamic therapy appear to be effective for improving well-being and quality of life.[92–94] Education about amplification of visceral symptoms and the vicious circle of anxiety, increased vigilance for symptoms, and resultant increase in symptoms and pain; relaxation training; and stress management techniques are helpful to both individuals and groups.

Multiple Chemical Sensitivity

According to the most widely used definition of multiple chemical sensitivity (MCS), it occurs after a documented environmental exposure that may have caused objective evidence of health effects, causes symptoms in multiple organ systems that vary predictably in response to environmental stimuli and occur in relation to measurable levels of chemicals below those known to harm health, and leads to no objective evidence of organ damage.[95] There is no exclusion for other medical or psychiatric syndromes. Common symptoms include fatigue, depression, memory loss, weakness, dizziness and headaches. Most new patients are women between the ages of 30 and 50, though many reports of MCS occurring in Gulf War veterans can be found in the literature. Environmental challenge testing, though sometimes advocated for, is not recommended as part of the work-up.

In contrast to the FSS discussed above, no published trials exist on the use of psychiatric medications in MCS. A recent study of mindfulness-based cognitive therapy showed positive effects on emotional and cognitive representations but no change in overall illness status.[96]

TREATMENT OF THE SOMATIC SYMPTOM DISORDERS

The first step in treatment is to make the diagnosis. Since patients may seek care in different places and physicians may not make the effort to understand the past medical history, the pattern of excessive illness behavior may not be recognized and the diagnosis delayed. Legwork to get records and to talk with the patient about their past may be necessary to reveal a larger longitudinal pattern. It is only if the physicians really know the medical data that they can offer gentle words of clarification. The way a patient adapts to illness and the way they experience pain or other symptoms often begins early in life in a family and sometimes traumatic context. Whether the symptom is fatigue or pain, the principle is to treat comorbid depression, anxiety disorder, and substance abuse and to be mindful how use and misuse of addictive medications add to the symptoms. Better function in daily life is the relevant outcome measure not the symptoms *per se*. The capacity of the patient to function in spite of symptoms[97] and gradual re-engagement in physical and social activities, is an important dimension. Listening to what patients believe about their symptoms and to what makes them mad, sad, or scared, allows them comfort and respect. Power is in the details of knowing what makes them overdo and what makes them avoid activities.[98,99]

Prognosis and Treatment

Somatic Symptom Disorder

The management of somatic symptom disorder, as extrapolated from somatization disorder and undifferentiated somatoform disorder, in many different organ systems, has been well formulated by Murphy.[100] It is best carried out by primary care physicians (PCPs) according to a conservative plan based on being a consistent care provider, preventing unnecessary or dangerous medical procedures, and inquiring in a supportive manner about the areas of stress in the patient's life. The last occurs during the physical examination, without inferring that the real cause for the increase in the patient's somatic complaints is psychosocial stress (which is what most authors believe). The basic goal is to help the patient cope with the symptoms rather than to eliminate them completely. In short, the aim is palliation, rather than outright cure.

Smith and associates[101] codified treatment recommendations in a letter to the PCPs of somatization disorder patients. These included regularly scheduled appointments (e.g., every 4 to 6 weeks); a physical examination performed at each visit to look for true disease; the avoidance of hospitalization, diagnostic procedures, surgery, and the use of laboratory assessments, unless clearly indicated; and advice to avoid telling patients, "It's all in your head." In a randomized controlled trial (RCT), this intervention reduced quarterly healthcare charges by 53%, largely as a result of decreases in hospitalization.[102] Neither the health of the patients, nor their satisfaction with their care, was adversely affected by implementation of the advice.

Cognitive-behavioral therapy (CBT), when compared with standard medical care, has also reduced symptoms, ratings of disorder by evaluators, and healthcare costs. The intervention focused on stress management, activity regulation, emotional awareness, cognitive restructuring, and interpersonal communication,[103] and the value has been established in multiple randomized controlled trials.[104] The benefits of antidepressant medications have not been as thoroughly studied, but data suggest their benefit and one meta-analysis suggested that added low-dose atypical antipsychotics also could have a role.[105] A variety of short-term psychodynamic psychotherapies have been reviewed[106] and a multidisciplinary treatment of severe somatoform disorder in hospital in the Netherlands has combined multiple individual and family approaches with art and physiotherapy.[107]

Guidelines for care of somatoform disorders have suggested a collaborative stepped care approach. Such a network in Germany connected 41 primary care physicians, 35 psychotherapists and 8 mental health clinics. They identified patients at risk, facilitated access to psychotherapy if needed, and recommended time-limited and low-dose antidepressant medication but no benzodiazepines to the primary care physicians. After 12 months, more of these patients discussed psychosocial distress with their physicians, who prescribed more antidepressants and fewer benzodiazepines.[108] There was no difference in the use of psychotherapy.

Conversion Disorder or Functional Neurologic Symptoms

The literature supports an optimistic outlook for these patients, at least in the first few years. Folks and co-workers[109] recorded a complete remission rate of 50% by discharge in those with conversion disorder in a general hospital. However, a fraction of these patients develop recurrent conversion symptoms (20% to 25% within 1 year). Unilateral functional weakness or sensory disturbance diagnosed in hospitalized neurological patients persisted in more than 80% (of 42 patients over a median of 12.5 years).[110] Patients with one conversion symptom may also develop other forms of somatization.

The most common form of treatment is to suggest that the conversion symptom will gradually improve. This ordinarily begins with reassuring news that tests of the involved body system show no damage and therefore that recovery is certain. Predicting that recovery will be gradual, with specific suggestions (e.g., vague shapes will become visible first; weight-bearing will be possible and then steps with a walker; standing up straight will come before full steadiness of gait; strength in squeezing a tennis ball will be followed by strength at the wrist and then elbow joints; and feeling will return to the toes first) usually succeeds, provided that the diagnosis is conveyed with serene confidence and the suggestions provided with supportive optimism. Lazare[111] pointed out that the psychiatrist should also discuss the patient's life stresses and try to detect painful affects to assess the non-verbal interpersonal communication embodied by the symptom. If patients are willing, their concerns with emotional valence can be heard out over time, even as they are offered respect for their strengths and the confidence that they will cope.

Confrontation is seldom helpful. Patients are particularly sensitive to the idea that an authoritative person has dismissed their suffering; their anger and sensitivity may be based on a history of abuse or neglect. Stonnington and associates[112] suggested that the best context for discussion of the diagnosis of pseudoseizure comes after the patient and the family have agreed that key representative events have been captured by video EEG monitoring. Co-morbid psychiatric diagnoses should be treated and precipitating and perpetuating factors identified. Behavioral interventions, physical therapy, and reassurance are crucial, particularly for less verbal patients.[112]

Some patients sense that there is a relationship between the stressful psychosocial conditions and the conversion symptomatology. An approach acceptable to some of these individuals has been to say that the body, mysterious in many ways, can be smarter than we are; it may tell us something is wrong before we realize we need help. When the stress in our lives becomes excessive, especially when our nature is more to overlook it or to grit our teeth and prevail, our body, by its symptoms, may blow the "time-out" whistle, forcing us to stop, to take a rest, and to get some help. This approach invites the patient to greater insight. A CBT-based guided self-help therapy, which explained changes in nervous system function as influenced by psychological and behavioral factors has been feasible and helpful for unselected neurology patients with conversion.[113]

Some hospitalized patients fail to improve with suggestion. Because they occupy a non-psychiatric bed, they must be told that if they insist that they are not well enough to leave the hospital, transfer to a psychiatric hospital or to a psychiatric unit will be arranged. Symptoms that have not responded to earlier suggestion may then improve sufficiently to permit discharge. One would have to entertain in such a patient, the possibility that the correct diagnosis is malingering. In general, a favorable outcome depends more on the patient's psychological strengths and on the absence of other psychopathology than on the specific nature of the conversion symptom itself.

Illness Anxiety Disorder

Extending from the literature on hypochondriasis, illness anxiety disorder (IAD) can be a chronic and disabling disease (note: we recognize that DSM-5 framers expect that SSD will subsume many patients formerly diagnosed with hypochondriasis, and we use the terms somewhat interchangeably, since much of the literature referred to is on hypochondriasis). Barsky and Ahern[33] note a time course of approximately 11 years in the group they studied. There may be some room for optimism, however, particularly when the illness has lasted less than 3 years and is not co-morbid with a personality disorder.[114]

When confronted with IAD, a treater's first step should be to screen for co-morbid affective and anxiety disorders (including obsessive–compulsive disorder, OCD). These are likely easier to treat, and their resolution may greatly diminish or bring an end to exaggerated disease fears. Isolated IAD is more difficult to cure. Several studies have suggested a role for selective serotonin reuptake inhibitors (SSRIs)[115,116] in those who met criteria for IAD. Persistent improvement was also related to continuation of SSRIs in the period after treatment; however, as many as 60% may remain disabled.[117] The factors that have been associated with a chronic course are severity of symptoms, functional impairment, childhood physical punishment, a longer duration of illness, and being more harm-avoidant and less cooperative.[117,118]

The most successful psychiatric interventions for primary IAD are cognitive, behavioral, and educational.[119] The treatment combination of education of the PCP and time-limited CBT for the patient improves a range of hypochondriacal symptoms, with modest treatment effect.[33] The manualized treatment for the patient targets cognitive and perceptual mechanisms of illness, including *hypervigilance* to visceral experience; *beliefs* about symptom etiology; *context* in which the hypochondriasis occurs; sick role *behaviors*; and *mood*. Randomized controlled studies have shown the benefit of mindfulness-based and other cognitive therapy adapted to focus on symptoms of health anxiety.[120–124] Both exposure therapy and cognitive restructuring have value.[125] Individual and group treatment have been combined,[126] and group acceptance and commitment therapy has been shown to be effective.[127] Tailored CBT for severe health anxiety has been adapted to the Internet.[128]

Patients with IAD tax the general physician. Such patients are difficult to reassure; their care is both time-consuming and expensive; and they often provoke strong negative reactions in their frustrated providers. Psychiatrists can be instrumental in easing anxieties and offering management recommendations. An internist's goals when treating a patient with IAD should be three-fold:[129] to avoid unnecessary diagnostic tests and to obviate overly aggressive medical and surgical intervention; to help a patient tolerate the symptoms, rather than striving to eliminate them; and to build a durable doctor–patient relationship based on the physician's interest in the patient as a person and not just in the symptoms. Once a physician views his or her task as palliative, not curative, the doctor–patient relationship becomes less contentious and adversarial. Further, patients are more likely to loosen the grip on their concerns when they feel that the physician has acknowledged and accepted them as "real."

Several practical measures may be helpful. The physician can forge a personal connection with the patient by paying particular attention to social history and by complimenting the patient on the ability to persevere despite great discomfort. Rather than providing as-needed appointments, the doctor can schedule meetings at regular intervals, thereby decoupling professional attention from symptom severity. Patients with IAD tend to develop iatrogenic complications and treatment side-effects. This has given rise to the clinical maxim, "Don't just do something, stand there." In other words, the best medical interventions are modest, simple, and benign.

DECEPTION SYNDROMES

The term "Deception Syndrome" has been used to describe patterns of behavior in which patients engage in willful deceit of providers. It encompasses factitious disorders and malingering, which differ in the motivation for the deceptive behavior.

Factitious Disorders

Factitious disorders are marked by the conscious production of symptoms with the unconscious goal of obtaining the sick role and being cared for. Patients may fake, exaggerate, intentionally worsen, or simply create symptoms. They do not admit to self-harm, but rather hide it from their doctors. The paradox, then, is that those with factitious illness come to healthcare providers requesting help, but intentionally hide the self-induced cause of their illness.

The DSM-5[13] no longer distinguishes between factitious disorders with physical symptoms and those with psychological features, though this remains a helpful distinction clinically. In a factitious disorder with physical symptoms, the most common presentation is that of a general medical condition. The types of physical symptoms and diseases that have been faked are limited only by the imagination of those who feign them.[130–134] Table 16-3 lists some common categories. Laboratory tests and diagnostic modalities may be particularly useful in distinguishing factitious symptoms from true medical illness. For example, in the case of suspicious infection, polymicrobial culture results that indicate an uncommon source (e.g., from urine or feces) is highly suggestive. Those who inject insulin to produce hypoglycemia will have a low C-peptide level on laboratory analysis, whereas glyburide can be measured in the urine of those suspected of taking oral hypoglycemics. Laxative abuse to cause ongoing diarrhea is confirmed by testing for phenolphthalein in the stool.[135] Finally, diagnostic studies in cases of suspected thyrotoxicosis (from surreptitious ingestion of thyroid hormone) reveal elevated serum total or free thyroid hormone levels, undetectable serum thyrotropin levels, low serum thyroglobulin concentration, normal urinary iodine excretion, suppressed thyroidal radioactive iodine uptake (RAIU), absence of goiter, and absence of circulating antithyroid antibodies.[136]

Detection of other types of physical factitious illness may require more astute physical examinations or observational skills (not to mention catching the patient "in the act"). For example, fever of unknown etiology may be caused by warming thermometers on light bulbs or radiators, or with a flame (though this is more difficult with modern thermometers). Hematuria may be produced by bloodletting from another body area (commonly from a finger prick) into the urine sample. With non-healing wounds where self-excoriation or "picking" behavior is suspected, witnessing the act either directly or with the use of video monitoring

TABLE 16-3 Typical Clinical Presentation of Factitious Disorder

TYPE	CLINICAL FINDINGS OR SYMPTOMS
Acute abdominal (laparotomaphilia migrans)	Abdominal pain; multiple surgeries may lead to true adhesions and subsequent bowel obstruction
Neurologic (neurologic diabolica)	Headache, loss of consciousness, seizure
Hematological	Anemia from bloodletting or use of an anticoagulant
Endocrinologic	Hypoglycemia from exogenous insulin; hyperthyroidism from exogenous thyroid hormone
Cardiac	Chest pain or arrhythmia
Dermatologic (dermatitis autogenica)	Rash; skin eruptions
Febrile (hyperpyrexia figmentatica)	Thermometer manipulation to produce fever
Infectious	Wound infected with multiple organisms (often through fecal material)

Adapted from Viguera AC, Stern TA: Factitious disorders. In Stern TA, Herman JB, editors: *Massachusetts General Hospital psychiatry update and board preparation*, ed 2, New York, 2004, McGraw-Hill, pp 145–147.

is diagnostic. Of note, the latter brings up ethical considerations, unless done with the consent of the patient. Finally, among the numerous other possible physical manifestations, those that rely on more subjective reports (including joint or muscle pain, headache, renal colic, or abdominal pain) may be present for months or years before a factitious etiology is even considered, much less proven.

Although the majority of published cases of factitious disorder involve physical symptoms, many patients primarily feign psychological symptoms. Psychological complaints encompass a broad spectrum of symptoms (including depression, anxiety, psychosis, bereavement, dissociation, posttraumatic stress, and suicidal and homicidal ideation).[137–141] In the case of factitious bereavement, for example, the patient may report a dramatic or recent loss of a child or other loved one with a display of emotion that invokes significant sympathy from medical treaters. When the truth is discovered, the reported deceased may either be still alive, have died long ago, or perhaps did not really play a major role in the patient's life. Another common feature of factitious disorder with psychological features is pseudohallucinations—perceptual disturbances that the patient recognizes as unreal and explicitly describes as hallucinations.

Whereas the term *Munchausen syndrome* is often used interchangeably with factitious disorder, the classic Munchausen syndrome is reserved for a subset of patients (approximately 10% of those with factitious disorder) exhibiting the most severe and chronic form, which is marked by the following three components: recurrent hospitalizations, travel from hospital to hospital (peregrination), and *pseudologia fantastica*.[134] Pseudologia fantastica is the production of intricate and colorful stories or fantasies associated with the patient's presentation. It is a form of pathologic lying characterized by an overlapping of fact and fiction (with a repetitive quality, grandiosity, or an assumption of the victim role by the storyteller).[142] Impostorship, though not a hallmark of Munchausen's syndrome, is also a common feature, with patients claiming to be a war hero or former professional athlete. Munchausen patients often make a career out of their illness. Serial hospitalizations render employment or sustained interpersonal relationships impossible. Moreover, patients who produce significant self-trauma or develop untoward complications from medical or surgical interventions become further incapacitated. The prognosis is generally poor in these cases, and patients may die prematurely from complications of their own self-injurious behavior or from iatrogenesis. Patients with Munchausen subtype are more likely to be male, to exhibit antisocial and dependent personality traits, and display average to above-average intelligence.[142]

Whereas Munchausen syndrome is the most dramatic form of factitious illness, common factitious disorder is more frequently encountered.[142] As opposed to those with Munchausen syndrome, patients with common factitious disorder do not typically use aliases or travel from hospital to hospital, but rather frequent the same physician. They are well known in their healthcare system because of numerous hospitalizations. Risk factors for common factitious disorder include female gender, a history of abuse, being unmarried, having experience in the healthcare profession, and having borderline personality disorder and masochistic personality traits.

Factitious disorder imposed on another is a subtype of factitious disorder recognized by DSM-5 and formerly called "factitious disorder by proxy," in which persons falsify symptoms or induce illness in another person.[143] The perpetrator in this case is most often the biological mother of a young child, although the elderly and those under the medical care of others are also at risk for being victimized. This disorder has two characteristic forms. The classic form involves a parent or caregiver intentionally inflicting injury or inducing illness in a child while deceiving treating clinicians with false or exaggerated information. The other, perhaps more common and potentially insidious, involves a caregiver embellishing or fabricating symptoms in order to cause overly aggressive medical evaluations and interventions. In contrast to standard factitious disorder, the motivation here is to satisfy the caregiver's psychological need to care for a chronically or severely ill individual. In a review of 451 cases of factitious disorder imposed on another, Sheridan found that victims are typically 4 years old or younger, with equal percentages of males and females. She further discovered that an average of 21.8 months elapsed between the onset of symptoms and diagnosis, and 6% of victims died. Perhaps even more alarming, is her finding that 61% of siblings had illnesses similar to those of the victims, and 25% of the victims' known siblings were dead.[144]

Much like general factitious disorder, the symptoms in factitious disorder imposed on another are more commonly physical than psychological, and may involve any symptom within the scope of imagination. The most common presentations seem to be apnea, anorexia, feeding problems, diarrhea, and seizures.[143,144] These may be induced in a variety of ways, from smothering the child to feeding the child laxatives or ipecac. Perpetrators often have some medical training or exposure to the illness that affects the child (e.g., a mother who has a seizure disorder herself). Other clinical indicators or red flags include a patient who does not respond to appropriate treatments, symptoms that improve when the mother does not have access to the child, unexplained illnesses with other children in the family, a mother who becomes anxious when her child improves, or a mother who encourages invasive tests.[145]

In the past two decades, a new variant of factitious disorder has emerged, known as Munchausen by Internet. Although not included in DSM-5, the syndrome has been described in several journal articles.[146,147] Rather than presenting to hospitals with symptoms, sufferers seek attention from other Internet users by feigning illness in chat rooms or on blogs, or social media sites. The expansion of the Internet has made it much easier for persons to gain a nuanced understanding of certain medical diseases in order to appear more convincing. Classic patterns of behavior in this variant of the syndrome include verbatim recapitulation of textbook descriptions of illnesses, with a description of recurrent, worsening illness followed by miraculous recovery, and a reported duration of severe illness that conflicts with the Internet user's behavior, such as blogging about being in the intensive care unit with septic shock. Some patients even fake their own deaths in this syndrome as the ultimate ploy for sympathy.

Diagnostic Approach

As previously suggested, making the diagnosis of factitious illness is often difficult. However, there are several elements of a general strategic approach that may be helpful. Early suspicion is important to avoid colluding with the patient in ordering unnecessary tests and subjecting the patient to further risk of iatrogenic injury. When suspecting factitious illness, one should first obtain information from all pertinent collateral sources. These may include previous or current caregivers, family members, current and old medical records, and laboratory and diagnostic studies. Technology may be making it easier for clinicians to detect factitious disorder. The expansion and unification of medical records through centralized databases means that many practitioners have access not only to records in their own hospital system but also to records in hospital networks and community health services, and many states have prescription monitoring programs which provide a central database for controlled substance prescriptions. Verification of the "facts" presented by the patient is critical.

Next, one should look for historic elements suggestive of factitious disease. Some of these are outlined in the DSM-5.[13] Recognition of typical presentations (including all of those outlined in Table 16-2) may provide further clues. Typical hospitalizations for those who feign medical or psychiatric illness share common characteristics. First, patients often come to Emergency Departments (EDs) after hours (at night or on the weekend), when staffing is decreased and senior-level staff are likely absent. Patients use medical jargon and generally know which diagnoses or conditions will merit hospitalization. Their histories are often quite dramatic and convincing, and such patients persuade their physicians to provide care by appealing to narcissistic qualities, such as omnipotence. Once hospitalized, treatments are marked by demands for specific interventions (e.g., surgery or particular medications) and by increasing needs for attention. When the demands are not met, patients become angry. In many cases, the patient correctly predicts worsening of the disease and complains to the staff about mistreatment or misdiagnosis. The patient may play on the clinician's fear of liability to drive further unnecessary testing and treatment. If staff uncovers the deception, strong countertransference feelings of hatred ensue. Patients are then rapidly discharged or elope from the hospital only to seek "treatment" at another facility soon thereafter.

When one is lucky enough to find medical paraphernalia or to observe the patient intentionally inducing his or her own symptoms, the diagnosis is assured. Of note, room and personal belonging searches without the patient's permission are controversial and, in many cases, considered an invasion of privacy. Before embarking on such an endeavor, it is prudent to consider the potential ramifications carefully and to seek legal counsel. There is no doubt, however, that in most cases the diagnosis relies on significant detective work based on a high level of suspicion.

True physical disorders (especially rare or unusual diseases with few objective findings) may mimic factitious disorders. It is essential to consider this possibility before prematurely diagnosing factitious illness. SSD and conversion disorder (see above) may also be mistaken for factitious disorder. These diagnoses, however, are distinguished from factitious illness, in that their symptoms are not under voluntary control.

As with all factitious illnesses, diagnosis of factitious disorder imposed on another may prove difficult unless one directly witnesses a perpetrator harming the victim. When the victim is a child or is elderly, both legal obligations and privacy rights may differ from those of a typical adult patient. This is particularly pertinent with regard to mandated reporting (which varies by state), as well as when video surveillance is proposed as a mechanism to uncover intentional harm. In general, whenever diagnostic or treatment strategies outside the usual standard of care are considered, it is best to consult with both professional medical and legal colleagues before undertaking them.

Malingering

Malingering involves the conscious feigning, induction, or exacerbation of physical or psychological symptoms for conscious gain. This so-called secondary gain is the hallmark of the phenomenon and can include obtaining something desired (such as food, shelter, or medication, especially controlled substances) or avoiding responsibility (such as missing a court date or obtaining time off from work, release from the military, or relief from child care or elder care obligations). The DSM-5 includes malingering under "other conditions that may be a focus of clinical attention."[13] Though the prevalence of malingering is unknown, it may be detected in up to 10% of psychiatric inpatients and up to 40% of patients applying for disability.[148] It is thought to be more common in men than women and is often co-morbid with antisocial personality disorder, though it has been observed in psychologically normal adults.

Malingerers most often pick symptoms that are highly subjective and difficult to prove (or disprove). Vague pains, such as headache, tooth pain, or back pain, are common. The goal may be to obtain narcotics or to be placed on disability from work. Psychiatric symptoms are often easier to fake than physical symptoms, and patients may claim that they are suicidal or are suffering from hallucinations or delusions.

Involvement in the legal system is a risk factor for malingering, particularly among patients who are referred for examination by an attorney. The presence of a lawsuit after a reported injury should also raise suspicion that the patient is malingering. In general, like those with factitious disorder, patients who malinger tend to have poor coping skills and to use immature defense mechanisms. As a group, they tend to seek medical or psychiatric care frequently, but they vary in terms of their personalities from charming and glib, to dependent and needy, to irritable and demanding.

Another common feature of malingering is a long list of claimed allergies. Malingerers tend to have a list of allergies that precludes the use of whole classes of medications and is structured to guide the physician toward prescribing desired medications, often controlled substances. Because they are desperate to have their needs met, patients who malinger frequently exhibit the "black cloud" phenomenon, in which the number and degree of bad things that have happened to them recently may strike the interviewer as implausible. Finally, perhaps the most consistent telltale sign of malingering is the escalation of symptoms in response to not having demands met.

The presence of clearly identified secondary gain is not absolute evidence of malingering—one must be careful not to miss the diagnosis of a true medical condition in this population. Many patients with true medical or psychiatric illness stand to benefit in other ways from treatment. The diagnosis of malingering is ultimately based on a combination of inconsistencies in the history, the presence of secondary gain, a history of suspected deception, and other associated features outlined above. Patients with a history of malingering remain at risk for real medical or psychiatric illness and should be granted a reasonable evaluation at each visit.

When malingering is suspected, certain interview techniques, such as asking repeatedly about details to establish inconsistencies, using gentle assumption to ask about secondary gain (e.g. "When is your next court date?"), and asking about low-frequency symptoms to highlight exaggeration of distress, can be helpful in building a case for the diagnosis. In some cases, formal psychological testing may also be useful. The Minnesota Multiphasic Personality Inventory-2 (MMPI-2) may pick up distortions or exaggerations in both physical and psychological symptoms via its embedded scales for faking good and faking bad.[149]

Management of Deception Syndromes

No specific psychiatric treatment has been shown to be effective in the management of deception syndromes. There are, however, a few principles that generally prove helpful. The first is to avoid premature confrontation, which may result in defensiveness, increased elusiveness, or flight from the hospital. Being aware of negative countertransference is also essential if one is to avoid being judgmental or acting on the hostility so often evoked by these patients. Because deception syndromes are often highly treatment-resistant, placing an emphasis on management over cure helps to reframe the treatment goals. Clear and open communication between the psychiatrist and medical and surgical colleagues is essential in this regard.

There is debate about whether it is useful or therapeutic to confront someone believed to be exhibiting a deception syndrome. Certainly, confrontation is likely to damage the therapeutic relationship and is often met with defensiveness and denial. Some recommend a gentle confrontation that allows the patient to save face, though this may be difficult to achieve if the deception is blatant. Strategies for gentle confrontation include reframing the desire for medical attention as an indicator of psychological distress and discussing the full range of possible diagnoses, including factitious disorder and malingering, with the patient. Because malingering and factitious disorder may not only harm the patient by generating unnecessary tests and work-up but also jeopardize the care of other patients through misallocation of limited resources, others advocate direct confrontation in cases where the diagnosis is clear. If the provider chooses to confront the patient about his behavior, it may still be possible to engage the patient in a discussion of motivations for the deception and alternative options for further treatment, including psychotherapy in the case of factitious disorder and referrals to outpatient resources, such as homeless shelters and substance abuse hotlines in the case of malingering.

In some cases, a decision may be made to discharge the patient who has been diagnosed with factitious disorder or malingering. The term "therapeutic discharge" is sometimes used to describe the circumstance in which continued hospitalization is felt to be counter-therapeutic and detrimental with respect to resource management. Because factitious disorder and malingering are diagnoses of exclusion, this approach is typically reserved for patients who have repeatedly engaged in deceptive behavior.

The first consideration once a diagnosis of factitious disorder imposed on another is made is that of protecting the victim. In many cases this means placing the child in a foster care situation (at least temporarily). Treatment then addresses both the victim and perpetrator. Although no effective treatment for victims has been established, it is generally thought that therapy to address co-morbid psychiatric diagnoses is a good place to start. Legal interventions are often required. Therapy for perpetrators is generally the mainstay of treatment; however, because many perpetrators never admit to wrongdoing, this often proves difficult.

THREE SHARED PARAMETERS OF PSYCHOSOMATIC CONDITIONS

In Figure 16-2, the somatic symptom and related disorders (excluding psychological factors affecting medical illness, where unexplained symptoms are not manifested), functional somatic syndromes, and malingering are depicted according to how they fall along three parameters that are discussed individually below. Each parameter is non-binary, such that

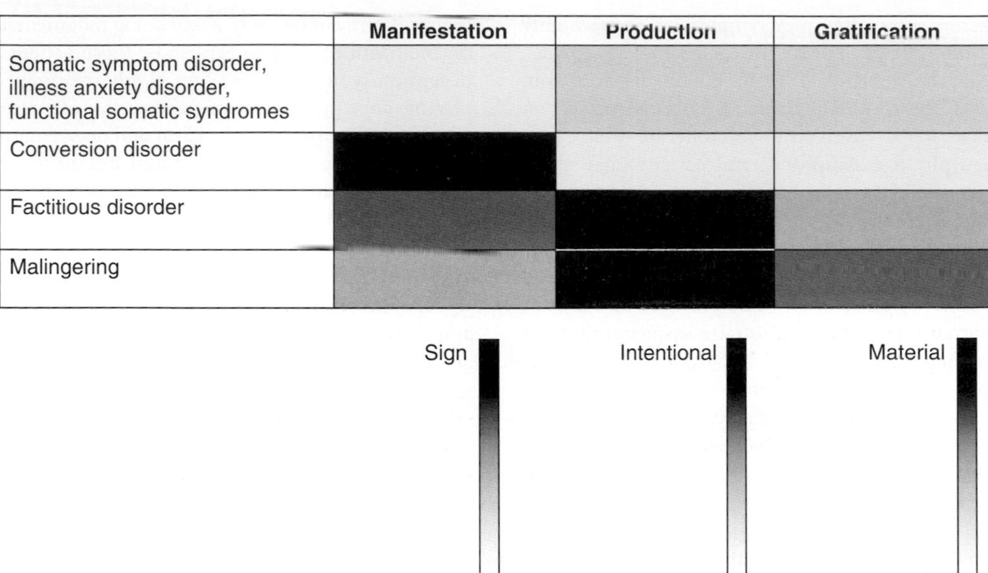

Figure 16-2. Three parameters of somatically focused syndromes.

most boxes in Figure 16-2 are, quite literally, "shades of gray." Breaking down these presentations in this manner offers some coherence to disparate categories that otherwise only share the vague quality of having a somatic focus. The figure and corresponding discussion are not a diagnostic scheme, but rather a way of thinking about what is going on in these complex situations.

Manifestation

Disease is revealed to physicians through symptoms and/or signs. *Symptoms* are "any morbid phenomenon... *experienced by the patient* and indicative of disease." *Signs* are "*discoverable on examination of the patient.*"[150] Both often occur together, and the line between the two is not always clear. DSM-5 incorrectly indicates that the Somatic Symptom and Related Disorders "share a common feature: the prominence of somatic symptoms associated with significant distress and impairment"[13] (see conversion and factitious disorder discussions above and below).

Many diseases are discoverable only by their signs. This may be due to the nature of the disease (e.g., early stages of hypertension), or the nature of the patient's temperament and culture (e.g., a thigh melanoma brought before an allopathic physician only once it interfered with walking).[151] Somatic symptom disorder, illness anxiety disorder, and the FSS are all marked by the amplification or fear of symptoms insufficiently associated with signs and diagnostic test results. The FSS patients included in this category are only those who also exhibit abnormal illness behavior, though this may represent a self-selected or even iatrogenic[27] majority of those for whom a diagnosis is made or extracted.

Symptoms may be significant in conversion disorder, but this diagnosis itself is dependent on neurologic signs. With sensory manifestations of conversion disorder, the distinction can be particularly blurred. However, these patients do not merely complain of blindness or weakness; he or she is presumed to "have" them. While conversion disorder's signs may not come "as advertised" (e.g., are inconsistent across time or circumstance, lack an anatomically coherent distribution), they should be discernible on exam or observation in the absence of patient commentary.

Most instances of diagnosed factitious disorder involve striking self-inflicted disease. As such, factitious disorder is usually manifest by signs of disease such as sepsis, hypoglycemia, and anemia. It has been noted, however, that this manner of presentation is likely preceded and/or overlapped by more subtle, undetected phases of elaboration and fabrication of symptoms without actual physical morbidity.[152] The opposite seems to be the case in malingering, with symptom fabrication being seen more often than sign induction.

Production

The historic influence of psychodynamic theory on psychosomatic medicine gives us terms such as "somatizing" and "conversion" that imply unconscious transformations of psychological states into physical ones. Cognitive-behavioral models also involve automatic processes that go on outside of awareness. It is more encompassing to describe the manifestations of somatically focused conditions on a spectrum of intentionality.

Patients with somatic symptom disorder, illness anxiety disorder, and the FSS are genuine in their identification of the symptoms of which they complain. That these symptoms seem exaggeratedly portrayed might speak to their actual perceived severity, to the desperation of people who fear that doctors do not take them seriously, or to intentional exaggeration of actual distress. The signs of conversion disorder are similarly unintentionally produced. DSM-5's aforementioned removal of the intentionality criterion notwithstanding, when conversion disorder is diagnosed, the signs are presumed, even if not proven, to be unintentionally produced.

By definition, intentionality and lying are at the heart of symptom and sign production in factitious disorder and malingering. Thus, in the production column, they receive the only outright black (or white) squares in the table. It is important to note, however, that the volitional falsification is of first causes rather than of biological correlates of signs. The intentional deception lies in *how* the patient became septic. When mere symptoms are falsified intentionally, the patient's untrue medical statements are simply called *lying*.

Gratification

Primary and secondary gain are sometimes used to describe how symptom and sign production satisfy patients' needs. Secondary gain refers to gratification derived from material items (e.g., for food, shelter, money, illicit substances) or to the items themselves. Primary gain refers to gratification derived from the relief of intrapsychic tension,[153] or to the means used to relieve that tension; in the somatic domain, that means is sometimes vaguely referred to as the "assumption of the sick role."

As already noted, privileges of the sick role include blamelessness for the products of sickness, relief from duties incompatible with the sickness, and entitlement to care.[24] Taking some liberties with the sick role concept, we expand the latter to include not just medical care but also social nurturing. The psychological benefits of blamelessness, relief, and care for those feeling unworthy, beleaguered, and unloved, brings some clarity to the nebulous concept of primary gain. Of course, blamelessness and legal culpability, relief and disability payments, and care and shelter, can all blur into one another, reminding us that the distinction between primary and secondary gains, beyond the outer margins, is unsubstantiated.[152]

When it comes to gratification, somatic symptom disorder, illness anxiety disorder, and FSS cluster together, with immaterial sick role privileges seeming to dominate. Sick role status depends on social and medical validation of one's sickness. This contingent aspect of sick role privilege may partially explain the desperate, sometimes hostile, way that these patients can pursue or cling to the medical legitimacy of their distress. These efforts to legitimize distress can eclipse patients' stated desires for relief, possibly explaining findings such as diminished placebo responses and the powerful negative prognostic effect of support group participation for patients with chronic fatigue syndrome.[154,155]

Patients with FSS, somatic symptom disorder, or illness anxiety disorder may eventually bring before their doctors disability paperwork or other requests for medical excusals, but these are secondary pursuits. Still, they straddle the types of gratification delineated here. Similarly, depending on one's belief in and "discovery" of a trigger (e.g., an impending divorce hearing, an unacceptable revenge fantasy), it can be difficult to determine for what type of gratification the signs of conversion disorder are mobilized.

Similar gratifications inherent to somatic symptom disorder, illness anxiety disorder, FSS, and conversion disorder, can inform treatment. Sick role privileges are balanced by a duty to at least pursue health.[156] Claiming sick role privileges without accepting the corresponding duty may be the shared characteristic of "heartsink patients."[157] The idea of bringing patient duty into the picture, allows for communication and limit setting that embraces rather than challenges the patient's sick role status, hinges it to healthier behavior, and reins in what patients can expect from physicians (and others) while clinging to invalidism.[158]

For the deception syndromes, of course, this rationale falls apart, since these patients pursue their sick role status disingenuously. Note that if the difference between immaterial/primary and material/secondary gain is sufficiently blurred, and if this is the main distinguishing characteristic between factitious disorder and malingering, then there are two superficial possibilities. One extends the disorder status of factitious disorder to malingering; the other extends the quasi-criminal status of malingering to factitious disorder. Instead, both conditions might be better understood as behaviors arising and distracting from broader problems. For example, malingering can be part of the broader patterns of non-pathologic criminality, sociopathy, or desperation; factitious disorder as maladaptive management of attachments in patients with borderline or other character disorders.[159,160]

CONCLUSION

Psychosomatic presentations are a nearly universal experience and symptom amplification is a major problem for a large subset of patients and the physicians who attempt to understand and treat them. DSM-5 has re-organized many of these presentations within the category of Somatic Symptom and Related Disorders, but to date, the rest of medicine has typically not used DSM classifications of these patients.

Ultimately, symptom amplification descriptions and names may be less important than the associated illness behaviors.[161] Addressing abnormal illness behaviors[22,23] through co-morbidity identification, strategic primary care approaches, psychotherapies, better navigation of the sick role status, and conservative use of medications, consultations, and diagnostic tests, is critical in the management of these patients.

REFERENCES

Access the reference list online at https://expertconsult.inkling.com/.

Patients With an Eating Disorder

17

Jennifer J. Thomas, Ph.D.
Esther Jacobowitz Israel, M.D.
Lazaro V. Zayas, M.D.
Kristin Russell, M.D., M.B.A.
Kathryn Coniglio, B.A.
Rosanna Fox, M.B.B.S.

OVERVIEW

Eating disorders are serious psychiatric illnesses, with high rates of morbidity and mortality. They are most common in young women, but affect people of all ages, genders, races, ethnicities, and socioeconomic statuses. Individuals with eating disorders can develop serious medical complications, requiring multidisciplinary treatment. Given these risks, early detection and treatment of an eating disorder can increase the likelihood of recovery. Medical stabilization is key before beginning mental health treatment, both to ensure the patient's safety and to enhance treatment efficacy.

EPIDEMIOLOGY

Overall, eating disorders are most common in adolescent and young adult females. In a national, cross-sectional survey of 9282 adults, the life-time prevalence was 0.9% for anorexia nervosa (AN), 1.5% for bulimia nervosa (BN), and 3.5% for binge eating disorder (BED) among females; and 0.3% for AN, 0.5% for BN, and 2.0% for BED among males.[1] Further, in an 8-year old prospective study in an all-female ethnically heterogeneous sample, the life-time prevalence by age 20 was 0.8% for AN, 2.6% for BN, and 3.0% for BED.[2] Sub-threshold or atypical presentations, categorized in the *Diagnostic and Statistical Manual of Mental Disorders*, 5th edition[3] as other specified feeding or eating disorder (OSFED) are also common. One community study of adolescent female twins showed that the prevalence rates for OSFED (5%) were comparable with full-threshold eating disorders (5.4%), with no significant difference in impairment between the two groups.[4]

Although eating disorders are most prevalent in westernized societies, they affect a diverse range of individuals. More broadly, eating disorders affect people in many different cultures and countries across the world. For example, individuals from Hong Kong with eating disorders had diagnostic classifications that corresponded well with life-time eating disorder phenotypes observed in the United States and Europe.[5] Lifetime prevalence rates of eating disorders range from 0.9% to 3.5% for White women;[1] 0.14% to 2.36% for African-American women;[6] 0.12% to 2.67% for Asian-American women;[7] and 0.12% to 2.31% for Latina women.[8]

ONSET AND COURSE

The etiology of eating disorders is largely unknown, with likely contributions from genetic, biological, psychological, and sociocultural factors. General risk factors for developing an eating disorder of any kind include low self-esteem, body dissatisfaction, and dieting.

AN typically begins during adolescence and/or young adulthood, with recent data showing a trend toward a decreasing age of onset.[9] Children as young as 7 years old may express body dissatisfaction and a desire to lose weight.[10] The onset of BN is usually later, in late adolescence and young adulthood, with a peak age of onset between 16 and 20 years.[11] The onset of BED is often later still, with an onset at 17 years or later.[12]

The heritability of eating disorders has been well-established. Family studies have shown a higher prevalence of AN,[13] BN,[14] and BED[15] among relatives of individuals with the same disorder. Longitudinal twin data suggest that genetic influence on the development of an eating disorder may be particularly activated during puberty.[16]

A recent longitudinal study of AN and BN showed recovery rates at 31.4% and 68.2%, respectively, after 9 years, and 62.8% and 68.2% after 22 years.[17] The remainder followed a chronic course.[17] Similarly, a 6-year longitudinal study of BED found that 43% of individuals with BED continued to be symptomatic.[18] Longitudinal studies have also illustrated patterns of diagnostic crossover, in which individuals move away from restrictive eating and towards bingeing and/or purging.[19]

Eating disorders are also associated with serious medical complications and a high mortality rate. In a longitudinal study of 246 women with AN, 16 eventually died due either to medical complications of AN (such as cardiac arrest, gastrointestinal hemorrhages, esophageal ulceration, or substance overdose) or by suicide.[20] A recent meta-analysis found that individuals with AN were 5.2 times more likely to die prematurely from any cause, and 18.1 times more likely to die by suicide, than 15–34-year-old females in the general population.[21]

Because nearly half of eating disorder cases are not detected in primary care settings,[22] more specialized outpatient medical services can provide other opportunities for diagnosis. Furthermore, early detection and intervention are crucial to improving prognosis.

CASE 1

Ms. D, a 21-year-old Caucasian college student without a psychiatric history, was brought to the clinic by her mother who was concerned that her daughter was exhibiting abnormal eating habits since her return home for summer break. Her mother described Ms. D as visiting the bathroom with increasing frequency after family meals and she had noticed food disappearing from the fridge and cupboards on several occasions. Her mother was concerned about Ms. D's "secretive" behavior and had witnessed her eating large quantities of chocolates and cookies in her room alone.

On interview, Ms. D was oriented, lucid, and avoided eye contact. On mental state exam, she was moderately depressed and quiet. She perceived her weight to be higher than she desired, and described low self-esteem; basing her self-worth almost entirely on her shape and weight. She denied any suicidal ideation but reported she had considered self-harm several times.

Ms. D first binged and purged following a set of disappointing exam results. Over the following 5 months, these episodes increased to 3 to 4 times per week. Following a binge, she described immediate feelings of guilt and shame. She denied using diuretics or diet pills, but reported taking laxatives 5 to 6 times each week. She became increasingly socially anxious and was afraid to eat around others for fear of losing control, and friends observing her behavior. At home she had begun to store food in her room or binge in the kitchen alone at nighttime.

On examination her BMI was 20.2, she had mild parotid swelling and signs of dental erosion. Russell's sign was absent and there was no abdominal bloating or tenderness. Ms. D reported occasional palpitations, generalized fatigue, and regular menstruation. Laboratory tests revealed a mild hypokalemia (3.1 mmol/L); other electrolytes were within normal limits.

Given that her weight was in the normal range and she was medically stable; Ms. D was diagnosed with BN and offered outpatient care and potassium supplementation. The team liaised with her PCP who prescribed 60 mg of fluoxetine daily. She was started on a 4-stage 20-session CBT program to interrupt the binge–purge cycle and reduce over-valuation of shape and weight.

Within the first 4 weeks of treatment, Ms. D was able to reduce her episodes of binging and purging to once every other week, and by completion of CBT, she had not binged or purged in several weeks. Her mood also improved.

DIFFERENTIAL DIAGNOSIS AND INITIAL ASSESSMENT OF EATING DISORDERS

Given the considerable overlap in symptoms across eating-disorder diagnoses (see DSM-5),[3] differential diagnosis can be challenging. Nonetheless, an accurate and specific diagnosis is crucial in order to select the optimal treatment strategy. Two specific challenges clinicians may face are: (1) not having the time or expertise to screen for an eating disorder, and (2) misattributing physical complaints to a specific medical abnormality, rather than an eating disorder. This is particularly true for symptoms associated with gastrointestinal (GI) distress, weight loss, or dental abnormalities. Patients may initially present to a medical doctor or to a dietitian, and subsequently be referred for psychiatric consultation after an extensive evaluation.

Clinical Detection of an Occult Eating Disorder

Detection of an eating disorder can be challenging, in part due to the reluctance of many patients to acknowledge and receive care for their illness.[23] Thus, some individuals may come to medical attention for an eating disorder only after they arouse clinical suspicion on a medical or pediatric service due to unexplained weight changes or symptoms, or when family members report concerns.

Given the prevalence and associated mortality and morbidity of eating disorders, clinicians should ask sensitive yet direct questions about weight and dieting history in order to detect body image disturbances and weight fluctuations. A national eating disorders screening program study indicated that 91% of individuals who had not previously volunteered eating and weight concerns to a health professional ultimately disclosed such concerns when asked directly.[24]

Because clinical history does not always elicit accurate or complete data, collateral history, physical signs, observable behaviors, and longitudinal clinical course should be used when possible as part of the evaluation. Physical signs may include low weight, parotid hypertrophy, excoriations on the dorsum of the hand (Russell's sign), or characteristic dental erosion. Laboratory studies may yield data suggestive of purging or nutritional compromise but do not have sufficient specificity or sensitivity to be useful in screening. Collateral data can sometimes be helpful, although often, family members are not aware of symptomatic behaviors.

Differential Diagnosis

The DSM-5 characterizes AN by restriction of food intake leading to a significantly low weight (i.e., a weight less than minimally normal for adults, and less than minimally expected for children); fear of gaining weight; and body image disturbance. Clinicians can further specify whether the patient has mild (BMI ≥ 17 kg/m^2), moderate (BMI 16–16.99 kg/m^2), severe (BMI 15–15.99 kg/m^2), or extreme (BMI <15 kg/m^2) AN. An important revision from DSM-IV to DSM-5 was the exclusion of the amenorrhea criterion, given that individuals without amenorrhea may have just as severe an eating disorder as those who are amenorrheic.[25] Individuals who do not endorse a fear of gaining weight, and thus are considered to be "non-fat phobic,"[26] may still be diagnosed with AN in the setting of low weight and persistent behavior that interferes with weight gain. There are two subtypes of AN: restricting (AN-R) and binge eating/purging (AN-BP).

BN is defined in DSM-5 as the presence of recurrent episodes of binge eating and inappropriate compensatory behaviors at least once per week for 3 months or more, in order to control weight. During a binge episode, an individual consumes an objectively large amount of food, coupled with a feeling of lack of control. Individuals with BN also overvalue the importance of shape and weight in ascertaining self-worth. Of note, a key difference between AN-BP and BN is weight status; individuals with BN are not underweight, and are normal weight or even overweight. Patients may utilize a range of inappropriate compensatory behaviors in order to purge calories consumed. Self-induced vomiting is a common purging method, although it is an inefficient means of ridding the body of calories. One study found that individuals retain over half the calories they consume after vomiting.[27] Individuals who purge may also use laxatives, diuretics, or enemas. While these are not as common as vomiting, many of these products are readily available over-the-counter, and can cause serious medical consequences. Patients with co-morbid insulin-dependent diabetes should also be assessed for inappropriately withholding their insulin. This behavior places them at risk for diabetic ketoacidosis, as well as long-term complications of poorly controlled blood sugars, and may necessitate inpatient care for stabilization and safety. The severity rating for BN is based on compensatory episodes per week (mild: 1–3; moderate: 4–7; severe: 8–13; extreme: ≥14) but the clinician is given freedom to increase the severity rating given the levels of other symptoms.

BED is characterized primarily by episodes of recurrent binge eating (at least once per week for 3 months) without compensatory purging. The binge episodes must be associated with three or more of the following: eating rapidly; eating until uncomfortably full; eating large amounts despite lack of hunger; eating in solitude to avoid embarrassment; and/or feelings of disgust or guilt following the episode. If the individual who is bingeing is also underweight or is using compensatory purging behaviors following a binge, a diagnosis of AN or BN (respectively) is more appropriate. Although BED is sometimes associated with obesity, not all individuals who are obese have BED, and not all individuals who have BED are obese.

The DSM-IV diagnosis of eating disorders not otherwise specified (EDNOS) was replaced in DSM-5 with OSFED. As with EDNOS, OSFED serves as a diagnosis for individuals who clearly have a clinically impairing eating disturbance but do not meet criteria for another eating disorder. OSFED comprises five example presentations, including atypical AN (all criteria for AN met, except the patient is not low weight); sub-threshold BN (bingeing and/or purging occurs less than once per week or for less than 3 months); sub-threshold BED (bingeing occurs less than once per week or for less than 3 months); purging disorder (purging without binge episodes); and night-eating syndrome (an individual awakens from sleep and consumes food). DSM-5 also includes a diagnosis called unspecified feeding or eating disorder (UFED) for instances in which there is insufficient information to confer a specific eating-disorder diagnosis, but symptoms are clearly causing distress or impairment.

Medical and other psychiatric causes of poor appetite and weight or vomiting should be excluded with appropriate history, examination, and diagnostic tests. Medical illnesses that the practitioner needs to differentiate from eating disorders include endocrinologic disorders (such as diabetes mellitus and hyperthyroidism), brain tumors, cancer, occult infections, and multiple GI disorders, such as celiac disease, peptic ulcer disease, and gastritis. Moreover, because eating disorders are frequently co-morbid with mood and anxiety disorders, personality disorders, and substance use disorders, a complete assessment of mental status and psychiatric history should be conducted. Finally, a careful assessment of suicide risk is essential.

Weight Assessment

Weight assessment is not only integral to the diagnosis of AN but it is also necessary for therapeutic management across the spectrum of eating disorders. Weight and height should be measured during the initial assessment. Because some patients may attempt to disguise a low weight by adding weight through jewelry, clothing, and hidden items, weights should be measured with the patient in a hospital gown only. If water loading is suspected, patients can be asked to void prior to weighing; urine specific gravity may be informative if it is relatively low.

BMI is the clinical standard for weight assessment for adults. The formula is as follows:

$$\text{BMI} = \text{height (in meters)} \div \text{weight (in kilograms)}^2$$

For children, the BMI generally increases with age, and therefore BMI centiles are a more accurate measure. They can be assessed by measuring height and weight and plotting on the U.S. Centers for Disease Control and Prevention BMI-for-age charts.[28]

INTERVENTIONS

Although acute treatment of medical complications, nutritional compromise, and associated acute psychiatric symptoms can begin in the general hospital setting, treatment is likely to eventually require transfer to a psychiatric specialty or outpatient setting. Therefore, the consulting psychiatrist has a critical role in establishing a diagnosis and the level of severity to guide inpatient management, disposition, and a comprehensive care plan. Additional potentially useful interventions in a general hospital setting include: (1) education of the clinical staff caring for the patient; (2) patient engagement in treatment and psychoeducation; (3) identification of referral resources for either specialized inpatient eating disorder care or for an outpatient multidisciplinary clinical care team; (4) implementation of behavioral strategies to control symptoms, when appropriate; (5) initiation of pharmacotherapy, when appropriate; and (6) implementation of a plan for nutritional rehabilitation, as appropriate. Education of the clinical staff on the general medical or pediatric service is essential to ensure that a thorough targeted work-up is complete, and that nutritional and medical complications of restrictive eating, binge eating, and inappropriate compensatory behaviors are addressed.

Engaging the Reluctant Patient

For the patient who is unable to admit the extent of the symptoms or to acknowledge that symptoms are problematic, gentle confrontation is recommended. This may include psychoeducation about clinical signs that are worrisome, availability and efficacy of treatment, and the substantial risks of not pursuing treatment.

Additionally, collaboratively creating a cognitive-behavioral formulation that highlights the predictable and self-defeating links among eating-disordered behaviors can be illuminating for patients who perceive symptoms as disparate or uncontrollable. Many patients believe their symptoms have an important primary gain (controlling their weight) and unduly base their self-worth on their body shape, weight, and appearance. Sometimes, an initial experience of positive social feedback and self-efficacy is so reinforcing that it induces them to continue to lose weight. Not infrequently, the restrictive eating gives way to bouts of binge eating, which in turn can segue to purging and other inappropriate compensatory behaviors. This binge eating can be further complicated by a preoccupation with food—so extreme that many patients report a constant distraction concerning the tally of calories they have consumed or that they plan to consume during the day. Thus, a viciously self-reinforcing cycle ensues.

Engaging a patient in eating-disorder treatment can be challenging because the patient may perceive this as a threat to all the gains he or she experiences from the symptoms. For instance, many patients experience distraction and emotional numbing as a result of their restrictive and binge-pattern eating and purging behaviors that can serve as a self-soothing mechanism and coping strategy for individuals who cannot readily access higher-level defenses. Moreover, most patients are convinced that they will gain weight if they establish normal dietary patterns, and extremely low weight AN patients often manifest cognitive inflexibility that can undermine insight and therapeutic engagement.

For general hospital inpatients reluctant to discuss or allow treatment of their symptoms, engaging the patient around mutually identified goals and identifying key points of leverage are key strategies. Even if the patient provides a seemingly off-target reply (e.g., an AN patient hopes to get her parents "off her back," or a BN patient would like to lose weight), the stated rationale can prompt the development of specific goals with which to ally with the patient, such as autonomy or health. In addition to informing the patient and family about medical complications and risks associated with the disorder, concrete evidence about adverse health impacts of the disorder can be presented as a strategy to motivate treatment engagement.

When appropriate, clinicians should work collaboratively with parents, teachers, coaches, or school administration to identify incentives for patients to meet therapeutic goals. For example, patients may be required to meet specific clinical benchmarks to be eligible to participate in school or extracurricular activities.

Especially when motivation or treatment adherence is in question or risk of decompensation is high, a treatment agreement specifying interim goals and the patient's responsibilities provides clarity to the team and the patient. For example, the patient may be asked to agree to attend all appointments, to allow weighing and laboratory work at intervals specified by the team, and to consent to communication among all members of the treatment team. In addition, parameters to be used in considering a higher level of care should be specified, so that if a patient's weight is unstable, all team members and the patient are in agreement about the point at which an increased intensity of care (e.g., adding a group, adding medication, or being admitted to an inpatient unit for eating disorders) is necessary. To be maximally therapeutic, non-negotiable outcomes—such as inpatient hospitalization at low body weight—should have a sound rationale, be consistently implemented throughout treatment, not take the patient by surprise, and provide clear opportunities for the patient to prevent implementation by altering undesirable behaviors.[29] Of course, involuntary hospitalization may be necessary when patients are at imminent risk for self-harm or are unable to care for themselves (e.g., as evidenced by ongoing untreated serious medical complications).

Considerations in Initiating Treatment

Goals of hospitalization for those with eating disorders are guided by the severity and duration of the disease as well as its medical complications. Initial goals generally encompass stabilization of medical parameters and behavioral symptoms, safety and containment (when appropriate), and a plan for nutritional rehabilitation.

A behavioral protocol can be implemented on a general medical or pediatric service to promote re-feeding or control inappropriate compensatory behaviors. Some services have standardized protocols, and in others, the consulting psychiatrist and staff can develop a plan to meet the needs of individual patients. A description of such protocols is beyond the scope of this chapter, but they include medical and nutritional monitoring and may also include supervised regularly scheduled meals, expectations for participation in meal selection with a nutritionist, expectations for duration of meals, restrictions of bathroom trips within an hour of meals, privileges (e.g., leaving the floor) contingent on meeting a dietary plan and weight goals, and restriction of physical activity.

Some patients who have been hospitalized on a medical service because of complications of their eating disorder will benefit from, or require transfer to, an inpatient setting for specialty psychiatric care. Others who are well stabilized, or for whom the eating disorder was an incidental finding, will be discharged home for outpatient care. Table 17-1 shows criteria for inpatient-level care of patients with an eating disorder.

Generally, treatment benefits from the inclusion of the primary care clinician, a mental health clinician, and, if needed, a psychiatrist and/or dietitian. A clear demarcation of responsibilities and roles (e.g., who will monitor weight, if necessary, or who will monitor frequency of purging behaviors that may require medical monitoring) and frequent and open communication about the treatment plan, progress, and concerns is optimal. Clinicians should strongly encourage patient consent to communicate all clinical information relevant to treatment planning among members of the team and should carefully scrutinize how exceptions will have an impact on treatment. Because splitting and miscommunication are both strong possibilities in such treatment situations, the team should make every effort to reach a consensus about the treatment plan and contingencies for changes depending on patient progress or difficulties and should present a unified front to the patient.

When evaluating an ongoing treatment or the development of a new treatment plan, clinicians should bear in mind that medical, nutritional, and psychological goals are integral to treatment; sometimes, progress with psychological symptoms is predicated on medical and nutritional

TABLE 17-1 Clinical Signs and Criteria Warranting Inpatient-Level Care to Stabilize or Treat an Eating Disorder

DOMAIN	GENERAL SYMPTOM[a]	EXAMPLE[b]
Weight	Substantially low weight for height and age Rapidly falling weight	<75% to 85% expected body weight for height and age
Behavioral	Acute food or water refusal Episodes of bingeing and purging of very high and/or escalating frequency Compensatory behaviors likely to result in acute and severe medical complications	Bingeing and/or vomiting multiple times per day resulting in social or occupational impairment and/or serious medical complications; inappropriate withholding of insulin
Other medical compromise	Abnormal vital signs reflecting nutritional compromise Severe medical complications	Severe hematemesis Severe neutropenia and/or thrombocytopenia Severe hypokalemia Uncontrolled type I diabetes Syncope
Psychiatric co-morbidity and risk of self-harm	Substantial risk of self-harm or suicide Co-morbid psychiatric illness resulting in safety risk or seriously undermining treatment Inability to adhere to treatment plan that will sustain minimal level of safety	Co-morbid substance use escalating in the setting of treatment for the eating disorder
Treatment-related	Lack of clinically meaningful progress in an outpatient setting resulting in social or occupational impairment or medical risk Necessity of close supervision to maintain symptom control Previously agreed-on criterion for hospitalization based on patient history	An adolescent's low weight poses risk for decreased peak bone mass or short stature Sustained or persistent inability to eat without supervision or to abstain from intractable purging after food intake Reaching a threshold weight at which the patient repeatedly has rapidly deteriorated

[a]These criteria may be sufficient but do not necessarily need to be present to indicate inpatient care.
[b]Weight, vital signs, metabolic, and other parameters for hospitalization are best interpreted in the context of the patient's overall health, medical and psychiatric history, support systems, and engagement in treatment.

stabilization. Similarly, if psychological symptoms are not addressed, medical complications and nutritional compromise can recur. With respect to the mental health component of treatment, psychosocial therapies and pharmacotherapies both have a role, but the former appear to be more effective. Thus, pharmacotherapy is more appropriately used as an adjunctive treatment to psychotherapy or when access to psychotherapy is otherwise limited.

Medical Intervention for Eating Disorders

Medical complications of eating disorders are common, can affect every organ system, and are potentially severe and even lethal (see Table 17-1). Complications are associated with behaviors that can occur across the spectrum of eating disorders. Medical therapeutic considerations for the comprehensive care of patients with BN, and patients with AN and OSFED who purge, include a plan to monitor for and address the most common and serious medical complications, including hypokalemia and cardiac dysrhythmias.

Poor nutrition associated with a restricted diet and a low body weight in AN can result in serious medical complications. Fluid and electrolyte disturbances require immediate attention. Potassium losses occur in the setting of chronic purging behaviors associated with either BN or AN (e.g., induced vomiting, laxative abuse, diuretic abuse). Laxative abuse results in diarrhea accompanied by cramping abdominal pain and, at times, rectal pain. Fecal electrolyte losses can be very high as the daily output increases considerably. Large amounts of sodium may be lost, but hyponatremia is uncommon because of the concomitant loss of water. The resulting picture of dehydration with hypotension, tachycardia, postural dizziness, and syncope needs to be addressed acutely, usually with intravenous (IV) fluids and electrolytes. Chronic deficiency of sodium and water may lead to increased renin secretion and secondary hyperaldosteronism that may then become autonomous, persisting after the laxatives are removed, a pseudo-Bartter's syndrome. Hypokalemia, as a result of laxative-related losses and purging, may appear as generalized muscle weakness and lassitude. More profound levels of hypokalemia may be life-threatening with cardiac arrhythmias. Of particular note, hypokalemia can, and often does, appear asymptomatically, so patients with chronic losses through vomiting, laxative abuse, or diuretic abuse must be routinely monitored with serum electrolytes, even in the absence of symptoms. Hyperphosphatemia, hypermagnesemia, and hypocalcemia can also be seen as a result of excessive purging with laxatives and replacement needs to be done to maintain homeostasis and organ function.

Cardiac consequences of AN and BN may be asymptomatic or lethal. It is imperative to obtain vital signs including orthostatic signs as well as a baseline EKG. Dizziness, palpitations, orthostasis, or syncope may herald cardiovascular danger.[30] Myocardial hypotrophy can occur, with reduced left ventricular mass and output.[31] Hypotension occurs early and orthostasis follows, possibly enhanced by volume depletion. Bradycardia is common in patients with AN, and it probably reflects cardiac impairment associated with reduced stroke volume. QT prolongation, can be unrelated to[32] or a consequence of, hypokalemia in AN and BN. Both QT dispersion and QT interval prolongation are predicted by low BMI and weight loss in patients with eating disorders. These electrocardiographic abnormalities require immediate medical intervention because they increase the risk of ventricular arrhythmia and sudden death.[33] Patients who use ipecac to induce vomiting are at risk of a life-threatening cardiomyopathy caused by the emetine in this product.[34]

GI symptoms most commonly seen in BN include bloating, flatulence, constipation, abdominal pain, and nausea. Constipation brought on by dehydration, or by long-term laxative abuse, often responds to stool softeners and to bulk-forming agents. These symptoms are sometimes accompanied by evidence of delayed gastric emptying and intestinal transit time. Although they may resolve with conservative treatment (including nutritional rehabilitation and establishing routine meals), they may also persist and exacerbate cognitive symptoms that maintain the eating disorder. Although GI signs and symptoms are frequently attributed to an eating disorder, primary GI illness should be evaluated in the entire clinical context. Most of the GI symptoms associated with disordered eating improve with conservative management (nutritional rehabilitation).

If motility is stimulated enough with the cathartic laxatives, absorption of nutrients may be impaired because of decreased transit time. Although laxatives may cause changes in the intestine itself, such as melanosis coli from pigment-laden macrophages in the submucosa of the colon secondary to anthraquinones, there does not appear to be any functional consequence to this. However, the preference is to manage frequent complaints of constipation with stool softeners as opposed to cathartic agents (so as not to iatrogenically reproduce the purging behavior, promote caloric loss, or waste potassium). Polyethylene glycol solutions, and other osmotic agents, such as lactulose, are used to ease evacuation.

Osteopenia and osteoporosis are among the most serious clinical concerns accompanying amenorrhea and weight loss in AN. The peak bone mass achieved as a young adult is the major determinant of bone density and fracture risk. AN is associated with markedly reduced bone density, especially at the lumbar spine, but also at the proximal femur and the distal radius. The importance of nutritional factors, lean body mass, and BMI in determining bone mass cannot be overstated. The duration of estrogen deficiency does not determine the severity of the osteopenia, and hormone replacement has not significantly increased bone mineral density in patients with AN,[35] and it may in fact be detrimental in that it creates a false sense of security from the monthly withdrawal bleeding without any tangible benefits to the bone. The primary therapy is weight gain. The most appropriate recommendations include a plan for nutritional rehabilitation, supplementation with 1500 mg/day of calcium and 800 IU/day of vitamin D. If the vitamin D level is low, a higher dose of 50,000 IU can be given weekly for 6 to 12 weeks. DXA scanning at the initial medical assessment of a patient with an eating disorder and at varying intervals every 12 to 24 months can assist in counseling those at high risk for fractures and bone loss.

Dental hygiene in eating-disordered patients with vomiting should also be addressed. Dental erosion and caries in patients with self-induced vomiting may occur because of the effects of gastric acid on teeth enamel. Preventive techniques to protect from further dental erosion include fluoride application and good brushing techniques. Patients who engage in vomiting should routinely be referred for dental care.

The comprehensive care of patients with BED includes addressing the medical co-morbidities and sequelae of the condition. Co-morbidities of BED include disorders associated with excess weight such as an elevated risk of type 2 diabetes, hypertension, cardiovascular disease, hypercholesterolemia, osteoarthritis, sleep apnea, gall bladder disease, and certain malignancies.

TREATMENT OF PATIENTS WITH ANOREXIA NERVOSA

Nutritional Rehabilitation

The most appropriate initial treatment strategy for patients with AN addresses weight restoration. Most patients with eating disorders will recover menses within 6 months of reaching 90% of their ideal body weight.[36] Orthostasis has been observed to remit after several weeks, at about 80% of expected body weight (EBW) in adolescents. However, a return to full health requires restoration of normal weight. Low BMI at referral predicts a poor prognosis[37] and is associated with significantly higher chronicity and mortality for patients with AN.[38] Relapse rises steeply as the percent of EBW at discharge falls, with 100% minimizing immediate relapse and readmission rising rapidly as discharge weight falls to 95%, 90%, and 85% of EBW.

Under-nutrition is also suspected to underlie some of the neurocognitive features of AN that may contribute to poor treatment response. For AN patients without severe nutritional compromise, weight management can begin in the outpatient setting with nutritional counseling and behavioral reinforcement for meeting weight goals.

Patients benefit from nutritional consultation, as they are often overly preoccupied with minor details of nutrition (such as calorie counting or carbohydrate avoidance), and their dietary knowledge may emanate from dubious sources, such as fad diet books or websites. Nutritional counseling can also be framed as an activity to assist judgment and motivation. Especially with underweight patients, establishing a caloric requirement and developing a dietary plan to meet the weight goals that are set are highly useful. Minimally, this plan includes three meals daily to establish expectations of eating in alignment with social norms and nutritional adequacy, and it generally includes snacks or caloric supplements (or both). If a patient is still unable to gain weight (e.g., the patient requires more calories or more help to adhere to the plan or needs to reduce physical activity), the need for additional measures can be assessed.

If patients are severely underweight (e.g., ≤75% of expected body weight), or remain chronically underweight with medical complications, they may require inpatient or partial hospitalization care. Patients may benefit from hospital-level care at a higher percent EBW if they have, for example, ongoing psychosocial stressors, a history of a pattern of rapid decompensation, or medical compromise. An inpatient hospital setting for nutritional rehabilitation offers diagnostic and therapeutic opportunities. For example, it promotes assessment of, and rapid response to, medical complications, and it allows dietary intake to be more carefully monitored, purging and exercise to be controlled, and behavioral reinforcement to be more easily implemented. In addition, if the patient withstands all feeding efforts, nasogastric feedings or parenteral feedings can be considered when there is extreme malnutrition and recalcitrance to treatment. Patients who require inpatient-level care to gain weight, but who recurrently relapse after discharge, may be best served in a residential care setting for an extended period to achieve and stabilize an adequate weight.

Calories should be increased incrementally, but rapidly, to achieve desired weight gains of 1 to 2 pounds weekly for outpatients and 2 to 3 pounds weekly in hospital settings. Caloric requirements for weight restoration vary, but may require up to 4000 calories a day as re-feeding progresses. Approximately 1 g of weight is gained for every five calories in excess of output, so 5000 extra calories beyond maintenance is necessary for a weight gain of 1 kg. Weight gain may occur rapidly at first because of fluid retention and the baseline low metabolic rate.[39] Intake levels usually begin at 30 to 40 kcal/kg (1000 to 1600 kcal/day). As the patient begins to gain weight, metabolic demands increase, and the intake needs to be increased considerably to continue to achieve ongoing weight gain.

Great care needs to be taken during nutritional rehabilitation to anticipate and avoid the re-feeding syndrome, a potentially catastrophic treatment complication that can result in heart failure, delirium, and death in under-nourished patients who are being re-nourished. In this syndrome, the demands that a re-filled circulatory system places on a nutritionally depleted cardiac mass result in cardiovascular collapse. This can be seen whether the nutrition is provided orally, enterally, or parenterally. Patients most at risk are those who are the most under-nourished. Prolonged starvation results in a reduced cardiac mass and output. During re-feeding, ventricular volume returns to normal while left ventricular mass remains reduced, potentially leading to fluid retention and congestive heart failure. Sodium and fluid retention compound this problem. Serum phosphate levels may drop precipitously, leading to depletion of phosphorylated compounds, with impaired energy stores resulting from a decrease in intracellular adenosine triphosphate, and tissue hypoxia secondary to reduced levels of erythrocyte 2,3-diphosphoglycerate. Phosphate depletion, in turn, produces widespread abnormalities, including cardiac arrest and delirium.[40] Potassium and magnesium also become depleted during starvation and upon re-feeding these are deposited intracellularly and serum levels may fall if no supplementation is provided. Although re-feeding syndrome generally emerges during the first 2 weeks of re-feeding, delirium associated with re-feeding can occur even later in the course.

Therefore, nutritional rehabilitation of the severely malnourished patient requires close monitoring for re-feeding syndrome; the greatest caution is required during the first weeks after commencing the nutritional support. Specifically, vital signs and physical examination for signs of edema or congestive heart failure should be followed closely during this period—and daily for at least a week. Some patients develop edema without heart failure and may experience rapid weight gain in the first few days of re-feeding. Phosphorus, magnesium, and serum electrolytes should be closely monitored during at least the first 2 weeks of re-feeding (e.g., it is recommended that this begin within 6 to 8 hours of feeding, continue daily for a week, and then continue at least every other day until the patient is stable). Cardiac telemetry is recommended during the first 2 weeks, and subsequent monitoring for complications of re-feeding should continue until the patient stablizes.[41]

Due to concerns regarding re-feeding syndrome, patients are cautiously re-fed with incremental increases of 200 to 300 kcal/day every 3 to 4 days as tolerated and as determined by individual weight gain. As patients near their target weight, they frequently require large amount of calories, upward of 3000 calories/day. Energy needs may be greater in young, growing adolescents. Supplements may be required. Sodium at 1 mmol/kg per day; potassium at 4 mmol/kg per day at least; and magnesium at 0.6 mmol/kg per day should be given. Phosphate, up to 1 mmol/kg per day intravenously, and oral supplements up to 100 mmol/day can be given to try to avoid the hypophosphatemia associated with re-feeding. Extra calcium may need to be given because hypocalcemia may occur during phosphate supplementation. Thiamine should be provided because acute thiamine deficiency can occur with re-feeding.[42] Folic acid, riboflavin, ascorbic acid, pyridoxine, and the fat-soluble vitamins A, D, E, and K should be supplemented as well.[43] Trace elements, including selenium, may also be deficient. A good rule of thumb is to provide a multivitamin with minerals on a daily basis.

Psychological Therapies

For adolescents with AN who are underweight but medically stable, manualized family-based treatment (FBT) has the strongest empirical support. This three-phase outpatient treatment spans 20 sessions over approximately 1 year and is based on the premise that the patient cannot control his or her symptoms, so the parents must temporarily claim responsibility for re-nourishment.[44] In phase one, parents are asked to correct the patient's malnutrition by providing an energy-dense meal plan and empathic but firm encouragement for increased calorie consumption. After steady weight gain, food choices are gradually returned to the patient during phase two, and the family is invited to explore the ways in which the AN has affected family dynamics. In the final phase, when the patient has reached a stable weight, therapy focuses on orchestrating a smooth return to normal adolescent development. As with many behavioral therapies, early change is critical to FBT success. In one study, adolescents who gained at least 1.8 kg by session 4 reached a significantly higher percent expected body weight at the end of treatment (99% vs 93% EBW), and exhibited significantly greater remission rates (46%

vs 11%), compared with those who gained less weight in the first 4 weeks.[45] Longitudinal follow-up studies suggest that approximately three-quarters of patients receiving FBT achieve good outcome (normal weight and menstruation) at 5-year[46] follow-up.

There are fewer empirical findings to guide psychological treatment selection in adults with AN. When distinct individual therapies are compared in randomized controlled trials (RCTs), treatments produce only modest weight gain, and many patients remain symptomatic. For example, in one study of adults with AN, focal psychodynamic therapy, enhanced cognitive-behavioral therapy (CBT), and optimized treatment-as-usual (i.e., non-manualized psychotherapy and medical monitoring) all produced small end-of-treatment weight gains of 0.73, 0.69, and 0.69 BMI points, respectively.[47] Similarly, a study comparing the Maudsley Model of Anorexia Nervosa Treatment for Adults (MANTRA) with specialist supportive clinical management (SSCM, a combination of supportive therapy and case management) did not identify any difference in weight gain (1.06 BMI points for MANTRA, and 0.80 for SSCM) between groups.[48] Another study found that adults with AN who received enhanced CBT gained an average of 2.77 BMI points, but that study lacked a comparison group.[49]

Modest results from individual therapies for adult AN have prompted some treatment researchers to change therapeutic approach or alter therapy goals. Uniting Couples (in the treatment of) Anorexia Nervosa (UCAN) is a couples-based intervention in which the patient's partner supports the patient in eating appropriate meals and snacks and encourages the patient to restore weight, but in a less authoritative and more developmentally appropriate way than would parents in youth FBT.[50] Results of an ongoing RCT comparing UCAN with family supportive therapy have not yet been published. Given that patients with longstanding AN are often reluctant to engage in treatment, a recent study evaluated the efficacy of a specialized form of CBT focusing on quality of life rather than weight restoration for patients with AN who had been ill longer than 7 years. Results indicated that patients who received quality-of-life-focused CBT scored significantly higher post-treatment on social adjustment and lower on eating disorder psychopathology compared to patients who received SSCM. However, neither group gained significant weight.[51]

Pharmacologic Management

Although there is some evidence to support the use of pharmacologic agents for the treatment of BN and BED, pharmacologic management of eating disorders in general, and AN in particular, should be considered as an adjunctive treatment. To date, most efforts to identify pharmacologic agents to treat the primary symptoms of AN have been disappointing, as treatment study trials for AN are characterized by small sample sizes, poor response rates, and attrition. As such, there is insufficient empirical support to recommend any single pharmacologic agent for AN.

There have been eight small RCTs that have evaluated the efficacy of the use of atypical antipsychotics for the treatment of AN, including olanzapine, risperidone, and amisulpride. Results from a meta-analysis combining the data from these studies reveal that when compared with placebo, use of atypical antipsychotic medications was associated with a non-significant increase in BMI.[52] In addition, the use of these agents had no effect on drive for thinness or body dissatisfaction and were even associated with an increase in anxiety and overall eating disorder symptoms.[53] As such, available data do not support a recommendation for the first-line or routine use of atypical antipsychotics in AN.

Empirical support for efficacy of serotonin selective re-uptake inhibitors (SSRIs) in the treatment of AN is also limited. Fluoxetine and citalopram are the only two SSRIs that have been tested in RCTs for the treatment of AN, with largely negative findings. Citalopram may have some efficacy in improving depression, obsessive-compulsive symptoms, and impulsivity in this population.[54] Fluoxetine has been studied for stabilization in weight-recovered patients with AN in two RCTs. One of these demonstrated some efficacy (when adjunctive to elective psychotherapy) at a dosage of 20 to 60 mg/day,[55] whereas the other failed to show efficacy compared with placebo when added to CBT (at a target dosage of 60 mg/day).[56] Whereas fluoxetine may have a role in stabilizing weight-recovered patients, it does not appear effective in addressing AN symptoms in underweight patients.

Other classes of pharmacologic agents have also been studied in AN. One small RCT from the early 1980s revealed average greater weight gain on lithium than placebo in the treatment of AN. Given the risk of lithium toxicity in patients with AN who may have reduced lithium clearance as a result of sodium and fluid depletion, the use of lithium in AN is not recommended.[57] In one small crossover study of the use of dronabinol in patients with AN, adjunctive use was superior to placebo for weight gain, though it did not result in any changes as compared with placebo on Eating Disorder Inventory-2 (EDI-2) scores.[58]

AN is frequently co-morbid with other psychiatric illnesses or symptoms that can benefit from pharmacologic management, but may have limited efficacy in severely underweight patients. Agents that promote weight loss or diminish appetite should be avoided if possible. In addition, when agents that can prolong the QT interval or cause orthostatic hypotension are deemed essential, they should be implemented with extra caution along with appropriate monitoring and instruction to the patient. Finally, medications that promote appetite or weight gain can have the inadvertent effect of triggering binge episodes and should therefore be used judiciously—and with full transparency to the patient—if indicated for other symptom targets for patients with AN.

TREATMENT OF PATIENTS WITH BULIMIA NERVOSA

Psychotherapy, with appropriate medical monitoring and intervention, is the first-line treatment for BN. Among psychotherapeutic interventions studied, CBT has the strongest evidence supporting its efficacy.

Psychological Therapies

Enhanced CBT (CBT-E) is a manualized outpatient therapy designed for use across eating disorder diagnoses.[59] For patients who are medically stable and not underweight (e.g., those with BN), CBT is designed to span 20 sessions over 4 stages. In Stage 1, patients are introduced to a model in which shape and weight concerns and strict dietary restraint promote binge eating and purging in a self-perpetuating cycle. The patient is asked to self-monitor intake to identify individualized triggers for binge eating and purging. The therapist assists the patient in developing a schedule of regular eating (three meals and two snacks daily), and uses the information gained in the self-monitoring records to help the patient identify alternative pleasurable activities to distract from urges to binge. Stage 2 involves taking stock of progress and identifying maintaining mechanisms to be addressed in Stage 3. In Stage 3, the therapist assists the patient in reducing factors that maintain eating disorder psychopathology, particularly body image disturbance. Specifically, the therapist may assist the patient in reducing body-checking and avoidance behaviors that exacerbate body dissatisfaction, and cultivating alternative aspects of self-evaluation other than shape and weight. In Stage 4 the patient develops a relapse-prevention plan by identifying stressful situations that may trigger future symptoms, and problem-solving potential solutions.

An RCT comparing CBT-E to wait-list control for individuals with BN or OSFED found that over half the sample endorsed eating-disorder features within standard deviation (SD) of the community mean at a 60-week follow-up.[60] At the start of treatment, 63.6% of the sample was engaging in binge eating and 62.3% in self-induced vomiting. By post-treatment, the proportion had reduced to just 33.8% and 36.4%, respectively. Remission rates for CBT are even more impressive when compared with other therapies. One study comparing 5 months of CBT-E to 2 years of psychoanalytic psychotherapy found binge/purge remission rates nearly 3 times higher in the CBT group (44%) than the psychoanalytic psychotherapy group (15%) at the end of treatment.[61] As in FBT, early change is critical to treatment success. In one study, patients who exhibited at least a 65% decrease in purge frequency by week 4 of enhanced CBT were significantly more likely to remit by the end of treatment.[62]

Although CBT-E is clearly the therapy of choice for BN, clinical judgment is required for those who do not respond to CBT or do not wish to participate. With regard to alternative psychotherapeutic modalities, interpersonal psychotherapy is as effective but generally takes longer to achieve results than does CBT, thus increasing the length of time the patient is exposed to bulimic symptoms.[63] Other therapies that have some empirical support for BN include integrative cognitive-affective therapy,[64] dialectical behavioral therapy,[65] and, for adolescents, FBT.[66]

Pharmacologic Management

Several pharmacotherapies have modest short-term efficacy for BN, but remission rates are low and medication management is generally considered as an adjunctive strategy.[67] Fluoxetine is the only FDA-approved agent for the treatment of BN, and the use of other agents is therefore considered off-label.

The decision to augment a psychosocial therapy with medication in the treatment of BN hinges on co-morbid illness, severity, past response to medication, patient preference, and patient commitment to adherence to a medication regimen. Choice of medication is guided by side effect profile, history of response, and expense, because the data are insufficient to support greater efficacy for any particular agent. However, data do support consecutive trials if a patient does not respond to the first agent. If an agent is prescribed, it is essential to ensure that the dosing schedule is arranged so that the drug is sufficiently absorbed before the purging behavior.

Fluoxetine 60 mg/day is the first-line pharmacologic agent for BN. It has shown efficacy in the reduction of symptoms of BN compared with placebo in two large RCTs, is generally well tolerated among individuals with BN, and shows efficacy in maintenance therapy over the course of a year.[68] Monotherapy with fluoxetine has also been found more effective than placebo for treatment of BN in a primary care setting.[69]

Sertraline was found to be effective in reducing the number of binge eating and purging episodes among patients with BN in one small RCT.[70] Fluvoxamine was evaluated in two clinical trials with inconsistent findings. One of these trials reported grand mal seizures among some study participants on active drug, although causal association is unknown.[71,72] As such, fluvoxamine should be used with caution in patients with BN and should not be considered first-line.

Other classes of agents also show promise. Topiramate was found to significantly reduce symptoms when compared with placebo in two 10-week RCTs, in doses up to 250 mg/day in one study and 400 mg/day in the other.[73,74] In addition, although naltrexone is not in routine clinical use, one study demonstrated that it had short-term efficacy at 200 to 300 mg/day versus standard dosages (50 to 100 mg/day) for patients with BN who had not previously responded to antidepressant therapy.[75] Higher doses of naltrexone, however, were associated with significant elevation in hepatic transaminases and should, therefore, be used cautiously in patients with BN. One RCT demonstrated short-term efficacy of ondansetron (24 mg/day divided into six doses) in severely symptomatic BN.[76] Similarly, a small RCT suggested efficacy of flutamide for reduction of binge episodes (but not vomiting) in BN. However, given limited support for its clinical use and the associated risk of teratogenicity and hepatotoxicity with this agent, it cannot be recommended for the management of BN.[77]

Several agents should not be used for the treatment of BN. The risk of serious adverse events associated with both bupropion (seizures) and monoamine oxidase inhibitors (spontaneous hypertensive crises) in patients with BN contraindicates their use for the management of BN.[78–81] The use of these medications to manage co-morbid depression in the setting of BN is relatively contraindicated as well and warrants careful consideration of risk-to-benefit ratios in the context of each patient's individualized needs.

TREATMENT OF PATIENTS WITH BINGE-EATING DISORDER

Patients with BED are often quite willing to seek and accept treatment because of their high levels of distress and their eagerness to combat the co-morbid obesity (if present). Because BED is frequently co-morbid with obesity, patients often seek treatment for weight reduction specifically rather than reduction in eating disorder symptoms.

Psychological Therapies

CBT has the strongest empirical support for BED. Because BN and BED share clinical features and CBT-E is meant to be transdiagnostic, CBT for BED is quite similar to that for BN, featuring psychoeducation, self-monitoring, normalization of eating, reducing the extent to which self-evaluation is based on shape and weight, and relapse prevention. In an RCT comparing CBT to pharmacotherapy for BED, 61% of patients who received CBT plus placebo and 50% of patients who received CBT plus fluoxetine abstained from binge eating after treatment. Both CBT treatments were superior to fluoxetine (22%) or placebo (26%) alone.[82] CBT can also be delivered in a brief guided self-help format with promising results.[83] Unfortunately, despite efficacy in the reduction of binge eating, CBT is not associated with significant weight loss in obese patients with BED,[84] prompting researchers to evaluate the efficacy of targeting weight loss and binge eating simultaneously. In one study comparing psychological therapies for BED, guided self-help CBT and interpersonal therapy (IPT) were more effective than behavioral weight loss treatment (BWL) in reducing binge eating at 2-year follow-up.[85] Although BWL patients lost significantly more weight than the other two groups immediately post-treatment, there were no differences in BMI at the 2-year follow-up. Furthermore, in another study comparing group CBT and group BWL, CBT produced a greater reduction in binge eating (44.4% vs 37.8% post-treatment and 51.1% vs 35.6% at 12 month follow-up). BWL was superior at producing short-term weight loss. Sequencing CBT and BWL did not produce any further benefit.[86]

As in behavioral therapies for the other eating disorders, early change is integral to treatment success in CBT for BED. In one trial, patients who exhibited rapid response (defined as at least a 70% reduction in binge frequency in the first 4 weeks of treatment) to CBT-guided self-help were significantly more likely to achieve remission at the end of treatment, compared with patients who did not show rapid response.[87] Interestingly, rapid and non-rapid responders did equally well in IPT, highlighting the possibility of offering IPT as a second-line treatment for patients who do not rapidly respond to CBT.

Pharmacologic Management

BED is more commonly associated with obesity as compared with the other EDs. This association with obesity informs pharmacologic management, as clinicians should assess the effects medications have on appetite and weight control, while also targeting binge episodes and other co-morbid psychiatric conditions. As a result, many agents, including stimulants, anti-obesity agents, antidepressants, and anti-epileptic drugs have been studied in the treatment of BED.

Lisdexamfetamine dimesylate (50–70 mg/day) is the only FDA-approved medication for BED. Three large RCTs found that lisdexamfetamine dimesylate led to fewer binge episodes per week and led to a decrease in obsessive-compulsive binge eating behaviors as compared with placebo.[88] The safety profile and tolerability of lisdexamfetamine dimesylate in this population was consistent with previous findings of adults with ADHD. Given the risk of potential recreational abuse and/or diversion, this agent should be used with caution in individuals with a history of a substance use disorder.

The use of anticonvulsants in the treatment of BED reveals some promising findings. In a multi-center RCT, topiramate (with dosing titrated from 25 mg/day over a period of 8 weeks to a maximum tolerated dose, up to 400 mg/day) reduced BMI, binge days, binge episodes, resulted in greater weight loss, and led to remission in 58% of participants in adults with BED and co-morbid obesity.[89] An additional 21-week RCT demonstrated that, in combination with CBT, topiramate (with dosing gradually titrated upward as tolerated from 25 mg/day to a maximum of 300 mg/day) enhanced the efficacy of CBT with regards to rate of weight change and binge eating remission.[90] Some patients do not tolerate the side effects (impaired cognition, paresthesia, taste perversion) of topiramate. In a single-center RCT, zonisamide (with flexible dosing between 100–600 mg/day) was superior to placebo at reducing binge frequency and at inducing weight loss, though it was poorly tolerated.[91]

SSRIs and SNRIs have been studied in several RCTs as an adjunctive therapy or monotherapy for BED. Of these, sertraline (flexible dose of 50 to 200 mg/day) and atomoxetine 40 to 120 mg/day have each shown efficacy for the reduction of BED symptoms compared with placebo in one RCT.[92,93] Data on other SSRIs cannot support a general recommendation for their efficacy in the treatment of BED. Although one RCT demonstrated efficacy of citalopram, the study used a mean dosage in excess of current FDA recommendations for this drug.[94] Fluvoxamine was not found to be more effective than placebo in an intention-to-treat analysis as part of a multi-center RCT nor in a second single-center RCT after 9 weeks.[95,96] In aggregate, RCT data evaluating fluoxetine do not support its efficacy in the treatment of BED either as a monotherapy or adjunctive therapy with CBT.[97] Duloxetine (mean dose 78.7 mg/day) was found to be superior to placebo in another RCT in reducing the weekly frequency of binge eating days and binge eating episodes, global severity of BED symptoms, and global severity of depressive symptoms.[98] In another RCT evaluating bupropion (300 mg/day) against placebo, there was no significant difference in reducing the frequency of binge eating.[99] Although RCTs evaluating the SNRI, sibutramine, were positive for reducing binge-eating and promoting weight loss as compared with placebo, it has since been taken off the market due to safety concerns.

Two RCTs evaluating orlistat, a pancreatic lipase inhibitor, in the treatment of patients with comorbid BED and obesity do not support that it is effective in sustaining a reduction of binge eating, although it is associated with promoting greater weight loss as compared to placebo or dietary modifications alone.[100,101]

SUMMARY

At the Massachusetts General Hospital, and in many general hospital settings, patients with eating disorders frequently present with a serious, chronic, medically complicated, or co-morbid illness. For patients with previously unidentified or untreated eating disorders, an inpatient admission can present opportunities to coordinate a multidisciplinary team and provide crucial psychoeducation. Inpatient assessment should ascertain the scope and severity of cognitive and behavioral symptoms associated with the eating disorder as well as other psychiatric co-morbidities. Assessment of nutritional compromise and medical complications is also essential to therapeutic planning. Interventions typically include assisting the medical team to complete an appropriate diagnostic work-up and address potential medical and nutritional complications as well as develop a plan for any behavioral interventions to be implemented during the admission and beyond.

REFERENCES

Access the reference list online at https://expertconsult.inkling.com/.

18

Pain Patients

Shamim H. Nejad, M.D.
Menekse Alpay, M.D.

OVERVIEW

Of all human experience, pain is, as long as it lasts, the most absorbing; it is the only human experience that when it comes to an end, automatically confers a sense of relief and joy. Moreover, by its very nature it is solitary. Despite its intensity and its unequalled power over mind and body, pain can be difficult to recall once it subsides.[1]

The International Association for the Study of Pain (IASP) has defined pain as "an unpleasant sensory and emotional experience associated with actual or potential tissue damage or described in terms of such damage."[2,3] This definition recognizes the fact that pain has both an acute nociceptive aspect and an emotional-affective dimension; these factors suggest that psychiatrists can have a significant role in the treatment of the pain patient. Conceptualizing pain in this manner underscores the fact that pain is an important and complicated sensation, one that may present in a multitude of ways.

In this chapter, the pathophysiology of pain, along with common pain syndromes and terminology are reviewed. In addition, the role of the psychiatric consultant along with psychiatric assessment of the pain patient will be discussed. Furthermore, general principles of pain therapy, including medications commonly used for symptomatic pain management, as well as approaches to the treatment of pain behavior are outlined.

PATHOPHYSIOLOGY OF PAIN

To understand pain one needs to know about the pathophysiology of nociception and to realize that the threshold, intensity, quality, time course, and perceived location of pain are determined by CNS mechanisms.[3] For example, neurosurgeons have shown that interruption of the specific pain pathways often does not eliminate pain; numbness does not confer analgesia. Peripheral nerve damage may result in changes in the receptive fields and recruitment of neurons at multiple levels of the nervous system (from the dorsal horn to the brainstem, and to the thalamus and cortex). Somatic therapies directed only at nociceptive input may be ineffective.[4]

Detection of noxious stimuli (i.e., nociception) starts with the activation of peripheral nociceptors (somatic pain) or with the activation of nociceptors in bodily organs (visceral pain). Somatic pain is usually well localized, attributable to certain structures or areas, and described as stabbing, aching, or throbbing. In contrast, visceral pain may be poorly localized, not necessarily attributable to the involved organ (i.e., as is the case with referred pain), and is characteristically described as dull and crampy.

Tissue injury stimulates the nociceptors by the liberation of prostaglandins, arachidonic acid, histamine, and bradykinin. Subsequently, axons transmit the pain signal to the spinal cord (to cell bodies in the dorsal root ganglia; Figure 18-1).

Three different types of axons are involved in the transmission of a painful stimulus from the skin to the dorsal horn. A-β fibers are the largest and most heavily myelinated fibers that transmit awareness of light touch. A-δ fibers and C fibers are the primary nociceptive afferents. A-δ fibers are 2–5 μm in diameter and are thinly myelinated. They conduct immediate, rapid, sharp, and brief pain (first pain) with a velocity of 20 m/second. C fibers are 0.2–1.5 μm in diameter and are unmyelinated. They conduct prolonged, burning, and unpleasant pain (second pain) at a speed of 0.5 m/second. A-δ and C fibers enter the dorsal root and ascend or descend one to three segments before synapsing with neurons in the lateral spinothalamic tract (substantia gelatinosa in the gray matter).

Substance P, an 11-amino-acid polypeptide, considered to be a major pain neurotransmitter, is released from the fibers at many of these synapses. Capsaicin, which is extracted from red hot peppers, inhibits nociception by inhibiting substance P. Inhibition of nociception in the dorsal horn is functionally quite important. Stimulation of the A-δ fibers not only excites some neurons but also inhibits others. This inhibition of nociception through A-δ fiber stimulation may explain effects of acupuncture and transcutaneous electrical nerve stimulation (TENS). The lateral spinothalamic tract crosses the midline and ascends toward the thalamus. At the level of the brainstem more than half of this tract synapses in the reticular activating system (in an area called the *spinoreticular tract*), in the limbic system, and in other brainstem regions (including centers for autonomic nervous system). Another site of projections at this level is the periaqueductal gray (PAG; Figure 18-2), which plays an important role in the brain's endogenous analgesia system. After synapsing in the thalamic nuclei, pain fibers project to the somatosensory cortex, located posterior to the Sylvian fissure in the parietal lobe (Brodmann's areas 1, 2, and 3).[5]

Developments in imaging technology have been helpful in understanding the relationship between pain pathways

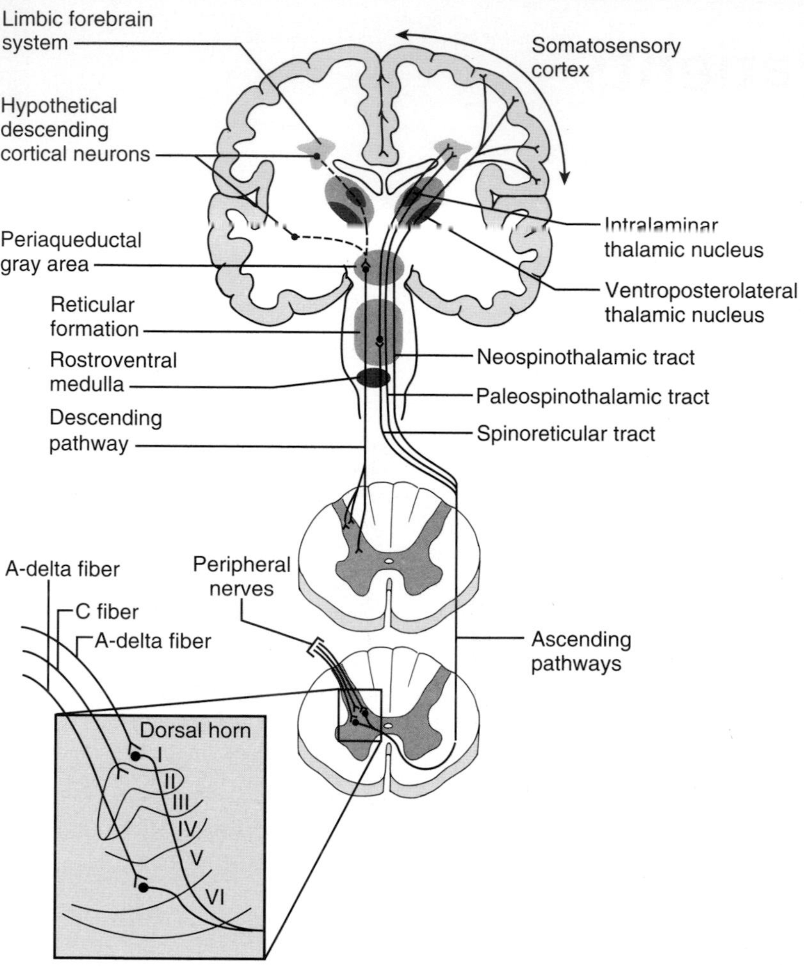

Figure 18-1. Schematic diagram of neurologic pathways for pain perception. *(From Hyman SH, Cassem NH:* Pain. *In: Rubenstein E, Federman DD, eds.* Scientific American medicine: current topics in medicine. Subsection II. *New York, Scientific American; 1989. Originally from* Psychiatry Update and Board Preparation, *Stern TA, Herman JB, (eds). McGraw-Hill, 2004.)*

and cortical and limbic areas. These findings may help explain the relationship between emotions, cognition, and pain modulation that we observe in clinical practice as heightened pain perception in depressed patients and high rates of depression in those with chronic pain. Functional imaging studies utilizing both functional MRI (fMRI) and positron emission tomography (PET) study have shown that acute traumatic nociceptive pain activates the hypothalamus and the PAG in addition to the prefrontal cortex (PFC), insular cortex, anterior cingulate cortex (ACC), posterior parietal cortex, primary motor/somatosensory areas, supplementary motor area (SMA), thalamus, and cerebellum.[6] Additionally, functional imaging studies have helped clinicians understand cognitive and emotional modulation of pain perception. Researchers have shown that with hypnotic suggestion the activity in the ACC is dependent on the intensity of the suggestion (i.e., same stimulus with the suggestion of "highly unpleasant" induces significantly more ACC activation than when suggestions are less unpleasant).[7,8] In another study, when subjects were distracted during a painful stimulus, pain perception was attenuated in somatosensory regions and the PAG.[9] The short-acting opioid, remifentanil, as well as placebo analgesia, have been shown to activate the ACC, which is rich in opioid receptors.[10] It is of interest that analgesia induced by both opioids and placebos was reversed with the opioid antagonist naloxone.[11] These findings suggest that cortical areas may exert control over lower brain areas involved in opioid analgesia.[10]

Endogenous analgesic systems involve at least 18 endogenous peptides with opiate-like activity in the CNS (e.g., endorphins, enkephalins, and dynorphins). Different opiate receptors are involved in different effects of opiates.

Mu (μ)-receptors are involved in the regulation of analgesia, respiratory depression, constipation, and miosis. Mu receptors (located in the PAG, rostral ventral medulla, medial thalamus, and dorsal horn of the spinal cord) are the receptors that are mainly responsible for supraspinal analgesia.

Kappa (κ)-receptors are involved in spinal analgesia, sedation, and miosis. They are located in the dorsal horn (spinal analgesia), deep cortical areas, and other locations; pentazocine preferentially acts on these receptors.

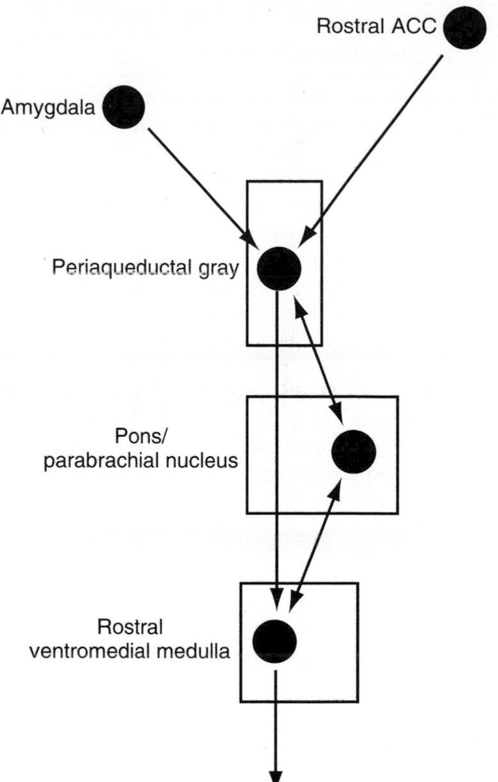

Figure 18-2. Endogenous opioid systems. *(From Petrovic P, Ingvar M: Imaging cognitive modulation of pain processing.* Pain, *95: 1–5, 2002.)*

Delta (δ)-receptors, like κ-receptors, mediate spinal analgesia, hypotension, and miosis. Enkephalins have a higher affinity for these receptors than do opiates. They are located in the limbic system, the dorsal horn, and other locations unrelated to pain. δ-Receptors also mediate psychotomimetic effects (i.e., psychosis) in the CNS. Their effects are not reversed by naloxone, an opiate antagonist.[5]

In terms of anatomic organization, the centers involved in endogenous analgesia include, in addition to PAG, the rostral ACC, amygdala, parabrachial plexus in the pons, and rostral ventromedial medulla.[10]

The descending analgesic pain pathway starts in the PAG (which is rich in endogenous opiates), projects to the rostral ventral medulla, and from there descends through the dorsolateral funiculus of the spinal cord to the dorsal horn. The neurons in the rostral ventral medulla use serotonin to activate endogenous analgesics (enkephalins) in the dorsal horn. This effect inhibits nociception at the level of the dorsal horn since neurons that contain enkephalins synapse with spinothalamic neurons.

Additionally, there are noradrenergic neurons that project from the locus coeruleus (the main noradrenergic center in the CNS) to the dorsal horn and inhibit the response of dorsal horn neurons to nociceptive stimuli. The effect of tricyclic antidepressants (TCAs) and other newer antidepressants is thought to be related to an increase in serotonin and norepinephrine that inhibits nociception at the level of the dorsal horn.[5]

PAIN TERMINOLOGY

Acute pain is usually related to an identifiable injury or to a disease; it is self-limited, and resolves over hours to days or in a time frame that is associated with healing. Acute pain is usually associated with objective autonomic features (e.g., tachycardia, hypertension, diaphoresis, mydriasis, or pallor).

Chronic pain (i.e., pain that persists beyond the normal time of healing or lasts longer than 6 months) may have a neurologic origin, involving lowered firing thresholds for spinal cord cells that modulate pain (triggering pain more easily); anatomic plasticity and recruitment of a wide range of cells in the spinal cord (so that touch or movement causes pain); convergence of cutaneous, vascular, muscle, and joint inputs (where one tissue refers pain to another); or aberrant connections (electric short-circuits between the sympathetic and sensory nerves that produce causalgia). Muscle pains often add to the pain experience. Vascular and other visceral mechanisms share features with neurologic mechanisms, however these mechanisms involved are not mutually exclusive.[12,13] Table 18-1[14–26] summarizes the clinical implications of the mechanisms of chronic pain. Characteristic features include vague descriptions of pain and an inability to describe the pain's timing and localization. Unlike acute pain, chronic pain lacks signs of heightened sympathetic activity. Depression, anxiety, and premorbid personality problems are common in this patient population. Usually the major issue is a lack of motivation and incentive to improve. It is usually helpful to determine the presence of a dermatomal pattern (Figure 18-3), determine the presence of neuropathic pain, and assess pain behavior.

Continuous pain in the terminally ill tends to originate from well-defined tissue damage due to terminal illness (e.g., cancer). It is a variant of nociceptive pain. Stress, sleep deprivation, depression, and premorbid personality problems may exacerbate this pain.

Neuropathic pain is caused by an injured or dysfunctional central or peripheral nervous system; it is manifest by spontaneous, sharp, shooting, or burning pain that is usually distributed along dermatomes (Figure 18-3). Neuropathic pain is often observed in deafferentation pain, complex regional pain syndrome (CRPS), diabetic neuropathy, central pain syndrome, trigeminal neuralgia, or postherpetic neuralgia.

Terms commonly used to describe neuropathic pain include: hyperalgesia (an increased response to stimuli that are normally painful); hyperesthesia (an exaggerated pain response to noxious stimuli, e.g., pressure or heat); allodynia (pain with a stimulus not normally painful, e.g., light touch or cool air); and hyperpathia (pain from a painful stimuli with a delay and a persistence that is distributed beyond the area of stimulation).

CRPS is a syndrome of sympathetically maintained pain, or pain in an extremity that is mediated by sympathetic overactivity. The syndrome is usually caused by injury; however, the cause is unknown in approximately 10% of cases. Any type of trauma, such as a sprain, a fracture, or a contusion, may cause it; iatrogenic causes include amputation, lesion resection, myelography, and intramuscular (IM) injections. CRPS may be disease-related (e.g., due to myocardial infarction, shoulder-hand syndrome, herpes

TABLE 18-1 Chronic Pain: Nervous System Pathophysiology[14–26]

NEUROLOGIC MECHANISMS	PHYSIOLOGIC EFFECTS	CLINICAL IMPLICATIONS
Neuroplasticity[14,15]	Recruitment of cortical and subcortical neurons so wide dynamic range cells can be activated by low-threshold mechanoreceptors Allodynia Allesthesia	Early, concurrent, multi-modal treatment of nociceptive, central, vascular, sympathetic and psychiatric aspects of the pain Block glutamate, substance P Early use of anti-epileptic drugs, membrane stabilizers, sympatholytics NMDA antagonists
NMDA excess and glutamate–GABA imbalance[16–19] Glutamate up, GABA down	Opioid tolerance Central hyperalgesia Hyperexcitability of peripheral and central pain cells	Normally non-painful light touch, muscle and joint movements are painful Treatment options: benzodiazepines, baclofen, anti-epileptic drugs, substance P antagonists, or other NMDA antagonists (e.g., ketamine), GABA agents
Neurotoxins[20]	Excitotoxic (e.g., quinolinic acid) Neuropathy	AIDS pain: anti-epileptic drugs, serotoninergic/noradrenergic agents, free radical scavengers
Opioid "off" mechanisms[21,22] Off cells in the medulla Morphine 3G/morphine up Side effect intolerance	Hyperalgesia as opioids increase (particularly intrathecal) Tolerance as morphine 3G increases Side effects greater than benefit	Maintain steady blood levels of opioids, or decreased opioids may increase pain Switching to a different opioid if one does not work Trial off opioids if minimal response
Sympathetic pain[15]	Mechano-allodynia, swelling Dystrophic changes	Sympathetic blockade and/or α-blocking drugs may be useful in CRPS, trauma, facial pain, arthritis
Monoamines (5-HT, NE, dopamine)[23–26]	5-HT increase lessens opioid analgesia 5-HT1 dysregulation leads to vascular pain 5-HT1 involved in affective disorders/suffering of pain	Full dosage, early use of antidepressant drugs, including tricyclics, SSRIs, and dopamine agonists, alone or in combination NE re-uptake inhibitors (e.g., desipramine, venlafaxine) useful for pain whether depressed or not Pergolide and methylphenidate are useful adjuvants
Psychiatric illness	Decreased sleep Decreased muscle relaxation Alienation, anxiety	Differential diagnosis of psychiatric conditions and appropriate treatments

NMDA, *N*-methyl-D-aspartate; GABA, γ-aminobutyric acid; CRPS, complex regional pain syndrome; 5-HT, 5-hydroxytryptamine; NE, norepinephrine; SSRIs, selective serotonin re-uptake inhibitors.

zoster, cerebrovascular accidents, diabetic neuropathy, disc herniation, degenerative disc disease, neuraxial tumors or metastases, multiple sclerosis, or poliomyelitis). CRPS is divided into two types. In type I CRPS, which typically develops after minor trauma or fracture, no overt nerve lesion is detectable. In type II CRPS, a definable nerve injury is present. Per diagnostic criteria set forth by the IASP, the diagnosis of CRPS can be made if the following criteria are met:[27]

1. Preceding noxious event without (CRPS I) or with obvious nerve lesion (CRPS II);
2. Spontaneous pain or hyperalgesia/hyperesthesia not limited to a single nerve territory and disproportionate to the inciting event;
3. Edema, skin blood flow (temperature) or sudomotor abnormalities, motor symptoms, or trophic changes are present on the affected limb, in particular at distal sites;
4. Other diagnoses are excluded.

The clinical course (which may last up to 6 months) starts with an acute phase that involves pain, edema, and warm skin. Subsequently, dystrophic changes dominate the picture with cold skin and trophic changes (3–6 months after the onset of the untreated acute phase). Irreversible atrophic changes (atrophy and contractures) eventually occur. There may be symptom improvement with inhibition of sympathetic output; sympathetic blockade may be both diagnostic and therapeutic.[28]

Idiopathic pain, previously referred to as "*psychogenic pain*," is poorly understood. The presence of pain does not imply or exclude a psychological component. Typically, there is no evidence of an associated organic etiology or an anatomical pattern consistent with symptoms. Symptoms are often grossly out of proportion to an identifiable organic pathology.

Jurisigenic pain results from perceived physical or emotional damage related to medical, personal, work, or product injury. Patients with this pain syndrome usually maintain the sick role for as long as possible to maximize financial return. It is important to recognize the existence of a conflict and to educate patients and attorneys; maintenance of a helping and neutral posture is critical.

Phantom-limb pain refers to severe and excruciating pain in the body part that is no longer present following

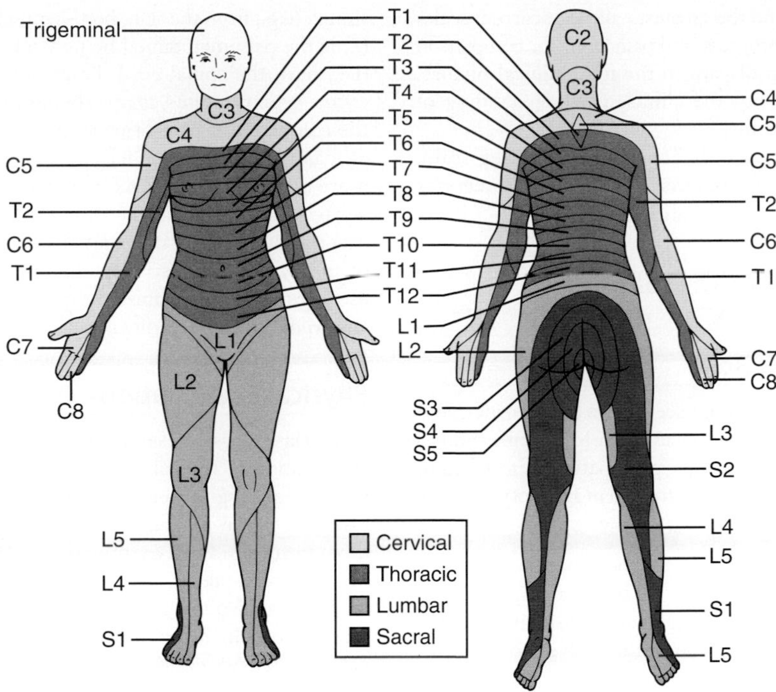

Figure 18-3. Schematic diagram of segmental neuronal innervation by dermatomes. *(From Hyman SH, Cassem NH:* Pain. *In: Rubenstein E, Federman DD, eds.* Scientific American medicine*:* current topics in medicine. Subsection II. *New York, Scientific American; 1989. Originally from Psychiatry Update and Board Preparation, Stern TA, Herman JB, (eds). McGraw-Hill, 2004.)*

amputation. The amputation of a limb is commonly followed by sensations that the deafferented body part is still present. These may include non-painful phantom sensations in specific positions, shapes, or movement, sensations of warmth or cold, itching, tingling, or electric sensations, and other paraesthesias.[29] However, pain may also be present, and occurs in 50% to 80% of all amputees.[30] Although this condition is most common after amputations of limbs, it can also occur after the surgical removal of other body parts such as the breast, rectum, penis, testicle, eye, tongue, or teeth.[31] The pathophysiology of this pain is poorly understood, however it is likely secondary to CNS[32–34] and peripheral factors (e.g., nociceptive input from the residual limb),[35] with psychological factors influencing the course and severity of the pain.[36] Consistent with the impact of the psyche on pain, one study showed that it is possible to induce pain in an amputee with hypnotic suggestion.[37]

Myofascial pain can arise from one or several of the following problems: hypertonic muscles, myofascial trigger points, arthralgias, and fatigue with muscle weakness. Myofascial pain is generally used to describe muscle and connective tissue sources of pain. Myofascial pain can be a primary diagnosis (e.g., fibromyalgia) or, as more often is the case, a co-morbid diagnosis (e.g., with vascular headache or with a psychiatric diagnosis). Psychiatric symptoms are common in patients with muscle pain; other symptoms often involve decreased energy, impaired sleep, and changes in psychomotor activity. Myofascial pain syndromes may involve muscle trigger points, hypersensitive skin, a subjective sense of swelling and numbness, somatic symptom disorders, affective and anxiety disorders, non-restorative sleep, as well as pain of the head and neck. The diagnosis should be considered if there are multiple muscle trigger points in the temporalis, sternocleidomastoid, rhomboids, or trapezius muscles; if the person cannot get at least 5 hours of uninterrupted sleep; and if chronic fatigue is present.[38] Deficient Stage 4 sleep is thought to underlie the lack of deep muscle relaxation, aching muscles, arthralgias, and general malaise.[39–41]

PAIN MEASUREMENT

The experience of pain is always subjective. Objective measurement of the patient's subjective response, however, is possible. Several sensitive and reliable clinical instruments for pain measurement are available. These include:

1. *The pain drawing*. This involves having the patient draw the anatomic distribution of the pain as it is felt in his or her body. The patient draws the outline of the body, labels where the pain is, and keeps this document as part of the medical record. The drawing serves as a clue to the anatomy of the problem, to the psychological state of the patient, and to the patient's level of knowledge.
2. *The visual analog scale*. A 100-mm visual analog scale (with 0 signifying no pain and 100 representing severe pain) is readily understood by most patients. It is also exquisitely sensitive to change; consequently, the patient can mark this scale once a day or even hourly during treatment trials, if desired. Two separate scales can be

kept for the least and the greatest pain. Concurrent scales for mood, overall progress, and pain allow for comparison of the relationship of pain to the total clinical picture, thereby rounding out the clinician's understanding of the patient's syndrome.

3. *Categorical rating scales. Ad hoc* categorical rating scales may be devised that comprise three to five categories for the ranking of pain severity.

THE PSYCHIATRY CONSULTANT AS PAIN PHYSICIAN

The Psychiatrist's Role

Physicians and patients alike seek knowledge, order, and relief when dealing with pain's chameleon-like manifestations; some of the common reasons pain patients or treating physicians seek consultation and treatment from psychiatrists include:

- To separate functional from non-functional factors. Unfortunately, the request to separate psyche from soma is often vexing. Through such consultations some physicians wish to absolve themselves of further responsibility
- To resolve inconsistencies between symptoms and physical findings (or the lack thereof): "No anatomic lesion could account for this." The referring physician wonders if a psychiatric disorder or central nervous system (CNS) pain is present or if he or she is missing something
- To assess the patient for depression, anxiety, or some other co-morbid neuropsychiatric disorder and its relation to the experience of pain
- To address a patient's or physician's fear or misunderstanding of opioids (e.g., use of high-dose analgesics, maintenance treatment, or toxicity)
- To determine if the use of psychopharmacologic agents might help alleviate pain and suffering
- To satisfy the referring physician's personal desire to punish a "hateful" patient, one who will not take yes or no for an answer and who interferes with normal medical decision-making.

The psychiatrist begins with a clarification of the reason for the consultation, creates some initial hypotheses, and examines the patient. If possible, the psychiatric consultant should be brought into the case early on and introduced as a member of the medical team. The referring physician should take care to ensure that the patient does not interpret the referral as a sign that he or she is not believed, and the physician should state that a psychiatrist is routinely asked to evaluate patients with longstanding pain. When the referring physician is comfortable using the services of a psychiatrist, the patient typically accepts the examination without protest. When the psychiatrist is called in at the end of a long and frustrating stand-off, the patient typically balks.

Gathering Important Preliminary Information

The psychiatric consultant's job begins by answering five questions: (1) Is the pain intractable because of nociceptive stimuli (e.g., from the skin, bones, muscles, or blood vessels)? (2) Is the pain maintained by non-nociceptive mechanisms (i.e., have the spinal cord, brainstem, limbic system, and cortex been recruited as reverberating pain circuits)? (3) Is the complaint of pain primary, as occurs in disorders such as major depression or delusional disorder? (4) Is there a more efficacious pharmacologic treatment? (5) Have pain behavior and disability become more important than the pain itself? Answering these questions allows the mechanism(s) of the pain and suffering to be pursued. Table 18-2 is a useful guideline to organize the questions, to test hypotheses, and to determine the diagnosis.

Physical Examination

A clinician's physical examination of the pain patient includes examination of the painful area, muscles, and sensation to pinprick and light touch (Table 18-3). The examination is essential to the psychiatric evaluation for pain and serves three purposes. First, examination of the patient allows for better history-taking, therapeutic alliances, and integration of data; it also helps to eliminate the physical–mental dichotomy, which, left unspoken, often contributes to the patient's defensiveness. Second, the psychiatrist can search for signs of different types of pain and distinguish them from symptoms of a conversion disorder. Third, inconsistent findings suggestive of somatic symptom disorder may be uncovered.

Psychiatric Examination

Interviewing the patient with chronic pain demands close attention to both what was said and what was not said, as well as to mindfulness of the patient's style of discourse. Because patients with an extensive history of pain often delight in regaling the examiner with their odysseys through clinics, spas, and hospitals, it is helpful to ask them to write detailed accounts of their pain from its onset to the present. A detailed history of when and how the pain began, inquiring about the various treatments received, and the patient's relationships with other physicians are also important in the evaluation of the pain patient. Throughout the history, look for fluctuations in the course of the pain. Why did it improve? Did the medication help, or was it some other factor that proved palliative? In addition, one should explore the patient's past and present mental state and consider the family history and cultural beliefs. Open-ended questions may include: Have you ever suffered like this before? What do you do think about in the early morning hours when you cannot sleep? What do others think is the nature of the problem? The psychiatrist also plays an important role in the treatment of the pain by his or her ability to recognize co-morbid psychiatric conditions that may present with pain.

Depression

Major depressive illness can be diagnosed in approximately 25% of patients who suffer from chronic pain. Recurrent affective illness, a family history of depression, and psychiatric co-morbidity (with anxiety and substance use) are often present. More often than not, depression pre-dates the pain; overall, 60% to 100% of pain patients have depressive

TABLE 18-2 Questions to Ask When Pain Persists

PAIN SYNDROMES: WHAT IS THE PROBLEM?	SELECTED DIAGNOSTIC CONSIDERATIONS	CONSIDER:
Is there an ongoing physical disease? (e.g., infection, cancer)	MRI for anatomic pathology Gallium scan for infection ESR for infection, cancer PSA, CEA, p24 testing Pelvic, breast, prostate, gastrointestinal examination	Progression of disease Metastatic disease Visceral pain: adhesions, referred pain, central pain
Is there a problem with the use and response to opioids? (e.g., misuse, lack of efficacy)	Central pain Opioids masking a psychiatric problem Opioid dosing error or inconsistency Opioid toxicity	Intravenous agents Antidepressants, anxiolytics, or sleep medications Opioid potency P450 2D6 codeine or oxycodone/SSRI interaction Meperidine toxicity
Is there a psychiatric disorder associated with pain? Depression Anxiety Somatic symptom disorder Psychosis Does CNS pain exist? (e.g., neuropathic pain)	Loss of all pleasure and mid–late insomnia Panic depersonalization, benzodiazepine failure, anxiety not relieved by analgesics Hypochondriasis Increased sensory threshold, decreased pain threshold Non-dermatomal distribution of pain Hyperpathia Allodynia, often opioid-resistant	Depression often masked by opioids or anxiolytics Co-morbid somatoform, mood, or anxiety disorders Pain drawing and explanation helpful for diagnosis Sharp sensation perceived as light touch is common Light touch is painful and sustained and has a delayed crescendo Tuning fork/moving a hair examinations detect allodynia best
Is it a pain behavior syndrome?	Somatic symptom disorder; rule out depression, substance use disorder, physical/sexual abuse, missed physical disorder	Anger and anxiety: denied Counter-dependent, demanding style Passive and endearing
Is the patient faking? Malingering Factitious disorder	Malingering for drugs/disability Factitious deception to maintain the sick role	Malingering or factitious disorders with physical symptoms are rare, much more likely to be something else
Is an unusual problem responsible for pain? Myofascial pain Porphyria Gastrointestinal pain Pelvic-visceral pain Neuropathic pain Sexual pain disorder	Muscle trigger points absent, deep sleep Laxative abuse, anorexia/bulimia Adhesions Hypoesthesia, allodynia Wasting illness, subcortical deficits/AIDS Conversion symptom, especially pelvic, gastrointestinal head pain	Myofascial pain often comorbid with other pain syndrome Visceral pain is diffuse, non-dermatomal, with sympathetic symptoms and may mimic psychiatric presentations Physical/sexual abuse antidote pain

MRI, magnetic resonance imaging; ESR, erythrocyte sedimentation rate; SSRI, selective serotonin re-uptake inhibitor.

symptoms. Although some depressive syndromes are secondary to pain itself (e.g., adjustment disorder with affective symptoms), many patients have major depression masked by denial or by medications that promote sleepiness. Denial of affect, particularly anger, is observed in many chronic pain patients referred for consultation. Diagnosing an affective illness when abnormal mood is minimized by the patient may be difficult, but the following tactics can be used to help find out affective disorders.

Ask questions about neurovegetative symptoms. Examples of questions to be posed include: How often do you wake from sleep at night? How long does it take you to return to sleep? Do you have early-morning awakening? When was the last time you really enjoyed yourself? Does food taste the same as it always has? Do you enjoy eating? What do you do for fun? Can you still smile? Do you have an interest in people, such as your grandchildren or friends? Do you have difficulty with decision-making? What do you do when you are angry? Do you sometimes feel you would rather be dead?

Evaluate the person's limbic (i.e., genuine and uncensored) response to emotionally charged stimuli. Look for denial of any strong emotion, particularly anger or sadness, and note if the patient answers affective questions with affective responses or only with avoidance and denial. Denial, displacement, or suppression of emotions suggests psychopathology. One could ask questions, such as, "Can you laugh at a joke at your own expense? Can you acknowledge anger at yourself and others?" The Minnesota Multiphasic Personality Inventory (MMPI) may be of particular use in refining the differential diagnosis when denial or repression is suspected. Covert hostility is typically elevated, which adds some validity to the label of denier. The so-called "conversion V" is present in many patients, and it occurs more often among those in denial. Patients with other chronic illnesses are more likely to have an "inverted V" configuration.

TABLE 18-3 General Physical Examination of Pain by the Psychiatrist

PHYSICAL FINDING	PURPOSE OF EXAMINATION
Motor deficits	Does the patient give-way when checking strength? Does the person try? Is there a pseudoparesis, astasia-abasia or involuntary movements suggesting a somatoform disorder?
Trigger points in head, neck, shoulder, and back muscles	Are any of the common myofascial trigger points present, suggesting myofascial pain? Presence of evoked pain (such as allodynia, hyperpathia, or anesthesia) suggests neuropathic pain
Evanescent, changeable pain, weakness, and numbness	Does the psychological complaint pre-empt the physical?
Abnormal sensory findings	Detection of lateral anesthesia to pinprick ending sharply at the midline Presence of topographic confusion Presence of non-dermatomal distribution of pain and sensation suggests either a somatoform or CNS pain disorder Presence of abnormal sensation suggests neuropathy or CNS pain
Sympathetic or vascular dysfunction	Detection of swelling, skin discoloration, or changes in sweating or temperature suggests a vascular or sympathetic element to the pain
Uncooperativeness, erratic responses to the physical examination	Detection of an interpersonal aspect to the pain, causing abnormal pain behavior, as in somatoform disease

Anxiety Disorders

In the pain patient, denial of fear, worry, or nervousness is a more ominous sign than is the mere expression of modulated fear or worry about pain. Given that it is normal to worry about a painful threat to the body and the mind, pathologic denial of any affect may be suggestive of psychosis, hypochondriasis, conversion, factitious disorder, or personality disorder. Questions, such as the following, may help glean important information: "Does the pain make you panic? Do you feel your heart beating fast, have an overwhelming feeling of dread or doom, or experience a sense of sudden high anxiety that overwhelms you?"

Anxiety disorders occur in approximately 30% of patients with intractable pain (usually in the form of generalized anxiety or panic disorder). More than 50% of patients with anxiety disorders also have a current or past history of major depression or another psychiatric disorder. Alcohol and substance use disorders are the most common co-morbid diagnoses; consequently, recognition and treatment of co-morbid depression and substance use is critical to long-term treatment outcome.

A variety of agents, including TCAs, selective serotonin re-uptake inhibitors (SSRIs), serotonin norepinephrine re-uptake inhibitors (SNRIs), mirtazapine, and clonazepam, alone or in combination, improve panic, anxiety, and depression as well as neuropathic pain, muscle tension, and sleep. Anxiety that results from disruptions of bodily integrity, sense of self, or attachment to caregivers occurs in one-third to one-half of chronic pain patients. This type of narcissistic injury can block efforts at physical and emotional rehabilitation and requires a pragmatic treatment approach. Anger is often linked to anxiety, although it is typically denied and expressed in terms of somatic symptoms. One can provoke affect quickly by holding up a clenched fist and asking the patient what he or she would do with it. The response will often be telling regarding denied anger. SSRIs are helpful with anger, anxiety, and mood disorders. Existential anxiety may increase when cancer is first diagnosed, when death nears, or when pain engenders feelings of helplessness. Spending time with the person, telling the truth, accepting the situation, and re-connecting with family members (parents and children) often decreases existential anxiety.

Somatic Symptom Disorders

Somatic symptom disorder occurs in 5% to 15% of treated chronic pain patients, and somatizers account for 36% of all cases of psychiatric disability, as well as 48% of all sick-leave occasions.[42]

Among those with a history of somatic complaints, pain in the head or neck, epigastrium, and limbs predominates. Visceral pain from the esophagus, abdomen, and pelvis associated with psychiatric co-morbidity, especially somatoform disorders, can be challenging to diagnose.[43] Missed ovarian cancers, central pain following inflammatory disorders, and referred pain are often over-looked because of the non-specific presentations of visceral pain. Moreover, in one study, 64% of women with chronic pelvic pain reported a history of sexual abuse.[44] Those that experience somatoform disorders often have painful physical complaints and excessive anxiety about their physical illness. Most of their pain complaints to physicians do not have a well-defined cause, and a psychiatric diagnosis is often particularly difficult to establish (Table 18-4).

Functional Neurologic Symptom Disorder

Functional neurologic symptom disorders (FND) may be manifest as a pain syndrome with a significant loss or alteration in physical functioning that mimics a physical disorder. Conversion symptoms may include paresthesias, numbness, dysphonia, dizziness, seizures, globus hystericus, limb weakness, sexual dysfunction, or pain. If pain or sexual symptoms are the sole complaints, the diagnosis is pain disorder or sexual pain disorder rather than FND. Pain, numbness, and weakness often form a conversion triad in the pain clinic.

TABLE 18-4 Somatoform and Related Disorders

DISORDERS	DIAGNOSTIC TIPS
Somatic symptom disorder	Physical symptoms that suggest physical illness or injury—symptoms that cannot be explained fully by a general medical condition, or by the direct effect of a substance, and are not attributable to another mental disorder Central and visceral pain, especially pelvic pain, can mimic somatic symptom disorder(s) Pain may improve with psychopharmacologic medications or psychological interventions without clear psychiatric diagnosis
Conversion disorder	Identifiable physical illness and conversion symptoms often co-occur An undiagnosed medical condition may underlie the psychiatric diagnosis Deciding if psychological factors are causative or a response is often impossible in chronic pain patients Culturally determined stress responses, numbness, total body pain, weakness, astasia-abasia, fainting, voices, and non-epileptiform seizure activity are transient and not included as conversion disorders
Hypochondriasis	Transient hypochondriasis is particularly common in the elderly Psychosis and depression may be concealed because of the patient's fears
Malingering/factitious disorder	Pseudomalingering with dissociative features (Ganser syndrome) presents with malingering, but also underlies real psychiatric illness. Some classify it as a conversion, dissociative, or factitious disorder

Psychological factors are judged to be etiologic for the pain when a temporal relationship between the symptoms and a psychosocial stressor exists—the person must not be intentionally producing their symptom. A mechanism of primary or secondary gain needs to be evident before the diagnosis can be confirmed. *La belle indifference* and histrionic personality traits have little value in making or excluding the diagnosis of conversion. A conversion V on the MMPI denotes the hypochondriacal traits and relative absence of depression that accompany conversion. Evoked responses, electromyogram (EMG), electroencephalogram (EEG), MRI, PET scans, and repeated physical examinations are useful for identification of patients who had been diagnosed erroneously as "hysterical."[45]

Factitious Disorder With Physical Symptoms

Factitious disorder with physical symptoms involves the intentional production or feigning of physical symptoms. Onset is usually in early adulthood with successive hospitalizations forming the life-long pattern. The cause is a psychological need to assume the sick role, and as such, the intentional production of painful symptoms distinguishes factitious disorder from somatic symptom disorders, in which intention to produce symptoms is absent. Renal colic, orofacial pain, and abdominal pain are three of the common presenting complaints in factitious disorder; of these, abdominal pain and an abdomen with scars herald the diagnosis most often. Despite the seeming irrationality of the behavior, those with factitious disorder are not psychotic.

Pain may be described as occurring anywhere in the body, and the patient often uses elaborate technical detail to intrigue the listener with *pseudologia fantastica*. Opioid medication-seeking behavior, multiple hospitalizations under different names in different cities, inconclusive invasive investigations and surgery, lack of available family, and a suave truculence are characteristic of this disorder. An assiduous inquiry into the exact circumstances of the previous admission and discharge leads to a sudden outraged discharge against medical advice. There is typically no effective treatment. If the patient were willing to receive care; however, psychotherapy would be the treatment of choice, coupled with addiction recovery services if there is an underlying substance use disorder.

Malingering

In malingering, the patient feigns a complaint, although no pain is felt, because of an external incentive, such as obtaining money, drug, or the avoidance of work. The conscious manipulation by malingerers precludes much diagnostic help from amytal interviews or hypnosis because of the willful withholding of information by the patient. The patient typically refuses psychological tests; this raises suspicion even before a diagnosis is made. Even when agreeable to testing, the MMPI can be skewed to normality by some patients, although differences (>7) between obvious and subtle scale scores and high L, F, K scale scores (T >70) may be suggestive nonetheless. The mnemonic for suspicion of the diagnosis is WASTE (*W*ithholding of information; *A*ntisocial personality; *S*omatic examination inconclusive and changeable; *T*reatment erratic with non-compliance and vagueness; *E*xternal incentives exist, such as occur in a medicolegal context). The psychiatrist's familiarity with the neurologic examination is always useful, but it is of critical importance for the diagnosis of malingering when nonanatomic findings arise. Once a non-functional etiology has been excluded, careful scrutiny of old records and calls to previous physicians may unearth evidence of similar behavior in the past. Similar to lying, malingering tends to be a character trait used in times of stress from early adolescence through the senium. Once revealed, psychotherapy can be offered; unfortunately, non-compliance is typical and prognosis guarded.

Dissociative States

Dissociation is caused by psychological trauma, and it involves a disturbance or alteration in the normally integrative functions of identity, memory, or consciousness. Pelvic pain, sexual pain disorders, headache, and abdominal pain are the most common pain complaints in developmentally traumatized individuals. Walker and associates[44] reported that in 22 women with chronic pelvic pain, 18 experienced childhood abuse. Of the 21 women selected as controls (i.e., without pelvic pain), nine had childhood abuse ($P<0.0005$). Dissociation, somatic distress, and general disability were more frequent in the group with pain. Denial makes the diagnosis of dissociative disorders in pain patients a longitudinal process, because truth is shared slowly with the physician only when the patient can tolerate it. Signs of an underlying dissociative disorder are periods of amnesia, nightmares, and panic, as well as anxious intolerance of close personal relationships.

GENERAL PRINCIPLES OF PAIN THERAPY

Pain Is Not Psychological by Default

The patient should not have his or her pain called "psychological" or "supratentorial" merely because it is not understood or because it is unresponsive to treatment. The physician should assure the patient that there is no question about the degree of suffering involved. Furthermore, psychological factors may play a role, but this by no means diminishes either the quality or the quantity of pain the patient endures. Education about the close relation of "psyche and soma" in CNS is often useful to establish an effective doctor–patient relationship.

Longstanding pain is difficult to assess largely because what we learn about pain is based on our concept of acute pain. The patient with acute pain moans, writhes, sweats, begs for help, and gives every appearance of being in great distress. Those nearby someone in acute pain typically feel an urge to help. When pain persists over days and weeks, the individual adapts to it, often without realizing it. The patient becomes able to sit in the physician's examining room and complains of agonizing pain while giving little or no evidence of actually being in agony. This adaptation means that the pain has become bearable, although there seems to be no change in intensity. This may be accounted for by several explanations: the sensation may become intermittent; the CNS inhibits the pain; or the patient becomes more capable of using distraction. It is ironic that the capacity to adapt to severe pain is often the patient's undoing because it causes the examiner to doubt the patient's veracity. The pain patient now is in the position of having to prove that he or she is in pain. The patient may feel himself or herself to be "on trial." To counter this end, the physician must know the pathophysiology of pain and employ the full range of neurologic, pharmacologic, and psychological therapies available.

Care Does Not Only Involve Symptom Management

An important principle of pain management is to assure the patient that treatment will continue, even if there is no immediate improvement. The physician should also guard against being affected by the patient's sense of discouragement. One of the fears expressed by many patients who suffer from chronic pain is that of abandonment; they believe that if they do not improve, the physician will no longer see them. In this case, an endless series of medications, without continuing examination, psychotherapy, or critical thinking, is tantamount to non-involvement or to abandonment. Education about relaxation techniques, yoga, acupuncture, TENS, ultrasound, and massage, all have their place in the therapeutic armamentarium. The value is not only in soothing the pain but also in helping the person to feel more in control, that is, less of a victim, and to become an active, educated participant while under the physician's care.

Caveats in Using Placebos

Few phenomena are as misunderstood as the placebo trial. A placebo trial shows whether or not the patient is placebo-positive; it does not prove that the pain is not real or that the person is either an addict or a malingerer. Similarly, it does not demonstrate that the patient would not benefit from an active medication. The trial is of no assistance in separating psychogenic from organic pain because the placebo response cannot be linked with any type of psychopathology. In fact, patients with depression, a somatic symptom disorder, or other varieties of emotional disturbance are no more apt to be placebo-responders than are so-called "normal" people.

Whether the pain is from a metastatic lesion or is part of a mood disorder, relief is experienced by the placebo-responder. Following surgery, about one patient out of three obtains pain relief from saline or from some other inert substance and is therefore considered placebo-positive. For instance, Evans and Hoyle[46] used sodium bicarbonate to treat individuals suffering from angina pectoris. In 38% of their subjects, they found this agent to be as effective as nitroglycerin. If a shot of sterile saline is substituted for a dose of opioid medication and the patient responds by obtaining relief, the nature of his or her pain may be questioned, even though relief is based on the conditioned response. Moreover, placebo effect and true effects are not independent. The mechanism for the placebo response is possibly the endogenous opioid pain-inhibiting system and is therefore influenced by psychological expectation. Placebo analgesia has been shown to be reversed with the opioid antagonist naloxone.[11]

In a valid placebo trial, the inert substance must be given to the patient in a randomized manner along with the usual opioid under double-blind conditions. Without this control, the placebo trial is limited. The only place for a placebo trial is an informed blinded experiment in which both the patient and the physician have discussed the intention and methodology and are in agreement to find the best treatment for a patient's pain disorder. One of the chief hazards of placebo use is that the patient may feel tricked if he or she discovers that a placebo has been administered to him or her. In this case, it is natural for the patient to feel on trial and wrongly accused, and there is no psychiatric fix for this error once it has happened. The physician who ordered the placebo needs to discuss it with the patient.

Deafferentation Surgery Is Usually Not the Answer

An abiding principle in the treatment of chronic pain is to avoid surgery whenever possible. Few surgical procedures on the CNS are persistently definitive in the cure or control of pain, and most carry with them a tax that is sometimes worse than the pain itself. In particular, CNS pain is notoriously refractory to surgery that interrupts afferent pain pathways. The pain is often made worse by procedures, such as a neurectomy, rhizotomy, tractotomy, and cordotomy. Surgery, with the one exception of cingulotomy, is not a treatment for depression that manifests as pain. A central procedure, such as cingulotomy, performed stereotactically using radiofrequency lesions, may be useful for intractable pain, especially because it has a low risk of psychiatric and physical morbidity. Personality changes, mental dulling, and memory impairment are rare. Unfortunately, even when pain is reduced with cingulotomy, it can return within 3 to 6 months. To exemplify this multiform plasticity of pain, consider the following account of an extraordinary case.

CASE 1

Mr. C, a 28-year-old mechanic, was thrown from his motorcycle en route to his wedding. Injury occurred to his brachial plexus and arm, requiring an amputation at the shoulder. He then developed severe phantom limb pain. Six months later, the stump was revised and a neurectomy performed; the pain, however, remained unaltered. The nerve was then severed further into the stump with similar result. An unsuccessful rhizotomy was then performed, followed by a chordotomy with the same outcome. He engaged in individual psychotherapy for a year, but there was no improvement. After six sessions of electroconvulsive therapy (ECT), the pain was only intensified. A higher cervical chordotomy was performed without success, and then a mesencephalic tractotomy; again, there was no relief. He next had both dorsomedial thalamic nuclei ablated using stereotactic electrocautery. He emerged from this procedure with his personality intact but still with his original pain. Then electrolytic lesions were made bilaterally in the inferior mesial quadrant of the frontal lobe in stages; still, the pain remained. Following this, he had a left radiofrequency amygdalotomy followed by a left cingulotomy. Nonetheless, the pain continued as before. The pain remained for 4 years after the accident, as pristine as it was 2 weeks after the injury.

Talking and Listening

A strategy to evaluate the feelings and behaviors observed in the pain patient is as necessary as the strategy for evaluating physical aspects of the pain. The skill required is not only a matter of diagnosing the major psychiatric illnesses that can present with pain—these patients often have a maladaptive style of interaction that requires a different kind of interpretive skill—but also a question of the physician's ability to relate to the long-suffering pain patient who shows poor judgment of surgical risk, denies anger, and rapidly alternates between idealizing and denigrating the medical caretaker. The fluctuations of both mood and cooperation frequently encountered in the clinical interview are symptomatic of the patient's damaged self-esteem or his or her injured narcissism. Chronic pain patients invariably feel damaged not only in the body part afflicted with discomfort, but also in self-image and spirit—a phenomenon known as narcissistic injury.[47] The techniques for interviewing the narcissistically injured pain patient are designed to establish a diagnostic working relationship. They allow for an accurate medical history to be elicited, mistrust between physician and patient to be avoided, an effective treatment plan to be developed, and the outcomes through compliance and education to be enhanced.

The interviewer should allow the patient to tell his or her own story. An initial degree of catharsis may be helpful in decreasing the patient's anxiety and in giving the physician a sense of the patient's character. The physician must actively facilitate an alliance with the patient while still maintaining neutrality and avoiding misplaced sympathy. The patient's underlying feelings of fear, anger, resentment, and mistrust are best uncovered by asking how others view the situation, essentially a counter-projective method. This approach sometimes bares unpleasant affects without the use of intrusive questions from the physician. Labeling overt and covert roles assigned by the patient to the physician is an important early intervention. Specifically, this means that the physician should point out when the patient is attributing unrealistic curative powers to him or her or appears to believe that the physician is indifferent to the patient's suffering. The longer one waits to confront these fantasies, the less effective any intervention will be. Expression of affect should be encouraged, and the physician should help the patient express the feelings he or she is having but does not want to acknowledge. The physician's assertive pursuit of the patient's true feelings avoids giving the appearance of unqualified support to feelings that need expression. Too much support not only bypasses psychological problems but also may actually increase conflicted feelings over withholding, control, dependence, and frail self-esteem. The physician's kindness should not be allowed to become a problem for the patient.

Optimal care of intractable pain patients requires the ability to process neurologic and psychiatric data while delineating and responding to the phrase-by-phrase manifestations of suffering and pain behavior. In essence, being able to get patients to talk about what they are angry about is just as important as discussing their insomnia or disc herniation. Progress occurs with these needy, angry patients, only when there is clear processing and separation of the reality-based facts of the case from unrealistic expectations. In that way, every clarification of an unrealistic idea can be an introduction to a more realistic alternative. The overall goal is to improve the patient's self-awareness and capacity for insight, thereby gaining control.

MEDICATION FOR PAIN: ANALGESIA AND ADJUVANTS

Judicious and effective use of medicine in patients with chronic pain rests on the concise evaluation of the four main components of the pain complaint: nociceptive pain, CNS mechanisms of pain, suffering, and pain behavior. In its most elemental form, the medical management of these four components employs opioids, anticonvulsants, antidepressants, and behavioral treatment. Non-steroidal antiinflammatory drugs (NSAIDs), aspirin, and nerve blocks are often helpful in the early stages of these illnesses. Opioids are, however, the most effective medicine for these pains when the severity increases.

Non-Steroidal Antiinflammatory Drugs

The World Health Organization (WHO) has established a three-step guideline for pain treatment (Figure 18-4). Step 1 involves the use of NSAIDs, aspirin, or acetaminophen. Step 2 adds codeine to the NSAID, with other adjuvants (e.g., TCAs, antidepressants, anti-epileptic medications, stimulants). Step 3 employs opioids with adjunctive medication. Conceived for cancer pain, and reporting efficacy in 90% of cancer patients, the three steps are a useful template for many kinds of acute pain, adjusted for the particular pain mechanism being treated. NSAIDs are useful for acute and chronic pain, such as inflammation, muscle pain, vascular pain, and post-traumatic pain, or when the physician wants to use a potent non-opioid analgesic. NSAIDs are generally equally efficacious and have similar side-effects.[48]

Side-Effects

Most NSAIDs can cause bronchospasm in aspirin-sensitive patients, induce gastric ulcers, interact with angiotensin converting enzyme (ACE) inhibitors (thereby contributing to renal failure), precipitate lithium toxicity, and impair renal function in the long term. NSAIDs can elevate blood pressure in patients treated with β-blockers and diuretics. The exception to this general rule is the non-acetylated (non-aspirin) salicylates that do not inhibit the synthesis of prostaglandins. These include choline magnesium trisalicylate and diflunisal; these agents do not cause bronchospasm in aspirin-sensitive patients, precipitate renal failure, or inhibit platelet aggregation. Certain NSAIDs, however, have features that make some preferable over others in particular situations. The discovery of the enzyme cyclooxygenase (COX) isoforms (1 and 2) led to the increased use of selective COX-2 inhibitors. COX-2 tends to facilitate the inflammatory response selectively and it has been argued that the use of new agents (parecoxib, etoricoxib, lumiracoxib, and celecoxib) may increase gastrointestinal safety.[49]

Based on currently available data, the US Food and Drug Administration (FDA) has concluded that an increased risk of cardio- and cerebrovascular events has been demonstrated for all of the cyclooxygenase-2 (COX-2) selective NSAIDs including rofecoxib, valdecoxib, and celecoxib.[49] Rofecoxib was voluntarily removed from the market in 2004 following the finding of increased cardiovascular events compared with placebo in a long-term study. Valdecoxib was voluntarily withdrawn from the market in 2005, after the FDA concluded that the overall risk versus benefit profile for the drug was unfavorable. Although an increased risk of cardiovascular events has also been demonstrated with celecoxib, the FDA has found that the benefits of celecoxib outweigh potential risks in properly selected and informed patients.

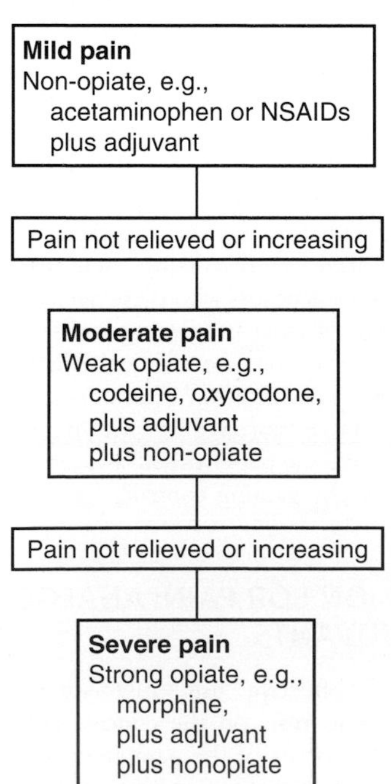

Figure 18-4. The analgesic ladder. *(From Borsook D, Lebel AA, McPeek B [1995]. MGH handbook of pain management. Boston, MA, Little Brown.)*

Special Features

Synergistic combinations of acetaminophen, aspirin, and caffeine are the cornerstone for temporary relief of pain (e.g., headaches and muscle pain) and potentiation of the effects of opioids. They do, however, have a limit on dosing and have only moderate potency; they are also not well tolerated by those who are very sick. NSAID variations then need to be considered. Choline magnesium trisalicylate (1000 to 1500 mg) is safe in aspirin-sensitive patients, and it does not prolong bleeding. Misoprostol can reduce gastrointestinal erosions in patients on maintenance NSAIDs, but its use can be limited by diarrhea, pain, and flatulence in about one-third of patients. Ibuprofen (800 mg) is a rapid-release agent that produces higher blood levels over the first half hour than the other preparations at equal dosage. Ketorolac (up to 30 mg every 6 hours) intramuscularly followed by oral dosing has a rapid onset and a high potency, enabling it to be substituted for morphine (note: 30 mg of ketorolac is equivalent to 10 mg of morphine). It should be used for no more than 5 days. Extended-release preparations can be useful when long, steady analgesia and simple dose regimens are needed (e.g., nabumetone, oxaprozin, ketoprofen, piroxicam). Naproxen (375 to 500 mg twice a day with enteric-coated, delayed-release tablets) can be well tolerated over time. Ketoprofen (200 mg) extended-release tablets can be taken once a day, but they are not intended for patients with renal disease or for those over 75 years of age. Ibuprofen works well as an opioid adjuvant for bone pain. Naproxen (up to 1500 mg a day), but not flurbiprofen, has also had positive results for bone pain. The newer COX-2 inhibitors may cause fewer gastrointestinal problems compared with other NSAIDs. Celecoxib does not impair platelet function. Parecoxib, etoricoxib, or lumiracoxib are not currently available in the United States. (For a list of NSAIDs, see Table 18-5.)

TABLE 18-5 Properties of Aspirin and Non-Steroidal Antiinflammatory Drugs

DRUG	DOSE (mg)	DOSAGE INTERVAL (h)	DAILY DOSE (mg/day)	PEAK EFFECT (h)	HALF-LIFE (h)
Aspirin	81–975	4	4500	0.5–1	0.25
Celecoxib	100–200	12	1200	1	11
Diclofenac	25–75	6–8	200	2	1–2
Diflunisal	250–500	12	1500	1	13
Etodolac acid	200–400	6–8	1600	1–2	7
Fenoprofen	200	4–6	3200	1–2	2–3
Flurbiprofen	50–100	6–8	300	1.5–3	3–4
Ibuprofen	200–400	6–8	3200	1–2	2
Indometacin	25–75	6–8	200	0.5–1	2–3
Ketoprofen	25–75	6–8	300	1–2	1.5–2.0
Ketorolac[a]					
Oral	10	6–8	40	0.5–1	6
Parenteral	60 load, then 30	6–8	120	0.5	6
Meclofenamic acid	500 load, then 275	6–8	400	1	2–4
Mefenamic acid	500 load, then 250	6	1250	2–4	3–4
Nabumetone	1000–2000	12–24	2000	3–5	22–30
Naproxen	500 load, then 250	6–8	1250	2–4	12–15
Naproxen sodium	550 load then 275,	6–8	1375	1–2	13
Oxaprozin	60–1200	24	1800	2	3–3.5
Phenylbutazone	100	6–8	400	2	50–100
Piroxicam	40 load, then 20	24	20	2–4	36–45
Sulindac	150–200	12	400	1–2	7–18
Tolmetin	200–400	8	1800	4–6	2

[a]Use no longer than 5 days.

Source: Adapted from Borsook D, Lebel AA, McPeek B. *MGH Handbook of Pain Management*, Boston, 1995, Little, Brown Publishers.

Opioids

Opioids help some cancer patients as well as those with non-cancer-related chronic pain.[50,51] Cancer pain is the most common indication for maintenance opioid medications.[52] Acute, severe and unremitting pain also requires opioid treatment, as outlined in the WHO analgesic ladder. At times, opioids may be the only effective treatment for chronic, non-malignant pain, such as the pain associated with degenerative disorders, and vascular conditions.[53] Bouckoms and colleagues[54] demonstrated that non-malignant pain treated with long-term oral opioids provides effective pain relief in about two-thirds of those treated. Nociceptive pain, absence of depression, and absence of any substance use were all significantly associated with long-term opioid treatment efficacy. Patients with neuropathic pain or major depression fared especially poorly; a bad outcome was four times more likely than a good outcome. Even when patients were carefully selected (i.e., lack of previous addiction or gross personality disorder), one-third of patients developed tolerance or addiction over a 3-year period. Even so, those patients with substance use disorders with chronic pain may still benefit from closely monitored physician-prescribed opioids for their physical pain if it stops them from turning to illicit supplies. These patients may require specific non-opioid strategies for their neuropathy and depression if gains are to be made. The use of buprenorphine products may be helpful given its less harmful potential versus opioid medications, coupled with its ability to also provide analgesia.

Opioid Potencies

Codeine is a good opioid for mild to moderate pain, but it has limited efficacy for severe pain. Morphine is the medication of choice for acute and chronic pain because of a long history of safety and decreased cost. Beyond these starting points, the basic principles of opioids are as outlined in Table 18-6.

Principles of Opioid Administration

Potency and Administration

Potency and administration are consistent with the characteristics of the drug, its half-life, and absorption by different routes; such knowledge helps to ensure that the dosage schedule is consistent with these parameters.

Oral Potency

Oral potency must be high so that parenteral use can be avoided if possible. Methadone is a good first choice because of its oral potency and relatively slow clearance. Morphine and hydromorphone, may be useful alternatives for initial treatment. Once oral doses have been initiated and titrated to a satisfactory level (e.g., 4-hourly dosing of morphine or methadone), the analgesic effect needs to be sustained by minimizing fluctuations in blood levels and the variable effects of dosing schedules. Morphine sulfate controlled-release (MSC) is ideal for this homeostasis because it is released more slowly than conventional oral morphine. Furthermore, morphine's effect is not significantly affected by minor hepatic disease. Only 50% of the morphine in its

TABLE 18-6 Potencies and Special Features of Opioids

DRUG	PARENTERAL (mg equivalent)	ORAL (mg)	DURATION (h)	SPECIAL FEATURES
Morphine	10	30	4	Morphine sulfate controlled release has 12 h duration
Codeine	120	200	4	Ceiling effect as dose increases, low lipophilic
Oxycodone	4.5	30	4	Oxycodone controlled release has 8–12 h duration (10, 20, 40 slow release mg)
Hydromorphone	2	8	5	Suppository 6 mg = 10 mg parenteral morphine
Levorphanol	2	4	4	Low nausea and vomiting, low lipophilic
Methadone	5	10	2	Cumulative effect; day 3–5 decrease respiration
Meperidine	100	300	3	κ, proconvulsant metabolite, peristaltic slowing and sphincter of Oddi dysfunction
Fentanyl	0.1	25 μg SL	1 (patch 72 h)	50 μg patch = 60 mg/day morphine IM/IV
Sufentanil	Not recommended	15 μg SL	1	High potency with low volume of fluid
Propoxyphene	Not available	325	4	High dose leads to psychosis
Pentazocine	60	150	3	κ, σ agonist–antagonist, nasal 1 mg q1–2 h
Butorphanol	2	Not available 3 (IM), 2 (NS)	μ, κ, σ, agonist–antagonist, nasal 1 mg q1–2h	
Buprenorphine	0.3	0.3	4–6	μ-Partial agonism; κ-antagonism; may precipitate withdrawal in patients already on chronic opioids
Tramadol	Not available	150	4	μ-Agonist, decreased reuptake 5-HT and NE, P450 metabolism
Nalbuphine	10	Not available	3	Agonist–antagonist

SL, sublingual; IM, intramuscular; IV, intravenous; 5-HT, 5-hydroxytryptamine; NE, norepinephrine; NS, nasal.

controlled-release formulation reaches the CNS after 1.5 hours, three times longer than it takes conventional oral morphine to reach the CNS. Steady-state is reached with MSC in about 1 day. A steady state with MSC at any fixed dose and dosing interval has a lower maximum blood concentration than does conventional morphine, thereby reducing fluctuations in blood levels. Note that MSC does not release morphine continuously and evenly, so that a dosing schedule of every 12 hours has more peaks and troughs than conventional oral morphine given every 4 hours. It is also important to be aware that chewing or crushing MSC further increases erratic release. MSC should not be given less than every 12 hours.

Avoid As-Needed Dosing

A steady-state opioid blood level requires approximately four half-lives to achieve consistency, and a steep dose–response curve makes pain relief erratic (e.g., if one dose is missed, it can take 23 hours to return to therapeutic analgesia). Dosing on an as-needed basis makes steady relief impossible. It also predisposes the patient to medication-respondent conditioning and to subsequent behavior problems.

Toxicity

Morphine and dihydromorphine uncommonly cause toxicity and hence are prescriptions of choice. Even so, when the glomerular filtration rate is poor and morphine or hydromorphone doses are high, toxicity may occur, even when equivalent doses of morphine are used without signs of toxicity. Meperidine hydrochloride should be avoided in difficult cases because of its short duration of action (2 to 4 hours) and because even at normal doses, its principal metabolite (normeperidine) can cause irritability, auditory and visual hallucinations, agitation, confused thinking, disorientation, hypomania, paranoia, and muscle twitches, in addition to partial and generalized seizures.[55,56] This CNS excitement is more likely to occur in patients with malignancy or renal impairment, or when the drug is given intravenously and the dose exceeds 300 mg/day for more than 3 days—all conditions in which there may be significant accumulation of the pro-convulsant normeperidine with repeated dosing. Methadone, once initiated, may accumulate in the body given its longer half-life, and care should be taken to ensure there is no excessive sedation or other signs of toxicity. Trouble-shooting checklists for opioids may be required when the basic principles mentioned above have not worked.[57]

Are Opioids the Drugs of Choice in Our Case?

Unduly long clinical trials and ongoing patient suffering may be avoided by giving the patient 10 mg of IV morphine as a single-blinded test dose. This is a diagnostic procedure designed to determine if opioids will relieve the pain. If there is a positive result with relief of pain, one concludes that morphine works well enough to continue its use. A negative outcome might result in a repeat dose of morphine at 20 mg to ensure that it was not just tolerance that failed to produce a benefit at 10 mg. In a doubtful case, one can give 0.4 mg of IV naloxone to confirm the lack of an opioid effect on pain. If there is neuropathic pain, for example, opioids may not produce a good enough response at normal doses. In about 50% of patients with intractable pain, opioids do not have a good enough analgesic effect. In a minority, it is the anxiolytic effect rather than the analgesic effect that is helpful.

Dosing

Prescriber fear and inexperience are the usual reasons that analgesics are given at inadequate dosage and frequency. Appropriate dosing requires knowledge of the potency and half-life of the drug. Common errors that occur at critical moments include failure to adjust the dosage when switching from parenteral to oral use (e.g., not increasing the dose of opioid medication when switching from IM/IV to oral dosing); failure to administer the drug at longer intervals than its half-life (e.g., methadone's analgesic half-life is 4–8 hours; consequently, methadone is usually needed at least three times a day when it is given for pain, not once a day as when it is given for opioid use disorder); and under-dosing when beginning MSC or fentanyl patches because both require at least 24 hours to reach steady-state (supplementary opioids are required for the first 24 hours).

Drug Delivery

An important question to bear in mind is whether the method of administration and type of opioid have been optimized. The most common problem in severe pain is the three-fold to eight-fold variability of IM absorption. This can be decreased by using agents that are hydrophilic (e.g., morphine and hydromorphone) rather than lipophilic (e.g., fentanyl, methadone, and meperidine). When more lipophilic agents, such as methadone, are used intramuscularly, injections into the deltoid rather than the gluteus muscle are preferable. If an erratic response occurs, it might be due to inconsistent drug delivery. Alternative methods include delivery of the drug intravenously, sublingually, intrathecally, ventricularly, or transdermally. For example, Kunz and co-workers described the innovative use of sublingual sufentanil, 25 mg every 3 minutes (for three doses) for severe but episodic pain.[58] The drug and route were preferable to patient-controlled analgesia (PCA), fentanyl sublingually or MSC because the volume of fluid was small, speed of onset was within 1 minute, and the half-life was short (and therefore not sedating the rest of the day); in addition, the cost was comparable with PCA, albeit more expensive than sublingual fentanyl. The patient could get out of bed and remain alert and comfortable with a low-tech intervention that is ideal for hospice or for home care.

Tolerance or Excessive Sedation

The age of the patient is an important factor in the efficacy of the drug. The duration of effect may double as age increases; as it does, so does the analgesic effect in a 70-year-old versus a 20-year-old. Opioid adjuvants (e.g., methylphenidate) may decrease or increase (e.g., with antidepressants) sedation.

Mixed Agonists and Antagonists

Pentazocine and butorphanol are commonly used opioids because of their mixed antagonist–agonist properties. Not only are they less potent than standard opioids, but also if combined with them during a period of transition, they may cause the patient to develop withdrawal symptoms, an acute confusional state, or even psychosis. Older people are particularly susceptible. Avoidance of mixing agonist opioid drugs with agonist–antagonist agents obviates this problem.

Addiction

The risk of opioid addiction in a population of medically ill patients is approximately 0.3%. Therefore, considering the patient as an addict on the basis of difficulties with managing opioids should be done cautiously. Acute sympathetic symptoms from drug withdrawal or tolerance are more likely to be the problem than addiction *per se*. Rather than addiction, unrecognized depression alone or co-morbid with anxiety is a more frequent, immediate explanation for the excessive need for opiates.

In recent years, oxycodone has attracted significant attention in the media due to its addiction potential. Clinical practice and research trials show that it is a good medication for pain due to its efficacy, fairly good side effect profile, and short onset of action. In patients who cannot tolerate or respond to other opioids it remains a good option.[59] The change of oxycodone to a new formulation has largely decreased its misuse potential.

Recent data suggest however, that the risk of prolonged administration of opioid medication can be as high as 3% in patients following major surgery, and thus the use of careful prescribing guidelines, distribution of small controlled amounts, along with informed consent of risk to the patient are advised.[60]

Opioid Adjuvants

Opioid adjuvants are indicated when toxic or pharmacokinetic factors limit further increases in the patient's opioid dosage or when pain remains uncontrolled by opioids in combination with other secondary treatments, such as decompression surgery, nerve blocks, or anxiolytic drugs. The choice of adjuvant should be individualized; one should aim for the simplest and most potent combination of drugs. The selection of the adjuvant depends on the symptoms associated with the pain; the character of the pain; and the physician's knowledge of any special issues, risks, drug interactions, or special mechanisms.

Guidelines for Opioid Maintenance Adjuvants

- Maintenance opioids should be considered only after other methods of pain control have been proven unsuccessful. Alternative methods vary from case to case but typically include NSAIDs; oral, transdermal, intravenous,

intrathecal, or epidural opioids; membrane-stabilizing drugs; anti-epileptic drugs, monoaminergic agents, local nerve blocks; nerve stimulation; and physical therapy.
- Opioids should not be prescribed for those with opioid use disorders unless there is a new major medical illness with severe pain (e.g., cancer or trauma). In such cases, a second opinion from another physician is suggested for all opioids used for longer than 2 months.
- If opioids are prescribed for longer than 3 months, the patient should have a second opinion consultation, ideally with a formal pain specialist, plus a follow-up consultation at least once per year.
- There should be one pharmacy and one prescriber designated.
- Opioid dosage should be defined, as should expectations of what will happen if there are deviations from it. For example, misuse leads to rapid tapering of the drug and a detoxification program, if necessary. There should be no doubt that the physician will stop the medication if there is concern for safety.
- Informed consent as to the rationale, risks, benefits, and alternatives should be documented. In addition, the patient should always be instructed to lock up medications, including the risk it may pose to children at home.
- The course of treatment, in particular, the ongoing indication(s), changes in the disease process, efficacy, the presence of tolerance, or emerging signs of a use disorder should be documented.

Justification for maintenance opioids, given the mixed benefits and risks, involves humanitarian and public health principles. If opioids are the only effective treatment for intractable suffering, they should be used for humanitarian reasons. The risk of episodic misuse may be justified in certain patients with high-risk histories or those with chronic pain, if use of medication lessens functional disability and illicit drug use. For example, a patient with a history of an opioid use disorder with chronic pain may benefit from a methadone maintenance program, which may also provide some level of pain management; furthermore, it may be an effective public health means of reducing the risk of human immunodeficiency virus (HIV) infection.

Analgesic Adjuvants

Pain may be refractory, despite the most judicious application of traditional anti-nociceptive measures, such as surgery, nerve blocks, and opioids. Stimulants, dopamine antagonists, tricyclic monoaminergic agents, benzodiazepines, anti-epileptic drugs, antihistamines, peptides, and prostaglandin inhibitors also have roles as non-opioid pain treatment adjuvants[61] (Table 18-7). The type of pain is as important as its cause in guiding the choice of an adjuvant. The pain may be characterized as a constant aching somatic pain, as in a fracture, or as a paroxysmal burning deafferentation sensation, as in phantom limb pain. The primary cause of the pain, however, does not necessarily determine its type or character. For example, the pain of metastatic cancer may be either neuropathic or visceral (and may or may not respond well to NSAIDs). Neuropathic pain is often refractory to opioids, and it covers a diverse group of conditions, which range from herpetic neuralgia to atypical facial pain. Patients suffering from this type of pain may respond to anti-epileptic drugs or TCAs. In the most difficult or ambiguous cases, a valuable technique is to use an IV dose of the drug to gain a rapid and accurate assessment of its effectiveness for the long term. IV morphine, lidocaine, and lorazepam can be used in this way to see whether or not any of these classes of drugs are worth pursuing.

Antidepressants for Pain

The mechanisms of action of TCAs are multiple and probably co-modulate the pain-relieving effect.[62] First, they have an effect in augmenting the descending periaqueductal spinal inhibitory control of pain mediated by serotonin and norepinephrine. In the spinal cord, the dorsolateral funiculus is a serotonergic inhibitory descending spinal pain pathway that modulates 80% of the spinal analgesic effect of opiates. Second, they potentiate naturally occurring or administered opiates. For example, desipramine, 8-OH-amoxapine, and imipramine are twice as potent as amitriptyline and four times as potent as trazodone and clomipramine at binding to opiate receptors. Third, antihistamine and α-receptor effects may be important with regard to potentiation. Fourth, there may be membrane-stabilizing anesthetic, anti-kindling anti-epileptic effects, which may also give secondary symptom relief of insomnia or anxiety.

The pain relief obtained from antidepressants is often independent of their effects on mood or the alleviation of major depression.[63,64] In fact, the greatest response to antidepressants in patients with pain may occur in those who are not depressed.[65] Antidepressants as analgesics are best thought of as monoaminergic cell stabilizers rather than just antidepressants. Serotonin, norepinephrine, and dopamine all modulate pain via their actions in the periphery to the CNS.

Serotonin presents a paradox because more serotonin is not necessarily better, yet function must be intact for pain to be inhibited. One type of peripheral serotonin receptor, 5-HT_{ID}, is found in cerebral blood vessels. Sumatriptan, a selective 5-HT_{ID} antagonist, acts to produce vasoconstriction and migraine headache relief. The raphe and mesolimbic structures are important sites of subcortical serotonin receptors, mainly types 1A, 2A, and B. These areas modulate pain and mood—the neurobehavioral sites of action. Despite the important role serotonin plays in pain, there are a number of exceptions to the simplistic notion of more serotonin, less pain.[66] For example, buspirone, fluoxetine, and trazodone have all been shown to be ineffective in attenuating certain pain syndromes.[67–69]

Norepinephrine-modulating medications also have value in treating chronic pain. Desipramine (average dose of 200 mg daily) relieved pain in diabetic neuropathy, in both non-depressed and depressed patients,[70] and also relieved post-herpetic neuralgia.[71] Duloxetine, a serotonin-noradrenergic re-uptake inhibitor (SNRI), has become the first antidepressant to have a specific pain indication for the treatment of painful diabetic neuropathy.[72] Duloxetine has also been studied in a number of large studies for the treatment of fibromyalgia and found to be efficacious, not only in pain reduction, but also in reduction of tender points and stiffness scores, while also increasing the tender-point pain threshold when compared with placebo.[73] These results

TABLE 18-7 Analgesic Adjuvants

AGENT	DOSAGE	INDICATIONS	SPECIAL ISSUES
Prostaglandin Inhibitors	Variable, limited by side effects and medical co-morbidity	Metastatic bone pain Inflammation Vascular pain	NSAID risks: gastrointestinal bleeding, renal impairment
Dopamine Antagonists Phenothiazines Butyrophenones	Antipsychotic D_2 receptor blocking doses	Post-herpetic pain Cancer pain Diabetic neuropathy Adjunct to TCAs Co-morbid anxiety or delirium	Haloperidol binds to opioid receptors Membrane stabilizing
Stimulants			Stimulants decrease pain and sedation
Methylphenidate Dextroamphetamine Pergolide	5–50 mg/day (t½: 2–7 h) 5–20 mg/day (t½: 4–21 h) 0.05 mg TID (t½: 6–72 h)	Postoperative pain and pain in pediatric and cancer patients respond well to analgesic stimulant combinations	Appetite and cognition improve; methylphenidate shows better long-term efficacy than does amphetamine
Steroids			
Prednisone Methylprednisolone	15+ mg/day PO 15 mg/kg IV boluses	Bone metastases Brain swelling Spinal cord compression Anorexia and pain Sickle cell pain	Risks: mood lability, withdrawal, anxiety, insomnia, gastrointestinal upset
Peptides			
Calcitonin	100–200 IU SC BID nasal 200 IC/day	Paget's, metastatic, and myeloma pain	Intrathecal, nasal, and SC are used
Somatostatin	500 µg	Vascular headaches	Somatostatin inhibits SP
Capsaicin crème	0.075%	Neuralgia, cancer pain Hyperalgesia, post-herpetic neuralgia, cluster headache, CRPS, inflammatory dermatoses, itching secondary to dialysis, psoriasis	Capsaicin effect peaks 4–6 weeks, for diabetic, post-mastectomy and arthritic pain
Antihistamines			
Diphenhydramine	150 mg	Opioid adjunct	Decreased inflammation, 5-HT, NE, dopamine, SR spasm, opiate clearance increased opiate binding
Hydroxyzine	100 mg		
Benzodiazepines			
Clonazepam Lorazepam	1–4 mg/day 2–16 mg/day	Adjuvant tricyclics Allodynia	Not a substitute for diagnosis of depression or substance abuse
Anti-Epileptics			
Phenytoin	300–450 mg/day	Cancer pain	Paroxysmal pain responds best to anti-epileptic drugs
Carbamazepine	400–1600 mg/day	Headaches, neuralgia	
Valproate	500–2000 mg/day	Central pain	
Gabapentin	900–1800 mg/day	Neuropathy	
Lamotrigine	100–300 mg/day	Migraine headaches	
Oxcarbazepine	300–1600 mg/day	Neuropathy	
Pregabalin	600–1200 mg/day	Neuropathy; PHN	
Topiramate	200–400 mg/day	Neuropathy	
Tricyclics Desipramine Imipramine	25–300 mg/day	Neuropathy Post-herpetic neuralgia	Burning Deafferentation pains respond best to the tricyclic drugs Increased side effects with amitriptyline

Table continued on next page

TABLE 18-7 Analgesic Adjuvants—cont'd

AGENT	DOSAGE	INDICATIONS	SPECIAL ISSUES
SSRIs		Diabetic neuropathy	
Paroxetine	20–60 mg/day		
Citalopram	20–60 mg/day		
SNRIs		Diabetic neuropathy	
Duloxetine	60–120 mg/day	Diabetic neuropathy; fibromyalgia	
Venlafaxine	75–375 mg/day	Fibromyalgia	

NSAID, non-steroidal antiinflammatory drug; TCAs, tricyclic antidepressants; IV, intravenous; SC, subcutaneous; SP, substance P; CRPS, complex regional pain syndrome; 5-HT, 5-hydroxytryptamine; NE, norepinephrine; PHN, post-herpetic neuralgia.

have also been reproduced by other SNRIs, with milnacipran and venlafaxine also having been shown to be efficacious for the treatment of pain associated with fibromyalgia.[74,75]

Reviews of Efficacy

Earlier reports of Lindsay and Wyckoff showed an efficacy of 70% to 80% for antidepressants for the treatment of chronic pain patients with depression.[76] Stein and associates reported that amitriptyline (150 mg/day) was more effective than acetaminophen 2 g/day in a controlled, double-blind study, with mild depression being one of the predictors of pain relief at the end of the 5-week study.[77] Blumer and Heilbronn showed twice the improvement (60%) in outcome and a halving of the dropout rate (25%) in those pain patients treated with antidepressants.[78]

Pain syndromes that may be responsive to antidepressants include those associated with cancer, post-herpetic neuralgia, arthritis, vascular and tension headaches, and facial pain. The literature reports a wide range of generally positive but poorly designed studies. Feinmann reviewed the 11 largest and best-designed studies on pain relief from antidepressants when depressive symptoms were present.[79] TCAs (amitriptyline hydrochloride) and MAOIs (phenelzine sulfate) were used, and the results demonstrated that these antidepressant drugs were beneficial in the treatment of chronic pain associated with depression.

A review by Goodkin et al. found that 37 of 53 trials (70%) of heterocyclic antidepressant drugs for chronic pain syndromes failed to meet minimum criteria for adequate design.[80] Of the remaining 16 trials that met design and protocol criteria, seven evaluated headache pain and documented positive effects with low-dose regimens. Complicating these findings was that smaller than typical antidepressant doses were used in many studies. In this same review, another non-random series of 17 studies was selected, of which five (29%) met minimum design and protocol criteria (i.e., clear protocol, placebo-controlled, and defined outcome measurements); only two of the five trials showed positive results. One study was for low-dose amitriptyline in mixed pain syndromes, and the other study was for desipramine in post-herpetic neuralgia. Max found that in 13 well-designed, randomized trials, antidepressants reduced pain in diabetic neuropathy and post-herpetic neuralgia, particularly the mixed serotonin and norepinephrine agents (e.g., imipramine, desipramine, and amitriptyline).[81]

Saarto and Wiffen, in a Cochrane-based review, reviewed available randomized clinical trials of antidepressants in neuropathic pain.[25] In total, 61 RCTs were included and it was found that TCAs were effective, with a number needed to treat (NNT) of 3.6 for the achievement of at least moderate pain relief. Venlafaxine had an NNT of 3.1 and there was limited evidence for the effectiveness of the SSRIs based on current available data.

In a meta-analysis conducted to assess the efficacy of antidepressants in treating back pain in adults, it was found that antidepressants were more effective than placebo in reducing pain severity but not functional status in chronic back pain.[82] TCAs have been shown to be an option for patients with chronic back pain, with SSRIs showing limited effectiveness. To date, SNRIs have not been studied for the treatment of chronic back pain.[26]

When is it worth trying a monoaminergic agent? A trial of an antidepressant medication is useful in any intractable pain condition whether or not depression is present, because analgesic effects are at least partly independent from antidepressant effects. Furthermore, the size of the analgesic effect does not differ significantly in the presence of depression.

There is no clear evidence for the superiority of any one antidepressant over any other. Amitriptyline, desipramine, and doxepin hydrochloride have been used most often in clinical studies. Even though sedating and non-sedating properties of drugs have no significant association with analgesic effect, the antihistaminic profile of an antidepressant correlates with effect.[83] Potent serotonin re-uptake blockade is not essential to pain relief; moreover, there is doubt about the efficacy of purely serotonergic drugs for neuropathic pain (e.g., fluoxetine, zimelidine, and trazodone).[84,85] Buspirone does not appear to relieve pain. With the exception of paroxetine, all antidepressant drugs studied in placebo-controlled trials of neuropathic pain have some inhibition of norepinephrine re-uptake (i.e., amitriptyline, desipramine, nortriptyline, imipramine, and maprotiline).[70] Venlafaxine has some agonist–antagonist opiate activity as well as norepinephrine, 5-hydroxytryptamine, and dopamine-reuptake effects, but it has yet to be rigorously proven as an analgesic.[86]

MAOIs may be particularly helpful in the attenuation of atypical pain associated with atypical depression. Both MAOIs and TCAs, however, may require a trial of at least 6 weeks for the full benefit to be evident.

Dopamine agonists can also augment analgesia. Dopamine has been associated with pain in clinical and experimental trials, and has also been shown to co-modulate opioid and substance P effects in the CNS. Psychostimulants can potentiate the effects of opioid analgesics.[87,88] Methylphenidate has been studied as adjuvant therapy for cancer patients receiving opioids. In a randomized, double-blind, placebo-controlled crossover trial of 32 patients with advanced cancer receiving chronic opiate therapy, statistically significant reductions in pain intensity and sedation were seen with the use of methylphenidate.[89] In another study of 50 patients with advanced cancer and opiate-induced sedation, 44 had a decrease in sedation after initiation of methylphenidate.[90] Patients with incident cancer pain (mild or no pain at rest, severe pain during movements) showed better pain control, and they tolerated higher doses of opioids when supplemented with methylphenidate.[91] A placebo-controlled trial demonstrated that the addition of oral methylphenidate resulted in improved cognitive function in 20 patients receiving continuous subcutaneous opioids for cancer pain,[92] and similarly, 5 of 11 adolescent cancer patients receiving opiates exhibited improved interaction with family or decreased somnolence when methylphenidate was added to their medication regimen.[93] While classified as a dopamine reuptake inhibitor, bupropion also has noradrenergic activity. Evidence of an analgesic effect is still very limited, although in one double-blind, placebo-controlled, crossover trial, 73% of 41 subjects with neuropathic pain obtained pain relief with bupropion treatment.

Monoaminergic agents in combination with clonazepam, valproate, or opioids, for cancer pain, are often safe and desirable.

Although some patients may respond to low doses of antidepressants for pain, a complete trial of antidepressants in pain patients requires a full dose of an antidepressant, the same as is used in major depression. The placebo-controlled study of McQuay and colleagues found that low doses of antidepressants (25 mg of amitriptyline) did not have the efficacy of higher doses.[94] The best results in the largest number of people are obtained, however, when the usual antidepressant dosage of drug is used (e.g., 300 mg/day of imipramine hydrochloride or its equivalent). Other pointers include:

- Depression should not be rationalized as appropriate
- Treatment of the depressed pain patient is no different than treatment of any other depressed patient
- Education of the patient as to the rationale for antidepressant treatment is advised for good compliance
- Maintenance treatment for 3 to 6 months is usually necessary for the best results.

Anti-Epileptic Drugs

Anti-epileptic drugs (AEDs) have a long history of effectiveness in the treatment of pain, especially neuropathic in origin, dating back to case reports for the treatment of trigeminal neuralgia with phenytoin in 1942 and carbamazepine in 1962.[95] Blocking abnormally high-frequency and spontaneous firing in afferent neurons in the dorsal horn and thalamus are the putative mechanisms for the efficacy of anticonvulsants with regard to pain. The consequence of blocking the hyperexcitability of low-threshold mechanoreceptive neurons in the brain leads to pain relief.[96] Phenytoin, carbamazepine, valproic acid (VPA), benzodiazepines, along with some of the newer AEDs including gabapentin, pregabalin, lamotrigine, topiramate, and oxcarbazepine are agents used to treat pain. These drugs have a number of shared cellular effects, which include antagonism of excitatory amino acids, γ-aminobutyric acid (GABA)-receptor agonism, sodium and calcium pump stabilization, and antagonism of adenosine. Indirectly, they all antagonize the effects of excitatory amino acids, which are believed to kindle hyperexcitability of CNS neurons.

Phenytoin has been shown effective in alleviating pain associated with various neuropathies, particularly trigeminal, diabetic, and post-stroke pain. Sharp, shooting, lancinating pain has been shown to respond especially well to this drug. It has more behavioral toxicity, however, and is less effective than carbamazepine, thus making it a second choice for analgesia.

Carbamazepine is generally superior to phenytoin for pain. The effect of carbamazepine on pain suppression is likely mediated by central and peripheral mechanisms. The ability of carbamazepine to block ionic conductance appears to be frequency dependent, which enables the drug to suppress the spontaneously active Aδ and C fibers responsible for pain without affecting normal nerve conduction. Since Blom[95] reported the analgesic properties of carbamazepine for patients with trigeminal neuralgia in 1962, carbamazepine has been shown to be effective also for post-herpetic pain, post-sympathetic pain, diabetic neuropathy, multiple sclerosis, and assorted neuralgias.[97] Higher levels (8 to 12 μg/L) are typically necessary for optimal efficacy.

The first reports of VPA used in neuropathic pain appeared in the early 1980s. VPA prolongs the repolarization of voltage-activated Na^+ channels, and also increases the amount of GABA in the brain, enhancing the activity of glutamic acid decarboxylase and inhibiting GABA degradation enzymes. VPA has been shown to decrease post-herpetic neuralgia, episodic and chronic cluster headaches, migraine, and postoperative pain, as well as various neuralgias. It has also been demonstrated that VPA is effective in treating migraine headaches in two double-blind, placebo-controlled trials.[98,99] These demonstrations of efficacy in pain reduction are in addition to the traditional place for VPA in the treatment of psychiatric disorders (bipolar and schizoaffective disorders). VPA sprinkles, in particular, are well tolerated and can substitute for carbamazepine and lithium in pain states, although no head-to-head comparisons have been completed.

Benzodiazepines have been controversial in the alleviation of pain, but they do have a definite place as safe and effective agents.[100] Combinations of benzodiazepines with antidepressants or opiates may be particularly useful clinically. IV lorazepam was superior to morphine, lidocaine, and placebo in a single-blind study of neuropathic pain,[101] however, these results were not reproduced in a randomized, double-blind trial in which lorazepam was less effective than amitriptyline in patients with post-herpetic neuralgia.[102] Orally, clonazepam is the drug of choice. It binds more slowly to central than to peripheral benzodiazepine receptors, and it is synergistic with serotonergic pain mechanisms, a factor that distinguishes it from other benzodiazepines. A useful diagnostic test for benzodiazepine-sensitive pain (BSP) is to administer lorazepam 2 mg IV in a single-blind manner evaluated by visual analog scale (VAS) monitoring. Positive results (>3 cm decrease in VAS) signify relief of ongoing pain. If positive results are achieved, it is recommended to give sequential IV lorazepam doses to break the pain cycle (in severe cases) or clonazepam (e.g., 2 to 4 mg orally at bedtime, and 1 mg twice a day).

Of the new generation of AEDs used for treatment of neuropathic pain, gabapentin is perhaps the best studied so far. Developed as a structural GABA analogue, it has no direct GABAergic action. It is believed that gabapentin acts on the α-2-δ type of Ca^{2+} channels. Gabapentin has been shown to relieve pain and associated symptoms in patients with both peripheral diabetic neuropathy, post-herpetic neuralgia, HIV-related neuropathy, and cancer-related neuropathic pain.[103–106] The dosages used in these studies typically ranged from 900–3600 mg daily in three divided doses. Additional studies are required to evaluate if gabapentin has efficacy in other pain states.

Topiramate works via multiple mechanisms, including prolongation of voltage-sensitive sodium channel inactivation, $GABA_A$ agonism, and non-N-methyl-D aspartate glutamate receptor antagonism. Topiramate has been found to be useful in the treatment of trigeminal neuralgia, along with diabetic neuropathy. As with any of the newer AEDs, continued studies will be required to determine the overall efficacy.

Oxcarbazepine is a keto-analog of carbamazepine, with the analgesic mechanism likely due to inhibition of voltage-dependent Na^+ channels and also, to a lesser extent, K^+ channels. While studies seem to show mixed results for the use of oxcarbazepine for diabetic neuropathy, it seems to have similar efficacy to carbamazepine in the treatment of trigeminal neuralgia; however, there are limited data regarding the efficacy and safety of this drug in the treatment of other neuropathic pain syndromes.

Pregabalin is a GABA analog believed to exert its analgesic effect by binding to the α-2 delta subunit of voltage-gated calcium channels on primary afferent nerves, and reducing the release of neurotransmitters from their central terminals. Evidence seems to show that pregabalin is effective for reducing the intensity of pain associated with diabetic polyneuropathy and post-herpetic neuralgia.[107,108]

Lamotrigine is a direct glutamate antagonist that also inhibits sodium channels. While initial case reports seemed to show some promise for use of lamotrigine in neuropathic pain states, most randomized, double-blind studies to date have not shown any significant efficacy.[109–113]

Sympathetically Maintained Pain

Sympathetically maintained pain (SMP)—regardless of whether it is due to RSD, opiate tolerance, hyperalgesia, inflammation, vascular headache, post-herpetic neuralgia, trauma, facial pain, or arthritis—may respond to sympathetic blockade.[114] Sympathetic efferent fibers release norepinephrine, which in turn activates α-adrenergic receptors. Activation of these receptors, either directly or indirectly, excites nociceptors. Activity in the nociceptors then evokes pain, and causes further discharge of nociceptors. α-Adrenergic receptor supersensitivity has been postulated as a likely mechanism for both the hyperalgesia and the autonomic disturbances associated with SMP.[115] The clinician can consider the early use of sympathetic blockade in any chronic pain syndrome with features of sympathetic dysfunction. SMP is diagnosed and treated using the method of injecting or transdermally applying an α-adrenergic blocking agent selected from the group consisting of an α-1-adrenergic antagonist, α-2-adrenergic agonist, or other drug that depletes sympathetic norepinephrine. One method to assess for SMP is to infuse 500 mL of one-half normal saline before putting phentolamine into an ischemic regional block, then administer phentolamine 10 mg IV over a 10-minute period. A positive test result is marked by relief of evoked pain stimulated by light touch or a tuning fork.[116] α-Blocking drugs (e.g., phentolamine, α-blocking antidepressants) and α_2-agonists, such as clonidine, given with or without opiates, are all potentially useful in patients with chronic pain. Intrathecal, epidural, and systemic administration of clonidine also produce analgesia and clonidine is often useful in patients who have developed tolerance to opiates and who have some types of vascular or neuropathic pain.[117,118] Transdermal clonidine (0 to 3 mg/day) is sometimes useful in neuropathy, although the results on the treatment are mixed.

The mechanism of action of dexmedetomidine resembles that of clonidine, although its affinity for the α-2 adrenoceptor is approximately eight times that of clonidine,[119] and it has a significantly higher α-2/α-1 selectivity ratio than does clonidine.[120,121] Besides its analgesic effects, its sedative effects are thought to be secondary to action on α-2-adrenoreceptors located in the locus coeruleus. Similar to clonidine, dexmedetomidine decreases the requirement for opioids in patients undergoing a variety of surgical procedures[122] and in a clinical trial where it was administered as a single agent for sedation, it reduced by approximately 60% the number of patients who needed opioids for the control of pain.[123] Dexmedetomidine was approved in the United States in 2000 for up to 24 hours of pain treatment in surgical patients, and is currently in clinical trials for the control of postoperative pain in thoracotomy patients.

β-Blockers are not efficacious in the treatment of sympathetically maintained pain except in their use for alleviating migraine headaches. Guanethidine, bretylium, reserpine, and phentolamine have been used successfully to produce a chemical sympathectomy.[124,125]

TREATMENT OF CENTRAL NEUROPATHIC PAIN STATES

The clinical hallmark of central pain is that it persists without an obvious nociceptive stimulus; the physiologic goal of treatment is to stabilize hyperexcitable neurons. Table 18-8 outlines some clinical approaches to central pain.

Carbamazepine has been shown to be among the most effective agents for some facial neuralgias, which can be so agonizing that some patients actually look forward to death. Within 24 hours of attaining steady state, it is effective in 80% of patients with trigeminal neuralgia, making it clinically superior to phenytoin. Other types of lancinating pain, such as post-herpetic neuralgia, post-sympathectomy pain, and post-traumatic pain, may also respond to AEDs. IV trials offer a quick, definitive way of identifying drug responders in complex or pressured situations. For routine CNS pain, clonazepam is well-tolerated for pain syndromes, especially when allodynia is present. It facilitates both pre-synaptic and post-synaptic inhibition, increases recurrent inhibition, and decreases the firing rate of normal and epileptic neurons

TABLE 18-8 Pain Management and Treatment

PAIN CHARACTERISTICS	WHAT TREATMENT IS NEXT?	COMMENTS
Nociceptive element present?	Nerve block for diagnostic and therapeutic reasons Imaging: MRI, looking for lesion	Even in pain that appears central (e.g., trigeminal neuralgia), nociceptive triggers can initiate pain and peripheral deafferentation
Allodynia present? (vibration, cold, or light touch)	Low-dose clonazepam (1–4 mg/day) if the person can tolerate benzodiazepines alone or in combination with desipramine 50 mg at bedtime (up to 300 mg eventually, if necessary) Mexiletine 150–400 mg TID	Allodynia predicts response to clonazepam Clonazepam relaxes muscles, improves sleep and anxiety Membrane stabilizers useful but cardiotoxicity needs to be checked Peptides useful
Paroxysmal attacks? (lightning-like)	Anti-epileptic drugs (AEDs) Carbamazepine 400–1600 mg/day (serum 8–12 g/L) Valproate 500–2000 mg/day Gabapentin 300–1200 mg TID Lamotrigine 100–300 mg/day	Clonazepam should usually be tried first, but works well synergistically with the AEDs listed Valproate for vascular headache Gabapentin: few drug interactions
Central pain— Allodynia Paroxysmal attacks Sharp perceived as light touch Decreased pain threshold Non-dermatomal distribution of pain Hyperpathia	Definitive trial is a single-blind random assignment of IV lorazepam (2–4 mg) vs lidocaine (100 mg) vs morphine 10 mg, rated on a VAS pain Amitriptyline 25 mg IV infusion as test dose with VAS pain	Careful physical examination essential Is sharp perceived as light touch? Light touch is painful, sustained, and has a delayed crescendo Tuning fork/moving a hair examination best for allodynia
Comorbid central pain? Vascular and myofascial pain	Valproate 250–2000 mg/day Physical therapy Monoaminergic prescription antidepressants Nasal calcitonin 200 IU/day Capsaicin 4–6 week trial Topical preparation	Common in head, neck, and face pain Mixed results with SSRIs Rule out sympathetically maintained pain
Psychiatric component? Rule out or treat	Co-morbid psychiatric and CNS pain: consider prescription with dual efficacy for pain and psychiatric diagnosis Benzodiazepine for allodynia and anxiety Antidepressants for neuropathy, depression, and anxiety Neuroleptics for neuralgia, anxiety, psychosis, and nausea AEDs for lancinating pain and mood stabilization	Rule out depression and anxiety, consider mimics of central pain, such as somatoform, factitious, or psychotic disorders Pain drawing by the patient is a good tool to uncover psychosis and myofascial pain Rule out akathisia, restless leg syndrome

MRI, magnetic resonance imaging; IV, intravenous; VAS, visual analog scale; SSRIs, selective serotonin re-uptake inhibitors; AEDs, anti-epileptic drugs.

in the brain; it also enhances sleep, relaxes muscles and blood vessels, and treats anxiety symptoms. It is the drug that exemplifies the need to select prescriptions based not only on their efficacy and tolerability but also on their mechanisms of action for disease processes that have multiple pathophysiologies.

ECT has been used in longstanding pain accompanied by depression. The rationale is that treating the depression eases the suffering associated with pain. Unfortunately, ECT is effective for major depression, but it does not relieve pain. The assumption that there must be chronic depression with chronic pain and that it will be amenable to ECT is usually untenable.

TREATMENT OF PAIN BEHAVIOR AND THE USE OF MULTIDISCIPLINARY PAIN CLINICS

Guidelines

Medicare guidelines offer one set of standards for multidisciplinary pain management. The pain must be of at least 6 months' duration (resulting in significant life disturbance and limited functioning); it must be attributable to a physical cause; and it must be intractable to the usual methods of treatment. Desirable characteristics for pain treatment facilities and standards of care in pain management have now been published (in response to skepticism about cost, quality, control, and diversity of pain treatment facilities).[116] Quality control guidelines developed by the Commission on Accreditation of Rehabilitation Facilities (CARF), under the umbrella of the Joint Commission on Accreditation of Healthcare Organizations (JCAHO), have led to the certification of more than 100 chronic pain management programs nationwide. Behavioral treatments, however, are not primarily for pain relief; they merely extinguish the behaviors associated with pain.[126] Furthermore, proof of the cost-effectiveness of inpatient multidisciplinary treatment is nascent and consequently still ill-defined.

Reasons for Referral to an Inpatient Multidisciplinary Pain Clinic

Inpatient multidisciplinary pain clinics should be considered in the following circumstances:

- When the diagnosis of the physical and psychiatric pathology is already complete or is so obscure that intensive observation is necessary (e.g., malingering)
- When consultation from an independent physician who is an expert in the treatment of chronic pain is necessary to confirm that no single modality of outpatient treatment is likely to work
- When the patient has already obtained maximum benefit from outpatient treatments (such as NSAIDs, nerve blocks, antidepressants, and simple physical and behavioral rehabilitation)
- When intensive daily interventions are required, usually with multiple concurrent types of therapy, such as nerve blocks, physical therapy, and behavior modification
- When the patient exhibits abnormal pain behavior and agrees to the goals of improved coping, work rehabilitation, and psychiatric assessment
- When medications for pain relief are so complex or compliance management so difficult that direct supervision of medical therapy is necessary
- When a self-medication program is required (typically with a written schedule of medications, a contract, and strategies mutually acceptable for patient and physician).

Hypnosis

The use of hypnosis in chronic pain syndromes is well-known. Self-hypnosis is particularly helpful, but only about one in four subjects are able to achieve a state of concentration of sufficient magnitude for lasting pain control. Hypnosis is a method worth considering, provided that the physician knows its limitations and how to apply it to the individual patient's needs.

Rehabilitation

Rehabilitation of patients who have chronic pain syndromes may require some combination of input from specialists in psychiatry, physical therapy, physical medicine and rehabilitation, behavioral psychology, and neurology. It is important to bear in mind that no special therapy, including exercise therapy, spinal manipulation, bed rest, orthoses, acupuncture, traction therapy, back schools, and epidural steroids, works well. Successful rehabilitation aims to decrease symptoms, increase independence, and allow the patient to return to work. A positive, rapid return to light-normal activities and work is essential if disability is to be minimized. Psychologically, this is the key to coping with acute trauma. Even with patients who experience low back pain, 50% of whom have a recurrence within 3 years of the initial episode, there is no evidence that a return to work adversely effects the course of the pain syndrome.[127]

Treatment of myofascial pain syndromes may be challenging. It involves restoration of Stage 4 sleep, aerobic conditioning (which could include physical therapy or yoga), and avoidance of drugs, such as caffeine and alcohol. Trigger point analgesia, behavioral modification of maladaptive sleep habits, and the treatment of anxiety and depression may be necessary if chronic muscle pain is to be relieved. Monoamine oxidase inhibitors (MAOIs) are often effective. TCAs (e.g., desipramine and imipramine) may also be effective and are easier to use than MAOIs because dietary restrictions are not needed. Response to SSRIs has been unpredictable for myofascial pain, at times provoking muscle spasms and not helping the myofascial pain.[128] Cyclobenzaprine and S-adenosyl-methionine (SAMe), however, have resulted in some modest adjunctive efficacy.[129] Eight weeks is the duration of an optimal trial for any of these agents.

Education

Education is needed for the caregivers as well as the patient. In the past, medical professionals, be they physicians or nurses, viewed the patient who is in constant need of pain medication with suspicion. Physicians often under-estimated the medication's effective dose, over-estimated the medication's duration of action, and had an exaggerated notion of the danger of addiction. Rarely were physicians told to vary the amount of drug prescribed based on the patient's body weight, renal function, and previous tolerance for the drug. The physician's *ennui* with failure, suffering, and death could also have led to flight from pain. When the amount of medication a patient requires for the management of pain becomes a *cause celebre* on the ward, the consulting psychiatrist should call a meeting of the housestaff, attendings, and nurses, so that all biases and suspicions can be brought into the open. Medical personnel are far more apt to under-estimate the amount of opioid required for a given pain than to over-estimate it. In either case, their opinions are usually based more on misinformation or folklore than on fact. Once these judgments are aired, the patient usually benefits.

Cognitive and Behavioral Therapies

Cognitive-behavioral therapy (CBT) has been shown to be effective in patients who suffer from either continuous or chronic pain. Negative, or catastrophic, thoughts are often present in patients with pain disorders. Such thoughts are highly correlated to the intensity of pain complaints. CBT focuses on re-structuring this negative cognitive schema into a more realistic appraisal of the patient's current condition. When a realistic perspective regarding the past, present, and future can be gained, patients may be able to more easily deal with their pain. Relaxation training is often a component of CBT for pain patients. Progressive muscle relaxation, stretch-based relaxation, deep breathing, and autogenic training are all relaxation techniques that may be learned.[130]

Coping and Psychotherapy

Coping with chronic pain always threatens two fundamentals of survival: attachment behaviors and intrapsychic defenses. To cope means to have people of quality around to fortify one's courage and to have adaptive defense mechanisms to negotiate the thoughts and feelings that arise in one's head. Helping the patient develop cognitive-behavioral coping skills is more effective for decreasing pain and psychological disability than is education alone.[131] Coping is also context-dependent and is most effective when the focus includes the couple or family.[132,133]

The psychodynamic aspects of coping involve conflicts over autonomy and care. Old conflicts about nurturance suggest there may be mixed feelings about recovery. Shame may mimic depression, trigger conservation-withdrawal, and produce counter-dependent behavior. Regression, some of which is normal, can be manifest as non-compliance, help-rejecting behavior, complaining, and behaviors akin to the metaphoric "cutting off your nose to spite your face." The hateful patient and the hateful physician are often compatriots in partnership with chronic pain, and a task of the psychiatrist is to clarify how these problems become played out in the physician–patient relationship. One should understand that the physician is a protective figure who is the recipient of both idealized and angry feelings when a cure is not forthcoming. Modern health care, with its fragmentation, multiple caregivers, and bureaucracies, guarantees rifts in the physician–patient relationship. To help the patient cope, the psychiatrist must be sensitive to the unconscious feelings of the patient and be prepared to manage denial and to employ family counseling, relaxation, exercise, physical rehabilitation, and pharmacotherapy, while still functioning as a teacher and physician.

REFERENCES

Access the reference list online at https://expertconsult.inkling.com/.

Patients With Seizure Disorders

19

Taha Gholipour, M.D.
Felicia A. Smith, M.D.
Jeff C. Huffman, M.D.
Theodore A. Stern, M.D.

OVERVIEW

The structure and function of the central nervous system (CNS) is altered by many neurologic disorders. Because the CNS controls affect, behavior, and cognition, neurologic disorders can lead to neuropsychiatric symptoms that resemble those found in primary psychiatric conditions. Therefore, the general hospital psychiatrist is frequently called on to assess patients who have classic psychiatric symptoms caused by an underlying neurologic condition (e.g., a seizure disorder).

In this chapter, we will review the management of patients with neurologic conditions that are commonly associated with neuropsychiatric phenomena. We will discuss seizure disorders and describe the diagnosis and management of non-epileptic seizures (formerly called *pseudoseizures*).

CASE 1

Ms. A, a 23-year-old woman, was admitted to the medical floor after she presented to the Emergency Department with a self-reported "big seizure" a few days earlier at home, and two weeks of recurrent brief spells of "panic" and out-of-body experience. A psychiatric consultation was requested given her extensive psychiatric history and suspected psychogenic non-epileptic seizure.

She reported having bipolar disorder, post-traumatic stress disorder (related to childhood sexual and physical abuse by a relative), and being a victim of physical assault as a teenager (involving a skull fracture and reported seizure). She endorsed smoking marijuana on a daily basis to control her anxiety symptoms, and a history of heavy drinking. She was currently unemployed and struggled with keeping her current living situation. She stopped her lamotrigine, which she was prescribed as a mood stabilizer, around a month ago. On exam she appeared anxious, but was euthymic. Other than a report of out of body (autoscopic) visual hallucinations along with the "panic spells" there were no other positive findings on the exam. She denied suicidal ideation or violent thoughts. The toxicology screen was positive for marijuana, and her alcohol and lamotrigine levels were undetectable. A head CT scan was reported as unremarkable.

The consultant confirmed the psychiatric history, provided input regarding management during the hospitalization, and expressed concern about the etiology of the spells; a neurology consultation was recommended as well as a video-EEG during the admission. An extended bedside EEG with video recording captured three identical events during which Ms. A remained conscious but appeared fearful. These were accompanied with slowing of the heart rate lasting for approximately 10 seconds, after which she reported the event to her nurse. Review of the EEG showed focal seizures arising from the right posterior temporal region.

The diagnosis of focal seizures with impairment of awareness from the right temporal lobe with presumed occasional secondary generalization and associated ictal bradycardia was made. The history of significant head trauma was considered the most likely etiology. Ms. A was re-started on lamotrigine, with levetiracetam as a second antiepileptic drug (AED) to protect her from generalized seizures while lamotrigine remained sub-therapeutic. As well as addressing co-morbid psychiatric diagnoses, the treatment team counseled Ms. A about medication adherence, contraception, avoidance of driving, and the risk of mood symptoms, aggression, or suicidal ideation with her new medication, levetiracetam. A neurology follow-up appointment was also made to address her new diagnosis, consider further work-up, and consider stopping the second AED.

THE MANAGEMENT OF PSYCHIATRIC SYMPTOMS IN PATIENTS WITH SEIZURE DISORDERS

Approximately half of all patients with seizure disorders have co-morbid psychiatric syndromes;[1] therefore, the general hospital psychiatrist should have a working knowledge of seizure disorders and the neuropsychiatric syndromes that are commonly associated with these disorders. Patients with seizures may have psychiatric symptoms that occur during a seizure (*ictal* symptoms), immediately before or after a seizure (*peri-ictal* symptoms), or between seizures (*inter-ictal* symptoms). Some medical and surgical treatments for this condition are also associated with psychiatric symptoms.

By way of definition, a clinical seizure is an abnormal paroxysmal discharge of cerebral neurons sufficient to cause clinically detectable events that are apparent to the patient or an observer.[2] Patients with a chronic course of repeated, unprovoked seizures are said to have epilepsy. Seizures can be *focal* (starting in a particular area of the brain, i.e., the focus) or *generalized* (involving both hemispheres simultaneously). Focal seizures (formerly called "partial seizures") may remain limited to their focus on the same brain hemisphere, or propagate throughout the rest of the cortex, often called *secondary generalization*. Consciousness is often fully or partially preserved as long as the seizure activity is restricted to only limited parts of the brain. Clinical symptomatology may be variable in this setting, correlating with the involved brain areas. Generalized seizures are associated with loss of consciousness, ranging from seconds of staring spells in *absence* seizures (formerly called *petit mal*) to *generalized tonic–clonic* convulsions (*grand mal*). Generalized tonic-clonic (GTC) seizures can occur after an immediate or delayed spread of focal seizure activity to the rest of the brain, or so-called *secondary generalization*. A *primary* generalized seizure happens in the absence of a suspected focus and in the setting of a genetic/idiopathic epilepsy syndrome, or due to metabolic disarray (such as hypoglycemia, hyponatremia, toxic exposure). GTCs are characterized by a sudden loss of consciousness with a brief tonic phase marked by contraction of skeletal muscles and upward deviation of the eyes. A more prolonged clonic phase (characterized by rhythmic movements and jerking of the extremities) follows.[3] These seizures are almost always followed by a *post-ictal* state with decreased responsiveness and a state similar to deep sleep that lasts minutes to hours. *Absence* seizures are characterized by brief (usually 5 to 10 seconds) lapses in consciousness and by motionless staring, without loss of muscle tone, and without any post-ictal change in consciousness. These seizures occur primarily in children and are rare after puberty. *Myoclonic* seizures are characterized by brief and sudden, often bilateral, muscle contractions that may occur singly or repeatedly; these are seen in a variety of epileptic syndromes in children but also occur in adults with advanced neurodegenerative diseases. *Atonic* seizures ("*drop attacks*") are a type of generalized seizure characterized by sudden loss of muscle tone leading to falls, without clonic activities seen in tonic-clonic seizures.

The terminology for focal seizures has changed repeatedly over the last decade which has caused some confusion. Focal seizures are generally described based on how they affect consciousness. Focal seizures with impairment of consciousness or awareness (formerly complex partial seizures, also known as focal unaware seizures) deserve special mention, insofar as they are the most common type of seizure in adults and are commonly associated with neuropsychiatric phenomena.[4] Particular types of focal seizures that also have a high prevalence of neuropsychiatric symptoms during and between seizures include *temporal lobe epilepsy (TLE)* and *psychomotor seizures*. On the other hand, focal seizures without impairment of consciousness or awareness (formerly simple partial seizures, also known as focal aware seizures) have symptoms limited to the area of cortex that are stimulated, such as simple motor seizures with twitching of corresponding muscle groups, or simple visual seizures with occurrence of visual experiences in the visual field corresponding to seizing cortex.

Focal seizures may involve sensory, affective, perceptual, behavioral, or cognitive symptoms. They may include hallucinations of any sensory modality; they can be olfactory (e.g., a noxious odor, like burning rubber), gustatory (metallic or other tastes), auditory, visual, or tactile. The most common affective symptoms are fear and anxiety, although depression may also occur; rage is uncommon. Such affective symptoms usually have a sudden onset and offset.

Behavior during focal seizures with impairment of awareness may also be abnormal; *automatisms* are common and may include oral or buccal movements (e.g., lip smacking or chewing), picking behaviors, or prolonged staring. Cognitive symptoms associated with focal seizures include *déjà vu* (a feeling of familiarity), *jamais vu* (a feeling of unfamiliarity), macropsia, micropsia, and dissociative, or "out-of-body" experiences. Patients with neuro-psychiatric symptoms secondary to seizures may be mistakenly diagnosed with a primary psychiatric disorder because the symptoms are often similar to those of psychiatric disorders, and because the inter-ictal (and even ictal) scalp electroencephalograms (EEG) may appear normal due to deep localization of involved cortices. Therefore, the general hospital psychiatrist must be particularly astute in differentiating patients with focal seizures from those with primary psychiatric disorders.

In the following discussion, the phenomenology and treatment of neuropsychiatric symptoms among patients with seizure disorders is outlined. The ictal, peri-ictal, and inter-ictal neuropsychiatric symptoms will be discussed, as will ways to delineate how these symptoms differ from those seen in patients without seizure disorders.

Ictal Neuropsychiatric Phenomena

Ictal psychiatric symptoms are most commonly associated with focal seizures, although they can also occur with generalized seizures.[1] Anxiety, fear, and psychosis are the most common psychiatric symptoms experienced during a seizure. Up to one-third of patients with focal seizures with impairment of awareness have anxiety or fear as part of their seizures;[5,6] the anxiety is often intense and may last throughout the course of the seizure. It is important to keep in mind that subtle focal seizures, such as a stereotyped anxiety, might be described as an "aura" (a term no longer recommended for describing these seizures) by patients and some physicians. Such symptoms may resemble those of panic attacks with autonomic symptoms, nausea, intense anxiety, and depersonalization. Therefore, patients with epilepsy may have both ictal anxiety and inter-ictal panic attacks that are difficult to distinguish. The more circumscribed the symptoms are to associated seizure phenomena (e.g., automatisms or hallucinations during an episode, or confusion or severe lethargy after the event), the more likely it is that the anxiety is ictal.

Ictal psychosis has also been seen in patients with focal seizures. Ictal psychotic symptoms are most often associated with temporal lobe foci, but nearly one-third of patients have non-temporal lobe foci.[7] Hallucinations during a seizure are much more likely to be olfactory or gustatory; auditory hallucinations (common in primary psychotic disorders) are less common, but simple auditory symptoms, such as echoing, might happen in the setting of a simple focal seizure involving auditory perception cortices. Paranoia is uncommon and usually short-lived. In contrast to patients with primary psychosis, consciousness is usually impaired during ictal psychosis, and affected patients are usually amnestic for the episode.[8]

Ictal depression is uncommon; it occurs as part of the aura in approximately 1% of patients with epilepsy.[9] Such depressive symptoms, as with other ictal symptoms, appear abruptly, in a stereotypical manner, and without obvious psychosocial precipitants. Although depressive symptoms often disappear abruptly, some authors have noted that ictal depressed mood may extend beyond other ictal or post-ictal symptoms.[9,10] Ictal crying (so-called *dacrystic seizure*) has been described in seizures with involvement of limbic structures.

Ictal anger, agitation, and aggression have also been reported, but appear to be exceedingly rare (fewer than 0.5% of patients in one large series[11]). Furthermore, ictal aggression is poorly directed and does not involve significant interactive behavior. Stereotyped shouting and pushing are among the most common manifestations, while patients rarely perform intricate, directed acts of violence during a seizure.

Determining whether anxiety, depression, or other psychiatric symptoms are ictal events or part of primary psychiatric conditions can be difficult. Table 19-1 describes some distinguishing characteristics of ictal and non-ictal symptoms. In general, ictal symptoms are more often abrupt in onset and offset, occur in concert with other stereotyped manifestations of seizures, and are frequently short-lived, usually lasting less than 3 minutes.[1] The most convincing evidence for the ictal nature of a symptom is a more or less stereotyped pattern; that is, a patient will not experience fear with one seizure and depressive symptoms with another—the pattern of symptoms will generally be the same.

Prolonged or frequent focal seizures, sometimes qualifying as *status epilepticus*, may result in prolonged ictal psychiatric symptoms that further complicate the diagnosis. Therefore, the EEG remains a key tool for establishing whether symptoms are ictal. Since most focal seizures have an identifiable *focus* such as an ischemic, neoplastic, or vascular lesion, brain imaging should be considered early if ictal symptoms are suspected. A patient's history, such as history of systemic malignancy, cerebrovascular risk factors, or suspicion for an inflammatory or infectious process in the brain, should decrease the threshold for imaging. Unfortunately, CT scans have low sensitivity and specificity for detecting many etiologies, despite their ready availability and lower cost; a magnetic resonance imaging (MRI) protocoled and reviewed by a radiologist for finding seizure foci, is strongly recommended.

Treatment of ictal psychiatric symptoms requires a careful evaluation. Primary psychiatric symptoms and ictal psychiatric symptoms are similar, frequently co-morbid, and have different treatments. Therefore, working with a neurologist for careful clinical evaluation, EEG monitoring, and when indicated, other diagnostic procedures should be followed to distinguish these phenomena. Once symptoms have been identified as ictal, treatment of the associated psychiatric symptoms requires treatment of the seizure with anticonvulsants. Treatment of ictal psychosis with antipsychotics or ictal anxiety with non-anticonvulsant anxiolytics is generally not indicated. Measures to reduce the risk of falls or other injury are crucial for patients whose seizure disorders remain active.

Peri-ictal Neuropsychiatric Phenomena

Despite the above-mentioned rarer ictal neuropsychiatric phenomena, the majority of neuropsychiatric disturbances happen in peri-ictal, and mostly post-ictal phases of seizures. They usually occur several hours after a seizure. Pre-ictal symptoms can occur and include psychosis, mood changes, or aggression in the hours or minutes before a seizure have been described and should not be confused with focal seizures that are sometimes called *auras*.[5,12] These symptoms tend to increase until the onset of the clinical seizure[13] and,

TABLE 19-1 Clinical Characteristics That Help Distinguish Epileptic From Non-Epileptic Events

	EPILEPTIC SEIZURES	NON-EPILEPTIC SEIZURES/EVENTS
Onset	Sudden onset and offset	Often gradual
Duration	Often <3 minutes	Variable
Perception	May experience olfactory, gustatory, visual hallucination; déjà vu; derealization	May experience auditory hallucinations; paranoia
Eyes during event	Open	Closed
Incontinence	Common	Rare
Awareness	Often impaired; can stay aware during some focal seizures	Variable; may be responsive during parts of the event
Recall of event	None or limited (e.g. aura)	Usually intact
Ictal EEG	Almost always abnormal	Unchanged from baseline
Inter-ictal EEG	Normal or abnormal	Often normal
Tongue bite	Lateral tongue	None or tip of tongue
Injury	May be present	Rarely present (suggestive of serious psychopathology)
Incontinence	May be present	Rare
Post-ictal state	Confusion or drowsiness is common	Rare
Prolactin	Elevated; or normal	Normal; rarely elevated from baseline

depending on the time course and nature of the symptoms, may be conceptualized as prodromes separate from the ictus or as ictal events.

Post-ictal neuropsychiatric symptoms are relatively common. Approximately 8% to 10% of patients with seizures have post-ictal behavioral disturbances.[14] These symptoms may occur in the context of a diffuse post-ictal suppression of the cortical activity that involves disinhibited, sub-cortical behavior (such as moaning, crying, laughing, cursing, sexual behavior, or rage). Autonomic instability may contribute to what is observed as a post-ictal behavior as well. Patients are often amnestic to these events, and difficult to control. Neuropsychiatric symptoms may also arise post-ictally, despite the presence of a clear consciousness. Patients may remember parts of events or even try to justify their behavior. By definition, post-ictal symptoms should remit spontaneously and are often short-lived, and persistence of symptoms beyond 72 hours should be considered as a possible inter-ictal symptom. However, such symptoms may persist for days or even weeks. Patients with well-defined, prolonged post-ictal neuropsychiatric syndromes may be more likely to develop persistent inter-ictal symptoms.[15]

Psychosis is the most common post-ictal neuropsychiatric symptom, occurring in up to 7.8% of epilepsy patients,[16] and often appears after a non-psychotic post-ictal period. It occurs most commonly in patients with focal-unaware seizures that become secondarily generalized,[9] especially in those with temporal lobe or bilateral foci. Psychotic symptoms vary widely, and affective symptoms (depressive or manic) may also be present. Symptoms can include paranoid or grandiose delusions and hallucinations in a variety of sensory modalities; Schneiderian first-rank symptoms of schizophrenia are rare.[15] Symptoms tend to resolve spontaneously but recur an average of two to three times per year. In a minority of patients, such symptoms become chronic, even in the absence of clear clinical seizures.

Post-ictal depression is also associated with focal-unaware seizures but is less common than post-ictal psychosis.[17] Patients with post-ictal depression may have flattened affect and anhedonia more often than sadness, and post-ictal depression is commonly associated with delirium and other post-ictal cognitive disturbances. Kanner and Balabanov found that symptoms last an average of 24 hours, although symptoms may be more prolonged.[17] In most cases, post-ictal depressive symptoms do not just represent a reactive response to the stress of having a seizure. Other post-ictal symptoms are less common. Acute post-ictal anxiety is relatively infrequent and is usually associated with post-ictal depression. Post-ictal mania and hypomania occur infrequently. Post-ictal aggression can also occur; however, it is generally associated with delirium, psychotic symptoms, or abnormal mood states.

The management of patients with post-ictal neuropsychiatric symptoms has a number of tenets. First, enhanced treatment of the seizure disorder is crucial; patients whose seizure disorders are poorly controlled appear to have a greater tendency toward post-ictal affective and psychotic symptoms. In addition to anticonvulsants for seizure prophylaxis, other psychotropic medications may be indicated, especially if symptoms are prolonged, present a risk to the patient or to others, or adversely affect the patient's ability to receive appropriate treatment. Such situations occur most commonly with psychosis, and low doses of antipsychotics can reduce agitation and diminish psychotic symptoms. If such symptoms are limited to the post-ictal period, these medications can be discontinued once symptoms resolve, because the best prophylaxis against recurrence of psychosis is treatment with anticonvulsants to prevent seizures. Antidepressants are uncommonly indicated for depressive symptoms limited to the post-ictal period.

In addition to medications, behavioral treatments can be instituted to facilitate coping and to maintain the patient's safety. Such interventions may include the use of restraints or observers, frequent re-orientation, or the presence of familiar family members. Finally, it is important to know the patient's post-ictal pattern of symptoms to prepare caregivers and family members for what lies ahead. Seizures and their neuropsychiatric sequelae are commonly stereotyped; that is, patients tend to have the same post-ictal symptomatology from seizure to seizure. If a patient is known to become psychotic or dangerous after a seizure, the treatment team can be prepared with antipsychotic treatments or other safety-enhancing measures.

Inter-ictal (Chronic) Neuropsychiatric Phenomena

Psychiatric syndromes are also common in the period between seizures; patients with seizure disorders have chronic psychiatric disorders at substantially higher rates than do those in the general population and those with similar quality of life burden from other chronic medical conditions. Depression, anxiety, and psychosis are all common with depressive disorders being the most prevalent. In contrast, inter-ictal hypomanic or manic symptoms are uncommon and often point to a possible primary mood disorder.

Inter-ictal depression is common and can be disabling. Rates of depression and suicide among patients with epilepsy are four to five times greater than those in the general population,[1,18,19] and up to 80% of patients with epilepsy report having some feelings of depression.[20] A constellation of biological and psychosocial factors likely coalesce to result in these elevated rates of depression, but risk factors for depression that are specific to seizure disorders include poor seizure control and focal seizures with impairment of awareness,[21,22] especially with left-sided temporal lobe seizure foci. In fact, suicide may be 25 times more likely among patients with TLE than among those in the general population.[23] Prior history of depression has also been associated with the onset of seizures, given that a history of depression increases (by three-fold) the risk of developing a seizure disorder.[17,24] Some have hypothesized that depression and epilepsy share neurotransmitter abnormalities (e.g., reduced noradrenergic, dopaminergic, and serotonergic activity), and that these shared abnormalities may explain the link between the two conditions.

The symptoms of inter-ictal depression are often distinctive. Atypical features are common,[20] and many patients have depressive symptoms that are more consistent with dysthymia than with major depression.[25] Blumer et al.[26] have described a clinical syndrome called *inter-ictal dysphoric disorder*, which is characterized by inter-ictal dysthymic symptoms with intermittent irritability, impulsivity, anxiety, and somatic symptoms. Some people with epilepsy and their family may report that worsening of these behavioral symptoms is predictive of a breakthrough seizure in the upcoming hours to days.

Inter-ictal anxiety disorders vary in frequency. Anxiety symptoms are more common in patients with epilepsy than they are in the general population, and, of the anxiety disorders, panic disorder appears to be the most common. Inter-ictal panic disorder is present in approximately 20% of patients with epilepsy,[5] with symptoms that differentiate the panic attacks from the feelings of panic that occur during a seizure. The treating neurologist may want to capture some of these events on video-EEG monitoring, preferably in an inpatient epilepsy monitoring study, to ascertain the non-ictal nature of these panic symptoms, especially in epilepsy with a temporal lobe focus. Other anxiety disorders, such as generalized anxiety disorder (GAD) or obsessive–compulsive disorder (OCD) are less common.[1] Inter-ictal personality disorder however, may involve prominent obsessive traits.

Inter-ictal psychosis can be intermittent (with brief, recurrent episodes), but more commonly it is continuous and chronic. Psychotic symptoms are approximately 10 times more likely to occur in patients with epilepsy.[1] Psychosis is also more common in epilepsy with a temporal focus, and also in patients with multiple seizure types, a poor response to seizure treatment, or a history of status epilepticus.[27] Clinically, inter-ictal psychotic symptoms most often consist of paranoid delusions with associated visual or auditory hallucinations. Affective blunting, a lack of motivation, and catatonia are also common.[27] Compared with patients with primary schizophrenia, patients with inter-ictal psychosis have a greater preservation of affect and more visual hallucinations.

An inter-ictal personality change among patients with TLE was described several decades ago and repeatedly reported by practicing epileptologists. The TLE personality syndrome, reported primarily by Gastaut and co-workers[28] and detailed by Geschwind,[4] has features that include moral rigidity, hyper-religiosity, hypergraphia, hyposexuality, and hyperviscosity ("a sticky personality"). However, some authors have questioned the existence of such a syndrome.[29]

The management of inter-ictal psychiatric phenomena is similar to the treatment of primary psychiatric disorders. However, there are a number of special considerations in this population. Given that most inter-ictal psychiatric symptoms are more common when seizures are poorly controlled, effective treatment with anticonvulsants is of vital importance. Treatment of psychiatric symptoms associated with epilepsy should also include behavioral and educational interventions that reduce the risk related to their seizure disorder (e.g., having family ensure that depressed patients take their anticonvulsants or keeping manic or psychotic patients from driving when this is unsafe).

One caveat in the treatment of patients with co-existing neuropsychiatric symptoms with antiepileptic drugs (AEDs) is the potential behavioral side effects of some of these drugs. The Federal Food and Drug Administration (FDA) has issued a class label change, asking AED manufacturers to warn patients and providers about a possible increased risk of suicidal thoughts and behavior, even when used for indications other than seizure control. This warning was issued in response to a large meta-analysis which shows an association, but not looking into the possible causality from underlying conditions in patients who are prescribed an AED.[30] Some AEDs are better known to affect patient's underlying or co-morbid behavioral symptoms in both positive and negative ways. Lamotrigine, valproate, and carbamazepine have long been used as mood stabilizers and are generally favored by neurologists when mood disorders or disturbances are established (or even perceived) in a patient with epilepsy. Phenobarbital may cause increased irritability in children with epilepsy, but not in adults. Topiramate (particularly at higher doses), zonisamide, phenobarbital, and vigabatrin can cause depressed mood. Lamotrigine and felbamate are generally considered stimulating and may produce anxiety or insomnia.[31]

Perampanel is a new broad-spectrum AED that targets the central glutamate AMPA receptors. During pivotal clinical trials, an increased risk of psychiatric adverse effects, consisting of alteration of mood and hostility was noted. This led to a black box warning for aggression and homicidal ideation. The behavioral side effects seem to be dose dependent and improved in most patients with decreasing dose.[32,33]

Levetiracetam, one of the most frequently used first-line AEDs has a great medical safety profile, but has become infamous for affecting mood and behavior. Different studies suggest around 10%[34] of patients started on levetiracetam report change in their mood or behavior in the form of irritability (most common), aggression, depression, or worsening depression, and labile mood, and rarely suicidality. Some patients will need to switch AEDs due to this side effect. There are observational studies suggesting that supplementation of pyridoxine (vitamin B_6) may improve the behavioral change in a group of pediatric epilepsy patients.[35]

Treatment of psychiatric symptoms with psychotropics is frequently indicated, but the effects of these agents on the seizure threshold should be considered. The risk of seizure with most antidepressant agents is quite small when these agents are used at standard doses.[36] Citalopram,[37] sertraline,[36] venlafaxine,[17] and tricyclic antidepressants (TCAs)[26] have all been used successfully in patients with epilepsy without significantly exacerbating the underlying seizure disorder. Given their relative safety with regard to seizure exacerbation and their overall safety and tolerability, selective serotonin re-uptake inhibitors (SSRIs) should be considered as first-line treatment for patients with inter-ictal depression. In general, starting with a low dose and increasing the dose gradually should minimize the risk of seizure in these patients. Bupropion and maprotiline are more strongly associated with the development of seizures. Among the TCAs, clomipramine may be associated with a greater risk of seizure and should probably be avoided as well. Monoamine oxidase inhibitors (MAOIs) have not been associated with an elevated risk of seizure, although they have not been studied in patients with seizure disorders. Finally, electroconvulsive therapy (ECT) can be used to treat patients with epilepsy and severe depression;[38] ECT appears to increase the seizure threshold between treatments,[39] and it has been used safely in patients with epilepsy.[40]

Patients with anxiety disorders can be treated with antidepressants or with benzodiazepines; buspirone, sometimes used for the treatment of GAD, can lower the seizure threshold and generally is not recommended for this population.[41] Patients on rapid dose escalation of buspirone may present with new-onset or breakthrough seizures, some of them a symptom of an underlying epilepsy.

Inter-ictal psychosis can be treated with antipsychotics. It appears that all antipsychotics may modestly lower the seizure threshold; however, low-potency antipsychotics, such as chlorpromazine, may have greater effects on the seizure threshold than higher-potency agents.[42] Clozapine has been associated with an elevated seizure risk and, in general, should be avoided. Therefore, when needed, recommended agents are atypical antipsychotics, such as risperidone, or high-potency typical antipsychotics. Again, titrating the dosage slowly and using the lowest effective dose should minimize the risk of seizure in this population.

In summary, virtually any psychiatric symptom can occur before, during, or after the seizure. However, anxiety is most common during a seizure, psychosis is most common post-ictally, and depression is the most common chronic symptom between seizures. All behavioral symptoms are more common in patients with focal seizures with impairment awareness (formerly complex partial seizures) than with other types of seizure disorders. Treatment of ictal phenomena involves treatment of the seizure, whereas post-ictal and inter-ictal phenomena may require the use of antipsychotics, anxiolytics, or antidepressants for optimal symptomatic relief. Careful attention to the patient's safety is always an important consideration (whether from seizure or suicidality), and a knowledge of the patient's pattern of symptoms associated with their seizures helps caregivers and family members prepare for sequelae.

NON-EPILEPTIC SEIZURES

Patients who appear to be having epileptic seizures may, in fact, be having abnormal movements as the result of another medical or neurologic problem or, most often, as a consequence of psychological factors (e.g., a conversion reaction). These events, called *psychogenic non-epileptic seizures (PNESs)*, pose a common and important problem. The terms *pseudoseizure* and *hysterical seizures* have been used in the past and are antiquated, and discouraged for reasons that should be obvious to mental health providers, to avoid assumption of these being voluntary events by family and other providers. The incidence of PNES is higher in people with a personal history of seizures as well as in those with a history of knowing or taking care of patients with seizures, such as a family member or a healthcare provider at any level. The prevalence of PNES increases significantly within outpatient and inpatient referral centers for epilepsy.[43] Clarification of the nature of events (epileptic vs non-epileptic, often psychiatric, non-epileptic seizures) are a common reason for admission to an epilepsy monitoring unit or inpatient video-EEG monitoring. Patients with PNES are often significantly disabled by these events. When they have concurrent epileptic seizures, these may be easier to control with AEDs or surgical procedures.[44]

As with other conversion disorders, the presence of PNES imposes a high burden on the patient's health, as well as on the healthcare system, and is often hard to diagnose and treat. Even after a diagnosis of PNES has been made, affected patients continue to be disabled by recurrent convulsive events.[43,45]

The general hospital psychiatrist is frequently called on to assess patients suspected of having PNES. Knowledge of the epidemiology, differential diagnosis, clinical features, and relevant diagnostic studies that may suggest the presence of PNES can significantly facilitate making the diagnosis. Once the diagnosis of PNES is suspected, it is important for the psychiatrist to be able to discuss the diagnosis of PNES with the patient in a way that is validating, reassuring, and supportive.[43,46,47]

PNES is common, occurring in approximately 10% of outpatients with intractable seizure disorders and in approximately 20% of patients with intractable seizures referred to epilepsy monitoring units.[43] About three-fourths of those with PNES are women, and they most often exhibit symptoms when they are between the ages of 15 and 35.[45] A history of sexual abuse is common among patients with PNES, occurring in at least 25% of those with the condition.[48,49] Roughly 25% of patients with PNES also suffer from epileptic seizures.[50] Unfortunately, sometime patients with either epileptic seizures (or cardiovascular events) are mistakenly diagnosed with PNES without adequate work-up, sometimes by a provider biased by the pre-existing psychiatric diagnosis or substance use, psychosocial history, and (as discussed earlier in this chapter) undiagnosed ictal or inter-ictal neuropsychiatric phenomena. Other non-epileptic events without a presumed psychiatric nature are less frequently, but occasionally, presented to the consulting psychiatrist, and it is important to recognize them. Syncope and undiagnosed cardiovascular causes with unusual symptoms are probably the most important to recognize. Table 19-2 displays a number of conditions that can be mistaken for epilepsy. Among PNES semiologies, recurrent unconscious, psychologically mediated hypermotor spells (essentially conversion GTC seizure-like spells) are the most common. Other causes of functional somatic symptoms, such as factitious disorder and malingering, are more extensively covered in Chapter 16.

TABLE 19-2 Differential Diagnosis of Non-Epileptic Events
General Medical Conditions
Transient ischemic attack (TIA)
Complicated migraine
Syncope
Hypoglycemia
Parasomnia (e.g., rapid eye movement [REM], behavior disorder, or night terrors)
Narcolepsy
Myoclonus (from metabolic disturbance)
Psychiatric Causes
Conversion disorder
Somatic symptom disorder
Dissociative disorder
Panic disorder (simulating partial seizures)
Volitional Deception
Factitious disorder (goal is to maintain the sick role)
Malingering (goal is to obtain secondary gain, e.g., disability income)

Clinical Considerations

This section addresses the approach to diagnosis of PNES. Although almost all of the features suggestive of PNES (discussed later) can also occur in true seizure disorders, certain clinical features of the peri-ictal and convulsive phases can help distinguish these two, although a single clinical feature taken in isolation should not be used to confirm a diagnosis of NES. It is useful to know the usual characteristics of GTC seizures, and careful observation throughout the seizure can be very useful in the diagnostic assessment. This is why inpatient admission and prolonged video-EEG to capture the event on video for review is considered the current best way of making the diagnosis.

GTC seizures are usually sudden in onset; although there may be an aura before the seizure, there is usually a sudden loss of consciousness, followed by a brief tonic period of <30 seconds. A more prolonged period of convulsive, clonic activity follows. This activity is characterized by bilateral, symmetrical, and rhythmic jerking of the upper and lower extremities; trunk activity and pelvic thrusting are uncommon. Loss of continence, tongue-biting, and other injuries may occur. The patient remains unconscious and unresponsive throughout the event and is amnestic for the episode. After the event, the patient may be confused or drowsy or complain of headache; the patient is rarely completely lucid in the immediate post-ictal period. Most GTC seizures are quite brief, lasting less than 3 minutes, and they have a stereotyped pattern in a given individual. On the other hand, Table 19-3 lists the clinical features that suggest PNES. It should be emphasized again that certain types of seizures are marked by symptoms that appear to suggest PNES. For example, focal motor seizures may involve asymmetrical jerking with preserved consciousness. Focal seizures with impairment of awareness can manifest with only behavioral or psychiatric symptoms. Frontal lobe seizures may cause pelvic thrusting and pedaling movements, but characteristically tend to occur in sleep. Automatisms during focal seizures with impairment of awareness may result in acts that appear volitional. However, a combination of atypical features suggest that PNES is the more likely diagnosis.[43,45]

TABLE 19-3 Features That Suggest Non-Epileptic (Conversion) Seizures
Historical Features
History of sexual abuse
History of other unexplained neurologic symptoms occurring during stress
Seizures despite multiple adequate trials of anticonvulsants at therapeutic levels
Features of Event
Events occur with suggestion/provocation
Gradual onset and offset of symptoms
Responsiveness during event
Weeping, speaking, or yelling during the event
Asymmetrical clonic activity
Head bobbing or pelvic thrusting
Rapid kicking or thrashing
Prolonged duration of symptoms (>3 minutes)
No EEG abnormalities during the event
Post-Event Features
Lucid during immediate post-ictal period
Able to recall event
Lack of incontinence, tongue biting, or physical injury despite numerous events
Post-ictal prolactin is normal
Neuropsychological testing suggestive of conversion symptoms

The use of video-EEG monitoring allows one to correlate EEG changes (or the lack thereof) during a convulsive event. If a patient experiences a typical event and the EEG remains normal, this suggests PNES, especially when there are other clinical features that are inconsistent with epilepsy. However, it should be noted that focal seizures may give rise to normal EEGs in 10% to 40% of cases.[51–53] The EEG capture of multiple events reduces the likelihood of such false-negative EEG findings. If the patient reports multiple semiologies, there is always a chance that the unwitnessed etiology is indeed a seizure, even if one other type of spell is determined to be PNES.

In addition to using video-EEG monitoring, use of suggestion or provocative stimuli may provide evidence for the diagnosis of PNES. The use of provocative stimuli was practiced regularly in the past, but has been a topic of ethical controversy as they are considered deceptive; examples include injection of normal saline or placement of a tuning fork on the head after a suggestion has been given that the procedure will likely cause a seizure. Much discussion has ensued about the ethics of deception under these circumstances; researchers have found that such provocative testing can be approached honestly with the patient with high rates of suggestibility and little adverse effect on the patient–physician alliance.[50] However, these techniques are now generally discouraged, while use of hyperventilation, photic stimulation, and verbal suggestion without creating explicit misinformation for the patient are commonly used.[54]

In terms of laboratory studies, the usefulness of prolactin levels to distinguish between epileptic and non-epileptic events is questionable, given that in more than 10% of patients with GTC seizures, 30% of patients with temporal lobe seizures, and 60% of patients with frontal lobe seizures, prolactin is not elevated.[55] Other diagnostic laboratory values, such as creatine phosphokinase (CPK), may be even less sensitive and specific, especially when taken in isolation.

Neuropsychological testing can be a useful adjunct to a clinical and laboratory evaluation. Such testing can provide information about co-morbid psychiatric diagnoses, personality styles, and tendency toward conversion reactions. Some studies demonstrate that patients with PNES, when compared with patients with epilepsy, exhibit less objective evidence of cognitive impairment and are more likely to show impairments that are a function of poor effort rather than real deficits.[56,57] Also, some studies of patients with PNES using the Minnesota Multi-phasic Personality Inventory (MMPI) report an association with the "conversion V" profile with elevations in scales 1 (Hs, hypochondriasis), 3 (Hy, hysteria), and 2 (D, depression).[55] However, such testing cannot definitively make or exclude a diagnosis of PNES, and there is significant overlap of results, particularly on cognitive testing, between patients with PNES and those with epilepsy.[58]

SUMMARY

Making a definitive diagnosis of PNES can be difficult. As presented in the clinical vignette at the beginning of this chapter (Case 1), there are characteristic features of epidemiology, clinical events, laboratory values, and EEG monitoring that may suggest PNES, but for each individual thought to have PNES, there are others in whom true epilepsy can result in a diagnosis of PNES. However, a thorough evaluation using each of these domains—with EEG-video monitoring being the best diagnostic test—can help the psychiatrist determine whether PNES is more or less likely. Finally, it is important to allow for the possibility that one's diagnosis of PNES may be incorrect; but this should not prevent clinicians from moving forward on the basis of their clinical findings. It should simply serve as a reminder to maintain an open mind about the diagnosis.

General medical providers often feel that once the diagnosis of PNES has been made, treatment is over. However, fortunately *and* unfortunately, treatment is truly just beginning. After the diagnosis is made, patients with PNES continue to have frequent and disabling PNES events; only about 30% will stop having convulsive events.[43,45] However, early diagnosis is associated with a better outcome,[59] and presentation of the diagnosis and a treatment plan in a way that is acceptable to the patient is critical.

Table 19-4 lists the important features of NESs diagnosis and the treatment plan for patients with the disorder. In general, the tenets of revealing the diagnosis are similar to those outlined for conversion disorder in Chapter 16. First of all, the diagnosis should be framed in a positive way: it is tremendously reassuring that these events are not due to abnormal electrical discharges in the brain, and there is no need to take anticonvulsant medications and deal with their side effects. If a patient feels as if he or she is being told that there is nothing wrong, it can be useful to emphasize that although there is not a *structural* or *electrographical* abnormality present, it is clear that there is an abnormality of *function* of their nervous system that will require integrated treatment. Furthermore, the physician should make it clear that he or she understands that these events are having a significant impact on the patient's life and obviously require ongoing efforts to reduce their negative impact.

Next, the physician should describe the impact of mood, anxiety, and stress on these symptoms and inform the patient that reduction of these symptoms is absolutely imperative to help the patient improve his or her function and quality of life. However, rather than simply making a referral to a psychiatrist, the physician should also emphasize that the patient will continue to see his or her neurologist or primary care physician on a regular basis as a crucial part of the treatment. The regularity of this follow-up is important: the patient should have an appointment with the caregiver, regardless of whether he or she is having active symptoms, thus disconnecting the link between symptoms and medical attention.

In one of the few controlled trials conducted to compare treatment options for PNES, LaFrance and colleagues conducted a small, randomized study.[47] Patients in this study were fairly motivated and had some insight into their PNES diagnosis, which is not always the case. The study had the following arms: medication (flexible-dose sertraline) only, cognitive-behavioral therapy informed psychotherapy (CBT-ip) only, CBT-ip with medication

TABLE 19-4 Guidelines for Presenting a Diagnosis of Non-Epileptic Seizures and Developing a Treatment Plan

PRESENTATION OF THE DIAGNOSIS	TREATMENT PLAN
1. Frame the diagnosis in a positive way: Symptoms are not due to abnormal electrical activity, and risks of anticonvulsants need not be undertaken.	1. The treatment plan should include as much psychiatric care as the patient will allow. Weekly psychotherapy to assess unconscious motivation, to allow psychoeducation, and to provide support is ideal.
2. Explain that symptoms are likely due to a problem with the *function* of the nervous system, rather than electrical or structural abnormalities.	2. Psychotropic medications should be used to treat co-morbid psychiatric symptoms (e.g., associated with major depression).
3. Explain that these symptoms are common and are likely to improve gradually over time. Give specific suggestions regarding how they will improve (e.g., episodes will become less prolonged, then become less frequent, then have fewer symptoms during each episode, and so forth).	3. Regular follow-up from other caregivers is a key component of the treatment plan. Appointments should be scheduled at regular intervals, whether or not the patient is symptomatic, and patients should receive positive reinforcement (and not a decrease in frequency of follow-up) when symptoms subside.
4. Acknowledge the disability that such symptoms have caused and the importance of developing a treatment plan that will improve the function of the nervous system and reduce disability.	4. Physical examinations should be done regularly, but diagnostic studies should be avoided unless clearly indicated.
5. Introduce the idea that anxiety, stress, and mood significantly affect the frequency and severity of these events and that reduction of these symptoms is crucial in the patient's treatment.	5. Despite the diagnosis of non-epileptic seizures, all caregivers should remain vigilant for the possibility that an organic diagnosis has been missed or that non-epileptic seizures and epilepsy are both present.
6. Describe a treatment plan that includes integrated, consistent treatment from providers in psychiatry, neurology, and primary care.	

(sertraline), or treatment as usual. The results showed significant seizure reduction and improved co-morbid depression and anxiety symptoms, as well as global functioning with CBT-ip both without and with sertraline, while medication alone and treatment as usual did not show any improvement.[47] This study and similar studies, despite the limitations regarding study population and study size, suggest that there might be more effective treatments for this group of patients.

REFERENCES

Access the reference list online at https://expertconsult.inkling.com/.

Patients With Cerebrovascular Disease and Traumatic Brain Injury

20

Felicia A. Smith, M.D.
Jeff C. Huffman, M.D.
Theodore A. Stern, M.D.

The structure and function of the central nervous system (CNS) is altered by many neurologic disorders. Because the CNS controls affect, behavior, and cognition, neurologic disorders may lead to neuropsychiatric symptoms that resemble those found in primary psychiatric conditions. Therefore, the general hospital psychiatrist is frequently called on to assess patients who have classic psychiatric symptoms caused by an underlying neurologic disease. In this chapter, we review the management of patients with neurologic conditions that are commonly associated with neuropsychiatric phenomena, including cerebrovascular disease and traumatic brain injury (TBI).

CEREBROVASCULAR DISEASE

Given that cerebrovascular accidents (CVAs) result in brain areas with reduced or absent function, it is not surprising that abnormalities of affect, behavior, and cognition are common after a CVA. This section discusses the prevalence, diagnosis, and management of patients with psychiatric symptoms after a CVA.

Each year, 16 million people worldwide suffer new strokes, and stroke is one of the leading causes of disability in the Western world.[1] According to the Global Burden of Disease Study in 2010, there were approximately 33 million people alive worldwide after strokes, with 70% of all stroke patients remaining with residual symptoms.[2,3] Cognitive impairments and neuropsychiatric syndromes, including depression and apathy, are frequent impairments after stroke,[4,5] and have an impact on the long-term prognosis (higher mortality and more disability) and quality of life of stroke survivors.[6,7] Such neuropsychiatric sequelae of strokes have been recognized for decades. More than 50 years ago, both Kraeplin[8] and Bleuler[9] noted an association between cerebrovascular disease and depressive illness. Ironside,[10] in 1956, was the first to describe pathologic crying and laughing associated with cerebral infarction, now a well-described post-stroke syndrome termed *pseudobulbar affect*. Despite the high incidence of these disorders and their frequent description in the literature, acute emotional and behavioral sequelae of stroke go largely unrecognized and untreated.[11]

One way to conceptualize certain neuropsychiatric syndromes caused by stroke is on the basis of lesion location. Whereas our understanding of brain circuitry has become much more sophisticated than prior models postulating that certain cortical lobes performed specific cognitive functions, it remains true that lesions in specific cortical areas are more likely to cause characteristic cognitive and neuropsychiatric deficits. For example, strokes in the left frontal lobe are more likely to result in a non-fluent aphasia, and strokes affecting the right parietal lobe most frequently cause anosognosia, an unawareness of illness or of neurologic deficits. Table 20-1 provides a list of some correlations between neuropsychiatric deficits and lesion locations.

Neuropsychiatric syndromes caused by strokes can also be discussed with regard to symptomatology. The following section discusses post-stroke cognitive impairment and delirium, depression, mania, psychosis, anxiety, and other common neuropsychiatric sequelae of stroke.

CASE 1

Mrs. B, a 75-year-old widowed executive with a history of generalized anxiety disorder, was admitted to the hospital with a right middle cerebral artery cerebrovascular accident (CVA). Her presentation was marked by left hemiplegia and a non-fluent aphasia. Because more than 3 hours had elapsed since the onset of her symptoms, she was not eligible for tissue plasminogen activator (tPA). Over the course of her hospitalization, she was diagnosed with atrial fibrillation and was placed on an anticoagulant. She worked with physical therapy and made slow gains in terms of motor function. Psychiatry was consulted at the rehabilitation facility 2 weeks after the stroke, to assess her for depression.

On interview, Mrs. B was alert and lucid, sitting upright in her hospital bed. She had prominent broken speech and she became frustrated quickly with her lack of ability to communicate, slamming her fist on the bedside table. Language comprehension was intact. Discussion with nursing revealed that the patient was experiencing poor sleep, poor appetite, and poor energy. The physical therapist added that while Mrs. B had been very motivated to participate in the rehabilitation exercises at the beginning of her stay, she had started to decline to take part over the past few days. The speech therapist noted a similar pattern when working with Mrs. B to improve her speech.

When asked if she felt depressed, Mrs. B nodded her head "yes." She quickly teared up when asked if she felt hopeless, and appeared quite distressed when asked if she found pleasure in anything. She also endorsed significant loneliness, as she had lost her husband 2 years prior and her grown children lived out of state. Finally, Mrs. B admitted to feeling more anxious than usual, and was especially fearful about the significant changes in store for her given that she had always been proudly independent and now was having difficulty with her activities of daily living (ADLs) in addition to communication. Despite feeling depressed, anxious, and hopeless, Mrs. B denied suicidal ideation and was amenable to treatment.

The consultant diagnosed Mrs. B with depressive disorder due to a CVA, with major depressive-like episode (post-stroke depression) in addition to her ongoing generalized anxiety disorder. She was restarted on an SSRI, fluoxetine, as it had helped her anxiety in the past. Mrs. B was also referred for close follow-up with a psychiatrist given her increased risk of poor outcomes both in terms of post-stroke functional improvement and higher-than-usual suicide risk in the setting of post-stroke depression and anxiety.

TABLE 20-1 Correlations Between Cortical Lesion Location and Neuropsychiatric Symptoms

CORTICAL AREA	POTENTIAL NEUROPSYCHIATRIC SYMPTOMS
Frontal Lobes	
Orbitofrontal region	Disinhibition, personality change, and irritability
Dorsolateral region	Executive dysfunction: poor planning, organizing, and sequencing
Medial region	Apathy and abulia
Left frontal lobe	Non-fluent (Broca's) aphasia, post-stroke depression (possibly)
Right frontal lobe	Motor dysprosody
Temporal Lobes	
Either side	Hallucinations (olfactory, gustatory, tactile, visual, or auditory), episodic fear, or mood changes
Left temporal lobe	Short-term memory impairment (to verbal or written stimuli), fluent (Wernicke's) aphasia (left temporoparietal region)
Right temporal lobe	Short-term memory impairment (non-verbal stimuli, e.g., music), sensory dysprosody (right temporoparietal region)
Left parietal lobe	Gerstmann's syndrome (finger agnosia, right/left disorientation, acalculia, and agraphia)
Right parietal lobe	Anosognosia, constructional apraxia, prosopagnosia, and hemineglect
Occipital lobes	Anton's syndrome (cortical blindness with unawareness of visual disturbance)

Cognitive Impairment and Delirium

Approximately 30–40% of patients experience delirium in the first week after a stroke[12,13] with those who suffered a hemorrhagic stroke at higher risk. Since delirium may be difficult to differentiate from cognitive deficits that result from focal brain lesions, it is essential to assess for waxing and waning symptomatology that is characteristic of delirious states. Risk factors for delirium include older age, impaired vision, impaired swallowing, and prior history of stroke.[14,15] The presence of delirium post-stroke confers a poorer overall prognosis and is associated with longer length of hospitalization, increased risk of dementia, and increased overall mortality.[16]

Cognitive impairment is also common post-stroke and occurs in about one-fourth of patients examined at 3 months after the event.[16,17] The term "vascular cognitive impairment (VCI)" includes the full spectrum from mild to severe cognitive impairment both in people with cerebrovascular disease and those with vascular (post-stroke) dementia.[2] Post-stroke risk factors of VCI include: severity of infarct, large size of lesion, older age, low education, history of diabetes or atrial fibrillation, and number of recurrent strokes.[2,18] The first year after stroke confers the highest risk of developing dementia, with an estimated incidence of 20–30%.[2,18]

Post-Stroke Depression

Post-stroke depression (PSD) is the prototypical acute psychiatric manifestation of stroke. It is common; approximately 30% of patients meet criteria for major depression in the first 3 months after stroke, and this often develops into a chronic remitting–relapsing condition.[19,20] Stroke-associated depression may reduce survival and increase the risk of recurrent vascular events as well as of cognitive impairment.[21–23] Risk factors for PSD include a history of depression, pre-stroke functional impairment, living alone, post-stroke social isolation, and possibly female gender.[24]

Both biological and psychological theories of etiology have been studied. Biological hypotheses include lesion location (e.g., of the left frontal region and left basal ganglia),[25–27] neurotransmitter mechanisms (decreased serotonin and norepinephrine), inflammatory cytokine-mediated (increased interleukin, IL-1β, IL-18, IL-6 and tumor necrosis factor, TNF-α), and gene polymorphism mechanisms (e.g., short variant of serotonin transporter gene-linked promotor region).[28,29] A recent study also showed an association between elevated serum levels of neopterin both in the acute post-stroke phase and in those with PSD at 6-month follow up.[30] Psychological factors, largely related to the various functional and personal losses associated with stroke, also contribute to the development of PSD. The correlation between location of stroke and the likelihood of developing PSD has been controversial; some studies have demonstrated positive correlations, and a large meta-analysis of 143 studies by Carson and co-workers[31] found no correlation between lesion location and the risk of PSD.

PSD is associated with significant long-term negative effects on social function, motor abilities, and quality of life.[32] Moreover, the negative effect of depression on functional impairment continues well beyond the period of abnormal mood symptoms.[33] Such extended functional disability may be due to poor initial rehabilitation efforts by patients with PSD that limit the recovery of strength and mobility.

Diagnosis of PSD is straightforward in many cases, although certain situations can make diagnosis quite challenging. A number of non-depressive neurologic stroke sequelae may resemble symptoms of depression. Patients with expressive aprosodias have monotonous speech that may make them appear sad or withdrawn, and their affect may appear blunted. The presence of anosognosia (neurologically mediated unawareness of illness usually associated with right parietal lesions) may look like denial associated with depression, and this symptom can itself lead to frustration and anger when others insist that the patient has a problem that he or she simply cannot recognize. Finally, aphasias can make the diagnosis of depression—or any diagnosis—more difficult because of the difficulty of communicating with such patients. By being aware of these potential neurologic sequelae and by carefully using criteria from the *Diagnostic and Statistical Manual of Mental Disorders*, 5th edition (DSM-5),[34] with particular attention paid to depressive symptoms that overlap less with concurrent medical and neurologic symptoms (e.g., feelings of guilt, worthlessness, hopelessness, suicidality), in most cases the psychiatrist can verify the presence or absence of PSD.

Despite the significant consequences of PSD (both because of under-diagnosis[11] and the fear of intolerable side effects from antidepressant medications), it is often under-treated. However, early and effective treatment of depression is perhaps even more crucial in this patient population than it is in other populations, given the need for full mobilization for occupational and physical therapy and other functional re-training early in the course of recovery.

A number of placebo-controlled trials have demonstrated that antidepressants are effective in the treatment of PSD. SSRIs[35–38] and nortriptyline[39] have been shown to relieve symptoms of PSD; another study of nortriptyline found that treatment of depression resulted in improved cognitive outcome.[40] A study by Robinson and associates[41] found that nortriptyline was more effective than either fluoxetine or placebo in treating PSD and improving functional outcomes. Studies of PSD have found disruptions of both noradrenergic and serotonergic pathways;[37] the effectiveness of venlafaxine was demonstrated in a case series by Kucukalic and colleagues,[42] and only 2 of 30 patients studied had mild elevations in blood pressure, which would be a side effect of concern with venlafaxine in post-stroke patients. Finally, a 2008 systematic review of 12 pharmacotherapy trials found that antidepressant therapy is modestly beneficial for remission of PSD; however adverse events were more common with antidepressants.[43] More studies are needed to fully assess the risks versus benefits in this regard.

Psychostimulants have also been used in the treatment of PSD. Retrospective studies using psychostimulants (methylphenidate and dextroamphetamine) to treat PSD found these medications to be effective, with response rates of 47–80%.[44,45] Response to psychostimulants was rapid (usually within 48 hours), and adverse events were rare. However, unlike SSRIs and TCAs, psychostimulants have not been studied under placebo-controlled, double-blind conditions for the treatment of PSD.

ECT also appears to be an effective treatment for PSD, with high rates of response and low rates of medical complications.[46] ECT is more extensively discussed in Chapter 37. In addition to the somatic treatments of PSD, there is evidence to suggest that care management programs, which include education, antidepressant treatment guided by algorithm, and close monitoring of therapy may be more effective than somatic treatments alone.[47] In addition to this, group and family psychotherapy have also been reported to safely and effectively treat PSD,[48,49] but there are few randomized and controlled trials of individual psychotherapies for PSD. One study found that problem-solving therapy reduced the incidence of depression and also delayed the time to onset, compared with placebo, for post-stroke patients.[50] Although there is some positive evidence for cognitive-behavioral therapy (CBT) as a treatment of PSD,[43] other studies have found no significant difference between CBT, attention placebo, and standard care.[51] More studies are needed in this area.

Administration of psychiatric medications to at-risk populations to prevent the onset of psychiatric illness is an increasingly popular area of study. Several recent studies have evaluated whether antidepressant medication can prevent PSD.[50,52–54] Although initial studies demonstrated differences in rates of depression in post-stroke patients who received medication compared to placebo, they were not statistically significant and were under-powered.[52,53] A more recent and methodologically sound study by Robinson and associates[50] evaluated 176 non-depressed patients within 3 months of stroke and randomized them to three groups, a double-blinded escitalopram and placebo group and a non-blinded problem-solving therapy group. Rates of major and minor depression were statistically significantly lower for both escitalopram and problem-solving therapy, though escitalopram remained significant only with an intention-to-treat analysis. The potential clinical impact of these studies is impressive, but more studies are needed to definitely direct clinical care.

For most patients with mild to moderate PSD, SSRIs are the treatment of choice, given their proven efficacy, favorable side effect profile, and cardiovascular safety. However, TCAs, despite higher rates of side effects than SSRIs, might also be considered first-line agents for PSD because of their potentially superior efficacy. For more severe depression that impairs decision-making capacity, nutritional intake, or ability to participate in rehabilitation, psychostimulants should be strongly considered; methylphenidate or dextroamphetamine can be started at 2.5 to 5 mg in the morning, and a protocol for dosing and patient monitoring can be followed (Table 20-2). ECT can also be considered in patients with incapacitating depression. Prophylactic treatment with antidepressants to prevent depression is supported by preliminary studies and may be prudent in patients with numerous risk factors; careful analysis of risks and benefits for the individual patient is still required.

Post-Stroke Apathy

Apathy is a disorder of diminished motivation and initiative that is characterized by restricted social engagement, lack of emotional response, and diminished cognitive abilities. In the post-stroke period, apathy was historically seen as a

TABLE 20-2 Guidelines for the Use of Psychostimulants to Treat Depression

1. Consider possible (relative) contraindications to psychostimulant use:
   a. history of ventricular arrhythmia
   b. recent myocardial infarction
   c. congestive heart failure with reduced ejection fraction
   d. poorly controlled hypertension
   e. tachycardia
   f. concurrent treatment with MAOIs.
2. Initiate treatment with a morning dose of 5 mg methylphenidate or dextroamphetamine (2.5 mg in frail elderly or medically tenuous patients).
3. Check vital signs and response to treatment in 2–4 hours (the period of peak effect).
4. If the initial dose is well tolerated and effective throughout the day, continue with a single daily morning dose.
5. If the initial dose is well tolerated and effective for several hours, with a loss of effect in the afternoon, give the same dose twice per day (in the morning and the early afternoon).
6. If the initial dose is well tolerated but is without significant clinical effect, increase dose by 5 mg per day until a clinical response is achieved, intolerable side effects arise, or 20 mg dose is ineffective (i.e., a failed trial).
7. Continue treatment throughout the hospitalization; stimulants can usually be discontinued at discharge.

symptom of other syndromes, such as depression or dementia, but emerging evidence suggests that it might be a distinct entity.[1,2,55,56] Post-stroke apathy (PSA) is as frequent as PSD and is also associated with poor functional recovery and low QoL.[5,21] PSA has been associated with right hemispheric sub-cortical lesions with a particular focus in the basal ganglia and anterior cingulate circuit which is involved in motivation.[2,57] Although more studies on treatment of PSA are needed, early work suggests the same treatment as PSD, including SSRIs and particularly psychostimulants.

Other Post-Stroke Psychiatric Phenomena

Other psychiatric syndromes that occur in the post-stroke period include anxiety, mania, and psychosis. Post-stroke anxiety is common, and usually arises in concert with PSD. Approximately one-fourth of patients meet criteria for generalized anxiety disorder (GAD) (except for duration criteria) in the acute post-stroke period; at least three-fourths of these patients with post-stroke GAD symptoms have co-morbid depression.[58,59] Post-stroke anxiety has a negative impact on the functional recovery of stroke victims and has been associated with impairment in activities of daily living (ADL) up to 3 years after the event.[59] The functional impairment of PSD and post-stroke GAD appear to be additive, insofar as patients with both GAD and PSD have greater ADL impairment at follow-up than those with isolated PSD.[60]

Post-stroke mania occurs in fewer than 1% of patients. Symptoms of post-stroke mania are similar to those of primary mania (with flight of ideas, pressured speech, a decreased need for sleep, grandiosity, and associated psychotic symptoms). Lesions in the right orbitofrontal cortex, right basal temporal cortices, dorsomedial thalamus, and head of caudate appear to be associated most often with post-stroke mania.[61–66] Stroke in the right hemisphere, compared with the left, has led to increased serotonin binding, and it is hypothesized that this may result in post-stroke mania.[67]

Post-stroke psychosis is also uncommon, occurring at a rate of approximately 1–2%.[68] Such patients usually have right temporoparietal lesions and a high rate of associated seizures.[68,69] This suggests that temporal lobe damage that leads to complex partial seizures (CPS) and to associated psychosis may account for symptoms in a significant percentage of these patients.

Finally, there are two other clinical neuropsychiatric syndromes that are common in the post-stroke period. The first is termed *catastrophic reaction*, a collection of symptoms involving patient desperation and frustration. This syndrome is relatively common—especially in the acute phase; rates of post-stroke catastrophic reaction are 3–20%.[70,71] Catastrophic reactions are strongly associated with PSD, with roughly three-quarters of patients with catastrophic reaction having PSD.[71] Catastrophic reactions are also associated with a personal and family history of psychiatric disorders.[70]

Catastrophic reactions also appear to be associated with anterior sub-cortical lesions and with left cortical lesions.[70–72] Given the strong association of catastrophic reactions and depression, some feel that such a reaction is a behavioral symptom of depression (provoked by anterior sub-cortical damage) rather than a discrete syndrome. Others feel that catastrophic reactions result from damage to left hemispheric areas involved in the regulation of emotions related to social communication.[71]

The second of these clinical syndromes is *pseudobulbar affect*, also termed *pseudobulbar palsy*. This syndrome (which consists of frequent and easily provoked spells of laughing or crying) occurs to some degree in approximately 15% of post-stroke patients.[73,74] The pathophysiology is unknown but is thought to involve frontal release of brainstem emotional centers.[75] It is usually seen in a mild form, with brief fits of crying or laughing linked with appropriate changes in mood; however, in more serious cases, it may involve frequent and spontaneous fits of laughing and crying inappropriate to the context. It can cause embarrassment, curtailment of social activities, and a decreased quality of life.[76]

Treatment of these post-stroke phenomena generally parallels the treatment of primary psychiatric syndromes. Post-stroke anxiety can be treated like any primary anxiety syndrome. SSRIs are effective in the treatment of a variety of anxiety disorders, including GAD, and, given that most patients with post-stroke anxiety have co-morbid PSD, these agents are often the treatments of choice. Benzodiazepines can also be given for isolated anxiety, but they can lead to ataxia, sedation, and paradoxical disinhibition; therefore, they must be used with caution in this population. Furthermore, these agents do not treat co-morbid depression.

Treatment of post-stroke mania follows the same rules as does the treatment of primary mania. Mood stabilizers and adjunctive antipsychotic medications or benzodiazepines are used to control symptoms. Treatment studies of post-stroke mania have found lithium, valproic acid, carbamazepine, neuroleptics, and clonidine variably efficacious, though none of these treatments has been examined in placebo-controlled, double-blind trials for this condition.[62,67,77–79] Post-stroke psychosis can be treated symptomatically with antipsychotics. However, anticonvulsants (especially valproic acid and carbamazepine) should be used when psychotic symptoms are the result of CPS, because psychotic symptoms should improve with better seizure control.

Finally, pseudobulbar affect and catastrophic reaction may respond well to antidepressants. A few trials of TCAs and SSRIs, some of which were placebo-controlled, have demonstrated efficacy in reducing symptoms of pseudobulbar affect.[80–83] Additionally, the combination of dextromethorphan and quinidine has been shown to reduce laughing and crying spells due to pseudobulbar affect in patients with amyotrophic lateral sclerosis (ALS)[84] and may also be of benefit in the post-stroke setting. Symptoms of catastrophic reaction may also improve with antidepressant treatment of co-morbid PSD.

In short, psychiatric symptoms after stroke are common and have a significant impact on the long-term outcome of post-stroke patients. Awareness of neurologic symptoms that may mimic psychiatric illness (e.g., anosognosia) and careful diagnostic interviews can allow accurate diagnosis and prompt treatment. In general, psychiatric symptoms secondary to stroke are treated in the same way as are non-stroke-related psychiatric syndromes with similar symptoms.

THE MANAGEMENT OF PATIENTS WITH TRAUMATIC BRAIN INJURY

Traumatic brain injury (TBI) is a leading cause of death and disability in the United States, contributing to 30% of injury deaths each year.[85] In 2010, TBI was associated with 2.5 million Emergency Department visits and 50,000 deaths.[85,86] Permanent neuropsychiatric disabilities affect an estimated 80,000 to 90,000 patients who suffer a TBI.[86] Of this group, psychosocial and psychological impairments lead to substantial disability and cause significant stress to their families. The consulting psychiatrist plays an important role in the evaluation and treatment of these patients. In this section the epidemiology and pathophysiology of TBI will be addressed; this will be followed by a discussion of the clinical features and treatment of the affective, behavioral, and cognitive aspects of TBI.

Epidemiology

Disorders that result from TBI are more common than any other neurologic disease, except for headache. Falls cause the majority: 28% of TBIs, and motor vehicle accidents (20%); assaults (11%); having one's head struck against an object (19%); other trauma (13%); and unknown trauma (9%) account for the remaining TBIs.[85] Among adults, alcohol is a contributing factor in 40–56% of cases.[85,87] The highest rates of hospitalization and death after TBI are found in persons older than 75 years.[85] Individuals who have had one brain injury are three times as likely, compared with the general population, to sustain a second, and after a second TBI the risk of another is 10 times higher.[85] It should be noted, however, that even more mild TBIs (i.e., without an associated hospital stay) may result in neuropsychiatric sequelae.

Pathophysiology

TBI can be divided into primary and secondary brain injuries. Primary injury consists of focal and diffuse lesions. Focal TBI generally results from a blow to the head that produces cerebral contusions or hematomas. Epidural hematomas, subdural hematomas, and cerebral contusions are all types of focal lesions. The location, size, and progression of the injury determine the resultant morbidity and mortality.[87] Most injuries occur in the polar temporal lobes and on the inferior surface of the frontal lobes as a result of contact with the bony prominences along the base of the skull, often a result of a coup–contrecoup mechanism of injury. All are diagnosed by computed tomography (CT) scanning or magnetic resonance imaging (MRI) of the brain. An epidural hematoma is usually caused by head trauma that is associated with a lateral skull fracture and with tearing of the middle meningeal artery and vein and therefore is most often located in the temporal or temporoparietal region.[87] There is often loss of consciousness followed by a period of lucency, and then neurologic deterioration. Prompt surgical evacuation of the hematoma is essential. Subdural hematoma is more common than epidural hematoma and generally results from tearing of a bridging vein between the cortex and a venous sinus. Much of the force of an impact is often transmitted to the brain, and the underlying brain injury actually determines the outcome in approximately 80% of cases.[87] Treatment also involves surgical evacuation. Finally, traumatic cerebral contusion is often associated with an initial bout of unconsciousness, generally followed by recovery. Edema may cause fluctuations in the level of consciousness, seizures, or focal neurologic signs. Surgery is rarely undertaken for cerebral contusions.

Diffuse lesions, or *diffuse axonal injury*, is seen more commonly in injuries that involve rapid acceleration, deceleration, or rotational forces.[88] The sites most prone to such injury are the reticular formation, basal ganglia, superior cerebellar peduncles, limbic fornices, hypothalamus, and corpus callosum.[88] Patients who suffer diffuse axonal injury have high rates of morbidity and mortality. The diagnosis, often missed on CT, may be made by use of diffusion-weighted MRI, which is sensitive to the axonal swelling seen after injury. Lack of radiographic evidence of injury does not translate into an absence of damage. Deficits in arousal, attention, and cognition (i.e., processing speed) often result from diffuse axonal injury.

Whereas primary brain injury (focal and diffuse) results from mechanical injury at the time of the trauma, secondary brain injury is caused by the physiologic responses to the initial injury. This is thought to involve a cascade of events, with edema and hematomas leading to increased intracranial pressure, which leads to compression and deformation of surrounding brain tissue and further damage. Neuronal damage is also mediated by release of neurotoxic substances. Although a full discussion of each of these is beyond the scope of this chapter, each substance must be considered when evaluating the status of a brain-injured individual in the acute care setting.

Clinical Presentation

TBI is often divided into three categories according to the severity and the duration of altered mental status; however, there is no definitive breakdown of specific types of sequelae that may be affiliated with each. Whereas more severe injuries are often thought to have more persistent and pervasive consequences, there are certainly instances of significant morbidity even with mild TBI. The severity of the injury is classified by the Glasgow Coma Scale (GCS; Table 20-3). Mild head injury correlates with a GCS score of 13 to 15, moderate injury with a GCS score of 9 to 12, and severe head injury corresponds to a GCS score of less than 8. Lower scores are associated with more severe injury and poorer recovery outcomes.[86]

Other factors that may increase morbidity include the following: lower intelligence quotient (IQ), a concomitant substance abuse disorder, older age, and a history of brain injury. Moreover, the DSM-5[34] suggests the following criteria to establish the severity of injury significant enough to cause Neurocognitive Disorder (NCD) due to traumatic brain injury (one or more of the following): (1) loss of consciousness; (2) post-traumatic amnesia; or (3) disorientation and confusion; (4) neurologic signs (e.g. neuroimaging demonstrating injury; a new onset of seizures; a marked worsening of pre-existing seizure disorder; visual field cuts; anosmia; hemiparesis). The neurocognitive disorder must present immediately after the TBI or immediately after recovery of consciousness and persist past the acute post-injury period. Diagnostic features of this disorder also include cognitive disturbances as well as fatigue; disordered sleep; headache; vertigo or dizziness; irritability or aggression; anxiety, depression, or affective lability; changes in personality; and apathy or lack of spontaneity. Of note, this syndrome is known to neurologists and the lay public as post-concussive syndrome.

TABLE 20-3 Glasgow Coma Scale

Eye Opening	
Spontaneous	4
To voice	3
To painful stimulus	2
None	1
Verbal Response	
Oriented	5
Confused	4
Inappropriate words	3
Unintelligible sounds	2
None	1
Motor Response	
Follows commands	6
Localizes pain	5
Withdraws from pain	4
Flexor response	3
Extensor response	2
None	1

These features are representative of the three major categories of neuropsychiatric sequelae that may be seen with TBI: cognitive impairment, changes in personality and behavior, and Axis I psychiatric disorders (e.g., mood, anxiety, and psychotic disorders). Each of these is outlined briefly.

Cognitive Impairment

Cognitive difficulties in acute care settings following TBI may be due to the brain injury itself, delirium, or other factors. As recovery progresses, deficits related to the TBI (e.g., attentional impairment, associated with the reticular activating system and prefrontal white matter) become more apparent.[89] Impairments in language and executive function (those skills necessary for independence in the world) as well as memory, often follow TBI.[89] Examples of executive dysfunction include poor planning, impaired abstraction, and difficulties with calculations. Neurocognitive testing is essential to further specify and quantify deficits. Moreover, neuropsychological testing is invaluable in designing an individualized rehabilitation program to meet the specific needs of each patient.

Personality Changes

Personality change due to TBI is a DSM-5[34] diagnosis characterized by a persistent personality disturbance that represents a change from the individual's prior personality; it is a direct consequence of the injury and is not better explained by delirium, dementia, or another Axis I disorder. The disturbance must also cause clinically significant distress or impairment in occupational or social function.[34] The terms *frontal lobe syndrome* and *organic personality syndrome* are often used to describe these personality changes.[90] Personality changes and behavioral manifestations often include labile affect, disinhibition, poor social judgment, apathy, lewdness, loss of social graces, perseveration, aggressive behavior, paranoia, and inattention to personal hygiene. In a 30-year follow-up study of patients with TBI, Koponen and colleagues[91] found that 23% of injured adults manifested an Axis II diagnosis. These changes may be a direct result of the TBI but also may be exacerbated or caused by delirium, seizures, or use of medications or substances. When evaluating personality changes, the physician should note that the patient may have little insight into the change, so including supportive family members in the evaluation and planning of treatment is essential. Additionally, families may need significant support to cope with changes present in their loved ones.

Mood and Anxiety Disorders

As many as 40% of patients with TBI will develop an Axis I disorder, most commonly major depression, an alcohol-use disorder, panic disorder, a specific phobia, or a psychotic disorder.[91] Depression occurs in 26–77% of those with mild TBI, whereas higher rates of depression are associated with more severe injuries.[92–95] These individuals have higher risk because of the neuroanatomic and physiologic changes that occur and because of lost capabilities, changes in roles, and financial and other losses that have occurred.[96] Pre-morbid substance abuse, poor functioning, lower education, and an unstable work history predict depression after TBI.[97,98] Because there may be significant overlap with cognitive impairment and personality changes, the diagnosis must be made with care. Major depression is associated with poor outcome across multiple domains; this makes its early diagnosis and treatment particularly important. Prominent signs and symptoms include fatigue, distractibility, anger, irritability, and rumination. Neuropsychological testing may be helpful in these individuals. Finally, there is an increased risk of suicide after TBI; up to 15% of individuals make a suicide attempt in the 5 years after TBI. In this population, intense despair, hopelessness, worthlessness and loss of sense of integrity, as well as relationship breakdown and isolation, contribute to the risk for suicide.[96,99] Additionally, prominent insomnia and chronic headache often exacerbate the situation. The combination of depression and disinhibition associated with frontal lobe injury is also thought to contribute to higher rates of suicide.

Mania has also been shown to occur more often after TBI than it does in the general population.[95] Predisposing factors may include a family history of affective illness, right temporal lobe lesions, and right orbitofrontal cortex injuries; unfortunately, consensus is lacking. Furthermore, seizures seem to be more common in this group;[95] this makes the EEG an important diagnostic tool following TBI. For this reason, anticonvulsant medications are the preferred mood stabilizers after TBI (see Treatment, below).

Regarding anxiety disorders after TBI, GAD, and post-traumatic stress disorder (PTSD) appear to be the most common.[95–101] OCD, specific phobias, and panic disorder have also been reported.[102] GAD is co-morbid with depression in approximately 11% of patients. There is some evidence that early intervention with CBT for acute stress disorder may prevent PTSD after mild TBI.[100] Other investigators have shown a relationship between impaired memory of the traumatic event and lower rates of PTSD;[101] however, more research is needed in this area.

Psychosis

Psychosis as a consequence of TBI is thought to be relatively rare. Although some authors doubt that a correlation exists,[95] others argue that psychosis may appear immediately after brain injury or years later (with rates between 0.7% and 9.8%).[103] Frontal and temporal lobe injuries are associated with psychosis, as are post-traumatic seizures.[104] Cognitive impairment and behavioral changes (already described) may mimic the symptoms of schizophrenia. Because individuals with schizophrenia have also been found to have a higher incidence of brain injury than those in the general population,[104] it may be true that head injury predisposes these individuals to schizophrenia. Alternatively, it may be that individuals who are already predisposed to schizophrenia have a higher incidence of brain injury for other reasons. More research is needed in this area.

Treatment

Treatment of neuropsychiatric sequelae of TBI is best accomplished with a comprehensive, multidisciplinary, rehabilitative approach. This may include psychiatric, neurologic, psychological, behavioral, occupational, and vocational evaluations. Specific brain-injury centers are best equipped to undertake this; however, not all communities have such resources. Psychiatric evaluation and consultation generally focus on several areas of intervention: pharmacological, behavioral, cognitive, and social (family support). These are discussed in the following section.

Pharmacology

Generally, medications effective for primary psychiatric disorders in non-TBI patients are similarly effective in TBI patients. Because brain-injured patients are often more sensitive to certain medications and their side effects, several guidelines should be considered. The principle of "start low, and go slow" is wise; being overly cautious may lead to inadequate medication trials if therapeutic doses are not achieved or medications are not given sufficient time to work. Slow titration as tolerated by side effects and an adequate duration of trials should be the goal.

Although treatment of depression and anxiety in patients with TBI follows the same principles as those for the treatment of depression and anxiety in the general population, careful attention should be paid to medication side effects. Medications with a high potential for lowering the seizure threshold, causing sedation (typically mediated by antihistamine effects), and inducing anticholinergic side effects and hypotension (usually mediated by peripheral alpha antagonism) should be avoided or used with great care if no better alternative exists. TCAs and bupropion, which both lower seizure threshold, are generally avoided. SSRIs are usually well tolerated. Several studies (only one of which was a randomized controlled trial) with citalopram, fluoxetine, and sertraline have demonstrated improvements in mood and aggression.[105–108] Psychostimulants may be employed for depressive symptoms (irritability, apathy, and depressed mood), cognitive symptoms (arousal, processing speed, and attention), and fatigue,[109,110] although paradoxical dysphoria, agitation, and paranoia may be seen in the brain-injured patient. Improvements have also been seen in depression, anxiety, irritability, and aggression with buspirone; it has a more favorable side effect profile and less abuse potential than benzodiazepines.[111–113] Propranolol (a β-blocker) has been shown to reduce the intensity of agitation and aggression following TBI.[103] Amantadine hydrochloride is a treatment considered to have potential therapeutic value in this population and has been shown to accelerate recovery in patients with severe TBI.[114] Finally, ECT remains a good option and is often under-utilized. Care should be taken to assess memory and cognitive dysfunction before recommending ECT, given the potential side effects of this treatment.

Mania should be treated using standard agents. However, neurotoxicity from lithium may develop at higher rates in patients with TBI; anticonvulsant mood stabilizers, such as valproic acid or carbamazepine, may be preferable. For patients with co-morbid seizures, anticonvulsants are the treatment of choice.

Neuroleptics are frequently used for agitation and aggression in TBI patients, as well as psychosis. The use of neuroleptics in this population is controversial given research, largely conducted on animals, that indicates they interfere with neural plasticity and are associated with longer post-traumatic amnesia and worse outcomes.[109,115] That said, there is also evidence that antipsychotics may be effective for the management of agitation and aggressive behavior.[116] Because brain-injured patients are at increased risk for extrapyramidal symptoms (dystonias, akathisias, and parkinsonian side effects), high-potency agents should be used with care and atypical antipsychotics are generally preferred over typical antipsychotics. Antipsychotics with significant anticholinergic side effects (e.g., clozapine and low-potency typical agents) and antipsychotics that lower the seizure threshold, such as clozapine, should be monitored carefully.

Finally, benzodiazepines and barbiturates should be used sparingly in patients with TBI because of their potential for causing paradoxical disinhibition, sedation, and worsening of cognitive and motor impairments.[109] If rapid sedation is desired in an agitated patient, low doses may be used with caution.

Behavioral, Cognitive, and Social Interventions

Once deficits related to TBI have been delineated, a comprehensive plan of treatment can be instituted. Behavioral treatments are helpful for the management of maladaptive social behaviors (including aggression) and personality disorders. For patients with prominent mood or anxiety symptoms, who are easily agitated, or who have low thresholds to anger and aggression, environmental modification (e.g., increasing structure, simplifying tasks, reducing or increasing stimulation, and removing triggers and irritations) helps reduce symptoms.[117] Specific cognitive rehabilitation programs may be helpful, depending on individual deficits. These deficits are best assessed by administration of neuropsychiatric testing. Teaching about stress management and coping skills may also be particularly useful. Finally, psychotherapeutic and social interventions, including family education and supportive therapy, may prove useful given the sense of loss and distress often felt by family members and by loved ones.

CONCLUSION

TBI is an important cause of neuropsychiatric disability in the United States. A thorough assessment of mood, anxiety, personality change, and cognition should be a routine part of post-injury screening. The consulting psychiatrist plays an important role in the evaluation and treatment of these patients. Prompt diagnosis and treatment, as well as appropriate referral using a multidisciplinary approach, will greatly benefit patients and their families.

REFERENCES

Access the reference list online at https://expertconsult.inkling.com/.

Patients With Abnormal Movements

21

Oliver Freudenreich, M.D.
Alice W. Flaherty, M.D., Ph.D.

OVERVIEW

Psychiatrists encounter patients with abnormal movements in various clinical settings. Recognizing and correctly labeling motor phenomena in each setting helps to create a differential diagnosis that serves as the basis for optimal treatment, since abnormal movements can be the first indication of an unsuspected medical or neurologic disorder in a psychiatric patient treated for psychiatric symptoms. A solid understanding of prototypical movement disorders (e.g., Huntington's disease, Parkinson's disease) and of tremors will help psychiatrists to correctly categorize abnormal movements. All movement disorders, primary or drug-induced, contribute to morbidity (with loss of independence) and mortality (e.g., secondary to falls or choking). Many are stigmatizing, as abnormal movements are immediately obvious to others.

Movement disorders caused by basal ganglia damage all create trouble starting or stopping movements. They differ from cerebellar disorders, which affect movement targeting, and from stroke-related weakness. Neuroleptic malignant syndrome and catatonia are discussed in Chapters 12 and 23, respectively. Real patients and videos are excellent ways to learn to recognize abnormal movements. A word of caution: many of the free videos on the Internet show patients with functional movement disorders who have made videos of themselves and do not depict classic movement disorders; therefore, one should select reputable sources, such as a video atlas.[1]

PATIENT HISTORY AND PHYSICAL EXAMINATION

A movement disorder is a clinical diagnosis, based on history and physical examination; laboratory tests and brain imaging usually do not facilitate making the diagnosis. A family history can be informative for hereditary movement disorders. One should ask carefully about present and past medications as well as substance use, as these are the most common causes of abnormal movements.

The examination begins with unobtrusive observation, when meeting the patient in the waiting area or approaching the bedside. One should determine if the movements exist when unobserved, and if the patient shuffles or writhes when walking. A patient who lies stiffly in bed might be parkinsonian, or catatonic. The neurologic examination is focused on establishing deficits beyond their relationship to the motor strip and the basal ganglia, and includes cortical functioning and cerebellar function as well as on eliciting other motor signs. Muscle tone should be determined (e.g. rigid, spastic, or hypotonic). If you suspect catatonia, you should perform an exam for other signs of catatonia. Some patients cannot relax while their limb is being examined for muscle tone, and seem to (voluntarily) resist each passive movement. This is called *gegenhalten* or paratonia.

Table 21-1 summarizes common movement symptoms. Overall, it is helpful to determine if your patient moves too much (hyperkinetic) or too little (hypokinetic), or if there are rhythmic tremors or non-rhythmic twitches. Myoclonus or asterixis can appear somewhat rhythmic on first glance, so one must observe carefully. Asterixis can suggest a serious metabolic disturbance, whereas myoclonus is non-specific and may be benign. Other phenomena that mimic tremor include focal seizures and cerebellar dysmetria. Some movements defy easy categorization but should be considered in psychiatric patients (e.g., catatonic symptoms, stereotypies, mannerisms).

When examining a patient with a tremor the main question is whether the tremor occurs mainly at rest (resting tremor) or during action (action tremor). Postural tremors can occur with either action or rest and are not themselves diagnostic. Writing or drawing will reliably evoke an action tremor in that hand, whereas rest tremors can intensify with movement of the opposite hand. The phenomenologic description of the tremor is followed by an examination of other neurologic signs or symptoms to help refine the diagnostic possibilities. This matters, since treatment depends on the tremor's etiology, although the treatment of some tremors can be non-specific and based on its severity and the patient's tolerance of it.

Table 21-2 summarizes gait disorders. Observing a patient's gait and understanding the etiology of a gait disturbance are particularly important during a patient visit. Gait disturbances not only limit a patient's independence but can lead to dangerous falls (especially in the elderly). Hypokinetic movement disorders, including parkinsonism associated with use of antipsychotics, lead to falls because patients react too slowly when they stumble. Ataxia or hyperkinetic movement disorders lead to fewer falls. A potentially reversible cause of a gait disturbance is normal-pressure hydrocephalus (NPH) that is manifest by a triad of (parkinsonian) gait, incontinence, and dementia (the latter being a late-stage manifestation). If diagnosed early, placement of a shunt can be curative.

TABLE 21-1 Motor Symptoms

Tremor (Rhythmic Involuntary Alternation of Agonist and Antagonist Muscles)
Action tremor—triggered by voluntary movement
Rest tremor—stops during voluntary movement
Postural tremor—seen with either action or rest tremor, not itself diagnostic

Movements That Look Like Tremor but Are Not
Cerebellar dysmetria (intention "tremor")—worsens as limb approaches target
Myoclonus—involuntary non-rhythmic jerk, moves only one joint
Asterixis (negative myoclonus, "flapping tremor")—arrhythmic lapses of sustained posture
Focal seizures—non-rhythmic trains of unilateral twitching, lasting seconds to minutes.
Fasciculations—visible contractions within a muscle that do not move a joint

The Hyperkinetic–Hypokinetic Spectrum—From Fast to Slow, in Descending Order
Chorea and **Dyskinesia** are essentially synonyms—brief, unpredictable, semi-purposeful
Choreoathetosis—when you cannot decide if it is chorea or athetosis
Athetosis—slow but continuous movements
Dystonia—abnormal postures held for at least several seconds
Lead-pipe rigidity—constant resistance throughout range of passive motion
Bradykinesia—slow movements
Akinesia—sustained periods of no movement

Other Hyperkinetic Movements
Hemiballism—violent, unilateral repetitive but non-rhythmic jerks of proximal limbs
Stereotypies—repetitive self-soothing movements (e.g., tapping foot, biting nails)
Tics—semi-voluntary fast movement, often multi-joint, usually urge-driven

TABLE 21-2 Gait Syndromes

Parkinsonian: slow, shuffling, stooping with arms flexed, festinating (unable to stop); many falls
Choreic: posturing, writhing; fewer falls
Ataxic: wide-based, lurching; fewer falls
Neuropathic: Foot slaps, patient steps high to avoid tripping
Spastic: stiff, circumducted leg, toe-walking
Functional (astasia-abasia): wild, seemingly poor balance but no falls.

One should also ask about swallowing difficulties, which can result in aspiration pneumonia.

IDIOPATHIC MOVEMENT DISORDERS

Parkinson's Disease

Idiopathic Parkinson's disease (PD) is one of the hypokinetic syndromes characterized clinically by the triad of slow movement, rigidity, and tremor. The combination of tremor plus rigidity leads to the cogwheeling on exam. Although a resting tremor is often the first sign of PD, up to one-fourth of patients have no tremor. Difficulties initiating movements, like starting to walk, are called freezing, where a patient's feet seem to be glued to the ground.

The mainstay of treatment for PD is the dopamine agonist levodopa.[2] Bradykinesia responds better to levodopa than does tremor. Unfortunately, while levodopa is highly effective early in reversing the dopamine loss-related akinesia, its long-term administration is complicated by levodopa-induced dyskinesias due to striatal hyperresponsiveness to acute dopaminergic stimulation. In later stages of the disease, patients experience periods of immobility that alternate with good symptom control (on–off phenomenon). Some patients with PD are *atypical* in that their response to dopamine agonists is poor. Atypical Parkinsonian syndromes (Parkinson's-plus) refer to patients who experience not only parkinsonian symptoms but other symptoms as well. Such syndromes include Lewy body dementia (LBD) or multi-system atrophy (MSA), where, as the name implies, other brain systems are affected. We caution clinicians that one will only know if a patient is poorly responsive to levodopa if it is actually tried.

PD is, for most patients, a multi-faceted disease and more than a pure movement disorder, either due to the biological nature of the illness, the side effects of treatment, or the psychological effects of having a progressive illness. Table 21-3 summarizes its core clinical symptoms.

TABLE 21-3 Clinical Symptoms in Parkinson's Disease

Motor
Bradykinesia
Masked face
Stooped posture and festinating gait
Falls, especially backwards
Atypical parkinsonism: spasticity, eye movement abnormalities

Neuropsychiatric
Pre-morbid personality (conscientious, inflexible, risk-averse)
Depression: may precede motor symptoms
Dementia: if early, is a sign of atypical parkinsonism
Psychosis: if early, is a sign of atypical parkinsonism

Some patients later found to have PD have a pre-morbid (i.e., prior to the onset of abnormal movements) personality style characterized by high harm avoidance and low novelty.[3] Such patients are temperamentally conscientious, industrious, inflexible, and prone to dysthymia. A complication of disease progression is a dopamine dysregulation syndrome and impulsive behaviors that can take the form of gambling, hypersexuality, compulsive shopping, or binge eating,[4] all uncharacteristic for the patient. Punding (i.e., repetitive, prolonged, purposeless behavior) is another late complication that makes life difficult for PD patients and their families.[5] These problems are due, at least in part, to use of medications, and antipsychotics with partial dopamine agonist properties (e.g., aripiprazole) carry some risk of inducing compulsions and impulsive urges to shop, eat, have sex, or gamble.

Fatigue, apathy, insomnia and depression are very common in Parkinson's disease. Dementia and psychosis are late-stage problems; when they begin early, they usually indicate atypical Parkinsonism. Autonomic dysfunction, such as postural hypotension and drooling are severe in multiple system atrophy, but are also often problematic in Parkinson's disease. Muscle rigidity can cause pain, especially in the muscles of the shoulder and back.

At least one-third of PD patients have depression and apathy (*abulia*). Apathy can be the first symptom of PD; it needs to be differentiated from the treatable psychiatric syndrome of depression. Depression is often missed due to the symptom overlap with PD, including motor retardation and masked facies, poor sleep, and cognitive complaints. As in other medical disorders, depression, when present, is a major contributor to poor quality of life. Depression and motor fluctuation are poorly correlated. In a clinical trial that compared placebo, paroxetine, and a noradrenergic tricyclic antidepressant, nortriptyline was effective but paroxetine was not.[6] The role of selective serotonin re-uptake inhibitors (SSRIs) is therefore thought to be limited, perhaps best reserved for patients with pseudobulbar affect, as SSRIs can worsen motor symptoms. A recent placebo-controlled trial, however, showed benefit from paroxetine and venlafaxine without exacerbating motor symptoms.[7] Other antidepressants to consider are bupropion or a stimulant; the latter used for apathy. The dopamine agonist, pramipexole, has a direct antidepressant effect in PD patients and is yet another option.[8] In refractory depression, electroconvulsive therapy (ECT) and transcranial magnetic stimulation (TMS) can be tried, although post-ECT delirium complicates its use. Mirtazapine is a good choice for those with anxiety and poor sleep.

In a large epidemiologic study, almost 30% of PD patients receiving routine outpatient neurologic care met criteria for dementia, with higher rates of sub-syndromal cognitive impairment found.[9] Over time, most patients with PD develop dementia. In a cohort of newly diagnosed patients, 83% of patients who lived for 20 years with PD had dementia.[10] The dementia of PD is a subcortical dementia characterized by slowed mentation and processing (bradyphrenia), poor attention, and difficulties with executive function. The Mini-Mental State Exam (MMSE) is insensitive for detection of these problems and should not be used as a screening tool. However, co-morbidities with cortical dementias (e.g., Alzheimer's dementia, LBD) lead to mixed cortical/subcortical pictures. On autopsy, LBD and PD with dementia look alike. They may represent the same disease, with dementia preceding motor problems in LBD and the reverse in PD dementia. Very poor antipsychotic tolerability is a hallmark of both LBD[11] and late-stage PD dementia. The mainstay of treatment for PD with dementia is acetylcholinesterase inhibitors that are also frequently used in LBD.[12] Levodopa is ineffective and poorly tolerated and can cause hallucinations in both conditions.

Psychosis complicates PD in about 50% of patients.[13] Symptoms (which include vivid dreams, illusions, hallucinations, misidentification syndromes, and paranoid delusions) can result from both the treatment of PD and also from the disease process itself, particularly if dementia develops. Early-onset hallucinations are a predictor of dementia and they are primarily, but not exclusively, visual. They can be simple (seeing flashes), of the passage variety (seeing fleeting images in the periphery), or take the form of presence hallucinations (feeling somebody is close by). More complex hallucinations include seeing small animals or children. Both hallucinations and delusions predict nursing home placement, so attempts to treat are important. The first step is to exclude other causes of psychosis, including polypharmacy. Next, modifying the PD regimen by reducing polypharmacy and lowering the levodopa dose and giving it more frequently, can sometimes help. Last, antipsychotics should be tried, although the tolerability of most antipsychotics, including those with loose binding to the dopamine receptor (e.g., quetiapine), is poor, particularly in later disease stages. Moreover, efficacy has not been clearly established for quetiapine, an agent which is often used because of its perceived better tolerability. Low-dose clozapine (e.g., 6.25 mg or 12 mg/day) might be the best choice, that can be used when no other antipsychotics have been tolerated.[14] Pimavanserin is a new selective 5-HT_{2A} inverse agonist for PD psychosis. In clinical trials, it did not worsen motor symptoms or cause undue sedation;[15] however, its role in the management of psychosis in PD remains to be established, particularly regarding its efficacy when compared with clozapine.

Sleep disruption from restless legs syndrome (RLS) or obstructive sleep apnea are common in PD, can be debilitating, but are relatively treatable (with gabapentin and continuous positive airway pressure, CPAP, respectively).[16] Many PD patients have rapid eye movement (REM) sleep behavior disorder (RBD), which can greatly disrupt their caregivers' sleep and contribute to caregiver stress. Of patients with RBD without PD, 50% will develop PD within a decade, and most of the rest will develop another neurodegenerative disorder.[17]

Huntington's Disease

Chorea Huntington or Huntingon's disease (HD) is a rare autosomal dominant progressive neuropsychiatric disorder. It typically begins in the 4th decade of life and leads to death in about a decade. Psychiatrists should keep in mind, however, that 10% of HD (juvenile HD) begins during adolescence,[18] and such patients may be misdiagnosed as having schizophrenia or other psychiatric disorders when neuropsychiatric symptoms precede motor symptoms. The age of onset is inversely correlated with the number of CAG repeat expansions in the pathogenic gene, a phenomenon known as genetic anticipation.[19] Unfortunately, knowledge of the genetic mutation and its mechanism has not yet been translated into disease-modifying treatments for this single-gene disorder.

As the name chorea Huntington implies, HD is a hyperkinetic movement disorder with hallmark choreiform movements. Psychiatrists might encounter patients with stimulant-induced chorea, which is a complication of long histories of stimulant misuse and known as "crack dancing," either acutely during cocaine use or with chronic use.[20] The differential diagnosis of choreiform movements is provided in Table 21-4.

Other motor phenomena in HD include dysphagia, Parkinsonism, and dystonia, particularly as the illness progresses. In addition, almost all patients with HD

TABLE 21-4 Differential Diagnosis of Choreiform Movements

Inherited Disorders
Huntington's disease
Fahr's syndrome (idiopathic basal ganglia calcification)
Neuroacanthocytosis
Wilson's disease
Friedreich's ataxia
Spinocerebellar ataxia
Acquired Disorders
Focal striatal lesion
Post-infectious: Sydenham's chorea, PANDAS (pediatric autoimmune disorders associated with streptococcal infection)
Pregnancy: Chorea gravidarum
Lupus erythematosus
Thyrotoxicosis
AIDS
Paraneoplastic syndromes
Drug-Induced
Tardive dyskinesia
Phenytoin
Cocaine ("crack dance")
Levodopa
Oral contraceptives

experience neuropsychiatric symptoms, ranging from dysphoria and irritability to anxiety and psychosis. Depression is also frequent, and the suicide risk is high. The end-stage of HD is characterized by increasing immobility and dementia. Patients with juvenile HD experience difficult-to-manage seizures and early psychiatric and cognitive symptoms in addition to bradykinesia, dystonia, rigidity, and oropharyngeal dysfunction.[21] Purely behavioral problems, such as aggression, are other possible early signs. A diagnosis of HD can be suspected if hallmark imaging findings of caudate and putamen degeneration are seen. Genetic testing confirms the diagnosis.

There are no disease-modifying treatments. Death typically occurs within 10 to 15 years of initial diagnosis. Symptomatic treatments include use of SSRIs for depression, low-dose antipsychotics for psychosis, and tetrabenazine for chorea. All treatments carry a risk of worsening the disease (e.g., worsening dysphagia) and must be adjusted to the disease stage.

A family history allows for early diagnosis, including pre-symptomatic testing. However, in some families, the history might be unknown or the parent might not have expressed symptoms yet. Genetic testing poses ethical challenges, particularly the testing of asymptomatic family members who might still be children.[22] The risk of suicide after diagnosis needs to be considered.

Tourette's Syndrome

The hallmark of Tourette's syndrome (TS) is tics that start before the age of 18 years and that consist of both multiple motor tics (e.g., eye blinking or shoulder shrugging) and vocal tics (e.g., throat clearing).[23] Chronic tic disorders, where patients have either motor or vocal tics but not both, are likely a *forme fruste* of TS. The male-to-female ratio for tic disorders is 3 : 1. Many children who develop Tourette's in early childhood have complete resolution of their symptoms by early adulthood. Co-morbid psychiatric disorders, especially OCD and attention-deficit disorder (ADD) are common. Other problems include depression and secondary social phobia related to the tics. As with other movements, tics worsen with stress, excitement, or fatigue. Tics are somewhat voluntary and can be suppressed when patients experience a premonitory urge, at least for a while. These features differentiate tics from myoclonus. An individual tic may move several joints, unlike myoclonus. Complex tics, like repeating phrases (echolalia) or shouting obscenities (coprolalia), are rare, and often misperceived as volitional.

Treatment of tics is usually unnecessary unless they are persistent, impairing, or distressing. Social phobia that has developed in response to tics can be treated directly with therapy and SSRIs. Habit-reversal training is a psychological treatment for tics that can work.[24] ADD, which is highly co-morbid with tics, can probably be treated with stimulants without the risk of worsening tics, contrary to previous recommendations and fears.[25] Tic-suppressing medications include the two α_2-adrenergic receptor agonists, clonidine and guanfacine, and antipsychotics.[26] Clonidine or guanfacine should be tried first, as they are safer than antipsychotics, albeit not as effective as antipsychotics. Antipsychotics can cause tardive dyskinesia and rebound tics when they are withdrawn. While the high-potency antipsychotics haloperidol or pimozide have traditionally been used to manage patients with TS, they are apt to induce extrapyramidal symptoms (and in the case of pimozide, it can increase the QTc interval). Instead, clinicians should try aripiprazole or risperidone. In severe presentations, patients may consider deep brain stimulation (DBS).[27]

Wilson's Disease

Wilson's disease (WD) is a very rare disorder of copper elimination.[28] Its symptoms are the result of insidious copper accumulation in organs, most importantly the liver and the brain.[29] Depending on which organ is affected most, patients may present to hepatologists (because of liver enzyme abnormalities or frank cirrhosis); to neurologists (because of a mix of movement problems, including dysarthria, dysmetria, chorea, and tremor); or psychiatrists (because of mood and personality changes, or rarely psychosis or catatonia). Kayser–Fleischer rings together with serum ceruloplasmin of <100 mg/L are diagnostic for WD. However, 50% of WD patients do not have eye findings. A 24-hour copper excretion in the urine >100 μg per 24 hours, in the absence of cholestatic liver disease, is strong evidence for WD. Ultimately, the diagnosis of WD hinges not on one single test result but on taking into account all clinical information.[30]

Timely diagnosis is important, since eliminating excess copper from the body by means of chelating and depleting agents, such as penicillamine, while also preventing the addition of copper to the body by means of copper-absorption inhibitors (e.g., zinc) is only effective early, before tissue damage has occurred.[31] Psychiatric treatments are not well studied but similar to other disorders that affect the basal ganglia; antipsychotics tend to be poorly tolerated. Without treatment, WD is fatal.

Restless Legs Syndrome (Willis–Ekbom Disease)

Restless legs syndrome (RLS) is a common neurologic movement disorder affecting up to 10% of the general population. Core features of RLS are the urge to move the legs in response to an increasingly unpleasant (oft described as "creeping") feeling that builds in the legs when patients are at rest. Moving the legs relieves this sensation. For most patients, RLS is worse at night, making it difficult for them to fall asleep or to sleep soundly. RLS should not be confused with mere positional discomfort, leg pain, or leg cramps. An important differential diagnostic consideration for psychiatrists is akathisia. Periodic limb movement in sleep (PLMS) is distinct from RLS but almost all patients with RLS show such movements during polysomnography.[32] RLS can be primary or secondary to other medical disorders, most importantly iron deficiency anemia and renal failure.[33] One should consider measuring the ferritin level to rule out iron deficiency in cases of suspected RLS. RLS is frequently co-morbid with depression that can pose a dilemma since antidepressants can exacerbate RLS.[34,35]

The main treatment is with dopamine agonists (e.g., pramipexole or ropinirole) or alpha$_2$ delta ($\alpha_2\delta$) calcium-channel ligands (e.g., gabapentin or pregabalin).[36] Benzodiazepines and opiates can help in difficult cases of RLS, but clinicians need to use them judiciously to avoid falls in the elderly and to guard against misuse, respectively.[37]

TREMORS

The tremor frequencies of different types of tremors overlap too much to be helpful, unless they are unusually slow (e.g., 4 Hz in PD) or high (e.g., 18 Hz in primary orthostatic tremor). To complicate matters, different types of tremor can exist in the same patient. A so-called "intention tremor" (dysmetria) associated with cerebellar disorders is often accompanied by other cerebellar signs (e.g., an ataxic gait or ocular nystagmus); however, as noted earlier, it is not a true tremor. Seizures with retained consciousness would be a very rare cause of bilateral tremor.

Because stress-induced adrenaline itself causes tremor, anxious people often have a tremor, and their awareness of it can worsen their anxiety. It is important to appropriately reassure patients if they perceive a mild tremor to be disabling or a new-onset tremor as a sign of things to come (e.g., like a brain tumor or a disabling progressive neurological disease). The psychological responses to tremors need to be managed with support to help cope with the tremor; treatment includes appropriate management of both the tremor and the psychological response to it. A physiologic (i.e., normal) bilateral finger tremor can be made worse by stress, physical work, or anxiety and also from stimulants, such as nicotine and caffeine. Professionals with stage fright, for example, can use a beta-blocker prior to a public appearance to suppress their physiological tremor. Some people have a prominent ("enhanced") physiologic tremor independent from stress or another neurological disease.

A so-called "benign essential tremor" is an isolated action tremor in the absence of other neurological movements that almost always involves the upper limbs (95% of cases) although the head and voice among other body parts can be affected. The tremor is bilateral and symmetric and is said to respond well to alcohol and to run in families. However, it is usually over-diagnosed because additional neurological signs suggestive of other syndromes, like Parkinson's disease, are overlooked. Moreover, it is increasingly recognized as not "benign" in the sense that it can be progressive and include non-tremor symptoms.[38] Propranolol is first-line treatment. Primidone can help but it must be titrated very slowly because of its propensity to induce severe sedation. Up to half of patients with an action tremor will show no clear benefit from pharmacotherapy.

DRUG-INDUCED MOVEMENT DISORDERS

Iatrogenic movement disorders and tremors are secondary to medication treatment, most often, but not always, due to use of antipsychotics. For psychiatrists, the most important iatrogenic movement disorders are related to extrapyramidal side effects due to antipsychotics and drug-induced tremors. These side effects are important because they can be life-threatening (e.g., laryngeal dystonia); unpleasant (e.g., akathisia); or functionally impairing (e.g., parkinsonism), and socially stigmatizing (e.g., tremor, tardive dyskinesia). Tardive dyskinesia is further problematic, in that it is potentially irreversible, as opposed to the other drug-induced symptoms that usually subside once treatment with the offending agent is stopped. Last, current or recent drug use can lead to movement disorders and to tremors, either during intoxication or withdrawal, depending on the substance.[20] NMS, which is accompanied by motor abnormalities, is an iatrogenic form of malignant catatonia[39] (it is discussed in Chapters 12 and 23).

Drug-Induced Tremors

A very long list of medications, including but not limited to psychotropics, can cause a tremor. A complete medication review, including over-the-counter drugs as well as alcohol and stimulants (e.g., caffeine and nicotine), is therefore critical for patients with a tremor. All major psychiatric medication groups (e.g., antidepressants, antipsychotics, mood stabilizers including lithium) can cause a tremor at usual doses. Sedatives, including benzodiazepines and alcohol, can cause movements during withdrawal, typically with a coarse tremor.

A resting tremor is almost always parkinsonian, including its drug-induced variant. On the other hand, lithium, many anti-epileptic drugs (e.g., valproate, lamotrigine), and stimulants cause action tremors. The tremor due to lithium is an exaggerated physiologic tremor (postural tremor);[40] it is symmetric and related to the dose and blood level of lithium. A more prominent and coarser tremor is the most common symptom of lithium intoxication that should alert clinicians to search for other signs of lithium toxicity (e.g., confusion, diarrhea) and to check the lithium level. If missed, prolonged lithium toxicity can cause an irreversible, poorly treatment-responsive cerebellar tremor.[41] Using the lowest effective lithium dose and removing aggravating factors is often enough to manage lithium tremor. The most commonly prescribed beta-blocker, propranolol, at doses between 60 and 320 mg/day, is effective in cases that require treatment.

Primidone, gabapentin, or benzodiazepines (to reduce arousal) are other options.

Whenever possible, the tremors should be treated in the context of the psychiatric syndrome. For example, one can change an antipsychotic to clozapine in a patient with extrapyramidal symptoms; or avoid medications such as valproate that worsen a tremor in a depressed patient with a tremor.

Antipsychotic-Induced Extrapyramidal Symptoms

Patients who are treated with an antipsychotic can develop one of three main iatrogenic movement disorders in the form of extrapyramidal symptoms (EPS); each follows a different time course. Early complications, after only a dose or so, include akathisia and acute dystonic reactions. Parkinsonism usually does not become apparent until after a few weeks of treatment. By definition, a late-developing ("tardive") problem is tardive dyskinesia (TD). Tardive variants have also been described for akathisia and dystonia. The Pisa syndrome is a variant of dystonia that can also be medication-induced and as the name suggests leads to a sideways-leaning patient due to persistent truncal dystonia.[42] In populations with serious mental disorders, patients might display various admixtures of the three main complications from antipsychotic use. In a representative cohort of 99 chronically institutionalized patients with schizophrenia who received mostly first-generation antipsychotics, only about 40% were free from motor symptoms when carefully examined, while 60% suffered one of three side effects.[43] Despite an increased use of second-generation antipsychotics over the past decade, the same group found an almost unchanged number of movement-disorder-free patients in their cohort when they were able to repeat their cross-sectional assessment 8 years later.[44] Antipsychotic-induced EPS remains a major clinical concern for any psychiatrist who prescribes antipsychotics for longer periods of time. When you assess a patient who is taking an antipsychotic, one should examine for all three main manifestations of EPS, taking into account the possibility of overlap, as graphically depicted in Figure 21-1.

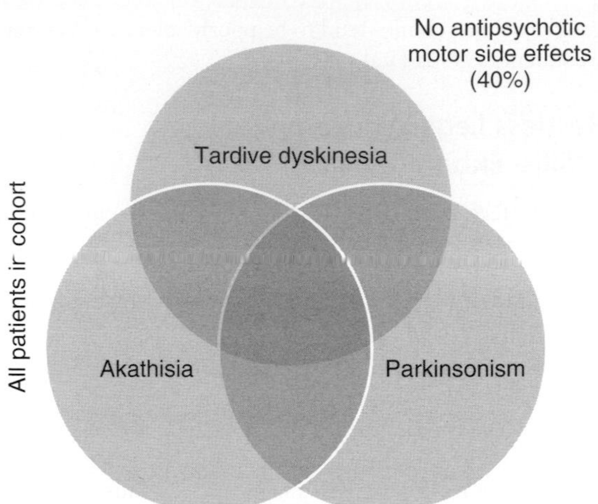

Figure 21-1. Overlap between antipsychotic-induced extrapyramidal symptoms (EPS) in a cohort of antipsychotic-treated patients. *(Based on Janno S, Holi M, Tuisku K, et al: Prevalence of neuroleptic-induced movement disorders in chronic schizophrenia inpatients.* Am J Psychiatry. *2004;161(1):160–163.)*

Acute Dystonic Reaction

Patients can have an acute dystonic reaction after only a single dose of an antipsychotic, with most cases occurring within a week. It classically takes the form of an oculogyric crisis (eyes rolling backwards), opisthotonus (body arching), torticollis, or trismus (jaw locking). These acute-onset problems are frightening and painful. Younger male patients are at highest risk. Many older patients with schizophrenia still remember and will tell you about the first time they received high-dose first-generation antipsychotics and had a dystonic reaction. Dystonic symptoms are rarely life-threatening, except when the dystonia affects the larynx.

One can treat acute dystonic reactions effectively with parenteral benztropine or diphenhydramine. When patients are sent home, they should receive a few days of oral benztropine or diphenhydramine to prevent a return trip to the ED. In addition, one should keep in mind that cocaine and PCP can cause dystonia. When starting a high-potency antipsychotic in a young, antipsychotic-naïve patient, an anticholinergic, like benztropine 1 to 2 mg twice daily, should be added as a prophylactic agent.[45,46] Tapering the anticholinergic after the first month of treatment is appropriate as it is no longer needed to prevent an acute dystonic reaction.

Akathisia

Akathisia is an inability to sit still: afflicted patients fidget and may get up during the interview to walk about. In mild akathisia, patients describe inner restlessness, but can, with effort, suppress visible movements. Very severe akathisia can induce suicidal and homicidal behavior. As with acute dystonic reactions, akathisia can occur after a single dose of an antipsychotic. It is important to distinguish akathisia from anxiety-driven stereotypies and from involuntary dyskinesias, by asking patients what drives their movements. Dyskinetic patients feel that their movements are involuntary. Akathisic and anxious patients both describe their movements as voluntary, but akathisic patients often feel irritable or bored, not frightened. If akathisia is misdiagnosed as psychotic anxiety, clinicians can worsen the patient's symptoms by increasing, rather than by decreasing, the antipsychotic.

Treatment of acute akathisia with a benzodiazepine (e.g., 10 mg diazepam) is reasonable, and, if possible, by lowering the antipsychotic dose. As with RLS, akathisia may respond to dopamine agonists and gabapentin. Although patients with akathisia can sometimes tolerate a switch to a more sedating antipsychotic with a lower propensity for akathisia (e.g., quetiapine, clozapine). However, all antipsychotics, including second-generation antipsychotics and clozapine, can cause akathisia. In very mild akathisia, low-dose mirtazapine,[47] and high-dose propranolol (at a high-enough dose, starting with 10 mg TID) can suppress akathisia. Of note, anticholinergics—while they are often used in the mistaken belief that they treat all EPS—are ineffective for akathisia.

CASE 1

John, a 22-year-old college student was brought to the Emergency Department (ED) by his friends, who had become increasingly concerned about him. He had been making illogical statements, not attending classes, and staying in his room all day. In the ED, he was found to be psychotic but neither depressed nor manic, and he was psychiatrically admitted. He had no medical problems and there was no substance use. Apparently, he had a similar episode 1 year ago, for which he was briefly admitted and treated with haloperidol.

On the unit, John was initially unwilling to start treatment because he had reacted badly to haloperidol. He remembered from his first hospitalization that he had "neck pulling" and "eyes rolling back into my head," which was frightening and painful. "Nobody warned me that this could happen." His treatment team told him he had an acute dystonic reaction and added benztropine to his haloperidol. He had stopped treatment shortly after being discharged because he "didn't feel right, kind of wired." With some hesitation, he agreed to try a different antipsychotic during this hospitalization. He was discharged on aripiprazole 10 mg/day, greatly improved after a 7-day hospitalization.

When John's outpatient psychiatrist saw him a week after discharge, John appeared visibly uncomfortable, and he was unable to sit still during the interview. He described general restlessness, and anxiety "all over" but he was not clearly psychotic. Walking helped transiently, but the restlessness was otherwise constant. His neurologic exam was normal with the exception of psychomotor agitation. He displayed no abnormal movement, had normal muscle tone and muscle strength, and there were was no tremor. There were no signs of catatonia.

To manage acute akathisia, the psychiatrist prescribed 5 mg of diazepam twice daily and stopped aripiprazole. The patient's sensitivity to extrapyramidal side effects suggested that he would need an antipsychotic with very low risk of akathisia, e.g. quetiapine, as opposed to trying to manage akathisia symptomatically with propranolol or low-dose mirtazapine. If quetiapine turns out to be insufficient to control the patient's psychosis, he might need clozapine to manage his illness. Unfortunately, the probability of adherence might already be compromised by having had an acute dystonic reaction and acute akathisia.

Parkinsonism

Parkinsonian symptoms from antipsychotics need to be managed if functionally impairing (e.g., increasing the fall risk or leading to difficulties swallowing) or distressing (e.g., tremor). Parkinsonian symptoms overlap with negative symptoms (the expressivity cluster) and can also easily be mistaken for depression. The drug-induced parkinsonian tremor is a coarse, low-frequency resting tremor that is indistinguishable from the idiopathic resting tremor of PD. Although psychiatrists often try to distinguish idiopathic parkinsonism from drug-induced parkinsonism by the predominance of unilateral tremor, in the former, their main treatment response should be the same in either case: lower any dopamine blockers, if possible. Parkinsonism can cause a lip tremor—sometimes called a "rabbit tremor" because of its resemblance to an eating rabbit—and is more rhythmic than the orobuccal dyskinesia of tardive dyskinesia. Unless a patient also has underlying Parkinson's disease, withdrawing the antipsychotic resolves drug-induced parkinsonism, but it may take months for the symptoms to resolve completely. Anticholinergics such as benztropine (1 or 2 mg twice daily), can suppress parkinsonism in patients with EPS who are unable to tolerate levodopa. Because anticholinergics can cause delirium in older patients, some clinicians try to use the milder drug amantadine (100 mg twice daily);[48] it is an NMDA receptor antagonist closely related to memantine. The risk of exacerbating psychosis is low in patients treated with antipsychotics.

Tardive Dyskinesia

By definition, tardive dyskinesia (TD) is a late complication from treatment with dopamine-blocking agents, usually antipsychotics. One should remember that metoclopramide, used widely to manage nausea and migraine headaches, can cause TD. Given the risk, metoclopramide should therefore only be used on a short-term basis.[49] Risk factors for TD include cumulative antipsychotic exposure, advanced age, and previous experience of EPS. The risk for developing TD from exposure to first-generation antipsychotics is estimated to be 5% per year in young adults.[50] It is somewhat lower for second-generation antipsychotics, but not negligible—even with quetiapine or clozapine.[51] Older adults have a much higher risk (25%) per year. Patients with mood disorders are more likely than those with schizophrenia to develop TD.

The classical movements of TD are involuntary, choreiform, movements that begin insidiously. Sometimes, a dystonic element can be present. As noted earlier, TD can also co-exist with residual parkinsonian EPS. TD movements most often affect the face, but can affect the limbs and trunk. TD symptoms fluctuate with one's level of arousal. Although TD often does not worsen after the first few months, even mild TD movements can cause social stigma. Voluntary movement can temporarily suppress mild TD; this should not be mistaken for the "distractibility" of a psychosomatic movement disorder. Severe TD is so disabling that its constant movements make patients unable to sit in a chair, feed themselves, or hold a book. TD can affect the diaphragm, interrupting breathing.

The best treatment for TD is prevention. A clear indication for the use of antipsychotics should exist and a low-risk antipsychotic chosen. Antipsychotics should be used judiciously in high-risk populations, such as the elderly patient with dementia, particularly since the use of antipsychotics in this population is of unclear benefit. The American Psychiatric Association recently published guidelines regarding the use of antipsychotics to treat agitation or psychosis in a patient with dementia.[52] Key recommendations included quantitative assessment of agitation and psychosis and periodic assessment of the need for ongoing treatment. Patients who receive antipsychotics in acute care settings to manage a delirium should not leave the hospital with an order for an antipsychotic unless ongoing treatment is indicated. Patients who are treated with a maintenance

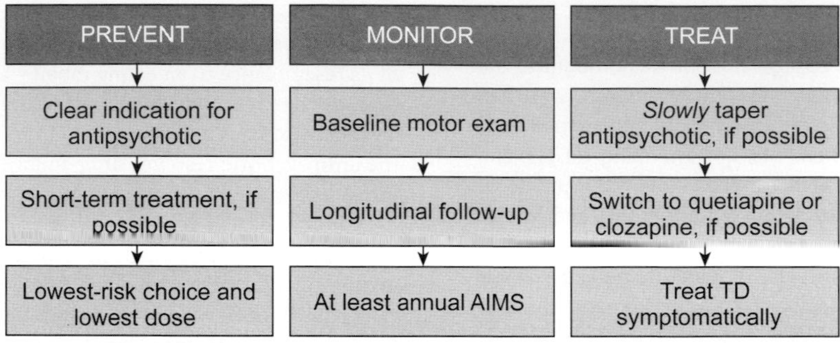

Figure 21-2. Prevention and treatment of tardive dyskinesia (TD).

antipsychotic need to be appropriately monitored. Clinicians must look for TD at every visit, as part of the mental status exam. In addition, a formal exam for TD with the Abnormal Involuntary Movement Scale (AIMS) should be documented periodically. The AIMS should be administered at least annually in routine care and more often in high-risk antipsychotic-treated patients. Instructions for the use of the AIMS are nicely summarized by Munetz and Benjamin.[53] Do not forget to obtain a baseline assessment for abnormal motor abnormalities before starting an antipsychotic to document either the absence or presence of any pre-existing motor abnormalities.

The best treatment for TD once it is recognized is to stop the offending drug—slowly. Abrupt antipsychotic discontinuation can induce withdrawal dyskinesias that can be severe, and even involve respiratory muscles. This point needs emphasizing: any patients with mild TD can convert to fulminant TD, with respiratory muscle involvement, because the clinician panicked and stopped the drug suddenly, causing serious rebound. When even gradual discontinuation worsens TD, the dopamine-depleting drug, tetrabenazine, can suppress TD during the taper, but it is sedating and can worsen mood.

If ongoing antipsychotic treatment is needed, clozapine is the best choice, followed by quetiapine. While the list of other potential treatments for TD is lengthy,[54] few have much benefit. Some treatments, such as vitamin E have shown promise in initial trials but failed to show benefit in subsequent larger trials.[55] The dopamine-depleting drug, tetrabenazine, is currently the most effective TD treatment.[56] It is, however, often not well tolerated, causes sedation, and has a short half-life. Improved analogs of tetrabenazine, such as valbenazine, are in clinical trials. For some patients with TD, particularly if there is a dystonic component or focal involvement (e.g., blepharospasm) botulinum toxin injections can help but they need to be repeated every 3 months.[57] Deep brain stimulation is a treatment of last resort for TD.[58] The basic management principles for TD are summarized in Figure 21-2.

FUNCTIONAL MOVEMENT DISORDERS

Up to 20% of patients in movement disorder clinics have functional movement disorders. Such movements can mimic any of the known movement disorders, but appear willful, or motivated. The diagnosis of functional movement disorder is problematic. All movement disorders affect willed action and the motivation to move—the line between "real" and "psychogenic" disorders is not so clear. The DSM-IV definition of somatoform disorders as having a "non-organic" cause reflects the intuitive dualism that even trained neuroscientists find hard to resist.[59] The DSM-5 definition of somatic symptom disorder avoids this error.

Observers typically suspect that patients with functional movement disorders are malingering or acting to obtain unconscious secondary gain. However, patients with functional movement disorders do not benefit from their symptoms; they typically are more disabled, more depressed, and more stigmatized than patients whose symptoms have a clear physical cause. Patients who malinger typically have symptoms that are more traditional and convincing than the apparently willful symptoms of functional disorders. Classic clues of "psychogenicity," such as *la belle indifference* (lack of concern for the medical problem) are highly unreliable. Clinicians should also not depend on the perceived "bizarreness" of the movements. Sudden unexplained onsets and full remissions suggest a functional movement disorder. Not falling despite wild flailing movements (astasia-abasia) suggests a functional disorder. Improvement of the symptom with distraction is often misdiagnosed, since most movement disorders are highly influenced by attention, anxiety, and movement of other body parts. A more reliable sign is entrainment of a tremor to the voluntary tapping of another body part at a new frequency.

Mass psychogenic illness is an interesting phenomenon that can produce epidemics of functional movement disorders. Such outbreaks are not only of historical interest (e.g., Saint Vitus dance in the Middle Ages during the Black Plague or hysterical illnesses in the Salem witch trials) but continue to occur. A recent outbreak for example affected about 20 teenagers in Le Roy, NY.[60] Mass psychogenic illnesses show us the important role of expectations and social learning and social networks.[61] In the specific context of a modern Western society, fears of toxins combined with distrust of industry and a cover-up by the state (all not necessarily unfounded) combine to produce psychogenic illness in a susceptible group where an initial index case allows for spread to occur in the social network. Recognizing mass psychogenic illness is as difficult at the level of a group as it is for individual patients as one can "never be sure" that there is no toxin, for example. Endless investigations can never clearly settle the case, just like more laboratory tests can never put to rest the idea that one might have a yet-to-be-discovered illness. Mass psychogenic illness requires recognition and prevention of spread. In many cases, opinion leaders need to be separated from the larger group. Media attention unfortunately makes containment next to impossible.

Neurologists typically perform exhaustive tests to rule out rare disorders that can cause abnormal movements, and wait until all are negative to discuss psychiatric factors that may contribute to the symptoms. It is better for both neurologists and psychiatrists to be involved from the start if a functional disorder is likely. Neurology needs to be involved, since it is difficult to ascertain the functional character of movements unless clinical experience is there to recognize hysterical unsteadiness (astasia-abasia) for example. Psychiatry on the other hand, can identify treatable psychiatric disorders and work with patients' psychological responses to their symptoms and build coping skills. However, quite frequently, patients resist referral to psychiatry and one could argue that the 50% or so without psychiatric psychopathology or distress have a point (i.e., there does not seem to be a conversion from psychological conflict to bodily expression). Unfortunately, these patients get stuck if neurologists in turn feel that they have little else to offer beyond diagnosis.

When and how should you tell a patient that his movements are "psychogenic?" One should not wait until "every possible test" has been done; instead, one should discuss anxiety and other psychiatric aspects of their symptoms at the beginning of their neurologic work-up. Most patients are firmly committed to finding a traditional medical explanation whose severity explains their subjective sense that there is something terribly wrong with their body. Rather than telling a patient "Don't worry, your tremor is just anxiety," consider re-framing your description physiologically, e.g., "past stress has raised adrenaline levels, and adrenaline causes tremor." Explain that "psychogenic" symptoms have "real" brain correlates (i.e., altered neurocircuitry) in functional neuroimaging studies.[62] Direct the patients to the website www.neurosymptoms.org, an excellent self-help website for patients who want to educate themselves about functional movement disorders.[63]

Doctors become frustrated by patients with functional symptoms when they do not know how to help them and if they believe that the patient does not truly want to get better. Cognitive-behavioral therapy, however, is one psychological treatment modality that can help.[64] Physical therapy is yet another, potentially helpful treatment that is safe and also allows for the gradual return to function as a goal, despite symptoms (which might improve in the course of this intervention).[65] Psychotropics can be used judiciously to address distress. A solid doctor–patient relationship that conveys sincere caring and a hopeful approach with symptom remission as a goal can prevent chronicity.

REFERENCES

Access the reference list online at https://expertconsult.inkling.com/.

Patients With Infectious or Inflammatory Neuropsychiatric Impairment

22

Jenny J. Linnoila, M.D., Ph.D.

OVERVIEW

While there has always been a close association between neurologic and psychiatric disorders, in the past decade, with the identification of a new class of autoimmune encephalitides that are associated with profound neuropsychiatric impairments,[1] and the realization that psychiatric disorders, such as schizophrenia, may be linked with deficient components of the immune system that are responsible for synaptic pruning,[2] the lines between the two disciplines are increasingly blurred. This overlap necessitates collaboration between neurologists and psychiatrists and an overall multidisciplinary approach to many shared patients. Similarly, there may be considerable overlap in the manifestations of infectious and inflammatory etiologies. The blending between "neurologic," "psychiatric," "infectious," and "inflammatory" disorders can make the diagnosis and treatment of these disorders a daunting task. This chapter aims to demystify some of these complex disorders and to offer a practical approach to the diagnosis and treatment of infectious or inflammatory disorders that present with neuropsychiatric impairment.

POTENTIAL ETIOLOGIES OF ACUTE AND SUB-ACUTE NEUROPSYCHIATRIC IMPAIRMENT

Encephalitis Versus Encephalopathy

In the hospital setting, neuropsychiatric impairment is most often secondary to similar, but distinct entities—encephalitis and encephalopathy. In general, *encephalitis*, or an inflammation of the brain, can be thought of as being due to direct involvement of the brain parenchyma itself, while *encephalopathy* is more of a general clinical term that refers to a non-specific confusional state that is not necessarily due to malfunction or inflammation of the organ itself. For instance, encephalopathy can stem from the dysfunction of other organs, such as the liver in hepatitis, the kidneys in uremia, and the body as a whole, as in sepsis. Encephalitis can also result in encephalopathy, but the opposite is not necessarily true; i.e., encephalopathy does not necessarily imply encephalitis. Encephalitis is commonly encountered in the hospital setting. Unfortunately, in the majority of cases, exact causes remain unknown. Even in cases where there is a high suspicion of an infectious cause, the causative microbe often goes un-identified. In the future, this may change with the incorporation of next-generation sequencing,[3] but this technology, which allows one to screen body fluids, including cerebrospinal fluid (CSF), for any known pathogen, is not widely available and is currently only available on a research basis. In recent years, it has become evident that many previously cryptogenic cases of encephalitis are autoimmune, mediated by pathogenic antibodies to neuronal cell surface antigens, such as N-methyl-D-aspartic acid receptors (NMDARs). Indeed, a retrospective analysis of nearly 500 cases of cryptogenic encephalitis demonstrated that about 1% of them were due to NMDAR encephalitis.[4] The pathophysiology underlying these autoimmune encephalitides remains unknown.

Causes of Encephalopathy

Encephalopathy has a relatively broad differential diagnosis. High on that list are toxic (both endogenous and exogenous) and metabolic causes. Infectious causes include hepatitis, systemic infections, and especially in the elderly, more common infections (such as pneumonia and urinary tract infections). Inflammatory causes, such as autoimmune hepatitis, primary biliary sclerosis, lupus, and immunoglobulin (Ig) A nephropathy, lead to encephalopathy primarily by leading to end-organ dysfunction or failure. There is recent literature that suggests that even celiac disease can lead to psychosis.[5] Encephalopathy typically manifests clinically as an altered mental status, or a delirium-type picture with waxing and waning confusion, disorientation, hallucinations, and sometimes seizures.

Work-Up for Encephalopathy

Blood and/or urine laboratory work-ups for encephalopathy commonly reveal abnormalities, such as metabolic or electrolyte derangements (for example hyponatremia, hypercalcemia, hypercapnia, hyperammonemia, transaminitis, elevated creatinine and/or blood urea nitrogen, hyper/hypoglycemia), elevated white blood cell count, and/or positive toxicology screening (positive drug screen and/or elevated anion gap). Electroencephalography (EEG) can reveal generalized triphasic discharges, which are classically seen in toxic/metabolic encephalopathy, or seizures. Brain magnetic resonance imaging (MRI) most often is normal or reveals symmetric changes, indicative of a generalized process that affects the brain. The work-up of altered mental status secondary to encephalopathy is not the focus of this chapter. The reader is referred to Chapters 10, 27, and 28. Rather, this chapter will focus upon infectious and inflammatory causes of encephalitis.

Encephalitic Neuropsychiatric Impairment

Clinical Features of Infectious Encephalitis

If encephalitis is suspected, distinguishing between infectious and inflammatory causes (Table 22-1) can be challenging, as there is often overlap in patients' initial clinical presentations. For the purpose of this chapter, inflammatory causes of encephalitis refer to autoimmune neurologic disorders, including those associated with cancer, termed "paraneoplastic disorders." In general, infectious causes of encephalitis are often associated with fevers,[6] but this may not always be true, especially in immunocompromised or elderly patients, who may not be able to mount a strong immune response. If present, headaches are more often noted in infectious, as opposed to inflammatory encephalitis. Additionally, infectious encephalitis usually results in a precipitous decline over the course of hours to days, as opposed to the decline seen with inflammatory causes of encephalitis, which more typically manifest over the course of weeks to months. Of course, exceptions exist. The neuropsychiatric decline noted in syphilis can manifest decades after initial infection. Also, a rapid decline may not be as prevalent for immunocompromised individuals. For instance, while acquired immune deficiency syndrome (AIDS) dementia has long been recognized, it is becoming evident that more subtle cognitive deficits similar to mild cognitive impairment, often a precursor to Alzheimer's disease, appear to develop slowly in patients with human immunodeficiency virus (HIV) over time.[7] This is true even for patients with what was thought to be relatively well-controlled HIV infection, as evidenced by low or undetectable serum viral loads. In recent years, it has become evident that even with well-controlled systemic disease, some patients with HIV infection may have progressive encephalitis, possibly due to "central escape" of the virus from medications that do not penetrate the CSF space well, or from persistent low-level central nervous system (CNS) inflammation.

In addition to encephalitis, infections can also trigger meningitis, or inflammation of the meninges, the protective coverings of the brain. Signs of meningismus include fever, headache, nuchal rigidity (which may produce positive Kernig's and Brudzinski's signs), and vomiting with or without photophobia.[6] Meningitis is much less frequently associated with autoimmune causes.

Clinical Features of Autoimmune Encephalitis

Regardless of the specific manifestations, there are a few features that raise suspicion for autoimmune disorders.[8] In general, there is a distinct change from a patient's baseline functional status over days to weeks. The patient's symptoms may have a fluctuating course. Family members often believe that the patient's behavioral or cognitive changes came "out of the blue" and are highly divergent from the patient's baseline personality. When considering psychiatric presentations, the patient's age is important; for example, it is highly

TABLE 22-1 Clues to an Autoimmune Versus Infectious Etiology for Encephalitis

CLUES TO AN AUTOIMMUNE ETIOLOGY	CLUES TO AN INFECTIOUS ETIOLOGY
Symptoms: predominantly psychiatric (especially early and at an unusual age for initial presentation)	**Symptoms:** broader, including fever,[a] headache, obtundation, meningismus
Onset: subacute (days to weeks)	**Onset:** often precipitous[a] (hours to days)
Medical history: personal or family history of organ- or non-organ-specific autoimmune disorder	**Medical history:** immunocompromised state
Serum: systemic markers of autoimmunity (e.g., elevated ANA or TPO antibodies) and/or identification of a neural autoantibody	**Serum:** markedly elevated[a] ESR and/or CRP, tests (cultures, ELISAs, PCR, western blots, antibodies, blood smears) identifying specific microbes
Cancer status: history of or concurrent malignancy	**Cancer status:** generally N/A, unless immunocompromised (e.g., from chemotherapy)
CSF studies: elevated WBC (usually <100 cells/μL), protein (usually <100 mg/dL), IgG index, oligoclonal bands, synthesis rate, and/or identification of a neural autoantibody	**CSF studies:** elevated WBC (usually >100 cells/μL[a]), protein (usually >100 mg/dL), elevated RBC and/or xanthochromia possible, decreased glucose, tests (cultures, ELISAs, PCR, western blots, antibodies, smears) identifying specific microbes
EEG: focal abnormalities	**EEG:** no particular pattern; could have triphasics
MRI brain: T2/FLAIR hyperintensities, rarely enhancement	**MRI brain:** T2/FLAIR hyperintensities (may be symmetric), more often has enhancement, may have leptomeningeal or spinal cord involvement, may have mass effect, may have blood
PET brain: areas of hyper/hypometabolism	**PET brain:** not typically done
Therapy: response to immunosuppression	**Therapy:** response to antimicrobials

[a]May not apply to immunocompromised patients.

ANA, antinuclear antibody; CRP, C-reactive protein; CSF, cerebrospinal fluid; EEG, electroencephalography; ELISA, enzyme-linked immunosorbent assay; ESR, erythrocyte sedimentation rate; FLAIR, fluid attenuation inversion recovery; IgG, immunoglobulin G; MRI, magnetic resonance imaging; N/A, not applicable; PCR, polymerase chain reaction; PET, positron emission tomography; RBC, red blood cell count; TPO, anti-thyroperoxidase antibody; WBC, white blood cell count.

unusual for hallucinations to occur in a young child and for schizophrenia to first manifest in a patient's 60s. Such circumstances would be less consistent with a primary psychiatric disorder and more consistent with autoimmune encephalitis. Additionally, a patient presenting primarily with isolated psychiatric symptoms is more likely to have an autoimmune disorder than an infectious encephalitis. Patients with autoimmune encephalitis may have a personal or family history of systemic autoimmune disease, such as Hashimoto's thyroiditis, rheumatoid arthritis, or celiac disease. Moreover, as with systemic autoimmunity, patients may have overlapping autoimmune neurologic diseases, such as neuromyelitis optica (NMO) and autoimmune encephalitis,[9] making diagnosis particularly challenging. Paraneoplastic disorders cause neurologic symptoms in patients with malignancy, commonly before the cancer is diagnosed.[10] A personal history of neoplasm in a patient with new neurologic symptoms should raise one's suspicion of a paraneoplastic disorder. However, especially early on into a patient's course, it can be difficult to differentiate infectious from inflammatory encephalitides, especially because many patients with autoimmune encephalitis present with a viral prodrome,[11] as in up to half of cases of NMDAR encephalitis.

Work-Up for Infectious and Inflammatory Causes

Bloodwork

Initial work-up for infectious and autoimmune causes of encephalitis should always include basic bloodwork, urinalysis, and toxicology screens, to exclude readily diagnosed causes of encephalopathy. Serum markers that raise the suspicion of an infectious or inflammatory encephalitis include an elevated erythrocyte sedimentation rate (ESR) and/or C-reactive protein (CRP). In general, markedly elevated values are more often associated with infectious, as opposed to inflammatory encephalitides. In autoimmune encephalitis, while ESR and CRP values can be elevated, they can also be normal. In the work-up for autoimmune encephalitis, elevated antinuclear (ANA) or thyroid peroxidase (TPO) antibodies, although non-specific, can be considered as helpful markers for an autoimmune tendency in a patient.[8] Specific infectious etiologies can be tested for in the serum, most often by growing cultures or testing for antibodies with enzyme-linked immunosorbent assays (ELISAs) or western blots or nucleic acids with polymerase chain reactions (PCRs).[6] A blood smear may be useful for detecting organisms and/or abnormal blood cells. Testing should be chosen based on a patient's presentation and personal risk factors, taking into account their age, sex, medical history, location, behaviors, travel history, and immunocompromised status, if applicable. Consulting with an infectious diseases specialist, either general or neurologic, can be useful to determine the specific tests to order.

Neural Autoantibody Testing

The past decade has seen the identification of over 10 new neurally directed autoantibodies that have been linked with autoimmune encephalitides.[1] Many of these are now available for commercial testing and are available as part of panels that are grouped by symptomatology, including encephalitis, seizures, and dementia, in addition to more traditional paraneoplastic panels.[8] As there can be significant overlap in the clinical signs and symptoms associated with each neural autoantibody, it is prudent to order a comprehensive autoantibody evaluation, as opposed to testing for a single autoantibody or a small sub-set of them. Neural autoantibody testing is available for serum and CSF and it is important to analyze both of them, as they are not necessarily equivalent. For instance, some autoantibody tests, such as for voltage-gated calcium channel (VGCC) antibodies, have been validated only in serum. Additionally, testing for other antibodies, such as the aquaporin-4 antibodies associated with NMO, is more sensitive from the serum, as compared to NMDAR antibody testing, which is more sensitive from CSF. For example, an analysis of paired CSF and serum samples from 250 patients with NMDAR encephalitis showed that whereas all the CSF samples tested positive for NMDAR antibodies, between 6% and 13% (depending on the methodology used) of the corresponding paired serum samples tested negative for NMDAR antibodies.[12] Thus, testing both the serum and the CSF raises the overall sensitivity (and specificity) of the testing. It is important to note that neural autoantibody testing is not fool-proof; sometimes it can reveal the presence of antibodies that are poorly correlated with the patient's symptoms and other times the patient may test positive for a low level of an antibody, such as low-level glutamic acid decarboxylase (GAD-65) autoantibodies, which may only indicate an autoimmune tendency, as opposed to a specific autoimmune encephalitis diagnosis. Thus, the results of neural autoantibody testing must be interpreted carefully to determine whether they are clinically relevant. Table 22-2 lists neural autoantibodies commonly associated with autoimmune encephalitides.

Intracellular Versus Cell Surface-Targeted Neural Autoantibodies

Paraneoplastic disorders, such as myasthenia gravis linked with thymoma[31] (and acetylcholine receptors) and Lambert-Eaton myasthenic syndrome linked with small-cell lung cancer (and VGCC antibodies),[32] have long been recognized. In the past few decades, many more paraneoplastic disorders were identified, linked with conditions such as cerebellar degeneration and limbic encephalitis,[10] a disorder characterized by confusion, behavioral changes, and/or seizures. Many of these paraneoplastic disorders have been associated with antibodies that target intracellular proteins. Studies have shown that many of these neural autoantibodies, while serving as markers of paraneoplasia, do not appear to be pathogenic themselves. Rather, they seem to reflect cytotoxic effector T-cell-mediated CNS damage, which is generally poorly responsive to immunotherapy, resulting in limited neurologic recovery of patients, even with maximal treatment.[33]

However, the last decade has seen the identification of many new neural autoantibodies, especially ones associated with autoimmune encephalitis.[14,17,19,20,24,27,28,34–36] As opposed to many of the previously identified paraneoplastic antibodies, these antibodies' antigens are mostly on, or associated with, the neuronal cell surface. These autoantibodies are less often associated with malignancy. Moreover, many of them are themselves pathogenic.[14,28,35,37,38] The autoantibodies trigger processes such as receptor downregulation, which is often reversible, in large part explaining the responsiveness of patients' symptoms to immunotherapy. In general, these neural antibodies infer good responses to immunotherapy. However, brain atrophy and other irreversible damage can

TABLE 22-2 Neural Autoantibodies Associated With Autoimmune Encephalitides

ANTIGEN	INTRACELLULAR/ CELL SURFACE	CLINICAL FEATURES	TUMOR ASSOCIATION
AGNA[13] (SOX1)	Intracellular	Lambert-Eaton myasthenic syndrome (LEMS), limbic encephalitis, neuropathy	Highly associated with small-cell lung cancer, especially with LEMS
AMPAR[14]	Cell surface	Limbic encephalitis; may occur with pure psychiatric manifestations. Relapses common	~70% (lung, breast, thymoma)
Amphiphysin[15]	Intracellular	Wide clinical spectrum: stiff person syndrome, cerebellar degeneration, limbic encephalitis, encephalomyelitis, myelopathy, peripheral neuropathy, opsoclonus myoclonus	~85% (breast, small-cell lung cancer)
ANNA-1[16] (Anti-Hu)	Intracellular	Wide clinical spectrum: sensory neuronopathy, limbic encephalitis, cranial neuropathies, cerebellar degeneration, encephalomyelitis, partial epilepsy, status epilepticus, autonomic dysfunction including intestinal pseudo-obstruction, opsoclonus myoclonus	~80% (small-cell lung cancer, neuroblastoma, prostate cancer)
CASPR2[17]	Cell surface	Encephalopathy, Morvan's syndrome, neuromyotonia Relapses of encephalopathy common	~0–40% (thymoma)
CRMP-5[18] (anti-CV2)	Intracellular	Wide clinical spectrum: cerebellar degeneration, limbic encephalitis, optic neuritis, retinopathy, uveitis, chorea, encephalomyelitis, sensorimotor neuropathy	~75% (small cell lung cancer, thymoma)
DPPX[19]	Cell surface	Encephalopathy with CNS hyperexcitability: confusion, psychiatric manifestations, tremor, myoclonus, nystagmus, hyperekplexia, PERM-like symptoms, ataxia Diarrhea and profound weight loss common	Rare B-cell neoplasms reported
$GABA_aR$[35]	Cell surface	Prominent seizures, status epilepticus	Infrequent
$GABA_BR$[20]	Cell surface	Limbic encephalitis, prominent seizures, status epilepticus	~50% (lung, neuroendocrine)
GFAP[21]	Intracellular	Wide clinical spectrum: encephalopathy, tremor, headache, myelopathic signs, meningeal signs, optic disc edema, psychiatric symptoms, ataxia, autonomic dysfunction, seizures, meningoencephalomyelitis	~1/3 (teratoma ≫ adenoma, CNS glioma, lung cancer)
GAD-65[22,23]	Intracellular	Wide clinical spectrum: encephalopathy, stiff person syndrome, cerebellar ataxia, seizure disorder With cancer more likely to see opsoclonus myoclonus syndrome and encephalomyelitis	~10% (lung cancer, neuroendocrine tumor, thymoma, breast cancer)
GlyαR[24]	Cell surface	Wide clinical spectrum: stiff-person syndrome, PERM, limbic encephalitis, cerebellar degeneration, or optic neuritis	Infrequent
LGI-1[17,25]	Cell surface	Limbic encephalitis, faciobrachial dystonic seizures, REM sleep behavior disorder, myoclonus ~60% with hyponatremia	≤10% (small-cell lung cancer, thymoma)
Anti-Ma2 (Ta)[26]	Intracellular	Ma2 (only): limbic encephalitis, hypothalamic dysfunction, brainstem encephalitis	Germ-cell testicular cancer common
mGluR5[27]	Cell surface	Ophelia syndrome: limbic encephalitis, myoclonus Very few cases	Hodgkin's lymphoma; may occur without tumor
NMDAR[11] (GluN1)	Cell surface	NMDAR encephalitis: progression through psychiatric manifestations, insomnia, reduced verbal output, seizures, amnesia, movement disorders, catatonia, hypoventilation, autonomic instability, coma ~50% viral prodrome ~30% with "delta brush pattern" on EEG Relapses 12% at 2 years	Age-dependent: ~10–45%, most often ovarian teratomas, rarely carcinomas, rare in children

TABLE 22-2 Neural Autoantibodies Associated With Autoimmune Encephalitides—cont'd

ANTIGEN	INTRACELLULAR/ CELL SURFACE	CLINICAL FEATURES	TUMOR ASSOCIATION
Neurexin-3α[28]	Cell surface	Confusion, seizures, altered consciousness Often follows viral prodrome (fever, headache, GI symptoms) Patients can deteriorate rapidly Few cases reported	None reported
VGCC[29a] (N-type, P/Q type[29b])	Cell surface	N: variable; includes encephalopathy, seizures P/Q: cerebellar degeneration, seizures	Sometimes associated with small-cell lung cancer
VGKC complex[30]	Cell surface	Wide clinical spectrum: includes LGI-1 and CASPR2, but also dementia and pain syndromes	Variable, ≤10–40% (small-cell lung cancer, thymoma)

Percentage refers to percentage of patients with particular antibody that also have malignancy.

AGNA, antiglial nuclear antibody; AMPAR, alpha-amino-3-hydroxy-5-methyl-4-isoxazolepropionic acid receptor; ANNA, anti-neuronal nuclear antibody; CASPR2, contactin-associated protein-like 2; CNS, central nervous system; CRMP-5, collapsin response mediator protein 5; DPPX, dipeptidyl-peptidase-like protein-6; EEG, electroencephalography; GABAR, gamma-amino-butyric acid receptor; GAD-65, glutamic acid decarboxylase; GI, gastrointestinal; GluN1, ionotropic NMDA glutamate receptor 1; GlyαR, glycine alpha receptor; LEMS, Lambert-Eaton myasthenic syndrome; LGI-1, leucine-rich; glioma-inactivated 1; mGluR, metabotropic glutamate receptor; NMDAR, N-methyl-D-aspartic acid receptor; PERM, progressive encephalomyelitis with rigidity and myoclonus; REM, rapid eye movement; SOX1, sex determining region Y box 1 transcription factor; VGCC, voltage-gated calcium channel; VGKC, voltage-gated potassium channel complex.

also occur in these encephalitides, necessitating rapid diagnosis and treatment for the best possible clinical outcomes.

Overlap Syndromes: Parainfectious Autoimmune Encephalitis

In general, the identification of a neural autoantibody corresponds with a diagnosis of autoimmune encephalitis. However, reports of NMDAR encephalitis after herpes simplex virus (HSV) encephalitis (HSE) have complicated the diagnostic picture, as there appears to be overlap between infectious and autoimmune encephalitides.[39–45] Some patients who have been treated for HSE and either suffer a recurrence of neurologic symptoms or continue to deteriorate or fail to improve, rather than having a recurrence of HSE, as was originally thought, have now been found to have subsequent autoimmune encephalitis. It is important to recognize this, as autoimmune encephalitides are often immunotherapy-responsive and thus the high morbidity typically associated with HSE may be modifiable. Many adult patients with post-HSE NMDAR encephalitis have predominantly neuropsychiatric symptoms, including behavior changes, agitation, aggression, suicidal ideation, confusion, and delusions, that were previously understood as sequelae of HSE.[46] It is possible that these symptoms may instead be attributable to subsequent autoimmune encephalitis. Moreover, a recent analysis revealed that this phenomenon happens with other herpes virus encephalitides, which can trigger the production of non-NMDAR neural autoantibodies.[47] Thus, a clean distinction between infectious and inflammatory causes of encephalitis does not always exist.

CSF Analysis

In addition to testing for neural autoantibodies, it is important to examine other characteristics of a patient's CSF. Before performing a lumbar puncture (LP), it is imperative to do either computed tomography (CT) or MRI imaging of the head, to rule out masses or hydrocephalus, which are typically associated with infectious causes, and can create a risk for herniation from an LP. CNS infections can cause CSF to appear cloudy or yellow. Herpes infections are neurotropic[48,49] and both HSV and varicella zoster virus (VZV) can cause necrosis and hemorrhage, potentially resulting in pink CSF, elevated CSF red blood cell counts, elevated CSF protein counts, and/or the presence of xanthochromia. Both infectious and inflammatory encephalitides can result in elevations of protein and white blood cell (WBC) counts. However, the protein and WBC elevations are typically much higher with infections, for instance, with protein >100 mg/dL and a WBC count >100/μL, as compared with <100 for each, on average, for autoimmune encephalitides.[8] WBC differential is also important. Whereas infectious encephalitides (bacterial > viral) can be associated with elevations in polymorphonuclear leukocytes, autoimmune encephalitides are overwhelmingly associated with elevated lymphocyte counts. However, viral meningitides can shift from a polymorphonuclear to a lymphocytic predominance.[6] CSF glucose is only rarely abnormal in autoimmune encephalitides. In contrast, especially with bacterial meningitis and CNS tuberculosis, glucose is often decreased. In autoimmune encephalitides, initial CSF pleocytosis often resolves and is replaced with alternative markers of inflammation, including elevated immunoglobulin G (IgG) index and oligoclonal bands,[1] which are considered general markers of intrathecal antibody synthesis, and can also be elevated in infectious encephalitis. As with the serum (and other bodily fluids), microbes can also be tested for directly in the CSF. A Gram stain and smear may be useful for detecting organisms and/or abnormal immune cells. Consultation with an infectious diseases specialist can help to determine which cultures and studies to order based on the patient's presentation, CSF markers, and personal risk factors (e.g., age, sex, medical history, location, behaviors, travel history, and immunocompromised status, if applicable).

Electroencephalography

Infectious and autoimmune encephalitides can both cause seizures. In contrast with the generalized discharges (such as triphasics) often associated with encephalopathy, encephalitides commonly cause localized, or focal abnormalities on the EEG. It is important to recognize that seizure phenotypes are broader than generalized tonic-clonic, or "grand mal" seizures. This is particularly important when considering the neuropsychiatric manifestations of seizures; partial complex seizures can cause behavioral arrest, confusion, and a sense of "lost time"; temporal lobe seizures can lead to auditory hallucinations and behavioral changes (such as hyper-religiosity); seizures involving the amygdala can result in fear or anxiety; and occipital lobe seizures can present as visual hallucinations. Whereas it may be impossible to distinguish infectious versus autoimmune encephalitides based on the EEG alone, at least one distinctive EEG abnormality, termed "extreme delta brush" has been strongly associated with NMDAR encephalitis.[50] On the other hand, faciobrachial dystonic (FBD) seizures, brief dystonic contractions of the patient's face and/or arm (typically on the same side) that are often seen in autoimmune leucine-rich, glioma-inactivated 1 (LGI-1) encephalitis,[51] may not be picked up by standard EEG scalp electrodes, perhaps due to a deep seizure focus. If autoimmune encephalitis is suspected, it is important to make the interpreting neurologist aware, so that the patient's EEG can be interpreted in the appropriate context.

Brain Imaging

Brain imaging is an essential component of the work-up for encephalitis. Brain MRIs should be done with contrast, whenever possible. In general, MRI abnormalities, including T2/fluid attenuation inversion recovery (FLAIR) hyperintensities and contrast enhancement, are more often seen in infectious, as compared to autoimmune encephalitides. An exception can be seen with severe and/or frequent seizures, which can lead to T2/FLAIR hyperintensities, contrast enhancement, and diffusion-weighted imaging (DWI) positivity.[52] Autoimmune encephalitides do not typically cause hydrocephalus, meningitis, ventriculitis, and the accumulation of material (such as the cysts seen with cryptococcal infection) in the ventricles, all of which can be seen with infectious encephalitides. In fact, autoimmune encephalitides, especially early into their course, may not produce any abnormalities on brain MRI. In these cases, abnormalities may instead be visible on PET imaging, in the form of areas of hypo- or hyper-metabolism.[53,54] As with the EEG, whereas PET findings can be seen in both infectious and autoimmune encephalitides, there are particular PET patterns, such as a frontotemporal-to-occipital gradient, reported in severe cases of NMDAR encephalitis,[55] which raise the suspicion for autoimmune encephalitis. Additionally, whereas the FBD seizures noted in LGI-1 encephalitis may not produce abnormalities on EEG, in some cases, they are associated with changes in the basal ganglia in brain MRI and/or PET imaging.[56] Also similar to focal EEG findings, discussed above, focal imaging abnormalities, seen either via MRI or PET, may sometimes correspond well with a patient's neuropsychiatric impairments (e.g., hyperintensity or hypermetabolism in the amygdala corresponding with fearful preoccupations).

Malignancy Screening

As mentioned previously, some neural autoantibodies have been associated with neoplasms, particularly those targeted towards intracellular proteins. This necessitates a search for malignancy, guided by a patient's particular neural autoantibodies and their personal risk factors for cancer, such as age, family or personal medical history, and smoking status.[8] Neoplasms are much less frequent in children than in adults.[57,58] Because neurologic symptoms frequently present before malignancy in paraneoplastic disorders (in up to 70% of cases),[10] neoplasms associated with autoimmunity are often detected early into their course and thus they can be small and have limited regional spread, to a single lymph node, for instance. Therefore, they may be difficult to identify on conventional imaging and subtle imaging abnormalities, such as pulmonary nodules or enlarged lymph nodes, should be investigated further when autoimmune encephalitides are diagnosed or suspected. There is sometimes controversy as to whether PET scans of the body should be used routinely in autoimmune malignancy work-ups. A study examining the added benefit of PET in cases of suspected paraneoplastic disorders determined that PET detected malignancies in up to 20% of cases suspected to be paraneoplastic, but where computed tomography (CT) imaging was negative.[59] This included cancers of the thyroid (papillary), tonsil (squamous cell), lung (small-cell, non-small-cell, and adenocarcinoma), and adenocarcinomas of the colon, prostate, and breast. However, the imaging modality is important to consider, depending upon the targeted malignancy. For instance, for tumors of the testicles or ovaries, ultrasound and MRI are recommended, whereas for cancers of the gastrointestinal (GI) system, endoscopy and colonoscopy are preferred.[8] Certain neural autoantibodies are predictive of particular cancer types, and can help to direct the malignancy search.[60] For patients with autoantibodies that are strongly associated with malignancy, if no malignancy or a malignancy different from that which was expected is identified, it is prudent to do periodic cancer screening once or twice yearly for the next few years.

Figure 22-1 outlines an overall diagnostic scheme for the work-up of infectious and autoimmune encephalitides.

ILLUSTRATIVE AUTOIMMUNE ENCEPHALITIC SYNDROMES MANIFESTING WITH NEUROPSYCHIATRIC IMPAIRMENT

In general, while the symptoms of infectious encephalitides are usually non-specific (such as fevers), they are often reflective of underlying pathophysiology. Altered mental status and/or obtundation, headaches, and vomiting are frequently seen with increased intracranial pressure and hydrocephalus, as in CNS cryptococcal infections. However, headaches and vomiting can also be secondary to meningeal involvement, such as seen with herpes, Lyme disease, or tuberculosis. Seizures can be due to general electrolyte imbalances, inflammation, or to mass lesions, which can be seen in tuberculosis, toxoplasmosis, neurocysticercosis, or cryptococcal infections, among others.

What follows are examples of autoimmune encephalitides that can present with profound neuropsychiatric impairment.

NMDAR Encephalitis

NMDAR encephalitis (see Case 1) is the most common and likely the best known of the autoimmune encephalitides.

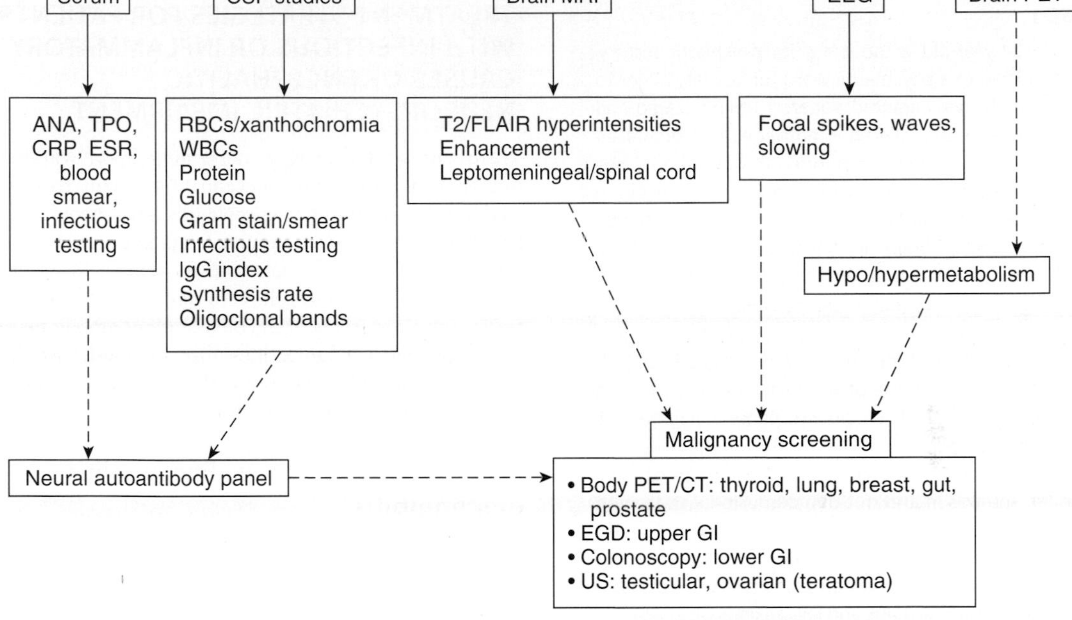

Figure 22-1. Diagnostic workflow for infectious and/or autoimmune encephalitis. Solid arrows indicate work-up done for both infectious and autoimmune encephalitides. Dashed arrows indicate additional work-up done for autoimmune encephalitides. ANA, antinuclear antibody; CRP, C-reactive protein; CSF, cerebrospinal fluid; CT, computerized tomography; EEG, electroencephalography; EGD, esophagogastroduodenoscopy; ESR, erythrocyte sedimentation rate; FLAIR, fluid attenuation inversion recovery; GI, gastrointestinal; IgG, immunoglobulin G; MRI, magnetic resonance imaging; PET, positron emission tomography; RBC, red blood cell count; TPO, thyroid peroxidase antibody; US, ultrasound; WBCs, white blood cell count. *(Modified with permission from: Linnoila J, et al.* Semin Neurol *2016; 36: 382–396).*

It was the first of the newer neuronal cell surface-mediated autoimmune encephalitides to be described, in 2007.[34] This disorder is most common in young adults, predominantly in females. In adults, the syndrome often starts with a viral prodrome, which progresses to psychiatric/behavioral changes and insomnia, usually followed by decreased consciousness, seizures, unusual movements, and autonomic instability that may result in central hypoventilation.[11] As patients recover, symptoms typically resolve in the reverse order. The psychiatric changes typically include paranoid delusions, hallucinations, behavioral disinhibition, catatonia, and anxiety. Oftentimes, patients' families seek out psychiatric care initially, and indeed many patients have ended up in inpatient psychiatric units, until they started suffering from seizures, autonomic instability, and obtundation. The syndrome in children is similar, but the first symptoms are often behavioral changes, seizures, or movement disorders.[61] In children who develop NMDAR encephalitis after HSVE, they often develop choreoathetoid-type movements, which are generally not observed in adults with the disorder.[41,43,46,62] In NMDAR encephalitis, the CSF often shows a lymphocytic pleocytosis with or without oligoclonal bands.[1] Only about one-third of patients have abnormal brain MRI findings, usually FLAIR hyperintensity in cortical or subcortical regions, or in the cerebellum and/or brainstem. However, they may have the frontal to posterior gradient on PET imaging. Approximately 30% of patients have the "extreme delta brush" EEG pattern. There is an age-related association with tumors, almost always ovarian teratomas, with a tumor found in 46% of all females, but in only 6% of those younger than 12 years.[11] In general, the best clinical outcomes are in cases where treatment is instituted early into the patient's course and where teratomas, if found, are resected.

Limbic Encephalitis

Limbic encephalitis is characterized by subacute short-term memory loss, confusion, sleep disturbances, and mood or behavioral changes, such as depression, irritability, and hallucinations occurring with or without seizures. Whereas initially thought to be associated with malignancy,[63] as historically many patients tested positive for paraneoplastic antibodies that have a strong correlation with cancer, it has recently become evident that many cell-surface targeted antibodies have also been linked with limbic encephalitis.[14,20,17] Limbic encephalitis is named based on the presenting symptoms, as well as on the underlying cerebral structures that are often disrupted, including the amygdala, hippocampus, and mesiotemporal lobes. Brain imaging often shows MRI T2 hyperintensity and/or contrast enhancement and/or PET hyper/hypometabolism in the mesiotemporal regions. If abnormal, the EEG often reveals focal temporal lobe seizures.

LGI-1 Encephalitis

LGI-1 encephalitis is the second most common autoimmune encephalitis after NMDAR encephalitis. LGI-1 antibodies are a subset of voltage-gated potassium channel (VGKC) antibodies, which are only rarely associated with malignancy (typically thymoma).[17] Patients with LGI-1 antibodies are predominantly men, usually in their 6th or 7th decade of

CASE 1

Ms. B, a 24-year-old without a prior psychiatric history, was admitted to a psychiatric ward for "anxiety". Prior to admission, she was paranoid, agitated, yelling, scared, and could not sleep. She called her mother with disorganized speech. She thought she responded through the TV. She was rigid and mute, with a mild fever, elevated blood pressure, and tachycardia; her parents took her to a nearby hospital. A head CT, brain MRI/A with and without contrast, an abdominal ultrasound, and two EEGs were normal. Toxicology and heavy metal screens were negative. An LP revealed 48 WBCs; 100% lymphocytes. ESR and CRP were mildly elevated. Infectious work-up was negative. Ms. B was given a 10-day course of acyclovir before HSV testing returned negative. She had a poor response to neuroleptics and benzodiazepines.

Ms. B's parents took her to a different psychiatric hospital. She was in and out of a confusional state, with labile emotions, bursts of seemingly volitional shaking episodes, disinhibited behavior, mutism, and preoccupations about dying. She had periods where she was more lucid, able to communicate, and less anxious. She had poor sleep, was noted to have jerky movements, and continued to run a low-grade fever. Ms. B was uncooperative with the neurologic examination and had intermittently unstable gait. She was transferred to a large tertiary care hospital.

Ms. B was catatonic and spoke of "walking with God". Repeat infectious work-up, toxicology screen, EEG, MRI, and LP (WBC 2) were normal. Brain PET showed posterior symmetric occipital lobe hypometabolism. NMDA receptor encephalitis was suspected; IVIg was administered. Shortly thereafter, CSF and serum NMDA receptor antibody testing returned positive. A search for a teratoma was unrevealing. Her catatonic symptoms were treated with benzodiazepines. Three weeks later, she was minimally improved. She received rituximab every 6 months for 2 years and had a slow but complete recovery.

life. LGI-1 encephalitis usually presents with limbic encephalitis, seizures, and sleep disruptions. Rapid eye movement (REM) sleep behavior disorder (RBD) has been described in patients with LGI-1 encephalitis.[64] Part of this dysfunction may be explained by antibodies binding to the hypothalamus,[65] which may also account for the hyponatremia seen in a little over half of patients. Some patients also have the brief myoclonic-like FBD seizures, which may be captured on the EEG. Less than half of patients have an abnormal CSF profile, although many of them have mesiotemporal FLAIR abnormalities on their brain MRIs.[1] Patients often have profound short-term memory deficits, which can vary from case to case, depending upon the extent of mesiotemporal involvement, whether it is unilateral or bilateral, and whether atrophy has occurred. A recent analysis of 76 cases of patients with LGI-1 encephalitis showed that, while many cases are responsive to immunotherapy including steroid treatment, treatment at sufficient doses (high-dose steroids, for instance) and for a sufficient amount of time (weeks to months) are necessary to prevent relapses.[25]

TREATMENT STRATEGIES FOR PATIENTS WITH INFECTIOUS OR INFLAMMATORY CAUSES OF ENCEPHALITIC NEUROPSYCHIATRIC IMPAIRMENT

Treatment strategies vary, depending upon whether an infectious or autoimmune encephalitis is being treated and whether the autoimmune encephalitis is paraneoplastic. For patients with multiple symptoms including seizures, behavioral and/or mood changes, and movement disorders, an interdisciplinary approach is often needed.[1] Successful treatment often stems from collaborations among neurologists, psychiatrists, infectious disease physicians and/or oncologists, in addition to physical, speech, and occupational therapists, as well as social workers.

Treatment of Infectious Encephalitis or Meningitis

In general, treatment of infectious encephalitides must proceed rapidly once they are diagnosed or even suspected, as by the time the patient reaches medical attention, these conditions can proceed quickly, resulting in significant morbidity and mortality. If an infection is suspected, empiric treatment with antibiotics and/or antivirals is commenced, until culture, PCR, and/or antibody results return.[6] Some of the morbidity associated with infectious encephalitis is secondary to a vigorous immune response, which can result in significant parenchymal edema. Thus, some infections, such as bacterial meningitis and neurocysticercosis are treated with steroids in addition to antimicrobials. The timing can be critical, however, as steroids are usually given before antibiotics for bacterial meningitis, and in HSVE, animal studies have shown that giving steroids too early can interfere with the body's ability to fight the herpes infection.[66] In theory, steroids should be given before neural autoantibodies develop. A clinical trial is underway to determine the optimal steroid treatment regimen for HSE.[67] In general, tuberculosis, fungal, parasitic, and opportunistic infections require treatment for months with multiple agents. Treatment of cryptococcal and cytomegalovirus (CMV) infections, for instance, requires different medications for the acute and maintenance phases. Some infections can co-exist, in particular HIV with CMV, syphilis, tuberculosis, toxoplasmosis, and/or *Cryptococcus*. Also, with institution of antiretroviral treatment for HIV infection, as the immune system is restored, patients can paradoxically worsen, as the immune system starts fighting infections that have been long dormant in the host, resulting in immune reconstitution inflammatory syndrome, or IRIS.[7] HIV will also require life-long treatment in order to maintain suppression. For infections such as *Cryptococcus*, which result in significant proteinaceous build-up and in hydrocephalus, frequent lumbar punctures or CSF shunts are required, to manage increased intracranial pressure. Only certain viral encephalitides are treated, including HSV, VZV, and CMV. In other viral infections co-morbidities are managed, but in general, many viral meningitides or encephalitides remain undiagnosed and resolve on their own. Consultation with an infectious diseases specialist is recommended.

Treatment of Autoimmune Encephalitis

Identification of Objective Measures to Follow Over Time

Treatment of autoimmune encephalitides often takes weeks to months. It is ideal to identify objective and validated markers of dysfunction that can be followed over time, to assess response to treatment (Table 22-3).[8] For instance, standardized bedside neuropsychological tests, such as the Mini-Mental Status Examination (MMSE) or Montreal Cognitive Assessment (MoCA) should be performed to provide objective measurements of cognitive deficits. EEGs and seizure diaries can be used to track seizure frequency, location, and/or duration. Video can be useful for tracking adventitious movements. In general, antibody titers are not particularly useful in assessing clinical responses to treatment, although baseline titers drawn after clinical recovery may be useful for diagnosing a potential relapse.

General Treatment Goals

In general, treatment should aim to maximize reversibility of symptoms and to maintain reversibility of symptoms while using a minimal therapeutic dose.[8] In order to maximize reversibility, it is imperative to make the diagnosis and to start treatment as early into the clinical course as possible. This may mean beginning treatment before antibody results are back, or treating despite negative antibody results, if there is a high suspicion for an autoimmune process. Having a neural autoantibody does not guarantee that the patient will respond to treatment, especially when it is an intracellular antibody. Successful treatment may be marked by stopping clinical progression, or deterioration, and not necessarily by reversal of symptoms. The overall initial goal in treatment is to determine whether there is a response to immunotherapy and then to maximize the reversibility of symptoms. To this end, a sufficient trial of immunosuppression must be undertaken. However, if multiple immunotherapies have been tried with no signs of objective improvement, the disorder may not be immunotherapy-responsive, and further trials may not be justified. Once a response to immunotherapy is demonstrated, the goal shifts to finding the minimal dose of immunotherapy that will best maintain the patient, if applicable. Whereas some autoimmune encephalitides appear to be monophasic, such as VGKC antibody encephalitis[30] (which can include LGI-1 encephalitis), others require longer-term treatment or maintenance immunotherapy to prevent relapse.

TABLE 22-3 Objective Measures for Monitoring Autoimmune Encephalitis Treatment Response

SYMPTOM/FINDING	OBJECTIVE TESTS TO FOLLOW
Cognitive decline	MMSE, MoCA, other neuropsychometric tests
Seizures	EEG (sleep deprived, EMU, or prolonged ambulatory), seizure diary
Brain inflammation	Brain MRI—T2/FLAIR, post contrast sequences Brain PET—track areas of hypo/hypermetabolism
Movement disorder	Movement lab studies,[a] video
Autonomic dysfunction	Autonomic reflex testing, thermoregulatory sweat testing,[a] gastric emptying study, GI transit study

[a]Specialized studies not available everywhere.

EEG, electroencephalography; EMU, epilepsy monitoring unit; FLAIR, fluid attenuation inversion recovery; GI, gastrointestinal; MMSE, Mini-Mental Status Examination; MoCA, Montreal Cognitive Assessment; MRI, magnetic resonance imaging; PET, positron emission tomography (modified with permission from: Linnoila J, et al. *Semin Neurol* 2016; 36: 382–396).

Treatment Strategies

The largest study of treatment outcomes for patients with a neuronal cell-surface antibody thus far came from an analysis of 501 patients with NMDAR encephalitis.[11] Most autoimmune encephalitides are treated similarly. These patients were generally treated with what were termed "first-line" therapy: steroids (typically intravenous, IV × 5 daily doses), IV immunoglobulin (IVIg; 5 daily doses), and/or plasmapheresis (5 sessions total, every other day), potentially followed by second-line therapies: rituximab and cyclophosphamide. This is a reasonable strategy for the inpatient treatment of many of the cell-surface-targeted neural autoantibodies, keeping in mind that recovery may take months. However, when there is little initial response to first-line agents, second-line therapies should be tried sooner rather than later, as opposed to trying multiple rounds of alternative first-line agents, particularly when the patient's symptoms are severe.[1,8] The second-line therapies are more likely to attack the pathophysiologic process underlying the patient's illness. For patients with intracellularly targeted antibodies, cyclophosphamide is generally preferable, as many of the other therapies have been found to be ineffective and there is an urgency to preserve brain function and structure, to attempt to prevent permanent brain atrophy.

Paraneoplastic Disorders

For patients with a co-existing malignancy, it is important to treat both the tumor and the paraneoplastic disorder concomitantly, if possible.[1,8] Working closely with an oncologist is advised. Many people assume that the cancer is more important to focus on initially. However, often malignancies associated with paraneoplastic disorders are small and localized. The longer the neurologic symptoms persist untreated and the more brain atrophy that occurs, the less likely it is that the patient will return to a reasonable level of neurologic function. Without prompt treatment of the neurologic symptoms, the patient may be cured of their cancer, but they may require institutionalization regardless, as paraneoplastic disorders can be quite severe, leaving some patients markedly disabled. It is presumed that the malignancy is the source of the antigen and thus removing the cancer, if possible, along with immunotherapy, is the best strategy for treating the neurologic symptoms and preventing a relapse. Unfortunately, in practice, tumor removal may not result in dramatic clinical improvement. If possible, adding cyclophosphamide to the chemotherapy regimen may be helpful.

Psychiatric Considerations in the Treatment of Patients With Infectious or Inflammatory Neuropsychiatric Impairment

As mentioned above, treating patients with infectious or autoimmune encephalitides is often a multidisciplinary team approach. While it is important to treat the etiology of their symptoms, if possible, for instance treating a co-existing malignancy, using antimicrobials to treat infections, and immunotherapy to treat autoimmune disorders to bring about a long-term resolution or remission of their disorder, many of the resulting symptoms require specialty management. Many patients with encephalitis are delirious and general delirium precautions (including frequent reorientation, surrounding the patient with familiar pictures or family members, and maintenance of a normal day/night light cycle) are needed. Some autoimmune encephalitides have a direct effect on the hypothalamus, resulting in disruptive sleep patterns that often require treatment. Patients may have a combination of seizures and mood disruptions, in which case choosing an antiepileptic drug, such as valproic acid or lamotrigine, which may have dual actions, may be ideal. Sometimes patients may have co-existing agitation and movement disorders, for example in NMDAR or LGI-1 encephalitis. In addition, some children with post-HSE NMDAR encephalitis and choreoathetoid movements have been reported to have anti-dopamine receptor antibodies.[43] In such cases, avoiding dopamine-blockers in favor of benzodiazepines may be preferred, as dopamine-blockers may result in rigidity, which, along with potential autonomic storming, may result in an incorrect diagnosis of neuroleptic malignant syndrome. Additionally, many patients with autoimmune disorders, including autoimmune encephalitis with catatonia and stiff person syndrome, can tolerate (and often need) high doses of benzodiazepines for successful symptomatic management, sometimes at doses that would ordinarily be sedating for most patients. Overall, while the patient's symptoms are being managed, it is also imperative to treat the underlying pathophysiology.

REMAINING QUESTIONS ON AUTOIMMUNE ENCEPHALITIDES

The field of autoimmune neurology is rapidly changing and with the seemingly constant identification of new autoantibodies, it is difficult to know how to interpret testing results and how best to apply that knowledge towards helping patients. Here follow some common questions encountered in the day-to-day course of diagnosing and treating autoimmune encephalitides.

What About Low-Titer Autoantibodies?

A common question is what to do about low-titer antibody results only slightly above the negative cut-off value?[8] Some antibodies, including GAD-65[68] and VGKC,[69] can be found at low values in normal patients without neurologic disease. This is particularly true for GAD-65, which can be elevated in patients with systemic autoimmune endocrinopathies, such as type I diabetes. Additionally, antibody results must be carefully interpreted after IVIg, as treatment can result in false-positives, which are typically present for weeks after the last dose. In general, results must be examined in the clinical context, with the caveat that sometimes antibodies are only rarely associated with certain symptoms; if the testing result is completely incongruent with the patient's presentation, it may be unrelated. However, sometimes low antibody results have been clinically relevant, as in the cases of some patients with low-value VGKC antibodies, yet positive for LGI-1 antibodies.[70]

What About Late Diagnoses?

Another question is whether to treat if the diagnosis has been only made after an extended period of time.[8] A corollary to this is whether there are cases of spontaneous remission. While spontaneous remissions have been reported, they are rare, as a large NMDAR encephalitis series showed.[11] This same analysis also noted that in paraneoplastic NMDAR cases, prompt tumor removal is important, as it speeds recovery and prevents relapses. Autoimmune neurologic disorders typically require treatment with immunotherapy. However, particularly in paraneoplastic cases that come to attention late, sometimes the neurologic symptoms have plateaued, remaining stable without deterioration for many months. Without evidence of ongoing decline, sometimes these patients are observed over time. While the best outcomes are seen with early diagnosis and treatment, even if a late diagnosis is made, if there is ongoing deterioration, a course of immunotherapy should be attempted, as responses to therapy are sometimes seen, and treating with immunotherapy addresses the etiology, as opposed to merely the symptoms of the disorder, which can be severe.

What Is Hashimoto's Encephalitis and Does It Truly Exist?

Antibodies against TPO have had an interesting trajectory in the history of autoimmune encephalitides.[1] This antibody, with or without anti-thyroglobulin antibodies, was initially thought to signify an autoimmune encephalitis known as Hashimoto's encephalitis,[71] although the range of clinical presentations was highly variable, making it difficult to describe a specific Hashimoto's encephalitis syndrome. Hashimoto's encephalitis was eventually re-named steroid responsive encephalitis with associated autoimmune thyroiditis (SREAT),[72] as Hashimoto's encephalitis patients were generally found to be responsive to steroids. However, this did not clarify the syndrome, as not all syndromes considered to be Hashimoto's encephalitis are responsive to steroids. With the identification of novel antibodies recognizing neuronal cell surface epitopes, as opposed to TPO antibodies that do not react with neurons, some patients with Hashimoto's encephalitis have been reclassified with specific syndromes, such as NMDAR or limbic encephalitis.[73] The TPO antibodies may be better interpreted as markers of autoimmunity. However, the boundaries of Hashimoto's encephalitis are unclear, and it should be considered only after excluding specific antibody-associated autoimmune encephalitides.[74]

Are Antibody Subtypes Important?

There have been many reports in the literature associating antibodies against neuronal surface antigens with several disorders, including neuropsychiatric lupus,[75] bipolar disorder,[76] and neurodegenerative conditions.[77] These antibodies must be distinguished from those that have been shown to be syndrome-specific or pathogenic. For instance, in NMDAR encephalitis, the associated antibodies are IgGs that target the ionotropic NMDA glutamate receptor 1, or GluN1, subunit of the NMDA receptor.[78] These are highly specific and pathogenic antibodies that, when well characterized in serum and particularly CSF, are not found in other disorders. Other NMDAR subunit-targeted antibodies or IgA or IgM antibody subtypes are unrelated to NMDAR encephalitis; they have been reported in the sera of patients with a myriad of neurologic and psychiatric diseases[79] at the same frequency as in healthy subjects (~10%),[80] without clear pathogenic effects. Part of the problem is the oversimplified use of the term "NMDA receptor antibodies" for all types of antibodies (IgA, IgM, IgG) and antibodies targeting different subunits. For all known (named) autoimmune encephalitides, pathogenic antibodies have been of the IgG class; these are the ones for which the commercial antibody panels test.

CONCLUSION

Common causes of neuropsychiatric impairment encountered in the hospital setting include encephalopathy, usually a consequence of end-organ failure, and encephalitis, which causes inflammation of the brain tissue itself. Encephalitis is often secondary to infections and/or inflammatory causes. The past decade has brought the realization that many inflammatory encephalitides are autoimmune in nature, associated with neural autoantibodies that serve as useful diagnostic markers, particularly in paraneoplastic cases. It has also been discovered that some infectious encephalitides can lead to subsequent autoimmune encephalitides, potentially clouding the diagnostic picture. Infectious and autoimmune encephalitides can have high morbidity. However, early diagnosis and treatment, usually from a multidisciplinary perspective, can improve outcomes.

REFERENCES

Access the reference list online at https://expertconsult.inkling.com/.

Catatonia, Neuroleptic Malignant Syndrome, and Serotonin Syndrome

23

Gregory L. Fricchione, M.D.
Scott R. Beach, M.D., F.A.P.M.
Anne F. Gross, M.D.
Jeff C. Huffman, M.D.
George Bush, M.D., M.M.Sc.
Theodore A. Stern, M.D.

OVERVIEW

Each of the syndromes described in this chapter involves a complex interaction of motor, behavioral, and systemic manifestations that are derived from mechanisms that are not fully clear. What *is* clear is that neurotransmitters, such as dopamine (DA), gamma-aminobutyric acid (GABA), and glutamate, are of major importance in catatonia and neuroleptic malignant syndrome (NMS), whereas serotonin (5-hydroxytryptamine, 5-HT) is centrally involved in serotonin syndrome (SS). Many now believe that NMS represents a malignant catatonic state that results from the use of DA-blocking medications and that SS may also be within the spectrum of catatonic disorders. Certainly, all of these syndromes have symptoms and treatments that overlap. As our psychopharmacologic armamentarium grows and as drugs with potent effects on modulation of monoamines proliferate, the diagnosis and management of these complex disorders becomes even more important.

CATATONIA

CASE 1 Catatonia

A 42-year-old man with a long history of complex partial seizures and a history of a left temporal lobectomy had intermittent seizures, despite the use of phenytoin and other anti-epileptics. After admission to the hospital following a seizure, he developed catatonic withdrawal. After administration of intravenous (IV) lorazepam, he became alert, agitated, and aggressive; moreover, he was paranoid, and reported nihilistic and religious delusions. After several more doses of lorazepam, a higher dosage of phenytoin, and a dose of an atypical antipsychotic (olanzapine), his psychosis gradually dissipated. At that point, he was able to state that he felt alone and dissociated, and he was unsure whether he even existed. "I feel separated from the human race, like I am on another planet," he said.

Definition

Catatonia comprises a constellation of motor and behavioral signs and symptoms that occurs in relation to neuromedical or psychiatric insults. Structural brain disease, intrinsic brain disorders (e.g., epilepsy, toxic–metabolic derangements, infectious diseases), a variety of systemic disorders that affect the brain, and idiopathic psychiatric disorders (such as affective and schizophrenic psychoses) have all been associated with catatonia.[1,2] Catatonia was first defined by Karl Kahlbaum in 1847.[3] It was among the first studies in the area of mental illness to use the symptom-based approach to diagnose disorders without a known etiopathogenesis.[1] Kahlbaum believed that patients with catatonia passed through several phases of illness: a short stage of immobility (with waxy flexibility and posturing), a second stage of stupor or melancholy, a third stage of mania (with pressured speech, hyperactivity, and hyperthymic behavior), and finally, after repeated cycles of stupor and excitement, a stage of dementia.[3]

Kraepelin,[4] who was influenced by Kahlbaum, included catatonia in the group of deteriorating psychotic disorders named dementia praecox. Bleuler[5] adopted Kraepelin's view that catatonia was subsumed under severe idiopathic deteriorating psychoses, which he renamed the *schizophrenias*.

Kraepelin and Bleuler both recognized that catatonic symptoms could emerge as part of a mood disorder or medical condition, but, as a result of a nosologic misconception, catatonia was overly associated with schizophrenia until the 1990s. Thanks in large part to the work of Fink and Taylor,[6] the *Diagnostic and Statistical Manual of Mental Disorders*, 4th edition (DSM-IV),[7] finally included new criteria for mood disorders with catatonic features and for catatonic disorder secondary to a general medical condition, as well as the catatonic type of schizophrenia. In DSM-5,[8] the catatonic subtype of schizophrenia was removed, leaving diagnoses of catatonia associated with another mental disorder, catatonic disorder due to another medical condition, and unspecified catatonia. According to DSM-5, a diagnosis of catatonia requires three or more of the following symptoms: stupor, catalepsy, waxy flexibility, mutism, negativism, posturing, mannerism, stereotypy, agitation, grimacing, echolalia, or echopraxia. In the case of catatonia due to another medical condition, the symptoms cannot occur exclusively during the course of a delirium.

Epidemiology, Risk Factors, and Potential Etiologies

Primary catatonia refers to catatonia associated with psychiatric etiologies. Prospective studies on patients hospitalized with acute psychotic episodes place the incidence of catatonia in the range of 7–17%.[9,10] In patients who suffer from mood disorders, occurrence rates have ranged from 13% to 31% over the past century, and catatonia appears to be particularly common in those with bipolar disorder.[11] Some have contended that the incidence of catatonia has diminished in cases of schizophrenia, but diagnostic and study design variations over the decades make this interpretation problematic. Personality disorders, post-traumatic stress disorder, and conversion disorder have also been cited as causes. Catatonia is more common in patients with neurodevelopmental disorders and in those with autism-spectrum disorders, with up to 17% of patients in the latter group displaying symptoms post-adolescence.[12] Catatonia is idiopathic in many cases.

Neuromedical "organic" etiologies account for up to 46% of cases in various series, and are referred to as secondary etiologies of catatonia. This underscores the need for a thorough neuromedical work-up when catatonic signs are present. Among all patients seen on psychiatry consultation-liaison services, up to 6% may have catatonia.[13] Table 23-1 includes an extensive list of neuromedical causes of catatonia; common etiologies include seizures, posterior reversible encephalopathy syndrome (PRES), central nervous system infections, Wernicke's encephalopathy, and systemic lupus erythematosus. In the case of lupus, all reported cases have occurred in females; common symptoms of catatonia include

TABLE 23-1 Modified Bush–Francis Catatonia Rating Scale[a]

Catatonia can be diagnosed by the presence of two or more of the first 14 signs listed below:

Sign	Description
1. Excitement	Extreme hyperactivity, and constant motor unrest, which is apparently non-purposeful; not to be attributed to akathisia or goal-directed agitation
2. Immobility/stupor	Extreme hypoactivity, immobility, and minimal response to stimuli
3. Mutism	Verbal unresponsiveness or minimal responsiveness
4. Staring	Fixed gaze, little or no visual scanning of environment, and decreased blinking
5. Posturing/catalepsy	Spontaneous maintenance of posture(s), including mundane (e.g., sitting/standing for long periods without reacting)
6. Grimacing	Maintenance of odd facial expressions
7. Echopraxia/echolalia	Mimicking of an examiner's movements/speech
8. Stereotypy	Repetitive, non-goal-directed motor activity (e.g., finger-play, or repeatedly touching, patting, or rubbing oneself); the act is not inherently abnormal but is repeated frequently
9. Mannerisms	Odd, purposeful movements (e.g., hopping or walking on tiptoe, saluting those passing by, or exaggerating caricatures of mundane movements); the act itself is inherently abnormal
10. Verbigeration	Repetition of phrases (like a scratched record)
11. Rigidity	Maintenance of a rigid position despite efforts to be moved; exclude if cogwheeling or tremor present
12. Negativism	Apparently motiveless resistance to instructions or attempts to move/examine the patient; contrary behavior; doing the exact opposite of the instruction
13. Waxy flexibility	During re-posturing of the patient, the patient offers initial resistance before allowing repositioning, similar to that of a bending candle
14. Withdrawal	Refusal to eat, drink, or make eye contact
15. Impulsivity	Sudden inappropriate behaviors (e.g., running down a hallway, screaming, or taking off clothes) without provocation; afterward, gives no or only facile explanations
16. Automatic obedience	Exaggerated cooperation with the examiner's request or spontaneous continuation of the movement requested
17. *Mitgehen*	"Anglepoise lamp": arm raising in response to light pressure of finger, despite instructions to the contrary
18. *Gegenhalten*	Resistance to passive movement that is proportional to the strength of the stimulus; appears automatic rather than willful
19. Ambitendency	The appearance of being "stuck" in indecisive, hesitant movement
20. Grasp reflex	Per neurologic examination
21. Perseveration	Repeatedly returns to the same topic, or persistence with movement
22. Combativeness	Usually aggressive in an undirected manner, with no, or only facile, explanation afterward
23. Autonomic abnormality	Abnormal temperature, blood pressure, pulse, or respiratory rate, and diaphoresis

[a]The full 23-item Bush–Francis Catatonia Rating Scale (BFCRS) measures the severity of 23 signs on a 0 to 3 continuum for each sign. The first 14 signs combine to form the Bush–Francis Catatonia Screening Instrument (BFCSI). The BFCSI measures only the presence or absence of the first 14 signs, and it is used for case detection. Item definitions on the two scales are the same.

(Modified from Bush G, Fink M, Petrides G et al: Catatonia—I: rating scale and standardized examination, *Acta Psychiatr Scand* 1996; 93:129–136.)

mutism, withdrawal and negativism, and patients need not have evidence of lupus cerebritis on imaging.[14]

Recent literature has highlighted that limbic encephalitis is frequently associated with catatonia. Etiologies of limbic encephalitis include infectious, autoimmune, paraneoplastic, and idiopathic causes. NMDA-receptor antibody encephalitis, often paraneoplastic secondary to an ovarian teratoma but also associated with other tumors and sometimes occurring in the absence of any identifiable tumor, is the form of limbic encephalitis most commonly associated with catatonic features.[15] A typical course begins with a viral-like illness including headache, fever, gastrointestinal and upper respiratory symptoms for up to 2 weeks. Anxiety commonly follows, often with new-onset panic attacks, and psychiatrists are frequently the first providers to examine such patients. Catatonic symptoms emerge later in the course, and are frequently accompanied by delirium, psychosis, behavioral disturbances, autonomic instability, and seizures.[16] These cases respond well to removal of the tumor, if present. Immunosuppressive therapies can often be very helpful. In some cases, the catatonia recurs cyclically following initial treatment and requires maintenance therapy. Cases of NMDA-receptor antibody encephalitis-related catatonia have been successfully treated with electroconvulsive therapy (ECT) prior to diagnosis, suggesting that ECT may represent a treatment alternative in these cases.[17]

Catatonia-spectrum symptoms are commonly described in the setting of hypoxia. Knowledge of this secondary cause of catatonia is critical, as ECT does not appear to be successful as a treatment for catatonia secondary to cerebral hypoxia. In such cases, other treatment modalities for catatonia should be pursued first, allowing for evaluation of delayed neurologic syndrome before administering ECT.[18]

Drug-related etiologies, including prescribed medications, have also been identified as secondary causes of catatonia. Dopamine antagonist medications (e.g., neuroleptics, metoclopramide) and dopamine-depleting medications (e.g., tetrabenazine) can lead to catatonia, as can the removal of dopamine agonist medications, sedative–hypnotic medications, and clozapine.[19,20] Some medications, including hydroxyzine, have mild dopamine-blocking properties, about which most practitioners are unaware. Withdrawal from gamma amino butyric acid (GABA)-ergic agents, such as alcohol or benzodiazepines, also represents a common etiology for catatonia. In the case of long-acting benzodiazepines, other signs of withdrawal may be subtle at the outset, and the presentation may be delayed. Recently, the literature has described cases of catatonia secondary to dexamethasone and pegylated interferon-alpha 2b and ribavirin.[21,22] Tacrolimus has also been identified as an offender in several case reports,[23] as has cyclosporine.[24] Disulfiram[25] and baclofen[26] have been implicated in multiple case reports, and antibiotics including macrolides and fluoroquinolones have been cited as causal.[27,28] Substances of abuse (e.g., phencyclidine, ecstasy) have also been identified as etiologies of secondary catatonia;[29] of late, catatonia secondary to synthetic cannabinoid use has been described[30] as has catatonia secondary to cannabis withdrawal.[31]

Although a genetic predisposition has not been clearly identified for catatonia, there appears to be increased familial transmission with periodic catatonia that shows a pattern of anticipation from generation to generation.[32–34] The disease locus for periodic catatonia maps onto chromosome 15q15.[35] There appears to be shared genetic susceptibility on chromosome 15 between catatonia in schizophrenia and autism.[36,37] In addition, Prader–Willi syndrome, a genetic disorder due to lack of gene expression from paternal chromosome 15q11–q13, is associated with catatonia[34,38,39] and data supports GABA dysfunction in Prader–Willi, schizophrenia, and autism associated with catatonia.[39] Catatonia has also been associated with other genetic disorders including fragile X[40] and DiGeorge syndrome.[41]

The 2′,3′-cyclic nucleotide 3′-phosphodiesterase (CNP) gene is oligodendrocyte/myelin-associated and found to be reduced in brains of patients with schizophrenia, bipolar disorder, or unipolar depression. A distinct phenotype that includes features of catatonia, such as posturing, emerges with aging in mice and patients with mental illness with reduced expression as CNP. Diffusion tensor imaging in these patients reveals axonal loss in the frontal corpus callosum.[42]

Subtypes of Catatonia

Motoric subtypes of catatonia include stuporous catatonia (catatonic withdrawal; characterized by psychomotor hypoactivity) and excited catatonia (characterized by psychomotor hyperactivity), which may alternate during the course of a catatonic episode.

Kraepelin, in 1908, identified a "periodic" catatonia with an onset in adolescence characterized by intermittent excited states, followed by catatonic stuporous stages and a remitting and relapsing course. More recently authors have argued that periodic catatonia supports the DSM-5 category of "unspecified catatonia," which can be used to diagnose idiopathic cases of catatonia not associated with primary psychiatric or secondary neuromedical causes. These authors highlight that periodic catatonia is defined by a longitudinal course of cyclical relapsing and remitting psychomotor symptoms interrupted by periods of mild residual symptoms and also report that periodic catatonia may respond better to treatment with antipsychotics rather than conventional treatment for catatonia.[43,44] In 1934, Stauder[44] described lethal catatonia, distinguished by the rapid onset of a manic delirium, high temperatures, and catatonic stupor; it was said to have a mortality rate of more than 50%. An overlapping syndrome, malignant catatonia, has been described more commonly in recent literature, typically involving fever, autonomic instability, and elevated creatinine kinase. Malignant catatonia, regardless of etiology, is considered a psychiatric emergency, and requires prompt treatment with early consideration of ECT.

Delirious mania is a syndrome with acute onset of excitement, grandiosity, emotional lability, delusions, and insomnia characteristic of mania and the disorientation and altered consciousness characteristic of delirium, as well as fever, tachycardia, hypertension, and tachypnea. It overlaps significantly with descriptions of lethal catatonia, and many would consider it a form of malignant, excited catatonia. Other hallmark features of delirious mania include denuding, water obsession, and inappropriate toileting.[45] The diagnostic evaluation, including careful assessment for catatonic symptoms, is essential; patients with delirious mania are often young females. The onset of mania tends to be more rapid than in classic bipolar disorder, and the mania tends to wax and wane with the delirium. The use of lithium and neuroleptics, common medications for the treatment of mania, may worsen the catatonic symptoms and lead to NMS. Higher-dose benzodiazepines are often needed at the outset, and ECT is considered the treatment of choice for patients with delirious mania.

Under the category of secondary causes of catatonia, some now argue that there should be a catatonia subtype associated with delirium, which would include excited forms (as can occur in delirious mania) and stuporous forms (as often seen in cases of encephalitis). Though the DSM-5 excludes the diagnosis of catatonia in the setting of delirium, there is no empirical basis for this exclusion and there is significant overlap between symptoms of catatonia and delirium. In fact, most cases of catatonia secondary to a neuromedical etiology co-occur with delirium. A recent review identified 13 cases from the literature and three cases from their consultation-liaison (C-L) service as meeting criteria for delirium and catatonia and the most common symptoms the patients presented with were mutism, withdrawal, posturing, and immobility.[46] Another recent study identified that 12.7% to 32% of patients with delirium met criteria for catatonic syndrome, and found that catatonia is more common in patients who had delirium prior to hospitalization, in the hypoactive subtype of delirium, and in women.[47] Further study of this subtype of catatonia is needed, as there are likely diagnostic and treatment implications.

Clinical Features and Diagnosis

Signs and symptoms of the catatonic syndrome are outlined in Table 23-1 (the Modified Bush–Francis Catatonia Rating Scale). The specific number and nature of signs and symptoms required to make a diagnosis of catatonia remains controversial. Some have contended that even one cardinal characteristic has as much clinical significance for diagnosis and treatment as the presence of seven or eight characteristics. The DSM-5 now requires 3 of 12 symptoms, while the widely used Bush–Francis Catatonia Rating Scale requires 2 of 14 symptoms for diagnosis and lists 23 symptoms for severity rating.[48] When assessing the etiology of the catatonia, the psychiatrist should consider secondary causes of catatonia related to underlying neurologic, toxic, or metabolic abnormalities, as well as primary psychiatric causes (Table 23-2). An approach to examining patients for catatonia is outlined in Table 23-3. Because catatonia is significantly under-diagnosed, it is important to maintain a high degree of suspicion and include a brief catatonia evaluation as part of all exams. A key is to differentiate catatonia from other syndromes with similar manifestations but with different etiologies, such as akinetic mutism, locked-in syndrome, and malignant hyperthermia.

In addition to routine studies to identify neuromedical causes of catatonia, the clinician can obtain a metabolic panel; serum and urine toxicologies; an infectious-disease work-up, including human immunodeficiency virus (HIV) and rapid plasma reagin testing; and autoimmune screening (erythrocyte sedimentation rate, C-reactive protein, antinuclear antibodies, paraneoplastic panel). Creatine phosphokinase (CPK) levels, though not indicative of etiology, should be monitored, as they may indicate a malignant subtype. Iron studies are also recommended, as low serum iron is a risk factor for catatonia and for conversion to malignant catatonia.

In cases of catatonia due to a psychiatric etiology, the electroencephalogram (EEG) will typically be normal, whereas neuromedical etiologies will often lead to an EEG with diffuse background slowing, consistent with delirium. Catatonia may also emerge as both an ictal and a post-ictal phenomenon. Neuroimaging, especially MRI of the brain, should be obtained, although a negative result does not rule out a neuromedical etiology.

When catatonic symptoms are associated with delirium and vital sign changes, limbic encephalitis must be considered as a potential cause.[15] Neuroimaging (e.g., MRI) may show enhancement in the limbic regions, but it is often normal. Though peripheral blood screening for paraneoplastic antibodies is often easier, strong consideration should be given to a lumbar puncture as the absence of antibodies in the cerebrospinal fluid is the only way to rule out this potential etiology. If suspicion is high, and abdominal and pelvic imaging do not reveal a tumor, consideration should be given to full-body positron emission tomography (PET) to locate a possible tumor.

Neuropathophysiology

Catatonia is thought to reflect a disruption in basal ganglia-thalamocortical tracts (including the motor circuit, rigidity; the anterior cingulate–medial orbitofrontal circuit, akinetic mutism and, perhaps through lateral hypothalamic connections, hyperthermia and dysautonomia; and the lateral orbitofrontal circuit, imitative and repetitive behaviors) (Figure 23-1).[9,10,49] Such disruption may lead to a relative state of hypodopaminergia in these circuits through reduced flow in the medial forebrain bundle, the nigrostriatal tract, and the tuberoinfundibular tract. Dopamine (DA) activity in the dorsal striatum, ventral striatum, and paralimbic cortex is thus reduced, perhaps secondary to reduced $GABA_A$ inhibition of $GABA_B$, substantia nigra, and ventral tegmental area interneurons. This would lead to a dampened DA outflow, whereas activation at $GABA_A$, through use of agonists such as lorazepam, would indirectly disinhibit DA cell activity.[2,50] Another possible site of pathophysiologic action involves reduced $GABA_A$ inhibition of frontal corticostriatal tracts, leading to *N*-methyl-D-aspartate (NMDA) changes in the dorsal striatum, and indirectly in the substantia nigra and ventral tegmental area.[2] Multiple etiologies, if they affect the basal ganglia, thalamus, or paralimbic or frontal cortices, will have the potential to cause those neurotransmitter alterations that will disrupt basal ganglia-thalamocortical circuits, leading to the phenomenology of catatonia.

In the mesostriatal and mesocorticolimbic systems, the long feedback loops from DA neurons are regulated by GABA pathways. Given its extensive projections on both limbic and motor structures, the nucleus accumbens (NAc) may be a hub for the linkage between motivation and movement.[51] By extrapolating from animal evidence (i.e., $GABA_A$ antagonists lead to catalepsy, and $GABA_A$ agonists protect against catalepsy), and from the hypothesis that neuroleptic-induced catatonia may result from reduced DA and $GABA_A$ activity in the mesostriatum, it has been proposed

TABLE 23-2 Potential Etiologies of the Catatonic Syndrome

Primary: Psychiatric
Schizophrenia-spectrum disorder
Mood disorder (major depression or bipolar disorder)
Dissociative disorders
Obsessive–compulsive disorder
Personality disorders
Conversion disorder
Autism spectrum disorders

Secondary: Neuromedical
Cerebrovascular
Alcoholic degeneration
Wernicke's encephalopathy
Cerebellar degeneration
Cerebral anoxia
Cerebromacular degeneration
Closed head trauma
Frontal lobe atrophy
Hydrocephalus
Lesions of thalamus and globus pallidus
Posterior reversible encephalopathy syndrome (PRES)
Parkinsonism
Postencephalitic states
Seizure disorders[a]
Surgical interventions
Tuberous sclerosis
CNS neoplasm

Poisoning
Coal gas
Organic fluorides
Tetraethyl lead poisoning

Infections
Acquired immunodeficiency syndrome
Bacterial meningoencephalitis
Bacterial sepsis
Syphilis
Malaria
Mononucleosis
Subacute sclerosing panencephalitis
Tuberculosis
Typhoid fever
Viral encephalitides (especially herpes)
Viral hepatitis

Metabolic and Other Medical Causes
Acute intermittent porphyria[a]
Addison's disease
Cushing's disease
Diabetic ketoacidosis
Glomerulonephritis
Hepatic dysfunction
Hereditary coproporphyria
Homocystinuria
Hyperparathyroidism
Idiopathic hyperadrenergic state
Multiple sclerosis
Pellagra
Wilson's disease
Peripuerperal
Systemic lupus erythematosus[a]
Thrombocytopenic purpura
Uremia
Paraneoplastic limbic encephalitis

Drug-Related
Neuroleptics
Other dopamine-blocking agents (metoclopramide)
Dopamine withdrawal (e.g., levodopa)
Dopamine depleters (e.g., tetrabenazine)
Sedative–hypnotic withdrawal
Alcohol withdrawal
Antidepressants (tricyclic antidepressants, monoamine oxidase inhibitors, and others)
Anticonvulsants (e.g., carbamazepine, primidone)
Aspirin
Disulfiram
Baclofen
Antibiotics (macrolides, fluoroquinolones)
Steroids
Tacrolimus
Cyclosporine
Interferon
Ribavirin
Lithium carbonate
Morphine
Cannabinoids
Hallucinogens (e.g., mescaline, phencyclidine,[a] lysergic acid diethylamide, cathinones)
Synthetic cannabinoids
Cannabinoid withdrawal

[a]Signifies the most common medical conditions associated with catatonic disorder from a literature review done by Carroll BT, Anfinson TJ, Kennedy JC et al: Catatonic disorder due to general medical conditions, *J Neuropsychiatry Clin Neurosci* 1994; 6: 122–133.

that primary psychogenic catatonia results from a similar destabilization.[50] $GABA_A$ agonists could be restorative by inhibiting the pars reticulata's inhibitory $GABA_B$ neurons, resulting in disinhibition of the neighboring pars compacta's DA cells with a resultant striatal DA agonism.[30,50]

The interactivity among the NAc, the ventral subiculum/hippocampus and medial PFC areas including anterior cingulate cortex (ACC) and medial orbitofrontal cortex (MOFC) is important for our understanding of catatonia given their common modulation by DA and their importance in value-based decision-making in the face of amygdalar-based threat. The NAc serves as a hub for the integration of cognitive information from the ACC/MOFC, affective information from the basolateral amygdala, and environmental context from the subiculum/hippocampus. It has this role primarily for the purpose of establishing a motivational valence (reward prediction error) in advance of translation into movement. The response selection itself is accomplished in the ACC–MOFC–supplementary motor area (SMA) network with the ACC serving as another transmodal hub for cortical and limbic information integration. This decision-making is mediated with the help of modulatory

TABLE 23-3 Standardized Examination for Catatonia

The method described here is used to complete the 23-item Bush–Francis Catatonia Rating Scale (BFCRS) and the 14-item Bush–Francis Catatonia Screening Instrument (BFSCI). Item definitions on the two scales are the same. The BFCSI measures only the presence or absence of the first 14 signs.

Ratings are based solely on observed behaviors during the examination, with the exception of completing the items for "withdrawal" and "autonomic abnormality," which may be based on directly observed behavior or chart documentation.

As a general rule, only items that are clearly present should be rated. If the examiner is uncertain as to the presence of an item, rate the item as "0."

Procedure

1. Observe the patient while trying to engage in a conversation.
2. The examiner should scratch his or her head in an exaggerated manner.
3. The arm should be examined for cogwheeling. Attempt to reposture and instruct the patient to "keep your arm loose." Move the arm with alternating lighter and heavier force.
4. Ask the patient to extend his or her arm. Place one finger beneath his or her hand and try to raise it slowly after stating, "Do *not* let me raise your arm."
5. Extend the hand stating, "Do *not* shake my hand."
6. Reach into your pocket and state, "Stick out your tongue. I want to stick a pin in it."
7. Check for grasp reflex.
8. Check the chart for reports from the previous 24-hour period. Check for oral intake, vital signs, and any incidents.
9. Observe the patient indirectly, at least for a brief period each day, regarding the following:
    - Activity level
    - Abnormal movements
    - Abnormal speech
    - Echopraxia
    - Rigidity
    - Negativism
    - Waxy flexibility
    - Gegenhalten
    - Mitgehen
    - Ambitendency
    - Automatic obedience
    - Grasp reflex

aminergic flow in the medial forebrain bundle. Disruption in these systems associated with $GABA_A$ and DA reductions and an up-regulation of glutamatergic activity primarily in the ACC/MOFC basal ganglia thalamocortical loop with nodes in the ventral striatum and medial dorsal nucleus of the thalamus will lead to pathological avoidance/approach decisions with catatonic overtones.

Haber et al.[52] have shown that the ACC/MOFC projects motivational messaging to the ventral striatum and then to the ventral tegmentum (VTA), while the premotor and motor cortex send motor information to the dorsal striatum and then to the substantia nigra pars reticulata.

The dorsolateral PFC sends frontal executive working memory and anticipated reward signal information into the central striatum and then to tegmental border zones between the ACA/MOFC (ventral) and motor cortical (dorsal) striatal and tegmental sites. There are non-reciprocal, feed-forward, components that link-up regions that are associated with different cortical-basal ganglia circuits. These feed-forward tracts serve an integrative function when all goes well resulting in complex goal-directed movement. These particular connections terminate indirectly on a DA cell via a GABA-ergic interneuron, resulting in disinhibition and facilitation of DA cell burst firing. In this way, ventral striatal (motivational) regions influence more dorsal striatal (motor) regions via spiraling striatal-nigral-striatal projections. $GABA_A$ and DA deficiency syndromes and glutamatergic excess will present a phenotype of catatonia and use of $GABA_A$ agonists will disinhibit DA flow altering terminal zone motivational state in NAc and ACC/MOFC.

ECT may be effective for catatonia on the basis of this GABA–DA interaction. Sackeim and associates[53] proposed that the neural state following ECT is produced by increased GABA transmission. They cited animal studies in which the concentration of GABA in the striatum became elevated after ECT. Some investigators believe that ECT may increase the sensitivity of post-synaptic DA receptors to available DA. An animal model of catatonia supports this hypothesis.

Neuroleptics reduce the conditioned avoidance response, which is thought to be secondary to decreased DA activity in the NAc and the striatum. Stress has been shown to increase medial prefrontal cortical DA release, which in turn is thought to reduce DA activity in subcortical DA terminal fields in the mesolimbic and mesostriatal systems.[54,55] Friedhoff and co-workers[56] were able to show that rats undergoing twice-daily tail-shock stress for 8 days displayed conditioned avoidance response inhibition, along with a reduction in NAc DA use. The findings provided support for a restitutive hypothesis involving an endogenous DA-dependent system that mimicked the effects of neuroleptics in the context of repeated stress-induced medial PFC hyperdopaminergia. When such a system downregulates too much because of neurologic or medical insult, primary psychiatric dysfunction, or neuroleptic medication, catatonic stupor may occur. Similarly, NMS has been postulated to be secondary to DA blockade in the mesostriatum (which is responsible for the motor disorder), the mesolimbic system (which is responsible for the mutism), and the preoptic anterior hypothalamus (which is responsible for the hyperthermia).[57]

Early work took a top-down approach to understanding catatonia pathophysiology, with a particular focus on deficits in OFC functioning.[58] Indeed, during working memory tasks and with emotional–motor activation, the OFC appears to be hypoactive in subjects who previously had been catatonic when studied with functional magnetic resonance imaging (fMRI) during provocative testing.[9] However, research on regional blood flow has also shown basal ganglia asymmetry with left-sided hyperperfusion, as well as hypoperfusion in the left medial temporal area, and decreased perfusion in the right parietal cortex.

It is probable, as Haber's work suggests, that bottom-up dysfunction is just as important in the integration of basal

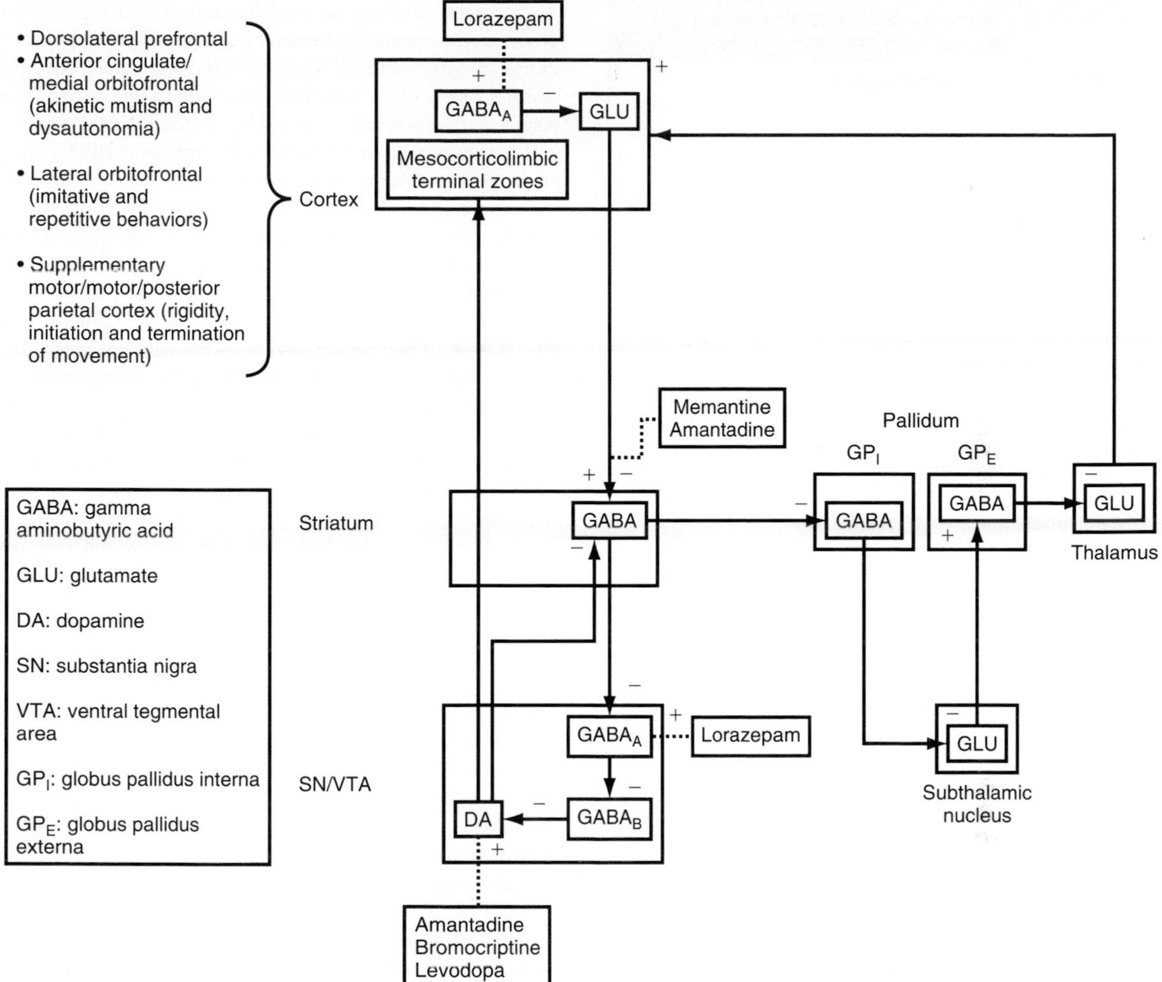

Figure 23-1. Basal ganglia thalamocortical circuits and catatonia: a candidate loop. *(From Fricchione GL, Huffman JC, Bush G et al: Catatonia, neuroleptic malignant syndrome, and serotonin syndrome. In Stern TA, Rosenbaum JF, Fava M et al, editors:* Massachusetts General Hospital comprehensive clinical psychiatry, *Philadelphia, 2008, Mosby, pp 761–771.)*

ganglia–thalamocortical circuit mediation of motivation and movement in the catatonic syndrome.[49] And, by examining the nature of basal ganglia thalamo–limbic–cortical loops, we can hypothesize why such a wide array of neuromedical and psychiatric etiologies can present with the catatonic syndrome and why the treatments (discussed later) may be therapeutic (Figure 23-1).

A more realistic and nuanced understanding of basal–ganglia–thalamocortical circuit dynamics may emerge as researchers develop testable hypotheses based on a more accurate understanding of this highly complicated circuitry. Such a strategy will be abetted by defining and controlling neurons based on directly observed input and output properties in the *in vivo* system.[59]

An evolutionary model for catatonia has been proposed, suggesting that catatonia in humans may be akin to "playing dead" behavior in primitive mammals (e.g., Virginia opossum, duck-billed platypus).[60] In this way,[61] catatonia may represent a maladaptive fear response in the setting of intense physiologic or psychological stress.

Fink and Taylor have proposed that catatonia may represent a form of limbic epilepsy.[61] Subtle ictal events involving the pre-frontal cortex and the basal ganglia have been postulated as causing catatonia. They note that the same medications used to treat complex partial status epilepticus (IV benzodiazepines) are also the treatment of choice for catatonia.

Management and Treatment

Whatever its etiology, catatonia is accompanied by significant morbidity and mortality from systemic complications (Table 23-4). In addition, many of the physical illnesses responsible for catatonia can be debilitating. Thus, timely diagnosis and treatment are essential. If a neurologic or medical condition is found, then treatment for that specific illness is indicated. Agents thought to exacerbate catatonia, including antipsychotic medications and other dopamine-blocking drugs (e.g., metoclopramide), should be discontinued. If dopamine agonists were recently stopped, they should be

TABLE 23-4 Some Medical Complications Associated With Catatonia

Simple Non-Malignant Catatonia
Aspiration
Burns
Cachexia
Dehydration and its sequelae
Pneumonia
Pulmonary emboli
Thrombophlebitis
Urinary incontinence
Urinary retention and its sequelae
Malignant Catatonia
Acute renal failure
Adult respiratory distress syndrome
Cardiac arrest
Cheyne–Stokes respirations
Death
Disseminated intravascular coagulation
Dysphagia due to muscle spasm
Electrocardiographic abnormalities
Gait abnormalities
Gastrointestinal bleeding
Hepatocellular damage
Hypoglycemia (sudden and profound)
Intestinal pseudo-obstruction
Laryngospasm
Myocardial infarction
Myocardial stunning
Necrotizing enterocolitis
Respiratory arrest
Rhabdomyolysis and sequelae
Seizures
Sepsis

Data from Philbrick KL, Rummans TA: Malignant catatonia. *J Neuropsychiatry Clin Neurosci.* 1994;6:1–13.

re-started, and withdrawal from GABA-ergic agents should also be treated appropriately.

Lorazepam is the first-line treatment for catatonia, regardless of etiology.[62] In 1983, Lew and Tollefson[63] reported on the usefulness of IV diazepam, and, at the same time, Fricchione and colleagues[64] reported on the benefit of IV lorazepam given to patients in neuroleptic-induced catatonic states (including NMS) and suggested its use in primary psychiatric catatonia. Rosebush and co-workers[62] reported that 80% of 15 catatonic episodes showed a complete and dramatic response within 2 hours of lorazepam treatment. IV lorazepam is preferred over other routes of administration because of its ease of administration, quick onset of action, and longer effective length of action.[65] With a drug distribution that is less rapid and less extensive, a relatively high plasma level can be maintained, thus prolonging the clinical benefit. Lorazepam also preferentially binds to the $GABA_A$ receptor, which may further account for its high efficacy. If IV access is unavailable, intramuscular (IM) or sublingual routes are preferred over oral medication. It is important to keep in mind that because the main affective response in catatonia is one of intense fear, repeated administration of IM medications may be traumatizing for patients. Nonetheless, given IM in the deltoids, lorazepam is more reliably absorbed than other IM benzodiazepines.

A typical starting dose of lorazepam is 2 mg. Lower doses may occasionally be used in pediatric populations or in frail, elderly patients, but are not recommended in adults because of the likely equivocal response. In many cases, the response to lorazepam 2 mg will be immediate and dramatic, with patients who were previously mute and rigid sitting up in bed and conversing normally. In other cases, the response may take 30–120 minutes and may be more subtle. A lack of response to an initial dose of 2 mg lorazepam does not rule out catatonia. If suspicion remains high, additional lorazepam should be given. Though patients with catatonia have a higher threshold for sedation, falling asleep after a dose of lorazepam also does not rule out catatonia. Many patients will awaken later with significant improvement in symptoms.

Once a positive response to lorazepam has been established, or if suspicion for the diagnosis remains high despite a positive response, lorazepam should be instituted in a standing regimen, generally at a dose of 2 mg every 6 to 8 hours. Because medications are often held when patients are asleep, and because catatonia has a very high likelihood of recurrence as the lorazepam wears off, nursing staff should be instructed to give the medication if the patient is asleep and to hold only for respiratory depression. Regular doses of lorazepam generally maintain the therapeutic effect, and standing benzodiazepines are recommended for at least the first 24 to 48 hours. If improvement is significant over that time, consideration can be given to a slow taper of benzodiazepines, in the order of a 10% to 25% decrease in total daily dose, each day. If lorazepam is unsuccessful within 5 days or if symptoms of malignant catatonia emerge, ECT should be considered.

ECT is considered the definitive and most effective treatment for catatonia in cases of partial or non-response to benzodiazepines, or in cases of lethal or malignant catatonia. Response to treatment is usually good for individuals with acute primary catatonia; 67% are improved by time of discharge.[66] Patients with manic features respond particularly well. Rates of long-term recovery range from 33% to 75%.[1] Two or three ECT treatments are usually sufficient to lyse the catatonic state, although a course of four to six treatments is usually given to prevent relapse, and 10 to 20 treatments are sometimes needed in difficult cases.

Bush and co-workers[67] studied the use of lorazepam and ECT in the treatment of catatonia. Of 21 patients (76%) who received a complete trial of lorazepam (11 received an initial 2-mg IV challenge), 16 had resolution of catatonic signs. All four patients referred for ECT (after failing lorazepam therapy) responded promptly. Mann and associates[68] found that in one series of cases of lethal catatonia where ECT was used, 40 of 41 patients survived. In another series,[53] although 16 out of 19 patients who had received ECT within 5 days of symptom onset survived, none of the 14 patients who received ECT after 5 days after symptoms did. The message is clear: when a patient presents with malignant catatonia of any type, ECT should be used expeditiously. Although an initial trial of lorazepam, a dopaminergic agent, or both, is reasonable for malignant catatonia, ECT should be instituted early if a medication trial is unsuccessful.

In the past, neuroleptics were frequently used to treat catatonia, and more recently, case reports have emerged of atypical antipsychotics being used to treat catatonia. Clinical experience suggests variable response to these drugs, however, and neuroleptics are well described as precipitating catatonic reactions and NMS.[69] Among the 292 patients with malignant catatonia reviewed by Mann and associates,[70] for example, 78% of those treated with a neuroleptic alone died, compared with an overall mortality rate of 60%. Use of typical or atypical antipsychotics as a primary treatment strategy for catatonia is therefore not recommended. If antipsychotic agents are needed to manage psychosis and agitation, low-potency agents in combination with benzodiazepines should be administered at the lowest effective dose.

Alternatives to ECT in simple catatonias include zolpidem 5 to 10 mg orally,[71] amantadine 100 mg twice a day orally, memantine 5 to 10 mg twice a day orally,[72,73] and topiramate 100 mg twice a day orally.[74] Amantadine and memantine have also been used successfully as adjunctive agents in many cases where lorazepam yielded only a partial response. Carbamazepine, valproate, calcium channel blockers, anticholinergics, minocycline, stimulants, lithium, thyroid medication, and corticosteroids have each had anecdotal success in catatonia.[75] Recent reports have also emerged of catatonia being treated with transcranial magnetic stimulation and transcranial direct current stimulation targeted to the right dorsolateral prefrontal cortex.[76,77] Adrenocorticotropic hormone and corticosteroids have also been reported to work in cases of lethal catatonia.[70]

Table 23-5 outlines recommendations for the treatment of simple and malignant (including NMS) catatonias, and Table 23-6 reviews management principles.

The treatment strategy for patients who have catatonia secondary to schizophrenia may be challenging, because the catatonia found in those with schizophrenia can at times be less responsive to lorazepam.[78,79] In these patients, amantadine and more recently memantine have shown some effectiveness in isolated cases, suggesting that NMDA antagonists may add some benefit.[80,81]

TABLE 23-5 Treatment of Simple and Malignant Catatonia

A. Test for catatonia. Lorazepam 2 mg IV (1 mg for adolescents or elderly patients) may result in temporary relief.
B. *Simple catatonia* (including neuroleptic-induced catatonia): lorazepam[a] 1 to 4 mg IV/IM/SL/PO trial followed by 3 to 20 mg/day in divided doses. Monitor for respiratory depression.
   → If still catatonic, consider adding dopamine (DA) agonist
   → If still catatonic, electroconvulsive therapy (ECT).[b]
C. Malignant catatonia (including neuroleptic malignant syndrome, NMS):
   1. Lorazepam IV trial expeditiously (effective in 75% of NMS cases). May add dantrolene ± DA agonist, but less evidence for these.
   2. If still catatonic and especially if temperature is higher than 102°F, or if there is severe encephalopathy, ECT should be instituted before day 5 of syndrome, if possible.

[a]Lorazepam effectiveness, 80% in one study,[25] 76% in another.[78]
[b]ECT effectiveness: 82–96% in five studies.
(Modified from Fricchione G, Bush G, Fozdur M et al: The recognition and treatment of the catatonic syndrome, *J Intensive Care Med* 1997; 12: 135–147.)

Prognosis and Complications

For patients with catatonia, the long-term prognosis is fairly good in almost half the cases.[9] Those with an acute onset and shorter duration of less than 1 month, diagnosis of depression, or a family history of depression have a better prognosis. Periodic catatonias can have good short- and long-term prognoses. However, given the potential morbidity and mortality, concerted efforts at supportive care are essential to avoid the myriad complications that are associated with simple catatonia, and more so with malignant catatonia (Table 23-4).

NEUROLEPTIC MALIGNANT SYNDROME

CASE 2 Neuroleptic Malignant Syndrome

A 56-year-old woman with a history of bipolar disorder was admitted to the hospital after arguing with her husband. She became agitated and combative and required haloperidol (5 mg IM) on two occasions in the emergency room. Her psychiatric history was notable for depression, suicidal ideation, and auditory hallucinations as a teenager that required ECT and long-term treatment with perphenazine, lithium, and sertraline. Soon after her admission, she became psychomotorically withdrawn, hypokinetic, mute, and rigid. Her temperature reached 101.6°F and her CPK level was elevated (2260 U/L). An EEG revealed generalized slowing. A diagnosis of NMS was made, and her medications were discontinued. Her catatonic symptoms responded to lorazepam (2 mg IV, twice). Divalproex sodium and olanzapine were started 2 weeks after the resolution of her NMS.

TABLE 23-6 Principles of Management of Catatonia

1. Early recognition is important. Once catatonia has been diagnosed, the patient must be closely observed and vital signs taken frequently.
2. Supportive care is essential. Such care involves hydration, nutrition, mobilization, anticoagulation (to prevent thrombophlebitis), and precautions against aspiration.
3. Discontinue antipsychotics or other drugs, such as metoclopramide, which can cause or worsen catatonia.
4. Restart recently withdrawn dopamine agonists, especially in patients with parkinsonism.
5. Institute supportive measures (e.g., a cooling blanket if hyperthermia is present, or parenteral fluids and antihypertensives or pressors if autonomic instability emerges and if malignant catatonia is suspected).
6. Maintain a high index of suspicion for the development of medical complications and for new medical problems.

Epidemiology and Risk Factors

By definition, NMS is temporally related to the use of a dopamine-blocking agent, or removal of a dopaminergic agent. Estimates of the risk for NMS have varied widely (from 0.02 to >3%). Different diagnostic criteria, survey techniques, population susceptibilities, prescribing habits, and treatment settings all contribute to the variance. In one center with a large number of patients treated with antipsychotics, 1 out of every 500 to 1000 patients was thought to develop NMS.[82] Age and sex do not appear to be reliable risk factors, though young adult men may be more prone to extrapyramidal symptoms (EPS). A history of catatonia is a major risk factor for progression to NMS. The period of withdrawal from alcohol or sedative–hypnotics may increase the risk of NMS because of aberrant thermoregulation and autonomic dysfunction. Agitation, dehydration, and exhaustion may also increase the risk. Basal ganglia disorders (e.g., Parkinson's disease, Wilson's disease, Huntington's disease, tardive dystonia) are thought to place patients at increased risk. Low serum iron appears to be a state-specific finding in patients with NMS, and patients with low serum iron in the context of catatonia may be at increased risk for NMS, if placed on neuroleptic medications. A history of NMS conveys the risk of recurrence, with up to one-third of patients having a subsequent episode when re-challenged. High-potency neuroleptics have been thought to produce an elevated risk and more intense cases of NMS. Nevertheless, use of atypical antipsychotics can cause NMS. IM injections and lithium have also been associated with an increased risk for NMS. Studies have not supported any particular genetic predisposition, although case reports have implicated an association with cytochrome CYP 2D6.[82]

Clinical Features and Diagnosis

Consideration of neuroleptics as potential causative agents is important because NMS is currently considered to be a severe form of neuroleptic-induced catatonia. NMS is a syndrome of autonomic dysfunction with tachycardia and elevated blood pressure, fever, rigidity, mutism, and stupor, associated with the use of neuroleptics. Hyperthermia, sometimes in excess of 42°C (108°F), is reported in 98% of the cases.[82] "Leadpipe" rigidity can occur. Parkinsonian features, including cogwheeling, may be present. Mental status changes occur in 97% of cases.[82] Most often, the NMS patient will be in a catatonic state; such patients may be alert, delirious, stuporous, or comatose. Diagnostic criteria for NMS remain under some debate, and various algorithms have been proposed over the years. Prior algorithms de-emphasized certain features of NMS, including altered mental status and fever. DSM-5 no longer lists specific criteria for NMS, instead favoring a descriptive approach. The latest criteria from the International Consensus study require recent dopamine antagonist exposure or dopamine agonist withdrawal; hyperthermia >100.4°F on at least two occasions; rigidity; mental status alteration; CK elevation at least four times the upper limit of normal; sympathetic nervous system lability including blood pressure elevation ≥25% above baseline, blood pressure fluctuation ≥20 mm Hg (diastolic) or ≥25 mm Hg (systolic) change within 24 hours; tachycardia ≥25% above baseline and tachypnea ≥50% above baseline; and a negative work-up for other causes.[83]

In 1985, Fricchione suggested that NMS is to malignant catatonia what neuroleptic-induced catatonia is to simple catatonia.[50] Goforth and Carroll also noted the overlap of catatonia and NMS.[84] All 27 of their cases of NMS met the DSM-IV diagnostic criteria for catatonia; 24 met stricter research criteria. The authors concluded that the two syndromes were identical, with NMS presenting as a more severe and iatrogenic variant of malignant catatonia. Fink also arrived at this conclusion.[85] Table 23-7 shows the symptoms of catatonia and NMS that overlap. Electroencephalograms (EEGs) are abnormal in roughly half of cases, most often with generalized slowing that is consistent with encephalopathy.[82] In contrast, CT of the brain and cerebrospinal fluid (CSF) studies are normal in 95% of NMS cases.[60]

In 1991, Rosebush and Mazurek[86] found decreased levels of serum iron in patients with NMS and suggested a role for lowered iron stores in the reduction of DA receptor function. Supporting the hypothesis of NMS as a severe variant of catatonia, Carroll and Goforth[87] reported a similar decrease of serum iron in three of 12 cases of catatonia, with NMS developing in two of the three cases. The third was without neuroleptic exposure and did not progress to NMS.[87]

Most commonly, NMS develops over a few days, often beginning with rigidity and mental status changes followed by signs of hypermetabolism. The course is usually self-limited, lasting 2 days to 1 month (once neuroleptics are stopped and supportive measures are begun).[82] Persistent cases are usually secondary to the use of depot neuroleptics, and ECT is highly effective in these cases. Although the mortality rate has been reduced through better recognition and management, there is still an approximately 6% risk of death, with acute respiratory failure being the biggest predictor of mortality.[88] Myoglobinuric renal failure and rhabdomyolysis may have long-term consequences.

TABLE 23-7 Catatonia and Neuroleptic Malignant Syndrome (NMS): Shared Features

	NMS	CATATONIA
Clinical Signs		
Hyperthermia	Yes	Often
Motor rigidity	Yes	Yes
Mutism	Yes	Yes
Negativism	Often	Yes
Altered consciousness	Yes	Yes
Stupor or coma	Yes	Yes
Autonomic dysfunction	Yes	Often
Tachypnea	Yes	Often
Tachycardia	Yes	Often
Abnormal blood pressure	Yes	Yes
Diaphoresis	Yes	Yes
Laboratory Results		
Creatine phosphokinase (CPK) elevated	Yes	Often
Serum iron reduced	Yes	Probable
Leukocytosis	Yes	Often

Atypical NMS is being more commonly described in the literature. The term was initially used to describe cases of NMS presenting with atypical features or lacking common core features, though many cases of so-called atypical NMS reported appear to actually represent cases of neuroleptic-induced catatonia, without significant malignant features. More recently, the term "atypical NMS" has been conflated to include cases of NMS arising secondary to the use of atypical antipsychotic agents. Evidence suggests, however, that most cases of NMS caused by atypical antipsychotics present with classic features, though clozapine may be less likely to induce rigidity and tremor.[89] A recent systematic review found that atypical NMS tends to have a lower clinical severity and less mortality.[90]

Benzodiazepines and ECT remain the cornerstones of treatment for NMS. Dopaminergic agents, bromocriptine, and amantadine anecdotally have been used successfully.[91] In a retrospective review of 734 cases, Sakkas and associates[92] concluded that these agents and the muscle relaxant dantrolene led to improvement; bromocriptine and dantrolene also were associated with a significant reduction in the mortality rate. However, in a prospective study of 20 patients, Rosebush and colleagues found that bromocriptine and dantrolene were not efficacious.[93] Bromocriptine in particular carries a significant risk of worsening underlying psychosis, and caution is therefore recommended. In clinical practice, it is rarely used, due to the high efficacy and lower rate of side effects with benzodiazepines.

Re-challenging a patient who has had NMS with an antipsychotic is controversial, as patients with a prior episode of NMS are at significantly increased risk for recurrence. Most investigators suggest that antipsychotics should not be given until at least 2 weeks after an episode of NMS has resolved, and that re-challenge should be with an atypical or with a typical of a lower potency.

SEROTONIN SYNDROME

CASE 3 Serotonin Syndrome

A 69-year-old woman with a history of depression partially responsive to paroxetine 40 mg/day had her dose increased to 60 mg/day; 2 weeks later, buspirone 5 mg TID was added, along with trazodone 100 mg for sleep. She became confused, diaphoretic, febrile (to 101.2°F), hyperreflexic, and mildly rigid and was admitted to hospital. Paroxetine, trazodone, and buspirone were discontinued. Over the next 2 days, her condition improved (with acetaminophen and supportive care).

Definition

Serotonin is a neurotransmitter involved in many psychiatric disorders, and many pharmacologic agents have been designed that affect central serotonergic tone. As the serotonin level increases, it is likely to have certain nervous system effects, including toxicity in excess. Heightened clinical awareness is necessary to prevent, recognize, and intervene when a toxic syndrome secondary to serotonin excess emerges. Though serotonin syndrome (SS) classically occurred as a result of an interaction between serotonergic agents and monoamine oxidase inhibitors (MAOIs), it is now far more common in cases of overdose on serotonergic agents or concomitant use of multiple serotonergic agents. Signs of SS include mental status changes (e.g., confusion, anxiety, irritability, euphoria, dysphoria); gastrointestinal symptoms (e.g., nausea, vomiting, diarrhea, incontinence); behavioral manifestations (e.g., restlessness and agitation); neurologic findings (e.g., ataxia or incoordination, tremor, myoclonus, hyperreflexia, ankle clonus, muscle rigidity); and autonomic nervous system abnormalities (e.g., hypertension, hypotension, tachycardia, diaphoresis, shivering, sialorrhea, mydriasis, tachypnea, hyperthermia).[94]

Epidemiology

The incidence of SS is unknown. There are no data to suggest that gender differences confer any particular vulnerability to the syndrome. Given the overlap of symptoms with NMS, SS is often mistaken for it and thus may be under-reported. The existence of the syndrome in varying degrees also may confound its recognition, as can unawareness on the part of the majority of physicians.[95] SS most often occurs in individuals being treated with psychotropics for a psychiatric disorder. It occurs in about 14–16% of SSRI-overdosed patients.[96]

Clinical Features and Diagnosis

As with NMS, taking a detailed history is crucial. Use of two or more serotonergic agents confers a greater risk of developing SS. Obtaining a history of neuroleptic use can be especially important, because NMS shares many clinical features with SS, as do other toxic syndromes (Table 23-8).

The syndrome ranges from mild to severe, with a mildly affected patient showing restlessness, tremor, tachycardia, shivering, diaphoresis, and the start of hyperreflexia. Moderately severe cases show tachycardia, hypertension, and fever, sometimes as high as 40°C (104°F). There are also mydriasis, strong bowel sounds, hyperreflexia, and clonus (greater in the lower extremities than the upper ones). Horizontal ocular clonus is also seen in moderately severe cases, as well as mental status changes of agitation, pressured speech, and autonomic hyperactivity. Head rotation movement with neck extension has also been reported. In severe cases, there are severe autonomic hyperactivity and severe hyperthermia with temperatures sometimes over 41.1°C (106°F). There is an agitated delirium accompanied by severe muscular rigidity, again greater in the lower extremities. This severe hypertonicity may obscure the appearance of clonus and hyperreflexia and thereby confound the diagnosis. Catatonic features are often present in SS, and may be more prevalent in cases of moderate to severe SS. Rigidity, mutism, and waxy flexibility are often observed. The syndrome can last from hours to days after the offending agents have been stopped and supportive treatment has been initiated. Based on his review of 38 cases, Sternbach[97] proposed the first operational definition of the syndrome in humans. In order to meet Sternbach criteria for SS, patients needed to have three of the following in the presence of recent addition or increase in dosage of a serotonergic agent: mental status changes, agitation, myoclonus, hyperreflexia, diaphoresis, shivering, tremor, diarrhea, and incoordination. Sternbach

TABLE 23-8 Comparison of Serotonin Syndrome With Neuroleptic Malignant Syndrome

FEATURE	SEROTONIN SYNDROME	NEUROLEPTIC MALIGNANT SYNDROME
Temperature	Hyperthermia variable	Hyperthermia
Mental status	Coma Confusion Delirium Stupor Euphoria Irritability Anxiety	Coma Confusion Delirium Stupor
Neurologic	Muscle rigidity variable Hyperreflexia Tremor Ankle clonus Myoclonus Incoordination	Muscle rigidity Hyperreflexia (uncommon) Tremor
Behavioral	Agitation Restlessness	Agitation Restlessness
Autonomic	Diaphoresis Hypertension/ hypotension Incontinence Mydriasis Sialorrhea Tachycardia Tachypnea Shivering	Diaphoresis Hypertension/ hypotension Incontinence Mydriasis Sialorrhea Tachycardia Tachypnea
Gastrointestinal	Diarrhea Nausea Vomiting	
Laboratory	Elevated (uncommon) Creatine phosphokinase (CPK) White blood cell count (WBC) elevated Liver function tests (LFTs) elevated	Elevated (common) CPK WBC elevated LFTs elevated

Modified from Keck PE, Arnold LM: The serotonin syndrome, *Psychiat Ann* 2000; 30: 333–343, p 339.

also emphasized distinguishing the syndrome from NMS by ensuring that a neuroleptic was not recently started or its dose increased. The Sternbach criteria were noted to be fairly non-specific, with 5 out of 10 symptoms being present in SSRI discontinuation syndrome, and 8 of 10 symptoms present in catecholamine excess. Criteria were also noted to have a high overlap with anticholinergic toxicity and substance withdrawal states. In response to these criticisms, the Hunter Serotonin Toxicity Criteria were proposed, establishing an algorithm for diagnosis.[98] If a patient has been exposed to a serotonergic drug within the past 5 weeks and spontaneous clonus emerges, the patient has SS. If there is inducible clonus or ocular clonus plus either agitation or diaphoresis, SS is present. If there are tremor and hyperreflexia, SS can be diagnosed. If there are hypertonicity, temperature >38°C (100.4°F), and either ocular or inducible clonus, SS is present. This approach to SS diagnosis may be more sensitive to serotonin toxicity and less prone to produce false-positive cases, though it may not detect mild cases of SS.

Laboratory abnormalities are mostly non-specific or are secondary to the medical complications of the syndrome. A complete laboratory evaluation is nevertheless essential to rule out other causes for the signs and symptoms that are shared with SS. Leukocytosis, rhabdomyolysis, and liver function test abnormalities have all been reported in patients with SS, along with hyponatremia, hypomagnesemia, and hypocalcemia. These latter disturbances are thought to be related to fluid and electrolyte abnormalities. Disseminated intravascular coagulation (DIC) has been reported in SS. Acute renal failure secondary to myoglobinuria can occur and has been associated with fatalities.

It is interesting to note that certain secreting tumors, such as carcinoid and small-cell lung carcinoma have been associated with SS. X-ray examinations and imaging of the abdomen and lung may sometimes be helpful in working-up SS. An EEG and neuroimaging are often useful in uncovering a seizure disorder or another neurologic condition as well. Drugs associated with SS are included in Table 23-9.

Because of the potential problems of using an MAOI and any medicine with serotonergic properties, caution on the part of the prescribing physician is required. A 2-week washout interval after discontinuation of an MAOI is required before starting any serotonergic medications. In the case of fluoxetine discontinuation, there should be a washout period of at least 5 weeks before an MAOI is initiated.

Pathophysiology

In both animal and human studies, the role of 5-HT has been implicated in the pathogenesis of SS. Nucleus raphe serotonin nuclei (located in the midbrain and arrayed in the midline down to the medulla) are involved in mediating thermoregulation, appetite, nausea, vomiting, wakefulness, migraines, sexual activity, and affective behavior. The animal model of SS seems to be associated with receptors in the lower brainstem and spinal cord. Ascending serotonergic projections are likely to play a role, particularly in hyperthermia, mental status, and autonomic changes. The 5-HT_{2A} and 5-HT_{1A} receptors appear to be overactive in this condition, which has led some to use 5-HT_{1A} antagonists in the management of SS.[96] There also appears to be CNS norepinephrine overactivity. This is clinically significant because clinical outcomes may be associated with hypersympathetic tone.[95] The roles of catecholamines and 5-HT_2 and 5-HT_3 receptor interactions are unclear, as are the contributions of glutamate, GABA, and DA.

Management and Treatment

No prospective studies have looked at treatment of SS. Recommendations for treatment are based solely on case reports and case series. SS is often self-limited, and removal of the offending agents frequently results in resolution of symptoms within 24 hours. Therefore, the initial step in managing SS is to discontinue the suspected offending agent or agents. The next step is to provide supportive measures

TABLE 23-9 Central Nervous System Serotonergic Agents

Antidepressants
Monoamine oxidase Inhibitors (MAOIs)
Isocarboxazid
Moclobemide
Phenelzine
Selegiline
Tranylcypromine
Tricyclic Antidepressants (TCAs)
Selective Serotonin Re-Uptake Inhibitors (SSRIs)
Fluoxetine
Sertraline
Citalopram
Escitalopram
Paroxetine
Fluvoxamine
Serotonin-Norepinephrine Re-Uptake Inhibitors (SNRIs)
Venlafaxine
Duloxetine
Desvenlafaxine
Other Antidepressants
Vilazodone
Vortioxetine
Mirtazapine
Nefazodone
Atypical Antipsychotics
Quetiapine
Olanzapine
Clozapine
Other Psychiatric Medications
Amphetamines
Buspirone
Lithium
Trazodone
Drugs of Abuse
Cocaine
Meta-chlorophenylpiperazine (mCPP)
Opioids and Opiate-Like Medications
Meperidine
Tramadol
Antibiotics
Linezolid
Other Medications
Dextromethorphan
Triptans
Bromocriptine
Pethidine
Supplements
L-tryptophan
Fenfluramine
Sibutramine
Dihydroergotamine (DHE)

to prevent potential medical complications. These supportive measures include the use of antipyretics and cooling blankets to reduce hyperthermia, monitoring and support of the respiratory and cardiovascular systems, IV hydration to prevent renal failure, use of clonazepam for myoclonic jerking, use of anticonvulsants if seizures arise, and use of hypertensive agents for significantly elevated blood pressures. The syndrome rarely leads to respiratory failure. When it does, it usually is because of aspiration, and artificial ventilation may be required.

Benzodiazepine management of agitation, even when mild, is essential for patients with SS. This is because benzodiazepines, such as diazepam and lorazepam, can reduce autonomic tone and temperature and thus may have positive effects on survival.[95] Physical restraints should be avoided if at all possible because muscular stress can lead to lactic acidosis and elevated temperature.

Specific 5-HT receptor antagonism has occasionally been advocated for the treatment or prevention of the symptoms associated with SS, though these are rarely used in clinical practice. Cyproheptadine (4 to 24 mg/day) has been used.[95] Ketanserin a 5-HT_2 antagonist and propranolol, which has 5-HT_{1A} receptor-blocking properties, have been used in a small number of cases. For the management of hypertension, nitroprusside and nifedipine, and for tachycardia, esmolol, have been advocated.[95] Dantrolene has also been used as a muscle relaxant. Because the rise in temperature is muscular in origin, antipyretics are of no use in SS, and paralytics are required when fevers are high.

Prognosis and Complications

SS occurs as a toxic state secondary to serotonin excess produced by high doses or combinations of serotonergic medications. This syndrome is often mild and goes unrecognized, so it may not be as rare as portrayed; it also is self-limiting. When severe, SS can rarely lead to death from medical complications, and supportive measures are required. Prevention, early recognition, and intervention benefit from a heightened clinical awareness of medications that can cause serotonin excess.

In SS, rhabdomyolysis is the most common and serious complication; it occurs in roughly 25% of cases.[82] Generalized seizures occur in approximately 1%, with 39% of these patients dying. Myoglobinuric renal failure accounted for roughly 5% of medical complications, as did DIC. Nearly two-thirds of those with DIC died.

REFERENCES

Access the reference list online at https://expertconsult.inkling.com/.

Patients With Disordered Sleep

24

Matt T. Bianchi, M.D., Ph.D., M.M.Sc.
Patrick Smallwood, M.D.
Davin K. Quinn, M.D.
Theodore A. Stern, M.D.

OVERVIEW

Scholars have long sought the cause and nature of sleep and sleep disorders, yet theories have far exceeded clear facts. Plato, for example, believed that sleep was caused by vapors arising from the stomach and condensing in the head, and Hippocrates believed that sleep was the result of blood and its warmth retreating into the body. Both 16th- and 17th-century scholars debated whether sleep was induced by oxygen deprivation, accumulated toxins, or the daily thickening of blood that impaired spirits from entering the nerves.[1] Despite these age-old theories, only in recent years have the mysteries of sleep been slowly unraveled. Indeed, we now know that sleep is an active biochemical process complete with various physiologic markers, stages, and patterns that, like vital signs, provide a basic indication of overall well-being. This chapter examines the biological and psychiatric aspects of normal and disordered sleep, followed by a brief discussion of the diagnosis and treatment of common sleep disorders.

SLEEP STAGES AND NORMAL SLEEP

Aserinsky and Kleitman (1953) were the first to investigate rapid eye movements during sleep. Kleitman postulated that depth of sleep could be assessed through eye motility, and he and Aserinsky began testing this hypothesis through direct observation of eye movements of infants during sleep.[2] They noted slow rolling eye movements during the early stages of sleep that disappeared as sleep progressed, and they saw periods of rapid eye movements associated with irregular breathing and increased heart rate.[2,3] They coined the terms *non-rapid eye movement* (NREM) to indicate the slow rolling rhythmic eye movements and *rapid eye movement* (REM) to indicate the fast erratic eye movements. In 1957, Kleitman and Dement discovered that REM and NREM sleep occurred cyclically throughout the night and named this overall NREM–REM pattern *sleep architecture*.[2,3]

Polysomnography

Polysomnography is the "gold standard" method for evaluating sleep physiology and many clinical sleep disorders. It involves simultaneously recording multiple physiologic variables in a standardized fashion known as the *polysomnogram* (PSG).[4] The parameters recorded by the PSG include, but are not limited to, the following:

- *Electroencephalogram (EEG)*: A recording of the electrical activity of cortical neurons via scalp electrodes that are placed in standardized positions, usually bilateral frontal, central, and occipital positions.
- *Electro-oculogram (EOG)*: A recording of eye movements bilaterally.
- *Electrocardiogram (ECG)*: A recording of heart rate and rhythm.
- *Electromyogram (EMG)*: A recording of the activity of the bilateral tibialis anterior muscles, and the submental (chin) muscles.
- *Respiration*: Recordings of nasal and oral airflow by means of pressure and thermal sensors, and recordings of thoracic and abdominal movements by means of respiratory inductance plethysmography.
- *Pulse oximetry*: A recording of blood oxygen hemoglobin saturation.
- *Snore monitor*: A detection and recording of snoring by means of a vibration sensor placed on the neck.

Through analysis of EEG, EMG, and EOG signals, the different sleep–wake stages are scored, typically by manual visual inspection by skilled technologists.[5] From the epoch-by-epoch scoring, various metrics are presented in typical PSG reports, such as sleep onset, NREM sleep, REM sleep, and awakenings that occur throughout the night.

The *waking state* is defined by the PSG in the following manner: the EEG reveals low amplitude and mixed high frequencies with eyes open, and an occipital predominant 8 to 13 Hz wave pattern known as *alpha waves* when eyes are closed; the EMG reveals muscle tone and activity; and the EOG demonstrates variable eye movements, including blinking.[2] *Sleep onset* is defined as the time elapsed from lights-out to the first epoch of NREM stage 1 sleep (N1).[2,5–8] The transition to N1 involves replacement of alpha waves with mixed theta frequency waves, slow rolling eye movements, and the EMG may register a modest decrease in muscle activity. Some patients at the transition to sleep may engage in *automatic behavior*, a phenomenon in which very complex cognitive and behavioral tasks are performed outside of awareness.[5,9]

Sleep is normally entered through NREM sleep. NREM sleep is divided into three stages identified by specific EEG criteria; REM is identified by a combination of findings on the EEG, EOG, and EMG.[5]

- *Stage N1*: Alpha waves, present during the waking state, account for less than 50% of an epoch (a 30-second

interval on the PSG). The EEG frequencies are mixed but lower than those seen during wakefulness, usually with emergence of theta waves (4 to 7 Hz).
- *Stage N2*: Theta activity continues in this stage, while two hallmark waveforms emerge: sleep spindles (rhythmic 12 to 14 Hz waves that last 0.5 seconds or more) and K-complexes (high-amplitude negative waves that are followed by a positive deflection, lasting 0.5 seconds or more).
- *Stage N3*: Delta waves (high-amplitude, slow-frequency 0.5 to 2.0 Hz waves) occur in at least 20% of an epoch. This stage is commonly called *delta sleep* or *slow-wave* sleep.

REM sleep, also known as *paradoxical sleep* owing to its similarity to wakefulness, is defined by three principal features. First, the EEG demonstrates low-amplitude high-frequency waves that may resemble those of wake or NREM stage 1. Second, the chin EMG reveals an absence of, or a marked decrease in, muscle activity. Finally, conjugate rapid eye movements become evident, often in bursts (phasic REM) separated by quiescent periods (tonic REM), on the EOG.[4]

Perception of sleep state, as well as sleep quality, is not as straightforward as it might seem. For example, the subjective experience of sleep-onset latency, of awakenings during the night, or total sleep time, often differ from objective measures. Healthy individuals, for example, who may feel that their sleep is consolidated, actually have multiple brief awakenings throughout the night when measured by EEG. Thus, they may over-estimate their total sleep time by 20 minutes or more. In contrast, patients with insomnia often have the opposite trend: under-estimating their total sleep, and over-estimating the time spent awake.[10] Another example of dissociation of physiology and symptoms may occur in patients with sleep apnea (discussed below), who may not have symptoms of sleepiness or disturbed sleep, even when their apnea is severe by objective measurements.

CASE 1

Mr. A, a 52-year-old man with chronic depression, managed with a stable dose of an SSRI, noted gradually worsening fatigue over the past year. Upon questioning about associated changes in his mood, he reported that he was concerned about the fatigue and could not be certain whether it was from worsening mood, or if the mild worsening in mood was from the fatigue. He had gained 10 pounds. Although he denied snoring and his wife has not noticed any breathing problems, he had an elevated body mass index and hypertension. You correctly surmised that he was at elevated risk of obstructive sleep apnea (OSA) and you recommended a polysomnogram (PSG). The test indeed revealed moderate OSA, and Mr. A agreed to a trial of continuous positive airway pressure (CPAP), but he found that he could not tolerate the mask. After consultation with a sleep physician to discuss alternatives, Mr. A was referred to a dental specialist who fitted an oral appliance. He returned to report that his mood and fatigue were substantially improved.

Sleep Cycle and Architecture

NREM and REM sleep do not occur randomly throughout the night; instead, they alternate in a rhythmic fashion known as the *NREM–REM cycle* every approximately 90 to 120 minutes.[2,5,6] N3 is most prominent in the first half of the night and diminishes thereafter. REM sleep shows the opposite pattern, with longer blocks as the night progresses. The time from sleep onset to the first REM is known as *REM latency*, which is usually 90 to 100 minutes. *Sleep efficiency* is the actual amount of sleep per total time in bed multiplied by 100, and is typically 85% or greater when measured by PSG in normal individuals. The average amount of sleep per night for adults is between 6 and 9 hours. The proportion of total sleep consisting of each sleep–wake stage in an average night are as follows: N1, 2% to 5%; N2, 45% to 55%; N3, 15% to 25%; and REM sleep, 20% to 25%.

Sleep Across the Life Span

Sleep quantity and sleep quality change across the life span.[11] Infants spend about two-thirds of the day sleeping, whereas in adulthood, this amount decreases to less than one-third. Sleep architecture becomes altered as people age. These changes include increases in sleep latency, nocturnal awakenings, time spent in N1 sleep, and decreases in N3 sleep, REM sleep, and overall sleep efficiency.[12,13]

NEUROANATOMIC BASIS FOR SLEEP

The actual neuroanatomic basis for the sleep–wake cycle remains uncertain, but current research reveals that specific regions of the brain are critical for wakefulness and for sleep. These neuronal systems are located in the brainstem, hypothalamus, and basal forebrain, and they project diffusely throughout the neocortex.[14–16] The major wake-promoting centers include the tuberomammillary nucleus (TMN; histamine), the reticular activating system (serotonin), the locus ceruleus (norepinephrine), the basal forebrain (acetylcholine), and the hypothalamus (orexin). The major NREM sleep-promoting nucleus is known as the ventrolateral preoptic nucleus (VLPO; GABA). The pedunculopontine and laterodorsal tegmental (PPT/LDT) nuclei of the brainstem, both cholinergic with projections mainly to the thalamus, play an important role in REM sleep circuitry.

The timing of sleep and of wakefulness is largely determined by an internal biological cycle known as the *circadian rhythm*.[17] This biological clock is an endogenous rhythm of bodily functions that is influenced by environmental cues, or *zeitgebers*, of which the main one is daylight. The average cycle is slightly longer than 24 hours for most people. The suprachiasmatic nuclei (SCN), in the anterior hypothalamus, is the brain region that controls human circadian rhythms. The SCN receives input from the eyes via the retino–hypothalamic tract, and it sends output to the hypothalamus and the pineal gland. Melatonin, a hormone secreted by the pineal gland during darkness (and production is suppressed by light), is associated with suppression of the SCN; it facilitates sleep in diurnal mammals.[18]

Sleep disorders related to the circadian rhythm emerge when a person's circadian rhythm clashes with environmental and societal expectations.

A second kind of "clock" exists, independent of the circadian rhythm discussed above that is controlled by the SCN. This homeostatic sleep system tracks how much sleep has occurred recently, such that over time spent awake, homeostatic pressure accumulates to increase the probability of sleep. The biological basis for this system is thought to reside in adenosine levels, which build during wakefulness and wane during sleep.[19,20] Caffeine is thought to improve wakefulness by blocking adenosine signaling.

SLEEP DISORDERS

Although several classification systems for sleep disorders exist, the *Diagnostic and Statistical Manual of Mental Disorders*, 5th edition (DSM-5)[21] and the *International Classification of Sleep Disorders*, 3rd edition (ICSD-3)[22] are the most widely used.

Insomnia

Insomnia is a repeated difficulty with sleep initiation, duration, consolidation, or quality, despite adequate opportunity for sleep, which produces daytime impairment. Patients complain of deficient, inadequate, or unrefreshing sleep; malaise; and fatigue. Sufferers often experience hyperarousal and anxiety at bedtime and have decreased daytime function with mild to moderate impairment in concentration and psychomotor function.[23–25]

Diagnosis

The diagnosis of insomnia is made exclusively based on the clinical history, which includes difficulty falling asleep or staying asleep, associated with non-refreshing sleep or some other daytime sequelae. The etiology of insomnia is often multi-factorial, but the final common pathway is postulated to be a state of increased arousal. There is evidence of increased arousal during sleep as well as during wakefulness in neuroimaging studies of patients with insomnia.[26] A PSG is not typically recommended for evaluation of patients with chronic insomnia, unless another sleep disorder, such as periodic limb movements of sleep (PLMS) or OSA, is suspected.

Psychophysiologic insomnia is caused by somatized tension and by learned sleep-preventing associations. Sufferers react to stress with increased physiologic arousal, such as increased muscle tension and vasoconstriction. Learned associations consist mainly of an over-concern with an inability to sleep, which results in a vicious cycle of over-concern, increased arousal, insomnia, and reinforcement of concern. Environmental cues also become associated with an inability to sleep, and sufferers often report sleeping better in unfamiliar surroundings, including sometimes even in the sleep laboratory.

Paradoxical insomnia, also known as sleep-state misperception, involves a dissociation between often severe complaints of inadequate sleep and objective findings on the PSG showing fairly normal duration and content of sleep. Patients with sleep-state misperception may under-estimate their total sleep time or over-estimate their sleep latency, or both. Theories to explain this discrepancy include excessive mentation during sleep and obsessiveness about sleep.[10]

Idiopathic insomnia is a chronic primary insomnia that develops in childhood and is most likely the result of an innate abnormality in the sleep–wake cycle. Prolonged sleep latency and poor sleep efficiency may be seen on PSG.[27] The presence of psychiatric or medical conditions that better account for the symptoms is called *insomnia due to a medical condition or mental disorder*.

Treatment

The approach to insomnia treatment begins with identifying and addressing potential root cause contributors, if possible. Often, medical or psychiatric co-morbidities are present, and it may be challenging to surmise causality by history, and instead simultaneously approaching sleep and its co-morbidities may be beneficial. Non-pharmacologic techniques are favored over use of medications, and the foundation of behavioral change is adopting sound sleep hygiene practices. Table 24-1 provides a guideline for proper sleep hygiene. Additionally, the approach known as cognitive-behavioral therapy for insomnia (CBT-I) is well validated as equivalent or superior in clinical effectiveness studies to use of prescriptions for the treatment of insomnia.[28] CBT-I involves techniques such as relaxation, and sleep-restriction therapy, a specific method of graded matching of time spent in bed to actual sleep. Although finding a CBT-I specialist can be challenging, validated on-line versions of CBT-I are increasingly available. Other behavioral techniques can be learned through self-help audio/visual programs or manuals or from consultation with a mental health clinician.

If behavioral techniques are unsuccessful, brief intermittent use of a sedative–hypnotic may be appropriate. Common sedative–hypnotic agents include several classes, such as sedating antidepressants, benzodiazepines, benzodiazepine receptor agonists, melatonin receptor agonists, antihistamines, and atypical antipsychotics. Trazodone is the most commonly used agent, although it is not FDA-approved for insomnia and it lacks clinical efficacy data; it is commonly used in patients with a history of substance abuse or hypnotic

TABLE 24-1 Basic Sleep Hygiene
Limit time in bed to the amount present before the sleep disturbance
Lie down only when sleepy, and sleep only as much as necessary to feel refreshed
Use the bed for sleep and intimacy only
Maintain comfortable sleeping conditions and avoid excessive warmth and cold
Wake up at a regular time each day
Avoid daytime naps
Exercise regularly, but early in the day
Limit sedatives
Avoid alcohol, tobacco, and caffeine near bedtime
Eat at regular times daily and avoid large meals near bedtime
Eat a light snack, if hungry, near bedtime
Practice evening relaxation routines, such as progressive muscle relaxation, meditation, or taking a hot, 20-minute, body temperature-raising bath near bedtime

abuse.[29] Tricyclic antidepressants (TCAs) are also used for insomnia, but they can be lethal in overdose, and they may induce anticholinergic-mediated side effects.

Second-generation antipsychotic agents, such as quetiapine and olanzapine, may also be helpful in resistant insomnia, but they can cause a metabolic syndrome, weight gain, orthostasis, extrapyramidal symptoms, and anticholinergic side effects.

The long-term use of benzodiazepines, although controversial, is a common practice, and it may be appropriate for patients who have insomnia secondary to an anxiety disorder. Benzodiazepines should either be used cautiously or avoided in patients with a history of alcohol or substance abuse, with a personality disorder, or with a sleep-related breathing disorder. To avoid dose escalation with these agents, prescriptions should be carefully monitored, when used for more than 4 weeks. Newer benzodiazepine receptor agonists (such as zolpidem, eszopiclone, and zaleplon) are often preferred, owing to their lower abuse potential, shorter half-lives, and approval for longer-term use (up to 6 months).[30,31]

Ramelteon, a melatonin receptor agonist, improves sleep latency and is effective for patients with poor sleep initiation. Melatonin is available over-the-counter and is commonly used, though it remains incompletely studied and the literature supporting its clinical efficacy is mixed.[32]

Sedating antihistamines are also available over-the-counter, either alone or in "PM" formulations combined with common analgesics. However, they can cause delirium in the elderly or in those with a compromised central nervous system (CNS). Chloral hydrate and barbiturates are not recommended given their risk profiles and the availability of safer alternatives.

Sleep-Related Breathing Disorders

The most common sleep-related breathing disorder is obstructive sleep apnea (OSA). Although OSA is a commonly encountered cause of hypersomnia, many patients with OSA have no objective or subjective sleepiness, which accounts in part for widespread under-diagnosis. OSA is characterized by repeated partial or complete obstructions of the airway in sleep, associated with oxygen desaturation and EEG arousal, as well as autonomic nervous system swings. The principal defect is repetitive occlusion of the upper airway at the level of the pharynx (which results from an abnormal decrease in oropharyngeal muscle tone), excessive tissue mass in the pharynx and tongue, malposition of the jaw or tongue, or a narrow airway.

The most significant risk factors for OSA include: male sex, age between 40 and 65 years, obesity, smoking, use or abuse of alcohol, poor physical health, and neck circumference greater than 17 inches.[33,34] Nocturnal signs and symptoms include snoring, gasping arousals, witnessed apneas, enuresis, reflux, hypoxemia, hypercapnia, and cardiac dysrhythmias. Daytime signs and symptoms include headaches, hypersomnolence, automatic behavior, neuropsychiatric abnormalities, and hypertension.[35–37]

Diagnosis

The PSG is the gold standard diagnostic test to identify OSA as well as related breathing syndromes, such as central apnea, or obesity-related hypoventilation. Manual scoring of the PSG allows quantification of the severity of OSA, based on the frequency of breathing events per hour of sleep. Several types of breathing pauses are identified. *Apnea* is defined as the cessation of airflow longer than 10 seconds. The most common form is obstructive apnea, based upon ongoing respiratory effort. These obstructions can be so complete and the effort so powerful that the chest and abdomen can move in opposite directions, a phenomenon known as *paradoxical breathing*. Central apnea, by contrast, has no respiratory effort. Mixed apneas contain features of both central and obstructive patterns. Hypopneas are partial reductions in airflow, of >30% amplitude, associated with 4% or more desaturation (Medicare definition).

Of all the sleep apnea spectrum disorders and disorders of excessive daytime sleepiness (EDS), OSA is the most common, accounting for the majority of all patients seen in sleep disorder centers.[33,38] The estimated prevalence of OSA is 5% to 15%, depending on the population demographics and the definitions used. Currently, the apnea hypopnea index (AHI) values in the mild range (5 to 15 events per hour) are felt to warrant therapy if symptoms attributable to poor sleep are present. For those with AHI values >15 per hour, treatment is recommended even if the patient is asymptomatic. This reflects an evolution in thinking about OSA, in light of data suggesting that the chronic health risks are linked to the AHI value, independent of symptoms, and the recognition that symptoms do not often correlate with the AHI.

Treatment

The treatment of OSA involves correcting the obstructive process, which can follow one of five main pathways. First, conservative measures can be undertaken, such as weight loss and avoidance of alcohol and sedatives that prolong apneas by increasing vagal tone, relaxing muscles, and preventing arousal for breathing. In addition, treating reflux and nasal congestion may be helpful. Second, because airway obstruction is facilitated by gravity for some patients, positional therapy can be used if PSG results document supine-dominant OSA with resolution or near-resolution while sleeping on one's side (lateral position). Third, oral appliances fitted by dental specialists may be used to alter the position of structures of the upper airway, and are currently recommended for those with primary snoring or mild to moderate OSA; and those with severe OSA who are intolerant of, or refuse, continuous positive airway pressure (CPAP) or surgical interventions.[39] Fourth, surgical interventions can be considered for appropriate cases. Uvulopalatopharyngoplasty (UPPP) aims to increase the volume of the oropharynx by removing the tonsils, adenoids, posterior soft palate, and redundant tissue on the sides of the pharynx by means of primary or laser-assisted surgery. The overall success rate for uvulopalatopharyngoplasty, as measured by at least a 50% reduction in apnea index, is only ~50%; moreover, there may be a gradual return of apneas to pre-treatment levels.[40] Maxillomandibular advancement (MMA) surgery has a higher success rate (~90%) but is a more involved surgery, requiring bone repositioning and 10 to 12 weeks recovery. A recent addition to surgical options includes placement of a hypoglossal nerve stimulator, acting much like a pacemaker, to move the tongue forward during sleep and thus open the airway. Fifth, the gold standard therapy for OSA remains CPAP, whereby purified humidified air is delivered via nasal or oronasal mask to stent open the airway during sleep and prevent obstructive events.[41] Bi-level positive airway pressure (BiPAP) operates on the same principle and can be helpful for comfort or when hypoventilation occurs in addition to OSA.

For a subset of patients with OSA who use CPAP or BiPAP, the breathing problem actually worsens, due to pressure-induced provocation of central apnea. This is sometimes known as "complex apnea." The treatment of choice is adaptive servoventilation (ASV), which is a special kind of pressure-delivery machine.

For patients who receive no treatment and who have an AHI of >20, the probability of a cumulative 8-year survival is reported at 63% ± 17%. With the use of nasal CPAP, regardless of the initial apnea index, the probability of a cumulative 8-year survival rises to 100%.[42]

Narcolepsy and Hypersomnias of Central Origin

Narcolepsy

Narcolepsy is a primary hypersomnia associated with a tetrad of symptoms:

- *Sleep attacks*: Irresistible and brief sleep episodes that occur several times a day, often at inappropriate times;
- *Cataplexy*: Sudden and brief loss of motor tone without impairment of consciousness, triggered by strong emotions (most often laughter, but also anger or surprise); the motor loss can be global or partial/unilateral;
- *Sleep paralysis*: Brief episodes of muscular paralysis associated with the transitions of sleep-onset or awakening; and
- *Hypnagogic* or *hypnopompic hallucinations*: Vivid visual and auditory phenomena that are associated with the transitions to sleep-onset or awakening.

Narcolepsy occurs in approximately 0.07% of the general population; it typically arises in the second decade of life. Symptoms usually begin with sleep and are associated with excessive sleepiness. Cataplexy occurs in approximately 50% of cases. The probability of developing narcolepsy is 40 times greater if an immediate family member suffers from it.[43] A strong association exists between narcolepsy with cataplexy and the human leukocyte antigen *HLA-DR2* and *DQ1* phenotypes. The most specific antigen associated with narcolepsy with cataplexy in all ethnicities is *HLA-DQB1*0602*.[44] Although 85% or more of patients with narcolepsy with cataplexy have this allele, fewer than half of patients with narcolepsy without cataplexy have it, and it is non-specific, being found in 25% of healthy controls.

Although the exact abnormality of narcolepsy is unknown, leading theories for narcolepsy with cataplexy implicate loss of neurons in the hypothalamus that synthesize the neurotransmitter *hypocretin*.[45] Also known as orexin, this neurotransmitter is produced in the posterior hypothalamus, has activating projections diffusely throughout the brain, and it inhibits activity in the sleep-inducing ventrolateral pre-optic area (VLPO). Hypocretin deficiency destabilizes sleep–wake partitioning, and in narcolepsy with cataplexy there is a loss of hypothalamic hypocretin-secreting cells.[46]

The diagnosis of narcolepsy is made on the multiple sleep latency test (MLST), a series of five scheduled naps with EEG, EOG, and EMG recordings, 2 hours apart during the day, typically following overnight PSG.[47] Short sleep latency (<8 minutes per nap), and two episodes of REM sleep or more during the naps are diagnostic for narcolepsy. Note that the MSLT cannot be properly interpreted in the presence of stimulants or REM-suppressing agents, such as antidepressants, which should be discontinued at least 2 weeks in advance, if clinically feasible.

Treatment is aimed at reducing both daytime sleepiness and at the REM-intrusion phenomena (including cataplexy, if present). Daytime sleepiness is effectively treated with psychostimulants, particularly members of the amphetamine class, such as methylphenidate (Ritalin), dextroamphetamine (Dexedrine), and others.[48] Modafinil (Provigil), a centrally acting stimulant, can promote wakefulness, has fewer side effects, and has a low potential for abuse.[49–51] Due to their ability to suppress REM sleep, antidepressants, particularly the TCAs but also selective serotonin re-uptake inhibitors (SSRIs) and serotonin-norepinephrine re-uptake inhibitors (SNRIs), are the treatment of choice for cataplexy, sleep paralysis, and hypnagogic hallucinations. Gamma hydroxybutyrate (GHB; Xyrem) is a gamma-aminobutyric acid (GABA) metabolite that can improve nocturnal sleep, EDS, and REM-intrusion symptoms including cataplexy, but it has high abuse potential. Prophylactic naps, when feasible, can reduce the total daily dose of stimulants.

Hypersomnias of Central Origin

Other hypersomnias of central origin include recurrent hypersomnia, or *Kleine–Levin syndrome*, a rare, often self-limiting condition that primarily affects male adolescents. Symptoms include hypersomnia, hyperphagia, and hypersexuality. Although the exact cause is unknown, it often follows an acute viral infection. Treatment includes the use of psychostimulants, SSRIs, and monamine oxidase inhibitors (MAOIs).

Idiopathic hypersomnia is characterized by constant or recurrent EDS, typically with sleep episodes lasting 1 hour or longer, despite normal nocturnal sleep patterns. *HLA-Cw2* is associated with this disorder.[22] In this disorder, fast-onset latencies are seen during MSLT, without the REM sleep occurrences typical of narcolepsy. Treatment of hypersomnia in idiopathic hypersomnia follows the recommendations for narcolepsy, i.e., amphetamine class agents, modafinil, or the related drug armodafinil.

Behaviorally induced insufficient sleep syndrome results from voluntary but unintentional chronic sleep deprivation. Patients do not appreciate the difference between the need for sleep and the amount they actually obtain. Prescribing longer periods of sleep reverses its symptoms.

Circadian Rhythm Sleep Disorders

Circadian rhythm sleep disorders emerge when societal expectations conflict with a person's endogenous sleep–wake cycle. Patients who have these disorders might complain of insomnia, hypersomnia, sleepiness, fatigue, or simply that their inherent timing of sleep does not align with social or work demands. Sleep that is misaligned with the endogenous circadian rhythm may suffer from reduced quantity and quality. The most commonly encountered circadian rhythm disorders include jet lag syndrome, shift-work sleep disorder, delayed sleep phase disorder, advanced sleep phase disorder, and non-24-hour day (or hypernychthemeral) syndrome.

Jet lag occurs when a person rapidly crosses several time zones, often from western to eastern time zones. This results in an advancement in the sleep–wake cycle, leaving the person feeling tired earlier in the evening.[52] *Shift-work sleep disorder* occurs when the circadian rhythm conflicts with a work schedule that does not coincide with a conventional day–night cycle.[52] *Delayed sleep phase disorder* occurs in persons whose circadian rhythm is set for a later time than the conventional sleep–wake cycle.[52] Considered "night owls," these persons are most alert in the evening and at night and become sleepy several hours after the conventional bedtime. If left undisturbed, they can sleep 7 to 8 hours, with problems arising when they are required to adhere to conventional daytime schedules.

Advanced sleep phase disorder occurs in persons whose circadian rhythm is set for an earlier time than the conventional sleep–wake cycle.[53] Considered "larks," these persons (who are often elderly) are most alert in the earlier morning, and they become sleepy several hours earlier than the conventional bedtime. Although they sleep for 7 to 8 hours, they might awaken at 2 to 3 a.m. complaining of an inability to stay asleep all night.

The *non-24-hour day syndrome* is a phenomenon seen most commonly in persons who are totally blind and who are unable to perceive visual *zeitgebers*. These patients, who function on a natural circadian rhythm of 24.5 to 25.0 hours, go to sleep and wake up about 45 minutes later each day, and thus are referred to often as "free running" phenotype.[52] As opposed to persons who follow a conventional sleep–wake schedule, their sleep–wake cycle will literally go "around the clock" in approximately 3 weeks, with increasing sleep complaints (insomnia) and daytime function complaints (fatigue) when their endogenous rhythm is anti-phase with conventional day–night scheduled activities or work.

The diagnosis of circadian rhythm disorders is based primarily on the history that can be obtained through a detailed sleep–wake diary maintained for several weeks. Common treatment options, often termed "chronotherapy," include gradually delaying sleep until the patient achieves a new schedule, receiving light therapy upon waking, or taking melatonin. The timing of light and melatonin is key. For example, delayed-phase patients should begin at their "natural" sleep zone, and then take melatonin 2 to 3 hours prior to bedtime, ensure avoidance of light until wake time (often after natural sunrise), and then obtain light exposure. Rapidly shifting the schedule and timing of light can paradoxically perpetuate the delayed phase. It is important to distinguish delayed sleep phase from onset insomnia, and advanced sleep phase from early morning waking forms of insomnia, because the treatments (chronotherapy) are specific to the circadian disorders.

Parasomnias

Parasomnias are a group of primary sleep disorders in which abnormal behaviors or physiologic events arise during specific sleep stages or during the transitions between wakefulness and sleep. These events occur across a spectrum from mild to bizarre, with clinical implications ranging from annoyance of bed partners to injurious behavior. Unlike with dyssomnias (insomnia and hypersomnia), children are more commonly affected by parasomnias than are adults. The parasomnias are subdivided into NREM arousal disorders, REM sleep disorders, and other parasomnias.

Arousal Disorders

In *sleepwalking disorder* or somnambulism, the patient experiences episodic motor behaviors while emerging from delta sleep, most often during the first third of the night. Some arousal disorder behaviors are simple (e.g., walking, sitting up in bed, or picking at bed sheets), but more complex and serious behaviors can occur (e.g., running, eating, driving, or committing violent attacks).[54] Patients are often unresponsive to efforts to wake them, confused and disoriented when actually awakened, and amnestic to the sleep-related event the next day. Sleepwalking is not uncommon in childhood; it is rare in adulthood, a fact that should prompt a search for a possible underlying medical, neurologic, or pharmacologic etiology. No definitive treatment for sleepwalking exists, but some patients respond to low-dose benzodiazepines or to sedating antidepressants. Adjunctive therapies include reassurance, hypnosis, and provision of a safe sleep environment.

As with sleepwalking disorder, *sleep terror disorder*, also known as *night terrors*, *pavor nocturnus*, or *incubus*, occurs during partial arousal from delta sleep, usually during the first third of the night. As in sleepwalking disorder, patients are difficult to awaken, they lack dream recall, and they are amnestic for the episodes. Caretakers are often bothered more by this disorder than are patients. Symptoms include repeated awakenings followed by intense fear, screaming, flailing, and autonomic hyperarousal (e.g., tachycardia, tachypnea, and mydriasis).[55] In adults, this disorder is associated with post-traumatic stress disorder (PTSD), generalized anxiety disorder, and borderline personality disorder. Treatment includes use of low-dose benzodiazepines, which suppress delta sleep. Adjunctive therapies include psychotherapy and stress reduction techniques.

Confusional arousals, also known as sleep drunkenness, occur when persons are awakened from delta sleep, from a nap, or induced to wake in the morning. They are characterized by disorientation, by amnesia, and occasionally by violent or sexual behavior. Allowing enough time for disorientation to wear off is usually sufficient treatment.

REM Sleep Disorders

The hallmarks of this group of parasomnias are the occurrence in REM sleep, dreaming, and awareness of the specific events. The most commonly encountered REM sleep disorders are nightmare disorder and REM sleep behavior disorder. The essential feature of *nightmare disorder* is repeated episodes of terrifying dreams that awaken the patient. In contrast to patients with sleep terror disorder, patients with nightmare disorder often have vivid recall of the events, are atonic during the experience, lack autonomic arousal, and experience the events in the latter half of the night when REM sleep is longest and most dense. The specific etiology for nightmares is often underlying emotional stress; treatment targets stress reduction, but it can include psychotherapy, rehearsal instructions, and reassurance. Nightmares associated with PTSD may respond to adrenergic blockage via prazosin.

REM sleep behavior disorder (RBD) presents as dream enactment ranging from simple to quite complex behaviors while asleep, including jumping out of bed, walking, running, or singing.[56] RBD events are typically accompanied by vivid dream recall. Patients with RBD lack the muscle atonia that normally accompanies REM sleep; this results in the literal acting out of dream content.[57] The disorder often occurs in isolation but longitudinal studies suggest that well over half will develop a parkinsonian syndrome over subsequent decades of life. RBD is also seen concurrently with other underlying neurologic processes, such as vascular and Alzheimer's dementia, and focal brainstem lesions of any cause. It is more common in the elderly, and it affects men nine times more frequently than women. Low-dose clonazepam is often used to suppress dream enactment, but should be used with caution with older age, fall risk, cognitive impairment, and potentially undiagnosed OSA. Melatonin, in isolation or in combination with clonazepam, may be helpful.

Other REM sleep disorders include *recurrent isolated sleep paralysis*, which involves the inability to move voluntarily at sleep onset or awakening. It can last up to several minutes, and it disappears spontaneously or with external stimulation.

Sleep-Related Movement Disorders

Periodic limb movements of sleep (PLMS), sometimes called *nocturnal myoclonus*, is a common finding in up to 40% of people older than 65 years of age and 11% of sleep disorder clinic patients who complain of insomnia.[58] PLMS manifests as brief (0.5 to 5.0 seconds), stereotypic, and involuntary contractions of the lower limbs (often the dorsiflexors of the ankle), at intervals of 20 to 40 seconds. Contractions appear more commonly during NREM stages 1 and 2. Although patients are typically unaware of them, the EEG may demonstrate nocturnal arousals and actual awakenings. Sleep is often unrefreshing, with hypersomnia being the most common complaint. When no other cause of sleep-related symptoms is present, besides the PSG-based finding of elevated PLMS, then the diagnosis of periodic limb movement disorder (PLMD) can be made.

Diagnosis is made by overnight PSG and is confirmed when the *myoclonus index* (the number of leg jerks per hour of sleep) reaches 15 or more. Although the pathogenesis of PLMD is unknown, it is associated with a variety of medical conditions (such as renal failure, diabetes, chronic anemia, peripheral nerve injuries, and even uncomplicated pregnancy). Medications, including antidepressants, neuroleptics, lithium, diuretics, and narcotic withdrawal may invoke or worsen PLMS. Treatment is symptomatic and includes use of dopaminergic facilitating agents (e.g., pramipexole, ropinirole), and in severe or refractory cases, benzodiazepines can be considered.

A disorder closely related to PLMD is the *restless legs syndrome*.[59] Restless legs syndrome is characterized by intense aching or crawling sensations inside the legs and calves that occur while sitting or lying; it causes an urge to move or rub the legs. Symptoms are typically worse at bedtime (or during the day at rest, such as in a car), and are relieved or improved by movement. For some, the symptoms interrupt sleep because the patient may repeatedly get out of bed to walk or stretch. As with PLMD, restless legs syndrome is associated with various medical problems, especially kidney failure, diabetes, iron-deficiency anemia, and peripheral nerve injury, as well as with the use of medications, particularly SSRIs and neuroleptics. Symptomatic relief may be provided by iron supplementation (oral replacement if serum ferritin <50), regular exercise, tapering offending medications, and avoidance of alcohol. Dopaminergic agonists, such as pramipexole and ropinirole, are effective options. Other agents that might provide relief include gabapentin enacarbil, and, in refractory cases, benzodiazepines, such as clonazepam, can be considered.[60,61]

Nocturnal leg cramps can occur multiple times a night, several times per week, and are often seen in the elderly. *Rhythmic movement disorder* involves stereotyped repetitive movements of large muscles, often of the head and neck, occurring before sleep and sustained into light sleep. A normal aspect of infancy, rhythmic movement disorder beyond childhood may be associated with intellectual disability, developmental delay, or psychopathology.

CASE 2

You have been following Ms. B, a 45-year-old woman with generalized anxiety and mild obsessive–compulsive disorder, managed with an SSRI as well as a PRN benzodiazepine. She also has chronic insomnia, and has noted that poor sleep can worsen her psychiatric symptoms, but also that when her anxiety is elevated, her sleep is negatively impacted. Because of her prominent sleep symptoms, you had aggressively attempted to control the insomnia, but over the years Ms. B has been refractory to multiple hypnotic trials. Although you recognized that cognitive-behavioral therapy for insomnia (CBT-I) is the gold standard for chronic insomnia, there were no specialist providers in her location. And although you also recognized that polysomnography is not routinely indicated for insomnia, her chronic and refractory nature prompted you to discuss such testing and she agreed. On PSG she was found to have a combination of sleep–wake state misperception and elevated PLMS. Although initially skeptical about the misperception finding, she was somewhat reassured after further discussion, though she still desired therapy. You alerted her to the growing options of validated online CBT-I options, and she agreed. You also recognized relative iron deficiency (based on ferritin level of 23), and you recommended iron supplementation, as well as moving her SSRI to the morning instead of night dosing to help reduce her leg movements. These interventions improved the proportion of good nights and she was able to avoid further hypnotic use.

Sleep Disorders Related to Another Medical Condition

Mood Disorders

Sleep abnormalities occur in up to 60% of outpatients and 90% of inpatients with depression. Consequently, more is known about sleep disturbances in depressed patients than in any other psychiatric illness. Most patients who have depression complain of initial, middle, and terminal insomnia and early morning awakening; in addition, they experience restlessness and fatigue. Hypersomnia and neurovegetative reversal, however, tend to occur in atypical depression.

A PSG is not recommended for the evaluation for mood disorders *per se*, except to the extent that a co-morbid sleep disorder of relevance may be diagnosed, such as OSA or PLMD. Prior work has suggested that a PSG in mood disorders may show prolonged sleep latency, decreased delta sleep, decreased REM latency, increased duration and density of the first REM period, and early morning awakening. Evidence suggests that these abnormalities can persist after remission and that they precede the onset of another episode. In addition, some studies suggest that decreased REM latency or decreased delta sleep can predict relapse in depressed patients.[62]

Sleep disturbance in bipolar illness depends on which phase of the illness the patient is experiencing.[63] During a depressed phase, for example, bipolar patients tend to experience hypersomnia and have an increased percentage of REM sleep, whereas during a manic episode they experience insomnia and have a lower percentage of REM sleep. Unlike other patients with insomnia, however, patients with mania rarely complain of their inability to sleep.

Psychotic Disorders

The most common sleep abnormalities in patients with psychotic disorders are difficulties with sleep initiation and sleep maintenance, which become apparent during the acute phase of these illnesses. Patients with psychosis, like those with depression, also have decreases in REM latency, total sleep time, sleep efficiency, and delta sleep. Because many of the medications used for treating psychosis can cause similar disruptions in sleep architecture, medication side effects must be ruled out. Current evidence suggests, however, that many of these sleep abnormalities, particularly delta sleep deficits, are the function of a psychotic disorder rather than the result of medication use.[64]

Anxiety Disorders

Although anxiety disorders are perhaps the most common cause of insomnia, their exact effect on sleep architecture is tenuous. As a general rule, patients with anxiety disorders often complain of disturbed sleep and have poor sleep efficiency.[65] Patients suffering from panic disorder can experience attacks during sleep, usually during the transition from NREM Stage 2 sleep and early delta sleep.[66,67] Patients with OCD report difficulties with initiating and maintaining sleep, which is often a result of pre-sleep anxiety and bedtime rituals before sleep onset. Of all the anxiety disorders, PTSD is the best studied. Sleep findings in patients with PTSD include easy arousability, nightmares, night terrors, and increased sleep-related movements.[68] In addition, total sleep time is often reduced owing to recurrent awakenings and impaired sleep maintenance.[65,68] Patients suffering from generalized anxiety have difficulty falling asleep and can awaken with anxious ruminations throughout the night.

Medical Disorders

Because pain, discomfort, and unremitting symptoms can interfere with sleep continuity, sleep complaints are common in a host of medical conditions. Patients who have pain syndromes often complain of symptoms that worsen at bedtime. Consequently, these patients often have disrupted sleep patterns, insomnia, early morning awakening, and daytime fatigue.[69–71] Polysomnographic features include increased NREM Stage 1 sleep, decreased delta sleep, and increased number of arousals.[70,72,73] Adequate pain control can substantially improve sleep for these patients. Sedating antidepressants or benzodiazepines, although they do not directly treat the pain, can help with sleep initiation and maintenance.

Patients who have respiratory conditions, such as asthma and chronic obstructive pulmonary disease (COPD), often complain of frequent nocturnal awakening, light sleep, early awakening, and daytime hypersomnia. In cases of severe COPD with nocturnal hypoxemia not explained by concurrent OSA, supplemental oxygen can improve the quality of sleep. Other polysomnographic features are similar to those found in patients with OSA, because many patients with primary respiratory disorders also suffer from co-morbid breathing-related sleep disorders.

Sleep complaints are common in other chronic medical problems, but they are less well investigated. Patients with angina and cardiac arrhythmias can experience exacerbations of their symptoms during sleep, most often during REM sleep. Patients in congestive heart failure often suffer orthopnea, paroxysmal nocturnal dyspnea, and nocturia, which may be confused with a primary sleep disorder, such as breathing-related sleep disorder, sleep terror disorder, nocturnal panic disorder, and sleep-related seizures.

Several neurologic disorders are commonly associated with sleep disturbance, including dementia, Parkinson's disease, and epilepsy. In cerebral degenerative disorders (e.g., Huntington's disease, spinocerebellar degeneration, and Rett syndrome) sleep fragmentation is common, as are periodic leg movements, reduced REM and delta sleep. OSA may be co-morbid in these disorders, with a subset exhibiting central apnea. Patients with dementia often experience sleep disturbance with delirium, agitation, wandering, and vocalizations. Their PSGs show sleep fragmentation and decreases in sleep efficiency, delta sleep, and REM sleep. Those with Parkinson's disease have similar PSG findings, including prolonged sleep latency, increased number of awakenings, and decreased REM sleep. They also demonstrate periodic leg movements, and may have tremors at sleep-stage transitions.

Epilepsy is classified as sleep-related if more than 75% of seizures occur during sleep. Suspicion for this condition is raised if a person experiences abrupt nocturnal awakenings, unexplained urinary incontinence, or abnormal movements during sleep. Epileptic discharges are typically activated by NREM sleep and suppressed by REM sleep. Sleep-related seizures are quite rare and are often confused with parasomnias, such as sleep terror disorder, REM sleep behavior disorder, sleepwalking disorder, enuresis, or nocturnal panic attacks.[74] Seizures occur predominantly during the first 2 hours of sleep and most often during light NREM sleep or in transitional states to and from REM sleep. Seizure type may be either generalized or partial, with temporal and frontal lobe seizures being the most commonly encountered variety of partial seizures.[75] The chief complaint is often non-specific and can include disturbed sleep, tousled bed linens, confusion, or muscle soreness. Some patients may be unaware that they have sleep-related seizures until someone observes a convulsion. The treatment for sleep-related seizures, as with most forms of seizures, involves use of anticonvulsants.

Substance-Induced Sleep Disorder

Substances, whether prescribed or illicit, can have profound effects on sleep. These effects can arise during regular use, acute ingestion, or withdrawal and can masquerade as any primary sleep disorder. As a general rule, if the substance is a CNS depressant, intoxication results in sedation and withdrawal results in insomnia. Similarly, if the substance is a CNS stimulant, intoxication results in insomnia and withdrawal results in sedation. Diagnosis of these disorders can only be made if the sleep disturbance is severe enough to warrant independent clinical attention, it is caused by the direct physiologic effects of a substance, if it developed during or within a month of intoxication or withdrawal from the substance, and if it is not the result of a mental disorder or delirium. Once a substance-related sleep disorder is suspected, a thorough substance-abuse history must be obtained to recognize the offending substance. Treatment consists of judicious discontinuation of the substance, management of any acute withdrawal, and treatment of any underlying co-morbid psychiatric problems that initiated or contributed to the substance abuse in the first place.

Alcohol is perhaps the most commonly used sleep aid, but its soporific value is limited by significant side effects, including dependence, addiction, and withdrawal. Its effects on sleep are well documented and depend on the pattern of use and the state of intoxication or withdrawal. During acute intoxication, alcohol alters sleep architecture by decreasing sleep latency, increasing delta sleep, and decreasing REM sleep for the first 3 to 4 hours of sleep. In the last 2 to 3 hours of sleep, wakefulness and REM are increased. OSA may be exacerbated by alcohol consumption. During acute withdrawal, however, its effects on sleep architecture are reversed; initial insomnia, decreased delta sleep, short REM latency, an increased percentage of REM sleep, decreased total sleep time, and decreased sleep efficiency all develop. Each of these features may be a contributing factor for alcohol relapse in dependent patients.[76–78] For recovering alcoholics, insomnia, poor sleep continuity, and decreased delta sleep can persist for several years after detoxification.[76,77] The definitive treatment for alcohol-related sleep complaints is detoxification and abstinence, in addition to treatment of co-morbid psychiatric conditions. Benzodiazepines, hypnotics, and sedating antidepressants should, in general, be avoided due to cross-tolerance, risk of alcohol relapse, and synergistic sedative effects that can lead to CNS depression should the patient relapse.

The effects of non-alcoholic substances on sleep are not as well established as are the effects of alcohol. In general, intoxication with either amphetamine or cocaine prolongs sleep latency, decreases the amount of REM sleep, disrupts sleep continuity, and shortens total sleep time. During the first week of withdrawal from these substances, patients often experience hypersomnia (a "crash") and excessive REM sleep, followed perhaps by several days of insomnia.[79]

Sedative–hypnotics, particularly benzodiazepines, shorten sleep latency, increase stage N2 sleep, and decrease REM sleep. Caution must be taken when prescribing benzodiazepines, particularly those with a short half-life, because 1 or 2 days of withdrawal-based insomnia can occur after just a few days of benzodiazepine use.[80] Opiates are also known to increase sleep and to reduce REM sleep, with rebound insomnia occurring upon their discontinuation. Chronic opiate use is also linked to central apnea.

SSRIs can produce arousal and insomnia in some patients and sedation in others. The effects of SSRIs on sleep architecture include decreased REM sleep and decreased delta sleep. They can also aggravate sleepwalking and REM sleep behavior disorder.[81]

APPROACH TO THE PATIENT WITH DISORDERED SLEEP

Once a sleep complaint has reached clinical attention, it is important to conduct a careful evaluation to correctly assess, diagnose, and treat any potential sleep disorder. Because this process can be complex and time consuming, the skills of a board-certified sleep specialist might be required. In addition, because some sleep disorders may not present with classic symptoms, if the patient has risk factors, active investigation may be considered. The following discussion is based on the general approach that many sleep specialists recommend for proper diagnosis and management of sleep complaints and disorders.

The initial step in the diagnostic process is to obtain a detailed sleep history, either through direct inquiry of the patient and his or her bed partner or by means of a sleep questionnaire. Table 24-2 provides a list of specific areas that should be addressed.[82] In addition to a detailed sleep history, patients are encouraged to keep a 2-week sleep diary that details the time and amount of sleep, the number and length of any naps, the number of awakenings, wake-up times, any medications taken, and subjective mood during the day. For patients in whom hypersomnia is the major complaint, an Epworth Sleepiness Scale—a simple, self-administered questionnaire that requires patients to rate their degree of sleepiness in a variety of routine situations)—is often given (Table 24-3).[83] In addition to the sleep history and screening examinations, a medical history including past medical history, current medications, alcohol and drug history, family history, and psychiatric history is completed.

After a comprehensive history, and if clinically indicated, the patient receives a detailed physical examination. For patients who have hypersomnia, this examination focuses on the distribution of obesity, the respiratory system, the cardiovascular system, and the oronasomaxillofacial region, with careful attention to the tongue, tonsils, uvula, and pharynx.[13,84,85] If indicated, laboratory examinations, including a complete blood cell count, blood gas analysis, pulmonary function tests, an ECG, thyroid function tests, serum iron analysis, and electrolyte count can be considered.

TABLE 24-2 Sleep History: Important Questions

- What time do you go to bed and wake up?
- How long does it take you to fall asleep?
- How often do you awaken overnight?
- Do you snore?
- Do you feel sleepy during the daytime?
- Do you experience any disturbing movement overnight including an urge to move the legs relieved by moving them? (RLS)
- Trouble moving or rolling over in bed? (rigidity)
- Abnormal postures? (dystonia)
- Do you act out your dreams overnight?

From Ashbrook, L. & During, E.H., Chapter 5 Sleep and Movement Disorders, Pages 89-113 (Table 5.1) in Miglis, M (ed.), Sleep and Neurologic Disease, First Edition. Elsevier 2017.

TABLE 24-3 Epworth Sleepiness Scale

How likely are you to doze off or fall asleep in the following situations, in contrast to feeling just tired? This refers to your usual way of life in recent times. Even if you have not done some of these things recently, try to work out how they would have affected you. Use the following scale to choose the most appropriate number for each situation:
0 = no chance of dozing
1 = slight chance of dozing
2 = moderate chance of dozing
3 = high chance of dozing

SITUATION	SCORE
Sitting and reading	______
Watching TV	______
Sitting inactive in a public place (e.g., a theater or a meeting)	______
As a passenger in a car for an hour without a break	______
Lying down to rest in the afternoon when circumstances permit	______
Sitting and talking to someone	______
Sitting quietly after a lunch without alcohol	______
In a car, while stopped for a few minutes in traffic	______
Total	______

From: Johns MW: A new method for measuring daytime sleepiness: the Epworth sleepiness scale, *Sleep* 1991; 14(6):540–545.

TABLE 24-4 Treatment Options for Commonly Encountered Primary Sleep Disorders

PRIMARY SLEEP DISORDER	NON-PHARMACOLOGIC TREATMENT	PHARMACOLOGIC TREATMENT
Dyssomnias		
Primary insomnia	Sleep hygiene Stimulus control Sleep restriction Biofeedback Relaxation training Paradoxical intention Cognitive therapy Psychotherapy	***Benzodiazepines*** Triazolam 0.125-0.25 mg hs Temazepam 7.5–30 mg hs Oxazepam 15–30 mg hs Lorazepam 0.5–2 mg hs Diazepam 2.5–10 mg hs Clonazepam 0.5–2 mg hs ***Imidazopyridines*** Zolpidem 5–10 mg hs Eszopiclone 1–3 mg hs ***Pyrazolopyrimidines*** Zaleplon 5–10 mg hs ***Antihistamines*** Diphenhydramine 25–50 mg hs ***Sedating Antidepressants*** Amitriptyline 10–75 mg hs Imipramine 25–100 mg hs Doxepin 3–6 mg hs Trazodone 25–200 mg hs ***Atypical Antipsychotics*** Quetiapine 12.5–200 mg hs Olanzapine 2.5–10 mg hs
Primary hypersomnia	Regular bedtime Avoid daytime naps	***Amphetamines*** Dextroamphetamine 5–60 mg/day Methylphenidate 5–80 mg/day Dexmethylphenidate 5–20 mg/day Amphetamine/dextroamphetamine 5–40 mg/day Lisdexamfetamine 20–70 mg/day ***Non-Amphetamines*** Modafinil 100–400 mg/day Armodafinil 150–250 mg/day

TABLE 24-4 Treatment Options for Commonly Encountered Primary Sleep Disorders—cont'd

PRIMARY SLEEP DISORDER	NON-PHARMACOLOGIC TREATMENT	PHARMACOLOGIC TREATMENT
Narcolepsy	Regular bedtime Daytime naps	***Amphetamines*** Dextroamphetamine 5–60 mg/day Methylphenidate 5–80 mg/day Dexmethylphenidate 5–20 mg/day Amphetamine/dextroamphetamine 5–40 mg/day Lisdexamfetamine 20–70 mg/day ***Non-Amphetamines*** Modafinil 100–400 mg/day Armodafinil 150–250 mg/day
Breathing-related sleep disorders	Weight loss Avoidance of sedating substances Positional therapy Oral appliance UPPP Maxillomandibular advancement Hypoglossal nerve stimulation Tracheostomy CPAP/BiPAP	Acetazolamide (for central apnea) No drugs have been reliably shown to improve obstructive sleep apnea
PLMD and RLS	None	***Dopaminergic Agents*** Pramipexole 0.125–1.0 mg hs Ropinirole 0.25–4 mg hs Rotigotine patch ***Benzodiazepines*** Clonazepam 0.5–2 mg hs ***Opioids*** Codeine 15–30 mg hs Oxycodone 5–10 mg hs ***Others*** Gabapentin enacarbil 100–800 mg hs
Parasomnias		
Sleepwalking disorder	Reassurance Maintenance of safe environment Psychotherapy Hypnosis	Diazepam 2.5–10 mg Clonazepam 0.5–2.0 mg
Sleep terror disorder	Reassurance Stress reduction	Diazepam 2.5–10 mg hs Clonazepam 0.5–2.0 mg hs
Nightmare disorder	Reassurance Stress reduction Psychotherapy Desensitization Rehearsal therapy	Prazosin
REM sleep behavior disorder	Reassurance Maintenance of safe environment	Clonazepam 0.5–2.0 mg hs Melatonin 3–12 mg hs

BIPAP, bilevel positive airway pressure; CPAP, continuous positive airway pressure; PLMD, periodic limb movement disorder; RLS, restless leg disorder; UPPP, uvulopalatopharyngoplasty.

Cephalometric x-rays of the skull and neck may be obtained by surgical colleagues to evaluate for skeletal discrepancies if craniofacial malformations are suspected as a possible etiology for any breathing-related sleep disorder.[13,84,85] PSG completes the evaluation and often confirms the diagnosis, and can be obtained with or without sleep specialist consultation.

Once a diagnosis has been confirmed, patients are offered appropriate treatment. Table 24-4 summarizes non-pharmacologic and pharmacologic treatments for the most commonly encountered primary sleep disorders.

REFERENCES

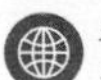

Access the reference list online at https://expertconsult.inkling.com/.

Sexual Disorders or Sexual Dysfunction

25

Linda C. Shafer, M.D.

OVERVIEW

A comprehensive psychiatric evaluation of any patient in the general hospital setting should include close attention to complaints, impairments, and deviations of sexual function. Although on occasion, sexual problems are the primary reason for consultation, more often they may provide important clues about an underlying medical or psychologic condition. Consider the "difficult" patient on obstetrics who repeatedly refuses gynecologic exams, the formerly mild-mannered elderly gentleman who now shouts obscenities and gropes at nurses, or the sexually provocative patient who evokes strong reactions from the medical team. Could the patient on obstetrics have a history of sexual trauma, the elderly man a frontal lobe tumor, or the provocative patient a personality disorder? These are a few of many examples that serve to highlight the role that understanding sexuality plays in caring for patients both compassionately and effectively.

The consulting psychiatrist should also be reminded of the importance that being able to maintain a healthy sexual life holds for many patients, regardless of the reason for hospitalization. Sexuality may take on even greater significance for patients suffering from illness that directly impairs sexual function, because of the difficulties both real and perceived. Psychiatric consultants should be alerted to high rates of sexual problems in patients with chronic diseases (especially cardiovascular disease, cancer, diabetes, neurologic problems, end-stage renal disease, and pain). Many chronic diseases result in depression, which in turn contributes to decreased sexual desire. Moreover, psychological reactions to existing illnesses run the gamut, from fear that sex can kill (post-myocardial infarction) to distress over low sexual self-image (post-disfiguring surgery), to avoidance of sex, to fear of pain during sex, to fear that sexual advances will be rejected, all leading to decreased sexual intimacy.[1]

When offering suggestions for patient management, such as prescribing a new psychotropic medication, care should be taken to minimize or treat sexual side effects as much as is possible. This may also help to improve patient rapport and compliance. In cases where sexual dysfunction appears to have a psychological component, or where longer-term behavioral, psychotherapeutic, or pharmacologic therapy may be warranted, referral for outpatient psychiatric care can be arranged. The consulting psychiatrist may be the first to diagnose a sexual problem and can facilitate the transition from inpatient to outpatient care.

EPIDEMIOLOGY AND RISK FACTORS

Sexual disorders are extremely common. It has been estimated that 43% of women and 31% of men in the United States suffer from sexual dysfunction.[2] In addition, lack of sexual satisfaction is associated with significant emotional (including depression and marital conflict) and physical (e.g., cardiovascular disease and diabetes mellitus) problems.[2–4]

Sexual disorders affect individuals across the epidemiologic spectrum. Risk factors include: female gender, older age, and co-existing psychiatric or medical (e.g., cardiovascular) disease.[2–5] It has been estimated that 10% to 54% of patients do not resume sexual activity after myocardial infarction (MI); 45% to 100% of patients with uremia or who are undergoing hemodialysis experience low sexual desire; and 26% to 50% of patients with untreated depression experience erectile dysfunction (ED).[6]

Among those with obesity and a sedentary lifestyle, weight loss and increased physical activity are associated with improved sexual function.[7,8] The association between race and sexual dysfunction is more variable.[2,9] There is a strong association between ED and vascular diseases.[10] In fact, ED may be the presenting symptom of cardiovascular disease.[11] ED may be more frequent among individuals with specific genetic mutations (e.g., polymorphisms in genes for nitric oxide synthase) in molecular pathways responsible for resisting endothelial dysfunction.[12] Sexual trauma for both sexes is associated with long-term negative changes in sexual function.[13] A strong association exists between paraphilic disorders and childhood attention-deficit/hyperactivity disorder (ADHD), substance abuse, major depression or dysthymia, and phobic disorder.[14,15] The prototypical patient with a paraphilic disorder is young, white, and male. Anxiety, depression, and suicidal thoughts or actions, as well as homosexual or bisexual orientation, are commonly associated gender dysphoria.[16]

PATHOPHYSIOLOGY

The ability to maintain adequate sexual function depends on complex interactions among the brain, peripheral nerves, hormones, and the vascular system. Disease states in these systems are associated with sexual dysfunction. However, no single comprehensive view has been established.

Brain regions involved in sexual arousal include the anterior cingulate gyrus, prefrontal cortex, thalamus, temporo-occipital lobes, hypothalamus, and amygdala.[17] The neurotransmitters dopamine and norepinephrine appear to stimulate sexual function, whereas serotonin may inhibit orgasm. Testosterone, estrogen, progesterone, oxytocin, and melanocortin hormones have a positive effect on sex, but prolactin is an inhibitor.[18]

Recent data suggest a central role for nitric oxide (NO) at the vascular level. In women, NO is thought to control vaginal smooth muscle tone; higher levels of NO are associated with increased vaginal lubrication. In men, NO allows for increased intrapenile blood flow, which facilitates erection. NO acts via the generation of cyclic guanosine monophosphate (cGMP), which has vasodilatory properties. Phosphodiesterase type-5 (PDE-5) inhibitors (the prototype of which is sildenafil) act to inhibit the degradation of cGMP, which prolongs the effects of NO.[19] Cholinergic fibers, prostaglandin E, vasoactive intestinal peptide (VIP), and possibly neuropeptide Y (NPY) and substance P may also improve vasocongestion.[20]

Sexual dysfunction may be best understood by having knowledge of the stages of the normal sexual response; these vary with age and physical status. Medications, diseases, injuries, and psychological conditions can affect the sexual response in any of its component phases, and can lead to different dysfunctional syndromes (Table 25-1).[21] Three major models of the human sexual response have been proposed.

Masters and Johnson[22] developed the first model of the human sexual response, consisting of a linear progression through four distinct phases: (1) excitement (arousal); (2) plateau (maximal arousal before orgasm); (3) orgasm (rhythmic muscular contractions); and (4) resolution (return to baseline). Following resolution, a refractory period exists in men.

TABLE 25-1 Classification of Sexual Dysfunctions

IMPAIRED SEXUAL RESPONSE PHASE	FEMALE	MALE
Desire	Female sexual interest/arousal disorder Other specified sexual dysfunction: sexual aversion	Male hypoactive sexual desire disorder Other specified sexual dysfunction: sexual aversion
Excitement (arousal, vascular)	Female sexual interest/arousal disorder	Erectile disorder
Orgasm (muscular)	Female orgasmic disorder	Delayed ejaculation Premature ejaculation
Sexual pain	Genito-pelvic pain/ penetration disorder	Other specified or unspecified sexual dysfunction

Kaplan[21] modified the Masters and Johnson model by introducing a desire stage; this model emphasized the importance of neuropsychological input in the human sexual response. The Kaplan model consisted of three stages: (1) desire; (2) excitement/arousal (including an increase in peripheral blood flow); and (3) orgasm (muscular contraction).

Basson,[23] who recognized the complexity of the female sexual response, more recently proposed a biopsychosocial model of female sexuality that consisted of four overlapping components: (1) biology, (2) psychology, (3) sociocultural factors, and (4) interpersonal relationships. Notably, this conceptualization suggested that women may be receptive to, and satisfied with, sex even in the absence of intrinsic sexual desire if other conditions were met (such as emotional closeness). The fact that physical measurements of female arousal (such as increased vaginal secretions) are poorly correlated with sexual satisfaction lends support for Basson's view.

Aging is associated with changes in the normal human sexual response. Men are slower to achieve erections and require more direct stimulation of the penis to achieve erections. Women have decreased levels of estrogen, which leads to decreased vaginal lubrication and narrowing of the vagina. Testosterone levels in both sexes decline with age, which may result in decreased libido.[24]

CLINICAL FEATURES AND DIAGNOSIS

The newly revised *Diagnostic and Statistical Manual of Mental Disorders*, 5th edition (DSM-5)[25] classifies sexual disorders into three major categories. *Sexual dysfunction* is characterized by a clinically significant disturbance in the ability to respond sexually or to experience sexual pleasure. *Paraphilic disorders* are characterized by recurrent, intense sexual urges that involve unusual objects or activities and cause personal distress or harm to self or others. *Gender dysphoria* involves conflict between one's assigned and experienced genders, resulting in personal distress or functional impairment.[25] The DSM-5 has made substantial changes to the classification of sexual disorders, as detailed later in this chapter.

The diagnosis of a sexual problem relies upon a thorough medical and sexual history. Physical examination and laboratory investigations may be crucial to identification of organic causes of sexual dysfunction. Primary psychiatric illness may present with sexual complaints (Table 25-2).[25] However, most sexual disorders have both an organic and a psychological component. Physical disorders, surgical conditions (Table 25-3),[21] medications, and use or abuse of drugs (Table 25-4)[26–30] can affect sexual function directly or cause secondary psychological reactions that lead to a sexual problem. Psychological factors may predispose, precipitate, or maintain a sexual disorder (Table 25-5).[31,32]

APPROACH TO SEXUAL HISTORY-TAKING

The sexual history provides an invaluable opportunity to uncover sexual problems (Case 1). Because patients are often embarrassed to discuss their sexuality with physicians or view sex as outside the realm of medicine, and because physicians are often reluctant to broach the topic of sex for fear of offending their patients, the need to make sexual history-taking a routine part of practice is paramount.

TABLE 25-2 Psychiatric Differential Diagnosis of Sexual Dysfunction

PSYCHIATRIC DISORDER	SEXUAL COMPLAINT
Depression (major depression or dysthymic disorder)	Low libido, erectile dysfunction
Bipolar disorder (manic phase)	Increased libido
Generalized anxiety disorder, panic disorder, post-traumatic stress disorder	Low libido, erectile dysfunction, lack of vaginal lubrication, anorgasmia
Obsessive–compulsive disorder	Low libido, erectile dysfunction, lack of vaginal lubrication, anorgasmia, "anti-fantasies" focusing on the negative aspects of a partner
Schizophrenia	Low desire, bizarre sexual desires
Paraphilic disorder	Deviant sexual arousal
Gender dysphoria	Dissatisfaction with one's own assigned gender and sexual phenotype, causing distress and/or harm
Personality disorder (passive–aggressive, obsessive–compulsive, histrionic)	Low libido, erectile dysfunction, premature ejaculation, anorgasmia
Marital dysfunction/ interpersonal problems	Varied
Fears of intimacy/ commitment	Varied, deep intrapsychic issues

Physicians should always attempt to be sensitive and non-judgmental in their interviewing technique, moving from general topics to more specific ones. Questions about sexual function may follow naturally from aspects of the medical history (such as introduction of a new medication, or investigation of a chief complaint that involves a gynecologic or urologic problem).

CASE 1

Ms. K, a 28-year-old administrative assistant without a psychiatric history, was admitted with lower abdominal and pelvic pain of unclear etiology. However, she refused a pelvic exam and pelvic ultrasound, which were deemed essential for her work-up. She threatened to leave against medical advice, and psychiatry was consulted to help elucidate her thought process and capacity to make this decision.

On interview, Ms. K was alert, oriented, lucid, and irritable. She stated, "The doctors have no right to do this to me. It's my body. They should find another way." Her angry words then gave way to tears and sadness. On taking a social and sexual history, Ms. K revealed that she had dated briefly several men, but her fears of sexual intimacy coupled with her partners' infidelities and physical and verbal abuse usually ended her relationships. Over the course of the interview, Ms. K revealed that she had been sexually molested by her stepfather beginning at the age of 12. She expressed resentment towards her mother, who "knew what was going on but stood by and did nothing."

After this history was revealed, the goal of the consultant was to gain the patient's trust and give the patient some control over her situation. The consultant took time to explain the importance of the pelvic exam and ultrasound in excluding potentially serious conditions. Eventually, the patient agreed to undergo the exams with the condition that only female providers be present and that a small speculum/ultrasound probe be used. With Ms. K's permission, the consultant brought Ms. K's suggestions to the team, who agreed with this plan. Ms. K underwent the exams uneventfully. Her work-up was unrevealing, and she was deemed medically safe to discharge home. The consultant checked back frequently during Ms. K's hospital stay and helped arrange for outpatient psychiatric care.

Screening questions include: Are you sexually active? If so, with men, women, or both? Is there anything you would like to change about your sex life? Have there been any changes in your sex life? Are you satisfied with your present sex life? To maximize its effectiveness, the sexual history may be tailored to the patient's needs and goals. Physicians should recognize that paraphilics are often secretive about their activities, in part because of legal and societal implications. Patients should be reassured about the confidentiality of their interaction (except in cases where their behavior requires mandatory legal reporting, e.g., as with child abuse).[33]

In taking a sexual history, the consulting psychiatrist should recognize that chronic illness often contributes to sexual dysfunction, whether by direct physical damage or associated psychological effects. Patients with cancer, end-stage renal disease, coronary artery disease, multiple sclerosis, and diabetes are all at increased risk of sexual problems. To explore the role physiologic illness may play in sexual dysfunction, consultants should ask questions about diseases, procedures, and medications that might affect hormone balance, disrupt normal anatomic genitalia, cause CNS dysfunction, damage vascular or peripheral nerve supply to sexual organs, or contribute to pain during sexual activity.[1]

With Internet pornography and "cybersex" activities now available on-demand, anytime, psychiatrists should be aware of increasing patient concerns about "sexual addiction." The sexual history-taker should feel comfortable exploring, as needed, the role of the Internet in the patient's sexual and non-sexual functioning and the potential for excessive and/or compulsive sexual activities. In fact, a new "hypersexual disorder" was proposed for inclusion in DSM-5, although ultimately not included in the text.[34] Yet, the possibility of impulsive, excessive sexual behavior causing distress to self or others remains. Thus, appropriate screening by a trained clinician is essential. "Hypersexuality" may be a primary problem. However, if behaviors are new or rapidly escalating, an underlying medical or neurological problem should be first excluded, particularly in the inpatient setting.

TABLE 25-3 Medical and Surgical Conditions Causing Sexual Dysfunctions

ORGANIC DISORDERS	SEXUAL IMPAIRMENT
Endocrine	
Hypothyroidism, adrenal dysfunction, hypogonadism, diabetes mellitus	Low libido, (early) erectile dysfunction, decreased vaginal lubrication
Vascular	
Hypertension, atherosclerosis, stroke, venous insufficiency, sickle cell disorder	Erectile disorder with intact ejaculation and libido
Neurologic	
Spinal cord damage, diabetic neuropathy, herniated lumbar disc, alcoholic neuropathy, multiple sclerosis, temporal lobe epilepsy	Sexual disorder—early sign, low libido (or high libido), erectile dysfunction, impaired orgasm
Local Genital Disease	
Male: Priapism, Peyronie's disease, urethritis, prostatitis, hydrocele	Low libido, erectile dysfunction
Female: Imperforate hymen, vaginitis, pelvic inflammatory disease, endometriosis	Genito-pelvic pain, low libido, decreased arousal
Systemic Debilitating Disease	
Renal, pulmonary, or hepatic diseases, advanced malignancies, infections	Low libido, erectile dysfunction, decreased arousal
Surgical Postoperative States	
Male: Prostatectomy (radical perineal), abdominal-perineal bowel resection	Erectile dysfunction, no loss of libido, ejaculatory impairment
Female: Episiotomy, vaginal repair of prolapse, oophorectomy	Genito-pelvic pain, decreased lubrication
Male and female: Amputation (leg), colostomy, and ileostomy	Mechanical difficulties in sex, low self-image, fear of odor

Physical Examination and Laboratory Investigation

Though history-taking is often the most important tool in the diagnosis of sexual disorders, the physical examination may reveal a clear medical or surgical basis for sexual dysfunction. Special attention should be paid to the endocrine, neurologic, vascular, urologic, and gynecologic systems. Similarly, laboratory studies may be indicated, depending on the degree to which an organic cause is suspected.[5,18] There is no "routine sexual panel."

Screening tests can be guided by the history and physical examination. Tests for systemic illness include: complete blood count (CBC), urinalysis, creatinine, lipid profile, thyroid function studies, and fasting blood sugar (FBS). Endocrine studies (including testosterone, prolactin, luteinizing hormone [LH], and follicular stimulating hormone [FSH]), can be performed to assess low libido and erectile disorder (ED). An estrogen level and microscopic examination of a vaginal smear can be used to assess vaginal dryness. Cervical culture and pap smear can be performed to investigate a diagnosis of dyspareunia. The nocturnal penile tumescence (NPT) test is valuable in the assessment of ED. If NPT occurs regularly (as measured by a RigiScan monitor), problems with erection are unlikely to be organic. Penile plethysmography is used to assess paraphilias by measurement of an individual's sexual arousal in response to visual and auditory stimuli. Genetic or chromosomal testing may be pertinent in the evaluation of gender dysphoria with ambiguous genitalia. For example, heritable disorders of abnormal sexual development (e.g., congenital adrenal hyperplasia, 5-alpha reductase-2 deficiency) are in some cases associated with gender dysphoria later in life.[25]

DIAGNOSTIC CRITERIA OF SPECIFIC SEXUAL DISORDERS

Male Disorders of Sexual Function

Erectile Disorder

ED (previously referred to as "male erectile disorder" and colloquially as "impotence") is defined as the inability of a male to obtain or maintain an erection sufficient to complete sexual activity in more than 75% of sexual encounters. Roughly 20–30 million American men suffer from ED; this symptom accounts for more than 500,000 ambulatory care visits to healthcare professionals annually. A number of risk factors for ED have been identified (see Table 25-6). Between 50% and 85% of cases of ED have an organic basis. Primary (life-long) ED occurs in 1% of men under the age of 35 years. Secondary (acquired) ED occurs in 40% of men over the age of 60 years; this figure increases to 73% in men who are over 80 years old. ED may be generalized (i.e., it occurs in all circumstances) or situational (i.e., it is limited to certain types of stimulation, situations, and partners). ED may be a symptom of a generalized vascular disease and should prompt further investigation.[2,10,35] Bicycle riding has also been linked to penile numbness (associated with perineal nerve damage) and to ED (due to decreased oxygen pressure in the pudendal arteries), although more research is needed.[36] Depression is a common co-morbidity in patients with ED.

Delayed Ejaculation

This disorder (previously referred to as "retarded ejaculation") is defined as a persistent infrequency of, delay in, or absence of ejaculation following normal sexual excitement in

TABLE 25-4 Drugs and Medicines That Cause Sexual Dysfunction

DRUG	SEXUAL SIDE EFFECT
Cardiovascular	
Methyldopa	Low libido, erectile dysfunction, anorgasmia
Thiazide diuretics	Low libido, erectile dysfunction, decreased lubrication
Clonidine	Erectile dysfunction, anorgasmia
Propranolol, metoprolol	Low libido, erectile dysfunction
Digoxin	Gynecomastia, low libido, erectile dysfunction
Clofibrate	Low libido, erectile dysfunction
Psychotropics	
Sedatives	
Alcohol	Higher doses cause sexual problems
Barbiturates	Erectile dysfunction
Anxiolytics	
Alprazolam, diazepam	Low libido, delayed ejaculation
Antipsychotics	
Thioridazine	Retarded or retrograde ejaculation
Haloperidol	Low libido, erectile dysfunction, anorgasmia
Risperidone	Erectile dysfunction
Antidepressants	
MAOIs (phenelzine)	Erectile dysfunction, retarded ejaculation, anorgasmia
TCAs (imipramine)	Low libido, erectile dysfunction, retarded ejaculation
SSRIs (fluoxetine, sertraline)	Low libido, erectile dysfunction, retarded ejaculation
Atypical (trazodone)	Priapism, retarded or retrograde ejaculation
Lithium	Low libido, erectile dysfunction
Hormones	
Estrogen	Low libido in men
Progesterone	Low libido, erectile dysfunction
Gastrointestinal	
Cimetidine	Low libido, erectile dysfunction
Methantheline bromide	Erectile dysfunction
Opiates	Orgasmic dysfunction
Anticonvulsants	Low libido, erectile dysfunction, priapism

MAOI, monoamine oxidase inhibitor; SSRI, selective serotonin re-uptake inhibitor; TCA, tricyclic antidepressant.

at least 75% of sexual encounters. It replaces "male orgasmic disorder," which was similar but substituted "ejaculation" for "orgasm." Delayed ejaculation is rare; fewer than 1% of men meet DSM-5 criteria. Risk factors include sexual inexperience and young age (under 35). Delayed ejaculation is usually restricted to failure to reach orgasm during intercourse. Orgasm can usually occur with masturbation and/or from a partner's manual or oral stimulation. The condition must be differentiated from retrograde ejaculation, in which the bladder neck does not close off properly during orgasm, causing semen to spurt backward into the bladder. Delayed ejaculation may also be an unsuspected cause of a couple's infertility problems. The male may not have admitted his lack of ejaculation to his partner.[37]

TABLE 25-5 Psychological Causes of Sexual Dysfunction

Predisposing Factors
Lack of information/experience
Unrealistic expectations
Negative family attitudes to sex
Sexual trauma: rape, incest
Precipitating Factors
Childbirth
Infidelity
Dysfunction in the partner
Maintaining Factors
Interpersonal issues
Family stress
Work stress
Financial problems
Depression
Performance anxiety
Gender dysphoria

TABLE 25-6 Risk Factors Associated With Erectile Dysfunction

Hypertension
Diabetes mellitus
Smoking
Coronary artery disease
Peripheral vascular disorders
Blood lipid abnormalities
Peyronie's disease
Priapism
Pelvic trauma or surgery
Renal failure and dialysis
Hypogonadism
Alcoholism
Depression
Lack of sexual knowledge
Poor sexual technique
Interpersonal problems

Premature (Early) Ejaculation

This disorder is defined as recurrent ejaculation with minimal sexual stimulation before, on, or shortly after penetration (within 1 minute) and before the person wishes it. Early ejaculation is common and was reported in nearly one-third of men ages 18–70 in an international cohort. However, less than 3% of men meet DSM-5 criteria, which specify that symptoms must cause clinically significant distress and occur for 6 months or more in at least 75% of sexual encounters. Prolonged periods without sexual activity increase the risk of premature ejaculation. If the problem is chronic and untreated, secondary erectile dysfunction may occur.[38]

Male Hypoactive Sexual Desire Disorder

This disorder, new to DSM-5, is characterized by persistent or recurrent absence of sexual thoughts or fantasies and desire for sexual activity. Symptoms must be present for 6 months or more. Unlike its DSM-IV predecessor, "hypoactive sexual desire disorder," the new DSM-5 diagnosis is specific to men, there is no "female" version. In men, sexual desire declines with increasing age. In fact, more than 2 in 5 men aged 66–74 report decreased sexual desire, compared with 6% of men aged 18–44. Yet, low sexual desire is usually not associated with clinically significant distress; less than 2% of men aged 16–44 meet DSM-5 criteria for male hypoactive sexual desire disorder.[39]

Female Disorders of Sexual Function

Female Sexual Interest/Arousal Disorder

This disorder (FSIAD) is new to DSM-5, and replaces the prior "female sexual arousal disorder" (FSAD). It is defined by reduced or absent sexual interest, thoughts, arousal, excitement, genital sensation and/or activity (with reluctant participation in and initiation of sex). Three or more of these components must be present for at least 6 months and cause significant personal distress to meet the criteria. The exact prevalence of FSIAD is not known; FSAD had an estimated lifetime incidence of 60%.[40–43]

Female Orgasmic Disorder

This disorder is defined as a recurrent delay in, or absence of, orgasm following a normal sexual excitement phase, in at least 75% of sexual encounters. Some women who can have orgasm with direct clitoral stimulation find it impossible to reach orgasm during intercourse; however, this is a normal variant. While as much as 35% of women experience difficulties with orgasm at some point in their lifetime, few report significant associated distress. The ability to reach orgasm increases with sexual experience. Claims that stimulation of the Grafenberg spot, or G-spot, in a region in the anterior wall of the vagina will cause orgasm and female ejaculation have never been substantiated, despite ongoing research. Premature ejaculation in the male may contribute to female orgasmic dysfunction.[41,44,45]

Genito–pelvic Pain/Penetration Disorder

This disorder, new to DSM-5, is defined as recurrent and persistent vulvovaginal pain or fear of pain during penetration or intercourse. It combines the DSM-IV entities *vaginismus* (involuntary vaginal spasm) and *dyspareunia* (painful intercourse), which clinically were difficult to distinguish, into a single diagnosis. Of note, genito–pelvic pain/penetration disorder can be diagnosed only in women, whereas dyspareunia was gender-neutral (albeit uncommon in men). Approximately 15% of North American women report recurrent pain with sexual intercourse, although the actual prevalence of the new disorder is not known. Contraction of the vaginal outlet as an examining finger or speculum is introduced during routine gynecologic examination may be a clue to the diagnosis. Sexual trauma and co-existing medical/pelvic conditions are important associations and potential precipitants. Lack of vaginal lubrication and other physiologic contributors to sexual pain should be first excluded.[46]

Sexual Dysfunction Disorders Affecting Both Genders

Substance/Medication Induced-Sexual Dysfunction

This disorder is characterized by clinically significant sexual impairment that is immediately temporally related to the ingestion of a specific substance or medication. The disorder should not be diagnosed during a state of delirium.[25]

Other Specified and Unspecified Sexual Dysfunction

These DSM-5 disorders replace the "sexual dysfunction not otherwise specified" designation in previous DSM editions and serve the same purpose. The "specified' modifier should be used if the clinician chooses to state the reason that criteria for another disorder are not met. Of note, DSM-5 has eliminated "sexual aversion disorder," which was characterized by marked disinclination towards partnered genital sexual contact; however, it can still be acknowledged as an "other specified" disorder.[25]

Paraphilic Disorders

Paraphilias refer to any persistent, intense sexually arousing fantasies, urges, or behaviors other than genital stimulation or fondling with a mature, consenting human partner. They may involve non-human objects or the suffering or humiliation of one's partner, children, or other non-consenting persons. Paraphilias may involve a conditioned response in which non-sexual objects become sexually arousing when paired with a pleasurable activity (masturbation). Some individuals always require paraphilic fantasies, while others rely on them during times of stress. Paraphilias run the gamut from exhibitionism (exposure of genitals to an unsuspecting stranger) to masochism (pleasure from abuse) to pedophilia (sex with a prepubescent child).[25]

Under DSM-5, paraphilias are considered disorders when they have been present at least 6 months; the individual has acted on the underlying urges; and the associated behaviors cause marked personal distress or harm to self or others. Most paraphilic disorders are thought to have a psychological basis. Individuals with these conditions often have difficulty forming more socialized sexual relationships. An interest in non-consenting partners may have legal and societal implications. Co-existent attention deficit hyperactivity disorder (ADHD), substance abuse, major depression or dysthymia, and phobic disorder are common.[25]

Gender Dysphoria

This group of disorders is characterized by discordance between one's assigned and one's preferred gender association, causing marked personal distress or impaired function for at least 6 months. It is subclassified into childhood and adult/adolescent forms, depending on the age of onset. The childhood form is typified by gender-atypical play and behavior. In contrast, adolescents and adults usually express a strong desire to rid oneself of assigned secondary sexual characteristics. By late adolescence or adulthood, 75% of boys with a history of gender dysphoria as a child will have a homosexual or bisexual orientation. Children with gender dysphoria may have co-existing separation anxiety, generalized anxiety, and depression. Adolescents and adults have a propensity for suicidal thoughts and actions as well as anxiety, depression, and paraphilic behaviors. Associated personality disorders are also common in male patients. One in 30,000 males and 1 in 100,000 females have gender-confirming (sex-reassignment) surgery.[16,25]

DIFFERENTIAL DIAGNOSIS OF SEXUAL DISORDERS

The differential diagnosis of sexual disorders includes medical and surgical conditions (Table 25-3),[21] adverse effects of medications (Table 25-4),[26–30] and other psychiatric disorders (Table 25-2).[25] Before a primary sexual disorder is diagnosed, it is important to identify potentially treatable conditions (both organic and psychiatric) that manifest as problems with sexual function. For example, treatment of depression may improve erectile function. Although paraphilic disorders often have a psychological basis, an organic cause should be considered if the behavior begins in middle age or later; there is regression from previously normal sexuality; there is excessive aggression; there are reports of auras or seizure-like symptoms before or during the sexual behavior; there is an abnormal body habitus; or there is an abnormal neurologic examination. See Table 25-7 for the psychiatric differential diagnosis of paraphilias.[25] Patients who present with gender dysphoria generally have normal physical findings and normal laboratory studies. The differential diagnosis includes non-conformity to stereotypical sex role behaviors, transvestic fetishism (cross-dressing), and schizophrenia (e.g., with the delusion that one belongs to the other sex).

TREATMENT

Organically Based Treatment

The essence of treatment for sexual disorders involves the treatment of pre-existing illnesses (e.g., diabetes); discontinuation or substitution of offending medications; reduction of alcohol, smoking, or both; increase in exercise; improvement in diet; and addition of medications for psychiatric conditions (e.g., depression). Although many medications for the treatment of hypertension inhibit sexual function, the angiotensin II-receptor blockers (e.g., losartan), are not associated with sexual side effects and may actually help prevent or correct sexual problems (such as sexual dissatisfaction, low frequency of sex, or ED).[47] Any hormone deficiency should be corrected (e.g., addition of testosterone for hypogonadism, thyroid hormone for hypothyroidism, estrogen/testosterone for postmenopausal females, or bromocriptine for elevated prolactin after neuroimaging of the pituitary). Many medical illnesses are associated with physiologic and psychological impairments that when treated improve sexual function; selected examples are shown in Table 25-8.[5]

Psychotropic Medication-induced Sexual Dysfunction

Antidepressants

Sexual dysfunction is a commonly reported side effect of selective serotonin re-uptake inhibitors (SSRIs). According to some estimates, as many as 30% to 40% of SSRI users experience anorgasmia, 10% to 20% of patients experience

TABLE 25-7 Psychiatric Differential Diagnosis of Paraphilias

- Intellectual disability
- Dementia
- Substance intoxication
- Manic episode (bipolar disorder)
- Schizophrenia
- Obsessive–compulsive disorder
- Gender dysphoria
- Personality disorder
- Sexual dysfunction
- Non-paraphiliac compulsive sexual behaviors
  - Compulsive use of erotic videos, magazines, or cybersex
  - Uncontrolled masturbation
  - Unrestrained use of prostitutes
  - Numerous brief, superficial sexual affairs
- Hypersexuality/sexual addiction

TABLE 25-8 Specific Treatments for Sexual Dysfunction Attributable to Medical Illness

DISEASE	ASSOCIATED IMPAIRMENT CAUSING SEXUAL DYSFUNCTION	TREATMENT
Coronary artery disease	Fear of recurrent MI	Reassure, encourage exercise
	Fear of nitrate–PDE-5 interaction	Switch from nitrate to trimetazidine (not FDA-approved)
	Concurrent depression	Treat depression
Renal failure	Low testosterone (men)	Consider testosterone
	Hyperprolactinemia	Try bromocriptine, 25(OH)D
	Low zinc levels	Consider zinc replacement
	Anemia	Erythropoietin
	Uremic menorrhagia	Consider cyclic or daily progesterone
	Concurrent depression	Treat depression
	Estrogen deficiency	Local estrogen therapy
Urinary incontinence	Urinary leakage during sex	Consider surgery
Diabetes	Hyperglycemia	Improve glycemic control
Elevated prolactin	Hyperprolactinemia	Treat underlying cause
Adrenal disease	Diminished adrenal hormones	Consider DHEA

TABLE 25-9 Treatment Strategies for SSRI-Induced Sexual Dysfunction

STRATEGY	COMMENTS
Decrease the dose	May diminish antidepressant effect Consider in patients on high doses
Switch SSRIs	Paroxetine linked to highest rates of sexual dysfunction Fluvoxamine may have fewer sexual side effects No clear evidence to support this strategy
Switch to a non-SSRI agent	Data support bupropion, mirtazapine, duloxetine (±), vilazodone, nefazodone (brand name Serzone withdrawn in the United States) Consider transdermal selegiline Not FDA-approved: tianeptine, reboxetine, moclobemide, agomelatine, gepirone Venlafaxine and desvenlafaxine *not* superior to SSRIs
Add "antidote" drug	Best evidence to support PDE-5 inhibitors (sildenafil, tadalafil, vardenafil, avanafil), next bupropion, then buspirone (high dose) PDE-5 inhibitors not only improve erectile dysfunction but also arousal and orgasm even in some women on SSRIs Small studies support maca root (herbal agent) Consider amantadine, dextroamphetamine, methylphenidate, ginkgo biloba, granisetron, cyproheptadine, yohimbine, atomoxetine (data mixed)
Take a drug holiday	Limited studies show no clear benefit to this approach May precipitate withdrawal and encourage noncompliance
Await spontaneous remission	Rarely occurs

decreased libido or ED, and 30% to 50% experience low desire.[5,48] Strategies to treat SSRI-induced sexual dysfunction are presented in Table 25-9.[48–58] Monoamine oxidase inhibitors (MAOIs) and tricyclic antidepressants (TCAs) also cause sexual problems. Because of their sexual side effects, the SSRIs have been used with success to treat premature ejaculation and reduce compulsive sexual acts associated with Alzheimer's disease,[59] paraphilic behavior,[60] and sexual obsessions in obsessive–compulsive disorder (OCD) spectrum patients.[61]

Antipsychotics

Typical antipsychotics (e.g., haloperidol, thioridazine) as well as atypical agents (e.g., risperidone, clozapine) are all associated with sexual dysfunction. Hyperprolactinemia may play a causal role. Most second-generation antipsychotics (e.g., olanzapine, quetiapine, aripiprazole, ziprasidone) are associated with fewer sexual side effects.[62] Antipsychotics have also been used to dampen sexually inappropriate behaviors and paraphilic behaviors.[63]

Premature Ejaculation

There is no Food and Drug Administration (FDA)-approved treatment for premature ejaculation. However, the SSRIs (e.g., fluoxetine, sertraline, paroxetine) used continuously or intermittently (2 to 12 hours before sex), can cause delayed or retarded ejaculation, which can treat premature ejaculation. Low doses may be effective. Clomipramine (a TCA) may be more effective in delaying ejaculation than the SSRIs.[64] Dapoxetine, an SSRI in phase III clinical trials with a rapid onset and short half-life, is being studied as an on-demand treatment for premature ejaculation.[65] Topical anesthetic creams (such as lidocaine derivatives) appear to be successful in slowing ejaculation without inducing the systemic side effects of antidepressants; however, they can cause local skin irritation and penile numbing that sometimes leads to erectile problems. The most popular of these agents is EMLA cream, a combination of lidocaine and prilocaine.[66] When the premature ejaculation is secondary to ED, PDE-5 inhibitors should be used to treat ED first.

Erectile Dysfunction

The mainstay of treatment for ED is the use of oral PDE-5 inhibitors (e.g., sildenafil, vardenafil, tadalafil, and most recently avanafil), which can help men with a wide range of conditions; they are easy to use, and have few adverse effects (Table 25-10).[19,57,67,68] An important absolute contraindication is the recent concurrent use of nitrates, which can lead to profound hypotension. Other potential risks include: hypotension with concurrent use of an α-blocker (e.g., for benign prostate hypertrophy or hypertension) and possibly hearing loss and development of non-arteritic anterior ischemic optic neuropathy (NAION). The PDE-5 inhibitors are effective in the treatment of antidepressant-induced ED and delayed ejaculation. Of note, the PDE-5 inhibitors are metabolized by P450 3A4 and 2C9 isoenzyme systems. Patients who take potent inhibitors (including grapefruit juice, cimetidine, ketoconazole, erythromycin, and ritonavir) of these P450 isoenzyme systems, should have a lower starting dose of a PDE-5 inhibitor. Statins may also help improve the efficacy of PDE-5 inhibitors.

Other oral agents are used to treat ED. Yohimbine (Yocon), an α_2-adrenergic inhibitor, has been available for many years and it may be useful in the treatment of psychogenic ED; however, its efficacy is uncertain. Phentolamine (Vasomax) is an α-blocker (not yet FDA-approved) that may produce erections by dilation of blood vessels. Apomorphine (Uprima) is a centrally acting D_1/D_2 dopamine receptor agonist administered sublingually (not yet FDA-approved). Although efficacious in the stimulation of erections, the drug is limited by its side effects, especially nausea and vomiting.[69] Centrally acting melanocortin

TABLE 25-10 First-Line Treatment for Erectile Dysfunction: Comparison of PDE-5 Inhibitors

MEDICATION	DOSE	ONSET	DURATION	FOOD INTERACTION	ADVANTAGES	SIDE EFFECTS	CONTRAINDICATIONS
Sildenafil (Viagra)	25–100 mg Max—one dose per day	30–60 min	4 h (up to 12 h)	Delayed absorption with high-fat foods	50–85% efficacy Longest track record	Headache, low BP, flushing, dyspepsia, vasodilation, diarrhea, visual changes (blue tinge to vision), hearing loss (rare) Non-arteritic anterior ischemic optic neuropathy (NAION)—not proven	Active CAD, hypotension No nitrates for 24 h after dose Caution with α-blockers
Vardenafil (Levitra)	2.5–20 mg Max—one dose per day	15–30 min	4 h (up to 12 h)	Delayed absorption with high-fat foods	75% efficacy No visual side effects Available as ODT preparation (Staxyn)	Headache, low BP, flushing, dyspepsia, vasodilation, diarrhea, visual changes, hearing loss (rare) Non-arteritic anterior ischemic optic neuropathy (NAION)—not proven	Active CAD, hypotension May prolong QTc May increase LFTs Avoid nitrates for 24 h after dose Avoid α-blockers (Hytrin and Cardura). Use cautiously with Flomax or Uroxatral
Tadalafil (Cialis)	5–20 mg	15–45 min	24–36 h	None	75% efficacy No visual side effects Can be taken with food More PDE5 selective	Headache, low BP, flushing, dyspepsia, vasodilation, diarrhea, back pain, myalgias, hearing loss (rare) Non-arteritic anterior ischemic optic neuropathy (NAION)—not proven	Active CAD, hypotension Avoid nitrates for 48 h after dose Avoid α-blockers (Hytrin and Cardura). Use cautiously use with Flomax or Uroxatral
Avanafil (Stendra)	50–200 mg Max—one dose per day	15 min	Up to 6 h	Delayed absorption with high-fat foods	Shortest onset of action Shortest duration Fewer drug interactions More PDE-5 selective	Headache, low BP, flushing, nasal congestion, dizziness, hearing loss (rare) Non-arteritic anterior ischemic optic neuropathy (NAION)—not proven	Active CAD, hypotension No nitrates for 12 h after dose (weaker and briefer effect compared with other PDE-5s) Start at lower dose (50 mg) if on (stable) α-blocker

CAD, coronary artery disease; QTc, corrected QT interval; LFTs, liver function tests.

receptor agonists (in development as an intranasal preparation) appear to be effective, but side effects (flushing, nausea) may limit their utility.[70] The amino acid L-arginine (an NO precursor) appears promising in men. Other agents under study include: naltrexone, an opioid antagonist, clavulanic acid (Zoraxel), a serotonin/dopamine modulator, and trazodone, a 5-HT_{2C} serotonin receptor. Herbal agents and supplements have shown limited benefit, with *P. ginseng*, *B. superba*, and *L. meyenii* (maca root) showing the most promise. Some "natural agents" in fact contain traces of PDE-5 inhibitors.

Non-approved topical agents include: alprostadil cream (Topiglan), minoxidil solution, and nitroglycerine ointment. In hypogonadal men, transdermal testosterone or clomiphene citrate may be considered. In fact, a recent large-scale set of randomized controlled trials showed improvement in erectile function, sexual desire, and sexual activity among elderly men with initially low testosterone who took testosterone therapy.[71] Second-line treatment for ED includes use of intra-penile injection therapy, intraurethral suppository therapy, and vacuum-assisted devices (Table 25-11). The third-line treatment for ED is surgical implantation of an inflatable or malleable rod or penile prosthesis. Endarterectomy or drug-eluting stents may correct ED in certain patients with underlying vascular disease.[72] Injectable gene therapies are in early investigational stages.

Female Sexual Dysfunction

The first medication for female sexual dysfunction, flibanserin (Addyi) was approved by the FDA in August 2015 after twice being rejected. It is indicated for premenopausal women with a DSM-IV diagnosis of hypoactive sexual desire disorder (HSDD); HSDD is not in DSM-5 but most closely resembles FSIAD. The drug remains controversial, given its only modest benefit with a potential for serious side effects, such as marked hypotension when combined with alcohol.[73] Besides flibanserin, the only other FDA-approved medication relevant to the treatment of female sexual dysfunction is ospemifene (Osphena), an oral selective estrogen receptor modulator indicated for postmenopausal dyspareunia (encompassed under "genito-pelvic pain" in DSM-5).[74] An alternative non-medication but approved intervention is EROS-CTD, a clitoral suction device, which is used to increase vasocongestion and engorge the clitoris for better sexual arousal and orgasm.[75]

Numerous drug trials are being done using medications approved for male sexual dysfunction (such as PDE-5 inhibitors), hormone-based therapies, and novel agents. In general, PDE-5 inhibitors are not effective in improving female sexual function, but they may benefit some women who exhibit greatly diminished genital vasocongestion.[76] PDE-5 inhibitors also appear to be effective for women with SSRI-induced sexual dysfunction. Bupropion (a dopamine and noradrenergic agonist) may increase arousability and sexual response in women. As in men, trials of yohimbine, apomorphine, and melanocortin agonists are ongoing. L-arginine may also enhance female sexual function.[41]

Testosterone (in a variety of forms), in combination with estrogen (Estratest), has been shown to improve libido, sexual arousal, and the frequency of sexual fantasies in surgically and naturally postmenopausal women.[77] However, it requires a relatively high dose, and because long-term estrogen use (including combination with progestin) is associated with risks, it is not routinely recommended. Recently, transdermal testosterone was shown to improve sexual function in postmenopausal women *not* taking estrogen, but long-term safety data are not available.[78] One agent in this category, Intrinsa, has been rejected by the FDA, while another, LibiGel, is in investigational stages. Tibolone, a steroid hormone with estrogenic, androgenic, and progestogenic metabolites, has been shown to increase vaginal lubrication, arousability, and sexual desire. However, it is also associated with an increased risk of stroke in women with osteoporosis over age 60 and has been rejected by the FDA.[79] In general, once fervent interest in hormonal

TABLE 25-11 Second-Line Treatments for Erectile Dysfunction

TREATMENT	EFFECTS	ADVANTAGES	DISADVANTAGES
Intraurethral suppository: MUSE (alprostadil)	Prostaglandin E_1 gel delivered by applicator into meatus of penis Induces vasodilation to cause erection	60% efficacy Less penile fibrosis and priapism than with penile injections Can be used twice daily	Not recommended with pregnant partners Mild penile/urethral pain
Penile self-injection: alprostadil (Caverject and Edex)	Prostaglandin E_1 injected into base of penis Induces vasodilation to cause erection	50–87% efficacy Few systemic side effects	Can cause penile pain, priapism, fibrosis Not recommended for daily use
Intracavernosal injection: vasoactive intestinal polypeptide (VIP) + phentolamine: aviptadil (Senatek)	VIP causes veno-occlusion while phentolamine increases arterial flow	Associated with less pain than alprostadil and therefore preferred by patients	Less effective than alprostadil
Vacuum constriction device (pump)	Creates vacuum to draw blood into penile cavernosa Elastic band holds blood in penis	67% efficacy No systemic side effects Safe if erection not maintained more than 1 h	May not be acceptable to partner Erection hinged at base; does not allow for external ejaculation

therapies has been tempered by associated risks of cardiovascular disease and breast cancer highlighted by landmark Women's Health Initiative (WHI) studies.

Additional novel therapies for female sexual dysfunction include intranasal oxytocin for improving sexual satisfaction. Onabotulinum toxin A (Botox) injections may help ameliorate vaginismus. Vaginal diazepam may also decrease sexual pain. In addition, sacral neuromodulation (Interstim), currently indicated for overactive bladder, has been shown in small pilot studies to increase sexual desire, lubrication, orgasm, and satisfaction.[80]

Paraphilic Disorders

Pharmacologic therapy for paraphilias is aimed at suppression of compulsive sexual behavior. The antiandrogen drugs, cyproterone (CPA) and medroxyprogesterone acetate (MPA, Depo-Provera), which act by competitive inhibition of androgen receptors, are used to reduce aberrant sexual tendencies by decreasing androgen levels (not yet FDA-approved). Treatment with a synthetic gonadotropin-releasing hormone analog (approved for prostate cancer but not paraphilia), including leuprorelin, triptorelin, and goserelin, decreases testosterone to chemically castrating levels (after an initial transient increase), and may completely abolish deviant sexual tendencies. The SSRIs and clomipramine may lower aberrant sexual urges by decreasing the compulsivity/impulsivity of the act and by decreasing aggressive behaviors. Psychostimulants, such as methylphenidate sustained-release, SR (Ritalin-SR), may be helpful when co-existing ADHD is present. Antipsychotics have also been used to treat paraphilias.[81,82]

Gender Dysphoria

The definitive treatment for gender dysphoria is gender-confirming surgery (formerly known as sex reassignment surgery), in combination with hormonal therapies to suppress secondary characteristics. Such hormonal agents include luteinizing-hormone releasing hormone (LHRH) agonists, gonadotropin-releasing hormone agents (GnRH), spironolactone, CPA, estrogens, and testosterone, with associated risks of cardiovascular and thromboembolic disease and osteoporosis. Of note, hormonal therapy alone is in general associated with significantly improved psychological symptoms and quality of life. In contrast, gender-confirming surgery is not uncommonly associated with significant regret and may actually not affect objective measures of psychological functioning.[16]

Psychologically Based Treatments

Sexual Dysfunction

General principles of treatment include improving communication (verbally and physically) between partners, encouraging experimentation, decreasing the pressure of performance by changing the goal of sexual activity away from erection or orgasm to feeling good about oneself, and relieving the pressure of the moment (by suggesting there is always another day to try). The PLISSIT model provides a useful framework for approaching treatment of sexual problems and can be tailored to the desired level of intervention. The stages are: (1) P, permission; (2) LI, limited information; (3) SS, specific suggestions; and (4) IT, intensive therapy. Permission-giving involves reassuring the patient about sexual activity, alleviating guilt about activities the patient feels are "bad" or "dirty," and reinforcing the normal range of sexual activities. Limited information includes providing basic knowledge about anatomy and physiology and correcting myths and misconceptions. Specific suggestions include techniques of behavioral sex therapy (Table 25-12). Intensive therapy may be useful for patients with chronic sexual problems, complex psychologic issues, or both. Whereas the first three stages (P, LI, SS) may be implemented by any health care provider, the last stage (IT) usually requires an expert with special training in sex therapy.[21,83]

Paraphilic Disorders

Paraphilic disorders are often refractory to treatment, and recidivism is high, but several non-pharmacologic modalities have been used with varying success. Insight-oriented or supportive psychotherapy is relatively ineffective. Cognitive-behavioral therapy (CBT) can be used to help patients identify aberrant sexual tendencies, alter their behavior, and avoid sexual triggers to prevent relapse. Aversive therapy, via conditioning with ammonia, is used to reduce paraphiliac behavior. Orgasmic re-conditioning is used to teach the paraphilic how to become aroused by more acceptable mental images. Social skills training (individual or group) is used to help the paraphilic form better interpersonal relationships. Surveillance systems (using family members to help monitor patient behavior) may be helpful. Lifelong maintenance is required.[84]

Gender Dysphoria

Individual psychotherapy is useful both in helping patients understand their gender dysphoria and in addressing other psychiatric issues. A thorough psychologic evaluation is generally required before gender confirming surgery can be performed. Marital and family therapy can help with adjustment to a new gender, including the possibility of intense and under-anticipated stigmatization and discrimination.[16,85]

CONCLUSION

Sexual problems are common in the general population, and in medically ill, hospitalized patients, the prevalence is even greater. Even when a sexual problem is not the primary reason for consultation, the consulting psychiatrist should feel comfortable and well-equipped to take a sexual history as a routine part of the evaluation. Although time and privacy are important limitations in the inpatient setting, the sexual history may reveal an unrecognized sexual concern; uncover an underlying medical or psychiatric illness; or at the very least help better understand the *patient* in a functional context, and in turn, improve the patient–doctor relationship.

With our population growing older, the potential for sexual problems is on the rise. Patients both in and out of the hospital are living with complex medical problems and taking multiple medications. At the same time, with the shifting focus of medicine from improving not only the length of life but also the *quality* of life, physician responsibility to recognize and treat sexual problems is ever greater. Consulting psychiatrists can be helpful in discerning the biological, psychological, and social factors that contribute

TABLE 25-12 Specific Behavioral Techniques of Sex Therapy

SEXUAL DISORDER	SUGGESTIONS
Male hypoactive sexual desire disorder	Sensate focus exercises (non-demand pleasuring techniques) to enhance enjoyment without pressure Erotic material, masturbation training
Female sexual interest/arousal disorder	Sensate focus exercises Lubrication: saliva, KY jelly for vaginal dryness
Other specified sexual dysfunction: sexual aversion	Sensate focus exercises For phobic/panic symptoms, use anti-anxiety/antidepressant meds
Erectile disorder	Sensate focus exercises (non-demand pleasuring techniques) Use female superior position (heterosexual couple) for non-demanding intercourse Female manually stimulates penis, and if erection is obtained, she inserts the penis into the vagina and begins movement Learn ways to satisfy partner without penile/vaginal intercourse
Female orgasmic disorder	Self-stimulation Use of fantasy materials Kegel vaginal exercises (contraction of pubococcygeus muscles) Use of controlled intercourse in female superior position "Bridge technique"—male stimulates female's clitoris manually after insertion of the penis into the vagina
Delayed ejaculation (during intercourse)	Female stimulates male manually until orgasm becomes inevitable Insert penis into vagina and begin thrusting
Premature ejaculation	Increased frequency of sex "Squeeze technique"—female manually stimulates penis until ejaculation is approaching, then the female squeezes the penis with her thumb on the frenulum. The pressure is applied until the male no longer feels the urge to ejaculate (15–60 seconds). Use the female superior position with gradual thrusting and the "squeeze" technique as excitement intensifies "Stop–start technique"—female stimulates the male to the point of ejaculation then stops the stimulation. She resumes the stimulation for several stop–start procedures, until ejaculation is allowed to occur
Genito-pelvic pain/penetration disorder	Treat any underlying GYN problem first Treat insufficient lubrication using, e.g., KY jelly Female is encouraged to accept larger and larger objects into her vagina (e.g., her fingers, her partner's fingers, Hegar graduated vaginal dilators, syringe containers of different sizes) Recommend the use of the female superior position allowing the female to gradually insert the erect penis into the vagina Practice Kegel vaginal exercises to develop a sense of control

to a sexual problem. Recognizing the sexual side effects of psychotropics and other medications is a key part of the evaluation. Fortunately, many effective treatment strategies now exist (e.g., use of PDE-5 inhibitors for SSRI-induced sexual dysfunction). With increasing understanding of the biological basis for sexual dysfunction, the opportunity to treat sexual problems should only continue to expand.

Some sexual problems may be the result of an acute illness or require only short-term treatment or medication adjustment. By seeing patients in the hospital setting and getting an appreciation of the psychological and physical limitations that patients face, consultant psychiatrists may offer creative solutions to facilitate a sexual life. The inpatient setting also provides a unique opportunity to get multiple specialists involved as necessary (e.g., urologist, gynecologist, and endocrinologist) to provide comprehensive care. Ultimately, the consultant psychiatrist may play a pivotal role in triaging the patient to an outpatient provider for longer-term management.

REFERENCES

Access the reference list online at https://expertconsult.inkling.com/.

The Psychiatric Management of Patients With Cardiac Disease

26

Scott R. Beach, M.D., F.A.P.M.
Christopher M. Celano, M.D.
Jeff C. Huffman, M.D.
James L. Januzzi, Jr., M.D., FACC, FESC
Theodore A. Stern, M.D.

OVERVIEW

Caring for cardiac patients can present a host of dilemmas for the general hospital psychiatrist. Patients with psychiatric conditions may exhibit cardiac symptoms, psychotropic agents can result in electrocardiographic abnormalities, and psychiatric manifestations may result from cardiac conditions. Because the overlap between psychiatry and cardiology is so great, knowledge of ways to manage specific problems can be of tremendous benefit. For instance, knowing how to deal with chest pain in the face of a psychiatric syndrome, an electrocardiographic complication from a psychotropic agent, or delirium due to cerebral hypoperfusion, can facilitate comprehensive and compassionate care.

This chapter focuses on three main psychiatric syndromes related to the cardiac patient: anxiety, depression, and delirium. For each of these syndromes, we will consider epidemiology, clinical manifestations, differential diagnosis, psychopharmacologic approaches, and practical management strategies for patients with cardiac disease in the general hospital. Additional information on the interface between psychiatric and cardiac care will also be provided in other chapters.

ANXIETY IN THE CARDIAC PATIENT

The assessment of anxiety in the cardiac patient in the general hospital is often complex. First, it may be difficult to ascertain whether the patient is experiencing distress as a result of a myocardial event, an acute confusional state, a primary anxiety disorder, or a complex interaction among these factors. Furthermore, there are many potential causes of anxiety for the cardiac patient, from an adjustment reaction to a serious cardiac event to the anxiogenic effects of cardiac medications administered to treat such events. Among inpatients, the threshold for treatment of anxiety tends to be lower than it is in the outpatient setting, insofar as the elevations in catecholamine levels and vital signs associated with mild to moderate anxiety may have profound cardiovascular effects in the patient who has recently experienced an acute coronary syndrome (ACS; myocardial infarction [MI] or unstable angina), coronary artery bypass grafting (CABG), or heart failure (HF).

Epidemiology

Anxiety Among Cardiac Patients

Anxiety is commonly experienced by patients with cardiovascular disease, such as coronary artery disease (CAD) or HF. Following an ACS, 20% to 30% of patients experience elevated levels of anxiety,[1] and 10% to 14% have anxiety levels higher than in the average psychiatric inpatient.[2,3] While this anxiety gradually improves in the months following ACS, 50% of those patients with elevated anxiety following ACS continue to have elevated anxiety 1 year post-event,[1] suggesting that a significant portion of patients with stable CAD may actually suffer from an anxiety disorder that warrants identification and treatment. Similarly, clinically significant anxiety is present in up to 25% of patients awaiting CABG, though in most cases this anxiety resolves in the three months post-procedure.[4] Anxiety is also highly prevalent in patients with more chronic cardiac diseases, such as HF. In patients with HF, 28% experience clinically significant anxiety, and 13% meet criteria for an anxiety disorder.[5]

Cardiac patients who are subjected to invasive technology, such as implantable cardioverter defibrillators (ICDs) or left ventricular assist devices (LVADs), may also experience anxiety, panic, and fear, oftentimes associated with these devices. A recent systematic review suggests that clinically significant anxiety is present in 27% to 63% of patients pre-implantation and 8% to 59% of patients post-implantation of an ICD.[6] Among patients who have undergone ICD placement, having received a shock from the ICD appears to increase the risk of anxiety,[6–8] though studies have not universally found this to be true.[6] The prevalence of clinically significant anxiety among patients receiving treatment with LVADs is somewhat lower, with 18% to 23% of patients reporting anxiety symptoms post-LVAD implantation.[9,10] This anxiety appears to improve as time passes following implantation.[9,11]

Anxiety Disorders in Cardiac Patients

In addition to high levels of free-floating anxiety, cardiac patients also experience elevated rates of formal anxiety disorders. Similar to the general population, generalized anxiety disorder (GAD) is commonly encountered in patients with cardiovascular disease. Among patients hospitalized for an acute coronary syndrome (ACS, arrhythmia, or HF), GAD was equally prevalent with clinical depression.[12] GAD also affects patients with stable CAD, with prevalence rates ranging from 5% to 24% in this population.[13–15]

Patients with cardiovascular disease also frequently experience panic disorder (PD), with some studies suggesting that patients with CAD have PD at approximately four times the rate of the general population.[16] Furthermore, approximately 20% of all patients who arrive at Emergency Departments with chest pain meet criteria for PD,[16] and up to 50% of patients who visit outpatient cardiology clinics for evaluation of their chest pain experience panic attacks or meet criteria for PD.[17] While some patients with PD and chest pain may not have underlying structural cardiac disease, some certainly do, and clinicians must remain open to the possibility of co-morbid cardiac illness in this patient population.[18]

Finally, cardiac patients who experience events as traumatic during their hospitalization may exhibit symptoms of post-traumatic stress disorder (PTSD). Recent studies have found that 8% to 16% of patients who have an MI develop symptoms of PTSD;[19–21] such PTSD symptoms also arise at a similar rate among patients who undergo CABG.[21,22] Studies of patients receiving intensive care for burn injuries and acute respiratory distress syndrome suggest that PTSD may be even more prevalent among cardiac patients in intensive care units (ICUs).[23,24] Finally, patients who have undergone placement of AICDs also appear to be at higher risk for PTSD. In this population, 10% to 25% have elevated PTSD symptoms,[25,26] and approximately 8% likely meet criteria for PTSD.[27] In one study, having more than five shocks from an ICD predicted higher post-traumatic stress symptoms at follow-up.[25]

Association Between Anxiety and Cardiac Illness

Anxiety and anxiety disorders may be associated with an increased risk for cardiovascular disease and poor cardiac outcomes, though the evidence for these relationships is not as strong as that for depression. Epidemiologic studies suggest that cardiac illness may lead to increased anxiety and that anxiety may also exacerbate cardiac illness. Acute and chronic emotional stress have been linked to the development of ventricular arrhythmias and to the exacerbation of silent myocardial ischemia.[28]

Among patients without pre-existing heart disease, anxiety has been associated with the development of CAD. In a recent meta-analysis involving 249,846 healthy individuals, anxious persons were at significantly elevated risk for the development of CAD and for cardiac-related mortality over the next 11 years, independent of health behaviors and sociodemographic and medical covariates.[29] This suggests that among healthy individuals, significantly elevated anxiety may be associated with physiologic changes in the body that predispose to a higher risk for the development and progression of CAD.

Among patients with CAD, the association between anxiety and cardiovascular outcomes is less clear. In a recent meta-analysis of 44 studies and 30,527 individuals, anxiety was associated with an increased risk of poor cardiovascular outcomes in unadjusted analyses; however, when controlling for sociodemographic, medical, and psychological covariates (often depression), many of these relationships became non-significant.[30] This would suggest that much of the relationship between anxiety and outcomes may be explained by other medical and psychiatric variables, such as depression. When examining specific subgroups of patients, anxiety was significantly associated with poor outcomes in patients with stable CAD but not in patients who recently had experienced an ACS.[30] It may be that a certain amount of anxiety is to be expected following ACS, and if this anxiety resolves quickly post-event, it may not have a significant impact on future cardiac health. In contrast, anxiety experienced in the setting of stable CAD may persist for longer periods of time and therefore may have more clinically significant effects on heart health. The links between free-floating anxiety and outcomes is equally unclear in patients with HF. Four recent prospective, observational studies failed to find a significant relationship between anxiety (as a symptom) and mortality, when controlling for relevant medical and psychological covariates.[31–34] However, similar to the studies in patients with CAD, some of these studies did find trends towards a significant relationship between anxiety and mortality in less-controlled analyses.[31,34] This suggests that while anxiety may be a useful marker for poor outcomes in patients with HF, its relationship with mortality may be accounted for by other psychiatric, medical, and socio-demographic factors.

While the relationship between anxiety and cardiac outcomes is not entirely clear, there is evidence that specific anxiety disorders are associated with adverse cardiac outcomes.[35] When anxiety reaches the threshold of a disorder, it is by definition more persistent, pervasive, and limiting, and carries a more significant risk in terms of cardiac outcomes. GAD has also been associated with higher rates of smoking, diabetes, and hypercholesterolemia, which may increase the risk of developing cardiovascular diseases.[36] Following MI, GAD has been associated with higher rates of mortality and cardiac re-admissions.[37] Similarly, in patients with stable CAD, GAD diagnosis predicted major cardiac events in the subsequent 2 years.[13]

PD also has been associated with the development and progression of cardiovascular disease. In a study of over 5,000 post-menopausal women, patients with a history of panic attacks in the past 6 months were at higher risk for subsequent MI, cardiac mortality, and all-cause mortality compared to individuals without a history of panic attacks.[38] Similarly, in a systematic review and meta-regression involving over 1 million patients, PD was associated with incident CAD, MI, and major adverse cardiac events.[39] These findings are supplemented by other studies that similarly have found PD to be associated with incident CAD,[40,41] though one study found that PD diagnosis was associated with a reduced risk of cardiovascular mortality overall.[41]

While there is less research available related to the relationship between PTSD and cardiac health, preliminary evidence suggests that PTSD may be harmful for cardiac health. PTSD has been associated with an increased incidence of CAD, independent of depression and other relevant factors.[42] In patients who have experienced an acute coronary syndrome, PTSD has been linked to a greater risk of major adverse cardiac events and all-cause mortality.[43]

In sum, cardiac patients have high rates of situational anxiety and formal anxiety disorders (e.g., PD, GAD, and

PTSD). While the links between anxiety (as a symptom) and cardiovascular outcomes is still unclear, anxiety disorders have been associated with an increased risk of developing cardiac disease, as well as worse cardiac outcomes and increased rates of mortality in patients with established disease. This highlights the importance of accurately identifying and treating these disorders when present in patients at risk for or with existing cardiovascular disease.

Differential Diagnosis of Anxiety in the Cardiac Patient

Anxiety in the general hospital is often a primary psychiatric problem caused by stressful medical events. However, anxiety in the cardiac patient can also be caused by a number of general medical conditions and medications commonly associated with cardiac care (Table 26-1).

Not uncommonly, cardiac events cause anxiety. Myocardial ischemia, arrhythmias, and HF can each cause anxiety owing to the sympathetic discharge associated with these conditions *and* because of what they may represent to the patient (e.g., the fear of dying, the worsening of medical illness, the loss of role identity). Other general medical conditions may cause or exacerbate anxiety in the cardiac patient; important among these is pulmonary embolism in the sedentary cardiac patient. Anxiety may also be a side effect of medications administered to cardiac patients, such as sympathomimetics. Anxiety can also result from substance intoxication or withdrawal that may be causing or exacerbating acute cardiac issues (e.g., cocaine intoxication, alcohol withdrawal). Finally, impaired sleep in the hospital (as the result of an unfamiliar setting, frequent nursing interventions, and significant noise) can lead to or exacerbate anxiety.

The general hospital psychiatrist should consider general medical causes of anxiety when evaluating cardiac patients; this is especially true when the anxiety has developed during an uneventful hospitalization, when the patient has no history of anxiety, or when anxiety persists despite appropriate treatment.

TABLE 26-1 Selected General Medical Causes of Anxiety Among Cardiac Patients in the General Hospital

Cardiac Events
Myocardial ischemia
Atrial and ventricular arrhythmias
Congestive heart failure
Other Medical Conditions
Pulmonary embolism
Asthma/chronic obstructive pulmonary disease (COPD) exacerbation
Hyperthyroidism
Hypoglycemia
Medications
Sympathomimetics
Thyroid hormone
Bronchodilators
Stimulants
Corticosteroids
Illicit Substances
Cocaine or amphetamine intoxication
Alcohol or benzodiazepine withdrawal

Psychopharmacologic Issues in the Anxious Cardiac Patient

Agents used to treat anxiety in the general hospital patient include benzodiazepines, antidepressants, and antipsychotics. Benzodiazepines are the medications most frequently used in the treatment of anxiety in cardiac patients. These medications rapidly relieve anxiety and appear to have a number of beneficial cardiovascular effects.

Benzodiazepines. Among patients with myocardial ischemia or infarction, benzodiazepines reduce catecholamine levels and decrease coronary vascular resistance.[44] Although β-blockers have similar effects, anxious patients tend to have elevations in vital signs, catecholamines, and coronary pressures as the result of their anxiety, despite the use of β-blockers; benzodiazepines can effectively treat these abnormalities. In addition, there is some evidence that benzodiazepines may inhibit platelet aggregation and raise the ventricular fibrillation (VF) threshold.[45] Furthermore, benzodiazepines are generally well tolerated by the general hospital population; low rates of hypotension, virtually no anticholinergic effects, and very low rates of respiratory compromise develop when standard doses of benzodiazepines are used. Benzodiazepines also appear to be safe even in seriously ill patients, with low rates of adverse events. Although clinicians may be concerned about the development of benzodiazepine dependence, when these agents are used in the acute care setting, at adequate doses and for appropriate indications, the risk of dependence is minimal. Benzodiazepines may even have beneficial effects on cardiovascular outcomes in specific populations, such as those with cocaine-induced chest pain.

One important caveat for the use of benzodiazepines is that they can exacerbate confusion and paradoxically worsen agitation in patients with delirium or dementia; therefore, other agents (e.g., antipsychotics) may be more appropriate for the treatment of anxiety, fear, and distress in the delirious or demented cardiac patient.

Antidepressants. Antidepressants can also be used in the treatment of anxiety in the general hospital. However, these agents often take several weeks to work and are best used to treat primary anxiety disorders, such as PD, GAD, or PTSD. For acutely anxious cardiac patients in the general hospital, when antidepressants are prescribed, it is often wise to co-administer a benzodiazepine to acutely reduce anxiety during a vulnerable cardiovascular state. Antidepressants will be discussed more extensively in the section on depression.

Antipsychotics. Antipsychotics can also be used for the treatment of heightened anxiety in the general hospital. Though no agents have specific approvals for anxiety disorders, the use of antipsychotics as adjunct treatment for anxiety in non-medical populations is now standard clinical practice. These agents have the additional beneficial effects of symptomatically treating co-morbid delirium, and they do not cause the paradoxical disinhibition that is sometimes associated with benzodiazepines. Antipsychotics, however, can cause orthostasis and anticholinergic effects (associated with low-potency typical agents and, to a lesser degree, some atypical agents) and may be associated with prolongation of the corrected QT (QTc) interval. Many atypical agents also carry a risk of weight gain, which may further predispose patients to adverse cardiac outcomes. Antipsychotics will be discussed more extensively in the section on delirium.

Other Agents. The anticonvulsant gabapentin has been used in the acute treatment of anxiety. Gabapentin is associated with essentially no risk of physiologic dependence, and does not cause orthostasis or anticholinergic effects. Its efficacy in the treatment of acute anxiety in hospitalized cardiac patients has not been formally studied. Gabapentin is also used at times to treat post-operative pain and alcohol withdrawal.

Approach to the Anxious Cardiac Patient

The psychiatric consultant is frequently called to cardiac floors to assess and treat anxiety. A careful, stepwise approach to these consultations can ensure an accurate diagnosis and appropriate treatment.

Consider a Broad Differential Diagnosis for the Patient's Distress. A primary role of the general hospital psychiatrist is to accurately characterize a patient's distress as anxiety, denial, depression, delirium, or another psychiatric phenomenon. Patients who appear anxious and tremulous may in fact be disoriented, paranoid, and frightened—that is, delirious. Therefore, the consultant should be careful in the interview to assess affect, behavior, and cognition.

If the patient's primary psychiatric symptom appears to be anxiety, the consultant should then consider the potential contribution of medications or medical symptoms to this anxiety. As noted earlier, there is a long list of conditions that can cause or exacerbate anxiety, and the consultant should carefully consider these and recommend appropriate diagnostic studies, if appropriate. It may be especially useful to note correlations between anxiety levels and the initiation or discontinuation of potentially offending medications or substances.

Evaluate Sources of Anxiety and Assess How the Patient Has Dealt With Difficult Situations in the Past. A careful psychiatric interview of the anxious patient will help determine what factors are causing his or her anxiety. Is the preoperative CABG patient anxious because a relative died during cardiac surgery years ago? Is the patient with an AICD fearful that his defibrillator will painfully discharge again? By determining the sources of anxiety, the consultant will be able to address these anxieties through education, reassurance, medication, or brief psychotherapy.

A related task is to determine the patient's coping style and coping strengths. How does he or she manage anxiety outside of the hospital? How has he or she managed difficult situations in the past? The consultant can use this information to identify the patient's strengths and determine the best approach to the patient's anxieties.

Another question for patients involves stimulation and control. Some cardiac patients crave control and wish to know every detail of their care; they feel anxious when they do not feel that they have comprehensive information about their illness and when they are not part of all treatment decisions. In contrast, other patients find such information and the pressure to make decisions over-stimulating and feel less anxious when told only the general details of their condition.

Recommend Appropriate Behavioral and Therapeutic Interventions. Having learned about the patient's sources of anxiety, coping strengths, and preferences regarding control, the consultant is in an excellent position to design a treatment plan that reduces a patient's anxiety. For example, if a patient reports that the hospitalization is overwhelming, members of the treatment team can be encouraged to limit detailed information and reassure the patient that they see this condition frequently (if true) and that they plan to provide excellent care to the patient. On the other hand, for the patient whose anxiety increases with the perceived lack of control, the treatment team can be encouraged to provide the patient with detailed information and written materials. The patient should also be included in treatment decisions; inclusion in even small decisions (e.g., the best time for dressing changes) can allay anxiety and allow the patient to feel in control.

In other cases, worried cardiac patients simply need to express their anxieties to someone. If the consultant, treating physician, and nursing staff can set aside short periods to reflectively listen to the patient's fears, this investment of time often results in significantly less anxiety, greater compliance with treatment, and less chaos for patient and staff alike. If the patient seems to have an insatiable desire to discuss his or her fears, staff can be taught to consistently set aside time to listen to the patient while setting limits on his or her time; for example, a nurse may tell the patient that she will sit with him or her for 5 minutes at the beginning, middle, and end of the shift to talk about his or her worries. If the patient attempts to engage the nurse in further conversation about this topic, the nurse can calmly tell the patient that they can discuss it at their next appointment.

Intelligently Use Psychiatric Medications for Specific Target Symptoms. Benzodiazepines are often the agents of choice for the anxious cardiac patient. If the anxiety appears to be short-term or situation-specific (e.g., whenever a procedure is performed), a short-acting benzodiazepine can be used on an as-needed basis, (e.g., lorazepam 0.5 to 1.0 mg as needed for acute anxiety). However, for most patients, longer-acting benzodiazepines given on a standing basis provide the smoothest and most consistent reduction of anxiety. Most anxious cardiac patients can be started on clonazepam 0.5 mg at night or twice per day; doses can be adjusted upward if this dose is well tolerated and anxiety persists. In general, these agents can be discontinued on discharge from the hospital if they were only used on a short-term basis.

Benzodiazepines may not be the agents of choice for patients with acute or chronic organic brain syndromes (e.g., delirium, dementia, traumatic brain injury), tenuous respiratory function (including obstructive sleep apnea), or a history of substance dependence. For these patients antipsychotics or gabapentin are often useful, alleviating agitation and confusion in delirious patients while also reducing anxiety.

We often start with doses of quetiapine at 12.5 to 25 mg at night or gabapentin at 100 mg three times daily.

Antidepressants may be useful in the treatment of primary anxiety disorders and when depression is co-morbid with anxiety; we sometimes co-administer a benzodiazepine to reduce initial anxiety associated with initiation of antidepressants.

Return Frequently to See the Patient. Anxious patients generally are relieved to see a familiar face, especially one that has attempted to understand and address their anxiety. Such frequent follow-up, therapeutic in itself, allows for careful monitoring of behavioral and pharmacologic interventions.

CASE 1

Mr. A, a 53-year-old executive without a psychiatric history, was admitted for CABG after his cardiac catheterization revealed three-vessel cardiac disease. Initially, he had an uneventful perioperative course. However, on the day after his operation, psychiatry was consulted to assess his capacity to leave the hospital against medical advice.

On interview, Mr. A was alert, oriented, lucid, and initially quite angry. He reported, "I have no assurance that I'm getting the right care; the doctors and nurses come in and out of my room and bark orders to one another but they don't include me at all. They haven't even listened to the fact that I always take my sleeping pill at 9 p.m. every night instead of 11 p.m. like they give it to me. I'm fed up." By the end of his tirade, Mr. A's anger had changed to fear and anxiety.

The consultant told Mr. A that he would bring his concerns to the team. The consultant met with members of the treatment team and encouraged them to provide as much information as possible about his care and to allow him to mandate his treatment when possible (e.g., getting his sleeping pill at 9 p.m.). The consultant, nurse, and Mr. A then met together so that Mr. A could express his concerns and the nurse and consultant could outline the ways their procedures would change so that he could have more information and more control. Mr. A agreed to this plan and also agreed to clonazepam 0.5 mg twice per day to reduce his anxiety.

The consultant checked back frequently with Mr. A to assess his response to this treatment plan. Small changes in the plan were instituted at his request, and his anxiety steadily decreased. He was discharged to cardiac rehabilitation and thanked the nursing staff for their "compassionate care."

DEPRESSION IN THE CARDIAC PATIENT

Over the past two decades, substantive research has firmly established a bidirectional link between depression and cardiac disease: Patients with depression are more likely to develop cardiac disease, and patients with cardiac disease are more likely to suffer from depression.[46] Multiple studies have also demonstrated that patients with depression and cardiac disease have worse outcomes than those without depression. These findings have underscored the importance of the general hospital psychiatrist's role in identifying depressed cardiac patients and considering appropriate treatments.

Depression in Patients With Established Cardiac Illness

Depression is common among patients with CAD, with prevalence rates of major depressive disorder (MDD) hovering around 20%.[47] This rate of MDD is greater than the prevalence of depression in the general population (approx. 15%), and is even higher for patients with more serious cardiac disease. Roughly 15% to 30% of post-ACS patients; 20% to 35% of patients with HF; and 24% to 33% of patients with an AICD meet criteria for MDD.[48–51] Rates of suicidal ideation are also increased among patients with cardiac disease.[52] Furthermore, studies indicate that most patients who are found to have major depression during a cardiac hospitalization have a history of MDD predating their cardiac event, and depressive symptoms often persist following discharge,[53,54] with more than half of patients with post-ACS depression remaining depressed after 1 year.

Despite the high prevalence of MDD and the risks it carries for cardiac patients, less than 15% of post-MI depressed patients are recognized as such.[55] Several factors likely account for these low rates of recognition. The pattern of depression (with hostility, listlessness, and withdrawal being more common than sad mood) is often somewhat atypical;[56] furthermore, depression is often seen as a normal consequence of a serious medical event, such as an ACS. Finally, most patients with ACS have brief inpatient stays, and it may be difficult to assess a patient's mood or to obtain psychiatric consultation during this limited time frame.

A review of post-MI depression delineated a number of putative risk factors for the development of post-MI depression.[50] These risk factors included smoking, hypertension, female gender, social isolation, medical complications during acute hospitalization, a history of depression, and first-time prescription of benzodiazepines (suggesting potential co-morbidity between anxiety and depression).

In short, depression is common among cardiac patients, and it has been best studied in those with recent ACS. Post-ACS depression is highly prevalent, poorly recognized, and frequently persistent.

Depression as a Risk Factor for Cardiac Disease

Evidence from many community studies over the past 20 years indicates that depression is an independent risk factor for cardiovascular disease. Several studies have found that patients with depressive symptoms are 1.5 to 3.5 times more likely to have an ACS than are those without such symptoms, while those with major depression have an even greater risk.[57–59] This increased vulnerability holds true for female patients as well as those over the age of 65, and has been demonstrated in studies with a follow-up period of more than 25 years.[48,60,61] In a meta-analysis, van der Kooy and colleagues examined 28 relevant studies comprising more than 80,000 subjects, and demonstrated that depression was associated with an increased risk of cardiovascular disease (RR 1.46).[62] This analysis found that the strongest association was made when patients were diagnosed by clinical interview and that studies using depression scales demonstrated a dose–response relationship between depressed mood and the development of cardiovascular disease.

In addition to predicting the development of CAD in healthy people, depression has also been associated with significantly higher rates of cardiac death and overall mortality among patients with established CAD. Numerous studies have found that depressive symptoms after ACS are associated with increased morbidity and mortality in the subsequent 5 years.[63–67] These effects on mortality appear to be largely independent of the severity of cardiac disease, demographic variables, medications, or other confounding factors. One early study found that depressive symptoms immediately after MI were associated with a four-fold to six-fold increase in risk of cardiac mortality in the next 6 to 18 months.[64,65] Bush and colleagues found that even minimal depressive symptoms were associated with an elevated risk of cardiac mortality, though more severe depressive symptoms more strongly predicted cardiac mortality.[66] The Stockholm Female Coronary Risk Study found that women with two or more depressive symptoms had a two-fold increased risk of future cardiac events (ACS, cardiovascular mortality, and revascularization procedures) over 5 years compared with women who had one or no depressive symptoms.[68] Similarly, a meta-analysis of 22 studies of post-MI subjects found that post-MI depression was associated with a 2- to 2.5-fold increased risk of negative cardiovascular outcomes.[69] Patients experiencing a first episode of depression in the aftermath of an ACS may be at the highest risk for negative cardiac outcomes.[70,71] In light of this overwhelming evidence, the American Heart Association in 2014 declared that depression was a risk factor for adverse events following an ACS.[72]

Depressive symptoms also appear to predict cardiac morbidity and mortality in other cardiac populations. In depressed patients hospitalized for cardiac illness, each additional point on the Patient Health Questionnaire-9 depression rating scale was independently associated with a 9% greater risk of cardiac re-admission over the next 6 months.[73] At least three studies have found that pre-CABG depressive symptoms have been associated with an increase in cardiac morbidity at 6- or 12-month follow-up.[74–76] Among patients undergoing cardiac transplantation, persistent depression was associated with increased rates of incident CAD and mortality.[77,78] Depression is a risk factor for incident HF, and several studies have shown that depression predicts higher mortality independent of demographic factors or clinical status.[48,79,80] Patients with depression at time of AICD placement have higher rates of all-cause mortality over the subsequent 4 years, and depressed patients with atrial fibrillation have higher rates of recurrence following cardioversion.[81,82]

Numerous mechanisms have been offered to explain the link between depression and cardiovascular disease. Behavioral hypotheses include continued poor health habits (e.g., smoking, lack of exercise) and non-compliance with medical care. Depressed patients appear to have decreased adherence to medication regimens, and depressed cardiac patients attend cardiac rehabilitation programs less frequently than their non-depressed peers.[83,84] Furthermore, patients who are depressed after ACS are less likely to follow recommendations about diet, exercise, and smoking cessation.[85]

Physiologic mechanisms that have been proposed in the link between depression and worsened outcomes in cardiac disease include inflammation, endothelial dysfunction, platelet activation and aggregation, and autonomic nervous system dysfunction. Two studies have suggested at least a minor contribution from inflammatory factors, including increased levels of C-reactive protein and interleukin-6 in both depression and cardiac disease.[86,87] Depression has been associated with impaired endothelial dysfunction in those with and at risk for heart disease.[59,88] Depressed patients with CAD appear to have increased platelet aggregation,[89] and this could increase vulnerability to myocardial ischemia.[90] In terms of autonomic system dysfunction, depressed patients, as well as those with CAD and HF, have been shown to have decreased heart rate variability (HRV). Further, depressed patients with CAD have greater decreases in HRV than patients with depression or CAD alone, and more severe depression correlates with a greater reduction in HRV.[91,92] Depressed patients also have increases in baseline levels of circulating catecholamines and exaggerated elevations in catecholamine levels during stress;[93] elevated catecholamine levels can result in increased myocardial oxygen demand and elevations in blood pressure and heart rate. Furthermore, elevated catecholamine levels have been associated with infarct initiation, infarct extension, and the development of VF in patients with MI. Perhaps the most obvious link between depression, increased sympathetic drive, and cardiac illness is seen in the phenomenon of Takotsubo cardiomyopathy, in which negative psychological factors, such as depression, grief, or acute loss can directly lead to a reversible cardiomyopathy that mimics an acute MI and can be fatal.[94]

The link between depression in cardiac patients and increased cardiac morbidity is likely mediated by multiple factors. One crucial question that remains unanswered is whether treatment of depression among cardiac patients improves cardiac prognosis. The vast majority of studies have not demonstrated a link between antidepressant therapy and improved cardiac outcomes, though the Enhancing Recovery in Coronary Heart Disease (ENRICHD) trial found a 40% lower risk of either death or non-fatal MI in patients treated with antidepressant medications.[95]

Differential Diagnosis of Depression in the Cardiac Patient

As with anxiety in the cardiac patient, there are a number of medical conditions and medications that can cause or exacerbate depressive symptoms. Table 26-2 lists a number of these medical influences on mood. Conditions associated with depressed mood that are common in the cardiac patient include hypothyroidism (both idiopathic and secondary to amiodarone, which is frequently prescribed to cardiac patients), Cushing's syndrome (Cushing's disease or symptoms secondary to steroid administration), neoplasm (especially pancreatic), vitamin B_{12} and folate deficiencies, and depression associated with vascular dementia.

A number of medications sometimes used in cardiac populations have been associated with depression. Steroids, methyldopa, and reserpine have each been linked with increased rates of depression. Substances can also influence mood; chronic alcohol use and withdrawal from cocaine or

TABLE 26-2 Selected General Medical Causes of Depression Among Cardiac Patients in the General Hospital
Medical Conditions
Hypothyroidism (idiopathic or amiodarone-induced)
Cushing's syndrome
Vitamin B_{12} or folate deficiency
Neoplasm (especially pancreatic, lung, or central nervous system tumors)
Vascular dementia
Movement disorders (e.g., Parkinson's disease or Huntington's disease)
Medications
Methyldopa
Reserpine
Corticosteroids
Interferon
Illicit Substances
Chronic alcohol or benzodiazepine abuse
Cocaine or amphetamine withdrawal

amphetamines commonly lead to depression. β-Blockers have long been associated with depression; however, a recent re-examination of the literature suggests a minimal association between β-blockers and depression.[96]

Because depression can have significant effects on cardiac and psychosocial outcome in cardiac patients and because the causes of depression are often reversible or treatable, the general hospital psychiatrist should consider these in all depressed cardiac patients.

Psychopharmacologic Issues in the Depressed Cardiac Patient

Antidepressants are effective in the treatment of depression for patients with cardiac disease. However, older antidepressants (i.e., tricyclic antidepressants [TCAs] and monoamine oxidase inhibitors [MAOIs]) have effects that make their use in cardiac patients difficult. TCAs have anticholinergic effects (including tachycardia) and can cause orthostasis. Even more concerning is the propensity of TCAs to prolong cardiac conduction and to have a pro-arrhythmic effect in some patients as a result of their quinine-like properties.[97,98] One study, controlling for medical and demographic factors, found that depressed patients on TCAs had more than a two-fold risk of MI, whereas selective serotonin re-uptake inhibitors (SSRIs) did not enhance risk of MI.[99] For these reasons, the use of TCAs is generally not recommended for patients with pre-existing cardiac disease.

SSRIs are now considered the best first-line medications for treating depression in patients with cardiac disease. None cause problematic orthostasis, and, with the exception of paroxetine, they are generally not associated with significant anticholinergic effects. The safety of SSRIs, particularly sertraline, has been well-established in post-MI populations. The multi-center Sertraline AntiDepressant Heart Attack Randomized Trial (SADHART) used a double-blind, placebo-controlled design to administer sertraline or placebo to 369 post-MI patients.[100] The investigators found that, compared with placebo, sertraline significantly improved depressive symptoms and was not associated with changes in ejection fraction, cardiac conduction, or adverse cardiac events. Two important limitations of this study were that patients did not begin treatment until an average of 34 days after their MI and that the patients were followed for only 24 weeks. The Canadian Cardiac Randomized Evaluation of Antidepressant and Psychotherapy Efficacy (CREATE) trial found citalopram safe and effective in treating depression in 284 patients with CAD.[101] More recently, the SADHART-CHF study found sertraline to be safe for treating patients with significant HF, though sertraline did not separate out from placebo in terms of reducing depressive symptoms or improving cardiac morbidity.[102] Our clinical experience with SSRI administration in cardiac patients has also found SSRIs to be safe, and we have safely prescribed SSRIs in post-MI patients earlier than 1 month after the MI when indicated by the severity of depression or the follow-up circumstances.

Though SSRIs had long been considered safe from the standpoint of cardiac conduction, the Food and Drug Administration (FDA) in 2011 issued a warning regarding the potential for citalopram to prolong the QTc interval and increase the risk for lethal ventricular arrhythmias such as *torsades de pointes* (TDP).[103] This warning was based on a thorough QT study ordered by the FDA, which showed a dose-dependent increase in QTc with citalopram, with an absolute increase of 18.5 msec at doses of 60 mg daily. Though a dose-dependent increase was also shown for escitalopram, the magnitude was smaller (10.7 msec at 30 mg), and no warning was issued. In 2012, the warning was downgraded to note that citalopram is not recommended at doses >40 mg in the general population, is not recommended at doses >20 mg in patients over the age of 65 or with pre-existing liver disease, is not recommended for patients with congenital long-QT syndrome, and should be discontinued in patients with QTc >500 ms. Several subsequent studies as well as a meta-analysis have suggested that citalopram does indeed separate out from other SSRIs in its propensity to prolong the QTc,[104,105] though not all findings have supported a dose-dependent relationship.[106] From a clinical standpoint, though the magnitude of increase is small and likely to be insignificant for most patients, many no longer use citalopram as a first-line agent in those with a history of or significant risk factors for heart disease, preferring sertraline instead, given its established safety.

Newer antidepressants are less well-studied than SSRIs. Venlafaxine can elevate blood pressure, which may preclude its use as a first-line agent in patients with cardiac disease. Duloxetine has not been associated with QTc-prolongation or other cardiac side-effects, and may be a reasonable second-line agent.[103] Bupropion, at therapeutic doses, does not have adverse effects on blood pressure, heart rate, or other cardiovascular parameters, and has been shown to reduce rates of smoking.[107] Furthermore, a study of bupropion in depressed patients with CAD found that this agent had a favorable cardiovascular side effect profile in this specific population.[108] Mirtazapine has few effects on cardiac conduction or vital signs, even in overdose.[109] The Myocardial Infarction Depression Intervention Trial (MIND-IT), a 24-week randomized, placebo-controlled study, found mirtazapine to be safe in 209 post-MI patients with depression, and mirtazapine often has more immediate effects on sleep than do other antidepressants.[110] However, mirtazapine is highly associated with weight gain as a result of its interaction with histamine receptors, limiting its use in patients with cardiac disease.

Psychostimulants have also been shown to be rapidly acting, efficacious antidepressants in medically hospitalized patients.[111,112] Though they may elevate blood pressure or heart rate, stimulants may be indicated in cardiac patients whose depression requires rapid treatment (e.g., depression that is severe, is negatively affecting rehabilitation owing to anergia or minimal oral intake, or is affecting the patient's capacity to make medical decisions). Stimulants are relatively contraindicated in patients with a history of ventricular tachycardia, recent MI, HF, uncontrolled hypertension or tachycardia. However, in many cardiac patients, psychostimulants can be used safely with slow dosage titration, beginning with 2.5 to 5.0 mg in the morning and increasing up to 20 mg per day.

Other Treatment Modalities for the Depressed Cardiac Patient

Several studies have also examined the efficacy of psychotherapy to treat depression in cardiac patients. Though both cognitive-behavioral therapy (CBT) and interpersonal therapy (IPT) have been shown to reduce depressive symptoms in patients with cardiac disease, effects are typically short-lived, and IPT in particular was shown to be inferior to clinical management in terms of depression scores.[95,101] One study suggested that CBT significantly improved depressive symptoms at 3 and 9 months in patients who had undergone CABG in the past year.[113]

Increasing evidence suggests that collaborative care, stepped care, and blended care models are highly effective in treating depression in cardiac populations. These programs use a non-physician care manager to identify and monitor psychiatric conditions while transmitting care recommendations from a study team psychiatrist to primary medical providers. Both pharmacologic and psychotherapeutic approaches are often utilized. Collaborative care programs have been successful for depressed patients undergoing CABG,[114] for patients with recent ACS,[115,116] and even when started in the hospital during an admission for acute cardiac illness.[117,118] In addition to improving depression, these programs have been shown to be cost-effective and possibly even cost-saving,[119] and have resulted in reduced rates of cardiac readmissions and death during the study period.[120]

Approach to the Management of the Depressed Cardiac Patient

The approach to the depressed cardiac patient is in many ways similar to the approach to the anxious cardiac patient. The consultant must first confirm that depression is the primary psychiatric symptom and evaluate for co-morbid psychiatric conditions. Furthermore, the psychiatrist must consider the presence of medical conditions or medications that can cause or exacerbate mood symptoms. Once these steps have been completed, an approach to treatment involves an identification of the patient's coping strengths and support network; it may also involve the weighing of the risks and benefits of antidepressant treatment.

Routine Screening. One of the biggest obstacles to diagnosing depression in patients with cardiac disease is failure to adequately screen. Since 2008, the American Heart Association has recommended routine screening for depression using the Patient Health Questionnaire-2 (PHQ-2) and PHQ-9 in patients with cardiac disease in all settings.[121] Given the resource burden and lack of evidence that screening alone improves outcomes, we recommend screening only in the setting of adequate treatment options. It is important to remember that cardiac patients are also at increased risk for suicidal ideation, and screening for thoughts of suicide is a crucial component of depression screening.

Consider Appropriate Psychiatric and Medical Differential Diagnoses. A positive screen for depression should be followed by consideration of alternative explanations. As with consultations on cardiac floors for apparent anxiety, we also find that consultations for apparent depression often reveal that a patient's distress is caused by another psychiatric syndrome, such as hypoactive delirium or somatic symptoms secondary to cardiac illness.

The consultant should also note the course of depressive symptoms to see if the onset or worsening of such symptoms correlated with the administration of a new medication or new physical symptoms or if there are other indications that a physical disorder might be implicated in the evolution of the depressive symptoms. The general hospital psychiatrist should also order laboratory tests and other studies as indicated.

Attempt to Identify the Patient's Coping Style and the Triggers for Depressive Symptoms. Determining the external factors that exacerbate depressive symptoms may help the consultant reduce the patient's stressors. The consultant can use this information to implement solutions that are psychotherapeutic in nature (e.g., discussing mortality and life goals) or more concrete (e.g., having family members call the patient to let him know he is missed and important to them). Identification of the patient's coping strengths—especially, how the patient has previously managed difficult situations—will inform the treatment team's approach to the patient.

Of particular interest to the psychiatric consultant are recent data indicating that patients with CAD who use a repressive coping style are at particular risk of adverse cardiac events and death.[122] Perhaps because these individuals report low levels of anxiety and depression, they were once thought to be at low psychological risk for clinical events. However, it is now thought that these individuals often fail to detect or report significant emotional distress, which could contribute to their increased risk of MI and death. The consultant should be particularly mindful of patients whose emotional cool seems at variance with the severity of their clinical circumstances.

Make Use of Existing Social Supports or Help Develop a Network. Social support has been associated with superior medical outcomes in depressed patients after MI;[123] therefore, if such social support does not exist, the consultant can work with the treatment team to consider options to improve the patient's support system. Such options could include participation in cardiac rehabilitation, having visiting nurses, or joining a support group.

Carefully Consider the Use of Antidepressant Medication. SSRIs, particularly sertraline, appear to be both safe and effective for patients with CAD, with few cardiovascular side effects. Citalopram may carry a slightly higher risk of QTc-prolongation and should therefore be used more thoughtfully in this population. Bupropion also has few drug–drug interactions and may be the agent of choice in patients with co-morbid MDD and a desire to stop smoking.

The risks and benefits of antidepressant medications should be more carefully considered in patients with recent MI and probably by extension all patients with severe cardiac disease. For most patients who have just had a MI or a CABG, we typically do not prescribe antidepressants for the onset of depressive symptoms within days after MI, both because such patients have not yet met criteria for MDD and because extensive data establishing the safety of these agents in the post-MI or post-cardiac surgery period do not exist. These patients should be encouraged to follow-up with a psychiatrist for further monitoring; alternatively, direct coordination with their primary care physician or cardiologist may allow for repeat screening in two weeks, with a plan for intervention if indicated. For patients who have evidence of pre-existing untreated MDD, however, initiation of an SSRI in the immediate post-ACS period may be indicated. Severe depression that impairs one's ability to adequately participate in rehabilitation or self-care, or the return of depressive symptoms in a patient with a prior history of severe depression, may also be indications for more aggressive treatment with medications. If available, involvement in collaborative care or blended care programs also appears to be an excellent treatment strategy for patients.

CASE 2

Mr. B, a 52-year-old gentleman with a history of MDD, was admitted to the hospital with chest pain. His electrocardiogram showed ST-segment depression in the anterolateral leads, his cardiac enzymes were elevated, and he was ruled in for an MI. Though he had not been depressed in the year before admission, he developed depressive symptoms in the days after his MI; psychiatric consultation was obtained.

On interview, Mr. B was dysphoric but alert, oriented, and able to actively engage in conversation with the interviewer. He reported depressed mood, anhedonia, and low energy, along with disturbed concentration and appetite; he denied significant anxiety. He denied feeling suicidal or being unable to care for himself. Mr. B reported one episode of relatively mild MDD 3 years earlier that responded well to sertraline (100 mg/day, for 1 year); he had also had several episodes of "feeling low" for 3 to 5 days that spontaneously resolved. He appeared to be invested in getting better, he had a strong social support network, and he planned to follow up with his cardiologist shortly after his hospitalization.

Given Mr. B's relatively mild current depressive symptoms, his history of having only one mild episode of MDD, and his ability and willingness to follow up with his cardiologist, the consultant decided to defer antidepressant treatment while Mr. B was in the hospital. The consultant contacted Mr. B's cardiologist and they agreed that sertraline should be started (given Mr. B's history of good response to this medication) if he continued to be depressed at his follow-up appointment in 2 weeks.

Mr. B had an uneventful medical course and was discharged 3 days after his MI. He followed up in 2 weeks with his cardiologist; he remained depressed and was started on sertraline. He tolerated the sertraline (100 mg per day) well, and his depressive symptoms subsided over the next 8 weeks.

DELIRIUM IN CARDIAC PATIENTS

Despite advances in the treatment of cardiac illness and the use of non-invasive procedures, general hospital patients with cardiac disease continue to suffer delirium at high rates (ranging from 3% to 72% depending on the specific illness and type of procedure).[124] The general hospital psychiatrist should be aware of the special issues in the diagnosis and management of delirium in cardiac patients.

Epidemiology

Delirium and Cardiac Disease

The incidence of delirium is 17% among those admitted to a cardiac floor,[125] 20% among those admitted for ACS,[126] up to 25% among those undergoing cardiac surgery,[127] and as high as 34% among those receiving IABP therapy.[128]

Reports of risk factors for the development of delirium in cardiac patients have varied, but it is universally agreed that the etiology of delirium in cardiac patients is multifactorial, with different factors varying in importance from patient to patient. Among biological and iatrogenic factors, there are multiple preoperative risk factors for delirium (including a history of MI or stroke, diabetes, aortic insufficiency, decreased cardiac output, dehydration, electrolyte imbalance, and the use of anticholinergic drugs).[127,129] Intraoperatively, the use of on-pump CABG surgery is associated with an increased rate of intracerebral microemboli and dysfunction of several neurotransmitter systems (serotonergic, noradrenergic, dopaminergic, and anticholinergic), both of which may contribute to delirium. Postoperatively, sleep deprivation, use of narcotic or sedative/hypnotic medications, and possibly some cardiac medications (e.g., digoxin) may cause or contribute to delirium.[124]

Delirium and Medical Outcome

Delirium in cardiac patients has been shown to be associated with longer intensive care unit (ICU) stays, ICU readmission, longer hospital stays, greater prevalence of falls, greater chance of discharge to a nursing facility, and increased mortality at 30 days and 1 year.[125,130–132] Older individuals who develop delirium in the setting of cardiac surgery have been found to have poorer short-term function in terms of independent activities of daily living.[133]

Differential Diagnosis of Delirium in the Cardiac Patient

In the delirious cardiac patient, a number of specific causes should be carefully considered (Table 26-3). Central nervous

TABLE 26-3 Selected Causes of Delirium Among Cardiac Patients in the General Hospital

Central Nervous System Hypoperfusion
Myocardial infarction/ischemia
Cerebrovascular accident (ischemic or hemorrhagic)
Hypovolemia (due to dehydration or bleeding)
Relative hypotension
Other General Medical Conditions
Electrolyte abnormalities (especially sodium with diuretic administration)
Thyroid abnormalities
Hypertensive encephalopathy
Hypoxia (during pulmonary edema)
Infections (e.g., pneumonia, urinary tract infections)
Alcohol withdrawal
Cardiopulmonary bypass
Medication-Related Causes
Digoxin toxicity
Narcotic analgesics
Benzodiazepines
Anticholinergic medications
H_2-blockers

system (CNS) hypoperfusion is a common mechanism of delirium in the cardiac population; this can result from poor cardiac output caused by HF or myocardial ischemia, from co-morbid carotid disease, from CNS bleeding (in the setting of anticoagulation), or from relative hypotension. The phenomenon of relative hypotension deserves special mention. Patients with baseline uncontrolled hypertension who are admitted with myocardial ischemia or another cardiac event are often placed on one or more antihypertensives, and blood pressure is run "low," with systolic blood pressure typically between 100 and 120 mmHg. Such patients are likely to have significant baseline hypertension, which may lead to stiffening of cerebral vessels with impaired ability to autoregulate. When these patients' blood pressure is lowered to "normal" (significantly below their baseline blood pressure), cerebral hypoperfusion and ischemia may result, leading to delirium.

Other common causes of delirium in the cardiac patient include hypoxia during HF, hypertensive encephalopathy, electrolyte abnormalities (e.g., hyponatremia in the context of diuretic therapy), and medication effects (e.g., digoxin toxicity). The general hospital psychiatrist should rule out each of these potential etiologies of delirium in the cardiac patient.

Psychopharmacologic Issues in the Delirious Cardiac Patient

The use of medications is an important component of a multi-pronged approach to the psychiatric management and treatment of delirium; such an approach also includes monitoring and ensuring safety, educating the patient and family regarding the illness, and implementing environmental and supportive interventions (e.g., placing the patient near the nursing station and frequently re-orienting the patient). This chapter will not discuss the treatment of delirium in depth, but it will touch on the topics relevant to the delirious cardiac patient.

In general, antipsychotic agents are used for the management of delirium. They can reduce agitation and psychotic symptoms and may help normalize the sleep–wake cycle. They usually are not the primary treatment for delirium, but they can reduce the risk of patient harm and alleviate patient distress until the etiology is identified and effectively treated. In general, they are quite safe.

Haloperidol has been the agent most widely used in the management of delirium. This agent can be given orally or intramuscularly, but the intravenous (IV) form is both more rapidly acting and much less associated with the development of extrapyramidal symptoms (EPS); prospective study and clinical experience have found the rate of EPS with IV haloperidol to be minimal.[134] Haloperidol generally has no significant effects on heart rate, blood pressure, or respiratory status, and it has essentially no anticholinergic effects.

Haloperidol has, however, been associated with the development of TDP. More than 70 cases of TDP have been reported to the FDA with IV haloperidol,[103] though TDP remains a very rare phenomenon, given the millions of delirious patients treated. Many of these cases were also confounded by the use of other QTc-prolonging medications and other risk factors for QTc prolongation. TDP appears more common at high doses (>35 mg/day) of haloperidol, though it has also occurred at low doses.[135]

Other typical antipsychotics sometimes used to manage delirium, such as chlorpromazine, are also associated with QTc prolongation and TDP. In the case of droperidol, concerns about its propensity to cause TDP have significantly reduced its availability and use.

More recently, atypical antipsychotics, especially risperidone, quetiapine, and olanzapine, have been used in the management of delirium. Though these agents are generally considered safe in cardiac populations, risperidone and quetiapine can cause orthostatic hypotension, and quetiapine and olanzapine have some anticholinergic effects. Many atypical antipsychotics also cause weight gain and predispose patients to metabolic syndrome, though the risk is likely lower with short-term use. There have also been concerns about the potential for atypical antipsychotics to cause QTc prolongation in patients with cardiac disease. In healthy volunteers, ziprasidone causes the greatest mean QTc prolongation of the atypicals, and although it has only been associated with TDP in a handful of cases, its use in cardiac patients is not recommended.[136] In a meta-analysis comparing side-effects of antipsychotic agents, ziprasidone and iloperidone caused the most QTc prolongation, while aripiprazole and lurasidone performed the best.[137] To date, there are no case reports of lurasidone causing QTc-prolongation or TDP. Finally, in elderly patients with dementia, atypical antipsychotics have been associated with mortality related to cardiac events (some of which may represent episodes of ventricular arrhythmia such as TdP); this has led to an FDA black box warning for these medications and highlights the caution needed when prescribing these medications in certain populations.[103]

Because hypokalemia and hypomagnesemia have been associated with the development of TDP, it is recommended that patients receiving antipsychotics for delirium have these electrolytes monitored and repleted as needed. If possible, an ECG should be checked prior to the initial dose of antipsychotic, and checked again 30–60 minutes following the dose. We recommend daily ECGs for at least two days for patients receiving standing doses of antipsychotics. If the QTc is >500 ms or increases by more than 25%, a careful risk–benefit analysis is recommended before proceeding with further dosing. Nonetheless, because TDP is a very low base-rate phenomenon and difficult to predict even in the setting of a prolonged QT interval, and because agitation in delirium may predispose patients to even greater risks, such as removing central lines and other devices, there may be an indication for ongoing use of antipsychotic agents even with significantly lengthened QTc intervals.

When QTc prolongation or other concerns preclude the use of antipsychotic medications, other second-line medications may be used for management of delirium in cardiac patients. Valproic acid is often helpful in reducing agitation and frontal disinhibition, and is relatively safe in cardiac populations. Increasingly, α_2 agonists, such as clonidine and dexmedetomidine, are being used to manage delirium. These agents should be used with some caution in cardiac patients, given their risk of hypotension and bradycardia, respectively. Trazodone is another agent sometimes used to mitigate agitation, though it also carries a risk of orthostasis. Finally, benzodiazepines are sometimes given in combination with an antipsychotic to reduce the dose of antipsychotic needed; though these agents may worsen confusion, they are effective in the short term, when sedation is urgently needed.

Emerging evidence has suggested a possible role for delirium prophylaxis in cardiac patients undergoing surgery or those with particularly high risk for delirium, though further studies are needed before this becomes common clinical practice. In a study of 126 patients undergoing cardiac surgery, those receiving risperidone after awakening post-operatively had significantly lower rates of delirium compared to those receiving placebo.[138] Dexmedetomidine, a potent and highly selective α_2 agonist, has been increasingly studied for delirium management and prophylaxis. A recent meta-analysis found reduced rates of postoperative delirium in patients receiving intraoperative dexmedetomidine, and other studies have shown lower delirium rates when dexmedetomidine was used for ICU sedation after surgery instead of propofol.[139,140]

The Practical Management of the Delirious Cardiac Patient

As with other conditions involving cardiac patients, the management of delirium involves careful diagnosis and the consideration of co-morbid conditions. Once diagnosis and etiology have been established, the general hospital psychiatrist can then implement optimal behavioral and non-pharmacologic strategies and intelligently use psychotropic agents that reduce medical risk while effectively decreasing symptoms.

Make an Informed Diagnosis of Delirium, and Carefully Consider Potential Etiologies. Delirium is characterized by an acute onset, disorientation, poor attention, fluctuation of levels of consciousness, and alterations in sleep–wake cycle. Psychotic symptoms, anxiety, worry, and reports of depressed mood may or may not be present. A careful review of the chart and cognitive evaluation (that considers orientation, attention, and executive function) can allow the consultant to use these factors to distinguish delirium from other psychiatric illnesses. Once a diagnosis has been made, the psychiatrist should work to consider all possible causes of delirium. The cause of delirium is frequently multifactorial; therefore, the identification of one potential contributing factor of delirium should not preclude the search for further potential abnormalities leading to an acute confusional state. The consultant should pay special attention to the initiation and termination of medications and their relationship to the onset of delirium; a careful review of nursing medication sheets often reveals a wealth of information that can provide important answers regarding a delirium of unknown etiology.

Aggressively Treat All Potential Etiologies of Delirium. Treating the core etiology of delirium is the only way to definitively reverse delirium; all other behavioral and pharmacologic remedies are symptomatic treatments that reduce risk and increase comfort until the primary etiologies of the delirium resolve. Therefore, treatment of urinary tract infections, vitamin B_{12} deficiency, mild metabolic abnormalities, and other seemingly minor contributing factors to delirium is absolutely crucial.

Use Non-Pharmacologic Strategies to Minimize Confusion and Ensure Safety. Having the patient situated near the nursing station or in other areas where the patient can be monitored frequently, can reduce the risk of falls, wandering, or other dangerous actions. Placing the patient in a room with a window and a clock—to help orient patients to day–night cycles—can also be useful. The use of mittens, sitters, or locked restraints may be required when a delirious patient's inability to safely navigate places him or her at risk; in almost all cases, medication should be given in combination with physical restraint to reduce discomfort and risk of harm while in restraints. The presence of reassuring family members or friends at the bedside can mitigate paranoia and agitation, whereas visitors that over-stimulate the patient may worsen symptoms. The consultant may recommend that the team either encourage or dissuade interaction with certain visitors depending on the response of the patient's symptoms to the visitors.

Use Antipsychotic Medications to Reduce Agitation and Psychotic Symptoms and Regulate the Sleep–Wake Cycle. Pharmacologic management should be strongly considered in those with hyperactive delirium or in those with significant psychotic symptoms, such as paranoia or hallucinations. IV haloperidol remains the "gold standard" for managing delirium. The protocol used at the MGH (Table 26-4) for the use of IV haloperidol considers risk factors for TDP and uses a progressive dosing schedule. An initial dose (from 0.5 to 10 mg based on the age and size of the patient and the extent of agitation) is selected and administered to the patient. If the patient is not calm within 20 to 30 minutes, the dose is doubled and continues to be doubled every 20 to 30 minutes until the patient is calm. This effective dose is then used when and if the patient again becomes agitated. Though most patients require standard doses of haloperidol (2 to 10 mg), some patients

TABLE 26-4 Massachusetts General Hospital Protocol for IV Haloperidol in Agitated Delirious Patients

Check Pre-Haloperidol QTc Interval

If QTc >450 ms, proceed with care.

If QTc >500 ms, consider other options.

Check Potassium and Magnesium, and Correct Abnormalities

Aim for potassium >4 mEq/L, magnesium >2 mEq/L.

Give Dose of Haloperidol (0.5–10 mg) Based on Level of Agitation and Patient's Age and Size

Goal is to have patient calm and awake.

Haloperidol precipitates with phenytoin and heparin; flush line before giving haloperidol if these agents have been used in the same intravenous tubing.

Wait 20–30 minutes. If patient remains agitated, double dose.

Continue to double dose every 30 minutes until patient is calm.

Follow QTc Interval to Ensure That QTc Is Not Prolonging

If QTc increases by 25% or becomes >500 ms, consider alternative treatments.

Once Effective Dose Has Been Determined, Use That Dose for Future Episodes of Agitation

Depending on likely course of delirium, may schedule haloperidol or give on as-needed basis.

For example, may divide previous effective dose over next 24 hours, giving every 6 hours.

Or may simply give effective dose as needed for agitation.

Consider small dose at night to regulate sleep–wake cycle in all delirious patients.

have required (and safely received) thousands of milligrams for agitation.[141]

If an agitated, delirious patient is or becomes unable to receive IV haloperidol (e.g., because of QTc prolongation), there are a number of other options. Atypical antipsychotics may be used, though it should be noted that they may also carry a risk for QTc prolongation and may be associated with other side effects, such as orthostasis. Consideration may be given to alternative agents discussed above, such as valproic acid, clonidine, dexmedetomidine, or trazodone, or to adding a small amount of benzodiazepine to the antipsychotic dose.

Once the agitated delirious patient has been safely and adequately sedated, there is often a question of whether to schedule antipsychotic medication or to use it on an as-needed basis for agitation. Such a decision may depend on the likely duration of the delirium, if this can be determined. For example, if the delirium is secondary to CNS hypoperfusion in a patient with low cardiac output on an IABP, such delirium may well be prolonged, and scheduling of an antipsychotic would be reasonable. In contrast, delirium in an elderly cardiac patient resulting from narcotic administration may be short-lived once the narcotic has been eliminated, and standing antipsychotics may not be needed. In most cases of delirium, we have found that it is often reasonable to schedule a low dose of IV haloperidol or an oral atypical antipsychotic at bedtime to help regulate the sleep–wake cycle, which is often seriously perturbed in delirious patients. We have found that by ensuring adequate sleep at appropriate hours, delirious cardiac patients have the best possible chance to recover.

CASE 3

Mr. C, a 64-year-old man with three-vessel CAD and no significant psychiatric history, was admitted for CABG. Though he was alert, oriented, pleasant, and cooperative before his surgery, he became angry and threatening 2 days later, reporting that the nurses were the "minions of the devil" and that he needed to leave the hospital immediately; notes revealed that he had not slept for 24 hours. Psychiatry was urgently consulted for "psychosis and capacity to leave against medical advice."

The psychiatrist found Mr. C sitting on his bed, wearing only his pajama top. He angrily reported that the nurses were stealing money from him and had injected "poisons" into him. He was disoriented to time and place, and he was unable to attend to conversation for more than a few seconds. He had pulled off his telemetry leads and not allowed the nurses to check his vital signs. The psychiatrist was able to get Mr. C to agree to stay for the moment, and after confirming a normal postoperative QTc interval and normal electrolyte levels, he persuaded Mr. C to accept an injection of 3 mg IV haloperidol. After 20 minutes, Mr. C became sedated, and he fell asleep after 45 minutes.

When Mr. C's leads were reattached and vital signs checked, he was noted to have new-onset atrial fibrillation with a rate of 119 beats/minute. His heart rate was slowed with the use of β-blockers, and he returned to normal sinus rhythm within 12 hours. He received two further doses of IV haloperidol, and 25 mg of quetiapine each night. His delirium slowly resolved over the next 6 days, coinciding with resolution of his atrial fibrillation and with treatment of a urinary tract infection, and the quetiapine was discontinued on his discharge to a cardiac rehabilitation facility.

REFERENCES

Access the reference list online at https://expertconsult.inkling.com/.

Patients With Renal Disease

27

Ana Ivkovic, M.D.
Kassem Safa, M.D.
Sean P. Glass, M.D.
Mary C. Vance, M.D.
Theodore A. Stern, M.D.

OVERVIEW

General hospital psychiatrists are frequently asked to consult on patients with renal disease, a patient population that accounts for approximately 4.5 million adults in the United States (cdc.org). Among these individuals, psychiatric consultation is most commonly requested for patients undergoing dialysis who develop depression and anxiety. However, a host of other neuropsychiatric conditions may be triggered by the psychological reactions to having renal failure, the need for renal transplantation, and the biological effects of renal impairment or its treatment. In addition, psychiatric consultation on patients with renal disease warrants particular attention to psychopharmacologic considerations involving the renal clearance of medications, the potential for renal toxicity, the neuropsychiatric side effects of medications (e.g., immunosuppressants), and the timing of medications in relation to hemodialysis (HD).

PATIENTS WITH NORMAL KIDNEY FUNCTION

Clearance of Toxins and Homeostasis

The kidneys serve to clear waste material from the bloodstream and maintain homeostasis of water, salt, and acid/base states. More than one-fifth of a person's cardiac output is delivered to the kidneys every minute, generating roughly 180 liters of filtrate every day. Only a small portion of this filtrate is excreted. This tight control is achieved by orchestrated structures called *nephrons*, the basic functional units of the kidney. Each nephron is composed of a highly differentiated vascular tuft, the glomerulus, which is entangled with a tubule that is lined by specialized epithelial cells arranged in a unique order. The glomeruli are in charge of filtering the blood through closely knit podocytes, which line the glomerular basement membrane and ensure that cellular elements as well as large macromolecules are not filtered. Renal tubules selectively re-absorb solutes and water, secrete toxins and acids, and concentrate the filtrate, resulting in a urine output that varies in volume and concentration according to one's daily intake of water and solutes. Levels of sodium, potassium, bicarbonate, calcium, phosphate, and magnesium are tightly maintained by these structures.

Volume Control

The ability of the kidneys to continuously filter a large blood volume each minute leads to its central role in controlling blood pressure.[1,2] The juxtaglomerular apparatus detects states of hyper- or hypofiltration and either decreases or increases the filtration rate via activity of the renin-angiotensin system. The collecting duct can further fine-tune the body's volume status via the epithelial sodium channels (ENaK), which are regulated by aldosterone secretion[3] that is triggered by a variety of stimuli (e.g., angiotensin II).

Endocrine Function

In addition to toxin clearance, electrolyte homeostasis, and volume status regulation, the kidneys also have an endocrine function. Interstitial fibroblasts within the kidney secrete erythropoietin in response to a decrease in oxygen tension in the blood,[4] which stimulates bone marrow erythropoiesis. Aldosterone secretion by the adrenal glands maintains euvolemia as an end-result of renin secretion by the kidneys. Additionally, the kidneys activate vitamin D (via the 1-alpha-hydroxylase enzyme), which is important for calcium and phosphorus absorption from the gut, serotonin activation in the brain, and mediation of the cross-talk between the kidneys and the parathyroid glands.[5]

All things considered—between toxin clearance, electrolyte homeostasis, blood pressure control, hypoxemia responsiveness, and vitamin D activation—it becomes clear that healthy renal function supports optimal brain function. Conversely, the presence of kidney disease should alert medical teams and consultants to the possibility of neuropsychiatric dysfunction.

KIDNEY DISEASE

Acute kidney injury (AKI), previously known as acute renal failure, is defined by an acute increase in the serum creatinine level; this abnormality is accompanied by a decreased urinary output.[6] Pre-renal, renal, and post-renal categorizations of the etiologies continue to be used. Pre-renal azotemia results from a decrease in the effective circulatory volume that is associated with hypovolemia, shock, as well as cardiorenal or hepatorenal syndrome. Intrinsic renal causes of AKI include ischemic or toxic acute tubular necrosis (ATN), vasculitis, glomerulonephritides, and tubulo-interstitial disorders.[7] Important causes of renal injury with particular relevance to the general hospital psychiatrist include drug-induced nephrotoxicity from non-steroidal anti-inflammatory drugs (NSAIDs) and certain drugs of abuse (e.g., heroin crystal nephropathy), as well as ATN secondary to rhabdomyolysis from a variety of causes (e.g., cocaine use, neuroleptic malignant syndrome, and other malignant catatonias). Post-renal etiologies of AKI include obstructive uropathy from nephrolithiasis, bladder outlet obstruction, pelvic tumors, or less commonly retroperitoneal fibrosis. AKI is widely associated with increased morbidity, length of hospital stay, as well as mortality.[8] In addition, AKI is a risk factor for the development of chronic kidney disease (CKD).[6]

CKD ranges from an increased risk status to end-stage renal disease (ESRD) and is defined by markers of kidney damage (i.e., albuminuria, abnormal urine sediment, abnormal imaging results) for more than 3 months or a glomerular filtration rate (GFR) <60 mL/min per 1.73 m^2 for ≥3 months, with or without kidney damage. ESRD or kidney failure is defined as a GFR <15 mL/min/1.73 m^2 or the need for dialysis.[9]

Epidemiology and Risk Factors

Kidney disease is a major public health problem. According to the United States Renal Data System's (USRDS) last annual report, the overall prevalence of CKD in the general population is 14%, and the prevalence of ESRD is 0.2%. Obesity, hypertension, and diabetes are the most common risk factors for developing CKD.[10] Genetics also play a role. For example, steroid-resistant nephrotic syndrome (SRNS), one of the most intractable kidney diseases, results from podocin mutations in about 25% of childhood cases and in 15% of adult cases.[11] Additionally, autosomal dominant polycystic kidney disease (ADPKD) affects 1 in 1000 individuals and results from mutations in *PKD1* and *PKD2* that affect renal tubular cell differentiation.[12]

Lithium and Kidney Disease

Widely and successfully used for the treatment of bipolar disorder, this alkali metal is known for its potential nephrotoxicity. Chronic lithium exposure is associated with an increased incidence of nephrogenic diabetes insipidus (NDI) and CKD; although both complications are uncommon, they are not rare. NDI results from lithium's inhibition of the translocation of aquaporin 2 to the apical membrane of the principal cell of the collecting duct, leading to decreased tubular permeability to water and the excretion of large volumes of dilute urine.[13] The accompanying hypernatremia stimulates thirst and polydipsia. Lithium-induced CKD manifests as a slowly progressing (over decades) kidney dysfunction with pathologic features of chronic tubulo-interstitial nephropathy including interstitial fibrosis, tubular atrophy,[14] and the development of microcysts.[15] The duration of lithium treatment is a principal factor in the development of kidney disease. In a Swedish population-based study it was found that the prevalence of ESRD was increased in patients treated chronically with lithium and that the mean duration of lithium treatment in these patients was 23 years.[16] Finally, lithium's narrow therapeutic window mandates frequent monitoring of lithium levels and educating patients about the risk of lithium intoxication. A recent Extracorporeal Treatments in Poisoning Workgroup (EXTRIP) systematic review of lithium poisoning recommended that hemodialysis is warranted when renal function is impaired and the lithium level is >4.0 mEq/L, or in the presence of a decreased level of consciousness, seizures, or life-threatening dysrhythmias (irrespective of the lithium level).[17] Of note, although lithium is contraindicated in acute renal failure, it may be used with caution in CKD. In fact, some patients who have required renal transplantation because of lithium-induced nephrotoxicity decide, in consultation with their nephrologist and psychiatrist, to resume lithium post-transplantation since it is often the only effective medication for their bipolar illness.

Paradoxically, recent data suggest that lithium may have nephro-protective properties in several animal models of AKI.[18] This is yet to be substantiated in clinical settings.

Complications of Kidney Disease

In addition to the increased morbidity and mortality associated with both CKD and ESRD, a wide array of symptoms and pathologies are linked with kidney disease. The most common cause of death in this patient population is related to cardiovascular disease (http://www.usrds.org.). Chronic inflammation, frequent shifts in hemodynamics, and disrupted calcium/phosphate metabolism are thought to contribute to the increase in cardiovascular events,[19] putting patients with CKD in the highest risk category for cardiovascular disease.[20]

Furthermore, kidney disease leads to a bevy of other complications. Anemia stems mainly from decreased erythropoietin synthesis by diseased kidneys but also from perturbed iron transport. Lower hemoglobin levels predict lower quality of life scores in patients with renal disease as compared with healthy controls.[21] Metabolic acidosis occurs frequently with progressive kidney disease, and it leads to loss of bone mass, potential acceleration of kidney disease, and altered metabolism leading to impaired nutritional status.[22] Perturbed calcium-phosphate metabolism and parathyroid hormone (PTH), vitamin D, and FGF-23 pathways are thought to contribute to vascular calcification and more frequent cardiovascular events in patients with CKD.[23]

Cognitive decline has also been associated with decreasing GFR[24] and is attributed to white matter lesions that have variable phenotypic presentations.[25,26] Furthermore, depression is highly prevalent in ESRD, and depressive affect has been related to death and cardiovascular disease in several reports[27–29] as well as non-adherence to dialysis.

Therapeutic Options for Advanced Kidney Disease

Once kidney disease progresses to ESRD there will likely be evidence of progressive anemia, acidosis, and a decreased functional and nutritional status that prompts the initiation of dialysis.[9] In 2013, according to the last USRDS data report, there were more than 660,000 cases of ESRD in the United States. Among these, 63.7% were receiving hemodialysis (HD), 6.8% peritoneal dialysis, and 29.2% had a functioning kidney transplant. Among new cases of ESRD, 88.4% initiated therapy with HD, 9% with peritoneal dialysis (PD), and 2.6% received a preemptive kidney transplant.

Dialysis

Hemodialysis (HD) became available after progress in the development of dialyzers (used primarily in war zones for AKI) in concert with the ability to create vascular shunts to access the circulation. In 1960, the first HD treatment was administered in Seattle to a patient dying from CKD. This was followed by a series of controversies (related to the selection of patients for dialysis), public attention, and finally the establishment of a Medicare program that provides universal coverage for patients with ESRD.[30]

More than 90% of patients who receive dialysis to treat ESRD are receiving HD. HD replaces kidney function by allowing the diffusion of small molecules across a semi-permeable membrane and at the same time by removing body water by ultra-filtration.[31] Access to the circulation is obtained by an arterio-venous fistula or synthetic graft that is typically placed in the non-dominant upper extremity or less often via an intra-jugular dialysis catheter. HD is most often conducted in dialysis units, three-times per week for 3 to 4.5 hours per session. More frequent HD with longer sessions, mostly provided overnight, has attracted attention over the last few years due to data that suggest better outcomes compared to standard HD.[31–33] Home-HD has also been gaining popularity over the last few years due to its convenience, flexibility,[34] and its potential for better survival rates[35] compared with in-center HD. However, it remains the least prevalent mode of dialysis. Peritoneal dialysis (PD), in contrast, is a popular home dialysis modality. It relies on the surface area and permeability of the peritoneal membrane to provide clearance and volume removal. Continuous ambulatory PD (CAPD) consists of instillation of dextrose-based solutions through a PD catheter with a dwell time of 3 to 4 hours before drainage, which is repeated 4 to 6 times per day.[36,37] It requires significant motivation on part of the patient. Automated PD consists of cyclers that assure dialysis at a pre-set frequency that is typically performed over the course of the night while the patient is sleeping, offering a convenient option especially for younger patients.[38] Unfortunately, PD is often limited to relatively short-term use, since it relies on preservation of the low but residual kidney function as well as the preservation of the integrity of the peritoneal membrane which can be affected each time PD is complicated by peritonitis.[39] The latter is a major source of morbidity and mortality in patients treated with PD, and interestingly depression has been shown to be a risk factor for its development.[40,41]

Overall, the time commitment of HD can be quite disruptive to a patient's life and it is frequently demoralizing. Depression frequently arises with HD treatments, prompting psychiatric consultation. The symbolism of being dependent on a machine for survival can also generate significant anxiety. Occasionally, patients refuse HD, prompting psychiatric consultation for capacity assessments, as illustrated by the following case.

CASE 1

Mr. C, a 62-year-old man with ESRD, was brought to the hospital by his family in the context of his refusal of HD for the past week; he was admitted for emergency dialysis in the context of a uremic encephalopathy. Upon clearing of his mental state, he informed the medical team that he wanted to stop HD, which prompted psychiatric consultation for determination of the "capacity to refuse HD."

The psychiatric interview revealed that prior to initiating HD several months earlier, he had been an active and independent man. He had hoped for a pre-emptive transplantation but he had no living donors, and his renal function deteriorated quickly, necessitating HD, which he had wanted to avoid. Although he was listed for a deceased donor, he knew that he could be waiting for several years before being transplanted. He described having a difficult time adjusting to being dependent on a machine, which was in marked contrast to the independence he valued about himself. He felt it was demoralizing to be surrounded by sick people on HD. In this context, he developed multiple neurovegetative symptoms of depression including anhedonia. In recent weeks, this had been intensifying, but he was too ashamed to seek psychiatric treatment and felt it would be easier to let nature "take its course." The consulting psychiatrist diagnosed him as having depression and initiated a trial of methylphenidate (for more rapid onset and his profound anergia) as well as sertraline. Mr. C felt better quickly, became more hopeful, and agreed to continue HD upon hospital discharge. With continued treatment of his depression, he remained adherent to HD and years later, was successfully transplanted.

Kidney Transplantation

Compared with dialysis, kidney transplantation is the best therapeutic modality for ESRD in terms of cost-effectiveness,[42] quality of life,[43] and survival.[44] It is also associated with improved cognitive function[45] compared with HD.

Currently in the United States, there are about 100,000 patients awaiting a kidney transplant. Annually, about 17,000 kidney transplants are performed across the nation; approximately two-thirds of these originate from deceased donors, and one-third from living donors.[46] As wait times on dialysis increase pre-transplantation they are associated with worse patient and graft survival post-transplant,[47] and as a result pre-emptive kidney transplantation is encouraged in patients with advanced stages of CKD for whom a living donor is available. The advantages of kidney transplantation come at the cost of life-long immunosuppressive medications required to prevent graft rejection. The most commonly used regimen is a triple immunosuppression with a calcineurin inhibitor (CNI; e.g., tacrolimus), an anti-proliferative agent (i.e., mycophenolic acid derivatives), and steroids.[46] Calcineurin inhibitors have a wide array of side effects, prompting the emergence of new CNI-sparing regimens with promising outcomes.[48,49] Steroid-free regimens are used in about 40% of patients after kidney transplantation[46] offering metabolic advantages[50] and neuropsychiatric benefits (e.g., decreased risk of affective psychosis by avoiding high-dose steroids post-transplant). Unfortunately, improved short-term outcomes with kidney transplantation are not yet paralleled by a similar improvement of long-term outcomes. As such, the half-life of a kidney allograft ranges between 11 and 16 years depending on whether it originates from a deceased or a living donor, respectively.[46] Most patients, particularly younger ones, have to cope with progressive CKD and they undergo kidney transplantation more than once during their lives. Non-adherence to immunosuppressive medications is prevalent in adolescent transplant recipients and is thought to be the cause of worse long-term outcomes in this age group.[51,52] Depression has been correlated to intentional non-adherence to immunosuppressive medication[53] and is a relative contraindication for kidney transplantation if untreated.

Psychiatric Disorders in ESRD

The general hospital psychiatrist should be familiar with the array of psychiatric syndromes that arise in patients with ESRD. Accumulating evidence points to the role of biological stress-mediators, especially hormones that affect the central nervous system (CNS) and hypothalamus–pituitary–adrenal axis, in precipitating and exacerbating mental disturbances in individuals with medical illnesses.[54] Patients with renal disease are no exception. Indeed, the abnormal peptide and steroid metabolism that occurs in ESRD creates a milieu of chronic stress. This, in conjunction with psychosocial factors, can precipitate and exacerbate psychiatric conditions that involve depression, anxiety, and cognitive impairment. Multiple treatments have been studied and continue to be assessed for their efficacy in treating psychiatric co-morbidities in the context of ESRD.

Depression and Anxiety

Depressive disorders and anxiety disorders are the best-studied and most common psychiatric illnesses in ESRD. One study of patients with CKD not on HD found that one-third had depressive symptoms and nearly one-third (31%) had anxiety symptoms,[55] although depression rates generally range from 20% to 30%[54] in patients with ESRD depending on the population assessed and questionnaire used; anxiety rates range from 12% to 52%.[56] According to a 2013 meta-analysis, the prevalence of depression in patients on dialysis was 22.8% as measured by clinician-administered scales, while it was 39.3% when measured by self-rated scales,[57] suggesting an over-estimation of depression when self-rated measures were utilized.

Of the numerous screening instruments available to assess depression, the Beck Depression Inventory (BDI) has been validated in patients on HD; a cut-off score of 14 to 16 has been suggested to have the highest sensitivity and specificity to make a depression diagnosis.[58] Multiple reliable instruments exist for the measurement of anxiety symptoms, but there is no consensus yet on a best screening tool for use in patients with ESRD.

Depression is a well-known condition linked with increased morbidity and mortality and it has been linked to poor outcome in CKD. Loosman and colleagues[55] recently showed that patients with CKD with depression were more likely to progress to adverse events (such as death, initiation of dialysis, and hospitalization) than were non-depressed patients with CKD. Patients with CKD and anxiety also trended towards progression to these outcomes, but results did not reach statistical significance. Although co-morbid depression and anxiety have been thought to compound the risk of a poor outcome,[54] the Loosman study did not demonstrate an additive effect of co-morbidity on clinical outcome.

The findings cited above apply to adults, but the impact of depression and anxiety on outcome of CKD has been assessed in children as well. In one Turkish study,[59] children and adolescents on dialysis had significantly higher depression scores than did healthy controls. Interestingly, pediatric transplant recipients also had significantly lower state anxiety scores than did healthy controls. Quality of life total scores were significantly lower for both children on dialysis and their parents than healthy control children and their parents. Moreover, quality of life scores were consistently higher for transplant patients than for dialysis patients, but the differences between these did not reach statistical significance.

The treatment options available to depressed individuals with ESRD mirror those for the general population and include psychotherapeutic and pharmacotherapeutic modalities. Few trials have been conducted to assess medications for depression in ESRD, and the data for therapy are even more limited. Selective serotonin re-uptake inhibitors (SSRIs) are recommended as first-line agents due to studies that demonstrate their efficacy in ESRD patients as well as their favorable side effect profiles compared with other antidepressants. Serotonin norepinephrine re-uptake inhibitors (SNRIs) are regarded similarly. Tricyclic antidepressants (TCAs) and monoamine oxidase inhibitors (MAOIs) should be used with caution, if at all, due to their potential adverse effects (e.g., arrhythmias, drug–drug interactions, orthostatic hypotension) that are exacerbated in dialysis patients. Additional details on psychopharmacologic considerations in renal impairment are reviewed later in this chapter. There are very few trials that have assessed treatment options for anxiety disorders in patients with ESRD. Clinical practice has shifted away from the use of older anxiolytics (such as benzodiazepines and barbiturates) with more severe side effects, and towards newer agents (such as SSRIs, SNRIs, and buspirone). The same cautions for dose adjustments in renal impairment exist as for depression.

Cognitive Impairment

Cognitive impairment in ESRD is common and under-recognized, with an estimated prevalence of 16% to 38%.[60] Disorders of cognition found in CKD range in acuity and severity from mild cognitive impairment (MCI) to dementia to delirium, and some manifestations (e.g., dialysis dementia) specific to ESRD are associated with aluminum toxicity, the delirium syndromes of uremic encephalopathy, and dialysis disequilibrium.

Many screening tools are available for the assessment of cognitive status, and one can be selected based on the amount of time it takes to administer and the degree of diagnostic accuracy required. The Mini-Mental State Exam (MMSE) and the Montreal Cognitive Assessment (MoCA) are two brief and popular instruments. Shorter exams tend to sacrifice specificity for sensitivity, and more extensive neuropsychological testing may be necessary when assessing complicated cases, decision-making capacity, or transplant candidacy.

Recognizing cognitive impairment in patients with chronic illness, including ESRD, helps to rule out and treat reversible causes of declining cognition. When the cause is not reversible, impaired cognition interferes with self-care and decision-making and should be taken into account in treatment planning, including planning for end-of-life care. Moreover, dementia is known to be associated with poor outcomes, including withdrawal from dialysis as well as increased morbidity and a higher mortality rate.[60]

Treatment options with disease-modifying potential in Alzheimer's dementia fall into two drug classes, the cholinesterase inhibitors (e.g., donepezil, rivastigmine) and the N-methyl-D-aspartate receptor antagonists (e.g., memantine). While the benefit of these medications is modest (i.e., delaying cognitive decline by perhaps 4 to 6 months), there is a paucity of data for their safety or efficacy in ESRD. Since memantine is excreted renally, it is important to reduce the dosing for patients with renal impairment.

Management of behavioral symptoms in patients with ESRD and dementia or delirium can also be gleaned from the literature and from other populations; it involves a stepped approach: environmental modifications; psychosocial interventions; and use pharmacologic agents. Based on studies that have shown an increased risk of stroke and death in patients with dementia treated with these medications, antipsychotics should be used with caution.

Specific to patients receiving HD, dialysis is known to reverse uremic encephalopathy, but it is unclear whether more extensive dialysis would further improve cognition. In general, treatment decisions in mild cognitive impairment, dementia, and delirium for patients with ESRD should be individualized, as there is a lack of relevant literature and clinical guidelines.

TREATMENT CONSIDERATIONS

When considering treatment options for patients with CKD, depression, and anxiety, pharmacotherapy and psychotherapy are the mainstays of treatment. Since psychopharmacologic considerations in CKD have been covered elsewhere in this chapter, here, we focus on other treatment considerations (including psychosocial factors that impact mental health in chronic illness).

Although depression, anxiety, and cognitive impairment are recognizable entities that often receive more attention from clinicians, the impact of "softer" psychosocial factors on well-being in the ESRD population should not be under-emphasized. Studies have shown that social support is linked to improved adherence and to greater survival rates in patients receiving HD.[61] The quality of marital relationships also differentially impacts the course of medical illnesses, with marital conflict related to worse outcome and marital satisfaction to better outcome.[62] Finally, societally and institutionally mediated factors should be kept in mind: minority race, lower socioeconomic status, and residence in poorer neighborhoods have been associated with worse outcomes in those with chronic illness as well as in those with ESRD.[63]

Beyond the provision of medical interventions, clinicians' efforts to address the psychosocial aspects of a patient's life directly may have a positive impact on his or her emotional well-being. A recent qualitative study[64] assessed the use of two low-cost interventions to elicit emotional issues during the clinical interview. These included the Patient Issues Sheet (asking about topics that patients wanted to discuss, such as "enjoying life," "worrying about the future," "diet") and direct questioning during the office visit about emotions. It was found that both of these interventions were feasible, acceptable, and generally positively regarded by patients and by clinicians.

Renal transplantation and the modality of renal replacement therapy have also been shown to impact depression, anxiety, and cognition in patients with ESRD. According to a study by Ozcan and colleagues,[65] measures of depression, anxiety, and cognition were better in patients following renal transplantation than in patients receiving PD or HD. Specifically for the cognitive functioning scale, renal transplant recipients scored significantly higher than did PD patients, who scored significantly higher than did HD patients.

Neurologic Complications in Renal Failure

Neurologic complications contribute to the morbidity and mortality in patients with renal failure and are related either directly to renal impairment itself or from its various treatment modalities (e.g., RRT, kidney transplantation, and associated immunosuppression).

Central Nervous System Complications

CNS dysfunction typically occurs when the glomerular filtration rate (GFR) drops below 10 ml/min. The most common and disabling CNS complication is encephalopathy. Encephalopathy in ESRD is often multi-factorial and results from a combination of uremic toxins (i.e., uremic encephalopathy), other metabolic abnormalities (e.g., acidosis, hyponatremia, hypocalcemia), and the underlying disorders that led to renal failure (e.g., hypertension).[66]

Uremic encephalopathy presents with a variety of changes in mental status, ranging from mild confusional states and personality changes to deep coma. Motor findings (e.g., asterixis, focal motor signs, and the "uremic twitch-convulsive" syndrome[67]) are often present.[68] Its presentation is most dramatic in the context of AKI, whereas milder, insidious forms that are manifested by subtle cognitive deficits and personality changes are more typical in CKD. Because chronic uremic encephalopathy presents more subtly and can resemble other conditions (e.g., hypertensive encephalopathy, medication side effects, or depression), the diagnosis is often missed.[68] Patients with uremic encephalopathy typically improve with dialysis; however, the degree of encephalopathy correlates poorly with degree of azotemia.[67] EEG findings in this condition are non-specific and typically include generalized slowing.[69] The diagnosis of uremic encephalopathy is made clinically and supported by improvement with dialysis or successful renal transplantation.

Other important causes of encephalopathy in renal failure include: Wernicke's encephalopathy (from accelerated loss of thiamine with dialysis); dialysis encephalopathy (or, "dialysis dementia," a now rare but progressive syndrome of dysarthria, mental status changes, myoclonus, and seizures arising from the use of aluminum-based phosphate binders or aluminum-containing dialysate); rejection encephalopathy (a confusional state occurring in the context of transplant rejection, presumably from excess cytokine production); hypertensive encephalopathy (characterized by confusion, headaches, nausea, and visual disturbances and rarely associated with the use of recombinant human erythropoietin for treatment of renal anemia); dysequilibrium syndrome (a short-lived state attributed to dialysis-related fluid and electrolyte shifts and characterized by altered mentation, headache, nausea, cramps, and seizures within 24 hours post-dialysis); other metabolic encephalopathies (e.g., from acidosis, hypercalcemia, hypermagnesemia, hypo- and hypernatremia); and drug toxicity (e.g., from accumulation of renally excreted drugs, altered protein-binding in renal failure, or neurotoxicity of immunosuppressive drugs in transplant patients).[67]

It is worth noting that Wernicke's encephalopathy often goes unrecognized since clinicians may overlook the diagnosis when the classical clinical triad is absent; Wernicke's encephalopathy often presents solely with confusion. For the renal transplant patient, immunosuppressant-related encephalopathy is another frequently overlooked cause of confusion that can be seen at both toxic and therapeutic drug levels. Other signs of toxicity (e.g., tremor, insomnia, headache, visual changes) help steer the clinician toward the correct diagnosis. Most importantly, posterior reversible leukoencephalopathy syndrome (PRES) may develop and is a clinical emergency.[70]

Once encephalopathy has been ruled out, the consulting psychiatrist should be mindful of other CNS disorders that occur commonly in patients with renal failure and mental status changes. As mentioned earlier, cognitive disorders, including dementia, are significantly more common in patients with renal disease than in age-matched controls, likely due to a combination of neurotoxic uremic toxins and vasculopathy. Patients with renal failure are more prone to developing atherosclerosis and are at increased risk for ischemic stroke. Anemia and ultra-filtration-related arterial hypotension that occurs with HD can result in cerebral hypoperfusion and ischemia. Additionally, because patients with renal failure have bleeding disorders (from a combination of anticoagulation and uremia that leads to platelet dysfunction), they are at increased risk for intra-cranial bleeding (e.g., subdural, subarachnoid, and intracerebral hematomas). Hemorrhagic stroke may also result from hypertension. Patients with polycystic kidney disease are also vulnerable to CNS bleeds due to their increased risk for cerebrovascular malformations.[67]

Hyponatremia is a common electrolyte derangement that develops in patients with renal impairment. If corrected too aggressively with dialysis, central pontine myelinolysis (CPM) (characterized by acute progressive quadriplegia, dysarthria, and altered consciousness) may arise. Extra-pontine regions of the brain can also be affected, and result in a varied clinical spectrum (e.g. parkinsonism with basal ganglia involvement or ataxia with cerebellar involvement).

Movement disorders are frequently co-morbid with renal failure. Most commonly, involuntary movements, including asterixis and myoclonus, seen in other forms of metabolic encephalopathy occur. The uremic "twitch-convulsive" syndrome consists of pronounced asterixis and myoclonic jerks accompanied by fasciculations and seizures. Dexmedetomidine has been reported to provide relief and should be considered for the agitated delirious patient with renal failure and this motor disturbance.[71] Choreiform movements in patients receiving HD have been associated with thiamine deficiency, possibly due to basal ganglia dysfunction.[72] Restless legs syndrome (RLS) occurs in approximately 25% of dialysis patients. If left untreated, RLS leads to significant psychological distress and insomnia, which often warrants psychiatric consultation. RLS is characterized by prickling, crawling, and aching sensations in the legs and an overwhelming urge to move the legs during rest, which can be relieved temporarily by movement. Treatment with dopamine agonists, benzodiazepines, gabapentin (typically 200–300 mg three times per week after dialysis), clonidine, or opioids is often useful.[67] Correction of iron deficiency, anemia, and vitamin D deficiency is also important. Kidney transplantation has been reported to result in significant improvement. The paresthesias of RLS can mimic uremic neuropathy (described later). Patients with RLS may also be confused and have akathisia, as the following case illustrates.

CASE 2

Psychiatric consultation was requested for Ms. K, a 57-year-old woman with bipolar disorder and ESRD on long-term HD who developed paranoid delusions directed toward staff at her HD center; this led to HD refusal. Although family members indicated that the delusions were present for at least several months, the delusions had never previously resulted in HD refusal. Her medication list was notable for quetiapine, sertraline, and ropinirole for "restless legs syndrome"; ropinirole had been increased weeks previously to a dose of 4 mg/day. On interview, Ms. K described her RLS as a constant feeling as if she needed to jump from her skin, and the sensation was not clearly relieved by rest. Akathisia from use of an SSRI and quetiapine was considered, prompting replacement of ropinirole with clonazepam. She reported subjective improvement on this regimen. Her paranoia eventually diminished, and she was able to resume HD at her previous HD center.

Renal transplant recipients are at increased risk of developing opportunistic infections and CNS neoplasms (see Chapter 29 for additional details.)

Peripheral Nervous System Complications

Peripheral nervous system (PNS) complications in renal failure include uremic polyneuropathy, mononeuropathies, and autonomic disturbances. Uremic polyneuropathy is a distal symmetric sensorimotor axonal neuropathy that typically occurs in patients with advanced renal failure, usually with GFRs <12 mL/min. The etiology is thought to be related to various nutritional deficiencies (thiamine, biotin, zinc) as well as to an accumulation of neurotoxic uremic toxins.[68] Sensory disturbances and decreased or absent tendon reflexes are common. Milder forms typically resolve with renal replacement therapy (RRT), whereas severe forms may not be reversible. Physical therapy and medications that target neuropathic pain can be useful as adjunctive agents. Renal transplantation is perhaps the most effective treatment.

Several mononeuropathies can be seen with uremic intoxication and as complications of RRT. Most commonly, nerves of the forearm are affected. Carpal tunnel syndrome occurs in nearly 90% of patients receiving chronic dialysis,[68] often on the side used in vascular access for dialysis (although the contralateral arm may also be affected).

Autonomic neuropathy is also common in renal failure. It is typically manifested by marked orthostatic hypotension and dialysis-related hypotension secondary to impaired baroreflex responses. There is some literature supporting the use of SSRIs in the management of dialysis-related hypotension. The best treatment, however, is successful kidney transplantation.

Finally, calciphylaxis arising with renal failure is a rare cause of painful myopathy that can significantly affect a patient's sleep and quality of life.

Pediatric Populations

Children with ESRD are also at increased risk for neurologic complications. A recent retrospective review of 68 children with ESRD revealed that neurological complications occurred in roughly one-third of children, with seizures being the most common event.[73] Uncontrolled hypertension was the leading cause of neurological events, indicating that more effective control of hypertension is needed in this population.

PSYCHOPHARMACOLOGIC CONSIDERATIONS

Renal disease can alter the pharmacokinetics of most medications.[74] Renal-induced changes in fluid balance and volume of distribution may change the bioavailability of hydrophilic medications. Uremic compounds may displace protein-bound drugs, thereby increasing the amount of free drug that circulates in the plasma. Renal disease may also modify hepatic drug metabolism by altering gene expression and function of cytochrome P450 enzymes.[74,75] Phase II metabolic reactions (such as glucuronidation, methylation, sulfation, and acetylation) aimed at making medications more water-soluble are impaired in renal disease.[76] Absorption of medications from the gastrointestinal (GI) tract are also seen in renal disease due to changes in gut motility (seen in gastroparesis due to diabetes) and edema in the GI tract due to volume overload.[75]

The ratio of free drug levels versus total drug levels (free drug plus protein-bound drug) is altered in renal disease. Furthermore, drug monitoring methods may only indicate the total drug level that is often reduced due to decreased protein-binding. Highly protein-bound medications, such as valproic acid, may therefore yield results that appear to be sub-therapeutic and doses may be erroneously increased, possibly to toxic levels. Therefore, free drug levels should be obtained whenever possible in patients with renal disease.[74,77]

Creatinine clearance (CrCl), as measured by the estimated glomerular filtration rate (eGFR), can be used to guide adjustments in medication dosage. Psychotropic medications that are primarily metabolized or eliminated by the kidney include: lithium, gabapentin, pregabalin, topiramate, risperidone, paliperidone, paroxetine, desvenlafaxine, venlafaxine, and memantine.[74,77–79] Duloxetine is also renally eliminated. Doses of these medications should be reduced depending on the level of renal insufficiency. Mild renal insufficiency is defined as CrCl >50 mL/min, moderate RI 10–50 mL/min, and severe RI is <10 mL/min.[74,76]

Whether a medication is effectively removed with HD or PD is determined by its level of protein-binding, lipophilicity, and volume of distribution. High amounts of lipophilicity and protein-binding, as well as a large volume of distribution make substantial removal by dialysis unlikely.[74,78] If dialysis clearance is <30% of the total drug clearance, it is likely that significant drug accumulation can occur and decreasing the dose of medication or avoiding it altogether may be warranted.[78] Dialysis will cause significant fluid shifts both during and after each treatment and it may take many hours to reach equilibrium. Medications associated with orthostasis should be used cautiously (or avoided when possible) in dialysis patients.[80] Dialyzable medications include: carbamazepine, gabapentin, lamotrigine, lithium, pregabalin, topiramate, and valproate.[74]

Most other psychotropic medications do not require drastic dose changes in patients with renal disease or even renal failure (Table 27-1).[77] However, consideration of possible accumulation or overlapping synergetic effects with other medications or organ failure should be considered. If renal clearance represents less than 30% of total drug clearance, then ESRD will unlikely affect drug pharmacokinetics and no dose adjustment is needed.[78] In this case, clinicians can use the "two-thirds rule" as advocated by Owen and Levenson.[74] Thus, for patients with renal insufficiency, two-thirds of the normal dosage is used (i.e., the total dose is reduced by one-third).

Indications and considerations for medication use in patients with renal disease by medication class are provided below.

Antidepressants

A recent review of antidepressant use for depression in patients with stage 3–5 CKD found that drug clearance was markedly reduced for selegiline, amitriptyline oxide, venlafaxine, desvenlafaxine, milnacipran, bupropion, reboxetine, and tianeptine.[79]

Bupropion's water-soluble metabolites, hydroxybupropion and threohydroxybupropion, are shown to be increased in patients with ESRD.[74,78,79] Toxic levels of bupropion may be associated with an increased risk of seizures, agitation, anxiety, and psychosis. In patients with renal insufficiency, the initial dose should be reduced and titrated with caution.

Mirtazapine's clearance is reduced in patients with renal insufficiency by 30% in moderate renal insufficiency and 50% in severe renal insufficiency.[77,78] It is also highly protein-bound and therefore not readily removed by dialysis. Initial and subsequent doses should therefore be reduced in patients with moderate to severe renal insufficiency.

TABLE 27-1 Medications Known to Require Dosage Adjustment in Renal Insufficiency Based on Estimated Glomerular Filtration Rate (eGFR)

	MILD RI (>50 mL/min)	MODERATE RI (10–50 mL/min)	SEVERE RI (<10 mL/min)
Antidepressants			
Mirtazapine	None	Reduce by 30%	Reduce by 50%
Paroxetine	None	Reduce by 25–50%	Max dose 40 mg daily
Venlafaxine	Reduce by 25%	Reduce by 50%	Reduce by 50%
Desvenlafaxine	None	Do not exceed 50 mg daily	Do not exceed 50 mg every other day
Antipsychotics			
Paliperidone	Start ≤3 mg daily Max dose ≤6 mg daily	Start ≤1.5 mg daily Max dose ≤3 mg daily	Start ≤1.5 mg daily Max dose ≤3 mg daily
Risperidone	Start 0.25–0.5 mg once or twice a day Beyond 1.5 mg, increase dose weekly or longer	Start 0.25-0.5 mg once or twice a day Beyond 1.5 mg, increases in dose should take place at weekly or longer intervals	Start 0.25–0.5 mg once or twice a day Beyond 1.5 mg, increases in dose should take place at weekly or longer intervals
Benzodiazepines			
Chlordiazepoxide	None	None	Reduce by ≥50%
Anticonvulsants			
Carbamazepine	None	None	Reduce by 25%
Gabapentin	CrCl >60 mL/min: max dose 1200 mg daily CrCl 30–60 mL/min: max dose 600 mg daily	CrCl 15–30 mL/min: max dose 300 mg daily	CrCl <15 mL/min: max dose 150 mg daily
Pregabalin	Reduce by 50%	Reduce by 75%	Reduce by 87.5%
Topiramate	None	Reduce by 50%	Reduce by 75%
Lithium	None	Reduce by 25–50%	Consider further decrease and dosing on alternate days
Cholinesterase Inhibitors			
Galantamine	None	Max dose: 16 mg daily	Use not recommended
Memantine	None	None	Max dose 5 mg twice a day

Data from Owen JA: Psychopharmacology. In, Textbook of Psychosomatic Medicine Psychiatric Care of the Medically Ill. Edited by Levenson, JL. Arlington, VA, American Psychiatric Publishing, 2010: 957–1019.[77]

There are very few data regarding the pharmacokinetics of trazodone in patients with renal disease.[74,78,79] No dose adjustments were suggested in patients with an eGFR >15 mL/min, whereas for patients with an eGFR <15 mL/min, it was recommended that doses should not exceed 150 mg.

There are very few data on the use of MAOIs in patients with renal insufficiency. Little or no data exist to inform prescribers on recommending isocarboxazid or phenelzine.[79] A 50% decrease in total daily dose was suggested for tranylcypromine in patients with an eGFR of <30 mg/mL. Similarly, the suggested dosing for selegiline was 50% that of the dose in normal renal function; 5 mg.

SSRIs have been found to be safe in patients with ESRD,[74,77–79] however, certain side effects as well as individual medications warrant special attention. SSRIs may be associated with serotonin-related platelet dysfunction and an increased risk of bleeding.[81] Moreover, bleeding risk may be elevated in patients with renal disease due to uremia-induced platelet dysfunction.[78] While not considered an absolute contraindication, bleeding risk should be monitored in patients with renal insufficiency receiving SSRIs.

Paroxetine clearance is significantly reduced in renal insufficiency (up to 50%) and doses should be reduced by 25% to 50% in moderate renal insufficiency.[74,77] Potential anticholinergic effects, such as urinary retention, orthostasis, and QT-prolongation, are also possible with paroxetine and its use should be limited in patients with severe renal disease. Citalopram doses >40 mg/day have been associated with significant QT interval prolongation.[82] Given the uncertainty and unpredictability of possible drug accumulation, electrolyte changes, and co-morbid cardiovascular disease, an alternative SSRI is advisable in patients with renal insufficiency.[78,82]

SNRIs (venlafaxine, desvenlafaxine, and duloxetine) are renally eliminated. Venlafaxine is not significantly removed by dialysis and may cause increased hypertension.[78] In mild to moderate renal insufficiency a 25% decrease in dosage is suggested,[74] for patients with an eGFR <30 ml/min a 50% reduction is recommended.[79] When discontinuing venlafaxine in patients with RI, a slow taper over 2 to 4 weeks is recommended to avoid withdrawal effects.[78] Desvenlafaxine is also not substantially removed by dialysis and dose reduction by 50% is recommended for mild, moderate, and severe renal insufficiency.[79] Duloxetine should be reduced by up to 75% of the total maximum dose in normal renal function, no higher than 40 mg/day for patients with an eGFR of <30 mg/mL.[79] Other sources suggest not prescribing duloxetine to patients with an eGFR <30 mg/mL.[79]

TCAs have been used in ESRD patients for decades, often with good effects. However, certain TCAs should generally be avoided due to anticholinergic properties, orthostatic hypotension, or QT-prolongation.[74,77] Nortriptyline and desipramine are less likely to cause these effects and can be considered in patients with ESRD.[74,83] No dose adjustments were recommended for nortriptyline or for doxepin regardless of the severity of renal insufficiency.[79]

Benzodiazepines

Use of benzodiazepines is common in patients with renal insufficiency due to higher rates of anxiety, restless legs syndrome, and sleep disorders.[78] Medications with active metabolites which are renally excreted (including chlordiazepoxide, diazepam, flurazepam, and clorazepate), should be avoided.[78] Drug accumulation is likely with most if not all benzodiazepines as these medications are not effectively removed by dialysis. In severe renal insufficiency, it has been suggested that chlordiazepoxide be reduced by 50%.[74,77] Lorazepam and oxazepam are the preferred agents of this class as they do not have active metabolites. Yet, levels of lorazepam and oxazepam may increase four-fold and smaller doses with increased interval of administration are recommended.[77,84]

Non-benzodiazepine sedative–hypnotics, such as zaleplon, zolpidem, and zopiclone, are generally under-studied in patients with renal disease.[74,77] While dose requirements may not be necessary, more data are needed.

Levels of the anxiolytic agent buspirone have been found to be increased up to four times in patients with an eGFR <60 mg/mL, and dose reduction is recommended.[74,77,78,84]

Mood Stabilizers

No dose adjustments are suggested for carbamazepine in mild to moderate renal insufficiency.[84] A 25% dose reduction is recommended in patients with severe renal insufficiency.[74,77]

No dose adjustment is necessary for valproic acid in patients with renal insufficiency though it is prudent to monitor the free level, as opposed to the total level as mentioned previously.

Gabapentin is extensively excreted by the kidney and dose reductions are recommended: for a CrCl of 30–60 ml/min a maximum dosage of 300 mg twice a day is recommended, for a CrCl of 15–30 ml/min a dose of 300 mg/day is recommended, and for a CrCl of <15 ml/min the maximum suggested dosage is 300 mg every other day.[74,77,84]

Lamotrigine levels have not been extensively studied in patients with renal insufficiency.

Oxcarbazepine dosing should be reduced by 50% in patients with an eGFR of <30 ml/min and initiation should not exceed 150 mg twice a day.[84]

Suggestions for dosing of topiramate are as follows: reduce the total daily dose by 50% in patients with moderate RI and reduce it by 75% in patients with severe RI.[74]

Lithium is almost entirely excreted by the kidneys. Its use is contraindicated in acute renal failure but not chronic renal failure.[77] Lithium is completely dialyzed and can be given as a single oral dose of 200 to 600 mg following HD, guided by levels checked immediately before dialysis.[85] Polyuria is common during treatment with lithium as evidenced by an incidence of 70% in otherwise healthy volunteers.[84] Severe polyuria, as seen in nephrogenic diabetes insipidus (NDI), may occur in up to 40% of patients taking lithium[86] and if present, discontinuation or starting the potassium-sparing amiloride (typically 5 mg twice a day) is recommended.[84] NSAIDs may be used cautiously to reduce urinary free water loss though this should be done in consultation with a nephrologist.

Autopsy studies demonstrate that lithium causes chronic tubulo-interstitial nephrotoxicity, especially in the distal and collecting tubules, as well as causing either segmental or global glomerulosclerosis.[14] The rates of renal insufficiency with chronic lithium use vary from 4% to 20% and are loosely defined in heterogeneous retrospective studies based on Cr levels >1.5 mg/dL.[84] Incongruity of findings as to the risk of developing renal failure with long-term use of lithium continues. In a recently published longitudinal randomized Danish population study, one cohort of patients with a diagnosis of bipolar disorder on maintenance therapy with lithium were found to be at an increased risk of developing CKD but not renal failure.[87] Another recently published study[88] examining the effects of long-term treatment with lithium (10 to 30 years) on development of renal disease found that there was a yearly increase in median serum creatinine levels from the first year of treatment. About one-third of the patients who had taken lithium for more than 10 years had evidence of chronic renal failure and 5% were in the severe or very severe category. A newly published article examined a stratification of risk strategy for the prevention of lithium-induced renal insufficiency.[89] Using regression models, they found that the features associated with risk included: older age, female sex, history of smoking, history of hypertension, overall burden of medical co-morbidity, and diagnosis of schizophrenia or schizoaffective disorder. Independent risk factors were the use of lithium more than once daily, lithium levels >0.6 mEq/L, and the use of first-generation antipsychotics.

During long-term treatment with lithium, creatinine should be monitored approximately every 6 months. If serum Cr is >1.5 mg/dL or increases >25% from baseline, further investigation is warranted,[84] including estimation of CrCl and eGFR or consultation with a nephrologist.

Antipsychotics

No dose adjustments are generally required for conventional or first-generation antipsychotics (including haloperidol, perphenazine, and chlorpromazine),[74,77] however, there are very few data on the use of conventional antipsychotics in patients with ESRD. Haloperidol undergoes extensive hepatic metabolism and only 1% is excreted unchanged in the urine. It is extensively bound to plasma proteins and has a large volume of distribution, making it difficult to remove by dialysis.[78] When prescribing conventional antipsychotics, it is pertinent to factor in relevant medication effects including the potential for QTc-prolongation, the development or worsening of movement disorders, and other side effects which patients with ESRD are more prone to experience.

Similar to conventional antipsychotics, most atypical or second-generation antipsychotics do not require dose adjustments in this patient population.[74,77,78] The notable exceptions to this include paliperidone and risperidone.[74,77] Paliperidone is a metabolite of risperidone and is extensively eliminated by the kidney. Its clearance is significantly decreased in all degrees of renal impairment.[74,77,78] If these agents are utilized in patients with advanced renal disease, they should be started at a low dose, titrated slowly and cautiously, and the target dose should be lower than in patients without significant renal disease.[74,78] For patients with mild renal impairment, paliperidone can be started at 3 mg daily with a maximum of 6 mg daily, whereas in moderate to severe impairment, it should be started at 1.5 mg daily with a maximum dose of 3 mg daily.[74] Risperidone can be started at 0.25 to 0.5 mg twice a day with slow titration and cautious monitoring.[74] As with conventional antipsychotics, patients with ESRD are at an increased risk for the development or exacerbation of class-related side effects and caution and close monitoring is warranted. For atypical antipsychotics, this usually includes: weight gain, hyperlipidemia, insulin resistance and hyperglycemia, cardiovascular morbidity, anticholinergic side effects, and movement disorders.

REFERENCES

Access the reference list online at https://expertconsult.inkling.com/.

Patients With Gastrointestinal Disease

28

Sean P. Glass, M.D.

INTRODUCTION

Psychiatric and gastrointestinal (GI) diseases have a bi-directional relationship that reflects a complex interplay between the central and enteric nervous systems. The assorted symptoms, sensations, and syndromes that result from this reciprocal relationship are associated with alterations in immune system functioning and modulation of neurotransmitters that are common to both systems. Psychological states of anxiety or fear may be experienced as "butterflies" in one's stomach, and high rates of depression are present in those suffering with inflammatory bowel disease, even in the absence of previous psychiatric illness. Psychotropic medications, aside from commonly causing GI side effects, are also made more or less effective depending on the integrity of the GI system's ability to absorb, metabolize, and distribute medications to the rest of the body. In the following sections, these complex relationships are explored with an emphasis on the relationship and treatment considerations that affect both disciplines.

DISORDERS OF THE OROPHARYNX, ESOPHAGUS, STOMACH, AND UPPER INTESTINES

Xerostomia

Xerostomia is defined by dry mouth, with or without decreased salivary production.[1] Psychotropic medications are a contributing cause in 10–50% of patients.[1,2] In a recent analysis that examined the relationship between xerostomia and psychotropic medications (first- and second-generation antipsychotics and anxiolytics) in patients with schizophrenia, Okamoto and colleagues[3] found a negative correlation between the number of antipsychotics and, especially, anxiolytics, and the degree of oral moisture. Mean oral moisture was decreased in patients as opposed to controls and there was no significant correlation with dose, whereas the number of medications used appeared to be significantly correlated with dry mouth. Benzodiazepines, lithium, carbamazepine, anticholinergics, and typical and atypical antipsychotics are all associated with xerostomia.[1,2] Antihypertensives, diuretics, and opioids are also associated with xerostomia.[2] Other causes include connective tissue disorders, such as Sjogren's syndrome, radiation therapy, anxiety, and depression.[1] Non-pharmacologic treatment includes frequent sips of water, using sugarless gums and candies, avoiding caffeine and alcohol, and using saliva substitutes.[2,4] Pilocarpine is an effective treatment,[4] though its use is contraindicated in patients with closed-angle glaucoma. Masters[4] reported its successful use in psychiatric inpatients in doses of 10–30 mg/day, divided into dosing of two or three times a day. Sweating and increased urination were the most common side effects. Another medication treatment option for xerostomia is sublingual bethanechol.

Dysphagia

Dysphagia has been reported to occur secondary to antipsychotic medications (first- and second-generation) as a result of drug-induced parkinsonism, dystonia, or tardive dyskinesia.[5] Case reports and case series have implicated various agents, including: haloperidol, loxapine, trifluoperazine, olanzapine, risperidone, quetiapine, clozapine, and aripiprazole. Treatment should address the suspected etiology. Thus, dysphagia due to drug-induced dystonia should be treated with IV or IM benztropine or diphenhydramine. Dysphagia due to drug-induced parkinsonism is typically not responsive to anticholinergic medication and is best handled with reducing or discontinuing the suspected agent.[2] For patients with dysphagia, regardless of primary etiology, care should be taken when prescribing sedating medications, as over-sedation in this population may result in aspiration and other dreaded events.

Globus Hystericus

The feeling that something is lodged in one's throat is an oft-reported symptom that requires medical attention. When pertinent diseases, including gastroesophageal reflux disease, airway masses, or esophageal masses have been ruled out, psychogenic causes are often considered. Functional dysphagia, classically known as *globus hystericus*, has a wide differential diagnosis as well as a high rate of co-morbidity with other medical conditions.[6] Management includes treating co-morbid conditions, and when applicable, psychotherapy and possibly medications for co-morbid anxiety.[6] If globus is thought to be due to a functional (or conversion) disorder, reassurance, psychoeducation, and psychotherapy is preferred.

Gastroesophageal Reflux Disease

Gastroesophageal reflux disease (GERD) is associated with increased rates of many psychiatric disorders. In a retrospective Taiwanese study, You and colleagues[7] found that GERD was associated with increased rates of depressive (HR = 2.91, 95% CI = 2.34–3.61, $p<0.001$), anxiety (HR = 2.75, 95% CI = 2.15–3.50, $p<0.001$), and sleep disorders (HR =

2.65, 95% CI = 2.02–3.47, $p<0.001$) versus controls without GERD. There did not appear to be a significant increase in rates of bipolar disorder or schizophrenia; however, in another Taiwanese study, Lin and colleagues[8] noted an increased incidence of bipolar disorder (incidence rate ratio, IRR 2.29, 95% confidence interval, CI = 1.58–3.36, $p<0.001$) among GERD patients than among controls. In another study that examined rates of GERD in patients with major depression, Chou and colleagues found that patients with major depressive disorder had a significantly increased rate of GERD (odds ratio, OR = 3.16; 95% CI = 2.71–3.68; $p<0.001$).[9] Various presumed mechanisms may account for the correlations between psychiatric illness and GERD, including increased production of pro-inflammatory cytokines from the esophageal mucosa and increases in autonomic (sympathetic) nervous system activation during coughing and arousal from sleep.[7] Most psychotropic medications can be used in patients with GERD without worsening symptoms; an exception is the use of anticholinergic medications that should be avoided if possible.[2] Benzodiazepines and SNRIs have been associated with improvements in sleep, a sense of well-being, and even reduction in core GERD symptoms.[2]

Nausea and Vomiting

Nausea is a common side effect of serotonergic antidepressants due to agonism of $5HT_3$ receptors in the gut.[10] Medications that antagonize $5HT_3$ receptors (especially mirtazapine, olanzapine, and ondansetron) are less likely to cause GI distress and may be useful in patients with nausea and co-morbid depression or anxiety.[10] Blockage of D_2 receptors, particularly in the chemoreceptor trigger zone, is also helpful in alleviating nausea and vomiting. Metoclopramide and prochlorperazine (a phenothiazine antipsychotic) are D_2 receptor antagonists marketed as antiemetics.[10] While they are often effective over the short-term, their use may be limited by extrapyramidal symptoms (EPS), such as akathisia, and long-term effects, such as tardive dyskinesia (TD). For patients with depression or anxiety and chemotherapy-induced nausea and vomiting (CINV), hyperemesis gravidarum (HG), and other conditions, the antiemetic properties of mirtazapine and certain antipsychotics (e.g., olanzapine, perphenazine, chlorpromazine, prochlorperazine, and other antipsychotics), and benzodiazepines can be considered if no other contraindications are present.

In a randomized, double-blind, placebo-controlled trial of patients scheduled to receive emetogenic chemotherapy, Mizukami and colleagues[11] demonstrated that the addition of 5 mg of olanzapine daily was associated with significant reductions in nausea and vomiting as well as with increases in quality of life over the control group. Lohr[12] reviewed treatment options for chemotherapy-induced nausea and vomiting and discussed potential treatment options. The psychotropic medications that have been shown to be efficacious in CINV include lorazepam (also found to be helpful, including systematic desensitization, hypnosis, biofeedback, imagery, and relaxation[13]), butyrophenone antipsychotics (including haloperidol and droperidol), phenothiazine antipsychotics (e.g., prochlorperazine and promethazine), olanzapine, and gabapentin.[12] Mirtazapine has also been found to be effective in treating nausea and depression in cancer patients.[2] Anticipatory nausea and vomiting may cause a considerable amount of distress in cancer patients who are receiving chemotherapy. Psychological models for chemotherapy-related anticipatory nausea and vomiting include classical conditioning (e.g., associating chemotherapy with environmental cues or other physical sensations), demographic factors (including younger age, female gender, and the propensity to experience certain physical symptoms such as dizziness), and beliefs and negative expectations related to treatment and symptom formation.[13] Adjunctive lorazepam has been shown to be helpful in anticipatory nausea and vomiting in this population.[13]

Although the belief that hyperemesis gravidarum (HG) is psychogenic has been discredited,[2] there is evidence to support the notion that this condition is associated with high degrees of psychological stress and with elevated rates of depression and anxiety disorders, even after pregnancy. In a study of 47 patients with HG, 25.5% had a mood disorder and the prevalence of any mood disorder was 14.9% in women in the first trimester. Psychiatric disorders continued throughout the pregnancy in two-thirds of the women with HG and a psychiatric diagnosis. In another study of 52 women with HG, Uguz and colleagues[14] found that the prevalence of mood disorders was 15.4% and that of anxiety disorders was 36.5%. A significant number of patients (36.5%) with HG had at least one personality disorder diagnosis (particularly an avoidant or obsessive–compulsive personality disorder). Furthermore, most of the mood or anxiety disorders occurred before the pregnancy in women with HG.[14] Treatment of HG typically involves vitamin supplementation (especially thiamine to avoid Wernicke's encephalopathy), pyridoxine (vitamin B_6) with or without doxylamine, and for more severe cases, use of metoclopramide or steroids.[15] Mirtazapine has been used successfully as has chlorpromazine.[2,15]

Cyclical vomiting syndrome (CVS) is a condition consisting of recurrent episodes of incapacitating nausea and vomiting that are interspersed with symptom-free intervals lasting anywhere from a few days to several months.[16] While most common in children, it also occurs in adults and may be associated with specific triggers or environmental cues (e.g., migraines, seizures, stress, menstrual cycles).[17] There have been many proposed etiologies; more recent plausible causes include sympathetic and parasympathetic dysfunction, stress/anxiety/depression, and a central mechanism of nausea/vomiting involving corticotropin releasing factor.[16] Treatment of CVS is multi-factorial, complex, and involves both pharmacologic and non-pharmacologic strategies. Interventions include identification and avoidance of any known triggers, use of prophylactic drug therapy to prevent recurrent episodes, use of abortive treatment and/or supportive care to ameliorate acute episodes, and provision of psychological support of the patients and family.[16] Various medications (including prokinetics, antiemetics, erythromycin, sumatriptan, TCAs, benzodiazepines, and anticonvulsants) have been used with varying success.[2] Acute vomiting episodes may require high-dose IV antiemetics and benzodiazepines. Long-term management with TCAs has been recently reviewed and found to be effective in most patients in decreasing the duration and frequency of episodes, emergency visits, and hospitalization in adults with CVS.[16] While side effects with TCAs are common,

Hejazi and McCallum[16] reported that they were generally mild and well-tolerated. The role of neuropsychiatric consultation and intervention may be particularly valuable in these patients; the major risk factors for non-response to treatment are co-existing poorly controlled migraine headache, a psychiatric disorder, and chronic narcotic and marijuana use.[16] Additionally, a personal or family history of migraine and the presence of co-morbid psychiatric disorders is thought to be associated with an increased risk (and likelihood if symptoms are present) of CVS.

Cannabis hyperemesis syndrome (CHS) is similar to CVS but it can be distinguished by pathognomonic behavior of frequently bathing in hot water and by chronic cannabis use.[18] Paradoxically, cannabis usually functions as an antiemetic, however, it is thought that with chronic use, toxic levels accumulate and activate CB_1 receptors in the gut. The peripheral CB_1 binding over-rides the common antiemetic properties on CB_1 receptors in the central nervous system and CB_2 receptors on glial cells. The result is decreased GI motility and emesis.[18] The mechanism related to hot water bathing is unknown but may include CB_1 activation by THC in the hypothalamus as well as a "cutaneous steal syndrome," which is thought to occur when blood flow is re-directed from the gut to the skin, resulting in emesis.[18,19] Management, other than replenishing fluids and nutrients, may involve the judicious and cautious use of benzodiazepines. Antiemetics have not been shown to be effective. The most effective treatment is likely the cessation of cannabis use; indeed, the diagnosis is supported by the fact that patients with CHS tend to have a remission of symptoms when stopping cannabis use and that symptoms tend to resume when cannabis is used again.[18]

Nausea and GI distress are the most common reason for discontinuation of SSRIs by patients.[2,20] SSRI-induced nausea is generally benign, transient, and if needed, can be managed with over-the-counter antiemetics. In addition to use of SSRIs, nausea is a common early side effect of psychostimulants, mood stabilizers, and anticholinesterase inhibitors.[2,10] Lithium is associated with nausea and vomiting but longer-acting formulations (e.g., Eskalith CR) or lithium citrate may reduce this effect (though lower GI symptoms are possible).[10] For patients taking sodium valproate, switching to divalproex sodium may help reduce nausea and vomiting.[20] For patients taking carbamazepine, dividing the total daily dose to twice daily may also alleviate nausea.[20] If nausea occurs in the setting of other side effects associated with drug toxicity, such as neurologic or other GI symptoms, consideration of drug toxicity and prompt evaluation should ensue.

Gastroparesis

Gastroparesis is characterized by delayed gastric emptying without an identifiable bowel obstruction. Patients with gastroparesis may experience symptoms including abdominal pain, nausea, vomiting, bloating, and early satiety.[21] Common causes include complications from diabetes mellitus, post-surgical complications, neurologic injury, and medication side effects. Anticholinergic medications worsen gastroparesis and should be avoided. This includes anticholinergic medications used for prophylaxis and/or treatment of extrapyramidal symptoms (EPS) or dystonic reactions, such as benztropine and Benadryl, as well as anticholinergic antipsychotic medications such as clozapine, chlorpromazine, and other low potency first-generation agents. Pharmacologic treatment for gastroparesis involves using prokinetic agents, such as erythromycin, bethanechol, and metoclopramide. Metoclopramide is a dopamine-$_2$ receptor antagonist that is used in a variety of GI disorders. Long-term use has been historically associated with an increased risk of tardive dyskinesia (TD) with rates ranging from 1% to 10% in different studies; however, a 2010 review by Rao and Camilleri[22] showed the risk of TD to be <1%. As with other D_2-receptor antagonists, metoclopramide may also be associated with other dreaded reactions including akathisia, dystonic reactions, and possibly, neuroleptic malignant syndrome.[2] A recent meta-analysis found that continuous IV administration is associated with a reduced rate of EPS when compared with bolus administration, and this may be an option for patients prone to these conditions.[23]

Gastric Bypass

CASE 1

Ms. A, a 62-year-old woman with a history of major depressive disorder and generalized anxiety disorder, successfully treated with fluoxetine (40 mg daily) and clonazepam (0.5 mg twice to three times daily), had successful Roux-en-Y gastric bypass surgery 2 months earlier and returned for a follow-up appointment. While she felt content and grateful with regards to her surgery, she also reported 1 month of worsening worry, muscle tension, difficulty falling and staying asleep, as well as decreased mood, energy, and motivation. Her fluoxetine and clonazepam were continued on the same doses after her surgery. No other medications were added or changed and her recent examinations and work-ups by her internist, gastroenterologist, and surgeon were unremarkable.

Fluoxetine and clonazepam levels were ordered, however, Ms. A did not get bloodwork drawn. She returned 2 weeks later, with worsening depressive and anxiety symptoms and she reported that she had not been as adherent with her diet and exercise recommendations and had been staying in bed for much of the day. She reported that she was adherent with her medications but stated that they were not working. Her current presentation was similar to her prior depressive episodes.

Fluoxetine was increased to 80 mg daily and clonazepam was increased to 0.5 mg in the morning and in the afternoon, and 1 mg at bedtime and she was referred for cognitive-behavioral therapy (CBT). She returned 2 weeks later with a slight, but noticeable, reduction in her symptoms of anxiety and depression. At this point, consideration was given to adding another medication and to increasing her doses even further, however, given that she was having a partial treatment response after 2 weeks, she was continued on her current psychopharmacologic regimen and psychotherapy.

She returned 2 weeks later and her symptoms were markedly improved. She had difficulty finding a good time for meeting with her therapist, so only attended two sessions. She continued her medications at higher doses and her only complaint was of some mild dizziness and feeling "jittery," which wore off.

Increasingly patients are receiving gastric bypass surgery with annual rates estimated at 350,000 worldwide in 2014.[24] This represents a 70% increase over the past two decades and increases are expected to continue.[24] Anti-obesity surgeries are typically classified into procedures that: promote intestinal malabsorption (e.g., jejunoileal and jejunocolic bypass), gastric restrictive surgeries (e.g., vertical banded gastroplasty, gastric band, gastric stapling, or sleeve gastrectomy), surgeries that combine restriction and malabsorption (e.g., Roux-en-Y gastric bypass), and surgeries that combine maldigestion, malabsorption, and gastric restriction (e.g., biliopancreatic diversion with partial gastrectomy, distal gastric bypass, or duodenal switch).[24] Regardless of the procedure, patients have less surface area to absorb nutrients and medications and have altered bowel transit times, often requiring adjustments in diet and medications.[25,26] The most common type of bypass surgery in the United States is the Roux-en-Y procedure. Roughly 20% to 50% of bariatric surgery patients have a history of a mood disorder[24] and the prevalence of other psychiatric disorders is unknown. Regardless of the prevalence of various psychiatric disorders, changes in GI physiology occur after surgical procedures and likely influences the type and amount of medications that can be effectively administered to patients post-procedure. This may have significant implications and adversely affect effective psychiatric treatment regimens.

In an analysis of medication absorption after Roux-en-Y gastric bypass surgery,[26] both lithium and bupropion led to increased absorption in patients versus controls, whereas many medications (e.g., amitriptyline, clonazepam, clozapine, fluoxetine, olanzapine, paroxetine, quetiapine, risperidone, sertraline, and ziprasidone) showed reduced absorption. Medications whose absorption did not change pre- and post-surgery included buspirone, citalopram, diazepam, haloperidol, lorazepam, methylphenidate, oxcarbazepine, trazodone, venlafaxine, and zolpidem.[2,26] In a retrospective study of 439 patients receiving the Roux-en-Y procedure, Cunningham and colleagues[27] found that 23% of patients showed an increase in use of antidepressant drugs after the surgery; 40% retained the same class of antidepressants; 18% started on a new class of antidepressants; and only 16% had a decreased need for antidepressant treatment. Hamad and colleagues[28] demonstrated that the bioavailability of SSRI medications was reduced in patients undergoing Roux-en-Y gastric bypass 1 month after surgery.

Patients with gastric bypass or gastrectomy are able to absorb medications dissolved in acidic solutions, whereas patients with significant alterations in their intestine are less likely to absorb alkaline-soluble medications.[24] Drug poisoning from highly lipophilic medications may also occur, as anti-obesity surgeries may result in significant changes and loss in body fat percentage and distribution.[24] Reductions in the size and area of the small intestine necessary for the absorption of nutrients, vitamins, and medications complicates the effective use of psychotropics in these patients. Medications dissolved in aqueous solution may help circumvent this, as they are absorbed faster than are medications in solid form.[2] Thus, dissolving medications in water before ingestion may result in improved absorption and in more predictable drug levels. Transit times through the intestine may be decreased; this limits the time that medications have in contact with the small intestine for proper absorption. When large portions of the stomach and proximal small intestine are removed, long-acting medications become less effective as they pass unchanged into the large intestine without losing their protective coating.[2] Therefore, immediate-release formulations are preferred over extended-release formulations in gastric bypass patients. Another strategy that may produce more reliable drug levels and hence treatment efficacy, is using medications that are available as orally disintegrating tablets, using liquid preparations of medications, using transdermal patches, or using intramuscular long-acting formulations for selected patients. Checking blood levels of medications may have more utility in this patient population than in non-bypass patients given the unpredictable absorption of many agents post-bypass.

DISORDERS OF THE LOWER GASTROINTESTINAL TRACT

Constipation

Constipation is a common side effect with anticholinergic medications, such as benztropine, tricyclic antidepressants (TCAs), many second-generation (atypical) antipsychotics, low-potency first-generation (typical) antipsychotics, such as chlorpromazine, and the SSRI paroxetine.[2,10] Paroxetine, which has high anticholinergic activity, as do many atypical antipsychotics (such as risperidone, quetiapine, olanzapine, and especially clozapine), may be associated with constipation in up to 25% of patients.[29,30] Medications with anticholinergic properties may cause constipation by a variety of factors, including alteration of duodenal motility, small and large bowel contractions, colon transit, and gastrocolic reflex.[29] Patients with medical and psychiatric conditions associated with a sedentary lifestyle or patients taking sedating medications (leading to sedentary lifestyle) may be at higher risk for medication-induced constipation.[29] FDA registration trials report rates of constipation between approximately 3% and 16% for SSRIs, SNRIs, bupropion, and mirtazapine.[10]

Constipation is a common side effect for patients taking clozapine with rates of 25% to 60% reported in the literature.[31] Studies examining colonic transit time on patients on clozapine (alone and/or with other antipsychotics) versus other antipsychotics, have shown that clozapine-treated patients have significantly more gut hypomotility than patients on other antipsychotics.[31,32] No associations were noted between objective findings of hypomotility with age, medication dose and duration of treatment, however, positive correlations were found with blood levels of clozapine. Median colonic transit time was 23 hours for patients not treated with clozapine, whereas for patients prescribed clozapine, the median transit time was 104.5 hours.[32] Because reduced motility, constipation, and pseudo-obstruction may lead to disastrous complications, such as ischemia or perforation, clozapine-treated patients should be treated with laxatives.[32]

Diarrhea

Diarrhea is reported to occur in approximately 6% to 20% of patients on SSRIs in FDA registration trials.[10] Rates of >1–2% (comparable with placebo) are found with bupropion XL, mirtazapine, and venlafaxine XL and rates with duloxetine and desvenlafaxine are approximately 10%.

Approximately 30% of patients experience diarrhea with vilazodone,[33] which is the highest rate among antidepressant users. While fairly common, SSRI-induced diarrhea is generally short-lived. Population-based studies of patients taking lithium and carbamazepine demonstrate high rates of diarrhea with these medications (33% and 25%, respectively) though the relationship to dose or duration of treatment is unclear. If persistent diarrhea occurs with lithium, carbamazepine, or divalproex, possible drug toxicity should be considered and evaluated, including obtaining drug levels.[10] Slow-release formulations may reduce the rates of diarrhea and slow-release lithium may reduce the likelihood of this side effect.[2]

Irritable Bowel Syndrome

CASE 2

Mrs. B, a 55-year-old married woman with mixed-type irritable bowel syndrome was referred for the evaluation of anxiety by her gastroenterologist. She had a history of major depressive disorder (MDD) in full-sustained remission, and likely had PTSD stemming from a sexual assault that occurred while in college 35 years earlier. Her only psychiatric treatment has been two or three brief trials with antidepressant medications prescribed by her PCP, that were not tolerated due to GI symptoms. She described longstanding patterns of frequent worry about various topics, multiple somatic symptoms and complaints, and insomnia; after further review of her history, it was clear that she met criteria for generalized anxiety disorder (GAD). She described having a "rough" childhood, though she also reported having good support from family and friends. Her parents, particularly her mother, were sick quite often, and she remembered someone in the household "always having a headache or back pain, or something." She struggled with various pain ailments in the past and for some time suffered from frequent migraine headaches. A successful attorney, she was happily married with three children in their teens and early twenties, and was in general happy with her life apart from her anxiety and GI symptoms. Work had been more stressful as of late however, and she reported worrying about her 18-year-old daughter going off to college. She stated that she experienced a considerable amount of abdominal cramping, bloating, nausea, and diarrhea lately. After reviewing potential treatment options, she declined an antidepressant trial, but was willing to be referred for cognitive-behavioral therapy (CBT) for generalized anxiety.

She returned to the clinic 2 months later. CBT had been helpful and she reported a "50%" reduction in symptoms. She wanted to reconsider embarking on a medication trial. After discussing the potential risks and benefits, she was started on fluoxetine (10 mg daily). She called 2 weeks later (as planned) and reported that while she experienced GI cramping and an increase in diarrhea, she thought the medication may be working and would like to increase the dose to 20 mg daily. She returned in 1 month and reported that her anxiety and GI symptoms were much improved. She also mentioned that her daughter would be attending a prestigious university that was close to home. Her CBT therapy was going well.

Irritable bowel syndrome (IBS) is a common functional GI disorder (FGID) that affects approximately 11% of the population worldwide;[34] it is the most common GI condition.[35] Diagnostic criteria for FGID, including IBS, are provided by the Rome Foundation, a panel of international experts that has been refining diagnostic criteria based on ongoing research since its inception in the late 1980s.[36] IBS has been classified based on the presence of abdominal pain with a prevailing irregular bowel movement pattern with three main subtypes: predominant diarrhea (IBS-D), predominant constipation (IBS-C), mixed (IBS-M), or an unclassified type. More recently, the definition of FGIDs (including IBS) is based on putative pathophysiologic features causing GI symptoms that include motility disturbances, visceral hypersensitivity and altered pain perception, altered mucosal and immune functions, altered gut microbiota, and altered central nervous system (CNS) functioning (altered brain–gut axis).[36] Additionally, environmental factors and triggers are prominent in the disease and include early life stressors (e.g., abuse and significant psychosocial stress), food intolerance, antibiotic use, and enteric infection (gastroenteritis).[35] The Rome criteria emphasize a biopsychosocial model approach to understanding the complex interplay of host and environmental factors in the pathogenesis and treatment of IBS.[36] IBS tends to be a relapsing–remitting illness and symptoms may vary over time.[35] Within 3 months after initial diagnosis, most patients experience symptoms on more than half of the days, with four distinct episodes occurring each month, each lasting 5 days or less.[34] After 1 year, approximately one-third to one-half of patients have prolonged periods without symptoms. With time however, this appears to fluctuate as 50% to 70% of patients report persistent symptoms after 10 years.[34] El-Serag[37] showed that during long-term follow-up of IBS patients, 2% to 18% worsened; 30% to 50% remain unchanged; and 12% to 38% improved. Psychiatric co-morbidity is high. Rates of Axis I disorders range from 40% to 94%, with depression as the most common disorder followed by anxiety and somatization disorders.[38] Other common co-morbidities in patients with IBS include chronic pain syndromes (including fibromyalgia and chronic pelvic pain), sleep disturbances, GERD, functional dyspepsia, and headache.[38] It is thought that the prevalence of celiac disease is increased in patients with IBS, though studies appear to be conflicting.[35] Inflammatory bowel disease, microscopic colitis, and bile acid malabsorption may be more prevalent in IBS patients, whereas recent studies suggest that the risk of colorectal cancer is <1% in IBS patients.[35]

Treatment for IBS includes both psychopharmacologic and non-psychopharmacologic interventions. CBT, psychodynamic psychotherapy, relaxation training, and hypnotherapy have been shown to be effective in various trials; however, considerable differences in study design and heterogeneity exist between studies.[35,38,39] TCAs and SSRIs are effective and positive studies have been demonstrated with various agents, including imipramine, amitriptyline, desipramine, doxepin, trimipramine, paroxetine, fluoxetine, and citalopram.[35,38,39] A recent systematic meta-analysis investigating the efficacy of antidepressants and psychological therapies in IBS demonstrated the pooled relative risk of IBS symptoms not improving with antidepressants or with psychological treatments was 0.67 (95% CI = 0.58–0.77) and 0.68 (95%

CI = 0.61–0.76), respectively.[39] TCAs may be preferred in patients with IBS-D due to possible constipating effects, and SSRIs may be more useful in IBS-C due to possible prokinetic effects. Similarly, for patients with anorexia, weight loss, or insomnia, TCAs may be preferred and SSRIs or TCAs may be helpful for patients with co-morbid anxiety or depression.[35] Pooled data indicate that the rate of adverse effects with antidepressants is 31.3% versus 16.5% for patients receiving placebo. No serious adverse effects occurred, while drowsiness and dry mouth were more common with TCAs.[39] Other medications that may be helpful in alleviating IBS symptoms include fiber, laxatives, anti-diarrheals, probiotics, anti-spasmodics, pro-secretory agents, antibiotics, and 5-HT_3 antagonists.[35]

Inflammatory Bowel Disease

CASE 3

Mr. C, a 31-year-old man with a 2-year history of an inflammatory bowel disease (with features of both Crohn's disease [CD] and ulcerative colitis [UC]) was admitted to the hospital for a (diagnostic) colonic resection. Considerable full-wall mucosal necrosis was detected in the descending colon and the distal portion of the transverse colon without any signs of rectal, anal, or other colonic or small bowel pathology. A large bowel resection was performed with placement of a colostomy. Pathologic diagnosis confirmed a diagnosis of UC. Psychiatric consultation was requested on postoperative day 3 for evaluation of depressive symptoms. Mr. C reported that he has been experiencing increasingly severe anxiety, worry, and physical tension, along with low mood, anhedonia, and feelings of hopelessness, over the past year. He had not received any psychiatric medications nor had he embarked on psychotherapy.

While Mr. C was relieved to learn that his GI symptoms would likely improve, he expressed considerable worry about the impact his illness and surgery would have on his life. He hoped that he would be able to resume a normal life, but he also worried about his ability to have a family and a successful career. Mr. C was also distressed about managing his colostomy.

Inflammatory bowel disease (IBD) is a chronic disease characterized by relapsing intestinal inflammation. It is thought to be due to genetic factors along with an atypical immune response to microbes in the intestines,[40] as well as to breakdown in the normal tolerance to gut microbiota.[41,42] The role of inflammation and abnormal levels of pro-inflammatory cytokines in various psychiatric disorders, particularly depression, is well-established and provides a putative link between many medical and psychiatric ailments, including autoimmune disease.[43,44] Environmental factors are also instrumental and include psychological stress, dietary factors (including low vitamin D levels), and air pollution.[45] Smoking, however, appears to have a protective effect on the development and relapse of UC.[46] The two main types of IBD are CD and UC. Both UC and CD are associated with extraintestinal manifestations (including: oral ulcers, oligoarticular or polyarticular non-deforming peripheral arthritis, spondylitis or sacroiliitis, episcleritis or uveitis, erythema nodosum, pyoderma gangrenosum, hepatitis and sclerosing cholangitis, and thromboembolic events) in up to 50% of patients. Current research indicates that both the incidence and prevalence of IBD are increasing all over the world.[47] In Europe, the prevalence of UC is 505 per 100,000 persons and the prevalence of CD is 322 per 100,000 persons. In North America the prevalence of UC is 249 per 100,000 persons, while for CD it is 319 per 100,000 persons.[47]

UC and CD are chronic debilitating conditions that are commonly associated with psychiatric symptoms, which in turn adversely affect disease course and severity. The prevalence of anxiety and depressive disorders in those suffering from GI problems is estimated to be between 24% and 27%; this rate is 2 to 3 times higher than that seen in healthy controls.[48,49] Anxiety and depressive symptoms are often found during relapses of IBD symptoms (up to 80% and 60%, respectively).[48,49] Rates of psychiatric co-morbidity in IBD are similar in UC and CD and differ from those in other chronic conditions, e.g., rheumatoid arthritis or diabetes.[50] Both anxiety and depression appear to increase after the diagnosis of IBD is made, possibly a consequence of the disease or a reaction to it.[50,51] While pre-morbid anxiety and depressive disorders have been thought of as risk factors for the development of IBD, the relative risk appears to be low and limited to the year before IBD was diagnosed, possibly representing an undiagnosed somatic illness.[50,51]

Some evidence suggests that both anxiety and depression negatively affect the course of CD.[38] Higher levels of anxiety and depressive symptoms have been associated with increased disease activity, including the number of relapses or failure to achieve remission with treatment. Furthermore, depression is considered to be a risk factor for failure of infliximab in patients with CD.[52] In a prospective study investigating the role of depression on disease course in patients with IBD, those with baseline ratings of depression had higher rates of relapse, relapsed more quickly, and had more severe relapses of IBD symptoms than did those with lower baseline depression scores.[53] Furthermore, a diagnosis of major depressive disorder (MDD) or generalized anxiety disorder (GAD) has been associated with higher rates of surgery in those suffering from CD vs patients with CD without these psychiatric co-morbidities.[54]

Due to the associations between psychiatric symptoms and IBD, a variety of psychotherapeutic interventions (including CBT, psychodynamic psychotherapy, relaxation training, and psychoeducation) have been tried. Studies have shown that psychotherapeutic interventions and psychoeducation do not positively impact the course of disease, but do help with psychological factors (such as coping, health-related quality of life, and anxiety related to the illness).[55] A recent randomized study looked at the efficacy of CBT that targeted anxiety, depression, and coping, and failed to show any benefit on disease activity (including remission) in UC or CD but did show positive effects on quality of life (QoL) scales.[56]

Additional evidence suggests that antidepressants (used for depression or anxiety) may have a positive effect on the course of illness in IBD patients. Patients with IBD and an anxiety or depressive disorder who were treated with an antidepressant for at least 6 months showed significant improvement in their QoL scores, CD activity index, as well as ratings of depression and anxiety on the Short

Form-36 (SF-36).[57] SSRIs, SNRIs, Wellbutrin, and Mirtazapine were used and were generally well-tolerated. Drowsiness and fatigue were the most common side effects. Approximately 7.5% of patients discontinued medications due to side effects, most commonly due to new-onset sexual dysfunction. Patients untreated or under-treated with antidepressants, with IBD and co-morbid depressive disorders or anxiety disorders, showed poorer QoL scores, and reported worse psychiatric and IBD symptoms. A retrospective case–control study involving 14 UC and 15 CD patients started on an antidepressant for a mood disorder showed reductions in relapse rates, use of steroids, and endoscopies in the year after their introduction versus matched controls.[58] A small study that assessed IBD patients' attitudes towards taking antidepressants showed that antidepressants are generally well-tolerated. Additionally, some patients attributed improvement in the course of IBD symptoms to the use of their antidepressants. [59]

Immunosuppressive medications used to treat core IBD symptoms may also be effective in treating depression in patients with IBD. Minderhoud and colleagues reported on 14 patients with IBD whose depressive symptoms improved after two infusions with infliximab.[60] Infliximab infusions have also been found to correspond to reduced depressive symptoms in a small cohort of patients with UC.[61] A recent retrospective study investigating the efficacy of immunosuppressive medication on depressive symptoms found significant decreases in the severity of depression as well as in overall depression scores in patients with IBD treated with immunosuppressive medications.[62] In this study, patients with active symptoms of UC (n = 16) and CD (n = 53) showed reduced PHQ-9 scores while treated with anti-TNF-α agents (including infliximab, adalimumab, and certolizumab). Patients also showed less depression when treated with azathioprine and methotrexate. It should be noted that the aforementioned findings should be viewed with caution, as the relationship between inflammation and psychiatric symptoms is complex and many potential confounders to the evaluation of treatment response exist. One such factor is the significant overlap of non-specific symptoms, such as fatigue and malaise, across many disorders which is often not accounted for in rating scales. Though more studies are needed, it is worth mentioning that many patients with IBD and co-morbid psychiatric conditions have appeared to find relief from psychiatric symptoms when immunologic treatment was aimed at their IBD symptoms and studies looking at immunologic treatment for psychiatric conditions are underway.

PSYCHIATRIC ISSUES RELATED TO CANCERS OF THE UPPER AND LOWER INTESTINES

GI Cancer

Psychiatric disorders are associated with poorer cancer detection and treatment, as well as an increased mortality rate. Approximately 50% of patients with advanced cancer meet criteria for a psychiatric disorder, most commonly an adjustment disorder, major depression, or an anxiety disorder.[2,63] Additionally, patients with psychiatric illness (particularly schizophrenia) often do not utilize preventative care and screening procedures, such as colonoscopy; this is associated with a poorer prognosis and outcomes.[64] A retrospective cohort study of 80,670 patients aged 67 or older with a diagnosis of colon cancer showed that patients with pre-existing mental illness were more likely to be diagnosed at autopsy, to be diagnosed at an unknown or later stage of cancer, and to receive no treatment at any stage of colon cancer.[65] Patients with pre-existing mental illness had a higher overall mortality rate and higher cancer-related mortality rate than controls. These findings were found with all major psychiatric diagnoses but were especially pronounced in those with dementia or psychotic disorders. The findings persisted after adjusting for sociodemographic factors, stage of diagnosis, and co-morbid conditions. Co-morbid depression was also an independent risk factor for lower survival rates and for increased rates of disease recurrence in a recent multivariate analysis of patients with oropharyngeal cancer.[66] In this study, Shinn and colleagues[66] implemented depression screening with the Physicians Health Questionnaire 9 (PHQ-9) and the Centers for Epidemiological Studies–Depression Scale (CES-D) at the beginning of their radiation treatment. Detecting depression at earlier illness stages, particularly in patients who may be otherwise overlooked (for instance, patients without pre-morbid psychiatric diagnosis), may lead to more successful detection, treatment, and overall outcomes.

Whether GI cancers and depression share common biological pathways that adversely affect outcomes is unknown. Poorer outcomes in depressed patients with cancer may be associated with abnormal chronic activation of the hypothalamic–pituitary axis, which is associated with prolonged inflammatory responses and weakened immunity, or via noradrenergic-driven tumor angiogenesis.[66] Other mechanisms may be that depression is linked with poorer health behaviors, such as decreased physical activity and tobacco and alcohol use.[66]

Consistent with the putative role of altered immunologic function, patients with advanced colorectal cancer with liver metastases and with increased levels of circulating interleukin-2R predicted higher rates of depression.[67] A recent prospective controlled study evaluated cytokine levels and ratings of depression and anxiety; they were compared in patients with colorectal cancer (who were admitted for tumor resection) and healthy controls.[68] A positive association was found between Hospital Anxiety and Depression Scale (HADS) scores and levels of IL-1β, IL-6, IL-8, and TNF-α, whereas a negative correlation was shown with IL-10. Antidepressants are typically effective in depressive and anxiety disorders that are associated with abnormal pro-inflammatory cytokine levels,[43,44] however, whether this holds true for patients with GI cancer is unknown.

Approximately 10% of cancer patients develop brain metastases; the vast majority of these occur with melanoma, lung, and breast cancer.[69] The incidence of brain metastases in cancers of GI origin is much lower (<1% in pancreatic and gastric cancer and <4% in esophageal and colorectal cancer).[69] Brain metastases associated with GI cancers are generally associated with a very poor prognosis; however, there are reports of prolonged survival after surgical resection of brain lesions. There is little information about the neuropsychiatric manifestations and sequelae of brain metastases associated with GI cancers.

LIVER DISORDERS

Hepatitis C

Hepatitis C virus (HCV) infection is associated with an overall reduced quality of life and overall functioning.[70] Approximately 50% of patients with HCV infection have a history of a psychiatric illness and approximately 90% have a history of a substance use disorder.[71] HCV is associated with multiple medical co-morbidities (including fibromyalgia, arthritis, peripheral neuropathy, and other numerous pain-related disorders).[72] Each of these may have bi-directional relationships as to causation and exacerbation of neuropsychiatric symptoms, further complicating successful management of these patients. Despite the high rates of co-morbid psychiatric and substance use disorders (SUDs) in patients infected with HCV, these patients are less likely to receive treatment of HCV infection (OR for psychiatric illness 9.45; OR for SUD 17.68).[71,73] Moreover, these patients have historically been excluded from research studies, despite having similar rates of treatment completion and sustained viral response (SVR) to those patients without co-morbid psychiatric or SUDs.[70,71] As discussed below, traditional therapies for HCV, most notably interferon-based treatments, are associated with higher rates of neuropsychiatric disorders and this has been of concern (and often served as a relative contraindication for treatment), as these therapies are associated with increased rates of depression or exacerbation of other underlying conditions, such as bipolar disorder.[70] Prophylactic antidepressant use, effective screening for psychiatric co-morbidity, and multidisciplinary team approaches have all been demonstrated to improve the treatment of many patients with psychiatric disorders (particularly depression and anxiety) receiving treatment for HCV.[70,74] In the past few years, HCV treatment strategies have changed to include the use of direct-acting antivirals and, thus far, these treatments have been associated with significantly fewer side effects, including neuropsychiatric side effects.[70,71,74] Given the high rates of HCV infection and the high rates of co-morbid psychiatric and SUDs, this may have a significantly positive effect towards the successful treatment of patients with HCV-infection.

Approximately 35 million people in the United States and approximately 3% of the world's population are infected with HCV.[70] The most common means of transmission is via intravenous drug use and, while less common, HCV can also be transmitted via sexual contact. Infants can also be infected by HCV-infected mothers.[70] Less common forms of transmission include blood transfusions, needle stick injuries, and application of tattoos;[70] fortunately, awareness, and prevention and treatment protocols have made these forms of transmission less common in the modern era.

Until recently, few options existed for treating chronic HCV infection. Treatment traditionally included the use of pegylated interferon-alpha (IFN-α) along with ribavirin for 24 to 48 weeks with response rates of approximately 55% as measured by SVR.[2,38,75] Treatment adherence was often difficult to maintain given the many side effects (e.g., anemia, leukopenia, fatigue, anorexia, thyroid disorders, insomnia, cognitive effects, and various psychiatric disorders) associated with IFN and ribavirin treatment.

As many as 70% of HCV-infected patients treated with IFN-α have suffered from mild-to-moderate depressive syndromes.[76] Some 20% to 40% of these patients have been diagnosed with MDD[76] and depression has been cited as the most common reason for discontinuation of drug treatment.[2] Onset of depressive symptoms usually occurs within 12 weeks of initiating IFN and typically resolves quickly upon discontinuation of treatment.[38] Although having a pre-existing psychiatric disorder confers a higher risk for developing a depressive disorder with IFN treatment,[77] other data suggest that the risk of IFN-associated depression is similar between patients with and without pre-morbid psychiatric disorders.[78,79]

While some studies have failed to show benefits of SSRIs over placebo,[72] more recent recommendations support the use of antidepressants for prevention of IFN-α-induced depression and treatment of depression in patients with chronic hepatitis C infection.[78,80,81] SSRIs and other antidepressants (including venlafaxine, mirtazapine, bupropion, and psychostimulants) in select populations are generally well-tolerated.[38,81] A 2014 systematic review and meta-analysis examined the efficacy of antidepressant pre-treatment of IFN-α-associated depression and found substantial decreases in the incidence and severity of depressive symptoms.[78] Benefits were found for all antidepressants, with the most benefit attributable to use of citalopram and escitalopram. Benefits of pre-treatment were observed, regardless of treatment duration or whether there were any pre-existing psychiatric disorders.

IFN-induced hypomania or mania have been reported at varying time points after initiating treatment (weeks or months), after major dose reductions, or after abrupt discontinuation.[38] In such cases, symptoms resolve with discontinuation of IFN along with starting psychotropic medications, most often an atypical antipsychotic. Mood lability or irritability are more common than are frank hypomania or mania, and may not require discontinuation or marked changes in treatment. IFN-induced psychosis is a rarely reported treatment side effect. For hypomania, mania, and psychosis, atypical antipsychotics are considered to be the best treatment option.[38] Despite this, in some instances, treatment with neuroleptics or other medications may not be effective without discontinuing IFN.[82] Patients with a pre-existing bipolar disorder and HCV infection are often not considered for antiviral treatment.[83] A retrospective analysis that examined the safety and efficacy of treatment of HCV infection in patients with bipolar disorder found that stable bipolar patients had similar rates of psychiatric complications as did patients with a history of depression; adherence and completion rates were similar between the groups.[83]

IFN-treated patients with HCV often report memory, concentration, and other cognitive problems.[2,38] These symptoms occur independently from depression or other psychiatric disorders and are thought to increase with the dose and duration of IFN treatment. Patients receiving IFN for HCV infection demonstrated notable decreases in multiple neurocognitive tasks, which generally were reversed after completion of treatment.[84] Frank delirium is a rarely reported side effect of IFN.[38]

Since 2011, the FDA began approving direct-acting antivirals for the treatment of HCV infection.[70,74] These medications do not act as inflammatory cytokines and do not appear to be associated with flu-like symptoms, depression, suicidal ideation, or other neuropsychiatric side effects classically associated with IFN-based therapies.[74] These medications, including the protease inhibitors boceprevir, telaprevir, sofosbuvir, and daclatasvir, have increased HCV treatment response rates, decreased the need for IFN-based therapy, and have not thus far been associated with significant neuropsychiatric side effects.[71] While the initial findings are promising, clinicians should remain cautious not to over-interpret these early discoveries as meaning that there are no associated risks. Protease inhibitors may inhibit cyclooxygenase P450 enzymes (especially CYP P450 3A4) and thus interfere with the metabolism of many medications. Furthermore, medications that stimulate P450 enzymes, such as carbamazepine, may reduce the levels of these medications, interfering with effective treatment.[71,74,85] Although these medications are better tolerated and the rates of neuropsychiatric effects are lower, caution should be exercised as pre-existing psychiatric and substance use issues may still affect therapy, including treatment adherence.[71] Thus, psychiatrists and other clinicians will still be faced with the task of understanding complex drug–drug interactions, monitoring treatment effects and outcomes, and optimizing psychiatric care before, during, and after treatment for HCV infection.

Hepatic Encephalopathy

Hepatic encephalopathy (HE) is characterized by the onset of neuropsychiatric symptoms and neuromuscular signs in patients with cirrhosis and/or portosystemic shunting. Afflicted individuals may present with mild neurocognitive deficits that may only be elicited by specific tests or with increasingly severe manifestations that include frank delirium or coma.[38] Psychometric tests that examine executive and other neurocognitive functions may be necessary for mild or subtle presentations, although there do not appear to be any gold standard bedside tests for this purpose and the validity of some tests is questionable. Serum ammonia levels are elevated in many, but not all patients with HE, and caution is required with interpretation of lab results, as some patients may have elevated and compensated levels at baseline.[38] An EEG may be of help in establishing the diagnosis, though findings of generalized slowing and triphasic waves, which are not always present, are non-specific indicators of delirium secondary to various toxic-metabolic pathologic states.[86] Neuromuscular manifestations can include myoclonus, asterixis, and focal neurologic deficits (such as hemiplegia in the absence of stroke).[38]

Common precipitating events for HE include: infections, GI bleeding, overuse of diuretics, electrolyte imbalance, and constipation.[87]

HE may also be the result of aberrant protein breakdown that leads to increased levels of serum ammonia.[87] Typically, protein is broken down into ammonia by gut bacteria, and ammonia is broken down into glutamine and urea by the liver; however, in the setting of severe liver disease, ammonia is not metabolized and a surplus of ammonia develops. In the brain, ammonia is metabolized by glutamine synthase to form glutamine.[87] Astrocytes play a prominent role in responding to increased levels of ammonia and glutamate. In acute liver disease, sudden increases in ammonia may lead to intracranial edema that leads to increased intracranial pressure. In chronic disease, astrocytes may adapt to elevated ammonia levels, resulting in a downregulation of glutamate.[87] Other mechanisms for HE include an increased blood–brain barrier permeability to GABA and other small non-lipid polar compounds, decreased activity of GABA-transaminase (resulting in increased GABA levels), and accumulation of endogenous compounds that bind to benzodiazepine binding sites on GABA receptors.[87]

Treatment of HE includes correction of precipitating factors (such as infections, electrolyte abnormalities, constipation, GI bleeding, and use of psychoactive medications). In addition, it is helpful to ensure regular bowel movements with non-absorbable disaccharide compounds (e.g., lactulose, vancomycin, rifaximin, ornithine aspartate, and sodium benzoate) which trap NH_3 in the gut lumen. Flumazenil has also been successful since endogenous GABA/benzodiazepine receptor ligands are increased in HE. The positive results with flumazenil are generally short-lived and its use does not appear to confer any benefit on the disease course or survival duration.[88] Flumazenil should be used with caution, as it may induce seizures in patients receiving benzodiazepines. Modification of nutrition and diet may include treatment with branched chain amino acids, acetyl-L-carnitine, and probiotics.[38]

DISORDERS OF THE PANCREAS

Pancreatic Cancer

CASE 4

Mr. D, an 85-year-old man with a history of hypertension and MDD was admitted to the inpatient psychiatric unit for elective electroconvulsive therapy (ECT) for an episode of MDD that had been refractory to conventional treatment with various antidepressants. He was taking sertraline (100 mg daily), bupropion sustained-release (100 mg daily), and lithium (300 mg daily). Other attempts to treat his depressive symptoms were limited by side effects, especially nausea, diarrhea, and fatigue. He had been hospitalized twice, once in the 1950s and once in 1980 for depressive episodes where he was successfully treated with ECT.

His wife and children reported that he had lost about 10–15 pounds over the past 2 months. He has been more despondent, sleeping more in the daytime, and sometimes not getting out of bed until the late afternoon. His appetite has been poor and his family stated that he looked like he has lost weight. He has been more "morose" and had not appeared to enjoy watching television, going for walks, or doing other activities that he normally enjoyed. His family was not aware of other symptoms and there have not been any known changes in memory or other cognitive functions. According to his wife, this is how he appeared in the 1950s and 1980s, when he was clinically depressed.

His admission examination and laboratory tests were unremarkable for acute or occult illnesses and ECT treatment was begun after discontinuing lithium (out of concerns for possible increased risk of delirium while receiving ECT treatment) and bupropion was decreased (to mitigate possible confounding changes on his seizure threshold).

After his third treatment, his mood began to improve; however, improvement typically lasted less than a day and rebounded entirely within 24 hours. He reported ongoing low energy and fatigue, loss of appetite and "no interest" in eating; in addition, he had insomnia, muscle aches, low motivation, and anhedonia. Sertraline was continued and quetiapine was started to target both insomnia and low appetite. After another three treatments, his symptoms continued and he began to report vague abdominal pain along with constipation. He reported intermittent nausea and was eating two meals a day without emesis or other reported or observed signs or symptoms. His physical exam was notable for mild mid-gastric and right upper quadrant tenderness without guarding or rebound. Labs showed mildly elevated total and direct bilirubin, AST, ALT, and lipase along with a mild decrease in his hemoglobin and hematocrit. Based on his continued complaints, physical exam, and laboratory findings, an abdominal ultrasound was ordered, which showed a large obstructing mass at the head of the pancreas. Abdominal CT and MRI confirmed the mass and Mr. D was diagnosed with pancreatic cancer. He was referred for an emergent oncology referral and was transferred to the oncology unit for further work-up and treatment planning.

Neuropsychiatric symptoms have long been associated with tumors of the pancreas. In 1931, Yaskin[89] reported that "nervous symptoms" appeared early in the course of pancreatic cancer and that disease manifestation was strongly linked to pre-morbid personality, socioeconomic, and psychogenic features. Clinical and academic findings have corroborated Yaskin's early report, and numerous studies have demonstrated an increased prevalence of psychiatric disturbances with pancreatic cancer.[90,91] Moreover, studies over the years have found that depressive symptoms and psychological distress may precede pancreatic cancer diagnosis by up to 6 months.[91,92] This points to a possible biological culprit linking these diseases, as depression related to psychological and coping reactions to illness would occur after a diagnosis is made. Interleukins, including IL-6, IL-18, TNF-α, as well other inflammatory cytokines, are elevated in pancreatic cancer.[93] Elevated IL-6 levels have been associated with various neuropsychiatric disturbances and in particular, with major depression.[44] Moreover, IL-6 appears to be particularly elevated in patients with pancreatic cancer and co-morbid major depression.[93,94]

As Case 4 indicates, patients who are ultimately diagnosed with pancreatic cancer may present a diagnostic challenge, particularly when presenting with depressive or other primary psychiatric features. Even when the diagnosis of pancreatic cancer is clear, patients who are depressed are less likely to have their cancers managed optimally than are patients who are not depressed,[95] thus necessitating close screening and monitoring of treatment interventions.

The prevalence of MDD in patients with pancreatic cancer ranges widely, from 10% to 75%, depending on which instruments were used for the evaluation and when patients were evaluated in their illness course.[96] Furthermore, the type and stage of pancreatic cancer is often not included in analyses of psychiatric symptoms that may impact the interpretation of self-reported or observed symptom severity and/or prognosis.

A 2009 study including 44 patients with neuroendocrine tumors of the pancreas that investigated rates of depressive symptoms with the Beck Depression Inventory-II (BDI-II), identified 17 (40%) patients with depressive symptoms: eight patients (18.2%) with moderate depression and nine patients (20.5%) with mild depression.[97] Utilizing the Public Health Questionnaire-9 (PHQ-9), a 2012 study including 22 patients followed over 6 months found that seven patients (32%) had reported mild depressive symptoms; five patients (23%) reported moderate depressive symptoms; and one patient (5%) reported moderately severe depressive symptoms.[96] More recent estimates indicate that approximately 10% to 20% of patients with pancreatic cancer suffer from depression.[95]

Somatic symptoms and neurovegetative symptoms (such as fatigue, low appetite, and pain), may be seen in various primary psychiatric disorders as well as in various clinical conditions. Numerous rating scales for depression and anxiety validated for screening primary psychiatric conditions (such as depression and anxiety) may not be as useful in certain patient populations due to the inclusion of various somatic markers that could be attributable to a primary medical condition. The Hospital Anxiety Depression Scale (HADS) excludes many of the somatic symptoms that may confound a more accurate diagnosis of anxiety or depression in the medically ill,[93,98] and it may be particularly useful in patients with pancreatic cancer, as many cancer-related symptoms are non-specific.[38]

Pancreatitis

Valproic acid (VPA) is rarely associated with drug-induced acute pancreatitis but does carry a black box warning for this reason. The exact mechanism is unknown but it may be related to the inhibition of histone deacetylases (that are primary targets of VPA) that results in impaired acinar cell proliferation and delayed regenerative reprogramming after injury.[99] A 2007 literature review noted that there were a total of 90 reported cases in the literature between 1979 and 2005.[100] The estimated prevalence is 1:40,000 and may develop at any time; however, it most commonly occurs within the first year of treatment or after a dosage increase.[101] There is no dose–response relationship.[38] Benign transient hyperamylasemia occurs in up to 20% of adult patients on VPA and does not confer greater risk of developing pancreatitis.[38,101] Routine screening of serum amylase or lipase is not recommended in the absence of symptoms suggestive of possible pancreatitis (abdominal pain, nausea, vomiting, diarrhea, and anorexia).[10] Discontinuation of the offending agent often results in resolution of symptoms within 10 days;[2] however, the mortality rate of VPA-induced pancreatitis is reported to be as high as 21%.[101] If drug-induced pancreatitis occurs, re-challenging with the same medication is absolutely contraindicated.[2,10,101]

MEDICATION CONSIDERATIONS IN GASTROINTESTINAL ILLNESS

Oral administration of medications may not be possible in patients with severe nausea or vomiting, esophageal disorders, or GI malabsorption syndromes. Challenges may also arise in patients who are delirious or unconscious, combative or uncooperative, or in surgical patients in the perioperative period. In such cases, alternative routes of administration are often required. However, many psychotropic medications are only available in oral form, thus making management potentially more complicated. While there are certain potential advantages or disadvantages to each type of administration route, certain patient factors including adequate tissue perfusion, venous access, and other factors need to be taken into account. Furthermore, side effect profiles of the same medication may differ between different routes of administration (e.g., increased QTc prolongation with IV haloperidol as opposed to less risk with oral formulations). Another key point is that the bioavailability and potency of medications may differ significantly between different administration routes and many medications require different dosing strategies among different formulations. Therefore, clinicians should refer to trusted sources in order to prescribe the correct dosing strategy. A summary of psychotropic medications available in IV, IM, sublingual, buccal, rectal, and transdermal formulations is summarized in Table 28-1. These data pertain to formulations available in the United States.

Liquid preparations or orally disintegrating formulations of psychotropic medication may be a viable option for patients who can tolerate oral dosing but who have difficulty swallowing tablets or capsules. Liquid formulations must still pass through the GI tract and undergo first-pass metabolism; thus, they still may not be suitable for patients with malabsorption, hepatic, or other GI diseases affecting drug metabolism. In the case of orally disintegrating tablets, this may be an option for some patients who are nonadherent, or who "cheek" their medication; once the tablet is placed on buccal or lingual mucosa, it will dissolve, thus making it difficult to spit out or hide.

While conferring certain advantages, liquid formulations and orally disintegrating tablets have some disadvantages. Doses for liquid formulations may be difficult to calculate and convert from capsule or tablet form, which may increase the risk of dosing errors.[102] Additionally, incompatibility problems, such as the formation of precipitate may occur when mixed with other liquids to increase palatability of these medications. Orally disintegrating tablets are often more expensive than tablets or capsules and this limits their use in many instances.[102] A summary of psychotropic medications available in liquid form or in oral disintegrating form is provided in Table 28-2. Clinicians should refer to packaging information or speak to a pharmacist, as many potential issues related to compatibility or incompatibility with other agents (such as caffeine, certain foods, other medications) may negatively impact treatment. Furthermore, many formulations contain other compounds that may cause side effects or be contraindicated in certain patient populations (e.g., alcohol, propylene glycol).[102]

SSRI-Related Upper GI Bleeding

A recent meta-analysis by Jiang and colleagues[103] reported that SSRIs are associated with an almost 55% increase in the risk for upper GI bleeding (UGIB). Bleeding is especially

TABLE 28-1 Non-Oral Preparations of Psychotropic Medication

MEDICATIONS	INTRAVENOUS	INTRAMUSCULAR	SUBLINGUAL	RECTAL	TRANSDERMAL
Anxiolytics	Diazepam Lorazepam Midazolam	Chlordiazepoxide Diazepam Lorazepam Midazolam		Diazepam	
Hypnotics			Zolpidem		
Antidepressants			Selegiline	Amitriptyline Doxepin	Selegiline
Typical antipsychotics	Chlorpromazine Haloperidol Perphenazine	Chlorpromazine Fluphenazine Haloperidol Loxapine Perphenazine Prochlorperazine Thiothixene Depot medications: Fluphenazine Haloperidol		Prochlorperazine	
Atypical antipsychotics		Aripiprazole Olanzapine Ziprasidone Depot medications: Olanzapine Paliperidone Risperidone	Asenapine		
Mood stabilizers	Valproate			Carbamazepine Valproate	
Psychostimulants				Dextroamphetamine	Methylphenidate
Cognitive enhancers					Rivastigmine

Medications that are available in the United States are listed.

Data obtained from Owen in Crone CC, Marcangelo M, Lackamp J, et al: Gastrointestinal disorders, in Clinical manual of psychopharmacology in the medically ill. Edited by Ferrando SJ, Levenson JL, Owen JA. Washington D.C. American Psychiatric Publishing, 2010, pp 103–148.[2]

TABLE 28-2 Liquid and Orally Disintegrating Formulations of Psychotropic Medications

MEDICATION	LIQUID FORMULATIONS AND DOSE (mg/mL)	ORALLY DISINTEGRATING FORMULATIONS AND DOSE (mg)
Antidepressants		
SSRIs	Citalopram 10 mg/5 mL (240 mL)	
	Escitalopram 1 mg/mL (240 mL)	
	Fluoxetine 20 mg/5 mL (5 mL, 120 mL)	
	Paroxetine 10 mg/5 mL (250 mL)	
	Sertraline 20 mg/mL (60 mL)	
TCAs	Doxepin 10 mg/mL (120 mL)	
	Nortriptyline 10 mg/mL (240 mL)	
NaSSA		Mirtazapine 15, 30, 45 mg
Antipsychotics		
	Aripiprazole 1 mg/mL	Aripiprazole 10, 15 mg
	Risperidone 1 mg/mL	Clozapine 12.5, 25, 100 mg
	Fluphenazine 2.5 mg/5 mL, elixir 5 mg/mL	Olanzapine 5, 10, 15, 20 mg
	Thioridazine 100 mg/mL	Risperidone 0.5, 1, 2, 3, 4 mg
Anxiolytics (Benzodiazepines)		
	Alprazolam 1 mg/mL (30 mL)	Alprazolam 0.25, 0.5, 1, 2 mg
	Diazepam 5 mg/mL (500 mL)	Clonazepam 0.125, 0.25, 0.5, 1, 2 mg
	Lorazepam 2 mg/mL (1 mL, 10 mL)	
Cholinesterase Inhibitors		
	Galantamine 4 mg/mL (100 mL)	Donepezil 5, 10 mg
	Rivastigmine 2 mg/mL (in 120 mL bottle)	
NMDA Receptor Antagonists		
	Memantine 2 mg/mL (in 360 mL bottle)	
Mood Stabilizers		
	Carbamazepine 100 mg/5 mL	Lamotrigine 25, 50, 100 mg
	Valproic acid 250 mg/5 mL (473 mL)	
Stimulants		
	Dextroamphetamine 5 mg/5 mL	
	Methylphenidate 5 mg/5 mL (500 mL)	

SSRI, selective serotonin re-uptake inhibitor; TCA, tricyclic antidepressant; NaSSA, noradrenergic and selective serotonin antagonist.
Data obtained from Muramatsu RS, Litzinger MH, Fisher E, et al: Alternative formulations, delivery methods, and administration options for psychotropic medications in elderly patients with behavioral and psychological symptoms of dementia. Am J Geriatr Pharmacother. 2010 Apr; 8(2): 98–114.[102]

more likely in patients who are also taking NSAIDs or anti-platelet medications, whereas the risk of bleeding is almost eliminated by the use of acid-suppressing medication.[103] Wang and colleagues[104] demonstrated that UGIB occurs soon after starting SSRIs with an adjusted odds ratios of 1.67 (95% CI = 1.23–2.26) for the 7-day window, 1.84 (95% CI = 1.42–2.40) for the 14-day window, and 1.67 (95% CI = 1.34–2.08) for the 28-day window. Anglin and colleagues[105] reported that there was an increased risk of UGIB with SSRIs and that the number-needed-to-harm for UGIB with SSRI treatment in a low-risk population was 3177, and in a high-risk population, it was 881. Furthermore, the risk of UGIB was further increased with the use of both SSRI and NSAID medications (OR = 4.25, 95% CI = 2.82, 6.42), consistent with other studies.[105] SSRI-induced GI bleeding is thought to be due to depleting serotonin in platelets, which do not synthesize their own serotonin and therefore require re-uptake from plasma. This results in decreased platelet aggregation and clotting.[38,103] SSRI use is normally safe in most patients, however, particular caution should be exercised in patients with pre-existing clotting or other bleeding disorders, as well as patients at risk for GI bleeding, particularly those taking NSAIDs.

MEDICATION CONSIDERATIONS IN LIVER DISEASE

Since most psychotropic medications are metabolized by the liver, impaired hepatic function will negatively impact various aspects of pharmacokinetics, including drug absorption (due to vascular congestion) as well as first-pass metabolism and biotransformation (due to damaged hepatocytes and altered cytochrome P450 enzyme function).[2] Oral bioavailability of medications may be increased due to prolonged biotransformation, metabolism, and clearance, and may also be increased in porto-systemic shunting where the medication is passed untransformed to the systemic circulation and brain. Changes in total body water and volume of distribution in moderate to severe liver disease result in altered distribution of water-soluble drugs and drug levels may shift drastically with fluid redistribution.[2]

Therefore, medications with narrow therapeutic windows, even those not metabolized by the liver, such as lithium, should be used with caution. Because moderate to severe hepatic disease results in decreased plasma proteins and interferes with protein-binding, total drug-level monitoring for medications that are highly protein-bound, such as valproic acid, may be misleading, and the unbound or free portion should be measured.

Regardless of the presence of hepatic dysfunction, many psychotropic medications can be continued unless liver enzymes exceed three times the upper limit of normal.[10] Initial doses of hepatically metabolized medications should be lowered and dose increases should occur over longer intervals. Medications that undergo complex multi-step biotransformation and those that are metabolized into active metabolites (such as amitriptyline, imipramine, venlafaxine, and bupropion) may pose greater challenges in this population than medications with more simple pharmacokinetics.[2] Medications with long half-lives (e.g., fluoxetine, aripiprazole) or extended- or slow-release formulations (e.g., venlafaxine XR) should be avoided if possible as their pharmacokinetics are less predictable.[2] Dosing changes and recommendations can be made while considering hepatic severity as measured by the Child–Pugh score (CPS) that considers total bilirubin, serum albumin, ascites, INR, and the presence or absence of hepatic encephalopathy.[2,10] According to Crone and colleagues,[2] patients with mild (CPS-A) liver failure can usually tolerate 75% to 100% of the standard medication dose, those with moderate (CPS-B) disease may require a 50% to 75% reduction in dose, and with severe disease (CPS-C) patients (particularly those with hepatic encephalopathy), conservative dosing schedules and close monitoring are required.

Certain psychotropic medications may be associated with drug-induced liver injury. Drug-induced liver injury is often idiosyncratic and cannot be predicted accurately by specific risk factors or drug dosage.[2,106] With the exception of carbamazepine and divalproex, there are no specific formal manufacturer's guidelines for monitoring liver enzymes.[10] Medication-induced hepatotoxicity is associated with alanine aminotransferase (ALT) levels in excess of aspartate aminotransferase (AST). Caution is required when interpreting laboratory results in patients who have pre-existing liver disease and in obese patients with steatohepatitis and non-alcoholic fatty liver disease.[10] Mild to modest increases in transaminases may occur with carbamazepine, divalproex, certain tricyclic antidepressants, serotonin norepinephrine re-uptake inhibitors, and atypical antipsychotics.[10] Voican and colleagues[106] recently reviewed data pertaining to antidepressant-induced liver injury and found that 0.5–3% of patients experienced asymptomatic and mild elevations of transaminases. Elderly patients and patients taking multiple medications confer the highest risk. Cases are generally not associated with dosage and the majority of reactions occur from several days to 6 months after initiating the medication. The highest risks of hepatotoxicity are associated with iproniazid, nefazodone, phenelzine, imipramine, amitriptyline, duloxetine, bupropion, trazodone, tianeptine, and agomelatine. Antidepressants with the lowest potential for hepatotoxicity were citalopram, escitalopram, paroxetine, and fluvoxamine.[106] Severe hepatotoxicity has been reported with duloxetine, nefazodone, carbamazepine, and divalproex; and divalproex and nefazodone both carry FDA black box warnings.[10] Valproate is associated with liver toxicity in 1 in 20,000 cases and in 1 in 6000 cases in patients under 2 years of age, or in patients receiving multiple anti-epileptic medications.[101] Cases of liver toxicity have been reported with lamotrigine and the risk of hepatotoxicity is roughly 16 cases per 100,000 treatment years.[101] Chlorpromazine and other phenothiazines may cause reversible cholestatic hepatotoxicity in up to 2% of cases; patients with primary biliary cirrhosis should not receive these medications.[2] Marwick and colleagues[107] assessed the pattern of liver function test (LFT) abnormalities associated with regular antipsychotic use. They found that a median of 32% of patients experienced elevated LFTs on any antipsychotic, with a range of 5% to 78%. The median percentage of patients with clinically significant elevations was 4%, with a range of 0% to 15%. Transaminases were most commonly elevated as opposed to bilirubin or alkaline phosphatase. Abnormalities were generally asymptomatic, arose within 6 weeks, and were either stably persistent or resolved with continued treatment. Consistent with other studies, chlorpromazine was the agent most associated with acute liver injury and this tends to show a cholestatic pattern, as opposed to a hepatotoxic pattern.

There are no specific guidelines for hepatic monitoring and it is likely that none is needed for the majority of patients receiving hepatically metabolized medications. If a patient has pre-existing liver disease, or develops symptoms after starting a medication, it is reasonable to investigate further. If no clinical symptoms accompany elevated serum transaminases up to 2 times the normal limit, watchful waiting with laboratory monitoring versus drug discontinuation is reasonable. If transaminase levels exceed 2–3 times the normal limit, it is advisable to discontinue the medication.[2,10] Certain medications known to be associated with severe hepatotoxicity (e.g., duloxetine, nefazodone, carbamazepine, and divalproex) should be discontinued even in more mild cases, as they are known to be associated with severe hepatotoxicity. Finally, if patients present with specific signs of liver disease, such as right upper quadrant pain, dark urine, lightly colored stool, itching, jaundice, nausea, anorexia, medications should be stopped immediately and expert consultation sought.

In contrast to ALT>AST patterns seen in drug-induced hepatotoxicity, in patients with alcohol-induced hepatotoxicity, AST:ALT ratios of 2:1 or 3:1 may be seen.[10] Carbohydrate-deficient transferrin and gamma-glutamyl transpeptidase (GTT) are both non-specific but sensitive markers of hepatic dysfunction and can be used to aide in the detection in recent (2-week) heavy drinking patterns. Elevated GTT distinguishes between liver-based as opposed to bone-based elevations in alkaline phosphatase, however it may also be elevated in congestive heart failure and may not be useful in this patient population.[10]

Some patients metabolize medications differently due to varying isoforms of cytochrome P450 genes. This may further complicate effective management in the presence of hepatic disease. At times, genetic testing may help indicate whether psychotropic medications are being metabolized differently in patients who can be considered rapid metabolizers, ultra-rapid (0–30% of the population) metabolizers, or poor (slow) metabolizers (0–14% of the population) due to the presence or absence of CYP P450 isoforms.[108] Additionally, medications which increase or inhibit the metabolism of medications (such as carbamazepine—a potent CYP P450 enhancer or paroxetine—a potent CYP P450 inhibitor) need to be taken into account as their presence may require further dosing adjustments in patients with or without liver disease. Knowledge of medications that are minimally metabolized or undergo no metabolism by hepatic CYP P450 enzymes can aid in appropriate medication selection. These medications include pregabalin, lorazepam, oxazepam, temazepam, desvenlafaxine, milnacipran, paliperidone, gabapentin, levetiracetam, lamotrigine, lithium, and memantine.[108]

REFERENCES

Access the reference list online at https://expertconsult.inkling.com/.

Organ Failure and Transplantation

29

Laura M. Prager, M.D.

OVERVIEW

Solid organ transplantation is an accepted, successful, and commonly employed treatment option for patients with end-organ failure. Transplantation recipients of a heart, liver, kidney, lung(s), pancreas, or small intestine now live longer with an overall improved quality of life. Transplantation now also offers hope to patients with severed upper limbs and to those who have suffered facial disfigurement. Progress in the development of immunosuppressive medications and in methods of organ procurement and distribution has also enabled transplantation. Former contraindications to transplant, such as a history of cancer or HIV infection, are no longer absolute barriers.

In the United States, the United Network for Organ Sharing (UNOS), a non-profit organization endowed by Congress but reporting to the Department of Health and Human Services, regulates the allocation and distribution of donor organs. UNOS has two branches: the Organ Procurement and Transplant Network (OPTN) and the Scientific Registry of Transplant Recipients (SRTR). The OPTN divides the country into 11 distinct geographic regions or donation service areas (DSA) and each region has its own waiting lists. Allocation of organs generally follows local, regional, and national progress, where local refers to the boundaries of the DSA. The length of time that a transplant candidate spends on a waiting list, regardless of organ, can differ greatly among regions.

The method of determination of a transplant candidate's place on a waiting list is organ-specific. For kidneys, "time served" on the waiting list is the primary determining factor. Potential pediatric recipients (age 18 years and younger) for both kidneys and livers take priority over adults. In 2014, OPTN/UNOS Kidney Transplantation Committee implemented new guidelines for adult transplant candidates taking into account a candidate's Estimated Post-Transplant Survival (EPTS) and creating a measure of kidney quality or the Kidney Donor Profile Index (KDPI) in an effort to optimize the match between donors and recipients.[1] The Lung Allocation Score (LAS) is a calculated score for patients over 12 years of age that identifies, among other things, the severity of illness and the likelihood of a successful transplant outcome. The score undergoes frequent modifications based on several factors, including shifts in the characteristics of the candidate cohort, with the consistent goal of reducing time spent on the waiting list. That score, in addition to other factors, includes age, blood type, and geographic location, and determines waiting-list placement for potential lung transplantation recipients. OPTN limits the allocation of lungs to patients less than 12 years of age to donors within the same age range. This policy has come under scrutiny due to a highly publicized case, in which the parents of a 10-year-old girl appealed to a federal judge to allow the patient access to lungs from the adult donor pool.[2] Increasingly, patients with acute respiratory failure have been placed on an extracorporeal membrane oxygenator (ECMO) as a bridge to transplant.[3] The Model for End-stage Liver Disease (MELD) is also a calculated score that predicts how urgently a patient over 12 years of age will need a transplant within the next 3 months. The only exception to the MELD system is a special category known as "Status 1." Status 1A patients have suffered acute hepatic failure and might die within hours or days without a transplant (Tables 29-1 and 29-2 list the LAS and MELD criteria). Since 1999, heart transplant recipients have received organs based on medical urgency; in 2005, UNOS/OPTN implemented a modification to that policy in terms of geographic sharing of organs. In 2012, it became clear that the current allocation policy was not sufficient based on the number of critically ill candidates who are not able to receive transplants. The heart subcommittee of UNOS/OPTN is now attempting to modify these guidelines and is engaged in an ongoing discussion about the most equitable way to distribute donor hearts.[4]

Several factors limit the success of organ transplantation. Allograft rejection and the complications of anti-rejection therapy also continue to limit successful transplantation. In addition, immunocompromised hosts are vulnerable to bacteria, viruses, and fungi that are not considered pathogenic in the normal population. Finally, the side effects of immunosuppressive medications that are used to manage rejection can be debilitating, disfiguring, or life-threatening, and increase the risk for neoplasm, problems with bone metabolism, a cushingoid body habitus, nephrotoxicity, posterior-reversible encephalopathic syndrome (PRES), and the development of diabetes mellitus.

The most pressing challenge, however, remains the shortage of available deceased-donor and living-donor organs. The scarcity of cadaveric organs creates a mismatch between the number of patients who need transplantation and the number who can undergo transplantation. In 2015, there were approximately 30,000 transplants performed in the

TABLE 29-1 Criteria for Lung Allocation Score (LAS) (Age 12 and Older)

Diagnosis
Age
Body mass index (BMI)
Presence of diabetes
New York Heart Association Functional Classification
Distance walked in 6 minutes
Forced vital capacity (FVC) % predicted
Pulmonary artery systolic pressure at rest
Central venous pressure at rest prior to exercise
Creatinine
Continuous oxygen requirement to maintain oxygen saturation at 88% or greater at rest
Requirement for ventilatory support
Current, highest, and lowest pCO_2

Adapted from United Network for Organ Sharing (UNOS): https://www.unos.org/wcontent/uploads/unos/lung_allocation_score.pdf

TABLE 29-2 Model for End-Stage Liver Disease (MELD) (Age 12 and Older)

Serum bilirubin (BR)
INR (international normalized ratio)
Serum creatinine
Need for dialysis twice within the past week or CVVHD
If MELD score >12, add serum sodium

Adapted from United Network for Organ Sharing (UNOS): https://optn.transplant.hrsa.gov/resources/allocation-calculators/meld-calculator/

United States; almost 25,000 were from deceased donors and 5000 from living donors. Kidney and liver transplants comprised the majority with approximately 18,000 and 7000, respectively. The remainder included heart, lung, and pancreas.[5] In recent years, transplant centers have attempted to expand the donor pool by harvesting organs from donors after circulatory death (DCD) in addition to harvesting organs from persons who have been declared dead by neurological criteria (i.e., brain death).[6] The recent changes in how deceased-donor kidneys are distributed, noted above, have helped to increase the number of patients who are "difficult to match" getting a transplant. But, there are still more than 101,000 patients on the national kidney transplant waiting list in 2017.

Organ donation by living donors is an increasingly important potential source of transplantable kidneys, livers, and lungs. This is especially true in Japan where there are no defined criteria for determination of brain death and therefore few cadaveric organs are available for harvest.[7] In the United States, living donors may be: related to the recipient; unrelated but emotionally connected; or anonymous, altruistic strangers. According to data from OPTN (from 2015) 24,980 transplanted organs came from deceased donors and 5989 organ transplants came from live donors.[5] Parent-to-child liver transplantation (of the left lateral lobe) is an option, as is adult-to-adult transplantation of the right hepatic lobe. Living-lung donation is also an option for carefully selected candidates, but it requires a lower lobe from two different donors for each single potential recipient. The source of the donated organ (i.e., from a deceased donor or living donor) does not affect recipient outcome.

Living organ donation raises several ethical questions: What is true informed consent regarding both short- and long-term risks for the donor? Is the donor's offer (be it from an emotionally connected or unrelated person) truly voluntary? It is difficult to determine what level of risk is acceptable for a healthy, altruistic donor.[8,9]

Several retrospective studies of the long-term medical and psychological sequelae in living organ donors have been conducted. Short-term risks for live kidney donors include the morbidity secondary to surgery and anesthesia (e.g., bleeding, infection) and salary loss during the weeks of recovery. For kidney donors, long-term health risks include the development of microalbuminuria and the potential for renal failure in the remaining kidney.[10] Very recently, researchers created a model to estimate a potential kidney donor's long-term risk of developing end-stage renal disease (ESRD) without donation that they hope will be helpful in advising potential donors.[11] The mortality rates for kidney donors is 0.03%;[12] with adult-to-adult liver donation there is a significant degree of morbidity, and mortality rate estimates approach 0.1% for left lateral donation and 0.5% for right lateral donation.[13] To date, no deaths have resulted from living lobar lung donation. One study found that donors lose 15% to 20% of their total lung volume and often experience a decrease in exercise capacity.[14] Another study demonstrated that both the forced vital capacity (FVC) and forced expiratory volume at 1 minute (FEV1) returned to 90% of baseline at 1 year post-lobectomy.[15]

PSYCHIATRIC EVALUATION OF THE TRANSPLANT PATIENT

Psychiatrists and other mental health professionals are involved in many different aspects of the transplantation process. In some centers, a designated psychiatrist works with a specific team: for example, the kidney transplant team. Other transplant centers rely on general hospital psychiatric consultation services, psychologists, or social workers to provide case-by-case consultation. The involvement of mental health professionals ranges from the preoperative evaluation of candidates and living donors, to the short- and long-term postoperative management of solid organ recipients.

The psychiatrist or other mental health professional plays an important role in the evaluation of the patient who is approaching a transplant. Initially, the psychiatrist conducts a thorough psychiatric evaluation of the potential recipient to determine suitability for transplant. The psychiatrist must be familiar with medical and surgical problems facing the patient (both before and after transplantation), in order to educate both the patient and the family members about the risks and benefits of transplantation.

The psychiatrist may also act as a liaison between the patient (and family members) and the transplant team. The patient will need support, direction, and clarification of the transplant team's expectations and concerns. The transplant team may require help interpreting a patient's behavior. The psychiatrist can direct the team's attention on ethical dilemmas that may arise, particularly in the area of directed living donation by a related or unrelated donor.

After transplantation, the psychiatrist will be instrumental in guiding the family through the patient's often difficult and unpredictable postoperative course, as well as in managing the neuropsychiatric sequelae secondary to graft rejection, infection, and immunosuppression.

Pre-Transplant Psychiatric Evaluation

There are no universally accepted guidelines for the psychiatric evaluation of potential candidates for organ transplantation and little reliable or predictive data regarding "suitability for transplantation." Some centers routinely offer a face-to-face clinical interview with a mental health provider, whereas other centers administer formal psychological testing or offer a structured or semi-structured interview. One of the most promising standardized psychosocial assessment tools is the Stanford Integrated Psychosocial Assessment for Transplant (SIPAT) developed by Maldonado et al., which can be used by any member of the transplant team as a way to determine patients' psychosocial risk factors and highlights current issues that might translate into problems post-transplant.[16] Transplant centers differ in their determination of who is an "acceptable" candidate and what degree of risk they are willing to assume.

Common psychosocial and behavioral exclusion criteria include active substance abuse, active psychotic symptoms, suicidal ideation (with intent or plan), dementia, or a felony conviction. Relative contraindications include poor social supports with an inability to arrange for pre-transplant or post-transplant care, personality disorders that interfere with a working relationship with a transplant team, non-adherence to a medication regimen, and neurocognitive limitations.[17] The pre-transplantation psychiatric evaluation should be primarily diagnostic, but it can also be both educational and therapeutic. General objectives of the psychiatric evaluation include screening of potential recipients for the presence of significant diagnoses that might complicate management or interfere with the patient's ability to comply with the treatment team's recommendations after transplantation. The diagnosis of a major depressive disorder, schizophrenia, or bipolar disorder should not be a contraindication to transplant if the patient has been stable for an extended period on appropriate medications and has adequate outpatient care and support.

CASE 1

Mr. A, a 40-year-old man with diabetes mellitus and end-stage renal disease, was referred for psychiatric evaluation of depression because he wanted to discontinue hemodialysis. There was no personal or family history of depression. He reported a depressed mood in association with chronic pain from diabetic neuropathy and from the severe headaches that often followed hemodialysis sessions. Mr. A agreed to a trial of an antidepressant and an analgesic after hemodialysis. His pain remitted, his mood lifted, and he subsequently chose to undergo renal transplantation.

Transplantation is possible even in those with an intellectual disability and with end-organ failure. Such patients may have family members who will assume legal responsibility for medical decision-making and oversee adherence to post-transplant protocols. The relationship between cognitive dysfunction secondary to end-organ failure and post-transplant function has not been well studied. Personality disorders are sometimes more difficult to diagnose in a cross-sectional interview, but, when present, can complicate the patient's interactions with members of the treatment team. Patients with borderline personality disorder or antisocial personality disorder are particularly problematic given their affective dysregulation, unstable personal relationships, and potential for impaired impulse control. Transplant psychiatrists must carefully assess the individual patient's history of interpersonal relationships, substance abuse, potential for self-injurious behavior, adherence to treatment recommendations, and interactions with caregivers, before making a decision as to whether such a patient can work successfully with the team.

Psychiatrists are often asked to predict a patient's motivation for transplantation and risk for non-adherence with medication regimens. Life following transplant requires consistent attention to, and compliance with, medical protocols. Post-transplant patients often take as many as 20 medications daily, attend regular clinic appointments, self-monitor blood pressure and blood sugar, maintain good nutrition, and frequently endure uncomfortable procedures and tests.

Evaluators may also wish to assess the patient's resilience and ability to persevere despite setbacks, as well as the availability of social supports that will allow for continued care in the community and easy transportation to and from the hospital. There is controversy as to whether or not the transplant team should explore social media sites in order to verify the patient's report of his/her lifestyle choices. Most mental health professionals who work with this population do not engage in what some have referred to as "patient-targeted googling,"[18] but others feel strongly that they must use whatever means they have in order to make a decision about a candidate's ability to comply with the demands of transplantation (personal communication, TransplantPsychiatry@googlegroups.com, 2013.)

Frequently, the question arises as to whether or not there is a conflict of interest if, as is often the case, the psychiatrist who conducts the initial screening for transplant candidacy is the same psychiatrist who works with the multidisciplinary transplant team to decide which candidates can be listed. Again, there are no national guidelines and individual transplant teams must address and resolve this ethical issue. The psychiatrist may choose to handle this situation by informing the patient and the family at the beginning of the evaluation that the information presented will be shared with other members of the team.

The issue of substance abuse in the pre-transplant population is particularly challenging because of the risk for relapse with possible non-adherence post-transplant. Most transplant programs require 6 months to 1 year of sustained sobriety before initiation of the transplant evaluation, although this policy has not been shown to affect outcome.[19] Some programs require patients to participate in a substance abuse counseling program in addition to Alcoholics Anonymous (AA) or Narcotics Anonymous (NA) as a prerequisite for listing if they appear to be at high risk for relapse. Cigarette smoking, any form of tobacco use, or use of nicotine-containing products is an absolute contraindication to lung transplantation. Patients must demonstrate sustained abstinence from cigarettes and undergo random measurements of urinary cotinine and/or serum carboxyhemoglobin as part of the evaluation process. In the end, individual transplant centers determine what degree of risk they are willing to tolerate.

PSYCHIATRIC CONSIDERATIONS IN PATIENTS WITH END-ORGAN FAILURE

Many psychiatric disorders (such as depression, anxiety, adjustment disorders, post-traumatic stress disorder [PTSD], and substance abuse) are common in the pre-transplant candidate population, regardless of the type of end-stage organ failure. Other disorders are unique to patients who suffer from a particular type of end-organ failure. Usually, there is a significant wait between the time of listing for transplant and the transplant itself. Many patients with heart failure must wait in a hospital's intensive care unit (ICU) attached to a cardiac monitor or an intra-aortic balloon pump (IABP); others live outside the hospital with left ventricular assist devices (LVADs). Years can go by while the patient with lung disease waits at home, sometimes far from a transplant center, becoming gradually sicker and more sedentary, all the while tethered to an oxygen tank. The wait is stressful. A call from a member of the transplant team saying that an organ is available can come at any time or not at all. Sometimes a patient arrives at the hospital only to learn that the quality of the harvested organ is not good enough—the so-called "false start" or "dry run." Loss of physical strength and productivity (with accompanying role change within the family or community) can lead to an adjustment disorder or to depression.

As many as 25% of dialysis-dependent patients with ESRD manifest symptoms of clinical depression.[20] Disorders of endocrine function (e.g., hyper-parathyroidism), and chronic anemia can also contribute to depression. The dialysis-dysequilibrium syndrome with resultant cerebral edema, as well as uremia, can precipitate a change in mental status or even a frank encephalopathy. Patients with renal failure are prone to delirium from the accumulation of toxins (e.g., aluminum) or prescribed medications that are normally cleared through the kidney.

Patients with cardiac failure are also at risk for depression and delirium. These patients can spend long periods in the ICU awaiting transplantation with little contact with the outside world. Delirium can be caused by decreased cerebral blood flow, by multiple small ischemic events, or by IABP treatment.[21] The development of the LVAD as a bridge to heart transplantation offers a chance for improved quality of life and functional status in this population. LVAD implantation as a bridge to transplant (BTT) confers a survival benefit for transplant candidates compared with those who are managed medically. LVAD can also be used as a bridge to candidacy (BTC) as implantation can stabilize a patient long enough for him/her to address other issues that preclude transplant candidacy, such as weight and possibly cardiac-induced pulmonary hypertension.[22]

Hepatic failure (e.g., from cirrhosis) is also associated with a high degree of depression and subclinical or frank encephalopathy. Treatment of the mood disorder can result in a more positive outlook and in better self-care. Suicide attempt by toxic ingestion (e.g., of acetaminophen) can result in sudden, drastic, hepatic failure and in an immediate need for transplantation. These patients are more difficult to assess because they are often on ventilators. The psychiatric consultant must therefore rely on collateral sources of information about the patient's pre-morbid function.

Patients with end-stage lung disease are likely to suffer from anxiety disorders, particularly panic disorder, in addition to adjustment disorders, depression, and delirium. Most patients who are not anxious pre-morbidly become anxious in the setting of increasing shortness of breath. They often describe anticipatory anxiety (in the setting of planned exertion), panic attacks, and agoraphobia, despite adequate oxygen supplementation. A decreasing radius of activity leads to both adjustment disorder and, sometimes, major depression, as patients struggle to cope with their relentless and progressive inability to perform even simple activities of daily living (ADLs).

CASE 2

Ms. E, a 21-year-old married woman with pulmonary fibrosis, was referred by her pulmonologist for lung transplantation. She had no other medical problems and had no formal psychiatric history. A college graduate, she had worked full-time for several years. During the year before her evaluation, she had to work fewer hours because of worsening pulmonary function. Although she described herself as "even-keeled," she had become increasingly anxious as her pulmonary function worsened. Even when her pulmonologist started her on continuous oxygen treatment, she remained anxious. At the time of her evaluation, she felt overwhelmed and was having panic attacks, particularly when she anticipated leaving her apartment to go to work. She also had trouble socializing with her husband and her friends. Her discomfort was so profound that she considered leaving her job. Panic disorder secondary to pulmonary decline was diagnosed, and a selective serotonin re-uptake inhibitor (SSRI) and a benzodiazepine (in a low dose) were prescribed. She did extremely well on this regimen, began a pulmonary rehabilitation program, kept her job, and resumed her social life with her friends.

Extremely compromised patients with pulmonary failure may become delirious from hypoxia or hypercapnia or from medications (such as IV benzodiazepines and narcotics) used to treat their anxiety and pain. Use of an extracorporeal membrane oxygenation (ECMO) as a bridge to lung transplant poses new challenges. Unlike mechanical ventilation, which has been considered a contraindication to transplant, ECMO allows patients to remain awake and alert and to participate in physical therapy.[23] However, patients on ECMO are often fearful of their tenuous condition and their total dependence on the machine and the staff. In this setting, they often become demanding and angry and deplete the energy and patience of the ICU team.

Psychiatric Care of the Pre-Transplant Patient

Psychiatric care of the pre-transplant patient is based on the bio-psycho-social approach. Psychotropic medications are often a mainstay of treatment. Psychotherapeutic intervention can be helpful as well. Enhancement of a network of social support from family members, neighbors, and friends is crucial. Substance abuse counseling may be required for at-risk patients. Transplant centers may offer support groups run by mental health professionals or clinical nurse specialists that welcome both pre-transplant and post-transplant patients. Psychopharmacologic management of the pre-transplant patient follows the adage, "start low and go slow." Choice of medication and dosage depends on the patient's diagnosis, as well as on the type and degree of organ failure.

The SSRIs are usually the first-line treatment of depressive disorders, given their generally benign side-effect profile and anxiolytic effects. For patients who also struggle to refrain from cigarette smoking, bupropion may be a good choice. Antidepressants are metabolized in the liver, and it is wise to use lower doses for patients with hepatic disease. In addition, there is some evidence to suggest that SSRIs can put patients at increased risk for upper gastrointestinal bleeding and therefore should be used with caution in patients with portal vein hypertension and with cirrhosis.[24] SSRIs must also be used with caution in patients with resistant bacterial infections who require the antibiotic linezolid (a weak monoamine oxidase inhibitor [MAOI]) because of the risk of serotonin syndrome.[25] With the exception of paroxetine, the SSRIs are well tolerated in patients with ESRD. Similarly, clearance of venlafaxine is reduced in renal failure and the metabolites of bupropion hydrochloride (which are excreted by the kidney) may accumulate and cause seizures in these vulnerable patients.[26]

Benzodiazepines are the mainstay of anxiety management; nonetheless, some transplant teams are unwilling to use them because of their addictive potential. Shorter-lasting agents (such as lorazepam) are preferable because longer-lasting agents (such as chlordiazepoxide) have active metabolites that can accumulate (particularly in patients with hepatic failure) and cause toxicity. Low-dose atypical antipsychotics (such as risperidone or olanzapine) can also be helpful in the treatment of anxiety in those patients who cannot tolerate benzodiazepines because of the risk of respiratory depression or abuse. Risperidone and olanzapine can worsen diabetes mellitus, which often occurs in patients with ESRD, and these agents should be used with caution.

Patients who require mood stabilizers (such as lithium, valproic acid, or carbamazepine) and neuroleptics can continue to take them before transplantation. Because the mood-stabilizing medications have a high level of plasma protein-binding, much lower doses are required in patients with ESRD. Lithium is completely eliminated by dialysis; therefore, serum levels should be obtained just before dialysis and a dose should be given just after dialysis. For patients with hepatic failure, one should adjust the dose of valproic acid or carbamazepine, both of which are metabolized in the liver.

Psychotherapy can also be an extremely important therapeutic intervention for patients approaching a transplant. Even the relatively brief psychiatric pre-transplant evaluation can serve as a good opportunity for patients to share their hopes and dreams for the future, as well as their fears of ongoing illness and of death either before or after transplant. Some psychiatrists will refer pre-transplant patients to other mental health providers for therapy because they feel that they cannot maintain the patients' confidentiality and continue to report to other members of the transplant team. Common issues raised in psychotherapy include grief over loss of productivity, guilt over dependent status, adaptation to a changing role within the family and community, potential for sexual dysfunction, concern about cognitive slowing secondary to immunosuppressive medications, and internal conflict between the reluctance to wish anyone ill and the desire for a deceased donor's organ.

Care of the Post-Transplant Patient

The postoperative period is unpredictable. Some patients recover rapidly and are able to leave the hospital within several weeks. Others can be less fortunate and spend many weeks or even months in the ICU, endure lengthy stays on the transplant unit, and face discharge to a rehabilitation facility. Common sequelae in the immediate postoperative period include delirium, anxiety, and depression. Over the long term, patients can manifest continued anxiety and depression, develop problems with body image, fail to adhere to post-transplant medication regimens, and even revert to active substance abuse.

Short-Term Care

The hallmark of the early postoperative period for almost all transplant patients is delirium. The etiology can be multi-factorial but it usually represents a combination of medication effects or withdrawal states, metabolic changes, or infectious processes. Heart transplantation patients are at risk for intraoperative cerebral ischemia that may predispose them to delirium in the very early postoperative period. Lung transplantation patients may become hypoxic. All of the immunosuppressive medications can cause psychotic symptoms (such as paranoid delusions and auditory and visual hallucinations, with or without accompanying delirium). Cyclosporine and tacrolimus can also cause posterior reversible encephalopathy syndrome (PRES). High-dose steroids can precipitate hypomanic or manic behaviors with or without psychotic symptoms (see Table 29-3).

Management of delirium demands a search for the etiology and treatment of the underlying disorder. Cautious use of neuroleptics (such as haloperidol) can offer relief from disabling and frightening symptoms. Haloperidol is usually the first choice because it can be given intravenously and it is primarily metabolized by the process of glucuronidation rather than by the cytochrome P-450 isoenzymes. If the patient can tolerate oral medications, olanzapine is also a good choice. Gabapentin can be helpful in the management of steroid-induced psychosis (if the patient can take oral medication), with dosage adjustment made for renal insufficiency. When patients are unable to tolerate haloperidol, infusion of dexmedetomidine, an alpha agonist, can be a good choice for management of refractory delirium. Resting the patient overnight with an IV infusion and then turning it off and waking him up during the day can help to reset a normal sleep/wake cycle and assist in management of delirium.

Early symptoms of depression (e.g., mood changes, sleep disturbance, irritability, poor concentration) may be secondary to medications (such as beta-blockers or steroids) or may represent a recurrence of a pre-morbid mood disorder.

TABLE 29-3 Psychiatric Side Effects of Immunosuppressive Medications

IMMUNOSUPPRESSANT AGENT	DESCRIPTION	POTENTIAL PSYCHIATRIC SIDE EFFECTS	LABORATORY FINDINGS
Cyclosporine *Neoral; Sandimmune*	Polypeptide fungal product	Delirium, auditory hallucinations, visual hallucinations, other psychotic symptoms, periventricular leukoencephalopathy	Side effects more prominent at high doses and serum values and tend to resolve as serum levels decrease, SSRIs may increase levels, carbamazepine may decrease levels, herbal agents such as St. Johns' wort may decrease levels
Tacrolimus *Prograf*	Also called *FK506* or *5FK*; macrolide antibiotic	Delirium, auditory and visual hallucinations, other psychotic symptoms, seizures, akinetic mutism	Side effects more prominent at high serum values and tend to resolve as serum levels decrease, MRI may reveal white matter changes in toxic patients
Mycophenolate *Mofetil CellCept*	Suppresses T and B cell proliferation as adjunct immunosuppressant or for patients who cannot tolerate cyclosporine or tacrolimus	Anxiety, depression, sedation	
Muromonab-CD3 *OKT3*	Given immediately postoperatively to prevent rejection, monoclonal antibody that suppresses CD3 T cell function	Aseptic meningitis, hallucinations during administrations	
Corticosteroids	Mainstay of most transplant regimens, usually started high and tapered over weeks to months, though many patients remain on low dose indefinitely	Increased appetite, anxiety, depression, hypomania, mania, paranoia	Often dose-related and resolve with lowered dose

Sometimes, new symptoms of depression herald the development of infectious processes (such as cytomegalovirus [CMV], or *Mycobacterium avium* complex [MAC]). Treatment with the SSRIs can be helpful both for their antidepressant and anxiolytic effects.

Anxiety symptoms in the early postoperative period can result from rapid adjustments in benzodiazepines or narcotics, from early immunosuppressive toxicity, or from sepsis. In lung transplant patients, anxiety can accompany acute rejection, pneumonia, or pleural effusion. Treatment strategies include a gradual tapering of high-dose IV or oral benzodiazepines and/or narcotics followed by maintenance with a low-dose, short-lasting benzodiazepine (such as lorazepam). Patients who have a pre-morbid generalized anxiety or panic disorder that recurs may be managed with a combination of an SSRI and a benzodiazepine.

Long-Term Care

Patients undergoing solid organ transplantation are effectively exchanging one set of problems: those related to end-organ failure, for another set: rejection of the allograft; side effects of immunosuppressive medications; and possible progression of an underlying systemic disease. Although transplant teams certainly inform potential recipients of the risks and benefits of the procedure, many of those recipients (and their families) have unrealistic expectations of their rate of recovery and their overall quality of life following transplantation.

Disappointment and dashed hopes can precipitate mood changes. Frequent medical setbacks, understood by the treatment team as part of the normal course of events, discourage patients and family members. Family members can aggravate the situation by expecting too much, too soon from the transplant recipient. Alternatively, family members or friends who have served as caretakers for many years may be unable to relinquish control, even when the recipient is clearly stronger and better able to care for himself or herself.

Transplant recipients have spent many years in and around hospitals. After a transplant, they gradually move back into their community. Initially, clinic visits can be bi-weekly. As time goes by, patients come into the hospital less and less often. Many transplant patients get anxious as they transition from the close monitoring provided by the medical and surgical teams to a more independent status. Phone contact with a member of the team can be helpful in such circumstances. These patients also benefit from regular attendance at a transplantation support group where, under the guidance of a knowledgeable team leader, they can share their experiences with other transplant recipients.

Almost all transplant recipients take steroids, and most have some visible changes in body habitus. Patients exhibit a cushingoid distribution of body fat and can suffer, among other things, hirsutism and easy bruising. Young women patients in particular struggle with these bodily changes and may be more likely than other transplant recipients to refuse to take the steroids as prescribed. This level of non-compliance is extremely worrisome because it can result in potentially life-threatening acute or chronic rejection. Prompt psychiatric evaluation of the non-compliant transplant recipient for the presence of an underlying mood or adjustment disorder is essential to prevent rejection of the allograft. Ideally, use of supportive psychotherapy might help such patients understand the potentially self-destructive nature of their actions and devise strategies that could ensure better adherence.

Substance abuse can also re-emerge in the post-transplant period, even though the patient may have had years of sobriety before transplantation. Members of transplant teams often have difficulty managing the liver transplant recipient who begins drinking again or the lung transplant recipient who picks up a cigarette, not only because of their concern regarding risk to the allograft but also because of their tremendous disappointment in the patient's behavior.

PEDIATRIC TRANSPLANTATION

In 2015, pediatric patients accounted for approximately 6% (1898) of all organ transplants done in the United States (30,969). Approximately 40% of those transplants were for children between the ages of 11 and 17 years.[27]

Pediatric transplant patients differ from adult transplant patients in a number of ways. A parent or appointed legal guardian makes the medico-legal decisions for the child; the children (infants, toddlers, and school-age children) are not responsible for the decision to proceed with transplant or for pre-transplant and post-transplant care. Most young patients require a transplant because of a congenital disorder (such as biliary atresia, cardiac malformations, or pulmonary atresia) and are not held responsible for their disease in the same way that adults who are chronic drinkers and who develop cirrhosis may be. A child's ability to understand the serious nature of his or her illness and the risks and benefits of transplant depends on the child's age and developmental stage. Many transplant patients have never had the chance to enjoy age-appropriate activities. The severity of their illness might have imposed limitations on school attendance and social interactions and bred a profound dependence on parents and other caregivers.

The primary goal of the psychiatrist who cares for a pediatric transplant patient is to help the child maintain a normal developmental trajectory in the face of life-threatening illness. The psychiatrist must also attempt to balance the needs of the child with the needs of parents, siblings, and involved members of the extended family. No one wants to deny a child the chance for a longer life. However, some children, like some adults, may not be appropriate candidates for transplantation. Sometimes a child is disqualified for transplantation because of the inability of adult caregivers to provide adequate monitoring or to follow the instructions of the treatment team. The psychiatrist who works with young patients with end-organ failure must also be able to understand and to withstand the anger and disappointment of members of the treatment team when faced with such a situation.

Pre-Transplant Evaluation

Unlike with adults, however, the order and style of the pre-transplant psychiatric interview depend on the child's age and developmental stage. With a pre-pubertal child, it is appropriate to meet first with the parents or guardians to obtain a coherent, chronological history and to assess the parents' understanding of the risks and benefits, as well as their history of compliance in obtaining care for their child. With an adolescent, it is helpful to interview the child alone, before speaking with the parents, in order to support his or her independence and wish for autonomy. Again, the psychiatric evaluation should address the following issues: presence of significant Axis I disorders (such as mood disorders, anxiety disorders, and learning disabilities) in the patient or in a caregiver; history of past or current substance abuse; relationship with caregivers; patient's and family's motivation for transplant; ability of the caregivers to comply with treatment recommendations (medication regimen and appointments); adequacy of social supports; and assessment of stressors within the family, such as marital discord or financial problems.

Although parents or guardians must be the ones to give "consent" for the surgery and postoperative care, a verbal child must be able to "assent" to the surgery and be willing to participate in treatment. Both parents and children must be fully engaged in preparation for transplant, as well as be able and willing to work together toward a common goal.

CASE 3

An 11-year-old boy with advanced cystic fibrosis (CF) and no past psychiatric history was brought by his mother for a living donor pre-transplantation psychiatric evaluation. His mother was worried that her son would die before his Lung Allocation Score would be high enough to allow him to qualify for transplant. She herself volunteered to be a living lobar lung donor and she aggressively pursued other potential donors until she found one. On initial interviews, the patient was cheerful and appeared to have a good understanding of why his mother and a friend each wished to donate a lung lobe. In his meeting with the transplant team psychiatrist, however, the patient was not able to talk at all about the potential for transplantation and did not appear to have any understanding of why the two adults would need surgery. Ultimately, the team decided that it was the patient's mother and not the patient who was the motivating force for transplant. The child clearly did not feel ready to have an elective transplant with his mother and a friend as a donor. The team put the process on hold and encouraged the family to wait for a deceased donor transplant.

The dilemma of the adolescent transplant candidate who abuses substances is particularly important. Adolescents are less likely than adults to have longstanding struggles with substance abuse, but they are often recreational users of alcohol or street drugs, particularly in social situations. The normal adolescent's need for autonomy and independence often leads to substance use, despite a cognitive understanding of the grave risks. Some teens with liver disease drink alcohol, and some teens with lung disease smoke cigarettes or marijuana. This behavior usually stops as the illness progresses and the patient becomes more medically compromised. It is difficult to know, however, whether this change reflects a true understanding of the risks, or whether it is simply a short-term response to the fear of jeopardizing their transplant candidacy.

In addition, adolescents often struggle to comply with medication regimens and treatment recommendations before transplantation. They are seeking to forge their own identity and to separate themselves from their parents. At the same time, they desperately want to be part of their peer group and to look just like everyone else. Often this translates into, for example, a teenager with cystic fibrosis who refuses to take enzymes at lunch in the cafeteria, or go to the nurse for an insulin injection in the middle of the day. Because non-adherence is a major cause of graft rejection, a history of this kind of behavior pattern in a pre-transplant adolescent candidate is worrisome—even though it is consistent with the patient's age and developmental stage.

In some instances, the evaluator may use the 17-item Pediatric Transplant Rating Instrument (P-TRI) to assess an adolescent's understanding of the transplant process; history of adherence to medication regimens and the recommendations of his/her treatment team; presence or absence of psychiatric problems and/or substance use; and degree of family engagement.[28] Although this screening tool can be helpful, it is important to remember that the P-TRI is not intended to determine eligibility for transplantation because the data linking patients' scores to transplant outcome are lacking.[29]

Post-Transplant Care

The postoperative care of the pediatric transplant patient is similar to that of the adult. Delirium is a common occurrence. The immunosuppressive medications can cause neuropsychiatric symptoms, and high-dose steroids can precipitate psychosis. Cautious use of IV haloperidol remains the mainstay of treatment.

Evidence suggests that the extent to which pediatric patients with life-threatening illnesses feel traumatized both by the procedure and by its sequelae correlates with the parents' sense of stress.[30] In fact, although parents (and primary care-givers) have a relatively high rate of PTSD in the first few years following their child's transplant,[31] the transplant recipients themselves experience symptoms of PTSD at rates comparable with those of children with other life-threatening conditions. Interestingly, the likelihood of experiencing such symptoms (e.g., re-experiencing, having flashbacks, or manifesting avoidance) does not seem to be related to the type of organ transplant and is more common in those adolescents with relatively mild complications, or in those whose organ failure occurred abruptly.[32] In one study, the authors found that children and parents differed in their assessment of psychological health following transplant. Children generally under-reported their psychological distress and parents reported that their children were more distressed than a normal cohort.[33] Regardless, it is extremely important to recognize and treat PTSD in pediatric and adult transplant recipients, as some feel that the presence of PTSD catalyzes an avoidance response that manifests as non-adherence and thus compromises outcome.[34]

In general, however, pediatric transplant patients do well. They feel better, return to school, and resume many of their activities. They do not demonstrate significant new psychopathology, although pre-morbid psychiatric illness may recur. Pediatric liver transplantation patients demonstrate significant neuropsychological deficits and developmental delays in intellectual and academic functioning, both before and after transplantation, thought to be related to the effect of elevated levels of bilirubin pre-transplant and total number of days in the hospital in the first year following transplant.[34] Other studies have shown persistent cognitive deficits in pediatric heart transplant recipients,[35] but a recent study found that 89% of children who underwent heart transplantation following LVAD bridging demonstrated normal cognitive function.[36]

CONCLUSION

The patient with end-organ failure who is approaching transplantation has few real options. These patients are profoundly physically disabled and emotionally drained. They are often depressed and anxious, and at times quite desperate. Recognition and treatment of psychiatric disorders, both before and after transplant, can improve their quality of life.

The role of the transplant psychiatrist is challenging but also immensely rewarding. It requires a sophisticated appreciation of the medical and surgical issues facing patients with end-organ failure, an understanding of the mechanism of action and side-effect profiles of their medications, and the ways in which those medications interact with psychotropic medications. As a member of a multidisciplinary team, the psychiatrist must act as a liaison to the patient, the family, and other medical providers, and serve as a resource for other team members. The transplant psychiatrist plays a central role in the selection of transplant candidates and potential living donors, necessitating an understanding of the ethical issues inherent in a system where resources are limited.

REFERENCES

Access the reference list online at https://expertconsult.inkling.com/.

Patients With Human Immunodeficiency Virus Infection and Acquired Immunodeficiency Syndrome

30

Scott R. Beach, M.D., F.A.P.M.
BJ Beck, M.S.N., M.D.
Jacqueline T. Chu, M.D.
Oliver Freudenreich, M.D.

OVERVIEW

Human immunodeficiency virus (HIV) infection and acquired immune deficiency syndrome (AIDS) are prevalent in disenfranchised populations, including substance users, men-who-have-sex-with-men (MSM), sex workers, ethnic minorities, and the seriously mentally ill, who all have particular difficulty advocating for and accessing adequate care. Not only is HIV infection more prevalent among the mentally ill,[1,2] but psychiatric illnesses are more prevalent in those who are HIV-positive.[3] Patients with personality disorders are also over-represented in the HIV-positive population,[4,5] likely because certain traits (e.g., impulsivity, reckless disregard for safety, affective instability, or chronic feelings of emptiness) can predispose persons to risky behavior and to HIV infection.

As recently as the 1990s, HIV infection was a terminal illness. However, the advent of highly active antiretroviral therapy (HAART) has made HIV a manageable, chronic illness for many,[6] although sometimes associated with a high medication side-effect burden. A new cohort of aging patients with HIV infection, a range of cognitive difficulties, and chronic diseases not necessarily related to HIV itself, is emerging, despite (or because of) improved overall survival.[7] Despite much progress, complacency, stigma, secrecy, and shame continue to interfere with HIV detection. Culture, lifestyle, and socioeconomic barriers to prevention and to appropriate HIV care persist.

HIV is a blood-borne, sexually transmitted retrovirus that contains RNA as its genetic material and the enzyme reverse transcriptase, which facilitates the (reverse) transcription of RNA to double-stranded DNA in infected human cells. This virion-derived DNA moves to the host cell nucleus, where it randomly integrates into host chromosomes, catalyzed by the virion-encoded enzyme, integrase. Once within the host chromosome, the pro-viral DNA can remain inactive (latent), or it can express a range of genetic activity, including functional virus production. Such now-functional viruses can go on to infect other cells, preferentially the CD4 subpopulation of T-lymphocytes, thereby causing severe (primarily cell-mediated) immune dysfunction for which the virus and the resulting syndrome were named. Immunodeficiency, a predilection for certain opportunistic infections, and AIDS-defining conditions correlate with a decline in CD4 lymphocyte count (Table 30-1). This infection cycle repeats billions of times, the host mounts an immune response, and a set point (or dynamic equilibrium) is eventually reached. The set point varies from person to person, and it has been found to be of prognostic significance.[8] Notably, the virus also invades the central nervous system (CNS) early, possibly within hours to days of the initial infection.[9,10]

Although the science behind HIV infection and its treatment is changing at a rapid pace, the general tenets of this chapter should provide a consistent framework for the safe and comprehensive psychiatric evaluation and care of adults at risk for, or infected with, HIV/AIDS. Four general questions help set the context for such an evaluation: At what stage of HIV infection is the patient in terms of symptomatic disease and CD4 lymphocyte count? Is there evidence of HIV-associated CNS infection? Does the patient have a pre-morbid psychiatric history? How did the patient become infected with HIV? The important implications of the first three questions might seem more obvious and should be clear by the completion of the chapter. The fourth question is often a highly personal story, one that reveals the patient as a person. The answer to this question foreshadows how the patient will relate to illness and to medical care. This knowledge informs not only the psychiatrist's evaluation but also the patient's individualized treatment and management plans.

EPIDEMIOLOGY

Despite the existence of effective therapies, HIV/AIDS remains a terminal illness in much of the world; it cuts across all ages and socioeconomic groups, each with specific characteristics and considerations.[11] The reported global

TABLE 30-1 AIDS-Defining Conditions That Emerge With Advancing Immunosuppression

CD4 CELL COUNT (CELLS/mm^3)	CONDITION
200–500	Thrush
	Kaposi's sarcoma
	Tuberculosis reactivation
	Herpes zoster
	Herpes simplex
	Bacterial sinusitis/pneumonia
100–200	*Pneumocystis jirovecii* pneumonia
50–100	Systemic fungal infections
	Primary tuberculosis
	Cerebral toxoplasmosis
	Progressive multi-focal leukoencephalopathy
	Peripheral neuropathy
	Cervical carcinoma
0–50	Cytomegalovirus disease
	Disseminated *Mycobacterium avium-intracellulare* complex
	Non-Hodgkin's lymphoma
	Central nervous system lymphoma
	HIV-associated dementia

Modified from APA: Practice guideline for the treatment of patients with HIV/AIDS, *Am J Psychiatry* 2000; 157S:1–62.

prevalence of HIV has increased from 33.3 million in 2010 to 36.7 million in 2015.[12] Women make up half of the infected adults worldwide, and roughly 1.8 million children younger than 15 years are infected.[12]

There has been a gradual decrease in the incidence of new infections since a peak in 1998, with a 2015 incidence of roughly 2.1 million, with 150,000 of those new cases diagnosed in children younger than 15 years. This incidence is only partially offset by the (declining) total number of AIDS deaths (1.1 million in 2015), which means the number of persons living with HIV will continue to rise, although the prevalence (measured over a growing global population) has stabilized. Eastern and Southern Africa remains the most heavily infected region, accounting for 52% of all people living with HIV, for 43% of all AIDS deaths, and for 46% of all new cases in 2015.[5] Nonetheless, these percentages have declined dramatically since the 1990s.

In the United States, among the most heavily infected industrialized nations, more than 1.2 million people are infected with the virus, of whom over 150,000 (13%) are unaware of their status.[13] The incidence of new infections is stable in the United States at about 50,000 per year. The advent of HAART in 1996 has decreased the incidence of AIDS onset and AIDS-related deaths, so more people in the United States are living with HIV infection than ever before.

HIV is an example of a concentrated epidemic, as the risk for contracting HIV is not evenly distributed across the population. A disproportionate number of the newly infected in the United States are ethnic and racial minorities (primarily Black and Hispanic; less so Asian and Pacific Islanders), and heterosexual women.[13,14] However, outbreaks of other sexually transmitted illnesses (STIs) in gay men raise the specter of a possible HIV resurgence in this population and suggest that the success of HAART may have led to complacency and the resumption of unsafe sexual practices in MSM,[15] to some degree fueled by the recreational use of methamphetamine (crystal meth).[16] Indeed, in 2011, the majority of new HIV diagnoses in the United States were among MSM (in all but one state), and the incidence among this group increased by 12% from 2008 to 2010.[13] Furthermore, unprotected anal sex at least once in the past 12 months increased from 48% in 2005 to 57% in 2011.[17] Up to 30% of patients with HIV disease are also infected with hepatitis C virus (HCV). These co-infected patients are rather different from HIV mono-infected patients with regard to risk factors and psychiatric illnesses; most patients have acquired HCV from injection drug use, which is the main mode of transmission for HCV.

MEDICATIONS FOR HIV INFECTION

Early treatment is now the gold standard in patients with HIV. ART initiation at the time of diagnosis, regardless of CD4 count, is recommended to reduce clinically relevant morbidity and mortality related to, and unrelated to, HIV/AIDS. In a large multi-site, multi-continent study known as the "START study," early treatment was shown to significantly reduce the risk of serious AIDS-related events, serious non-AIDS-related events, or death from any cause, compared with a deferred-treatment initiation arm, in which subjects were not treated until the CD4 count dropped below 350.[18] Since 2012, the United States Department of Health and Human Services (DHHS) guidelines have recommended immediate ART initiation;[19] with publication of the START study, the WHO has adopted the recommendation of ART for all as well.[20]

Goals of antiretroviral therapy are to achieve sustained virologic suppression of HIV, recover immune function (for which the surrogate marker is CD4 T lymphocyte cell numbers), and thereby reduce HIV-associated morbidity and mortality and reduce community transmission of HIV. There are currently six FDA-approved classes of antiretroviral medications: nucleoside reverse transcriptase inhibitors (NRTIs); non-nucleoside reverse transcriptase inhibitors (NNRTIs); protease inhibitors (PIs); integrase strand transfer inhibitors (INSTIs); entry inhibitors; and fusion inhibitors.[21] As described earlier, the complex process leading to successful viral replication and propagation involves several steps. Drugs target various stages of the HIV replication cycle: in the first four classes mentioned, they interfere with viral replication inside infected host cells; the latter two classes prevent viral entry into the host cell.[22,23] Antiretroviral medications are used in combinations, typically three agents from more than one class. Single-drug therapy is ineffective because of the rapid development of resistance to that agent and in turn, to an entire class of medications.[22–25] Similarly, incomplete adherence to a multi-drug combination regimen allows HIV-1 to continue replicating, again allowing for mutation to occur and class-wide resistance to develop, thus limiting the prospects for further effective treatment.[25] Therefore, the impression of importance of adherence to medications and engagement of patients in therapy is critical for treatment success.

TABLE 30-2 Antiretroviral Recommended First-Line Regimen Options

INSTI-Based Regimens	DTG/ABC/3TC[a,d]
	DTG/TDF/FTC
	EVG/c/TAF/FTC[b,d]
	EVG/c/TDF/FTC[c,d]
	RAL/TDF/FTC
PI-Based Regimens	DRV/r + TDF/FTC

[a]Only for patients who are HLA-B*5701-negative.
[b]Only for patients with estimated CrCl ≥30.
[c]Only for patients with estimated CrCl ≥70.
[d]One pill once daily regimen.
INSTI, integrase strand transfer inhibitor; DTG, dolutegravir; ABC, abacavir; 3TC, lamivudine; TDF, tenofovir disoproxil fumarate; FTC, emtricitabine; EVG/c/TDF/FTC, elvitegravir/cobicistat/tenofovir DF/emtricitabine; EVG/c/TAF/FTC, elvitegravir/cobicistat/tenofovir alafenamide/emtricitabine; RAL, raltegravir; PI, protease inhibitor; DRV/r, ritonavir-boosted darunavir; CrCl, creatinine clearance.
Adapted from Panel on Antiretroviral Guidelines for Adults and Adolescents. Guidelines for the use of antiretroviral agents in HIV-1-infected adults and adolescents. Department of Health and Human Services. Available at http://www.aidsinfo.nih.gov/ContentFiles/AdultandAdolescentGL.pdf. Accessed June 25, 2016.

The United States DHHS provides recommendations for the treatment-naive patient, of which first-line consists of two NRTIs plus either an INSTI or ritonavir-boosted PI. Of these, there are currently three one-pill once-daily options;[19] several studies and a meta-analysis have shown better adherence in populations receiving once-daily regimens (Table 30-2).[26]

Nucleoside (and Nucleotide) Reverse Transcriptase Inhibitors

Nucleoside and nucleotide reverse transcriptase inhibitors (NRTIs) are nucleoside analogs that inhibit the action of the enzyme reverse transcriptase which thereby slows or prevents viral replication. This class forms the backbone of most current combination regimens. While older NRTIs were associated with challenging pharmacokinetics requiring multiple daily doses, drug interactions, and complications, such as pancreatitis and bone marrow toxicity, or disfiguring lipodystrophy, newer drugs are better tolerated and easier to take. Currently, the two most commonly used NRTI combinations are: tenofovir disoproxil fumarate (TDF) with emtricitabine (FTC); and abacavir (ABC) with lamivudine (3TC). In 2015, tenofovir alafenamide, an oral prodrug of tenofovir, was approved by the United States FDA as a safer alternative to TDF, featuring less potential for adverse kidney and bone effects compared with TDF.[27]

Non-nucleoside Reverse Transcriptase Inhibitors

As with the NRTIs, the NNRTIs also interfere with reverse transcriptase. The NNRTIs are potent agents and have been shown to be active against viral strains of HIV that are resistant to NRTIs and sometimes PIs. However, if NNRTIs are used alone or with a single NRTI, resistance develops quickly, and it usually generalizes to the whole class (i.e., to all the NNRTIs). Drug interactions with other drugs can occur because of their metabolism by the cytochrome P450 (CYP) hepatic isoenzyme system.[24] Efavirenz is an NNRTI noteworthy for its greater potential for neuropsychiatric side effects (e.g., somnolence, agitation, insomnia, abnormal or vivid dreams, impaired concentration and attention, psychosis, and suicidality). Such side effects are thought to be related to plasma level and are pharmacogenetically predisposed.[28,29] Importantly, the risk of suicidal ideation or attempted or completed suicide may be up to twice as high for patients taking an efavirenz-containing regimen compared with efavirenz-free regimens.[30] The NNRTIs as a class can also cause a rash early on; it is thought to be more common and severe (including onset of Stevens–Johnson syndrome) with nevirapine, which is less commonly used in the United States but still is a component of regimens in developing countries.[24]

Protease Inhibitors

Protease inhibitors (PIs) are another potent class of medications, and unlike NNRTIs have a higher barrier to resistance. The initiation of 3-drug therapy (NRTI backbone and either NNRTI or PI agents) heralded the “highly active” antiretroviral therapy or HAART era. For the first time, HIV RNA was suppressed below the limit of detection, immune recovery occurred,[24] and patients' survival increased dramatically.[31]

PIs interfere with viral replication, maturation, and new infection of cells by inhibiting the enzymatic cleavage of necessary viral protein precursors. The PIs have undergone significant drug development and have matured from being handfuls of pills multiple times per day with prominent side effects to well-tolerated minimal once-daily regimens. PIs are metabolized by CYP enzymes, leading to the most significant drug interactions among antiretroviral agents. PIs can cause gastrointestinal (GI) side effects and liver transaminase elevations. In addition, PIs can worsen or cause diabetes, insulin resistance, lipodystrophy, and hyperlipidemia.[24]

Integrase Inhibitors

Integrase is the viral enzyme that catalyzes the integration of virally derived DNA into the host cell DNA in the nucleus, forming a provirus that can be activated to produce viral proteins. The initiation of integrase inhibitors in 2007 brought the first new class of medications in two decades, which was found to be an incredibly effective and well-tolerated class. A trial with treatment-naive HIV-1-infected patients demonstrated more-rapid decline in viral load (as compared with efavirenz) key data, which helped to make integrase inhibitors, initially used for multi-drug-resistant HIV, a key component of first-line regimens for treatment-naive individuals.[32]

Entry Inhibitors

Moving away from the replication cycle, the next two classes of agents prevent viral entry into the host cell. In order for the HIV virion to enter the CD4 cell, it must bind to the cell at two binding sites. Viral protein gp120 forms a complex with the CD4 receptor exposing CD4 cell co-receptors, either CCR5, CXCR4, or both. The virus can use either co-receptor to bind to gp120 to enter into the host cell, but some strains of virus are predisposed to CCR5, and others to CXCR4. Maraviroc selectively targets CCR5 and blocks the binding of HIV to CCR5 co-receptors in CCR5-tropic (R5 virus) HIV-1 infection. Hence, if the virus is able to use CXCR4 as a co-receptor instead, maraviroc is not effective. Therefore, prior to the use of maraviroc, viral tropism testing must be performed to determine if it is a solely CCR5 tropic virus. Though well-tolerated, this tropism makes maraviroc a limited option.

Fusion Inhibitors

Enfuvirtide interferes with viral fusion to the host cell membrane by inhibiting the necessary conformational change in a particular viral envelope protein (gp41) that would allow viral entry into a host cell. Administered subcutaneously, enfuvirtide requires twice-daily injections. It is commonly associated with injection-site reactions, an increased incidence of bacterial pneumonia, and rare hypersensitivity reactions. The drug is now rarely used for treatment-experienced patients who develop viral replication despite continuous antiretroviral therapy.[33]

HIV INFECTION AND THE CENTRAL NERVOUS SYSTEM

Within days of the initial infection, the virus is transported to the brain by monocytes that then differentiate into macrophages. These infected but not dead macrophages may be activated randomly, leading over time to excessive secretion of normal inflammatory substances and cell death without neuronal infection. That is, HIV infection causes neuronal destruction without infecting neurons.[34] The CNS appears to be an independent reservoir of HIV replication; CSF viral load does not consistently correlate with plasma levels.[35,36] HIV in the CNS might also have different characteristics, such as mutations with increased viral resistance or neurotoxicity, than those of the peripherally observed virus. Current antiretrovirals have variable blood–brain barrier penetrance, they may be less potent inhibitors of viral replication within the CNS, and some are themselves neurotoxic. The optimal antiretroviral drug regimen to combat HIV in the brain remains to be determined, but peripheral suppression of viral replication will need to be coupled with neuroprotection. New therapies might target regulatory human genes involved in viral replication,[37] the identification and exploitation of brain HIV-inhibitory factors,[10] and the enhancement of intrinsic brain defenses that favor neuroprotective, as opposed to neurotoxic, responses to the virus.[10]

HIV has a predilection for subcortical structures, such as the hippocampus and basal ganglia, with lower concentrations in the cerebellum and mid-frontal cortices.[38,39] This distribution, further differentiation of viral burden within particular basal ganglia regions, and concomitant structural changes in the brain (including ventricular enlargement, hippocampal atrophy, decreased basal ganglia volume, and white matter lesions), might explain the more characteristic cognitive and behavioral impairments associated with HIV infection of the CNS, as well as the sensitivity of patients with HIV to the extrapyramidal symptoms (EPS) of certain psychiatric medications.[34,40–42] These types of lesions in the base of the skull are better visualized by brain magnetic resonance imaging (MRI) than by computed tomography (CT) scanning.

When evaluating neurocognitive impairment in the HIV-positive patient, HIV infection of the CNS should always be a diagnosis of exclusion, made only after a thorough investigation of other possible etiologies for neurocognitive impairment, especially if symptoms are new or of acute onset.[43] Opportunistic infection, neoplasm, other systemic illness, medication side effects, drug–drug interactions, use of recreational drugs, withdrawal syndromes, and metabolic and nutritional derangements should be considered. Primary psychiatric disease should be at the bottom of the list, especially if there is not a significant pre-infection history.[44–46]

Although neuropsychologic testing might not be specific,[38] it helps to localize and quantify impairments. Recommended neuropsychological tests include an HIV-specific test battery based on measures found by the AIDS Clinical Trials Group (ACTG) and the Multicenter AIDS Cohort Study to be sensitive to HIV-related cognitive deficits. These measures include Trail Making A and B, WAIS-R (Wechsler Adult Intelligence Scale—Revised) digit span and digit symbol, grooved pegboard, finger tapping, Stroop color and word test, FAS test of verbal fluency, Odd Man Out test, and computer-based measures of complex reaction time.[47–50] Other measures are added as clinically indicated. Test battery times less than 60 minutes are less likely to produce patient fatigue, which confounds test interpretation and creates significant patient frustration or humiliation. Despite these recommendations, there is no ideal test, and it is important to keep in mind that mild deficits on testing can have significant functional consequences.

HIV-ASSOCIATED NEUROCOGNITIVE DISORDERS (HAND)

HAND encompasses three conditions, including HIV-associated dementia (HAD), HIV-associated mild neurocognitive disorder (MND), and asymptomatic neurocognitive impairment (ANI). HAND presents with executive dysfunction, memory impairment, attention deficits, and poor impulse control, and can be associated with motor dysfunction including bradykinesia, loss of coordination and gait imbalance. These conditions are all diagnosed using neuropsychological testing and functional status assessments, and are thought to affect 15% to 55% of HIV-positive individuals.[51]

HIV-associated Dementia

HIV-associated dementia (HAD), a subcortical dementia similar to that seen in Huntington's disease,[38] is severe enough to cause functional impairment and marked impairment (>2 standard deviations, SDs, below demographically corrected norms) in at least two cognitive domains. HAD is an AIDS-defining condition with a prevalence in the United States of 21% to 25% before the advent of HAART; since then, it has decreased to less than 5%.[51] Associated with reduced white-matter volume, atrophy of the basal ganglia (reduced gray matter volume), and cell death, HAD is characterized by slowed information processing, deficits in attention and memory, and impairments in abstraction and fine motor skills.[34,38,52] Though the prevalence has decreased dramatically, HAD is now seen in patients with less severe immunosuppression and less evidence of structural brain changes, such as HIV encephalitis, as compared with 20 years ago.

HIV-associated Mild Neurocognitive Disorder

Mild neurocognitive disorder (MND) is thought to affect 20% of HIV-positive patients. By definition, MND involves mild to moderate cognitive impairment (1 SD), in at least two cognitive domains, that at least mildly interferes with daily activities.[53] For patients in cognitively taxing jobs, however, even "mild" problems may be significant enough to interfere with, and to preclude, continued employment.

Asymptomatic Neurocognitive Impairment

By definition, ANI, which may affect up to 30% of patients with HIV infection and accounts for 70% of all HAND, also involves mild to moderate cognitive impairment (1 SD) in at least two cognitive domains but without obvious impairment in daily function.[54] It is extremely difficult to make the judgment that there are no obvious functional impairments without extensive third-person observation. ANI is a significant risk factor for progression to more severe forms of HAND, conveying a two- to six-fold increased risk.[55]

HAND in the Era of HAART

Ongoing HIV replication in the brain can persist even in the setting of systemic viral suppression. Early HIV infection of the CNS and persistent CNS HIV infection and inflammation probably contribute to the development of HAND, and it may be that neuronal dysfunction, rather than cell death, is the mediator. Chronic macrophage/microglial activation and associated oxidative stress, viral persistence in the CNS, and HAART-related toxicity may also play a role.[51] Markers that remain strongly correlated with the development of HAND include $CD4^+$ T cell count nadir and a history of clinically defined AIDS. Other risk factors for the development of HAND include older age, diabetes, hyperlipidemia, tobacco and other substance use, and HCV co-infection. Cognitive reserve is also important—those with a higher education level may be less likely to develop HAND.[56]

There remains no definitive treatment for HAND. Formerly, there was hope that early treatment with HAART would prevent the onset of HAND, but the recent START trial failed to show a major effect of early HAART treatment.[18] For patients not currently on HAART, initiation of medication can lead to dramatic improvements in a subset, but many patients on HAART will still develop HAND over time. However, maintenance on HAART conveys a much lower risk of progression of HAND, assuming viral load remains suppressed. Recently, a few small studies have suggested that the addition of maraviroc to an existing effective combination regimen may be associated with improved cognition in individuals with baseline impairment.[57] Importantly, the CNS penetration-effectiveness (CPE) of an antiretroviral medication into the CNS is not correlated with improvement in HAND. In fact, a large cohort study of over 50,000 patients found that those receiving a regimen with high CPE were 74% more likely to develop HAD compared to a regimen with low CPE.[58]

CSF Viral Escape

As many as 5% to 10% of patients on HAART may experience a phenomenon in which there is a discordant elevation of HIV RNA in the CSF despite relatively intact immune function correlates with incident neuropsychiatric symptoms. This phenomenon is known as CSF viral escape. Patients present acutely to subacutely, with symptoms of encephalitis, myelitis, or meningitis, and may experience psychiatric symptoms including depressive features. The CSF usually demonstrates a lymphocyte-predominant pleocytosis and mild to moderately elevated protein, while MRI often shows bilateral, confluent white matter hyperintensities.[51,59] CSF viral escape is thought to be influenced by either independent development of viral resistance in the CSF and/or inadequate CNS penetration of HAART.

DIFFERENTIAL DIAGNOSIS OF PSYCHIATRIC DISTRESS

Psychiatric symptoms are common in the HIV-infected population and can reach a level of severity to meet criteria for *Diagnostic and Statistical Manual for Mental Disorders*, 5th edition (DSM-5) disorders.[60] Or, as with neurocognitive impairments, psychiatric symptoms may be sub-syndromal; underlying causes should be identified and reversed when possible, although it might still be necessary to treat the psychiatric symptoms (Table 30-3).[61]

Mental Disorder Due to Another Medical Condition

Differential diagnosis should always begin with mental disorder due to another medical condition.[44,62] HIV CNS infection and HAND should be considered, along with opportunistic infections and neoplasms. Other considerations include side effects of medications; drug–drug interactions, such as herbal and OTC preparations; alcohol and recreational drugs; substance intoxication or withdrawal. Nutritional effects include nutritional deficits, such as thiamine, folate, zinc, cobalamin (vitamin B_{12}), and pyridoxine (vitamin B_6); poor intake resulting from medication or disease-induced nausea, painful oral lesions; poor absorption; abnormal losses, such as from gastritis, diarrhea, vomiting, or nephropathy; or increased demand resulting from hypermetabolic state due to infection, stress, or neoplasm.[46] Metabolic derangements (e.g., electrolyte abnormalities), renal or hepatic dysfunction, and endocrinopathies (e.g., glucose intolerance, hyperadrenalism, hypocalcemia, or thyroid dysfunction) can also cause psychiatric symptoms.

TABLE 30-3 Differential Diagnosis of Neuropsychiatric Symptoms in Patients With HIV Infection and AIDS

Psychiatric disorders
Psychoactive substance intoxication or withdrawal
Primary HIV-associated syndromes
• Seroconversion illness
• HIV CNS infection
• HIV-associated neurocognitive disorders (HAND)
CNS opportunistic infections
• Fungi: *Cryptococcus neoformans, Coccidioides immitis, Candida albicans, Histoplasma capsulatum, Aspergillus fumigatus*, and mucormycosis
• Protozoa/parasites: *Toxoplasma gondii* and amebas
• Viruses: CJ virus (progressive multifocal leukoencephalopathy, PML), CMV, adenovirus type 2, herpes simplex virus, and varicella zoster virus
• Bacteria: *Mycobacterium avium-intracellulare, M. tuberculosis, Listeria monocytogenes*, Gram-negative organisms, *Treponema pallidum*, and *Nocardia asteroides*
Other neurotropic infective agent
• Hepatitis C virus
Neoplasms
• Primary CNS non-Hodgkin's lymphoma
• Metastatic Kaposi's sarcoma (rare)
• Burkitt's lymphoma
Medication side effects
• Endocrinopathies and nutrient deficiencies
• Addison's disease (CMV, *Cryptococcus*, HIV-1, and ketoconazole)
• Hypothyroidism
• Vitamins A, B_6, B_{12}, and E deficiencies
• Hypogonadism
Anemia
Metabolic abnormalities: hypoxia; hepatic, renal, pulmonary, adrenal, and pancreatic insufficiency; hypomagnesemia; hypocalcemia; water intoxication, dehydration; hypernatremia; hyponatremia; alkalosis; and acidosis
Hypotension
Complex partial seizures
Head trauma
Non-HIV-related conditions

CJ, Creutzfeldt–Jakob disease; CMV, cytomegalovirus; HIV, human immunodeficiency virus.
Adapted from: Querques J, Worth JL: HIV infection and AIDS. In: Stern TA, Herman JB, editors: *Psychiatry update and board preparation*, New York, 2000, McGraw-Hill, p 208.

Delirium

Delirium is a common neuropsychiatric complication in hospitalized patients with AIDS, and it may be a predictor of significantly decreased survival.[63] In patients with asymptomatic HIV infection or CD4 lymphocyte counts greater than 500/μL, it is rare for an HIV-related condition to cause delirium; substance intoxication or withdrawal is a more likely cause. This includes drugs (such as steroids) used as alternative HIV therapies.

Among patients with symptomatic HIV infection or a CD4 lymphocyte count <500/μL, HIV-related conditions and iatrogenic causes (Table 30-3) should be high on the differential diagnosis for delirium and should be at the top of the list for patients at advanced stages of AIDS or when the CD4 lymphocyte count falls below 100/μL. There should be a continued high index of suspicion for substance intoxication and withdrawal. Seizure disorder should also be in the differential diagnosis because HIV-infected patients are at increased risk for new-onset seizures, especially partial complex seizures.[64]

A sudden change in mental status is not characteristic of HAD alone. Patients with advanced HAD experience symptomatic worsening with mild states of delirium during the late afternoon when they are increasingly fatigued or during the night (i.e., sundowning).

The primary goal in the management of delirium is the identification and treatment of causative factors. The need for laboratory tests, including brain imaging, electroencephalogram (EEG), CSF examination, and blood tests, must be guided by history and clinical examination. If delirium is a treatment-emergent adverse effect, the suspected medication should be discontinued or an alternative agent substituted.

Depression

The most common psychiatric complication of HIV infection or AIDS, depression, should never be considered appropriate. When a person suffers from clinical depression (i.e., experiences sufficient symptoms to meet DSM-5 criteria), the patient deserves to be treated.[65,66] The same criteria for a diagnosis of depression in a person without HIV infection should be used in a person with HIV infection. As is the case with certain other medical illnesses, it may be hard to interpret the more somatic neurovegetative symptoms (e.g., fatigue, loss of appetite, altered sleep patterns, or difficulty with concentration).

Low testosterone in HIV-positive men has been linked to symptoms of depression, including low mood, irritability, and decreased libido. Testosterone replacement has been found to be helpful in some men with HIV and depressive symptoms, even in the absence of hypogonadism.[67] Checking total testosterone levels in the morning should be considered in this population.

Fatigue

Clinically impairing fatigue affects at least one-third of patients with HIV/AIDS.[68] Although the etiology may be multi-factorial, a search for remediable causes is an important first step. Pain and sleep deprivation contribute to fatigue in many patients. Importantly, fatigue is not pathognomonic for depression. In fact, fatigue is associated with advanced HIV disease. It can also be disproportional to apparent disease status.

Bereavement

The patient with HIV infection or AIDS often suffers multiple losses (including friends, health, physical ability, career, income, housing, child custody, independence, or a sense of freedom or autonomy). Mood and related symptoms require careful evaluation in the setting of loss or bereavement. If the patient meets criteria for major depression and is not responding to supportive interventions, pharmacologic treatment is warranted.

Suicide

Suicidal thoughts should always be assessed; they are more prevalent in patients with asymptomatic HIV infection than in those with AIDS, and may be seen in the setting of a new diagnosis.[69] The incidence of suicide in patients with HIV infection or AIDS has decreased since the advent of HAART; it is now similar to that seen with other medical illnesses. The incidence of suicide in this population of HIV-infected persons and those with other medical illnesses, however, is still higher than in the general population. Risk factors include symptomatic depression, persistent pain, drug use (specifically injection drug use) or alcohol use, domestic violence, altered cognition (i.e., delirium or HAD), social isolation, multiple losses, hopelessness, being transgender, and personality disorders.[70–72] Serious thoughts of self-harm usually indicate the need for inpatient care. Electroconvulsive therapy (ECT) may be a life-saving procedure for patients who are severely depressed and suicidal, especially when they are medically compromised and unable to tolerate medications or the delay in their effectiveness.

Anxiety

Prevalent in HIV infection, anxiety runs the gamut from an acute response to a devastating diagnosis, to a full-blown anxiety disorder. Patients with a history of an anxiety disorder are at increased risk, as are those with few social supports and poor coping skills. In susceptible patients, onset or recrudescence of anxiety symptoms may be predictably related to disease milestones or to signs of disease progression, such as initial diagnosis, declining CD4 count, increased viral load, onset of opportunistic infections, chronic pain or paresthesias, wasting, or physical changes that make the disease more public. The somatic symptoms often associated with anxiety (e.g., tremor, muscle tension or spasm, shortness of breath, dizziness, headache, sweating, flushing, palpitations, nausea, vomiting, or diarrhea) need to be carefully investigated for possible medical causes, medication side effects, drug interactions, use of activating recreational drugs, or withdrawal from opiates or sedative–hypnotics.

Mania

Mania in the setting of a personal history of recurrent mood episodes is a core feature of bipolar disorder and is considered primary (idiopathic) mania. Without such a history or a strong family history of bipolar disorder, any first episode of mania in the setting of HIV infection should be considered secondary (organic) mania as a result of the physiologic effects of HIV CNS infection, opportunistic infections, neoplasm, medications, or substance use.[73] Zidovudine at high doses has also been associated with the development of mania.[74] A positive correlation exists between the manifestation of HIV-associated mania and the eventual development of HAND, although mean survival is not adversely affected. HIV-associated structural brain lesions might not be more common in patients who develop mania.[75] HIV-related mania is clinically distinct from primary mania, in that HIV-related mania typically manifests with more irritability and psychosis rather than euphoria, and patients are more cognitively impaired.[76]

Psychosis

A pre-existing psychotic disorder may be a risk factor for HIV infection, and it is positively associated with psychosis in HIV-positive patients. The literature somewhat suggests that a history of substance abuse, depressive episodes, or certain personality disorders might also correlate with the onset of psychotic symptoms in HIV-associated disease and that antiretroviral therapy may be protective against the development of psychosis.[77–79] Secondary causes include more immediate psychoactive substance use (particularly methamphetamine use), CNS HIV infection (usually a late-stage manifestation) or opportunistic infections, neoplasms, nutritional deficits, metabolic derangements, or delirium. HIV-infected patients with psychosis tend to exhibit greater cognitive impairment.[79]

Sleep

Sleep problems are highly prevalent (30% to 40%) in HIV infection for a variety of reasons.[80,81] They may be related to the stage of HIV disease, persistent pain (e.g., from peripheral sensory neuropathy), or psychosocial issues.[81] Lack of structure (e.g., from unemployment), daytime napping, and other contributions to disordered sleep hygiene can lead to reversal of the sleep–wake cycle. Other related medical conditions can include sleep apnea, congestive heart failure, paroxysmal nocturnal dyspnea, gastroesophageal reflux, polyuria, or delirium. Related movement disorders associated with sleep include restless legs syndrome (RLS) and periodic limb movement disorder (PLMD).

Medications, such as antivirals, interferon, psychostimulants, antidepressants, and bronchodilators and substances such as alcohol, caffeine, nicotine, cannabis, and opiates can interfere with restorative sleep. Psychiatric disorders, such as depression, anxiety, adjustment disorders, acute stress, and coping with life events, can also disrupt normal sleep. Few things in life seem better when one is sleep deprived. Insufficient or inefficient sleep negatively affects energy, mood, memory, cognition and cognitive speed, work performance, and quality, enjoyment, and safety. Insomnia and fatigue also appear to be associated with increased morbidity and disability. One-fourth of patients try OTC sleep aids (e.g., diphenhydramine, valerian root, or melatonin), 27% use alcohol, and less than 15% take prescribed sedative–hypnotics.

Substance Use

Although injection drug use is the second most common risk factor HIV infection in the United States, other modes of drug use and alcohol abuse also increase the risk of infection through unsafe sexual practices, drug-induced hypersexuality, disinhibition, impulsiveness, altered cognition, impaired judgment, or prostitution to obtain drugs or money for drugs. In the substance-abusing population, HIV infection is associated with youth, homelessness, being from an ethnic minority, and having a history of sexual victimization. Prior psychiatric illness is also common.

HIV infection tends to be diagnosed at a more advanced stage of the disease in injection drug users and may have a more rapid downhill course. Injection drug use is also seen as a bridge of infection through heterosexual and mother-to-child transmission. Continued drug use can speed the patient's decline in several ways: suppressed immune function, increased risk for infections (e.g., STIs, HCV, pneumonia, abscesses, endocarditis, and tuberculosis, TB), drug interactions with antiretroviral agents, poor ability to adhere to complicated medical regimens, and chaotic lifestyles that make scheduled medical follow-up difficult. This population has a high tolerance to medications and possibly a low tolerance to pain, discomfort, or inconvenience. It is also a population at risk for impaired cognitive function from neurotoxic substances, poor nutrition, metabolic encephalopathies, ischemia, stroke, seizures, and head trauma.

Among MSM with HIV infection, crystal meth use represents a major co-morbidity. Use of crystal meth fuels unsafe sex practices in a culture known as "party and play," leading to increased rates of transmission. Chronic crystal meth use can also lead to manic symptoms as well as psychosis, and these symptoms often develop with shorter lengths of use in HIV-positive individuals as compared to the general population. Long-term methamphetamine use can also lead to significant dyskinesias.

Pain

The evaluation of pain and its adequate treatment and management are essential in the care of patients with HIV infection or AIDS. In a systematic literature review of pain in HIV patients, the point prevalence of pain ranged from 54% (based on 1-week recall) to 83% (based on 3-month recall).[82] Pain is a common reason for psychiatric consultation and, rather than death, is often what patients fear most. Pain control is one of the cornerstones in the care of patients with end-stage AIDS. Pain syndromes, including neuropathy, myopathies, and headache, are common among patients with HIV infection, particularly those who have received certain older antiretroviral drugs (see later). The psychiatrist might need to intervene when hospital staff who care for a patient with a history of substance disorder fail to distinguish between the management of the patient's addiction and the adequate treatment of pain or fail to provide adequate pain relief to patients from a racial or ethnic minority.

Peripheral sensory neuropathy, the most common pain syndrome in patients with HIV-associated disease, affects up to 35% of patients with AIDS.[83] Most commonly, the neuropathy manifests as a distal, symmetric polyneuropathy that can be caused by HIV infection or particularly by the "d" antiretroviral drugs, ddI, ddC, and stavudine (d4T). Today, peripheral neuropathy due to antiretrovirals is typically seen in older patients who had been treated with these medications in the past. The diagnosis is confirmed on the basis of the neurologic examination and laboratory tests, including an electromyogram and nerve conduction studies. Treatment includes a change in the antiretroviral regimen to avoid nerve-toxic agents and the avoidance of other aggravating factors such as alcohol.

CASE 1

Mr. C, a 55-year-old male, diagnosed with HIV 10 years earlier and followed in the clinic for the last 4 years, on ART, presents with new-onset paranoia regarding his downstairs neighbor. He has started to believe that the neighbor is breaking into his apartment during the day and has placed recording equipment throughout the apartment. Mr. C reports that he is sleeping much less and not leaving the house. History is notable for depression, treated for many years with fluoxetine, and a past history of alcohol use disorder, in remission for the past 7 years.

Consultation with the patient's primary care physician reveals that his CD4 count has remained high and his viral load undetectable over the last 3 years on his current regimen. Cognitive testing reveals mild deficits in attention and focus, with some mild executive dysfunction also noted.

The differential diagnosis includes major depression with psychosis, a schizophrenia-spectrum disorder including delusional disorder, alcohol-induced psychosis in the setting of possible relapse, other substance-induced psychosis, an unrecognized bipolar disorder presenting as mania with psychosis, HIV-dementia with psychosis, opportunistic infection in the CNS, antiretroviral medication-induced psychosis, and CSF viral escape. Given that the medication regimen has not changed and the patient does not take any antiretrovirals associated with prominent neuropsychiatric effects, antiretroviral effect seems unlikely. As CD4 counts have remained high and there are no focal neurologic deficits, opportunistic infection also seems unlikely. The patient's bedside cognitive testing is not severely impaired enough to suggest an HIV-dementia; deficits are mild. Aside from insomnia, the patient denies other prominent symptoms of mania or depression. Prior to further neurologic work-up, a urine toxicology is obtained, and reveals the presence of amphetamines, which are not prescribed. On confrontation, the patient acknowledges a pattern over the last several years, of binge use of crystal meth in association with unsafe sexual practices. The diagnosis of amphetamine-induced psychosis is confirmed. Via counseling, engagement in a support group, and ongoing psychiatric treatment, the patient is able to achieve sobriety, and his psychotic symptoms gradually reduce in severity over the next several months, though he continues to have some lingering vague paranoia.

APPROACH TO PSYCHIATRIC CARE

Screening and Prevention

It is estimated that 13% of those infected with HIV in the United States are unaware of their seropositivity, that the unaware are responsible for the majority of new infections, and that many would take steps to change their risky behavior if they were informed of their status.[84] In 2006, the Centers for Disease Control and Prevention (CDC) Division of HIV/AIDS Prevention took steps to address this by issuing new recommendations advocating for universal (not based on risk factors) HIV screening in all healthcare settings: medical inpatient and outpatient, mental health, and substance abuse settings. The recommendations require no special patient consent for screening, which is performed once the patient is so notified, unless the patient specifically declines consent; this is universal opt-out screening.[85] However, two states (New York and Nebraska) still have statutes that require written informed consent. In 2013, the United States Preventative Services Task Force recommended universal screening for HIV, which resulted in insurance companies having to cover the screening.[86]

Psychiatrists should strongly consider screening patients for HIV, consistent with the CDC recommendations, especially given that they care for an at-risk population.[87] Screening is critical not just for secondary infections, but also to ensure that patients receive early treatment as recommended, when the immune system is not yet seriously damaged. In a study of patients in three different psychiatric facilities, 4.8% of patients were HIV-infected, a prevalence over four-fold greater than the general population.[88] Screening should also take place routinely at substance-use treatment sites. Studies have shown that patients at such sites often have not been tested recently for HIV, and a small but significant minority has never been tested.[89]

Of the 45,000 HIV transmissions in 2009, 91.5% were attributable to patients with HIV who were undiagnosed (18% of the population) or not retained in medical care (45% of the population).[90] These figures illustrate that screening is necessary but insufficient for prevention, as patients must know about their status and be retained in care for ongoing counseling. After screening, the next step in prevention is the assessment of the patient for risk factors and behavior. Patients must be able to perceive themselves as at risk in order for counseling to be effective. Prevention models with individuals and groups of chronically mentally ill and substance-abusing patients must be specific and tailored to the population being addressed. Programs with counselors whose cultural backgrounds are similar to those of the patient population have proved most effective. Programs geared toward the injection drug use community have enlisted community members as prevention leaders.

Pre-exposure prophylaxis (PrEP) was approved by the FDA in 2012 as a strategy to prevent new infections in patients engaging in high-risk behavior. Several randomized clinical trials as well as real-world observational studies have demonstrated a substantial decline in new infections when PrEP is used regularly.[91] Unfortunately, use of PrEP is correlated with decreased use of condoms and increased rates of transmission of other STIs. Psychiatrists should be aware of the option of PrEP for patients engaged in high-risk behaviors.

Collaboration

Although a number of demonstration projects have shown the efficacy of wrap-around services for HIV-infected patients,[92] it is the exception rather than the rule to have medical, mental health, and addiction services, including opiate replacement therapy, in one coordinated site.[93] More commonly, patients with multiple diagnoses have complicated treatment regimens and have multiple providers at diverse sites of care, a situation that can parallel the chaos in the rest of their lives. In the absence of single-site treatment, intensive management of care can keep all treaters informed, provide outreach to improve attendance at appointments, assist with concrete services (e.g., housing, transportation, child care), and help devise and implement an individualized medication adherence plan. The consultation psychiatrist has a unique opportunity to facilitate communication and to coordinate care among members of the patient's care team.

Adherence

Adherence is the cornerstone of successful therapy for HIV infection. Missed doses lead to treatment resistance and sometimes resistance to whole classes of medication. This, in turn, is correlated with increased morbidity and mortality, as well as the development of more treatment-resistant viral strains. Active substance use, homelessness, a lack of social supports, domestic violence, personality disorders, and psychiatric illness, especially major depression, have long been recognized as risk factors for poor adherence.[94–96] However, the presence of one or more of these factors is not justification for exclusion from antiretroviral therapy. Rather, these factors are challenges to be addressed in preparation for initiating HAART, which may be postponed for several months while active treatment is initiated for addictions or psychiatric problems, along with readiness for concurrent medications and education about adherence.[97] The patient hospitalized with HIV infection is a captive audience for the initiation or reinforcement of this preparation for HAART.

Effective adherence programs are tailored to the patient in terms of language, education, culture, lifestyle, and personality. Individualized adherence programs capitalize on or enhance the patient's social supports (e.g., family, intimate partners, friends, and groups), cognitive abilities, and personality style. They require accessibility, flexibility, and positively framed incentives (i.e., rewards, not punishments).[62,98] Adherence is further promoted when the patient has a high level of satisfaction with the physician, understands the importance of taking every dose, believes that missed doses lead to resistance, knows and recognizes each specific medication, and is informed of possible side effects.[98]

Simplifying the regimen (e.g., reducing the number of doses and food restrictions) and minimizing the pill burden helps fit the regimen into the patient's lifestyle. Clearly written instructions are helpful, if the patient is literate. Tying pill-taking to daily routines, along with pill boxes, alarms, pagers, directly observed therapy, or new smart-phone application reminder systems, can also increase adherence. Patients who are comfortable taking medications in front of other people also have an easier time incorporating HAART into their lives.[99]

Adherence is not static; it needs to be inquired about, and promoted by, each provider at every visit. Pill fatigue, complacency, transient or prolonged relapse of substance abuse or depression, onset of morphologic or metabolic side effects, onset or exacerbation of other medical conditions, hospitalization, or psychosocial stressors (e.g., financial, housing, insurance issues or changes, family or relationship issues, and travel) can interrupt or decrease the patient's previous level of adherence.

In addition to adherence to medication, adherence to appointments is also an important component of treatment. Adherence to scheduled medical appointments is associated with optimal viral suppression and might warrant appropriate outreach efforts.[100] A recent study showed an increase in all-cause mortality for patients who failed to achieve retention in clinical care, and missed visits independently increased mortality in those considered to be retained in care.[101]

TREATMENT

Non-pharmacologic Treatments

Case Management

Case management is often necessary to help with basic needs, such as food, shelter, transportation, child care, medical coverage, and other entitlements, which may be needed in this population and are powerful barriers to adequate treatment. In particular, patients with cognitive impairment (executive dysfunction and memory problems) are at risk for falling through the cracks unless appropriate help and supervision are provided.

Groups

Groups of various types, often provided in the community or by AIDS activist organizations, offer a supportive, social network and positive affiliations for members of an often disenfranchised and stigmatized population. Self-help, 12-step, and peer-counseling groups are examples of such community-based programs. Therapy groups and other more formalized groups might focus on aspects of living with HIV infection (e.g., disclosure, adherence, parenting), participant characteristics (e.g., women, particular ethnic minorities, MSM, substance abusers), or mission (e.g., risk reduction or prevention).[102]

Individual Psychotherapy

Individual psychotherapy can help patients cope with HIV infection or AIDS-related issues and distress with approaches, such as coping strategies, problem-solving, disclosure of HIV status, discrimination, relationships, sexuality, and bereavement. For patients whose infection was diagnosed more than a decade ago, issues of facing a foreshortened life span may be replaced by issues of living with a chronic illness. There may be themes of remorse and longing for missed opportunities referent to this erroneous life view. The focus and goals of therapy may be specific to the stage of HIV-associated disease; late in the course of AIDS, therapy may focus on end-of-life issues (such as concerns about ongoing childcare and guardianship, coping with loss, progressive disability, and unremitting pain).

For specific diagnoses, including depression or anxiety disorders, proven therapies, such as interpersonal psychotherapy or cognitive-behavioral therapy (CBT), have been shown to be effective in this population.[102–104] Self-hypnosis, guided imagery, meditation, muscle relaxation, massage, yoga, aerobic exercise, or acupuncture may be therapeutic for selected patients.

Adherence to medications for HIV infection and psychotropic medications should be reinforced or explored. It should be stressed that the therapist is a member of the patient's treatment team, and appropriate releases should be obtained to allow all team members to communicate and to coordinate care. The therapist, for instance, may spend more time with the patient and be the first clinician to suspect cognitive dysfunction that requires medical work-up and intervention.

Pharmacologic Treatment

Drug–Drug Interactions

Patients with HIV infection or AIDS may be taking HIV-related medications, psychotropic drugs, OTC and herbal preparations, alcohol or drugs of abuse, and drugs to treat those addictions. Such drug combinations are prone to interactions, overlapping side effects, and toxicities. Drug side effects, such as diarrhea (common to many antiretroviral agents), can decrease the absorption of other drugs. Potential drug interactions do not necessarily preclude the concomitant use of such medications but require a careful risk-to-benefit assessment, possible dose adjustment, periodic drug level monitoring, and monitoring for or treatment of side effects. Some general principles and frequently updated resources (Table 30-4) can aid in the safe pharmacologic treatment of these patients.

Effects on the CYP enzyme system in the liver account for many of the drug–drug interactions. Of the key CYP isoenzymes involved in the metabolism of psychotropics and antiretrovirals (1A2, 2C9/19, 2D6, and 3A4), 3A4 and 2D6 account for the majority of the metabolism of psychiatric medications. Allelic differences cause 10% of whites and 1% of Asians to slowly metabolize 2D6 substrates,[105] and 20% of African Americans and Asians and 5% of whites slowly metabolize 2C19 substrates.[106,107] Medications can rely on more than one metabolic pathway, which acts as a safeguard against drug interactions. *In vitro* studies of drug metabolism do not adequately portray the human experience that is complicated by individual genetic and nutritional differences and multi-drug and substance regimens.[105,108] As a rule of thumb, the PIs, followed by the NNRTIs, have the broadest effects on the CYP system; the NRTIs are mostly devoid of drug interactions. The PI ritonavir also induces glucuronyl transferase, a non-CYP metabolic enzyme.[108]

For a variety of reasons, patients with HIV infection are very sensitive to small doses of psychiatric medications, similar to what is seen in geriatric patients. Helping the patient tolerate medications is ultimately more important than is raising the dose quickly. The general principle is, "start low and go slow." However, patients still need to receive an appropriately high dose of any psychotropic. Because of the pill burden and complicated schedules patients with HIV infection must often endure, once-a-day medication therapy is generally preferable. Anticholinergic medications should be avoided or minimized because of their deleterious effects on cognition and the possibility of delirium or even seizures. Decreased saliva can also predispose to the development of thrush.[44]

Depression

The SSRIs remain the drugs of choice for depressive disorders in HIV patients because of established efficacy in this patient population and a favorable risk-to-benefit profile.[109] SSRIs are largely metabolized, though not exclusively, by 2D6 and 3A4. Ritonavir, and to a lesser extent indinavir,

TABLE 30-4 Clinically Useful HIV/AIDS Resources on the Internet

PROGRAM	URL	COMMENTS
AIDS Clinical Trials Information Service (ACTIS)	www.actis.org	Provides quick and easy access to information on federally and privately funded clinical trials for adults and children
The Body Pro	www.thebodypro.com	Provides news updates and latest treatment guidelines
Centers for Disease Control and Prevention (CDC)	www.cdc.gov/hiv/	Comprehensive database with epidemiology, guidelines, latest research, and advocacy
HIV/AIDS Treatment Information Service	www.hivatis.org	Allows you to view and download HIV treatment guidelines, general HIV treatment information, and more
New York State Department of Health AIDS Institute	www.health.ny.gov/diseases/aids/	Coordinates state programs, services and activities relating to HIV/AIDS
UCSF HIV InSite	hivinsite.ucsf.edu/medical	Includes a drug-interaction database by drug class, drug profiles, fact sheets, and links to treatment guidelines
United Nations Programme on HIV/AIDS	www.unaids.org	International epidemiology, news, and recommendations
United States FDA HIV/AIDS Program	www.fda.gov/oashi/aids/HIV.html	Includes information about approved antiretroviral drugs and treatment guidelines

inhibit metabolism of 2D6 substrates; all of the PIs inhibit 3A4 metabolism to varying degrees.[110] Inhibition of the metabolism of the SSRIs, venlafaxine, and mirtazapine by ritonavir and indinavir increases the levels of the antidepressants, which might allow a therapeutic response at a low or moderate dose. Although high doses of the antidepressants could lead to serotonin syndrome or other toxicities, a wide range of concentrations are generally well-tolerated.[111]

All SSRIs are associated with sexual side effects, akathisia-like activation, and GI symptoms. Fluoxetine, with the longest half-life, is a good option for patients who have tumultuous lives and who might miss doses. Use of fluoxetine weekly is also an option. Sertraline, citalopram, and escitalopram have the least potential for clinically significant drug interactions.[112,113] While citalopram was once considered the initial SSRI of choice for patients with HIV/AIDS, recent concerns about the potential for greater QT prolongation with citalopram, coupled with evidence suggesting HIV patients are themselves at higher risk for QT prolongation, has somewhat limited its use as a first-line agent.[114,115]

Serotonin–Norepinephrine Re-Uptake Inhibitors

Venlafaxine, its metabolite desvenlafaxine, and duloxetine are serotonin and norepinephrine (hence, "dual") re-uptake inhibitors. The extended-release form of venlafaxine is a reasonable first-line medication because of its once-a-day dosing and relative lack of drug interactions. Because of inhibition by ritonavir and indinavir noted above, lower doses are often sufficient. SNRIs can be initially stimulating, and some patients have difficulty tolerating them. SNRIs can raise blood pressure unacceptably in hypertensive patients, and blood pressure monitoring is required. Milnacipran is an SNRI marketed in the United States for fibromyalgia.

Bupropion

The antidepressant least likely to have sexual side effects, bupropion, does not treat anxiety. Bupropion's continued stimulant effect, if tolerable, can benefit patients with fatigue or apathy, although, unlike psychostimulants, bupropion tends not to improve HIV-related cognitive slowing.[44]

Bupropion lowers the seizure threshold in a dose-dependent manner, which is a concern in patients who have a history of seizures, poorly controlled seizure disorders, head trauma, or other threshold-lowering pathology (e.g., space-occupying lesions, infections, or alcohol or psychoactive substance use). Patients with eating disorders or metabolic derangements from drug side effects (such as vomiting or diarrhea) may be at increased risk for seizures. The slow-release forms may be safer with regard to seizure risk, and lower doses (100–300 mg) are often used in patients with HIV. The actual risk of seizures in HIV patients treated with bupropion seems much less than previously thought.[108] There has been one report of *in vitro* 2B6 inhibition by ritonavir, nelfinavir (PI), and efavirenz (NNRTI), causing significant interference with bupropion metabolism.[116] Whether this interference is significant *in vivo* is unclear. A prospective study that included the administration of bupropion to patients on PIs reported no serious adverse events and, specifically, no seizures.[117]

Trazodone

Primarily used for its major side effect, trazodone makes people very sleepy within 20 to 30 minutes of ingestion, usually at a low dose of 25 or 50 mg. In low doses, it is minimally anticholinergic. Men of all ages must always be informed of its rare but serious side effect, priapism (prevalence is about 1/7000).

Mirtazapine

At low doses, mirtazapine is useful for patients who have difficulty eating and sleeping, even in the absence of clear depression. At higher doses, it is also an effective antidepressant, albeit with major long-term management issues related to histaminergic side effects (e.g., daytime drowsiness and significant weight gain). Patients who receive mirtazapine should be weighed at regular intervals. Mirtazapine appears to have no significant drug interactions with ART.

Tricyclic Antidepressants

Tricyclic antidepressants (TCAs) are often used in small doses for neuropathic pain, insomnia, or headaches. TCAs have a narrow therapeutic window; metabolic inhibition at 2D6, from PIs (or most SSRIs), can lead to serious toxicity, including death. Safe concurrent use of these medicines requires therapeutic drug monitoring of the TCA levels (to determine the appropriate dose) and monitoring electrocardiograms (ECGs), particularly if the patient is on other QTc-prolonging medications.[108]

The side effect of constipation may be helpful in some HIV-infected patients with diarrhea. TCAs can be lethal with ingestion of a 2-week supply. The least anticholinergic ones, nortriptyline and desipramine, are recommended given that anticholinergia can worsen cognition.

Monoamine Oxidase Inhibitors (MAOIs)

Because of the myriad drugs patients with HIV infection might need over time, MAOIs are relatively contraindicated in these patients. They should specifically not be co-administered with zidovudine.

Psychostimulants

Psychostimulants, such as methylphenidate and dextroamphetamine, may be used to target co-morbid attention deficit hyperactivity disorder, augment antidepressant therapy, or to treat the symptoms of fatigue and cognitive decline associated with HIV infection.[118–120] Methylphenidate can inhibit 2C9 and 2C19 metabolism, leading to increased levels of certain TCAs (i.e., desipramine, clomipramine, and imipramine), barbiturates, and warfarin. Dextroamphetamine, however, is a 2D6 substrate that neither inhibits nor induces the CYP isoenzymes, though it can compete at active sites.[108]

In low doses, psychostimulants can improve appetite, energy, and mood. They work quickly, often within hours, and have few side effects or interactions. Especially useful in patients who are unresponsive to or intolerant of other antidepressants, stimulants also effectively improve the early symptoms of cognitive decline; they help patients attend and stay more focused and organized. In late HAD, however, they can become toxic. Stimulants should also be avoided in the presence of psychotic symptoms or in those with a history of seizures. Abuse is rare in patients who have no history of a substance disorder. A history of a substance disorder is not a contraindication to the use of stimulants but it does require that the prescriber be more cautious. Modafinil and armodafinil are related wakefulness-promoting non-stimulant psychotropic drugs that are sometimes used instead of a psychostimulant for HIV-related fatigue and depression.[121]

Anxiety

Anxiolytic Antidepressants

For prolonged use in anxiety disorders, the SSRIs as well as SNRIs are beneficial, and they decrease the needed dose of benzodiazepines when these medications are co-administered.

Benzodiazepines

For more time-limited episodes of intolerable anxiety, short- to medium-acting benzodiazepines without active metabolites and the least drug–drug interactions should be used. Benzodiazepines are primarily 3A4 substrates, with the exception of lorazepam, oxazepam, and temazepam, which are metabolized by glucuronyl transferase. For this reason, these three exceptions are the drugs of choice when patients on (3A4-inhibiting) PIs require treatment with a benzodiazepine. Other benzodiazepines would be expected to have increased levels when co-administered with PIs, leading to possibly dangerous sedation or respiratory depression. However, use of these glucuronyl transferase substrates with ritonavir can require higher doses of benzodiazepines.[108] The NNRTIs efavirenz and nevirapine, along with the PI ritonavir, have the potential to induce the 3A isoenzymes. This 3A induction may be delayed and cause a drop in previously elevated benzodiazepine levels, resulting in decreased efficacy or withdrawal. This unpredictability precludes the regular use of such short-acting agents (e.g., alprazolam) because of the risk that withdrawal will precipitate seizures.[122]

Buspirone

An option for patients on PIs, buspirone unfortunately takes several weeks to become effective. Concomitant use of benzodiazepines may be necessary to help the patient through the initiation and titration period. In advanced systemic illness, but not less symptomatic disease, buspirone has worsened cognition and triggered mania.[44]

Antipsychotics

Although generally not recommended for anxiety because of potentially serious long-term metabolic effects, low doses of atypical antipsychotics may be effective if fear or pain are prominent. See the section, "Psychosis" below for more information on the use of antipsychotics in patients with HIV.

Bipolar Disorder

Beyond optimizing the antiretroviral regimen, treatment of HIV-related secondary mania should be tailored to the patient's HIV status and general medical condition. In advanced HIV/AIDS, patients might find lithium or carbamazepine less tolerable. Although lithium does not interact with the CYP system, it should be avoided in HIV-positive patients with advanced illness because of its potential for toxicity with fluid and electrolyte shifts. Carbamazepine induces 3A4, lowering levels of the PIs and other antiretrovirals, a situation that could foster resistance, possibly to a whole class of medications.[108] It might be possible in certain instances to avert this resistance by using higher doses of the antiretroviral. However, carbamazepine is also relatively contraindicated in immune-suppressed patients because of its potential to cause leukopenia.

Valproate increases the risk of liver toxicity (especially in patients with chronic HCV or other liver disease) and bone marrow suppression (especially in combination with zidovudine, whose levels may be increased via glucuronyl transferase inhibition).[123] Nonetheless, valproic acid may be more effective for patients with secondary mania and brain abnormalities on MRI.[124]

Lamotrigine bypasses the CYP system, but it is a glucuronyl transferase substrate and needs to be titrated slowly to reduce the risk of Stevens–Johnson syndrome.[108]

Nonetheless, lamotrigine is often the mood-stabilizer of choice in patients with HIV and bipolar disorder, especially those with a history of recurrent depression and less severe mania.

Although benzodiazepines have anti-manic properties, they carry the risk of disinhibition, anterograde amnesia, and confusion; they are generally not considered to be primary pharmacologic treatment of mania. For medically complex patients with HIV disease, antipsychotics may be preferred over the standard mood stabilizers.

Psychosis

Antipsychotics are the treatment of choice for psychotic symptoms of almost any cause. Patients with HIV infection, however, are extremely sensitive to side effects of antipsychotics and are at risk for extrapyramidal symptoms (EPS) and neuroleptic malignant syndrome (NMS) with high-potency agents and confusion or seizures with low-potency agents.[79,125]

The second-generation antipsychotics are often chosen because of better tolerability, particularly with regard to EPS. Very low starting doses and cautious titration are recommended. Risperidone and olanzapine have each been used effectively for HIV-related psychosis without causing undue sedation or cognitive impairment.[126] The deleterious effect of many second-generation antipsychotics on glucose metabolism, however, can limit their usefulness, especially in patients already at risk for diabetes, such as those taking PIs.[127] Aripiprazole has fewer metabolic side effects but still causes weight gain, while ziprasidone and lurasidone also have good metabolic profiles. Metformin is increasingly used for metabolic syndrome induced by antipsychotics, and may be an option for HIV-positive patients who develop such side effects. Lurasidone toxicity has been reported in combination with atazanavir in at least one report.[128]

Plasma levels of clozapine, which has a complex metabolic pathway involving 1A2, 2C9/19, 3A4, and 2D6, can increase with concomitant use of PIs. Despite its relative contraindications given the potential for drug interactions and added bone marrow toxicity, clozapine may still be used, particularly because it is possible to monitor clozapine serum levels.[129]

Substance Use Disorders

The treatment and management of hospitalized patients with HIV infection and substance abuse disorders has five main features, depending on the patient's level of addiction or recovery: prophylaxis against or treatment of withdrawal; encouragement to enter a recovery program, including referral to a comprehensive addictions program; maintenance of recovery during the stress of hospitalization; adequate pain control, including the use of narcotic medications, if appropriate; and careful monitoring for drug–drug interactions, especially for patients on methadone maintenance.

Prescribed medications that are being abused might need to be discontinued. There are limitations to the model of harm reduction used in many addiction-treatment programs, and the psychiatrist should know that prescribing oral forms of abused injection drugs does not promote recovery from substance disorder. This practice might only introduce the problems of dependence on high doses of oral substances.[130]

If the patient is on methadone maintenance and opiate analgesia is required, an agent other than methadone should be used to maintain clear boundaries for the patient and the methadone maintenance program. For patients on methadone maintenance with symptomatic HIV infection or with $CD4^+$ lymphocyte counts below 500/μL, the initiation of some antimicrobial agents can have pharmacologic consequences. For example, methadone increases zidovudine serum levels, which can lead to increased toxicity. Treatment with rifampin can increase methadone metabolism and potentially precipitate acute opiate withdrawal. In this instance, the daily methadone dose needs to be increased. The discharge plan would need to include notifying the patient's methadone clinic of this dosage change. Methadone also has a tendency to prolong the QT interval, placing patients with HIV at increased risk for lethal ventricular arrhythmias, such as *torsades de pointes*, especially when administered with other QT-prolonging agents.

Patients prescribed Suboxone as opiate replacement therapy also face many challenges surrounding pain treatment. In some cases, Suboxone may block the effects of full μ-opioid agonists, leading to inadequate pain control with typical regimen. There are no definitive guidelines for management of the pain patient on Suboxone maintenance therapy, and recommendations range from continuing the Suboxone and adding in a short-acting opioid analgesic to discontinuing Suboxone during treatment.[131] Suboxone has been used safely in many patients with HIV.

Another important substance–medication interaction to be aware of is that ritonavir inhibits metabolism of ecstasy, ketamine, cocaine, and other stimulants, as well as γ-hydroxybutyrate (GHB). Fatal interactions between ecstasy and ritonavir have been reported.[108,132]

Pain

The treatment of HIV-related neuropathy is similar to the approach used with a chronic pain syndrome. Low doses of TCAs can be effective, either alone or in combination with other analgesic therapies. No systematic studies have been conducted to compare the effectiveness of different TCAs, and no evidence exists for the superiority of amitriptyline for HIV-related neuropathy. Desipramine and nortriptyline are better tolerated and appear to be as effective.

Anticonvulsants in low doses can be effective for neuropathic pain, either alone or in combination with other analgesic therapies. Both carbamazepine and valproic acid have been effective, but hematopoietic and hepatic side effects and drug interactions must be monitored. Gabapentin may be effective for neuropathic pain; its use avoids hematopoietic and hepatic side effects. Low-dose clonazepam can be particularly effective for hyperpathic pain. Lamotrigine has support for its use for HIV-related sensory neuropathy from a controlled trial.[133]

Some antiarrhythmics also have local anesthetic properties and can be useful for some types of pain syndromes. Postherpetic neuralgia can be highly disabling in HIV-infected patients, particularly those who have had multi-dermatomal herpes zoster. IV lidocaine can offer relief, often with once- or twice-weekly infusions, and a significant dose reduction in narcotic analgesics.

Opiates are beneficial for short-term use or for periods of pain exacerbation, but they can induce tolerance and abuse or dependence. A history of a substance disorder does not preclude the use of opiates required for adequate analgesia, but it requires careful monitoring to prevent unauthorized escalation of the dosage. In discharge planning for patients with advanced HIV disease, the psychiatrist should remember that cognitive impairment can make compliance with as-needed dosing schedules difficult, and patients can accidentally overuse analgesics. The use of a pill alarm or box can help. If long-term therapy with opiates is needed, the psychiatrist should consider long-acting oral or transdermal formulations. The latter are particularly helpful in the care of terminally ill patients, many of whom have odynophagia or dysphagia.

Opiates also interface with hepatic metabolism, affecting and being affected by interactions with antiretroviral medications. Meperidine may be cleared more quickly, leaving a higher concentration of its neurotoxic metabolite that causes delirium and possibly seizures. Clearance of fentanyl, a 3A4 substrate, is decreased by ritonavir, which can cause nausea, dizziness, and possibly respiratory depression. Codeine and its derivatives are prodrugs that need to be converted to analgesics. PIs can block this conversion and make pain control more difficult.

CONCLUSION

Neuropsychiatric symptoms are part of the HIV infection and AIDS and have multiple etiologies. HIV CNS infection and primary psychiatric disorders should always be considered. Other CNS infections or lesions, medications, drugs of abuse, drug–drug interactions, and metabolic derangements need to be explored. Whenever identified, underlying causes should be treated, but the psychiatric symptoms can require more immediate, symptomatic treatment.

Patients with HIV infection are often sensitive to small amounts of medication, and they should generally be given geriatric doses with careful monitoring and slow dosage titration; ultimately, however, an effective dose must be prescribed. The PIs, and to a lesser extent the NNRTIs, are responsible for the majority of the drug–drug interactions with psychotropic medications. These interactions occur largely because of interference with the hepatic CYP enzyme system. Having access to frequently updated and reliable resources assists with the choice of safe pharmacologic alternatives in this population. Optimal psychiatric care (e.g., effective remission of depression) can help patients achieve sufficient adherence to antiretroviral treatment and even improve their prognosis.

REFERENCES

Access the reference list online at https://expertconsult.inkling.com/.

31

Patients With Cancer

Carlos G. Fernandez-Robles, M.D.
Kelly E. Irwin, M.D.
William F. Pirl, M.D., M.P.H.
Donna B. Greenberg, M.D.

OVERVIEW

The seriousness of the diagnosis of cancer challenges the capacity to survive, sets a course in life, and dashes hopes and dreams. Over the 20th century, even as cancer treatments improved and some patients were cured, psychiatrists in the tradition of humane psychiatry used their skills to stand by patients who were overwhelmed and helped them make complex treatment choices by which they could shape the rest of their lives or their end-of-life care. Psychiatrists have offered expert diagnosis and management of co-morbid psychiatric syndromes and collaborated with oncologists so that treatable psychiatric illnesses have not stood in the way of oncologic care. Specific cancer-related or cancer treatment-related neuropsychiatric syndromes (Table 31-1)[1–5] can, and should, be recognized and treated. Additionally, psychiatrists can help patients to cope with physical symptoms, developmental losses, changes in relationships, and the effects of cancer on families.

Ever since Weisman and co-workers explored how to help patients cope with cancer who were demoralized,[6–8] psychiatrists have tried to understand who their patient was before the diagnosis was made in order to better comprehend the nature of the patient's existential predicament. The psychiatric interview can assess the personal past, present plight, anticipated future, regrets, salient concerns, physical symptoms, disabilities, coping strategies, and psychiatric vulnerabilities (Table 31-2)[7] of those who have received a cancer diagnosis.

Denial and "Middle Knowledge"

Patients often seem to know and want to know about the gravity of their illness, yet they often talk as if they do not know and do not want to be reminded about their cancer.[9] Weisman used the expression "middle knowledge" for the space between open acknowledgment of death and its utter repudiation. Patients may deny facets, implications, or mortal threat of an illness.[9] Middle knowledge is most apparent at transition points (e.g., when a cancer recurs). However, denial is an unstable state; it is almost impossible to maintain denial against even the most reluctant patient's inner perceptions. To preserve a relationship, patients often deny their knowledge of impending death to different people at different times.[10] Tactful discussions of mortality allow patients to be responsive to those closest to them for as long as possible.[9]

Hope and the Doctor–Patient Relationship

Physicians convey respect when they explore the patient's capacity to cope, help nurture courage and resiliency[11] and the attainment of a sense of control while appraising and reappraising available choices. Presenting the facts about an illness does not break the trust established between a patient and a doctor. Furthermore, hope is not merely related to prognosis. The patient's capacity to hope is also related to an ego ideal and the conviction of one's influence on the world. As the physician bolsters the patient's self-esteem, a sense of purpose adds value to life regardless of the time frame. The psychiatrist's capacity to listen non-judgmentally allows patients to express doubts and weaknesses and accept who they are and why they see things as they do. The physician's presence protects patients from abandonment and offers a place where they can explore what is meaningful to them.[11,12]

Medical Choices

The psychiatrist also clarifies with the patient which choices are feasible. Unfazed by personal shock, anxiety, and denial (and armed with a medical education) the psychiatrist is in an excellent position to understand (better than the patient) the individualized medical plan, and help the patient navigate through challenging decisions. Focusing on problems, setting priorities, making clear what the patient is doing and not doing about a problem, and exploring strategies are key elements of care. By doing so, patients can make the choices that are most important for them. Meanwhile, the psychiatrist, in collaboration with oncology staff, sorts through differential diagnoses as psychological symptoms develop and the medical condition and treatment progress. The psychiatric assessment involves an evaluation of affective, behavioral, cognitive, and physical symptoms, and the creation of a differential diagnosis. The work also includes education about how to support significant others and how to allow help or relinquish control to those who have shown themselves trustworthy. Honest communication allows for acceptance, a reduction of bitterness, and replacement of denial with the courage to confront what cannot be changed.[10]

Distress

Emotional distress is common following a cancer diagnosis and its treatment; incidence rates during all phases of the

TABLE 31-1 Neuropsychiatric Side Effects of Cancer Drugs

Hormones[1]

Anti-estrogens

Tamoxifen, toremifene: hot flashes, insomnia, mood disturbance; at high doses tamoxifen can cause confusion

Anastrozole (Arimidex), letrozole (Femara), exemestane (Aromasin): hot flashes, fatigue, mood swings, and irritability; cognitive effects are not known

Raloxifene (Evista): no cognitive side effects noted

Leuprolide (Lupron), goserelin (Zoladex): hot flashes, fatigue, and mood disturbance

Androgen Blockade

Leuprolide (Lupron), goserelin (Zoladex): hot flashes, fatigue, and mood disturbance

Flutamide (Eulexin), bicalutamide (Casodex), nilutamide (Nilandron): as above

Glucocorticoids

Dose-related, variable psychiatric side effects including insomnia, hyperactivity, hyperphagia, depression, hypomania, irritability, and psychosis

Treated by *ad hoc* antipsychotics easily with cancer patients

Other drugs with benefit: lithium, valproate, lamotrigine, and mifepristone

Dexamethasone (Decadron) 9 mg equals 60 mg of prednisone; psychiatric side effects are associated with this dose level

Steroids used as part of an antiemetic treatment with chemotherapy infusion, with lymphoma protocols as high as prednisone 100 mg for 5 days, with nervous system radiation treatment to reduce swelling, with taxanes to reduce side effects

Biologicals

Interferon-α[2,3]

Depression, cognitive impairment, hypomania, psychosis, fatigue, and malaise

Responsive to antidepressants, hypnotics, antipsychotics, stimulants, and antianxiety agents

Associated with autoimmune thyroiditis that may increase or decrease thyroxine; check thyroid function

May inhibit metabolism of some antidepressants by P450 enzymes CYP1A2, CYP2C19, CYP2D6

Interferon-β has less neurotoxicity

Interleukin-2

Delirium, flu-like syndrome, dose-dependent neurotoxicity, and hypothyroidism

Chemotherapy

Vincristine (Oncovin), vinblastine (Velban), vinorelbine (Navelbine)

Neurotoxicity is dose-related and usually reversible. Fatigue and malaise are noted. Seizure and SIADH are uncommon. Postural hypotension may be an aspect of autonomic neuropathy

Less toxicity is noted with vinblastine and vinorelbine

Procarbazine (Matulane)

Mild reversible delirium

A weak MAO inhibitor

Antidepressant use must consider the timing of procarbazine or risk serious interactions

Disulfiram-like effect; avoid alcohol

Asparaginase (Elspar)

Depression, lethargy, and delirium with treatment

Cytarabine (ARA-cell, Alexin)

High-dose IV treatment (over 18 g/m^2 per course) can cause confusion, obtundation, seizures, and coma, cerebellar dysfunction, and leukoencephalopathy. Older patients with multiple treatments are more susceptible. Delirium and somnolence can be seen 2–5 days into treatment. Those with renal impairment are more vulnerable

Fludarabine (Fludara)

Rare somnolence, delirium, and rare progressive leukoencephalopathy

5-Fluorouracil (5-FU)

The primary neurotoxicity is cerebellar, but encephalopathy with headache, confusion, disorientation, lethargy, and seizures has also been seen

Rare deficiency of enzyme that metabolizes dihydropyrimidine dehydrogenase (DPD) is associated with greater exposure and more toxicity

Fatigue is the most common side effect

Cerebellar syndrome and rarely seizure or confusion or parkinsonism may be noted

High-dose IV thymidine may be an antidote for toxicity

Capecitabine (Xeloda)

Related to 5-FU, but with less neurotoxicity

Methotrexate

Causes neurotoxicity particularly when the route is intrathecal or high-dose IV (usually over 1 g/m^2). The toxicity, which is usually reversible, is related to peak level and duration of exposure. Leptomeningeal disease or other conditions that break the blood–brain barrier may impair drug clearance. Prolonged exposure allows the drug to pass through the ependyma of the ventricles to cause leukoencephalopathy. The risk is greater in patients also exposed to cranial radiation. Intrathecal

TABLE 31-1 Neuropsychiatric Side Effects of Cancer Drugs—cont'd

methotrexate may also cause seizures, motor dysfunction, chemical arachnoiditis, and coma. Serum levels are followed closely; folinic acid (leucovorin) rescue is an antidote. Alkalinization may lower the serum level

There is a dose- and route-related risk of delirium

Pemetrexed (Alimta)

An anti-folate given with supplements of folate, intramuscular vitamin B_{12}, and dexamethasone. It is associated with a 10% rate of depression and fatigue

Gemcitabine (Gemzar)

Fatigue, flu-like syndrome, and a rare autonomic neuropathy

Etoposide (Eposin)

Postural hypotension and rare disorientation

Carmustine (BCNU)

Delirium, only at high doses, rare leukoencephalopathy

Thiotepa

Rare leukoencephalopathy

Ifosfamide (Ifex)

Transient delirium, lethargy, seizures, drunkenness, parkinsonism, and cerebellar signs that improve within days of treatment

Risk factors: liver and kidney impairment

Hyponatremia

Leukoencephalopathy

Thiamine or methylene blue may be antidotes

Cisplatin

Rare reversible posterior leukoencephalopathy, parietal, occipital, frontal with cortical blindness

Peripheral neuropathy, poor proprioception, and rarely autonomic

Hypomagnesemia secondary to renal wasting

Vitamin E (300 mg), amifostine may limit peripheral toxicity

Hearing is decreased due to dose-related sensorineural hearing loss

Carboplatin

Neurotoxicity only at high doses

Oxaliplatin (Eloxatin)

Acute dysesthesias of hands, feet, perioral region, jaw tightness, and pharyngo-laryngo dysesthesias

Paclitaxel (Taxol)

Sensory peripheral neuropathy not worse with continued treatment

Rarely seizures and transient encephalopathy, and motor neuropathy

Given with steroids

Docetaxel (Taxotere)

Like paclitaxel but less neurotoxicity

Inhibitors of Kinase Signaling Enzymes[4,5]

Specific inhibitors of kinase signaling enzymes, do not typically cause major behavioral side effects. However, their toxicity related to overlapping effects on several kinase pathways has not been fully defined. Hypertension has been an important side effect related to inhibition of the vascular endothelial growth factor (VEGF). Asthenia or feelings of weakness are commonly reported

Imatinib (Gleevec)

Can cause fluid retention and fatigue, rarely low phosphate; confusion and papilledema

Sunitinib (Sutent)

Hypothyroidism, TSH should be checked every 3 months

Sorafenib (Nexavar)

Fatigue and asthenia and rarely hypophosphatemia

Thalidomide

Drowsiness and somnolence improve over 2–3 weeks, dose-related, associated with dizziness, orthostatic hypotension, tremor, loss of libido, hypothyroidism, and rarely confusion

Bortezomib (Velcade)

Postural hypotension and asthenia; confusion, psychosis, and suicidal thoughts have been reported

---

Monoclonal Antibodies[4,5]

Rituximab (Rituxan)

Headache and dizziness

Trastuzumab (Herceptin)

Headache, insomnia, and dizziness

Bevacizumab (Avastin)

Fatigue, and rarely posterior reversible encephalopathy syndrome

Trastuzumab (Herceptin)

Asthenia, insomnia, and rarely posterior reversible encephalopathy syndrome

TABLE 31-2 Concerns of Patients With Specific Cancer Types

CANCER TYPE	POSSIBLE CONCERNS
Prostate cancer	Significance of serum prostate-specific antigen (PSA) test results: anxiety Once diagnosed, the initial choices are watchful waiting, surgery, or radiation treatment Side effects of surgery or radiation, including incontinence or erectile dysfunction Sexual function and dysfunction Androgen blockade and its effects on fatigue, mood, and sexual interest
Breast cancer	Body image related to mastectomy or to re-construction Adjuvant chemotherapy and its side effects, including alopecia, weight gain, fatigue, and impaired concentration As a result of adjuvant treatment, anti-estrogens, or aromatase inhibitors, menopausal symptoms, including insomnia, sexual dysfunction, and hot flashes The question of prophylactic mastectomy Sexuality and fertility In those with known genetic risk factors, health of loved ones
Colon cancer	Adjustment to surgery or an ostomy Body image and sexual function Bowel dysfunction In those with known genetic risk factors, health of loved ones
Lung cancer	Physical limitations of reduced lung capacity Post-thoracotomy neuralgia Cough Guilt about nicotine addiction (past and present)
Ovarian cancer	Anxiety about the tumor marker CA-125 Sexual dysfunction and infertility Pain and recurrent bowel obstruction
Pancreatic cancer	Maintenance of adequate nutrition Poor appetite Bowel function (and the need for pancreatic enzymes and laxatives) Pain Diabetes Depressed mood
Head and neck cancer	Facial deformity Dry mouth Poor nutrition A weak voice and difficulty with communication Post-treatment hypothyroidism Guilt about alcohol and nicotine addiction (past and present)
Lymphoma	Corticosteroid-induced mood changes The need for recurrent chemotherapy and its effects
Hodgkin's disease	Post-treatment hypothyroidism Fatigue
Osteosarcoma	Amputation/prosthesis vs bone graft Impaired mobility Post-thoracotomy neuralgia

illness are estimated at 29% to 50%,[13] and it occurs in up to 60% of those receiving specialized palliative care.[14] The National Comprehensive Cancer Network (NCCN) Distress Management Guidelines Panel defines distress as "a multifactorial unpleasant emotional experience of a psychological (cognitive, behavioral, emotional), social, and/or spiritual nature that may interfere with the ability to cope effectively with cancer, its physical symptoms and its treatment. Distress extends along a continuum, ranging from common normal feelings of vulnerability, sadness, and fears to problems that can become disabling, such as depression, anxiety, panic, social isolation, and existential and spiritual crisis".[15] Underlying psychopathology, difficulties with housing and finances, limited social support, substance abuse, troubled relationships, and poorer functional performance have been associated with higher levels of distress.[16] A person's capacity to cope with stress is put to test during the cancer experience, and strategies, such as avoidance, rumination, catastrophic thinking, and hypervigilance, often interfere with good adjustment. Weisman and co-workers defined a treatment to reduce distress, correct deficits in coping, re-claim personal control, and improve morale and self-esteem. They asked patients to examine their relationship to cancer (their current concerns), articulate their understanding of what might interfere with effective coping, and envision options that might lead to satisfactory solutions. Treatment focused on coping and adaptation rather than on psychopathology, conveying an expectation of positive change, a sense that options and alternatives are seldom exhausted, and an awareness that perceiving problems in a flexible fashion helped generate support.[7]

Screening

Since 2015, cancer programs seeking accreditation from the American College of Surgeons Commission on Cancer have been required to offer cancer patients screening for distress at least once at a pivotal medical visit and link patients in distress with psychosocial services offered on-site or by referral.[17] The widely used "distress thermometer," a simple visual tool developed by the NCCD, serves as a rough initial single-item question screen, which identifies distress that arises from any source, even if it is unrelated to cancer.[18] More efficient tools, such as the Brief Symptom Inventory (BSI) and the Functional Assessment of Chronic Illness Therapy, can help identify those factors contributing to distress.[19,20] Currently, newer and innovative programs are being developed; the Distress Assessment and Response Tool (DART) program is a screening tool used to detect physical and emotional distress and practical concerns and is linked to triaged inter-professional collaborative care pathways.[21]

Psychosocial Interventions

In addition to extending survival, the oncology community increasingly recognized the value of considering quality of life.[22] A principal goal of psychosocial care is to recognize and address the effects that cancer and its treatment have on the mental status and emotional well-being of patients, their family members, and their professional caregivers.[23] Analyses of clinical trials implementing psychosocial interventions (e.g., educational programs, cognitive-behavioral therapy, supportive-expressive group therapy, spiritually based interventions, relaxation training, and mindfulness) have shown its efficacy in reducing distress, positively impacting medical outcome, alleviating symptoms (such as pain and fatigue), and improving patients' quality of life.[23–26] Psychosocial interventions, particularly those based on cognitive-behavioral therapy, have proven cost-effective for improving health-related quality across all distress domains, compared with usual care.[27] As a strategy to improve the quality of psychosocial care provided, large cancer centers (e.g., Memorial Sloan-Kettering Cancer Center and Massachusetts General Hospital) have created integrative care programs that facilitate on-site access to complementary alternative services.[28–29]

ANXIETY SYNDROMES

Anxiety is part of the emotional reaction that accompanies a diagnosis of cancer. A common mistake among patients and providers is to consider anxiety as normal even when it is both excessive and impairing. Clinically significant anxiety is present in up to 34% of cancer patients.[30] Patients with high levels of trait anxiety are at most risk following a cancer diagnosis, and thus it is important to identify it early in their care.

Anxiety can arise from a wide variety of causes. In oncology patients, it can be classified into four separate categories: situational anxiety; anxiety secondary to a medical condition or its treatment; primary anxiety; and existential anxiety.[31] Patients anticipate the results of cancer markers and scans; their mood rises and falls with the results or news of progressive disease.[32] Most patients are vigilant to physical symptoms after treatment, and worry that such symptoms signify recurrent disease. A visit to the doctor can be reassuring for most; but for some, the alarm of danger does not turn off. Metabolic derangements such as hypercalcemia and hypoglycemia,[33] hypoxia related to parenchymal or mediastinal disease, pulmonary embolism, pleural effusions or pulmonary edema,[34] structural brain lesions leading to complex partial seizures,[35] and side effects of medications, such as steroids and antiemetics, can all be misdiagnosed as anxiety.[36]

Claustrophobia becomes clinically important when magnetic resonance imaging (MRI) is required for diagnostic purposes or when patients are trapped in bed by orthopedic care (e.g., after repair of a leg riddled with osteogenic sarcoma). Needle phobias also occur and can be problematic; they may be treated with rapid desensitization.[37]

Post-traumatic stress disorder (PTSD) is uncommon (occurring in 3% to 10%) in patients treated for cancer;[38] Pitman and colleagues[39] have shown that women with breast cancer have a physiologic response 2 years after hearing a narrative of the two most stressful experiences during their cancer treatment.

Specific cancer-related symptoms (e.g., embarrassment related to unexpected diarrhea) can exacerbate social anxiety and agoraphobia.[40] Disability and poor quality of life have also been associated with co-morbid anxiety disorders and physical conditions.[41] The management of anxiety symptoms should include both pharmacologic and non-pharmacologic interventions. Antidepressant medications suppress the chronic state of alarm and reduce chronic anxiety. Benzodiazepines are best used for specific anxiety-provoking procedures. Cognitive-behavioral therapy and stress management offer patients the opportunity to learn adaptive skills for coping with stressors.[42]

Nausea and Vomiting

Approximately one-half of cancer patients will experience nausea or vomiting during the course of their disease either because of the cancer itself or because of their treatment.[43] Delayed nausea, which comes after the first days of chemotherapy, significantly compromises quality of life even more than does vomiting.[44] As a result of chemotherapy-induced nausea and vomiting, patients can develop anticipatory nausea and anxiety associated with the smells and sights linked with treatment. They may have nausea and vomiting even before arriving at the hospital for treatment. Anticipatory nausea and vomiting are apt to occur in younger patients, in those who have had more emetic treatments, and in those who have trait anxiety.[45] Conditioned nausea morphs into anticipatory anxiety, insomnia, and aversion to treatment. The best treatment for anticipatory nausea is the control of chemotherapy-induced nausea and vomiting (CINV).[46] Addition of neurokinin$_1$ receptor antagonists to 5-hydroxytryptamine$_3$ [5-HT$_3$] receptor antagonists and/or steroids significantly reduces the occurrence of CINV.[47] Hypnosis, CBT techniques, and anti-anxiety agents (e.g., alprazolam, lorazepam) can reduce phobic responses as well as anticipatory nausea and vomiting (both during and after chemotherapy).[4,48]

DEPRESSION

In people with cancer, major depressive disorder (MDD) is associated with poor quality of life, worse adherence to treatment, longer hospital stays, greater desire for death, and an increased rate of suicide and mortality.[49–52] Major depression has been found to occur in approximately 16% of patients with cancer, with minor depression and dysthymia combined reported in almost 22% of patients.[53] These rates are at least three times as common as those found in the general population.[53] Additionally, people with a history of MDD are more likely to develop MDD after the diagnosis of cancer, and about half of those with MDD occur in those without a history of MDD.[54]

The diagnosis of MDD in people with cancer relies on the same *Diagnostic and Statistical Manual of Mental Disorders*, 5th edition (DSM-5) criteria as are used in those without cancer. However, the diagnosis can be complicated by symptoms that overlap with cancer and with cancer treatments. To address this issue, alternative criteria have been proposed, such as the Endicott criteria, that suggests somatic symptoms (e.g., anorexia, insomnia, fatigue) be replaced by non-somatic symptoms (e.g., tearfulness, social withdrawal, self-pity).[55] The Hospital Anxiety and Depression Scale (HADS) is a valid instrument in the assessment of emotional distress in cancer patients that follows a similar approach.[56]

Similar to the evaluation of other medically ill patients who appear depressed, it is critical to consider possible medical contributions in the differential diagnosis. Untreated pain, hypothyroidism, and medications (e.g., corticosteroids, chemotherapies, such as α-interferon, pemetrexed, taxane drugs) may contribute to MDD. Delirium, especially the hypoactive subtype, is often erroneously labeled as depression. Although mood symptoms may occur as part of delirium, key features of delirium include a generalized impairment of attention and cognition, symptom severity that waxes and wanes, and a disturbance of the sleep–wake cycle. Fatigue is a common cancer-related symptom that can be difficult to tease apart from MDD. Anhedonia may be one of the most surefire factors for MDD.[57] Apathy (e.g., that results from a lesion in the frontal lobes) can also be reminiscent of MDD. With apathy, there are delayed responses, cognitive impairment, and a loss of spontaneous action or speech.

The treatment (which consists primarily of antidepressant medications, psychotherapy, or both) of MDD in people with cancer is quite similar to the treatment of MDD in people without medical co-morbidities. Severe cases of MDD, especially those associated with wasting because of diminished appetite, may be treated with electroconvulsive therapy (ECT). Although complementary treatments (e.g., herbal preparations, acupuncture, massage) are available, little data exist supporting their efficacy in the treatment of MDD in cancer patients.[58]

Although antidepressants are commonly used to treat MDD that is co-morbid with cancer, placebo-controlled trials in cancer patients are scarce. A recent meta-analysis focusing exclusively on pharmacologic interventions reported that treatment with antidepressants was found to improve depressive symptoms more than placebo.[59] Furthermore, it found that sub-syndromal depressive symptoms may improve with antidepressants. No particular antidepressant class has been shown to be most effective for treating depression in patients with cancer,[60] and other factors, such as previous adequate response, side effects, and drug-interaction profile, should be taken into account when choosing an agent.[61] Gastrointestinal and anticholinergic effects can worsen pre-existing conditions or side effects from their cancer medications. Venlafaxine, duloxetine, and low-dose tricyclic antidepressants are helpful in the treatment of neuropathic pain;[62] bupropion can play a role in the treatment of fatigue, poor concentration, or nicotine dependence.[63] Mirtazapine has emerged as an effective treatment option in the management of depressed cancer patients with nausea, insomnia, and low appetite.[64] Some of the selective serotonin re-uptake inhibitors (SSRIs) (e.g., fluoxetine, fluvoxamine, paroxetine) as well as bupropion, can interfere with the use of chemotherapeutic agents, including tamoxifen (because of their effects on cytochrome P450 2D6).[65] If an antidepressant is necessary in the setting of tamoxifen use, venlafaxine, escitalopram, or citalopram (less potent 2D6 inhibitors) should be selected.[66] Stimulants (e.g., methylphenidate, dextroamphetamine) may also be beneficial for MDD (i.e., insofar as they may lift mood, increase appetite, and improve cognitive difficulties and fatigue) in the medically ill, especially when time is of the essence, but there is little evidence to support this practice.[67,68]

Although little research has been conducted on medications for MDD in people with cancer, several studies confirm the efficacy of psychosocial interventions.[69] Recently diagnosed patients with cancer with mild to moderate depression may benefit from psychoeducation, CBT, relaxation strategies, and problem-solving approaches, while those with advanced disease may benefit from supportive-expressive psychotherapy that focuses on processing fears associated with death and other existential issues.[53]

CASE 1

Mr. G, a 45-year-old man with a history of CML was treated with a stem cell transplant that was complicated by graft-versus-host disease (GvHD). His past psychiatric history included one episode of major depression that was treated with sertraline, but discontinued due to muscle twitching despite a good response. In addition, he had a history of ulcerative colitis. He was admitted with failure-to-thrive after a flare of gut GvHD complicated by cytomegalovirus infection; psychiatry was consulted for evaluation of depression.

On interview, Mr. G. was lying in bed with his eyes closed, and he provided only terse responses. While initially he coped well with his diagnosis, he was having difficulties more recently, and he was "just waiting for it to pass". His mood had "tanked" with significantly reduced energy and concentration, he was feeling pessimistic about his future, and had "lost faith in his team." Nurses reported that although his symptoms were responding to treatment, he had been apathetic, disengaged from care, and not participating in physical therapy, which had been interfering with his medical progress.

Mr. G. had been reluctant to engage in discussions about his options; the consultant held off from a discussion of medications or psychotherapy, and focused on examining the patient's plight. He learned that Mr. G had been a successful businessman and because of his illness he had not been able to provide for his wife and 1-year-old child and he feared that his child would not remember him after he died. He did not feel in control of his situation and he thought that he had to stop his fears. After a few visits, the consultant had established trust and Mr. G was more willing to discuss options to improve his symptoms. Mr. G agreed to try some medication, but refused to take an antidepressant given his previous experience. The consultant recommended methylphenidate; after titrating the dose Mr. G felt more energetic and started participating in physical therapy. After several days he was strong enough to be transitioned to a rehabilitation facility to continue his recovery.

FATIGUE

Fatigue is the most commonly reported symptom in people with cancer and the symptom that causes them the most functional impairment.[70] It is often confused with MDD.[71]

Although fatigue is not a psychiatric disorder, psychiatric conditions can cause fatigue; therefore fatigue could be considered a psychosomatic condition. A recent meta-analysis of cancer symptoms found a pooled prevalence of 77.8%.[72]

Diagnosis

Fatigue may occur before the diagnosis of cancer, during active cancer treatment, and into the survivorship years. Primarily asking questions about the presence and severity of the symptoms establishes the diagnosis. Although there are validated instruments for the measurement of fatigue (e.g., the Functional Assessment of Chronic Illness Therapy–Fatigue scale, FACIT-F),[71] administration of these questionnaires may not be feasible in busy clinical settings. The NCCN recommends screening for fatigue at visits with a one-item, 0-to-10 scale, similar to that used for the screening of pain, with 0 being "no fatigue" and 10 being "the most severe fatigue." Scores of ≥4 should prompt further evaluation. (The full set of guidelines also includes a review of the literature and can be viewed at www.nccn.org.[70])

The NCCN recommends that the primary evaluation include exploration of the modifiable causes of fatigue (e.g., anemia; pain; sleep disturbances, including insomnia, difficulty staying asleep, and sleep apnea; emotional distress, including MDD and anxiety; poor nutrition; inactivity or deconditioning; use of medications and chemotherapies that cause fatigue, e.g., gemcitabine, corticosteroids, narcotics, antiemetics, and β-blockers; and other medical conditions, e.g., hypothyroidism, hypogonadism, adrenal insufficiency, hypercalcemia, hepatic failure, and cardiovascular or pulmonary compromise). Fatigue may also be a side effect of radiation therapy.

Treatment

The primary treatment for fatigue is modification of its contributing factors; this should be done in conjunction with the patient's oncologist or primary care physician. Mental health clinicians can provide treatment for any underlying psychiatric disorder, as well as offer fatigue-specific interventions (e.g., use of stimulants, exercise, behavioral interventions).

Exercise

Abundant evidence supports aerobic exercise as beneficial for individuals with cancer-related fatigue during and post-cancer therapy, specifically those with solid tumors.[73] Mental health clinicians can encourage exercise through motivational interviewing and through behavioral changes. Because patients can have serious physical morbidities, such as large bone metastases that could lead to fracture, consultation with the oncologist is recommended before initiating exercise. The American Society of Clinical Oncology recommends that patients engage in moderate levels of physical activity including moderate aerobic exercise (150 minutes/week) and strength training (2–3 times/week).[74] Those patients with severe fatigue are encouraged to participate in frequent sessions of low-intensity exercise, 5 to 10 minutes, spaced throughout the day.[75] A physical therapist can assist in designing an exercise program that is appropriate for a person with physical limitations that result from cancer or cancer treatments. For more medically complicated patients, exercise might best be done in a cardiovascular or pulmonary rehabilitation center.

Behavioral Interventions

Behavioral interventions (e.g., CBT, energy conservation) may be beneficial as both primary and adjunctive treatments for fatigue in cancer patients. CBT emphasizes management of fatigue rather than attempting to cure it.[76] Energy conservation is similar to CBT in some respects; it focuses on prioritizing activities and delegating problem-solving difficulties caused by the fatigue, and improving organizational skills.[77] Furthermore, new web-based CBT programs that are less time-consuming are being piloted; these are more cost-effective alternatives, easily accessible to a larger number of patients who are too ill to come to weekly office visits.[78]

Stimulants

A Cochrane Review of drug treatment for cancer-related fatigue, after combining five randomized controlled studies, concluded that current evidence supports the use of psychostimulants for this condition.[79] NCCN guidelines recommend the use of methylphenidate after other non-pharmacologic approaches have failed.[70] However, stimulants can raise blood pressure and heart rate and increase the risk of sudden death. For these reasons they should be used with caution in patients with cardiac disease. Common side effects include constipation, sleep disturbance, anxiety, and (at higher doses) anorexia.

CONFUSION AND COGNITIVE IMPAIRMENT

In cancer, delirium is highly prevalent; its incidence ranges between 10% and 27% in early stages,[80] but it increases to 44% in patients admitted to a hospital;[81] it occurs in more than 85% in patients with terminal illness.[82] Common causes include infection, hypoxia, metabolic abnormalities, pain, substance withdrawal, and side effects of medications (e.g., anticholinergic agents, opioids). In the majority of cancer patients, delirium is multi-factorial, with a median number of three precipitating factors per delirious episode.[83] Older patients, as well as immobilized patients, or those with structural brain disease, vascular disease, or impairment of lung, kidney, or liver function, are predisposed to delirium.[84] The hypoactive motor sub-type of delirium is most prevalent among cancer patients[85] posing an additional treatment challenge, as diagnostic overlap with depression and dementia is not uncommon.[86] Specific cancer-related syndromes involving cognitive impairment in cancer patients are listed in the subsequent paragraphs.

Hypercalcemia

Hypercalcemia (in patients with metastatic lesions to the bone or with tumor-related ectopic production of parathyroid hormone-related protein) secondary to cancer can cause nausea, vomiting, constipation, progressive mental impairment, and if not corrected, may progress to coma and renal failure. A serum protein-bound calcium count below 11 mg/dL may initially appear normal when the free calcium is elevated or when serum albumin is low and not taken into consideration. Hypercalcemia is be treated with diphosphonates, hydration, and diuresis.

Hyponatremia

Hyponatremia may result from the syndrome of inappropriate antidiuretic hormone (SIADH) secondary to a paraneoplastic syndrome, (especially from small-cell carcinoma, non-small-cell lung cancer, mesothelioma, pancreatic cancer, duodenal cancer, lymphoma, endometrial cancer, leukemia, and other conditions). SIADH is also associated with lung infections, cerebral tumors, brain injuries, and use of many psychotropic medications (e.g., phenothiazines, SSRIs, carbamazepine, and tricyclic antidepressants [TCAs]). Lethargy and confusion are attributable to cerebral edema caused by the movement of water across the osmotic gradient created by a reduction in the serum sodium;[87] chronic hyponatremia is associated with falls and inattention in the elderly.[88]

Brain Tumors

The incidence of primary brain tumors is 6.6 per 1,000,000, but the rate of metastatic brain tumors is higher (ranging from 8 to 11 per 100,000). Virtually any tumor can metastasize to the brain, the most common being non-small- and small-cell lung cancers, breast cancer, and melanoma.[89] Brain metastases are less common but also occur with sarcoma and thyroid, pancreatic, ovarian, uterine, prostate, testicular, and bladder cancers. In patients with small-cell lung cancer, brain metastases are anticipated, and prophylactic cranial irradiation (PCI) is recommended in patients who achieve clinical response to systemic chemotherapy.[90] Isolated brain metastases caused by non-small-cell lung cancer may be treated surgically, and modern radiation techniques target small areas of the brain.

Deterioration in consciousness can occur in 33% to 85% of patients with space-occupying lesions, and agitation and delirium occur in 15% to 19%.[91,92] Tumors (particularly of the frontal, temporal, and limbic lobes) that affect the hardwiring of motivation, attention, mood stability, and memory come to psychiatric attention. Temporal lobe epilepsy can be associated with neuropsychological symptoms (e.g., memory dysfunction, anxiety, hypergraphia, viscosity). For these patients, neuropsychiatric consultation and formal testing may be of critical importance to define and treat the specific loss. Surgical resection or irradiation of the tumor can reduce the neuropsychiatric symptoms, however symptoms may persist and pharmacologic and psychotherapeutic measures can be instituted to improve functioning and quality of life. Antipsychotics may be used for treating agitation, hallucinations, delusions, or disturbances in thought associated with delirium or psychotic syndromes; while mood stabilizers are helpful in the management of impulsivity, irritability, and manic symptoms.[93] Stimulants, such as methylphenidate and modafinil, have been used in the treatment of cognitive dysfunction in this population, and while results have been mixed, recent studies have shown benefits in processing and executive function.[94] Programs that focus on attention re-training and compensatory skills training of attention, memory, and executive functioning, have shown a salutary effect on short-term cognitive complaints and on longer-term cognitive performance and mental fatigue.[95]

Leptomeningeal Disease

Leptomeningeal disease or carcinomatous meningitis, (seen most often in breast cancer, lung cancer, melanoma, and non-Hodgkin's lymphomas), can lead to diffuse encephalopathy due to changes in brain metabolism or reductions in regional cerebral blood flow. If there are no focal signs or findings on neuroimaging, the associated malaise may be considered (erroneously) as psychiatric. In addition to mental status changes, headache, difficulty with walking, limb weakness, and seizures are common. Dizziness and sensorineural deafness have also been noted. Malignant cells in the cerebrospinal fluid (CSF) confirm the diagnosis, but a sufficiently large fluid sample improves the chance for a positive diagnosis; 50% to 70% may be falsely negative. A magnetic resonance imaging (MRI) scan of the brain may be unremarkable in 20% but more likely will show hydrocephalus, brain metastases, or contrast enhancement of the sulci or cisterns.[96,97]

Delirium in Hematopoietic Stem Cell Transplantation (HSCT)

The incidence of delirium among patients undergoing HSCT is high, 35% to 50%, with most cases developing within the first 2 weeks post-transplantation.[98–100] Elevated alkaline phosphatase and blood urea nitrogen (BUN) levels, poor executive functioning, and high doses of opioid medications are risk factors for delirium during HSCT.[99] An engraftment syndrome may cause delirium with non-infectious fever, skin rash, pulmonary edema, and diarrhea, as well as hepatic and renal dysfunction. Usually this syndrome occurs when the neutrophil count is >500/mm^3 and pro-inflammatory cytokines (e.g., IL-1, TNF-α, and IFN-γ) and innate immune cells induce heightened antigen presentation and T-cell activation.[101] Finally, posterior reversible encephalopathy syndrome (PRES) is a rare but serious complication after allogeneic HSCT. Encephalopathy with headache, vomiting, focal neurologic deficits, altered mental status, visual impairment, and seizures characterize it. Immunosuppressive drugs (e.g., cyclosporine, tacrolimus), used in the prophylaxis of graft-versus-host disease, may promote the development of PRES.[102,103] Discontinuation of offending drugs and control of blood pressure reverse neurologic symptoms in most cases.[104] Replacement with the mammalian target of rapamycin (mTOR) inhibitor everolimus can effectively prevent severe GvHD without recurrence of PRES.[105]

Hyperviscosity Syndrome

Hyperviscosity syndromes, seen in multiple myeloma and lymphomas, present with the triad of focal neurologic changes, vision abnormalities, and bleeding. Diagnosis is made on a combination of clinical symptoms and evidence of venous dilatation, hemorrhages, exudates, or papilledema on fundoscopy, in conjunction with increased viscosity levels of ≥4.0 centipoise (normal viscosity is 1.4–1.8 cp).[106] Plasmapheresis promptly relieves the symptoms and should be performed regardless of the viscosity level if the patient is symptomatic.[107]

Idiopathic Hyperammonemia (IHA)

IHA has been defined as a plasma ammonia level greater than twice the upper limit of normal (with other liver function tests being relatively normal, and in the absence of inborn errors of metabolism or other identifiable causes); it may be associated with lethargy, confusion, ataxia, seizures, coma, and death in patients with cancer.[108] Although extremely rare, it occurs more often in those with hematologic malignancies who are neutropenic following bone marrow transplantation and it has also been reported in patients receiving chemotherapy with 5-fluorouracil (5-FU)[109] and in patients with multiple myeloma.[110] Management centers on limiting protein intake and on increasing ammonia excretion, both through use of ammonia-trapping agents and, if necessary, hemodialysis.[108]

Cushing's Syndrome

About 10% to 15% of cases of Cushing's syndrome result from ectopic corticotropin and/or corticotropin-releasing hormone (CRH) overproduction caused by lung or, more rarely, gastroenteropancreatic or other neuroendocrine tumors.[111] Psychiatric disorders, including mood, psychotic, and cognitive disorders are a feature of the syndrome of ectopic ACTH production in 53% of patients.[112] Surgery represents first-line treatment, however, different from pituitary corticotropin-dependent Cushing, cases with ectopic tumors are generally responsive to somatostatin analog therapy.[113]

Paraneoplastic Limbic Encephalitis (PLE)

PLE is a specific autoimmune encephalopathy that causes memory difficulties, anxiety, depression, agitation, confusion, hallucinations, and complex partial seizures. This syndrome has been most commonly associated with small-cell carcinoma of the lung, but it also occurs with Hodgkin's lymphoma, thymoma, and cancers of the testes, breasts, ovaries, stomach, uterus, kidney, thyroid, and colon.[114] Typical presentations consist of progressive confusion and deficits in short-term memory. Less commonly, patients experience visual and auditory hallucinations, delusions, or frank paranoia. Detection of antibodies directed against onconeural antigens in the serum or the CSF may assist in diagnosis. MRI findings, if present, include abnormal hyperintensity on the T_2-weighted image, sometimes completed with use of contrast. Removal is key to the treatment of the syndrome; first-line immunotherapy (steroids, IV immunoglobulin, plasmapheresis) minimizes autoimmune response and neural inflammation and can result in improvement in up to half of the cases.[115] Second-line immunotherapy (rituximab, cyclophosphamide) is usually effective when first-line treatments fail.[115] Anticonvulsants and neuroleptics have been used in the symptomatic treatment of psychiatric manifestations.

Toxic Leukoencephalopathy

White matter injury can be an early, a transient, or a late consequence of cancer treatment. Radiation and certain anti-cancer drugs cause myelin and axonal loss, spongiosis, white-matter gliosis, areas of necrosis, and fibrotic thickening of small blood vessels in the deep white matter.[116] Risk of leukoencephalopathy is related to patient age, total dose of radiation, fraction size, and timing of chemotherapy. Patients with vulnerable brains or delayed metabolism of the drug are at higher risk.

Patients with mild leukoencephalopathy may complain of difficulty with attention, concentration, and vigilance. Apathy, anxiety, irritability, depression, or changes in personality may be seen with memory loss, slowed thinking, and failure of executive oversight. In more severe cases, dementia, abulia, stupor, and coma are seen. Language, praxis, perceptions, and procedural memory are usually spared. Bedside tests on mental status examination can identify treatment-induced cognitive dysfunction, resembling features of subcortical dementias. Magnetic resonance imaging (MRI) scans usually disclose bilateral and symmetric white matter areas of hyperintense signal on T2-weighted and fluid-attenuated inversion recovery images.[117] A common example of this toxicity is seen in patients who have received high-dose methotrexate and radiation treatment for childhood acute lymphoblastic leukemia (ALL) or primary CNS lymphoma.

Chemotherapy-Related Cognitive Impairment (CRCI)

CRCI is commonly reported following treatment of patients with cancer. Cognitive impairments were found in delayed memory, verbal memory, delayed recognition memory, visual-spatial skill, selective attention, and attention capacity.[118] CRCI has a significant negative impact on self-esteem, self-confidence, work performance, and social relationships.[119] Symptoms are transient and reversible, but take at least several years to disappear.[120] Precise underlying mechanisms are poorly understood and are likely multi-factorial. Interventions to help alleviate CRCI include non-pharmacologic treatment, such as CBT and occupational therapy.[121] If these interventions are insufficient, consideration of psychostimulants, such as methylphenidate or modafinil, is reasonable, although data confirming the efficacy of these agents have yielded mixed results.[122]

Effects of Hormonal Therapy in Cancer Patients

Treatment of hormone-sensitive tumors involves use of medications aimed at reducing the availability of sex hormones. Patients who receive adjuvant treatment for breast cancer often develop menopausal symptoms because of a direct effect on the ovary that decreases hormone levels and hastens menopause. Menopause is a goal of treatment for those with estrogen receptor-positive tumors.

Two classes of drugs are used; tamoxifen, (a mixed agonist–antagonist of estrogen), and aromatase inhibitors, which reduce estradiol to barely detectable concentrations. There seem to be no differences in quality of life measures in women taking either class.[123] Vasomotor symptoms are the most frequent side effects and about 20% experience mood swings and irritability.[124] Men receiving androgen ablation for prostate cancer experience hot flashes that are more frequent, severe, and longer lasting.[125]

Gonadotropin-releasing hormone (GnRH) agonists (i.e., leuprolide and goserelin), have been associated with depression in non-cancer populations, however, in patients with prostate cancer, well-controlled prospective studies have yielded mixed results, and at least one has suggested that fatigue is more prevalent and may be mistaken for depression.[126–128]

Serotonin and norepinephrine re-uptake inhibitors (SNRIs) and SSRIs reduce the frequency and severity of hot flashes and improve mood, sleep, anxiety, and quality of life in patients undergoing hormonal deprivation therapy for hormone-sensitive tumors.[125,129] Gabapentin and pregabalin have also been beneficial in decreasing hot flashes in this patient population.[130]

Survivors of Childhood Cancer

Nowadays, childhood cancer is more commonly considered a serious chronic illness rather than a uniformly terminal illness. Child psychiatrists work side by side in the outpatient setting with the pediatric hematology–oncology teams to treat the emotional needs of the child in age-appropriate ways during active treatment and thereafter. With consideration of the child's stage of development, psychiatrists can judge what the child will understand and what he or she will want and need to know.

The most common consultation questions include evaluation of the child with anticipatory anxiety, sleep disturbances, behavioral problems, or mood changes. The child may feel anxious, nauseated, or vomit on approaching the hospital, clinic, or phlebotomist, despite advances in antiemetic medication. Behavioral interventions and medications are helpful. Sleep disturbances may be related to the child's worries about the illness or to medications, such as steroids. Child psychiatrists are also consulted for behavior problems in younger children who become more aggressive or difficult to manage. The emphasis in treatment of depression or withdrawn states is on the child's ability to enjoy life. Overall, children tend to be quite resilient; the large majority has reported levels of psychological health comparable with those in the general population; however, studies have found a subgroup experiencing persistent distress, including depression, anxiety, and somatization.[131]

Children are particularly prone to radiotoxicity in the first 2 years of life because of the rapid growth of the brain and white matter development in those years. MRI studies of long-term survivors of acute lymphoblastic leukemia (ALL) have demonstrated smaller volumes of multiple brain structures compared with healthy controls.[132,133]

Cognitive defects have been extensively documented, while intelligence, working memory, and processing speed are the domains more commonly affected.[134] The combination of radiation treatment and intrathecal methotrexate increases the risk of cognitive impairment. Children exposed to cranial irradiation may also suffer from hypothyroidism and growth hormone deficiency. Children who have been treated for leukemia or brain tumors should be monitored for cognitive and endocrine dysfunction.

CONCLUSION

Psychiatrists can help patients cope with affective, behavioral, cognitive, and physical symptoms associated with cancer and its treatment, as well as with developmental losses, changes in relationships, and the effects of cancer on families.

REFERENCES

Access the reference list online at https://expertconsult.inkling.com/.

Burn Patients

Sean P. Glass, M.D.
Shamim H. Nejad, M.D.
Gregory L. Fricchione, M.D.
Frederick J. Stoddard, Jr., M.D.

32

OVERVIEW

Burn injuries are as ancient as fire itself. All afflicted individuals need help and many require psychiatric consultation; their psychiatric care may be as challenging as their surgical care.[1] Depending on their experience, physicians, nurses, and trainees new to a burn unit may experience trepidation and fear, but these feelings moderate as they relieve pain, help patients survive, and see the repair of disfiguring scars. Nevertheless, the burn unit is stressful for all—viewing an acutely burned infant, child, or adult can satisfy the stressor criteria for post-traumatic stress disorder (PTSD) and evoke nightmares in staff and patients.

Burn units and clinics bring together specialists from several disciplines, and have long been practicing collaborative care. The Massachusetts General Hospital (MGH) Level 1 Trauma Center treats burned adults at the MGH and treats children at the affiliated Shriners Burns Hospital. Since 9/11, all burn centers in the United States have enhanced their disaster preparedness;[2] psychiatric education regarding disasters is important for staff on burn units in order to enhance resilience and increase preparedness.[3]

HISTORY

The current era of burn treatment and research began about 75 years ago at the MGH after the Cocoanut Grove fire on November 28, 1942. Cobb and Lindemann,[4] eminent early MGH psychiatrists, collaborated with other physicians and chronicled the deliria and post-traumatic reactions of the survivors of that tragedy in which 491 people died. Lindemann,[5] in a classic paper (based in part on his work with 13 bereaved disaster victims of the Cocoanut Grove fire and their close relatives, and with relatives of members of the armed forces), reported for the first time the symptoms and psychotherapeutic management of acute grief. Their studies involved psychiatric treatment of grief that would be applied to soldiers, civilians, and the bereaved.

Burn injuries challenge hospital staff and hospital systems. In 2003, as in the Cocoanut Grove fire, The Station nightclub fire in Rhode Island wreaked havoc. It resulted in 100 deaths and tested emergency and burn trauma disaster plans at the MGH, the Shriners Burns Hospital, and the entire region; fortunately, the triage system worked superbly. Unlike the September 11, 2001 terrorist attacks when staff readied for transfers to their burn units but were surprised by how few survived to be treated, scores survived this nightclub fire (despite severe burns to the lungs, face, hands, and upper body) because of the emergency response and advances in modern burn care. As described earlier by Cobb and Lindemann,[4] some of these survivors, their children, and other relatives developed and were treated for survivor guilt, traumatic grief, and what is now recognized as PTSD.[6]

In the last 40 years, strong leadership and new research have led to improved methods of resuscitation and transportation; excision and grafting;[7] anesthesia;[8] pain control and opiate management;[9,10] anxiety management;[11] pulmonary care;[12] cardiovascular and infection control; application of artificial skin and skin substitutes;[13] psychiatric assessment and treatment (Table 32-1); plastic surgery techniques;[14] and rehabilitative efforts that include interventions for those with disfiguring facial and body burns. Taken together, these innovations have dramatically improved both mortality rates and the morbidity associated with burn injuries in the United States.

Just as Cobb, Lindemann, and Adler did for adults, Bernstein[15] and others pioneered the psychiatric care of burned children and their families; moreover, they conceptualized consultations to the burn team. Childhood injuries, including burns, are now, after years of neglect, a priority for medical research and treatment.[16,17] Both adult and child injury rates have dramatically dropped.[16] A key resource regarding education and research for burn care is the American Burn Association,[18] which is linked to federal agencies, a variety of foundations, and the International Society for Burn Injuries. Many patients also benefit from self-help groups, like the Phoenix Society, which is the international self-help organization for children and adults with burns, and their families.[19] Its mission is to increase the understanding of burned individuals and to support their care.

EPIDEMIOLOGY

According to the American Burn Association Fact Sheet, approximately 486,000 people are seen and treated annually for burn-related injuries in the United States.[20] About 40,000 patients are admitted for treatment of burn-related injuries and approximately 30,000 of these are treated at designated burn centers. There are 128 designated burn treatment centers in the United States and the average number of admissions to these centers is approximately 200 annually. According to the National Burn Repository 2015 report, the overall survival rate for burn injuries is 96.8%.[19] Roughly

TABLE 32-1 10-Point Plan for Consulting With Burned Patients

1. Speak with the patient at the bedside and ensure the patient's safety.
2. Consult directly with the burn or trauma team, the surgeons and other physicians, nurses, social workers, and others about the patient, clarifying your time availability and role. Within psychiatry, arrange for supervision, peer consultation, and departmental support.
3. Obtain the history of the burn circumstances, psychopathology, or substance abuse, and social and family function.
4. Diagnose the patient: assess the developmental stage, burn severity, other stressors, mental status (including pain, stress, memory), psychiatric risk (delirium, suicide, child abuse), prognosis, medical and surgical issues including medications and their interactions, alcohol or drug withdrawal, current risk factors, language/cultural factors, legal status, and staff or family concerns. Recommend special studies or consultations as indicated.
5. Monitor, explain, and treat pain, delirium, stress, insomnia, and depression. Provide staff support and, for complex cases, plan a team conference.
6. Assess, treat, and support the dying child or adult and the family, and assist with the clarification and the resolution of ethical dilemmas.
7. When the patient has survived the acute phase, progress to treating residual mental disorders, substance abuse, and other problems.
8. Facilitate grieving and adaptation of the patient and family to cosmetic or functional losses.
9. Collaborate in planning plastic and reconstructive surgical follow-up if possible and communicate psychiatric findings and recommendations to the primary care physician. Support re-entry to school or work, including special education and rehabilitation services.
10. Remain available for follow-up consultation to the patient and caregivers, clarify the psychiatric issues, and assist the patient and family in obtaining psychiatric services.

two-thirds (68%) of burn victims are male.[21] The mean age of burn victims was 32 years; children under the age of 5 years accounted for 19% of the cases, while patients age 60 years or older accounted for 13% of the cases. Most burns occur in the home (73%). The remainder of burn injuries occur at work (8%), in the street or on the highway (5%), while recreational activities account for 5%, and the remaining 9% are designated as "other." Among inpatient admissions, the most common burn type is scald injury (34%), while other injuries are due to contact (9%), electrical (4%), chemical (3%), fire/flame (3%), and other.[21]

Between 2005 and 2014, the mortality rates for males increased from 3.1% to 3.2% while for females, rates decreased from 4.4% to 3.6%.[21] Advancing age and the presence of inhalation injury pose significant mortality risks. For patients under the age of 60 with a total body surface area (TBSA) burn between 0.1% and 19.9%, the presence of inhalation injury increases the likelihood of death by nearly 24-fold. The most common complications of burn treatment are pneumonia, respiratory failure, cellulitis, septicemia, and wound infection; these clinical complications are in large part a function of the number of days spent on the ventilator (with the risk increasing dramatically after ≥4 days). The average length of hospital stay for survivors is best approximated by figuring on one day per percentage TBSA burns.[20,21]

TYPES OF BURNS

Burns are classified by the depth of the injury (from first–fourth-degree burns).[22] First-degree burns are characterized by an intact epithelium (that is pink, dry, and painful); these burns require no specific care. Second-degree burns are wet, pink to red, and edematous; these changes signify that the dermis is damaged. These burns are further categorized into superficial and deep and they must be monitored closely. Laser Doppler imaging is a widely accepted method for early and accurate assessment of burn depth. Third-degree, or full-thickness (of dermis) burns are leathery, dry, and lack sensation; these burns require surgical treatment. The most severe burns are fourth-degree burns; these extend through the subcutaneous tissue to the tendons, muscles, and bones, and they require complex surgical reconstruction.

The operative treatment of burns includes wound debridement, escharotomy and fasciotomy (release of burned skin and muscle, respectively) and grafting. The non-operative treatment involves daily wound care (performed multiple times each day), and systemic care and management of associated medical and surgical problems.[22]

RISK FACTORS

Risk factors for burn injuries are different for children, adults, and the elderly, although poverty is a risk factor in all populations. A combination of developmental and familial factors contributes to the risk of burns in children. Increased exploration by young children, access to scalding or flammable liquids or flames, childhood depression, behavioral disturbances, and parental psychopathology each predispose children to burns. Burns to children should not be indiscriminately labeled as due to neglect or to abuse because, on careful assessment, they may be the result of a combination of developmental, environmental, and family variables. However, child neglect or abuse accounts for between 6% and 20% of pediatric burns; the age of maximum risk of abuse is 13 to 24 months, and scalds are the most common type of inflicted burn.[23] Factors suggestive of abuse include a burn distribution inconsistent with the history; a carer changing the story of what occurred (from one interview to the next); prior injuries or accidents; a parent who neither visits nor is attentive; a consistently awake but withdrawn child who appears immune to pain; and other signs of abuse, such as fractures.[24] Suspected abuse must be reported to the appropriate state agency in most states.

Among adults, risk factors for burns include drug and alcohol intoxication and dependence,[25] major mental illness, antisocial personality disorder, and exposure to occupational hazards (Tables 32-2 and 32-3).[25–32] Certain populations, such as the homeless and the elderly, have an increased risk of burns.[33] Homeless people are more likely to be assaulted

TABLE 32-2 Risk Factors for Burns in Adults

Alcohol use disorder
Substance use disorder
Depression
Suicide attempts
Antisocial personality disorder
Schizophrenia
Bipolar disorder
Chronic medical illness
Dementia
Abuse/homicide
Occupational hazards

TABLE 32-3 Risk Factors for Burns in Children and Adolescents

Poverty
Neglect
Abuse
Unsafe housing
Family discord
Risk-taking behaviors
Learning disabilities
Depression
Fire-setting

by burning and to have higher rates of substance abuse and psychiatric illness as compared with domiciled burn patients.[33] Demented elders are also at risk for burns; scalds are much more common than flame burns and typically occur during routine activities of daily living.[25]

PRE-BURN PSYCHOPATHOLOGY

Psychiatric illness is over-represented in individuals with burn injuries. Depressive symptoms are common after a burn.[34] Frequency rates within the first year vary, depending on measures and definitions of severity versus meeting diagnostic criteria. Weichman et al.[34] reported that prevalence ranges from about 4% at discharge to between 10% and 23% 1 year after injury, with increasing prevalence through the first year after discharge. These rates are much higher than in the general population. Few studies have examined depression for longer than 1 year, but one found that prevalence increased between the first and second year, and that up to 42% of survivors have moderate to severe depression 2 years after injury.[35] Female gender and facial burns were associated with more depression. Dyster-Aas and associates,[36] in a prospective case series of 73 patients with burns, used structured clinical interviews and found that two-thirds of patients had at least one life-time psychiatric diagnosis (i.e., major depression [41%]; alcohol abuse or dependence [32%]; simple phobia [16%]; and panic disorder [16%] were most common). Wisely and co-workers[37] looked at 72 patients admitted to a burn unit over a 5-month period and found that 35% had a psychiatric diagnosis before the burn; depression, drug and alcohol abuse, personality disorders, and psychotic disorders were the most often detected.

Individuals with self-inflicted burns often have a high prevalence of severe mental illness (e.g., schizophrenia or major depression).[38–40] One review of 582 patients with self-inflicted burns found that 78% had a psychiatric history,[39] an increased likelihood of psychotic symptoms, of being prescribed psychotropic medication at the time of the burn, and of being a psychiatric inpatient.[40] Our experience also shows that patients with bipolar disorder (while manic), schizophrenia, conduct-disorder, and alcoholism are at risk for self-immolation. Sometimes it is difficult to discern whether a burn was accidental, a parasuicidal gesture, or a *bona fide* suicide attempt. Attempts at suicide via self-immolation occur worldwide and often result in massive, disfiguring burns.[41]

A study of adolescent self-immolators revealed serious untreated or partially treated psychopathology (including drug abuse, psychosis, intense conflict with parents, and physical or sexual abuse). Studies of adults have similarly found elevated rates of alcohol use disorder, depression, psychosis, and personality disorder as pre-existing factors.[42–44] These patients tend to arouse intense feelings in caregivers and are among the most difficult surgical and psychiatric patients. Despite their burns and severe psychopathology, most patients cope well with psychiatric treatment that is initiated on the burn unit. Their prognoses are very guarded, since self-immolation, as with a severe overdose, is an indicator of affective or other disorder and ongoing suicide risk, although those who later commit suicide do not necessarily do so by burning.

Finally, suicide attempts may turn out to be homicide attempts as part of the "honor killing" or maiming, such as acid burns to the face of victims accused of incest or of seducing a rapist.[44] The psychiatrist, consulting to units where patients may be admitted from around the world, must be aware of patients' cultural and ethnic background, in order to understand the circumstances surrounding the burn injury. Unfortunately, because of barriers in reporting, including undiagnosed and unreported abuse, an exact estimate of prevalence of these injuries is not known.

ASSESSMENT AND MANAGEMENT OF PATIENTS WITH BURNS

Psychiatrists who work in the general hospital are frequently called to assess burned patients, as for any other surgical patients.[45] The role of the psychiatrist changes in parallel with the patient's recovery; in general, it begins with a brief assessment in the acute phase that focuses on management of delirium and pain, then it morphs to the evaluation and treatment of symptoms of PTSD in the months after the burn, and then it targets psychosocial adjustment to disfiguring burns in the years after the burn. These phases can be divided into acute, intermediate, and long-term recovery.

Diagnosis and Developmental Assessment

Setting the stage for a discussion of the acute, intermediate, and long-term management of burn patients, we will review a diagnostic approach that incorporates a developmental model; this aids in the formulation and treatment of all medical and psychological problems experienced by the burned patient. This is particularly important for assessing children; consideration of the developmental stage provides the necessary context for understanding children's responses to trauma.[46] A developmental model for the assessment of burned children follows;[47] it has been supplemented by a developmental model that is useful throughout the life cycle.[48] For infants through adolescents additional discussion relating to developmental stage is provided before the case example.

Developmental Stage and Burns: Case Examples

Infancy (Birth to 2.5 Years Old)

Infancy is the period from birth to emergence of language (typically until 2 to 2.5 years old). Infants experience the world in the moment and require immediate gratification of needs, whether related to pain, hunger, or absence of nurturance. For infants, there is little separation between them and their primary nurturer; burn injuries, with the necessary procedures and monitoring involved, inevitably disrupt this primary attachment. As much as possible, pediatric burn care minimizes the disruption by providing surrogates to mitigate the depressive reactions to absent parents and by providing as soothing and nurturing an environment as possible. Because of infants' cognitive immaturity and inability to make sense of what is happening to them, they take their cues largely from parents and caregivers, who (witnessing their infant in pain, and having fears of death and disfigurement) typically experience significant guilt and distress over the burn circumstances. Care of the burned infant is inevitably intertwined with care of the parents; the more stable the parents, the better the infant's recovery. Methods to provide parental interventions to reduce their stress improve post-traumatic outcomes.[49,50]

CASE 1

A 4-month-old girl was admitted with 20% TBSA scald injuries to the face, neck, and chest. Her parents felt intense self-reproach and feared future scars; intermittently they had difficulty soothing her because of their own distress. Psychiatric consultation was requested to deal with her refusal to eat, her crying in anticipation of painful dressing changes, and her anxiety that was aroused by her mother's departure for home to be with her older children. With support of nursing staff, social work, and child psychiatric staff, the mother roomed with the infant, pain was reduced by use of opiates, and the infant healed with skin grafting (over a 2-week period) and appeared to resume her normal developmental course. This case illustrated typical signs of distress in a burned infant, manifestations of parental stress, and an approach involving the parents and the child to intervention.

Pre-School Age (2.5 to 6 Years Old)

Egocentricism (belief that the world revolves around them and that others see the world from their perspective alone), magical thinking (inter-weaving of reality and fantasy such that medical events have magical causes), and preoccupations with body integrity, are the hallmarks of pre-school children. Children in this age group may develop notions of guilt and punishment during the hospitalization, and see injuries and painful treatments as punishment for bad deeds or thoughts. Some may regress, withdraw, and stop speaking. The child psychiatrist provides understanding and reassurance to relieve guilt-ridden parents. Similar to infants, pre-school children are generally interviewed with the parent present. As the children get older, therapeutic play with drawings, puppets, and games are central to recovery, and are often used as both diagnostic and therapeutic tools. Through play they can safely regain their cognitive skills, express their feelings and traumatic memories in ways that may not be permitted anywhere except in play therapy, and gradually work through their traumatic experiences with a psychotherapist towards resuming normal development.[51]

CASE 2

A 3-year-old boy with smoke inhalation and 30% TBSA burns, mostly partial thickness, became increasingly withdrawn, except when in his brother's company; when with his brother, he would play with toys and be more outgoing. He was interpersonally inhibited and afraid of wound dressing changes. His pain was only partially relieved by oral morphine and lorazepam; he clung to nursing staff, and he appeared to regress. His speech was indistinct; what he did say was repeated over and over. Consistently somber, he stared silently at staff and did not speak or interact in a meaningful way. Psychiatric assessment determined that he suffered from a combination of an acute stress disorder and a mild anoxic brain injury. These conditions,[52,53] and possibly depression, were the consequences of his burn.

School-Age (7 to 12 Years Old)

Ability to understand their bodies, curiosity, a rule-informed cognitive style, and continuous efforts to gain control are the hallmarks of school-age children. With respect to burn injuries, they will want to understand the injury and its treatment and seek to gain control over it. They benefit from having a schedule of the treatments and other activities.

CASE 3

A 10-year-old boy sustained 40% TBSA electrical burns when his kite got entangled on high-voltage electrical wires. His treatment involved frequent wound dressing changes, which he tolerated well initially. However, he refused to start physical therapy and this reluctance spread to his participation in wound care; he would yell and cry upon seeing medical supplies. On interview, he told the psychiatrist that he never signed up for physical therapy and that the exercises were very painful; he felt the assignments were unfair. With the surgeon and nurse, and child psychiatrist collaboratively taking time to explain the need for, and the prospected course of, these treatments (providing the duration of each session and their frequency) and eliciting his questions, he became visibly relaxed and ready to work out a schedule that allowed him to watch his favorite cartoons before and after his wound dressing changes and physical therapy sessions.

Adolescence

Although adolescents have the capacity to understand the injury, its treatment, and ramifications on their lives, they remain quite vulnerable. This stage of development is marked by striving for independence, while managing ongoing dependency on their parents. Additionally, fitting in with peers and maintaining one's body image, which is undergoing change, are of paramount importance to teenagers; therefore the potential disfigurement related to burn injuries can be particularly devastating to them, and to their parents and family.

CASE 4

A 15-year-old boy sustained 85% TBSA flame and inhalation injuries in a grease fire from a cookstove; a friend perished in the fire. Trouble sleeping, bad dreams, and flashbacks of the fire plagued him. Nightmares persisted for 6 weeks. He tried to think about "positive things during the day" so that his dreams would be positive. One month later, he described a different type of dream. He described romantic fantasies about a female staff member who was caring for him. He was relieved to hear from the psychiatrist that such dreams were not unusual when a close relationship develops between a patient and a caregiver. He became able to acknowledge age-appropriate emotions. Near discharge, his nightmares of the fire recurred, as did positive dreams related to returning home and resuming his life. This case illustrates how dreams of burned patients can evolve and how they can be useful in psychotherapy to adapt to severe injury.[51]

Young Adulthood

CASE 5

A 23-year-old father of two was admitted with 40% TBSA burns to his face, neck, upper torso, and arms following a house fire. He received morphine for pain and diazepam for anxiety. He became acutely delirious (with agitation, disorientation, and combativeness), which required physical restraints and 10 to 20 mg of IV haloperidol per day for the first few days of the admission. The delirium seemed secondary to smoke inhalation and cerebral anoxia. He healed well over a 2-week period, and all medications (except for morphine that was used for dressing changes) were tapered. He was observed to be inappropriate, "strange," and to be "more like a kid." Psychiatric reassessment also revealed terror and post-traumatic intrusive thoughts and nightmares of the fire. He faced several stressors (e.g., severe burns suffered by his wife, two young sons, and younger brother) and his grief was intense. He recalled, but was unable to cope with, images of the fire and the injuries to himself and his loved ones; they were all nearby, in various stages of recovery. He responded well to emotional support, to clarification, and to reassurance, as well as to tranquilizers that restored adequate sleep and reduced the intensity of his terror. This case illustrates the combined effects of anoxic brain injury, delirium, acute stress, and acute grief in a young adult.

Elderly

CASE 6

A 77-year-old woman caught her housecoat on a gas stove and sustained 15% TBSA first-degree and second-degree burns to her left side. Care providers called her "lovely" but cognitively impaired. She had a history of valvular disease with congestive heart failure (CHF), metastatic breast carcinoma (requiring bilateral mastectomies), and deep venous thrombosis (DVT). Confusion decreased when doses of diazepam and morphine were reduced. This case involved an ill, elderly woman who responded slowly, but well, to acute compassionate care.

Acute Phase: Assessment and Treatment

From the day of admission, assessment and treatment proceed hand in hand. Initial assessment is often difficult and history must often be obtained from others,[46] because the patient may be unable to communicate.[54] When reviewing the record, the consulting psychiatrist pays particular attention to all aspects of the initial presentation (e.g., police and emergency medical service records [that describe the circumstances in which the patient was found], toxicology screens [that yield important information about drugs and alcohol and risk for withdrawal], and chemistries and tests of kidney and liver function [that reveal current contributions to delirium]). Special studies, including brain imaging (when there is concern for head injury, stroke, severe hypoxic insult, or worsening mental status not explained by available data) and electroencephalography (EEG) (when there is concern for seizure or to verify presence of delirium) are often indicated.

Explanations about the burn and its treatment are followed by an assessment of the efficacy of these interventions. Communication should involve a vocabulary that the patient can understand and should be appropriate to the patient's developmental and cognitive levels and emotional ability. Because a burned patient may be confused, afraid of death or dismemberment, anxious about pain, or sedated, the initial history may need to be obtained from other individuals. Explanation, reassurance, and relief of pain help to reduce fear and confusion. A formal mental status evaluation is necessary to diagnose subtle changes in mental function. The patient's initial emotional reactions (e.g., denial, fear, guilt, grief, anger, or emotional withdrawal) should be noted. A history of developmental, mental, or substance abuse disorders; medical illness; and psychiatric treatment should be obtained; the social context should also be established. When family members understand, feel supported, and are reassured, they are better able to calm their loved one; however, when this support is absent the opposite is often true. As an alliance with the patient and family develops, additional history typically clarifies the circumstances of the injury.

During the acute phase after burn injury, adult patients may experience a variety of psychological responses to their injury, including survival fear and search for meaning.[54]

Survival Fear During the Acute Phase After Injury

Here, the patient is mainly focused on survival. As expected with survival-related fear responses, the patient is often hypervigilant, tremulous, and focused on physical recovery. Psychological processing of the injury is difficult in the context of hypervigilance and the patient is less able to process verbal content. Therefore, the patient will probably benefit from frequent re-orientation and repetition of basic information, including a realistic appraisal of their chance of survival, the severity of their injury, the physical phenomena being experienced, and the most likely course of recovery.[54]

Search for Meaning During the Acute Phase After Injury

Patients provide a detailed recounting of the events of their injury, while searching for explanations about what happened and why it happened to them. Patients may deal with helplessness; grieve the loss of limbs, certain functions, and their pre-injury appearance; and work on accepting their new disability, capabilities, and physical appearance.[54–56]

In the acute assessment of children and the elderly, the psychiatrist routinely assesses for abuse and neglect. Clinginess to nursing staff, exacerbation of a fear response in the presence of parents or caregivers, and co-existing injuries not explained by the burn (e.g., fractures, bruises, soft tissue contusion, cigarette burns), should raise concerns of child or elder abuse or neglect. Protective measures should be taken and mandatory reporting to social services completed.

Burn-Induced Delirium

Burn-induced delirium usually occurs soon after the injury and it may portend an increased risk of death. Confused, agitated, or aggressive patients can hit staff, attempt to leave the hospital, fall, self-extubate, and dislodge intravascular lines and skin grafts. Delirium occurs in 10% to 30% of all burn patients and in up to 80% of burn patients in the critical care setting. Specifically, one prospective study of burn intensive care unit (ICU) patients demonstrated delirium in 77% of ventilated burn patients. The majority of patients were identified as having hypoactive delirium.[57] Traditional risk factors for delirium include traumatic brain injury, advanced age, pre-morbid dementia, and substance use (including alcohol and tobacco), among others. Each of these factors is also associated with increased risk of sustaining a burn injury. Agarwal et al.[57] reported that delirium in patients who were mechanically ventilated, tended to be younger and have lower rates of cognitive impairment compared with those in the general hospital population. Risk was not associated with advanced age, cognitive impairment, substance dependence, burn type or severity, or presence of an inhalation injury. Instead, delirium was independently associated with medications used to target anxiety and pain control. Specifically, benzodiazepine exposure independently predicted the development of delirium (odds ratio [OR] 6.8, $p<0.001$). In contrast, receiving higher doses of IV fentanyl and higher doses of methadone were both associated with half the risk of delirium.[57] With severe burns, patients are often kept anesthetized and intubated until grafting is completed; thus, acute delirium is often masked. Prompt evaluation, the maintenance of safety (which may necessitate the use of restraints), treatment of the causative factors, and institution of environmental changes and supportive personal contact with staff and family are indicated.

Acute Stress Disorder and Post-Traumatic Stress Disorder

The *Diagnostic and Statistical Manual of Mental Disorders*, 5th edition (DSM-5)[58] criteria for acute stress disorder (ASD) include re-experience of the trauma, avoidance, and anxiety or arousal. The symptoms must last for at least 2 days and occur within 4 weeks of the trauma; the condition is not due to drugs or medications, or to the patient's medical condition. Some studies have found symptoms of acute stress occur in 11% to 32% of burn patients; the rates vary in part by virtue of the measurement methods used.[31,59–61] Risk factors for developing ASD include the scope of the burn, poor pre-morbid mental health, and the tendency to blame others for the burn.[62] Awareness and recall of the injury may be delayed until opiates and benzodiazepines are tapered, at which time the intrusive recollections, nightmares or night terrors, and associated arousal states may begin. The presence of ASD poses a significant risk for subsequent development of PTSD in adult patients from 1 month until 2 years after the burn.[54] Treatment strategies aimed at reducing or preventing the development of future PTSD are generally lacking.[53] Psychological debriefing after traumatic injury is contraindicated, but multi-session CBT is effective. The efficacy of beta-blockers, such as propranolol, is mixed. Benzodiazepines have consistently been shown to be ineffective and pose significant additional risks for delirium in this patient population.[54,59] The most effective pharmacologic strategy includes using stress doses of steroids, such as hydrocortisone, though clear guidelines as to safe and specific use in this population are absent.[59] Opiates may be effective at reducing the rates of subsequent PTSD, though results are mixed overall. Finally, early treatment with selective serotonin re-uptake inhibitor (SSRIs) for ASD has mixed results, whereas they are generally considered first-line in established PTSD.[59]

In children, emotional withdrawal or over-reactivity may occur in association with re-experiencing or with hyperarousal. They may become agitated or combative during wound dressing changes or other painful procedures; having parents leave the room during these treatments may exacerbate the child's reaction. Later in the recovery period, depression may develop, with interpersonal withdrawal and a decreased appetite. In children, anhedonia, sleep and appetite disturbances, emotional withdrawal, and irritability are the most common accompaniments of depressed mood. Brief supportive psychotherapy, alliance building, treatment of pain and anxiety, and provision of appropriate reassurance are of benefit.

PAIN ASSESSMENT

Pain is ubiquitous in burn patients; partial-thickness burns (with intact nerve endings) are more painful than are full-thickness burns (where nerve endings are largely destroyed). Although the burn itself is painful, a significant amount of the pain is associated with daily debridement and wound care. Pain is often under-estimated and under-treated, because staff fear that respiratory depression or death will result from treatment;[63] organizational approaches (implementation of pain management guidelines and educational programs) have reduced this problem. In responding to this, Szyfelbein and associates[64] and others have used self-rating scales and measured serum endorphin levels; they proved that high-dose IV opiates were needed to provide relief from pain for those with severe burns. Improving pain relief[65,66] and sharpening the focus on psychological as well as pharmacologic interventions is important to improve outcomes.[67]

The 0 to 10 visual analog scale is often used to quantify the patient's level of perceived pain when at rest, and before and after dressing changes, debridements, and physical and occupational therapy.[54] In general, for patients unable to communicate (e.g., owing to the use of paralytic agents or to intubation), much information about pain, anxiety, and fear may be gathered by noticing facial expressions (e.g., grimacing or wincing), body language (e.g., withdrawing, pushing away, or startle reactions), and autonomic signs (e.g., changes in heart rate and breathing rates with disturbing or soothing stimuli). When a patient is in a medically induced coma with no objective or subjective means to measure pain, estimates of maximum analgesic requirements for body weight are recommended.

The addition of short-acting IV and oral agents (especially opiates, midazolam, and propofol) to target acute pain and anxiety has dramatically lessened the suffering secondary to acute burns. Initially, the location(s), source, quality, intensity, course, and duration of pain are identified; then, with nursing staff, self-reported ratings of pain (from 0 to 10 with 10 equaling the most severe pain) are monitored in response to treatment. Burn pain correlates with endorphin levels and with the extent and depth of the burn.[68] Because infants cannot provide self-reports, behavioral measures (e.g., facial expressions, body movements, and crying) and physiologic parameters (e.g., heart rate, blood pressure, respiratory rate, oxygen saturation), and if available, levels of epinephrine, norepinephrine, growth hormone, and cortisol are useful in monitoring pain responses.[69] For children who are unable to communicate verbally, self-reported measures (such as the Faces Scale, the Visual Analog Scale, and the Oucher Scale) are useful; among staff-rated scales, the Children's Hospital of Eastern Ontario Pain Scale (CHEOPS) has utility.[70] The most easily used self-rating scales for burn patients are 0 to 10 visual analog scales;[71] these rate pain from 0 to 10, with 0 as no pain and 10 being the most severe pain experienced.

Psychological Treatment of Pain

It is widely accepted that emotional and cognitive states modulate the experience of pain, and vice versa. Psychological techniques to ease burn pain include: education, hypnosis, relaxation, patient participation in dressing changes, and biofeedback; these techniques do not predispose to side effects or toxic effects as do medications. Patients can be trained to use these methods,[67] and they can discover that they are capable of achieving self-control over pain.

Developmentally targeted psychological approaches to pain management are effective for both children and adults. Hypnosis for burn pain is effective and practical,[72–74] but it requires more staff time than when relying solely on the use of analgesics. Hypnosis[75] and simple and complex relaxation techniques (such as focused imagery) are in wide use and are practical for children (who are the most hypnotizable subjects) and for adults. Spiegel and Spiegel[76] described a method that is generally applicable for burn patients. Intriguingly, Ewin[77] has reported that hypnosis can acutely prevent the post-burn inflammatory response, thereby lessening burn severity. Patient-mediated methods involve the patient's active participation and are designed to shift the locus of control in burned children to themselves.[65,78] This involves preparation for painful procedures and increases the patient's ability to choose when, for how long, and who will perform invasive procedures by encouraging their participation at each step. This structured method can lead to fewer maladaptive behaviors, improved outcomes, and use of lower dosages of narcotics. Cognitive-behavioral therapy (CBT) has been shown to be effective at treating various chronic pain syndromes and is a viable treatment option for patients regardless of medical co-morbidity, however, data on the efficacy of CBT in acute pain syndromes in burn patients is scarce.

Pharmacologic Treatment of Acute Burn Patients

If pain symptoms are inadequately controlled, particularly related to procedures, the patient may anticipate that pain will be associated with each subsequent intervention, commonly referred to as an *anticipatory pain response*, which is a fear-based, as opposed to an anxiety-based, response.[54] This difference is crucial, as it dictates treatment. Fear is amygdalar in origin and treated with dopamine antagonists, while symptoms of anxiety are treated with benzodiazepines.

Preventing and reducing the often overwhelming and frightening reactions that patients have during wound care, repositioning in bed, and while working with physical therapy are crucial aspects of caring for burn patients. Co-administration of low-dose IV haloperidol with IV opioids 15 minutes before dressing changes can reduce the anticipatory fear response.[54] Alternatively, co-administration of oral olanzapine or other atypical antipsychotics with opioids (30 to 45 minutes prior to dressing changes) may bring about similar benefits.[54] In children and adolescents, risperidone is rapidly effective and usually well tolerated, and may be required through the acute phase of care.

Once a method is in place for tracking the patient's pain, a pharmacologic regimen is then designed to meet the patient's needs. In the intubated patient, or the patient with large-scale burns that necessitate frequent trips to the operating theater for excision and grafting (E&G), IV fentanyl is often utilized for basal control of pain, with bolus administration for intermittent pain symptoms. For smaller-scale burns or later in the course of a larger-scale burn patient, long-acting opiate analgesics, such as methadone, may be employed for basal pain control, with the short-acting narcotics, such as hydromorphone or morphine, used for intermittent pain and for procedural pain control.[54]

Pain control in the opioid-dependent patient with burn injury is also an important issue. Generally, patients with active or recent chronic opioid use, whether illicit or iatrogenic, will exhibit physiological tolerance to opioid medications, necessitating increased dosages or frequency of administration.[54] These patients will often respond better to use of a patient-controlled analgesia (PCA) pump for the first 24 to 36 hours, and achieve improved pain control versus nurse- or clinician-administered PRN approaches. Their previous 24 hours short-acting narcotic requirement can then be converted to a long-acting analgesic (e.g., methadone) with the goal of decreasing the amount of short-acting narcotic required by the time of discharge.[54]

Benzodiazepines are often used in hospitalized burn patients to induce sedation, reduce agitation, and decrease anxiety.[79,80] Given that alcohol use disorder (AUD) and intoxication are risk factors for burn injuries, alcohol withdrawal is commonly encountered and benzodiazepines (or phenobarbital) are used in the treatment of withdrawal. A host of benzodiazepines are available for use, including short-acting agents (e.g., midazolam [which has rapidly assumed a significant place for brief procedures],[81] lorazepam,[82,83] oxazepam, triazolam) and long-acting agents (e.g., chlordiazepoxide, diazepam, clonazepam, flurazepam). There is no consensus as to the best benzodiazepine to use; however, longer-acting benzodiazepines with active metabolites, such as diazepam, may allow a smoother course of withdrawal, lower the chance of recurrent seizure, and have greater efficacy in the prevention of delirium.[84] Benzodiazepines with an intermediate half-life, such as lorazepam, may have a safer profile in children and adolescents, and patients with co-morbid hepatic dysfunction. Alternatives to benzodiazepine management for alcohol withdrawal are finding increasing use. One such method is the use of the long-acting barbiturate phenobarbital, which is very often used with good success at the MGH.[54] In a retrospective analysis of benzodiazepine withdrawal (studying 310 patients treated over a 5-year period), the use of a phenobarbital taper showed significant efficacy and minimal adverse effects, the most common being sedation.[85] Their recommended dosing schedule involved a 3-day taper of phenobarbital starting with a one-time dose of 200 mg, then 100 mg q4h × 5 doses, then 60 mg q4h × 4 doses, then 60 mg PO q8h × 3 doses. Some patients received extra doses if they manifested persistent symptoms of withdrawal. This study supports the common clinical practice of substitution of various sedative–hypnotics in the treatment of withdrawal.

Neuroleptics or antipsychotics are frequently used to control delirium-related[86] agitation or severe insomnia in older adolescents and adults. Atypical antipsychotics are usually preferred for children due to hypotension and dystonia from haloperidol. IV haloperidol (although not approved by the Food and Drug Administration [FDA] for IV use) is the most widely studied and accepted neuroleptic for the management of delirium with adults in critical care settings.[87] Before using any neuroleptics, a baseline electrocardiogram (ECG) is obtained to measure the QTc (ideally <450 ms); serum potassium and magnesium levels should be within the normal range. For acute agitation in patients who are smaller, younger, elderly, neuroleptic-naive, or who have mild agitation, one should begin with small doses of IV haloperidol (0.5–2 mg) and titrate to an effective dose depending on the clinical response. A general rule of thumb when titrating IV haloperidol is to wait 20 to 30 minutes after giving the first dose; if it was ineffective, double the dose and repeat this until a dose is reached that calms the agitated patient. If a patient requires escalating doses of haloperidol, an ECG should be repeated to monitor the QTc, and one should also continuously re-evaluate whether other immediately reversible causes may be contributing to agitation (e.g., hypoxia or pain). Once an effective dose has been reached, that dose can be repeated every few hours as necessary to control agitation. Patients who are larger, have been on antipsychotics regularly, or have moderate to severe agitation, may need larger doses (5–10 mg) at the outset, after which a similar titration to an effective dose can be pursued. Very high doses have been used safely and with good results.[88] Extrapyramidal side effects (e.g., dystonia) may occur, but their incidence is exceedingly low,[89] and dystonia can be largely prevented by use of antiparkinsonian agents. Occasionally, when severe agitation occurs and when the goal is to enhance deep sedation, a propofol drip and/or IV haloperidol, lorazepam, and a narcotic may be necessary.[90] This state reduces the metabolic demand imposed by agitation, minimizes pain, and produces amnesia that may decrease the vulnerability to PTSD.

Atypical antipsychotics (e.g., risperidone, quetiapine, ziprasidone, olanzapine, paliperidone, and clozapine) are increasingly used for adult burn patients, adolescents, and (primarily risperidone) with some children, though they have not been systematically studied in burn patients. Olanzapine (IM and oral forms), risperidone (oral forms), and quetiapine (oral forms) are more commonly used for management of agitation secondary to delirium, intense fear, and severe insomnia. (See Chapter 10 for more information on management of delirium in the medically ill.)

Drug Side Effects, Toxicity, and Adverse Interactions

Side effects, toxicity, and adverse interactions can occur with just about any agent used in burn care. Given that the consultation psychiatrist most frequently employs opiates, benzodiazepines, ketamine (in children), and antipsychotics in the acute management of burn patients, we will review those medications.

With antipsychotics, side effects and adverse reactions can be grouped by the following receptors or channel interactions: potassium-delayed rectifier channel (QT prolongation); anticholinergic side effects (e.g., tachycardia and constipation); antihistaminergic effects (e.g., sedation and weight gain); alpha antagonism (orthostatic hypotension); and dopamine antagonism (e.g., akathisia, dystonia, tardive dyskinesia, and neuroleptic malignant syndrome [NMS]). Of these, the gravest and least common are NMS and torsades de pointes (associated with QT prolongation). These syndromes are described in other chapters.

Opiates have an array of side effects (including exacerbation of delirium, respiratory depression, and development of physiologic and psychological dependence and withdrawal) with which the consulting psychiatrist should be familiar. Burn patients who require high amounts of opiates over a matter of weeks will become physiologically dependent; tapering is recommended to prevent an uncomfortable withdrawal syndrome. Minor withdrawal symptoms may be managed with clonidine and dicyclomine (to reduce stomach cramps). The interaction of opiates and benzodiazepines may cause delirium, excess sedation, and respiratory depression.[91] Opiate toxicity can be reversed by naloxone.

Side effects and adverse reactions of benzodiazepines include paradoxical worsening of agitation, respiratory depression (which can be additive with other medications) and, similarly to opiates, development of tolerance and therefore withdrawal. In children, midazolam infusions are not associated with lactic acidosis believed to result from the accumulation of propylene glycol, a problem seen occasionally with lorazepam infusions.[92] Benzodiazepine toxicity can be reversed by use of flumazenil; however, seizures may be induced if this medication is administered to benzodiazepine-dependent individuals. Signs and symptoms of benzodiazepine withdrawal include anxiety, dysphoria, insomnia, abdominal cramps, nausea, vomiting, sweating, tremors, and seizures. Benzodiazepines must be tapered because the withdrawal syndrome can be life threatening due to the risk of seizure.

Ketamine, an *N*-methyl-D-aspartate (NMDA) receptor antagonist, is one of the most well-known psychotomimetic drugs.[93] It is frequently used for rapid sedation in children and adults; the long-term neurodevelopmental effects of it are unknown despite its extensive use. Though clinicians seek to balance the risks and benefits of aggressive pain management with ketamine, for years it has been in wide use in pediatrics because of its ability to manage procedure-related pain without major adverse short-term or long-term effects. The possibility that ketamine may rapidly reduce the emergence of depressive or post-traumatic symptoms in traumatized patients may add to its utility if confirmed for burn patients.[94–97]

Pharmacologic treatment of patients with burns is often complicated by prior substance use and abuse, the possibility that use of pharmacologically active agents will adversely alter mental state, the critical condition of the patient (especially with respiratory failure or renal insufficiency), drug interactions, altered pharmacodynamics, and the need to balance the benefits of the medication against the risks of unwanted side effects or toxicity.[98] When this is the case, reducing the dosage of medications or stopping medications in favor of psychotherapeutic interventions may be safest.

Of note, although patients with burns may develop a physical dependence to analgesics and anxiolytics, addiction is rarely caused by use of these agents in the context of burns. Additionally, substance abusers may at first require higher doses of opiates or benzodiazepines to effectively treat symptoms than do others without similar histories.

Intermediate Phase

The intermediate phase, during which the patient is healing, is less stressful. Lengthy hospitalizations, however, are the period for which the term *continuous traumatic stress* may be most fitting.[91] During this time, the psychiatrist may be called to see a burn patient with a pre-morbid psychiatric condition who is depressed, displaying symptoms of PTSD, or who is having special difficulty adapting to the frequent stresses of burn care. Even the most resilient of patients may have difficulty with body image disruption or a re-experience of trauma symptoms upon re-hospitalization for ongoing burn treatment. These patients benefit from individualized psychological and psychopharmacologic treatment. Watkins and colleagues described four staff interventions that can aid patients during their progression during this phase:[54]

1. Educating the patient about the expected course of recovery specific for the type of injury sustained.
2. Orienting the patient to the physical phenomena that will be experienced during this phase of recuperation (e.g., itching, nociceptive and neuropathic pain).
3. Creating a program for self-care and activities. Initially, goals should be realistic about the degree of physical impairment sustained by the patient, with gradual progression of goals once the patient begins to derive a sense of pride in his or her accomplishments.
4. Focusing on returning abilities versus remaining disabilities by verbal acknowledgment and praise of any improvements in autonomous functioning, no matter how small.

Psychological Interventions

A shift from the acute to the intermediate phase occurs when survival is assured, when most burn wounds are grafted, and when the patient approaches ambulatory status. At this time it is possible to assess more fully the mental status and to begin differentiating issues of mourning the prior body image, grieving the loss of loved ones, depression, and PTSD. In addition, assessment and diagnosis of neurologic or pre-existing psychiatric impairment becomes feasible. The patient's awareness of functional losses and disfigurement is eased by responsive staff and by supportive, informed family members. Psychotherapeutic interventions also focus on phase-related issues (e.g., forthcoming surgery, return to home, work and school, and rehabilitation).[99]

Adaptation of the family usually follows the course of the patient's recovery. Remarkably similar feelings and defensive responses are observed in the patient and his or her family. Psychotherapeutic support (often several sessions per week) during this phase, especially regarding guilt feelings and grief, assists the family and enables them to support the patient's coping through this phase.

Some hospitals provide groups that offer brief psychotherapy, education, and rehabilitation. Several types of group interventions have been used: a children's group structured to encourage expressive drawing and puppet play, an adolescent or adult group for hospitalized patients, and family groups for parents or families of acutely ill patients. These group interventions focus on education about treatment, grief, and one's response to hospitalization, surgery, stigmatization, discharge, and re-entry into society. In England, Rivlin and associates[100] conducted parent groups using a multidisciplinary approach, which the parents rated as helpful.

Body Image and Plastic and Reconstructive Surgery

After the acute treatment of burns, the intermediate phase often involves ongoing care with plastic and reconstructive surgeons. Although the surgeries they perform may begin early in treatment, they may continue for years after the initial burn. Many burn survivors with changed appearance have ongoing difficulties with psychological and social adaptation.[101] One longitudinal study of body image of survivors of severe burn injury found that 1 year after injury, body image satisfaction and distress was the most significant predictor of overall psychosocial function.[101] The more one defines one's self by physical appearance, the greater the self-consciousness about appearance.[102] Certain problems or mental disorders should prompt psychiatric consultation in those returning for post-burn plastic and reconstructive surgery. For children, lack of age-appropriate preparation, preoperative panic, PTSD, parent–child disturbances, attention deficit hyperactivity disorder (ADHD), depression, and enuresis or encopresis are not unusual. For adults, PTSD, psychosis, or substance abuse may occur. Certain burns that require cosmetic surgery (e.g., of the face and head, breasts, or genitalia) and are associated with functional deficits (e.g., burns to the mouth, hands, arms, and lower extremities), including amputations and revisions, require special consideration. These may also necessitate special expertise in preoperative psychological assessment and postoperative management.

Plastic surgeons develop psychological skills for the evaluation of burned patients and may seek psychiatric consultation for their patients.[103] Because much of acute treatment, even with recent improvements in care, is outside the control of the patient and the family, a central psychological goal at this point is to increase the patient's and the family's role in the treatment course. Although staff assist the patient to see himself or herself anew,[104] the consultant, in turn, becomes aware of the experience of being burned through the eyes of the patient. Body image revision occurs through plastic surgery, allowing another stage of reintegration of body image and healing of the damage to appearance and to self-image.[105,106] Focused, short-term supportive and educational psychotherapy is helpful, and protocols for these treatments have been developed.[107] Furthermore, helping patients accept untoward changes in their life is crucial during this stage, with a particular focus on acceptance of loss.[54]

As patients become more actively involved in their recovery and attempt to resume basic autonomous functioning, they begin to cognitively define and emotionally realize the long-term and often permanent losses that they have sustained from their burn injuries. While some losses may be immediately obvious (e.g., loss of ambulation, function of limbs, loss of limbs), others may not be as apparent. The loss of some ability to associate with friends and family, or the loss of the opportunity to live life in the manner they were accustomed to may be equally devastating. This initial realization is often expressed as "hurt," and perceived as feelings of sadness or "depression," and may be exhibited by social withdrawal, tearfulness, decreased appetite, impaired sleep initiation and/or maintenance, or decreased participation in physical therapy. The patients should be allowed the opportunity to talk about their perceptions regarding these issues and the emotional difficulties they are experiencing, in an effort to legitimize their situation and allow them to ventilate their perceptions and feelings regarding losses.[54] The capacity to tolerate fear and anxiety associated with re-hospitalization should be assessed before embarking upon plastic and reconstructive surgery. If there is significant psychopathology, review of records and a preoperative assessment are indicated to reduce postoperative complications. Preoperative problems include phobic reactions to surgery, unrealistic expectations of "perfect" surgical results, embarrassment or shame related to severe disfigurement, and resurgence of PTSD symptoms (e.g., flashbacks or nightmares). Reality-oriented preoperative psychotherapeutic interventions support the patient's coping and facilitate a positive attitude following surgery.

Occasionally, evaluation of emotional readiness for elective surgery results in a recommendation to postpone the surgery. Though such readiness should be part of pre-admission assessment, such reactions may not be apparent until the patient arrives for surgery and is immersed in the hospital environment. A patient who presents with panic upon admission and re-experiences prior burn-related trauma may require postponement of elective surgery until outpatient desensitization treatment for the phobia, treatment of panic disorder, or both, can be started (before undergoing surgery).

Acute Burns

Today, children and adults usually survive once they reach an acute burn unit, even with massive burns. Despite suffering severe burns to the bronchial tree, face, torso, or extremities (which may require deep, disfiguring excisions of fat and muscle, or amputations), people survive. In fact, in 1984, the percentage of burns associated with a 50% mortality was 65% and by the early 1990s, it increased to 81%.[108] Many of these survivors drew on personal strengths and family supports and were incredibly resilient, which is now confirmed in longitudinal follow-up and recovery curves, some for more than 10 years post-burn.[55,56]

Psychiatric treatment of those with massive burns initially focuses on the management of pain, stress, or delirium, then deals with grief and injury to body image. Next, treatment focuses on support, restoration of mobility, self-esteem, and hope. Finally, treatment helps the burn survivor resume educational, occupational, and social function. Encouragement, education, and advocacy for the massively burned patient is crucial to mobilize resources so that life, school, and work outside the hospital can be resumed and that the social stigma of disfigurement can be endured.

LONG-TERM PHASE AND OUTCOMES

In many ways, the long-term phase of post-burn treatment is a continuation of the intermediate phase, with ongoing assessment and treatment of recurrent or emerging psychiatric illness and reintegration of a patient's sense of self, having been forced to grieve various aspects of their body, function, and even life roles. The general hospital psychiatrist should be aware of this dynamic phase of recovery.

General Outcomes

Many small studies of varying quality and a few larger ones relate to outcomes after burns.[109–111] Very important findings of positive long-term outcomes of severely burned children in a well-designed study were cited above in a large longitudinal study.[55,56] Clearly, the quality of burn and reconstructive treatment has improved, as have the interventions to enhance burn recovery.[112] This makes conclusions based on earlier studies unreliable when attempting to predict current outcomes. These findings confirm the review[109] of child outcome studies, that "collectively, findings indicate that little empirical data exist to support the contention that the majority of pediatric burn victims exhibit severe poor post-burn adjustment." Others[110–112] essentially agreed with these conclusions for adults from a rehabilitation psychology perspective. They suggested that poor outcomes were mainly a result of severe pre-burn psychopathology, which is significant. In another study, Park and co-workers[113] conducted a cross-sectional survey of 686 patients with burns; they found that lack of family support and living expense burden were the two most significant risk factors for patients with acute burns; and those factors, in addition to medical expenses burden, were the risk factors associated with psychosocial problems in chronic burn patients.

Although there is much pre-burn psychopathology in adults and some in children, this theory under-emphasizes the severity and chronicity of post-traumatic reactions. Issues of vulnerability, resilience, and the effects of traumatic stress on emerging personality development[114] have been thoroughly summarized. Although pessimistic conclusions about outcomes are unwarranted, serious psychiatric and psychological morbidity after severe, disfiguring burns merit attention. For children, the multiple long-term consequences of exposure to traumatic stresses include learning and attachment disorders, depression, anxiety disorders, and trauma- and stressor-related disorders, among others.[115]

Post-Traumatic Stress Disorder (PTSD)

The largest risk factor for the development of PTSD following traumatic injury seems to be a previous history of psychiatric illness.[54] Additional risk factors for the development of PTSD following injury include acute pain symptoms, female gender, and personality characteristics such as externalization of blame, poor coping style, and high neuroticism. Characteristics of the burn, including higher percent of the TBSA and location on the face, head, and neck, have also been linked to the development of PTSD.

In child and adult studies, the prevalence of PTSD after burns ranges from 20% to 45%,[116–118] but partial PTSD is more frequent. In a longitudinal study of burn victims, van Loey and colleagues[119] showed that severe stress reactions immediately after injury are common and generally decrease over time; pain-related anxiety predicts post-traumatic stress symptoms 1 year after the burn; consecutive painful wound treatments related to burn severity have a cumulative effect and predispose towards post-traumatic symptoms in the long term; however, the absence of early post-traumatic stress symptoms did not necessarily prevent development of chronic post-traumatic stress symptoms. In adult burn survivors, PTSD occurred among 20% to 45% of patients, often with associated sleep disorders.[120] Roca and colleagues[121] followed 43 patients (from discharge to follow-up 314 months later); 7% initially fulfilled criteria for PTSD; this increased to 22% at 4 months. Perry and co-workers[122] also found an increase from 35% at 2 months to 45% at 12 months. Most studies and clinical observation indicated a gradual attenuation of PTSD symptoms, but these studies suggested that it might not be so. Behavioral, cognitive, and pharmacologic therapies all have a place in the treatment of PTSD;[123] new short-term treatments are being tested.[124]

Additionally, several studies of children, adults, and soldiers have found that early and aggressive treatment of pain is associated with reduced PTSD symptomatology in burn survivors.[125,126] Saxe and associates[127] demonstrated that early post-burn administration of IV morphine reduced the emergence of post-traumatic stress symptomatology in older children, and probably in 1–4-year-old children.[128] Perioperative administration of ketamine was associated with a reduced rate of PTSD in adult burn victims;[129] however, administration during the first 3 days was associated with an increased rate of ASD symptoms.[130] In a double-blind, placebo-controlled study, early post-burn administration of sertraline to acutely burned children to prevent PTSD did not favor the drug over placebo.[130,131]

Initiation of quetiapine for states of hyperarousal may be helpful, in addition to assisting in treating difficulty with sleep initiation and sleep maintenance, particularly when associated with nightmares. If nightmares persist, a trial of prazosin can be started and titrated to assist in symptomatic control.[54] CBT may also be helpful to challenge cognitive distortions or to treat underlying anxiety or depressive symptoms.

Depression

Depression is also found to occur at higher rates in post-burn patients compared with those in the general population. Several studies have sought to evaluate the prevalence of depression among burn patients. Similar to PTSD, patients with pre-morbid mood disorders and particular coping styles are more likely to develop depression. One study found that patients with pre-morbid affective disorder were five times more likely to develop a mood disorder in the first year following a burn.[117] A review by Thombs and associates[132] found that major depression was identified (using structured interviews) in 4–10% of adult patients 1 year after a burn. The prevalence of depressive symptoms varied depending on the scale used; the Hospital Anxiety and Depression Scale yielded rates of 4–13%, whereas the Beck Depression Inventory yielded rates of 13–26% for moderate to severe symptoms and 22–54% for mild symptoms.

Surgical reconstruction improves appearance and strikingly enhances social and emotional adjustment. One study demonstrated a prevalence of at least mild to moderate symptoms of depression in 46% of patients undergoing burn reconstruction;[133] depressive symptoms were largely predicted by body image dissatisfaction and by physical function. Outcome studies in adults suggest that a majority adjusted well to their burns over the long term, but that those with facial burns are more likely to experience social rejection, impaired self-esteem, and withdrawal. These results do not resolve the likelihood of severe burn-related emotional disability in burned adults. If there is no surgical contraindication, initiation of an SSRI, such as sertraline or citalopram, may be initiated to treat underlying symptoms. Use of selective noradrenergic re-uptake inhibitors (SNRIs), such as duloxetine, may also be employed, with the potential benefit of also helping to treat underlying neuropathic pain from burn-related injury. For patients with significant underlying apathy or abulia, initiation of a stimulant, such as dextroamphetamine or methylphenidate, may be indicated and useful.[54]

Chronic Pain

Although pain subsides once the burns heal, ongoing pain has been documented years following burns;[134,135] two studies found that about one-third of burn patients 1 to 9 years out from a burn continue to have significant pain, and the majority of these patients had sleep, work, or social disruption related to the pain. In addition to pain, itching, particularly in deep thermal burns with hypertrophic scars, is one of the more disturbing physical complaints endorsed by patients with burns, and it can become chronic in some patients.[136] A study by Van Loey in 2008[136] prospectively followed burn patients for 2 years and found that at 3 months, 87% of patients complained of mild to severe itching, and this decreased steadily over the next 21 months (such that at 2 years, 21% of burn patients had moderate to severe itching). The study showed that at 2 years, post-traumatic stress symptoms and the number of surgical procedures predicted itching. Although itching has a fairly well understood biologic basis, psychological factors may also contribute to the chronicity of itching. Psychoactive medications, including naltrexone,[137] gabapentin, and doxepin[138] have been tried with some success. More research is needed in this area.

Lastly, observations of patients who do well following burn injuries have led to insights about resiliency factors and a growing body of literature regarding predictors of success in recovery. Positive emotions, self-efficacy, resilience, ability to sleep during recovery, and baseline resilience at the time of injury have all been identified as protective factors.[139–142]

END-OF-LIFE CARE

The mortality rate on adult units is much higher than on pediatric burn units because of more extensive burns, severe medical and psychiatric risk factors, an increased mortality risk associated with being older, and the limits of what medical care can achieve. Elderly patients with burns are more likely to require ventilatory support, more intensive care, and have higher mortality rates.[25] Most burn-related deaths occur during the initial phases, but some patients survive for months before death arrives, and some patients survive within the acute burn care setting and then fail in less intensive rehabilitation settings.

The psychiatrist is often consulted to assist in the care of dying patients and their families to minimize pain and suffering and to assist in the process of decision-making at the end of life.[143–145] With massive burns, decisions whether to continue treatment may arise. This is challenging emotionally and spiritually to all involved; patients may benefit from pastoral care; burn teams may benefit from optimal care or ethics committee consultations. Some patients and families, in collaboration with the burn team, choose palliative care (or "comfort care") rather than enduring the pain and suffering of treatment and the cosmetic, functional, and psychological sequelae of burns.

Although it is often traumatic when an adult dies, it is always emotionally traumatic when a child dies from burns.[143–146] It is essential to provide accurate explanations about the risk of death to families and to patients when possible, as well as emotional preparation for this possibility. Support in their grieving is helpful to relatives of burn patients who die, especially from members of the burn team who worked closely with them. Many grieving family members are very grateful for the care their loved ones have received.

STAFF SUPPORT, STAFF STRESS

Psychiatric skills are especially valuable and valued by burn patients; stressed staff also know their benefits. It is useful to understand organizations in which one works, the rapid changes that affect hospitals and health care, and the virtues of developing a relationship with a multidisciplinary team to care for severely traumatized patients. One's introduction to the unit may be followed by shock, dismay, fear, frustration, and sadness as the full meaning of burn care takes hold.[19,145] Respect for the coping styles of the staff is crucial, since it may at times appear that individuals are harsh, regressed, or over-involved. The psychiatrist on the team, simply by his or her presence, encourages communication; a reflective attitude about staff members' feelings as well as those of their patients is helpful. By encouraging staff to ask questions, the psychiatrist can enable them to think diagnostically and therapeutically about their patients' and their own future, and provide them with a sense of satisfaction and hope. Gratitude for sharing the burden of tragic or irreversible situations and for lending an ear may be forthcoming. The psychiatrist is often able to place trauma in a positive perspective and to broaden and deepen the psychiatric knowledge of the entire burn team.

ETHICAL CONSIDERATIONS

Ethical issues stimulated by burn care may be a source of difficulty for staff and the family; these issues may be magnified by costs, which may exceed US$1 million for a single patient. Ethical issues[54] include consent to treatment, quality of life, prevention of intolerable pain, organ donation, decisions about resuscitation or withdrawal of life support, cost of care versus potential benefit, responsibility for long-term care of most severely burned, right to treatment, and determination of disability. Consultation by the ethics committee to the burn team in difficult cases is often helpful to provide optimal care to the patient and family.

Internet information sources are available online regarding burns (American Burn Association); pain (American Pain Society); psychopharmacology, traumatic stress (International Society for Traumatic Stress Studies; Dartmouth traumatic stress library); American Psychiatric Association, and American Academy of Child and Adolescent Psychiatry.

REFERENCES

 Access the reference list online at https://expertconsult.inkling.com/.

Chronic Medical Illness and Rehabilitation

33

Nasser Karamouz, M.D.
John B. Levine, M.D., Ph.D.
Gregory L. Fricchione, M.D.

OVERVIEW

Most of us take our ability to function physically (e.g., to open a tube of toothpaste, answer the telephone, tie our shoelaces, use the toilet, or comb our hair) and cognitively for granted. However, these capabilities can be lost suddenly after an accident (e.g., with a traumatic brain injury [TBI]; spinal cord injury [SCI]; an extensive burn); the onset of a debilitating chronic illness (e.g., cancer, multiple sclerosis, epilepsy); or an exacerbation of a pre-existing illness (e.g., an amputation associated with diabetes, seizures after an anoxic encephalopathy, stroke complicating lupus). For individuals with these conditions, rehabilitation is usually indicated to help restore lost function. However, despite rehabilitation, some aspects of everyday function never return.

Psychiatrists who consult such patients need to reconcile their need to offer such patients support with their limited personal experience with such sudden or chronic loss of function, as well as with the realism that complete recovery may not ultimately be obtained. This challenges the psychiatrist's ability to understand and to develop a therapeutic alliance with patients undergoing rehabilitation. In such cases, the psychiatrist needs to acknowledge this limitation and develop alternative strategies, such as recruiting assistance of others who have had personal experience with loss of function.

Further, the need to help patients maintain hopefulness, while accepting limitations and grieving losses of function, runs counter to the physician's typical focus on achieving a full recovery.

This chapter addresses such challenges faced by patients with chronic medical conditions and by the psychiatrists who treat them. The focus is on inpatient rehabilitation, though similar principles apply when consulting patients in other settings.

DIAGNOSTIC CONSIDERATIONS

While certain psychiatric conditions (depression, cognitive impairment, adjustment disorders, and behavioral difficulties) are more common in patients undergoing rehabilitation,[1,2] diagnostic criteria are often not met because the symptoms of DSM-5 and ICD-10 are often similar to those associated with the patient's injury. As a result, diagnosis in rehabilitation focuses more on symptom constellations than it does in other settings.

Typically, symptoms are myriad in the rehabilitation setting (Figure 33-1). When evaluating a patient undergoing rehabilitation, the psychiatric consultant should consider that the incidence rates of psychiatric syndromes are higher in this population. For example, depression, among amputees may be as high as 58%; for those with multiple sclerosis, it may be seen in up to 27%; and for those with cancer, it has been seen in up to 25%.[2] Further, the prevalence of suicide and of suicidal intent[3] is also substantially higher among patients undergoing rehabilitation. Individuals with cancer have suicide rates that are 15 to 20 times greater; those with spinal cord injuries have a rate 15 times greater; and those with multiple sclerosis have a rate 14 times greater, than those in the general population.[2,4]

Phases of Rehabilitation

The phases of rehabilitation help to contextualize symptom presentation. As outlined in Figure 33-1, patients' progression through rehabilitation can be viewed via a three-stage model. During the initial phase of inpatient rehabilitation (following one's transition from the acute medical hospital), psychiatric issues often arise, related to agitation and resolving states of physiologic hyperarousal.

During the middle phase, the rehabilitation patient's denial of a deficit related to his/her injury is the most common reason for psychiatric consultation. During this phase, patients often have difficulty accepting their deficit, either due to neurologically based anosognosia, or, more commonly, to anxiety about their deficits. This results in a need to re-visit the therapeutic contract and develop strategies to acknowledge deficits so that functional recovery can proceed. If denial of a deficit is not interfering with rehabilitation, it can generally be addressed later. Frustration related to the lengthy rehabilitation and uncertainty about long-term prognosis increases during the middle phase of treatment. Emotional stress in rehabilitation is typically highest during this phase and most discharges against medical advice (AMA) occur during this phase.

As rehabilitation progresses, patients start to focus on their anticipated loss of support from the hospital staff

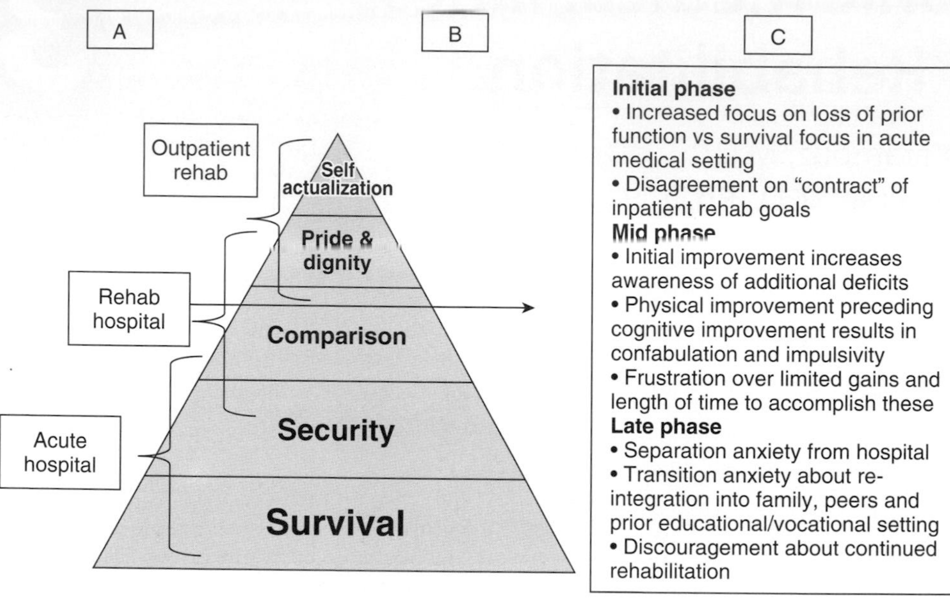

Figure 33-1. Rehabilitation settings (A) as related to Maslow's hierarchy of needs (B) and (C) psychiatric issues arising within the rehabilitation hospital setting.

following discharge, their need for increasingly independent function, concern about whether outpatient care will be adequate to manage residual deficits, and increased concerns about anticipated gains that have not been met. During this phase, interventions that help with discharge-related anxiety include: bridging discharge plans (through active communication between inpatient and outpatient rehabilitation staff prior to discharge), focusing on gains that have been met, and tailoring the discharge planning to the patient's and/or family's particular concerns.

The progression through different rehabilitation settings and the phases of physical and emotional recovery during inpatient rehabilitation, parallels movement through Maslow's hierarchy of needs (Figure 33-1).[5] Considering the questions listed in Table 33-1, can help to identify the basis for psychiatric symptoms seen during each phase of rehabilitation, whether they surround the formation of an initial contract, increased awareness of deficits during rehabilitation, or stress related to discharge.

While progressing through rehabilitative phases, the patient and family typically experience an iterative process involving relief and discouragement. As with other developmental transitions, enthusiasm about functional improvements is often followed by sadness associated with an increased awareness of the deficit being remediated (e.g., after the amputee has gained the ability to walk with a prosthetic device there is increased awareness of the lost limb). The degree of sadness associated with the increased awareness of improvements during rehabilitation varies with how vital that function was for a given individual. For example, awareness of the lost limb often has more impact on a patient who had been athletic compared with one who was more sedentary. Thus, the psychiatric consultant should anticipate a higher degree of sadness and demoralization[6] in the former patient than the latter. In contrast, for the patient with more sedentary and cognitively based interests,

TABLE 33-1 Key Questions in Developing a Treatment Plan for Psychiatric Symptoms Interfering With Goals of Rehabilitation

1. Is the patient in agreement with the goals that the staff has in mind for the patient's rehabilitation?
   → If yes go to question 2
   → If no address reason for disagreement with noted concern before addressing question 2
2. Does the patient agree that the proposed intervention will help resolve the identified goal?
   → If yes move to question 3
   → If no address reason for disagreement on usefulness of a rehabilitation intervention
3. Does the patient agree that a potentially useful intervention should be undertaken?
   → If yes move to question 4
   → If no address why the patient objects to pursuing a treatment even though they feel it would result in improvement, before addressing question 4
4. Is the patient motivated (does he/she want) to participate in the proposed intervention?
   → If yes go to question 5
   → If no address motivational issues for moving to question 5
5. Does the patient participate in treatment?
   → If yes, no further intervention is recommended
   → If no, address resistance to participation in planned intervention

increased awareness of deficits during the phases of rehabilitation after a TBI may carry a particularly strong negative valence. Furthermore, the consulting psychiatrist should anticipate that a patient's tolerance for feelings of discouragement that accompany progress during rehabilitation will vary with the patient's level of pre-morbid stress tolerance. Less resilient patients are usually prone to greater exacerbations of pre-existing psychiatric symptoms during their hospitalization.[7,8] Therefore, assessment of pre-morbid coping style and vocational/recreational interests will help the psychiatric consultant to contextualize levels of emotional distress during rehabilitation. These shifts in hopefulness that occur at the various stages are illustrated in the case example (Case 1).

CASE 1 Example of Psychiatric Consultation in a Patient With Traumatic Brain Injury

Ms. V, a 20-year-old woman, was admitted to the rehabilitation hospital following a severe motor vehicle accident (that led to multiple orthopedic injuries as well as TBI involving a frontal-temporal and thalamic intracranial bleed). Her presentation was complicated by a history of social service involvement and a history of disruptive behavior and substance use.

During the initial phase of recovery, psychiatric consultation focused on helping the family cope with anxiety as their focus shifted from relief that she had survived a near lethal injury to the fact that she was still minimally responsive 2 weeks after being brought out of a chemically induced coma. In addition to supportive interventions for the family, psychoeducation was provided to help them understand the steps that could be taken to help facilitate increased cognitive arousal. With their approval, amantadine was prescribed and gradually titrated to the maximum dose (150 mg BID), while a cognitive arousal protocol was implemented in speech, occupational, and physical therapy. On HD#3, the patient opened her eyes and began to show volitional eye tracking, non-verbal responses, and purposeful movements for the first time since the injury. Renewed relief ensued which was followed by discouragement that no verbal responses had returned. The patient was alert enough to participate in forming an initial contract about her treatment and both the patient and her parents, and family members agreed on the main goal in all three rehabilitation therapies. Further, agreement on addressing her still dysregulated sleep cycle and level of disorientation was agreed upon as part of the "initial contract". Trazodone and melatonin were prescribed and insomnia improved, and behavioral strategies to facilitate orientation were initiated. On HD#7, she began to whisper non-meaningful sounds that progressed to two-word responses by HD#10. Increased relief and hopefulness during this period was followed by renewed anxiety and some pessimism about her recovery, as getting to longer verbal expressions was difficult and as short-term memory impairments became more apparent in assessments (could only hold one object in memory).

During the middle phase of rehabilitation, the discrepancy between the increased alertness but still limited short-term memory and other cognitive capacities was associated with a period of increased agitation, impulsivity, and perseveration. Some hypersexual behaviors (exposure of genitals in public) were also noted. As is typical during this period, there was increased tension between patient and staff, among family members, and among staff about why progress had slowed and how to manage the increased impulsivity, agitation, and perseveration. These issues were addressed with new approaches in rehabilitation (increased sensory focus in occupational therapy [OT] and physical therapy [PT] and shifting the focus to short-term memory deficits in speech). The agitated behavior scale was charted 5×/day in order to objectively track the effect of interventions on the target symptoms of impulsivity, aggression, and sensory-seeking behavior. Behavioral strategies to help with these symptoms were instituted through nursing and social work (e.g., use of a netbed to prevent her trying to walk to the bathroom when she had not yet recovered this function; use of abdominal binder to protect the G-tube; presenting her with a daily schedule before starting the day, with this divided so the length of information provided was appropriate to her cognitive capacity, and asking the patient to repeat back the information). Pharmacologic interventions during this phase were cross-tapering trazodone (50 mg) to quetiapine (50 qhs and 12.5 am) to address agitation and insomnia, low-dose SA methylphenidate (weaned up to 5/2.5 due to sensory and sleep side effects at higher doses), and clonidine 0.5 TID, and fluoxetine 10 mg qd was started as the agitation subsided. As the periods of agitation resolved, the alliance with the treatment team improved and the patient was able to re-engage in further therapy. Substantial gains accrued during this phase (HD #20–30). In speech, short-term memory, processing speed, and confabulation improved (earlier in this phase she would respond that the physical therapist [PT] was her gym teacher when she couldn't remember her name between sessions). In PT, she started to stand and then walk for short distances with minimal assistance, and in OT she was able to become independent with transferring from her wheelchair to the bathroom. Her mood improved and while she had periods of tearfulness and sadness about residual deficits, she gradually become less overwhelmed by these and the frequency and duration of euthymic mood states increased, and her affective state dysregulation decreased.

During the late phase of her rehabilitation, she started to engage with other patients during recreational therapy and tolerated successful visits from her best friend. This was timed with increased discharge planning about re-entry to her home environment, outpatient rehabilitation supports that would be needed, and home renovations that had to be made for wheelchair accessibility, as the patient was only beginning to regain walking at the time of discharge. Significant residual deficits remained that were addressed in outpatient long-term rehabilitation, as she entered the late phase of rehabilitation. At this point, the focus shifted to planning the appropriate supports for discharge to outpatient rehabilitation. Psychiatric consultation was provided to support the many gains that she had made during her rehabilitation while validating anxiety and sadness about coping with continued functional deficits with less supports than they had within the inpatient hospital.

Developmental Factors

In addition to the patient's phase of progression through rehabilitation, certain stages of childhood and adult development helped to contextualize the diagnostic questions posed for the psychiatric consultant. For example, functional losses from illness or injuries that occur during critical developmental periods in childhood are particularly refractory to rehabilitation (e.g., aphasia from a stroke occurring during the peak of language development). In contrast, illnesses that result in physical losses that occur outside of critical developmental periods are more responsive to rehabilitation when they occur proximal to the developmental period of that function (limb amputation due to congenital conditions has less psychiatric co-morbidity than when they occur after functional use of that limb has developed).[9] Therefore, just as the patient with athletic interests may be more susceptible to distress associated with an amputation, an injury-based amputation will generally lead to greater emotional distress than in a patient whose amputation resulted from a chronic illness (such as diabetes) or a congenital abnormality.[9,10]

Symptom Type and Intensity

Symptom type and intensity help distinguish normal from problematic adjustment reactions. As in most other areas of consultation–liaison (C–L) psychiatry, distinguishing "normal reactions" due to injury-related stress or illness-related stress is often vital. While this determination can be subjective, some general guidelines help to make this distinction.

Criteria that distinguish normal grief and normal stress reactions from pathologic grief or a stress disorder, help to separate normal from problematic adjustments during recovery. Specifically, self-blame, guilt, refusal to participate in a therapeutic rehabilitation or recreational therapy, agitation (that involves physical or verbal aggression), panic attacks, psychotic symptoms, and suicidal or homicidal ideation, usually suggest an atypical and problematic adjustment.

Prioritizing non-somatic over somatic symptoms of depression, as identified by the use of the Hospital Anxiety and Depression Scale,[11] generally provides a more accurate assessment of depression and anxiety in rehabilitation patients. Still, a change in somatic symptoms, if it follows the trajectory of change in non-somatic depressive symptoms, should be part of this assessment.

Periods of sadness, tearfulness, anticipatory anxiety, resistance to participation in a therapeutic intervention (as long as it can be overcome with behavioral interventions), helplessness, and even hopelessness, are frequently normal reactions to the stress of adjusting to a physical impairment during rehabilitation. With regard to these latter symptoms, their frequency, intensity, and duration should decrease over time. While such symptoms wax and wane in intensity during treatment, they typically trend toward improvement as time passes. If symptom intensity is high or an overall trajectory of improvement is not apparent, then the consultant should consider whether an emotional response consistent with an adjustment reaction has developed into another syndrome.

Symptoms That Interfere With the Goals of Rehabilitation

Considering whether a particular symptom is impacting progression in rehabilitation helps to differentiate whether a symptom (such as tearfulness) is consistent with a normal adjustment reaction or at an intensity level that qualifies for a problematic adjustment. Asking rehabilitation staff about a change in a patient's motivation and their engagement in rehabilitation also helps in distinguishing normal from problematic adjustments. Finally, consideration of responses to reassurance, particularly from staff and/or family to whom the patient has previously responded positively, usually indicates that an adjustment reaction has evolved into something of greater concern.

Increased severity of symptoms during rehabilitation should be considered in light of the phases of rehabilitation (outlined in Figure 33-1). Namely, if symptoms of an adjustment reaction become more intense or impairing during the middle phase, they may be a response to issues during this phase, such as frustration about limited progress. If they appear in the mid-phase response, then the consulting psychiatrist would have a higher threshold for understanding symptoms as part of an evolving depression.

Psychiatric Look-Alikes

Psychiatric look-alikes are particularly important diagnostic considerations in rehabilitation. The psychiatric consultant needs to consider that symptoms (e.g., severe agitation, impulsivity, unprovoked aggression, or unusual levels of moaning) that indicate a problematic adjustment or another psychiatric syndrome have a higher-than-usual likelihood of arising secondary to a physiologic condition related to injury or illness.[12] Here, the phases of rehabilitation outlined in Figure 33-1 can also be helpful. An overview of the brain circuits involved in response to and recovery from a physical injury or illness is shown in Figure 33-2.

Aphasia

Fluent aphasia, such as Wernicke's aphasia, often seen after dominant hemisphere strokes, involves disordered speech that can be confused with the loose thinking found in schizophrenia or bipolar disorder. A history that confused speech had a sudden onset helps to differentiate fluent aphasia from loose thinking, suggestive of a pre-existing psychiatric disorder.

In patients with non-fluent motor aphasia after a dominant hemisphere stroke (i.e., Broca's aphasia), the slow, telegraphic speech, along with word-finding difficulties can suggest depression-based psychomotor retardation or a cognitive impairment. Through yes-or-no questions, visual communication strategies (selecting pictures of different affective states or clock-drawing to assess cognition), and examination of non-verbal affect (eye-contact, use of gestures) allow such patients to express their feelings and cognitive abilities and enhance assessment of co-morbid depressive and cognitive disorders.

Agitation

Agitation, sometimes with psychotic symptoms, can result from autonomic "storming" and persistent symptoms of a delirium that did not fully resolve prior to transfer from the medical to the rehabilitation setting. Moreover, after this initial phase resolves, it may re-present when other conditions arise (such as head injury). Overall scores, sub-scores, and item analysis of the Confusion Assessment Protocol (CAP), particularly the Agitated Behavior Scale (ABS) component, can help assess the intensity of symptoms and the

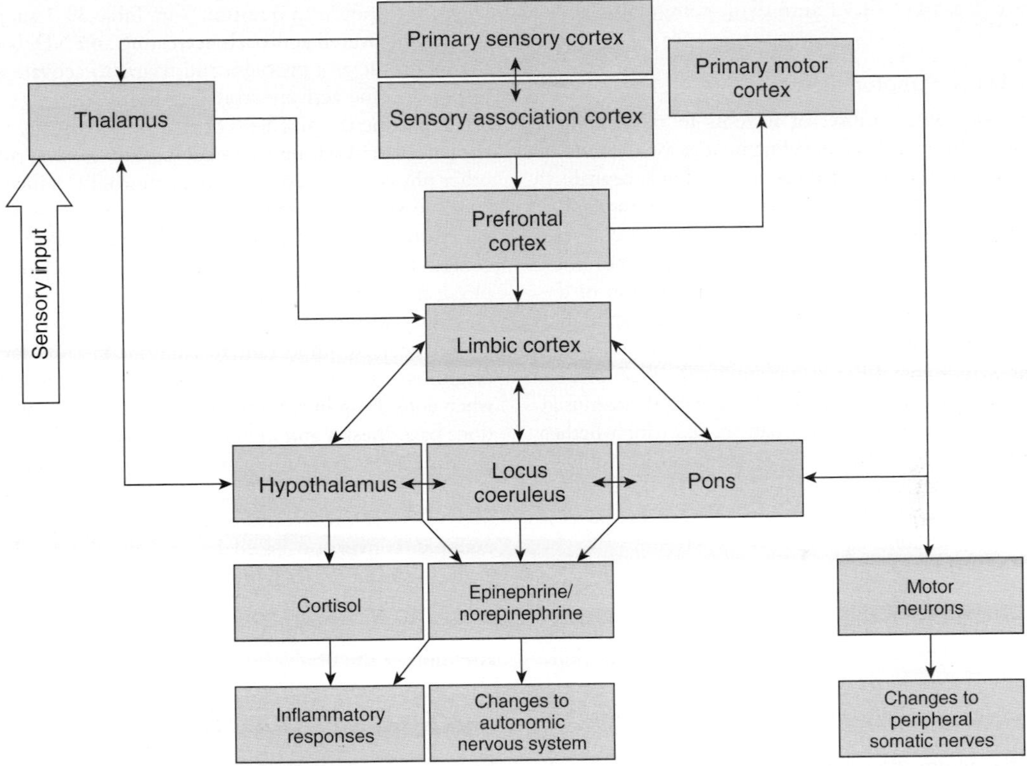

Figure 33-2. Impact of injury-induced sensory changes on brain pathways involved in healing during rehabilitation. *(Adapted from Fricchione and Levine.[17])*

differential diagnosis of agitation and associated confusional states.[13]

Pseudobulbar Affect

Patients who have chronic neurologic illnesses that cause upper motor neuron damage and adversely impact corticobulbar tract functioning may result in pseudobulbar affect (e.g., with vascular dementia or a lysosomal storage disease), moaning, or pathologic crying, that persists during rehabilitation, due to a neurologic not psychiatric etiology. Pseudobulbar affect responds to use of a selective serotonin re-uptake inhibitor (SSRI);[14] recently the combination of dextromethorphan and quinidine (Nuedexta) has been FDA-approved for this condition[15] (while secondary options include use of TCAs, noradrenergic re-uptake inhibitors, dopaminergic agents, and uncompetitive *N*-methyl-D-aspartate receptor antagonists).[14] However, it is important to consider that strong emotional outbursts in such patients may not be due to depression, mania, or another psychiatric condition. It is sometimes appropriate to treat such responses (because of their negative impact on the patient's ability to function in group settings) but it is important to identify the underlying diagnosis as a non-psychiatric condition (for coding purposes, the ICD 10 diagnosis of F09: major neurocognitive disorder with behavioral disturbance, can be used).

On the other hand, the presence of pseudobulbar affect does not rule out a co-morbid psychiatric diagnosis. In such cases, other symptoms of depression need to be used to make the diagnosis. For example, thought content that is congruent with the affective outbursts as well as co-occurring neurovegetative signs of depression signal a co-morbid psychiatric condition in patients with pseudobulbar affect.

Aprosodia

Lesions in the frontotemporal non-dominant hemisphere or in those post-TBI often present with aprosodia involving an impaired ability to receive or to convey affect,[16] that can also masquerade as the constricted affect of a patient with depression. To confirm the presence of aprosodia, the consulting psychiatrist can assess the patient's ability to repeat a neutral sentence, such as, "I am going to the store," with several different emotional tones (e.g., happiness, sadness, anger), as well as to detect changes in tonality when listening to the phrase (while not given non-verbal cues).

Sensory Abnormalities

Sensory deprivation in patients in rehabilitation recovering from an amputation, or exacerbation of an illness that impairs sensory input (such as multiple sclerosis) often is manifest by excessive responses due to the nervous system's attempt to make sense of the decreased input.[17] When motor responses are abnormally low, apathy and withdrawal should be considered.

When hyperactivity results from conditions with sensory deprivation, they can be seen as anxiety or behavioral agitation. The psychiatric consultant should search for other symptoms to identify depression, anxiety, or agitation. This distinction is particularly important in hypoactive states in patients who have an increased risk of developing major depressive disorder (MDD) in rehabilitative settings (about

30%), as well as when they return to the community (about 25%).[18]

Temporal Lobe Symptomatology

While uncommon, a subset of patients in rehabilitation following a TBI or with a demyelinating disease that affects the temporal lobe (such as acute demyelinating encephalitis) can develop new-onset psychotic symptoms, acute agitation, aggression, and impulsivity. Imposter delusions, such as seen in Capgras syndrome and other misidentification syndromes, are associated with injuries to the posterior region of the temporal lobe. Furthermore, such patients are at higher risk for temporal lobe seizures that can result in new-onset psychotic symptoms (14% of patients with TLE exhibit post-ictal and inter-ictal psychosis[19,20]). As with the confused verbal output of the fluent aphasic patient, clarifying whether the onset followed or preceded the temporal lobe injury, helps to distinguish whether the etiology of such symptoms is based on the temporal lobe lesion or exacerbation of a pre-existing condition.

Abulia

Damage to the frontal cortex after a TBI, stroke, multiple sclerosis, or Parkinson's disease can lead to MDD. Lesions in this area can also produce abulia, a syndrome featuring apathy, loss of motivation, and loss of goal-directed behavior. Abulia can lead to the misdiagnosis of depression as the cause of the amotivational state.

In addition to a more sudden onset than in amotivational states due to depression, patient's with abulia due to neurologic syndromes (such as multiple sclerosis and Parkinson's disease) do not complain of depressed mood, despite lacking motivation and they are less preoccupied with suicide. Furthermore, symptom endorsement on the Hamilton Depression Scale (HDS) and the Montgomery–Asberg Depression Rating Scale can help to distinguish apathy and slowed thinking due to Parkinson's disease from depression. On the HDS, item endorsement of suicidal thoughts and feelings of guilt are significantly higher in depression than those characterized by apathy,[21] while on the Montgomery–Asberg Scale, depression and anhedonia have been most strongly associated with apathy due to depression rather than an abulic syndrome.[22] Finally, appetite disturbance and early morning awakening can differentiate depression from abulia related to Parkinson's disease.[23]

Diagnosis Is Critical to Treating the Patient With a Somatic Symptom Disorder

While rehabilitation is considered the optimal setting for patients with an IDC-10 and DSM-5 diagnosis of somatic symptom disorder (SSD) (previously termed "somatoform disorder" in DSM-IV), the most important step in treating this condition is making the diagnosis, discussing it with the patient, and determining whether there is agreement on the diagnosis. Patients who do not accept this diagnosis will generally not improve in rehabilitation. While outcomes for SSD are not as good as for other patients in rehabilitation, framing the syndrome as a functional neurologic disorder (FND) and applying standard rehabilitation strategies leads to the best outcome. This involves identification of a set of neurologic signs (e.g., Hoover's sign).[24] In addition, a negative response to question 5 in Table 33-1 suggests an FND. The overall approach in treating an FND, is framing the syndrome as a problem and trying to activate a motor response while actively attending to it.[24]

As making the diagnosis of an SSD will usually fall upon the psychiatrist within the rehabilitation setting, ruling out other physiologic etiologies or co-morbidities is critical, as in some studies a high percentage of patients with SSD were subsequently determined to have a medical diagnosis consistent with a disability or a co-morbid psychiatric and physical condition.[25] Multiple sclerosis is a condition frequently misdiagnosed as SSD.[26,27] Paraneoplastic syndromes are particularly important to rule out in considering the diagnosis of somatic symptoms or other psychiatric disorder when consulting in rehabilitation settings, as in such conditions paresthesias and memory loss can be a *forme fruste* of a cancer, most commonly small-cell lung cancer or gynecologic tumors.[28,29] Finally, even if the primary symptom is due to an SSD, it can produce medical complications. For example, conversion-based lower-extremity paralysis that leads to disuse of that limb can lead to Achilles tendon contracture, a decubitus ulcer, or a pulmonary embolism. Psychiatric consultation for these patients should draw attention to the prevention of such complications.

TREATMENT STRATEGIES

As a general guideline for treating the symptoms and diagnoses discussed above, the psychiatric consultant should prioritize treatment of symptoms that impact rehabilitation ahead of other symptoms, whenever possible. Once a symptom has been prioritized, the sequence of questions outlined in Table 33-1 can help guide formulation of a treatment intervention for a symptom that is interfering with productive participation in rehabilitation. Finally, as with diagnosis, formulation of a treatment plan will benefit from contextualizing it in terms of the patient's phase of rehabilitation. Interventions for particular issues arising in rehabilitation are discussed below with reference to these general guidelines.

Addressing Denial

Addressing denial should be guided by clarification of its etiology and by understanding whether it is impairing participation in rehabilitation. Denial of a problem that has been identified by rehabilitation staff as a treatment goal needs to be addressed more promptly and directly in rehabilitation than in other settings. It often emerges when establishing the therapeutic contract in the early phases of rehabilitation, as a negative response to question 1 from Table 33-1.

When due to a neurologic condition, such denial is termed *anosognosia*, such as in right parietal lobe strokes or other injuries to the non-dominant hemisphere (e.g., left-sided neglect of a hemiplegic arm). In such cases, the neurologically based reason that an initial contract cannot be established is best addressed through OT and PT strategies that allow increased awareness of the neglected limb, with strategies such as constraint-induced movement therapy.[30]

Denial due to psychiatric issues can arise at any phase of treatment. For example, in the late phase, pragmatic factors, such as a patient's concern that acknowledging a problem will result in an excessive burden to the family, can result in avoiding effective discharge planning. In this phase, such denial should be addressed in family discharge meetings.

Denial related to efforts to avoid associated anxiety or depressive feelings is more difficult for a patient to maintain in rehabilitation than in other settings, because the nature of rehabilitation therapy involves confronting the patient with their deficits and using strategies to cope with them (e.g., having a weak lower limb is much harder to deny in daily OT and PT exercises that involve its use). As one cannot simultaneously deny and acknowledge a functional deficit, rehabilitation can become stressful for the patient who relies on denial to manage anxiety associated with the deficit being actively addressed with rehabilitation. In addressing stress that arises from this dilemma, the consulting psychiatrist should attempt to balance accepting adaptive aspects of such denial with challenging the more maladaptive aspects. However, in rehabilitation, this balance will be skewed toward challenging it, as optimal recovery from an injury can be significantly impaired when intensive rehabilitation is delayed.

Anxiety and Depression

Evidence supports treatment of anxiety and depression with both psychosocial and pharmacologic interventions. Cognitive-behavioral therapy (CBT) that re-directs patients to a here-and-now focus help to calm patients.[31] Problem-solving therapy involves more active and targeted approaches than CBT and has efficacy in the treatment of depression and anxiety during rehabilitation when combined with escitalopram treatment.[32,33] These approaches can help to address the tendency of patients in rehabilitation to spend a large portion of their time worrying about future difficulties that they will face, while adjusting to their new, more medically or cognitively compromised, lives.[34,35] For example, if a patient states that he or she is worried that they "will never walk again," it is helpful to empathically re-direct their question to a more present and problem-specific focus for which they can get "evidence" (e.g., directing the patient to questions about whether they made progress during the day's efforts to increase their ability to walk). Psychoeducation on how daily interventions in rehabilitation result in "remodeling" of physiologic pathways[36] that have been damaged can also help re-direct patients and their families from focusing on long-term unpredictable outcomes.

Pharmacotherapy with SSRIs for depression and anxiety in TBI and stroke patients, and for anxiety in stroke patients has a limited, but generally positive evidence base, and is considered first-line treatment in these conditions.[33,37,38] Further, there is also evidence of improvement in cognitive and motor functioning in stroke patients with motor impairment.[39]

In contrast, while the SSRIs have efficacy for depression in cardiac patients undergoing rehabilitation,[40] there is limited evidence that it positively impacts cardiac function, though participation in rehabilitation may be of benefit.[41] Still, given the sizable literature that depression is associated with worse cardiac outcomes,[42,43] treatment with SSRIs is indicated. There is limited evidence to support using manualized psychotherapy techniques (e.g., CBT or interpersonal therapy) in cardiac patients.

For patients with spinal cord injuries, gabapentin and pregabalin have demonstrated efficacy for anxiety and depression, in addition to its well established benefit for pain.[44] Prazosin should be considered for anxiety associated with PTSD symptoms in patients with TBI, and it may have a general benefit for anxiety.[37] Recently, both animal and clinical studies involving orexin neuropeptides suggest potential therapeutic benefit for post-stroke cognitive and depressive symptoms.[45]

Secondary agents for anxiety include trazodone,[10] beta-blockers, alpha agonists (particularly when agitation and anxiety overlap), and buspirone.[10,37] For TBI patients or in patients with other neurologic conditions, benzodiazepines are not recommended due to their potential negative impact on cognitive function and neuroplasticity.[37] For acute anxiety they are sometimes needed due to their fast rate of action. Their negative cognitive effects are limited when used in this way. Bupropion should be used with caution in patients with injuries that lower their seizure threshold.

Agitation

Agitation is a common symptom during the early and middle phases of rehabilitation and it responds to instituting a behavioral plan along with use of medications. Non-pharmacologic strategies should be implemented in all cases of acute agitation, in addition to medication management. Ongoing assessment of target symptoms with the agitation behavioral scale component of the CAP,[13] will help assess the effect of the planned interventions. Evaluation of potential physical problems, such as hyponatremia, new onset of delirium, constipation, and infections should also occur during the evaluation and treatment of agitation.

In general, agitation arising in the first phase of treatment (due to autonomic storming) is more likely to have a physical basis than it is later in rehabilitation, but infections obviously can arise at all phases. Assessing level of consciousness using the disorders of consciousness protocol (DoC),[46] particularly in the early phase of rehabilitation, will help develop an appropriate treatment plan for agitation associated with minimally conscious patients.

Behavioral strategies, when agitation is related to a communication deficit, should focus on finding alternative ways for the patient to express whether there is an underlying emotional distress. Interventions that allow the patient to use "yes/no" responses and non-verbal communication can result in acknowledgment of a concern the patient could not express due to aphasia and will usually result in reduced agitation. If the communication deficit involves expressive aphasia, use of a picture board to identify a possible source of agitation is helpful.

Safety management, depending on the level of agitation, often involves using protective physical barriers (such as a netbed, abdominal binders for patients picking at tubes, and a 1:1 sitter). Even when a patient has significant cognitive deficits related to their agitation, involving a familiar staff member, or a close family member, helps with re-direction from the agitated behavior.

Addressing memory deficits with verbal and non-verbal reminders of expected transitions helps to prepare the patient for the even minor changes in routine that can precipitate agitation. Such information should be "chunked" or divided at the level that the patient can effectively employ. Calendars help to reduce disorientation associated with agitation, not only to date, but to the day's schedule, and to an approximate discharge date. When agitation is related to the level of sensory simulation, it will often respond to sensory reduction (involving lower lighting, noise reduction, limiting the number of people in the room, and scheduling periods of rest in between the three main therapy sessions that occur during a given day, e.g., PT, OT, and speech therapy).

Overall, with agitation, the rule of getting ahead of a trigger for agitation is very important, so the patient can then feel rewarded with success about completing a task, rather than using reminders that arrive after a difficult transition; these are experienced as criticism.

Finally, scaffolding strategies that provide context for an activity help reduce agitation associated with an activity that a patient cannot place in the perspective of a goal they want to attain. For example, frustration and associated agitation with a particular OT activity involving upper extremity control may decrease by reminding the patients that the goal of this OT exercise is to help them feed themselves that evening.

As with behavioral interventions, medication for agitation should be initiated early to minimize the tendency for it to escalate quickly. Using standing doses as soon as possible so a symptom is not being "chased" with PRN dosing is recommended. Psychiatrists should err on the side of active pharmacologic treatment for overt agitation, as well as associated underlying anxiety or depression, given the risks associated with its under-treatment.

For patients with cognitive deficits, who are most at risk of having acute agitation, the typical antipsychotics are not routinely recommended due to their problematic effect on cognition. While there are also concerns about adverse cognitive effects of second-generation antipsychotic agents (SGAs), the benefits of SGA treatment outweigh this concern when an antipsychotic medication is needed. Clozapine should generally be avoided due to the higher seizure risk in many patients with neurologic disorders and impaired cognitive function.

In determining the risk:benefit ratio for prescribing an SGA for agitation, the psychiatrist should consider the potential safety risks to the patient and others on the unit against the side effect concerns, such as orthostatic hypotension, neuroleptic malignant syndrome, akathisia, dyskinetic movements, and QTc prolongation associated with the risk of arrhythmia-induced sudden death.

Pharmacotherapy for agitation associated with cognitive impairment should also consider medications that can facilitate cognitive function. Usually, these will be started after a medication that directly targets the acute agitation is started. Evidence supports the use of amantadine and methylphenidate as cognitive enhancers in brain-injured patients.

Non-antipsychotic medication available for the treatment of agitation in TBI and other cognitive disorders includes antidepressants (trazodone, citalopram, and sertraline), anti-epileptics (valproate, carbamazepine, gabapentin), buspirone, and anti-hypertensive agents (propranolol, pindolol, clonidine). Benzodiazepines are sometimes used but can worsen confusion and cognitive dysfunction and cause paradoxical disinhibition.

Managing Sexual Dysfunction After Spinal Cord Injury

Managing sexual dysfunction is important for a patient's emotional and psychological well-being after a spinal cord injury. Complete spinal cord lesions can cause genital anesthesia, but some patients retain some genital sensation, genital response, and even orgasmic capability (if the lesion is partial). Some men can ejaculate without pharmacologic assistance, but most cannot. Many women and men report the development of new areas of arousal above the level of the lesion, sometimes leading to satisfying "phantom orgasms" with caressing or other tactile stimulation.[47,48]

Men may be able to achieve reflex erections sufficient for intercourse, or they may respond to treatment with prostaglandin E_2 agents (with variable results). Patients treated with sildenafil have improved erection response rates, and a substantial number of individuals with complete lesions also benefit from it.[47] Women are similarly affected but can use supplemental lubricants if vaginal lubrication is insufficient and intercourse is desired.

Difficulties with positioning, bowel and bladder incontinence, autonomic dysreflexia, and spasticity during sexual activity can be a problem for both women and men. Some patients find that their sexual preferences evolve in a manner that supports their remaining physical capabilities (e.g., increased interest in providing the partner with oral–genital stimulation).[49]

Co-Morbid Medical and Psychiatric Conditions

Co-morbid medical and psychiatric conditions should guide pharmacotherapy and psychotherapy. Because of the many physical conditions being addressed in the acute rehabilitation setting, the psychiatric consultant needs to consider treatment recommendations in light of their interaction with psychosocial and pharmacologic treatments being administered by other specialists. For example, for agitation in patients with hypertension, a non-selective beta blocker, such as propranolol, is generally indicated ahead of other agents for agitation.[37] Conversely, in patients susceptible to orthostatic hypotension, medications with strong alpha-adrenergic affinity should be avoided (SGAs, TCAs, prazosin, and clonidine), particularly because rehabilitation therapies often involve significant positional changes. Finally, as movement disorders are common problems during rehabilitation, in some cases, benzodiazepines will be used for anxiety in spite of the concern regarding cognitive function, when movement disorders (such as athetoid movements or spasticity) has become a rate-limiting step for progress in rehabilitation.

Psychosocial treatments should also consider the issue of co-morbidity, particularly regarding which aspects of a patient's psychiatric presentation should be dealt with in which modality. In general, emotional stress that is amenable to a psychosocial intervention is usually most apparent to the rehabilitation therapists (from speech therapy, occupational therapy, and physical therapy) and nursing staff because they have the most intensive and frequent interactions with patients in this setting. These clinicians tend to ask for psychiatric consultation when they note difficulties in establishing a good working alliance, which are impacting their ability to make progress with the patient's rehabilitation goals.

At times, in this setting with three therapists actively working with the patient in rehabilitation daily, it may be difficult for the psychiatric consultant to know what role to take in counseling patients so as to be effective but not redundant with the other therapists. As a general rule, counseling interventions by consultants from psychiatry, psychology, and social work are most helpful when issues arise that rehabilitation staff find more complex than they can address during their rehabilitation session and/or that they need guidance on how to best address within such situations. Conversely, the consulting psychiatrist should obtain input from rehabilitation therapists about aspects of their cognitive and physical progress that will inform the component of psychiatric counseling the psychiatrist does.

REFERENCES

Access the reference list online at https://expertconsult.inkling.com/.

Intensive Care Unit Patients

34

John Querques, M.D.
Theodore A. Stern, M.D.

Including a chapter on the psychiatric care of patients in the intensive care unit (ICU) runs the risk of suggesting that the evaluation and treatment of patients differ depending on patients' location in the general hospital. Such a risk evokes the unfortunate misnomer "ICU psychosis," with its erroneous suggestion that a psychotic condition can be induced by a patient's mere residence in an ICU and the absurd corollary that transfer out of that environment can be curative. While we maintain that patients and their needs transcend geography, we also recognize that the critical nature of illnesses treated in ICUs creates a unique environment for patients, staff, and consultation psychiatrists alike. In this chapter, the serial presentation of a typical ICU psychiatric consultation highlights the distinguishing characteristics of this distinctive setting, the common reasons for consultation requests in the ICU, and the clinical approach to consultative practice in the ICU.

THE INTENSIVE CARE UNIT SETTING

The chief difference between the ICU and other hospital units is the severity of the morbidity treated there. Patients are admitted to ICUs when they require life support for organ system failure, close monitoring or treatment for potentially life-threatening complications, or careful observation and treatment that cannot be safely provided elsewhere in the hospital. Some of the conditions commonly treated in the ICU include stroke, myocardial infarction (MI), arrhythmias, severe pneumonia, sepsis, multisystem organ failure, trauma, and burns.

Commensurate with this degree of morbidity, the intensity of the treatment arrayed against these life-imperiling conditions contributes significantly to the ICU ambiance. The numerous "lines"—wires, catheters, and tubes—wending their way to and from critically ill patients attest to the high-technology care rendered in the modern ICU. Patients routinely require mechanical ventilation, which entails endotracheal intubation and sedation, and sometimes pharmacologic paralysis; use of vasopressors, cardiac monitors, pacemakers, parenteral nutrition, and several intravenous (IV) antibiotics is common. In more severe situations, renal replacement therapies, intra-aortic balloon pumps, left ventricular assist devices, and heart–lung machines become necessary.

The flashing lights, sounding alarms, and constant whirrings of machines in action create an almost surreal, de-humanized (and de-humanizing) atmosphere that is difficult for patients, families, and staff to tolerate. It seems odd that human lives hang in the balance in such a mechanized setting, the nature and purpose of which has been indicted for engendering delirium, anxiety, and depression in patients; tension and stress that can progress to fatigue and burnout in ICU staff; and feelings of hopelessness, helplessness, frustration, despair, and anger in family members, as well as in patients and staff. The acuity of illness and potential for rapid changes in clinical status create a tremendous pressure for the staff to stay ahead of the curve and a powerful stimulus for families to remain on high alert. When a patient succumbs to an illness that ultimately proves a foe mightier than the awesome therapeutic forces arrayed against it, the staff confronts death and their own personal feelings of weakness, imperfection, insecurity, and impotence that may be stimulated by the loss of a patient. Amid their own struggles, they must somehow comfort bereaved family and friends.

THE PSYCHIATRIST IN THE INTENSIVE CARE UNIT

The psychiatrist called to assess a patient in the ICU approaches the task with all of the preceding in mind. The consultant must brace himself or herself for the experience of intense pressure that surrounds the care of critically ill patients, lest he or she be disarmed by it. The consultant is aware of the strain borne by the physicians and nurses who toil in this environment daily and respects that they might be preoccupied or busy with a clinical matter more pressing than the consultant's own. In dealing with families, the consultant is cognizant that their extreme apprehension might color their account of the patient's history and their appraisal of the current situation. Family members may be unimpressed by the need for a psychiatrist when their loved one is seen as barely clinging to life; they may think of such a consultation as superfluous and they might even be insulted, annoyed, or angered by what feels like an intrusion. Even staff might not be immune to this reaction to the psychiatrist, feeling that the brain—let alone the psyche—is less important than the "real" problem.

The consulting psychiatrist anticipates the likely moribund state of acutely ill patients, their consequent inability to participate in the usual psychiatric examination, and the need to modify the examination accordingly. Even more than usual, the history from the patient may be vague and spotty, if not entirely non-existent. The consultant appreciates that the rapidity of clinical change in patients in the ICU necessitates frequent (probably daily, if not twice-daily) visits; careful review of clinical developments as discussed with the team, culled from the chart, and gleaned from laboratory results; and a degree of accessibility greater than that required on general medical–surgical floors.

In the account of a psychiatric consultation in the ICU that follows, we highlight each of these characteristics of the ICU setting and review three common reasons for psychiatric consultation requests in the ICU: depression, altered mental status, and decision-making capacity. The fictitious, but typical, case also demonstrates that the consultee's question often shifts as the patient's clinical status changes and that a single consultation in the ICU often is actually several consultations in one. The case is presented in segments, much as a real case typically unfolds.

CASE 1

Mr. A, a 70-year-old man with a history of diabetes mellitus, hypertension, a stroke, and an MI was admitted to the ICU with severe pneumonia. He was febrile, tachypneic, and hypotensive, and the team was concerned about the possibility of sepsis. IV antibiotics were started, and by the next morning, the chest film and Mr. A's clinical status had improved, although blood cultures were still pending and the possibility of sepsis still loomed.

Because Mr. A looked depressed, a psychiatrist was called to evaluate depression. When the psychiatrist arrived at the bedside, Mr. A was diaphoretic and taking 30 breaths per minute. In place were two IV catheters, a cardiac monitor, and a Foley catheter. Because his breathing was so labored, Mr. A initiated no speech and he kept his answers short; they were almost inaudible. At times, he appeared to drift off even though he remained awake, and the psychiatrist had to regain Mr. A's attention periodically. Though he was not feeling particularly "joyous," as he said with as much of a laugh as his shallow breath allowed, he denied feeling depressed, sad, or "down in the dumps." Given Mr. A's discomfort, the psychiatrist terminated the interview early; his family was too overwhelmed to talk to the psychiatrist.

The psychiatrist's impression was that Mr. A was delirious due to infection and hypotension. He also suspected an underlying dementia but could not be sure given the paucity of information in the history. In the face of Mr. A's denial of depressed mood, a demonstrable (albeit small) affective display, and inattention, a diagnosis of major depression could not be made. Because the delirium was mild and was not associated with agitation, the psychiatrist recommended checking and monitoring "the usual suspects" but not instituting a psychopharmacologic intervention. Some clinicians would have opted to suggest treatment with a dopamine-blocking agent, even in the absence of agitation.[1,2]

Consultation requests to "rule out depression" are common in the ICU. One reason for this is the notion held by some physicians and nurses that a patient in extreme clinical circumstances *must* be depressed. In this belief, such clinicians consider psychiatric diagnosis to be merely a matter of intuitive common sense rather than of expert clinical judgment.[3] One expects a patient with a serious illness to have certain feelings about his or her plight (e.g., sadness, worry, anxiety, dread, or anger). However, intuition alone is insufficient to make a diagnosis; careful clinical assessment is required. In this case, the observation that Mr. A looked depressed tipped the scale and prompted the consultation request for a more comprehensive examination and expert opinion.

Another reason consultations to assess depression are common in the ICU is mistaking *biography* for *history*,[3] as may have occurred if Mr. A had been asked if he was depressed and he answered affirmatively. The syndrome of depression is not just feeling depressed, sad, or blue, however, but rather a constellation of specific affective, behavioral, and cognitive symptoms and signs. *It is only after a patient's current affective state is embedded in the context of an historical perspective that a diagnosis of major depression can be made.* Under extreme pressure of time and stress, ICU teams often defer to a psychiatrist to elicit the requisite history and to rule depression in or out.

Mr. A's clinical state precluded a thorough elicitation of historical evidence for depression; it highlighted the need for flexibility in modifying the usual clinical examination according to the patient's needs. Faced with a paucity of historical detail, the consultant placed a high premium on the mental status examination; most importantly, he noted inattention, which a diagnosis of depression does not explain. Some might argue that the consultant should not have ruled out depression because he did not collect the data required by the *Diagnostic and Statistical Manual of Mental Disorders* (5th edition; DSM-5),[4] and depression might underlie the delirium. Others, as do we, contend that a diagnosis of depression in the face of delirium is difficult if not impossible to make and that even if it were feasible, the presence of delirium trumps it. If depression is still suspected after the sensorium clears, the consultant can re-interview the patient and also elicit history from family and friends.

The consultant noted the possibility of dementia underlying the delirium. This suspicion was based on a knowledge of Mr. A's history of diabetes and hypertension (both of which can cause microvascular changes in the cerebral circulation), as well as prior stroke and MI (evidence of disease in two separate vascular territories) and knowledge that a "bad" or "insulted" brain (one affected by age, trauma, structural lesions, extensive substance use, human immunodeficiency virus, or dementia) predisposes to delirium. Given the discomfort of Mr. A and the emotional state of the family at this point, the consultant did not yet have sufficient data to make this diagnosis definitively. It must await a change in the clinical circumstances.

A discussion of the "usual suspects" invoked by the consultant and the decision to forego pharmacologic treatment is beyond the scope of this chapter; the interested reader is referred to Chapters 10 and 11.

CASE 1, *continued*

When the consultant returned the following morning, he found that Mr. A had become agitated overnight and had removed both of his IV catheters, thus missing a scheduled dose of antibiotics. Whereas the day before the consultant believed that Mr. A had a quiet delirium, today he believed that the delirium was an agitated one. After ensuring that serum potassium, calcium, magnesium, and albumin levels, as well as the QT interval corrected for heart rate, were normal, he recommended haloperidol 1 mg orally twice daily.

This turn of events highlights the importance of frequent visits to the patient in the ICU. Given the development of agitation, the diagnosis shifted slightly from a quiet to an agitated delirium, which warranted a change in management (i.e., empirical treatment of the agitation with an antipsychotic). Moreover, the agitation in this case had already jeopardized Mr. A's treatment and would very likely continue to do so if not treated. While the team addressed the underlying causes of the delirium (infection and hypotension), empirical treatment with an antipsychotic was essential to quell the agitation.

Low serum levels of potassium, calcium, and magnesium and the administration of certain medications (including haloperidol and atypical antipsychotics) can prolong the QT interval, which heightens the risk of torsades de pointes, a potentially fatal polymorphic ventricular tachyarrhythmia. The QT interval varies with heart rate, age, gender, time of day, and a host of other factors. The proper measurement of the QT interval; the most accurate method for its correction for heart rate; and the relationship among QT prolongation, torsades de pointes, and antipsychotics are the subjects of considerable uncertainty and disagreement, even among experts. Several reviews of this complicated topic are available.[5–8] In short, the administration of haloperidol (or another neuroleptic medication) to an agitated or delirious patient often allows necessary medical treatment to proceed uneventfully. This benefit generally outweighs the risk of a cardiac dysrhythmia.

CASE 1, *continued*

When the psychiatrist returned later that day, Mr. A's respiratory status had worsened and the team was concerned about needing to intubate him. They had solicited his informed consent, but he had refused to give it. Given his altered mental status, they asked the consultant if Mr. A was competent to refuse intubation and mechanical ventilation.

Again illustrated is the propensity for clinical change in ICU patients, the consequent importance of frequent visits, and the broadening of the consultation question. In this way, the psychiatrist often becomes an integral member of the extended team, much as an infectious-disease or endocrine consultant would in this case.

The team mistook *competency* for *capacity*, the former being a legal notion that can be determined only by a judge. *Capacity*, on the other hand, is a clinical term that refers to a patient's mental capability to understand his or her situation (e.g., the illness, the recommended treatment, alternative treatments, and the risks and benefits of those interventions) and to accept or to refuse a treatment recommendation consistent with his or her own personal ideals and values.[9] Whereas any physician, regardless of training, is able to assess a patient's capacity (and, in fact, does so routinely any time he or she does even simple procedures, such as phlebotomy and IV insertion), given their special training in examination of affect, behavior, and thinking, psychiatrists are often called on to render these opinions.

These consultations often arise only when a patient *refuses* a recommended course of therapy. Paternalistic physicians tend to think that the patient's thinking process *must* be impaired if he or she disagrees with the treatment plan; if the patient accepts, his or her capacity is presumed to be intact. However, this common occurrence belies a fundamental misconception about decision-making capacity; that is, it hinges not on *what* the patient decides but on *how* the patient decides it. Whether the patient opts for the course of treatment recommended by the physician, or the therapy that the doctor would choose for himself or herself if the doctor were in the patient's shoes, is irrelevant. Rather, the patient must make a stable choice based on a full understanding of the facts and an appreciation of those facts as they pertain to him or her specifically, and that is consistent with his or her own goals and values.[9]

A layperson's understanding of the medical facts is sufficient. In this case, the consultant wants to assure himself that Mr. A knows and understands the following:

- He might stop breathing because of the pneumonia, an infection of the lungs.
- Should this happen, a machine can breathe for him by means of a tube inserted into his windpipe; without the tube and the machine, he will die.
- Generally, as pneumonia resolves, patients who require a breathing machine eventually resume breathing on their own.
- The risks of the tube include intubation of the food pipe, bleeding, infection, and hoarseness when the tube is removed.
- No alternative treatments exist.

In addition, the consultant must be sure that Mr. A appreciates what these facts mean for him specifically. The following are examples:

- His previous MI renders his heart more vulnerable to the stress of labored breathing and inadequate oxygenation.
- Although small, the risk of infection from the endotracheal tube is greater because he has diabetes.
- Although diabetes compromises his ability to fight the pneumonia, Mr. A does not have a terminal illness and his doctors expect him to recover, even if he requires mechanical ventilation.

Finally, the consultant looks for evidence that Mr. A's choice coincides with his values and goals. For example, if Mr. A repeatedly indicated that he wanted to live while steadfastly rejecting intubation (without which, as he has been told, he would most assuredly die if he stopped breathing on his own), the consultant would rightly detect an inconsistency between the patient's decision and his desire to live.

Because capacity is not global, a patient may have capacity to make some decisions but not others. The reason for this discrepancy lies in the risk-to-benefit ratio of the proposed diagnostic or therapeutic intervention.[10] When the benefit of a treatment far outweighs its risk, the standard for capacity to accept is low, but the standard for capacity to refuse is quite high. In Mr. A's case, the relatively small risk of bleeding, infection, and so on, compared with the overwhelming benefit of mechanical ventilation, establishes a high standard for capacity to refuse this treatment.

CASE 1, *continued*

The psychiatrist offered his opinion that Mr. A did not have the capacity to refuse intubation and mechanical ventilation. When his respirations became even more labored, he was sedated and intubated; mechanical ventilation commenced. He then could not speak and he had no enteral route. The consultant recommended administration of IV haloperidol.

Psychiatric examination and treatment of Mr. A became exceedingly difficult, but not impossible. The psychiatric consultant in the ICU must be creative, resourceful, and ready to accommodate to the changing clinical status of the patient. Lack of an oral route is easily circumvented, because medications can be crushed and delivered through a nasogastric tube or delivered parenterally. Although haloperidol is not approved by the Food and Drug Administration for IV use, widespread experience with this agent attests to its safe and effective use by this route in delirious patients, with the same caveats that apply to oral use.

Intubated patients can communicate in several ways: writing, mouthing answers, pointing to letters on a letter board, or responding to yes/no questions with head nods, eye blinks, or squeezes of the examiner's hand. Requiring practice for both the patient and the physician, these maneuvers can be time-consuming and frustrating, especially when the patient is sedated (which is the rule in intubated patients).

A psychiatric consultant can feel stymied by an obtunded patient's inability to engage in a verbal dialogue. However, a host of physical findings can be made by simple observation (e.g., diaphoresis, dry skin, flushing, mydriasis, miosis, tremor, myoclonus, facial asymmetry). Muscle tone, reflexes (primitive and deep tendon), and pupillary reaction to light are also assessable in a somnolent patient, as are the vital signs. Scoring of verbal, motor, and eye-opening responses according to the Glasgow Coma Scale[11] rounds out the examination of the lethargic patient.

CASE 1, *continued*

Over the next several days, the pneumonia and the delirium steadily improved. Mr. A was successfully extubated, and haloperidol was discontinued. Now able to speak in full sentences, albeit hoarsely, he provided the consultant with additional history. This information, added to collateral data obtained from the family, allowed the consultant to confirm his preliminary impression of the absence of major depression but the presence of an underlying dementia.

CONCLUSION

The successful denouement of this case highlights again the critical importance of flexibility, responsiveness, and resolve on the part of the ICU psychiatric consultant. First a competent physician, the psychiatric consultant must accept responsibility for the patient's care, see it through from initiation of the consultation to its end, and approach the patient and the family fully aware that the arc of each consultation is unique and unpredictable. Patients' beclouded sensoria and family members' taxed emotional states yield information in piecemeal fashion; history emerges only when the bits and pieces are stitched together. Attention to linguistic nuance and limbic music take a backseat to keenness of observation and physical and neurologic examinations. No place for premature diagnostic closure, the ICU adheres to an unfixed timetable and the clinical state of affairs largely resembles a moving target. In the ICU, one minute's certainty becomes the next minute's wild speculation, and the consultation psychiatrist assigned there must always be in "Condition Red."

REFERENCES

Access the reference list online at https://expertconsult.inkling.com/.

Patients With Genetic Syndromes

35

Tamar C. Katz, M.D., Ph.D.
Christine T. Finn, M.D.
Joan M. Stoler, M.D.

OVERVIEW

Genetic syndromes are disorders with a characteristic set of features that are due to an underlying common genetic mechanism, either an individual genetic mutation or a chromosomal abnormality. This chapter provides a brief overview of the genetics of major psychiatric disorders, genetic syndromes, and inborn errors of metabolism that the general psychiatrist may encounter in the hospital or clinic setting. It emphasizes several characteristics about the genetics of major psychiatric disorders. First, psychiatric disorders have a substantial genetic component and understanding the role of genetics in psychiatric pathology is therefore useful for understanding disease physiology and treatment. Second, the environment plays a substantial role in the expression of these disorders; significant interactions between the genetic background and the environment lead to disease expression. Third, this chapter explores several current approaches used to identify the genetic basis of psychiatric disorders and offers recent insights about psychiatric genetics. Finally, this chapter highlights the fact that psychiatric disorders, genetic syndromes, and metabolic diseases may all present with psychiatric symptoms as part of their observed presentation. In fact, behavioral manifestations may be as important as other clinical features for the identification of underlying genetic illnesses.

Knowing when to suspect that a genetic or metabolic issue may be contributing to the presenting condition of a patient is important in formulating a differential diagnosis. Proper identification of genetic and metabolic illness may allow for new opportunities for treatment or intervention directed at the primary process (e.g., correction of hyperammonemia in urea cycle disorders) rather than management of its downstream effects (e.g., delirium). For the most part, the disorders reviewed here may present in late childhood to adulthood; this chapter specifically excludes those disorders that are lethal in infancy or early childhood. When an underlying genetic syndrome or metabolic disease is suspected, a consultation by a geneticist may greatly benefit the patient and help direct clinical management.

Currently, there are no available treatments that can cure genetic syndromes or replace missing genetic material. For this reason, treatment is directed at symptomatic management, surveillance for associated medical conditions, and early developmental interventions. However, an improved understanding of the underlying genetic mechanisms of psychiatric illnesses vastly expands the potential for future targeted therapy, including targeted pharmacologic approaches, gene therapy, and pre-implantation genetic diagnosis, among others.

VARIED APPROACHES TO UNDERSTANDING PSYCHIATRIC GENETICS

Epidemiology of Psychiatric Disorders

Twin, family, and adoption studies can assess the magnitude of genetic versus environmental factors that lead to a phenotype.[1,2] Family studies usually measure the life-time prevalence of a disorder among first-degree relatives of the affected individual, known as the index case. Adoption studies can help further disentangle genetic and environmental influences by comparing rates of a disorder in biological family members with those in adoptive family members. In addition, comparing rates of a disorder in twins that were raised in the same household with twins reared in separate households can provide further evidence about the genetic and environmental influences that lead to expression of the disorder. For example, comparing concordance rates in monozygotic twins raised apart (in different environments) can provide an estimation of the *heritability* of a disorder, as these individuals have near identical DNA and differ primarily in their environment.

Heritability estimates the extent to which differences in the appearance of a trait *across a population* can be accounted for by genetic factors. Heritability is measured on an index from 0 to 1; a heritability index of 1 means that 100% of the variability between individuals in a population is due to genetic factors (i.e., there is no environmental contribution). It is an estimate of the additive sum of all the genetic influences on a trait in the population. A helpful conceptualization of the heritability index is that all traits exist on a continuum from "genetic" to "environmental," with most traits receiving influence from both factors.

Heritability says nothing about the likelihood of a particular individual to inherit a gene, nor about the number of genes that are involved in a trait or the effect size of a

TABLE 35-1 Epidemiology of Common Psychiatric Disorders[3–15]

	HERITABILITY	MONOZYGOTIC CONCORDANCE	DIZYGOTIC CONCORDANCE	LIFETIME RISK (GENERAL POPULATION)	INCREASED RISK IN INDIVIDUALS WITH FIRST-DEGREE RELATIVES
Bipolar disorder	60–85%	45%	5%	1%	10-fold increased risk
MDD	40%	23–49%	16–42%	6.7–17.1%	3-fold increased risk
Panic disorder	45%	24%	11%	4.7%	5-fold increased risk
Schizophrenia	70–89%	50%	15%	1%	10-fold increased risk
Alcohol dependence	35–60%	76%	61%	8–10% female 10–15% male	6–10-fold increased risk
Autism	>90%	70–90%	5–10%	0.66–1.5%	50–100-fold increased risk
ADHD	75%	82%	38%	8.1%	2–8-fold increased risk

MDD, major depressive disorder; ADHD, attention deficit hyperactivity disorder.

given gene. Thus, if the heritability of bipolar disorder is 0.75, this indicates that 75% of the variability observed in those with bipolar disorder is due to genetic causes but does *not* suggest that a particular individual has a 75% chance of developing bipolar disorder.

As Table 35-1[13–15] demonstrates, both genes and environment contribute substantially to the expression of psychiatric disorders, more so for major depressive disorder (MDD) than for schizophrenia or autism, and the relationship between genetic and environmental influences is far more complicated than a simple linear relationship. Environmental factors that contribute to the expression of these disorders include early life events, stressful life events, difficult family environments, exposure to toxins and infectious agents, and a dysregulated immune system.[15]

Gene-by-Environment Interactions

Gene-by-environment interaction is the tendency of two different genotypes to respond to environmental influences in different ways. In some cases, sensitivity to a particular risk factor for a disease may be inherited rather than the disease itself being inherited.

This gene-by-environment interaction was demonstrated in an often-quoted 2003 study of the interaction of the serotonin transporter gene and stressful life events in the onset of episodes of MDD.[16] The serotonin transporter is the target of selective serotonin re-uptake inhibitor (SSRI) antidepressants. There is a common polymorphism in the promoter of the serotonin transporter gene that leads to a "long" allele or a "short" allele lacking a 44 base-pair sequence. The short allele is associated with a reduced expression of the serotonin transporter. The 2003 study by Caspi and colleagues[16] examined a birth cohort of 1037 children followed to age 26 years for evidence of a linkage between the short or long allele of the serotonin transporter gene, stressful life events, and MDD.[17] Stressful life events included problems in employment, financial, housing, health, and relationships. In the absence of stressful life events, the presence of either the short or long allele of the serotonin transporter gene was not associated with depressive symptoms in these individuals. However, with an increasing number of stressful life events, individuals with the short allele of the serotonin transporter gene, compared with those with the long allele, have an increasingly greater number of major depressive episodes, depression symptoms, suicidal thoughts, and suicide attempts. In addition, individuals with the short allele had an increased probability of adult major depressive episodes with increasing childhood maltreatment, whereas individuals with the long allele did not have more adult depression with childhood maltreatment. In both of these examples, individuals heterozygous for the short and long alleles had an intermediate phenotype compared with individuals homozygous for the short or long allele. These experiments show how an environmental factor, such as stressful life events, interacts with the genetic background of an individual, in this case a functional polymorphism in the serotonin transporter gene, to lead to psychiatric disorders such as MDD.

A second study, also conducted by Caspi and colleagues,[18] highlights the effects of childhood trauma in the context of a functional polymorphism in the monoamine oxidase A (MAO_A) gene promoter.[18] The MAO_A promoter has been shown to moderate the association between exposure to early childhood trauma and the development of antisocial or aggressive personality traits. Among children with low MAO_A levels, childhood abuse is associated with higher levels of aggression and antisocial traits, whereas high levels of MAO_A appear to be partially protective against development of these traits even among childhood abuse victims.

Advances in Identification of Genetic Mutations that Underlie Psychiatric Disorders

A major current undertaking in psychiatric neurosciences is to identify genomic regions that influence psychiatric disorders and will provide opportunities for diagnostic accuracy, mechanistic clarification, and treatment precision.

While some disorders are due to single dominant genes, such as the role of the *methyl-CpG-binding protein 2 (MeCP2)*, which is implicated in 95% of Rett syndrome cases, a leading hypothesis for many psychiatric disorders is that multiple risk genes of small effect size interact with one another, and at times with environmental factors, to lead to the disease phenotype. Several approaches commonly used by scientists to identify genes linked to psychiatric disorders are elaborated here.

The *candidate gene approach* focuses on selecting one or a small group of genes believed to be implicated in a disease. This approach relies on a strong hypothesis that a gene's function is likely to be involved in a disease mechanism. For example, studies of the serotonin transporter gene and its role in MDD were derived from pre-existing knowledge that serotonergic function was implicated in depression. Targeted studies of this gene revealed that mutations in the serotonin transporter gene lead to higher rates of depression within the population. These studies focus on a small number of specific genes and as such, they are often faster and less expensive than whole genome studies (discussed below). However, this approach is often not effective for diseases without background knowledge, or for those caused by the combined effect of multiple genes. Candidate gene approaches may utilize techniques such as *fluorescence in situ hybridization (FISH)*, a cytogenetic technique that uses fluorescent probes designed to bind complementarily to any gene of interest. These probes can localize anywhere on the chromosome a gene is located and detect deletions and/or duplications within that gene. Similarly, sequencing or SNP analysis is used for identification of gene mutations other than deletions or duplications.

In contrast, in a *whole genome approach* scientists sequence a near complete copy of an individual's genome to elucidate all mutations present in affected individuals as compared to healthy controls. This approach may identify unexpected genetic mutations anywhere in the genome that are implicated in disease pathology without requiring *a priori* knowledge of a particular gene's function. This higher identification rate is a mixed blessing; while it is more likely to identify the full spectrum of mutations involved in an illness it also yields more false-positives or mutations of unclear clinical significance that may cloud treatment decisions.

Another approach that has become increasingly utilized is *genome-wide association studies* (GWAS), in which hundreds or thousands of genomes are sequenced from individuals with and without a disease and compared with one another to identify genomic variations between these populations. Genomes may be compared between unrelated individuals, biological or adopted relatives, individuals of similar or different ethnicity, environment, or any number of parameters.

GWAS take advantage of the fact that, while most genes are fixed within a population, some genes, known as *polymorphisms*, contain variants within a population. Most polymorphisms exist as single base-pair changes within the gene in which one of the four nucleotide bases is substituted for another. These variations, known as *single nucleotide polymorphisms (SNPs)*, occur approximately once every 300 base-pairs, accounting for healthy genetic diversity within a population. However, GWAS studies reveal that particular SNPs may be more prevalent in certain disease phenotypes, suggesting that a certain SNP may be "associated" with the disease phenotype. Because SNPs occur normally within the population, GWAS require thousands of patients to achieve statistical power to see an association, and must consider factors such as race, gender, and geography to reduce false-positives. GWAS have been instrumental in elucidating genes that are likely implicated in mental illness. For example, GWAS identified over 108 loci that meet genome-wide significance for schizophrenia with sample sizes in some studies exceeding 36,900 subjects.[19] Many of the identified genes are involved in regulatory functions that are impaired in schizophrenic patients including *DRD2* (D_2 dopamine receptor gene), *TCF4* (a transcription factor involved in neurogenesis), *NRGN* (a post-synaptic protein kinase substrate involved in learning and memory), and *ZNF804A* (a transcription factor involved in regulating neuronal connectivity). Multiple genes involved in glutamatergic neurotransmission and synaptic plasticity were also implicated.

In addition to studying SNPs, GWAS have identified over 1000 *copy number variants (CNVs)*, which are duplications or deletions of genomic segments ranging from 1 kilobase to several million bases that in some cases are enriched in patients with schizophrenia, autism, and bipolar disorders.[20] CNVs may be inherited from one or both parents, or may arise as new, or *de novo*, mutations in individuals. These CNVs may interrupt an implicated gene and may cause downshift mutations in later genes. A 2008 study showed that novel CNVs were present in 15% of 150 individuals with schizophrenia and only 5% of controls.[21] Most of the structural variants identified were different and rare, and these variants disrupted genes important for brain development. A larger study of 3391 patients with schizophrenia found a 1.15-fold increased burden of CNVs in patients with schizophrenia than in controls,[22–25] particularly rarer, single-occurrence CNVs. In addition, children with autism spectrum disorders have a significantly increased burden of *de novo* deletions and duplications.[26,27]

Another important finding of GWAS has been the identification of genes that are shared between psychiatric disorders. For example, microduplications of 1q21.1 are associated with both autism spectrum disorder and schizophrenia, and microduplications of 16q11.2 are associated with autism spectrum disorder, schizophrenia, and bipolar disorder, yet individuals who have any one of these disorders are unlikely to have all three.[28] These findings underscore the complex and polygenic etiology of many psychiatric disorders, and the current limitation of understanding how genetic susceptibility translates to phenotypic expression.[29] Another compelling example of the overlapping genetic etiology of varying psychiatric disorders is the discovery of the gene called *Disrupted-in-Schizophrenia-1 (DISC-1)* in a large Scottish family with a high incidence of schizophrenia. This family had a balanced translocation between chromosomes 1 and 11, and *DISC-1* was discovered at the breakpoint of this translocation. *DISC-1* is involved in regulating brain development, neuronal migration, and a signaling pathway important for learning, memory, and mood.[30–35] The translocation in this large extended Scottish family is associated with not only schizophrenia but with bipolar disorder and MDD.[34,35] Genes, such as *DISC-1*, that influence how the brain develops may impart a risk for multiple disorders. In the future, DSM diagnostic categories may be refined on the basis of findings about the genes involved in psychiatric disease.[36]

Once genetic loci of interest have been identified, *linkage studies* are used to generate a logarithm of the odds score (LOD score), which estimates whether two or more genetic loci are perturbed or inherited with higher frequency in affected individuals than would be expected by random chance. An odds ratio of 1000 : 1 (corresponding to an LOD score of 3) is the typical threshold of linkage determination.

These findings may be verified or determined by a recently developed technique, *multiple ligation dependent probe amplification* (MLPA), which allows for detection of differences in genetic copy numbers, and can detect up to 50 different genes that differ by as little as one nucleotide.

An alternative approach is to determine the genetics of intermediate phenotypes or "endophenotypes," in which symptoms manifest at a low level that does not meet criteria for acute mental illness. For instance, the polymorphism in the serotonin transporter gene discussed previously has been associated with increased amygdala reactivity and reduced coupling of corticolimbic circuits seen by neuroimaging. Another intermediate phenotype that is studied is the inhibition of P50-evoked responses to repeated auditory stimuli in schizophrenia.[37]

Assessment of the Patient for Genetic Syndromes

Certain features of the medical history, family history, and physical examination may indicate the possibility of a genetic syndrome that underlies observed psychiatric symptoms. In addition to the comprehensive review of systems and medical history during the initial assessment of patients, inclusion of questions about pregnancy and the perinatal period, birth defects, and surgeries in infancy or early childhood that may have been performed to correct congenital anomalies may provide valuable clues to an underlying genetic syndrome. In addition, careful review of the developmental history (with special attention paid to early developmental milestones) may reveal the presence of specific developmental delays, intellectual disability, or learning disabilities. When inquiring about family history, the clinician should ask specific questions about recurrent miscarriages; stillborn children; early infant deaths; and a family history of intellectual disability, seizures, or congenital illness, which may help in uncovering an underlying genetic disease, especially when the pattern of illness appears to be Mendelian (e.g., dominant, recessive, or X-linked inheritance). Some standard assessment questions are summarized in Table 35-2. In addition, careful physical examination may reveal abnormalities of growth, dysmorphic features, or involvement of various organ systems. Results of imaging studies may aid in the assessment of underlying malformations suggested by physical examination (e.g., echocardiogram to rule out structural heart defects when a murmur is appreciated, neuroimaging when neurological defects are detected).

Selected Genetic Disorders

CASE 1

Ms. A, an 18-year-old woman, presented to the psychiatric emergency room with auditory hallucinations and paranoid ideation. She had a history of attention deficit hyperactivity disorder (ADHD) and oppositional behavior. Her full-scale IQ was 78, and her verbal IQ was 15 points greater than her performance IQ, characteristic of a non-verbal learning disorder. Review of systems revealed surgery in infancy for correction of a congenital heart defect and frequent episodes of sinusitis, otitis media, and pneumonia. On physical examination, she was short with a flat facial expression. Facial features included a high-arched palate, a small chin, and a nose with a broad, square nasal root. Ms. A was admitted to the inpatient psychiatric service and treated with atypical neuroleptics with a good result. Consultation with the genetics service for her dysmorphic facial features and congenital heart defect, along with her cognitive and psychiatric symptoms, resulted in a diagnosis of velocardiofacial syndrome (VCFS).

Disorders Due to Chromosomal Abnormalities and Microdeletions

Velocardiofacial Syndrome/DiGeorge Syndrome

Velocardiofacial syndrome (VCFS) (including most patients previously diagnosed with DiGeorge syndrome), is due to a microdeletion on chromosome 22q11.2, resulting in the loss of up to 60 known and predicted contiguous genes.[38] VCFS has been called a "genetic subtype of schizophrenia," and it is estimated that as many as 2% of patients with schizophrenia may have this disorder and be undiagnosed.[39–41] This rate may be even higher among patients with childhood-onset schizophrenia. The spectrum of selected disorders with associated psychosis is summarized in Table 35-3. Psychiatric symptoms in those with VCFS and schizophrenia do not appear to differ from those without VCFS and schizophrenia. Roughly 60% to 75% of patients with VCFS have significant psychiatric morbidity, including mood disorders, ADHD, autism, substance abuse, anxiety disorders, and oppositional defiant disorder.[41–47] These behavioral difficulties can begin at an early age. The physical features of people with VCFS include: a characteristic facial appearance (broad and squared nasal root, mid-face hypoplasia, short palpebral fissures, retruded chin), cleft palate, and/or velopharyngeal insufficiency (which may manifest as hypernasal speech, nasal regurgitation in infancy, or frequent ear infections); congenital heart defects, aplasia/hypoplasia of the thymus (leading to immune problems); problems with calcium homeostasis; low muscle tone; and scoliosis.[48] Facial hypotonia may result in a somewhat flat, expressionless appearance. Learning disabilities, especially non-verbal learning disorder, are common. However, patients can exhibit only some of these features, and the spectrum of findings may vary even within families. Diagnostic testing is available on a clinical basis and involves testing for the microdeletion by FISH, chromosomal microarray (CMA), or multiplex ligation-dependent probe amplification (MLPA).

TABLE 35-2 Additional History and Physical Examination Assessment for Genetic and Metabolic Illness

Prenatal History
Any complications with pregnancy?
Timing of complication(s)?
Maternal diabetes, systemic illness?
Maternal hypertension, eclampsia, or toxemia?
Maternal infection or high fevers?
Toxic exposures (medications, illicit substances, alcohol, radiation, chemicals)?
Any abnormalities on ultrasound?
Any indications for amniocentesis/chorionic villus sampling (CVS)?
Amniocentesis/CVS results?
Birth/Perinatal History
Mode of delivery (vaginal vs cesarean section, natural vs induced vs emergent)?
Complications with delivery?
NICU or prolonged hospital stay in infancy?
Issues with feeding or growth?
Developmental History
Timing of major verbal and motor milestones?
History of speech, occupational or physical therapy?
Decline in school performance?
History of special education services, academic supports?
Family History
Ethnicity/race of parents?
History of consanguinity?
Patterns of illness in family members?
History of infertility, miscarriages?
History of infant/child deaths?
Family members with surgeries in childhood?
Multi-Organ Review of Systems
History of decompensation with illness?
Dietary history of food intolerances, or unusual food preferences?
Episodic neurologic symptoms?
Problems with linear growth or weight gain?
HELLP (*H*emolysis, *E*levated *L*iver enzymes, *L*ow *P*latelets)?
Physical Examination
Asymmetry of features?
Presence of dysmorphic features?
Signs of neurologic dysfunction?
Psychiatric Review of Systems
Non-specific behavioral problems (e.g., tantrums, violent behavior)?
History of developmental regression (outbursts, hyperactivity)?
Self-injurious behaviors?
Difficulties with sleep?

NICU, neonatal intensive care unit.

Smith–Magenis Syndrome

Smith–Magenis syndrome is due to a microdeletion of chromosome 17p11.2 or a mutation in the gene RAI1.[49] In infancy, these patients may exhibit failure to thrive and hypotonia. Physical findings, which may change over time, include short stature, scoliosis, eye abnormalities, renal problems, heart defects, peripheral neuropathy, and hearing loss (both conductive and sensorineural). Characteristic facial features include a square face with prominent forehead, deep-set and upslanting eyes, a broad nasal bridge with a short nose and fleshy nasal tip, full cheeks, and a "cupid's bow" tented upper lip. The jaw becomes more prominent with age. Although they may have hypersomnolence in infancy, a striking feature of this syndrome is marked sleep disturbance, with absence of rapid eye movement (REM) sleep in some patients. In addition, abnormalities of circadian rhythms and melatonin secretion have been documented.[49–51] Most patients have developmental delay, and their IQs may range from borderline intelligence to moderate intellectual disability. Patients have symptoms of ADHD, tantrums, impulsivity, and a variety of self-injurious behaviors, including onychotillomania (pulling out fingernails and toenails) and polyembolokoilamania (insertion of foreign bodies), head-banging, face-slapping, and skin-picking.[50–53] In addition, they may show stereotypies, most commonly a "self-hug" when happy.[54] The behavioral features may be seen as early as 18 months of age. Abnormalities of lipid profiles have been seen in these patients, with elevations of cholesterol, triglycerides, and low-density lipoprotein.[55] Diagnostic testing involves testing for the microdeletion with FISH, MLPA, and if negative, molecular testing of the RAI1 gene.[50,56]

TABLE 35-3 Selected Disorders With Associated Psychosis

GENETIC SYNDROMES	INBORN ERRORS OF METABOLISM
Velocardiofacial syndrome/DiGeorge syndrome	Acute intermittent porphyria
Prader–Willi syndrome	X-linked adrenoleukodystrophy
Huntington's disease	Niemann–Pick disease, type C
	Metachromatic leukodystrophy
	Tay–Sachs disease
	Wilson's disease
	Mitochondrial disease

Williams Syndrome

A microdeletion on chromosome 7q11.23 results in Williams syndrome. The loss of different genes within the deletion contributes to the phenotype: the elastin gene is thought to be responsible for the supravalvular aortic or pulmonic stenosis and other connective tissue features, while the LIMK1 may be responsible for the visuospatial difficulties.[57] Patients with Williams syndrome are described as having an elfin facial appearance with a broad forehead that narrows at the temples, a short nose with a fleshy nasal tip, large and prominent ear lobes, a wide mouth with full lips, and a small jaw. The iris of the eye has a stellate or lacy appearance. Other characteristics include a hoarse voice and hyperacusis (hypersensitivity to sounds). Intellectual disability in the mild to severe range is usually present, with an average IQ of 56. Specific learning deficits in visual–spatial skills are in marked contrast to strengths in verbal and language domains and are important for the identification and care of these patients. Psychiatric symptoms and conditions include autism, ADHD, depression, and anxiety. Patients with this syndrome may show circumscribed interests or obsessions and may be somatically focused. Despite being socially disinhibited and overly friendly, they tend to have difficulty with peer relationships and may become socially isolated. Affected individuals are described as overly talkative, a feature that may be, in part, reflective of generalized anxiety. Diagnostic testing involves the detection of the microdeletion with FISH or MLPA techniques.[58–61]

Prader–Willi Syndrome

Although several genetic mechanisms may result in Prader–Willi syndrome, the absence of a critical region of the paternally inherited chromosome 15q11–q13 is central to the disorder. This region of chromosome 15 undergoes the process of imprinting, by which genes are switched on or off depending on whether they are of maternal or paternal origin. In contrast to Prader–Willi syndrome, the absence of the maternally derived region results in Angelman syndrome (severe intellectual disability, seizures, ataxia, and characteristic behaviors). Prader–Willi patients may be hypotonic and show failure to thrive in infancy. Most have short stature and small hands, feet, and external genitalia; some have fair skin and hair coloring. A characteristic facial appearance with upslanting almond-shaped eyes and a thin upper lip is seen. The hallmark behavior of this disorder is hyperphagia, with resultant morbid obesity, which develops early in childhood. Behavioral interventions have been effective in controlling this behavior if started at an early age. Psychiatric symptoms and conditions include obsessional thoughts, compulsions, repetitive behaviors, mood disorders, anxiety, psychosis, ADHD, autism, skin-picking, and temper tantrums. Afflicted individuals may have a high pain threshold, and they rarely vomit. These patients may show decreased IQ and learning problems, although they also show areas of relative strength in visual–spatial skills (e.g., as with jigsaw puzzles). Diagnostic testing for Prader–Willi syndrome involves analysis of the critical region for methylation status (the process that determines whether genes are turned on or off) or the detection of the deletion by FISH, MLPA, or CMA.[62–65]

Down's Syndrome

The majority of individuals with Down's syndrome are diagnosed prenatally or soon after birth. This disorder is included in this chapter because of its known association with Alzheimer's dementia, in which cognitive decline or changes in behavior in adults with Down's syndrome may prompt psychiatric consultation. In 95% of cases, Down's syndrome is due to an extra free copy of chromosome 21; the remainder of cases are due to unbalanced translocations or duplications involving the Down's syndrome critical region on chromosome 21 or mosaicism. Down's syndrome is the most common genetic cause of intellectual disability; an increased incidence is observed with older maternal age. Most clinicians recognize the characteristic Down's syndrome face, which consists of eyes with upslanting palpebral fissures, epicanthal folds, and Brushfield's spots (white spots in the iris), a flat nasal bridge, low-set ears, and a protruding tongue. In addition, they have a short neck, short stature, and single transverse palmar crease. These patients may also have a variety of congenital malformations, including heart defects, duodenal atresia, and high rates of hypothyroidism. Intellectual disability is seen in the majority of patients, with an average IQ of 45–48 with a wide range. Social skills are usually more advanced than would be expected given the level of intellectual disability. Decline in cognition or changes in behavior in middle-aged adults with Down's syndrome may indicate Alzheimer's disease. The presence of an extra copy of the *amyloid precursor protein* (APP) gene (one of the causative genes in early-onset Alzheimer's disease) on chromosome 21 is thought to contribute to increased rates of dementia in these patients. Non-specific behavioral symptoms, depression, and anxiety may also be seen. Diagnostic testing for Down's syndrome involves karyotype analysis of chromosomes.[66–69]

Turner's Syndrome

Approximately 50% of cases of Turner's syndrome are due to the loss of an entire X chromosome, which is designated as 45,X. The other cases have other abnormalities of one of the X chromosomes or a mosaic karyotype with 45,X and another cell line. These patients are female, with physical characteristics of short stature, a webbed neck, and a flat, broad chest. Diagnosis may be delayed until adolescence, when these girls fail to develop secondary sexual characteristics (as a result of gonadal dysgenesis). Use of hormonal therapy can help afflicted girls achieve pubertal changes but will not result in fertility. These patients may also have involvement of other organ systems, including congenital heart or kidney disease. Psychiatric symptoms and conditions include ADHD, depression, anxiety, and problems with social skills. Specific learning disabilities (especially visual–spatial deficits) have been reported. Diagnostic testing for Turner's syndrome involves karyotype analysis of chromosomes.[70–72]

Klinefelter's Syndrome

Klinefelter's syndrome is due to the addition of an extra X chromosome, resulting in 47,XXY. These patients are male and usually described as tall, and they may be somewhat hypotonic and clumsy. They typically have a small penis and testes. Contrary to earlier descriptions, they have a male distribution of body fat and hair, although gynecomastia may be seen. They may be first diagnosed in adolescence, after they fail to enter puberty, or as part of an infertility work-up. Use of testosterone can help with the development of secondary sexual characteristics. An increased incidence of ADHD, immaturity, and depression has been reported in these patients. Cognitively, specific learning disabilities are seen. Diagnostic testing for Klinefelter's syndrome involves karyotype analysis of chromosomes.[73]

47,XYY

Males with an extra copy of the Y chromosome have been of interest to the psychiatric profession for many years because of reported increased criminality and antisocial behaviors in these patients. Although early studies conducted on criminal populations were limited by ascertainment bias, more recent studies have continued to show small increases in these behaviors in 47,XYY males compared with controls. However, increased rates of antisocial or criminal behavior appear to be related to the cognitive deficits seen in some of these patients.[74] Physical findings may include accelerated linear growth in childhood and tall stature as adults. They may have a lower than average IQ or specific learning disabilities, especially in reading and language domains. Psychiatric conditions include ADHD and conduct disorders.[75] Overall, the majority of these patients may never receive medical attention because they may lack any identifying features. Diagnostic testing for 47,XYY involves karyotype analysis of chromosomes.

Autosomal Dominant Single-gene Disorders

Huntington's Disease

Huntington's disease is due to an increased number of CAG triplet repeats in the *HD* gene on chromosome 4p16. The normal number of CAG repeats ranges from 10 to 26 in unaffected individuals, where patients with Huntington's disease have between 36 and 121 repeats. The number of repeats may expand from one generation to the next, and increased severity and earlier onset of illness (known as anticipation) may be seen in subsequent generations. Psychiatric symptoms are prominent in the early presentation of this disorder and may include changes in personality, depression, and apathy. Later, progressive cognitive decline and dementia occur. Mood lability and psychosis may also be seen. A high suicide rate is reported in these patients. Early physical findings include dysarthria and clumsiness with deterioration in both voluntary and involuntary movements and the development of chorea. The abnormal movements are often treated with high-potency neuroleptics, but there is no treatment that stops the progressive neurologic decline in this disease. Characteristic atrophy of the caudate and putamen may be apparent on MRI or CT of the brain. Changes in the volume of these structures may be seen on MRI prior to onset of symptoms.[76] Diagnostic testing involves molecular detection of an increased number of CAG repeats in the *HD* gene.[77–79]

Tuberous Sclerosis

Tuberous sclerosis is due to mutations in the *TSC1* (on chromosome 9q23) or *TSC2* (on chromosome 16p13.3) genes. Patients with tuberous sclerosis exhibit characteristic skin findings of flat hypopigmented macules (ash-leaf spots), shagreen patches (raised area with dimpled texture), and angiofibromas (red papular lesions). They may have small pits in their tooth enamel. Tumors occurring in different organ systems are seen, including central nervous system (CNS) tubers, retinal hamartomas, cardiac rhabdomyomas, and renal angiomyolipomas. Seizures are a common feature of this disorder. Patients with tuberous sclerosis have been reported to have symptoms of pervasive developmental disorder and ADHD. Intellectual disability may occur, depending on the extent of CNS involvement. The diagnosis is made using clinical diagnostic criteria and mutation analysis of the *TSC1* and *TSC2* genes.[80,81]

Neurofibromatosis Type I

Neurofibromatosis type I (NF1) is due to a mutation in the *NF1* gene on chromosome 17q11.2, which is believed to result in loss of tumor suppressor function. Abnormalities of skin pigmentation (*café au lait* spots, freckling in axilla or groin), Lisch nodules (small brown spots) on the iris, bony abnormalities, neurofibromas (cutaneous, subcutaneous, or plexiform), and macrocephaly are some of the physical findings in NF1. Complications may arise depending on the size or location of neurofibromas or because of the development of malignant tumors. Psychiatric symptoms may include learning disabilities and ADHD. Diagnosis is made using clinical criteria and mutation analysis of the *NF1* gene.[80,82,83]

X-linked Dominant Disorders

Fragile X Syndrome

In contrast to Down's syndrome, which is the most common *genetic* cause of intellectual disability, fragile X syndrome is the most common *inherited* (i.e., transmitted from a mother who carries the abnormal gene) cause of intellectual disability. Fragile X is the result of dysfunction of the *FMR1* gene at Xq27.3 caused by increased numbers of trinucleotide repeats. Normal alleles have approximately 5 to 44 repeats, and borderline alleles have approximately 45 to 58 repeats. Having greater than approximately 200 CGG repeats results in the full syndrome; a "premutation" allele with approximately 59 to 200 repeats may expand to the full syndrome when passed on from a mother to her children. The full syndrome is most often found in male subjects, but female subjects who carry a full-length mutation on one of their X chromosomes may have features of the disorder of variable severity. Approximately one-third of female subjects with a full-length mutation are thought to be normal, one-third are mildly affected, and the remaining one-third have findings similar to the full syndrome in males. In addition to intellectual disability in the moderate to severe range, physical features, such as large testes, connective tissue disease (loose joints), low muscle tone, and characteristic facial appearance (large head with prominent forehead and jaw, long face with large ears) may help identify males with this disorder. Of note, the facial features and testicular size may be more apparent after puberty. Psychiatric symptoms include autistic features, ADHD, oppositional defiant disorder, mood disorders, and avoidant personality disorder and traits. Premutation carriers (especially males) are at risk for FXTAS (fragile X tremor ataxia syndrome) with progressive ataxia, intention tremor, deficits in executive function and cognitive decline. Generalized anxiety disorders and phobias have also been noted in premutation carriers.[84,85] Diagnostic testing to determine the number of trinucleotide repeats in the *FMR1* gene is widely available.[86–88]

Rett Syndrome

Rett syndrome is due to a mutation in the *MECP2* gene on chromosome Xq28. This syndrome is described in girls who appear normal at birth and during the first several months or years of life. They then experience a progressive loss of developmental skills associated with acquired microcephaly. Additional features include impaired language, loss of purposeful hand movements (replaced by stereotyped hand movements), gait abnormalities, seizures, bruxism, and screaming spells. Girls with less dramatic regression, milder intellectual disability, and autistic-like features have been noted, referred to as variant Rett syndrome.[89] Mutations in the *MECP2* gene, once thought to be fatal in males, have been recognized as a cause of neonatal encephalopathy in males and also intellectual disability with manic-depressive psychosis and pyramidal signs in boys.[90] Diagnostic testing for analysis of the *MECP2* gene is available.[91,92]

METABOLIC DISEASE

Inborn errors of metabolism are a class of genetic disorders that result in dysfunction of production, regulation, or function of enzymes or enzyme co-factors. The disruption of normal metabolic processes may lead to a buildup of pathway by-products or production of alternate substances that cause toxicity. In addition, the absence of essential pathway end products may lead to disease states. Classically, disorders of metabolism have been described in children. However, presentation or recognition of disease may be delayed in patients with relative preservation of enzyme activity that is seen in milder forms of disease, and many disorders have later-onset forms. Metabolic disorders are most often classified on the basis of the abnormal substances involved or by the cell location where the enzyme dysfunction occurs.

Testing for metabolic illness begins at birth, by population screening for a variety of illnesses by state-mandated newborn screening programs. However, the number of diseases tested for varies widely by state, and even the most comprehensive testing has been available only for the past several years. Thus, it is unlikely that older children and adults would have benefited from these screening programs. Furthermore, even the most comprehensive state panels do not rule out all, or even most, genetic and metabolic diseases. For this reason, suspicion of a metabolic disease should be pursued vigorously. Early identification of metabolic illness is crucial to maximize good outcome.

Assessment of the Patient for Metabolic Illness

Essential to the evaluation for possible metabolic illness is careful history-taking. Questions about dietary history (e.g., food intolerances, unusual food preferences, colic or reflux), a history of decompensation associated with minor illness, or history of transient neurologic symptoms (e.g., lethargy, encephalopathy, ataxia, confusion) may lead to detection of an underlying metabolic illness. In addition, careful review of developmental history, especially a history of a developmental regression, loss of skills, or decline in cognition, is important. Because many metabolic illnesses are inherited in an autosomal recessive fashion, a review of family history should include questions about consanguinity and ethnicity. In addition, a history of stillbirths or early infant deaths may prove informative. For example, it is thought that many children who died of Reye's syndrome (manifested by vomiting, liver dysfunction with fatty infiltration, and hypoglycemia) may have had underlying problems with disorders of fatty acid oxidation.

Abnormal results of routine and specialized laboratory studies may be abnormal only during the period of acute illness or metabolic decompensation, thus prompt collection of indicated specimens is crucial for diagnosis. Some general laboratory tests to consider when evaluating a patient for metabolic illness are listed in Table 35-4. Abnormal results on preliminary testing may direct more specific assessment of certain metabolic pathways.[93] Thorough ophthalmologic examination may prove particularly helpful when evaluating metabolic illnesses because the retina provides a window through which to observe the metabolic processes in the brain.

TABLE 35-4 Laboratory Studies to Evaluate Metabolic Illness

LABORATORY TEST	METABOLIC STATE/DISORDERS TESTED FOR
Electrolyte panel	Acidosis, calculation of anion gap
Liver function tests	Storage of abnormal substances in liver
Blood gas	Determination of pH (acidosis vs alkalosis)
Ammonia (NH_3)	Urea cycle disorders—primary elevation Organic acidemias, disorders of fatty acid oxidation—secondary elevation
Lactate, pyruvate	Disorders of energy metabolism
Plasma amino acids	Amino acid disorders (e.g., urea cycle defects, homocystinuria)
Urine organic acids	Organic acidemias
Acylcarnitine profile	Disorders of fatty acid oxidation, organic acidemias
Very long-chain fatty acids	Peroxisomal disorders
Urine mucopolysaccharides	Lysosomal storage disorders
Urine oligosaccharides	Lysosomal storage disorders

Many metabolic illnesses affect the brain, either directly (e.g., via destruction of white matter in metachromatic leukodystrophy) or indirectly (e.g., as encephalopathy in urea cycle disorders). For this reason, neuropsychiatric symptoms associated with metabolic disease may vary widely. Conversely, many metabolic illnesses may have similar acute presentations (e.g., delirium). As is the case with genetic syndromes, some patients meet full criteria for psychiatric disorders, whereas others may exhibit non-specific behavioral findings.

Treatment of psychiatric and behavioral symptoms related to inborn errors of metabolism is typically symptom-focused and uses traditional psychotropic medications in a manner similar to treating symptoms in the general population. However, the ultimate treatment for some of these conditions may be prompt identification of the disorder and mitigation of disease progression via directly addressing the metabolic deficit. Further, the chance for a greater risk of side effects from psychotropic medication use, and the potential to directly impact the metabolic pathway (e.g. with porphyria below) must be considered.[94]

Selected Metabolic Disorders With Psychiatric Features

CASE 2

Mr. B, a 57-year-old man, was admitted to the medical service due to a change in mental status. He was reported to have prominent mood lability, disorientation, and disorganized and racing thoughts. His medical history was significant for hypertension, dental surgery, and a history of hepatitis 6 months previously (attributed to alcohol intake and medication side effects). Mr. B had been consuming six beers at a time, several times a week. His family history was unremarkable. On evaluation, he appeared anxious and restless, and a tremor was noted. He had difficulty with speech and had abnormal facial movements. He exhibited mood lability and had difficulty completing cognitive tasks. Laboratory studies showed a mild elevation of liver transaminases, a low serum ceruloplasmin, and a greatly increased urine copper excretion, which led to a diagnosis of Wilson's disease.

Autosomal Dominant Disorders

Porphyrias/Acute Intermittent Porphyria

The porphyrias are a group of disorders with dysfunction of heme biosynthesis. One of the more common porphyrias is acute intermittent porphyria (AIP), which results from mutations in the *hydroxymethylbilane synthase (HMBS)* gene on chromosome 11q23.3 that causes decreased activity of porphobilinogen (PBG) deaminase. AIP is inherited in an autosomal dominant manner. Episodic neurovisceral attacks are the predominant manifestations of AIP; they consist of recurrent abdominal pain, vomiting, generalized body pain, and weakness. Photosensitivity is not a feature of AIP as it is with some types of porphyria. Psychiatric symptoms and conditions, such as delirium, psychosis, depression, and anxiety, may accompany the acute attacks. Between attacks, constitutional and psychiatric symptoms resolve, although anecdotally these patients are often described as having a distinct personality with long-standing histrionic traits. Over time, indications of demyelination may develop. Of importance to the psychiatric consultant is that medications that upregulate heme biosynthesis may worsen attacks. For this reason, patients treated with medications that upregulate the cytochrome P450 system may make symptoms worse, because heme is an essential part of the cytochrome ring; these patients may be incorrectly labeled as treatment refractory. Offending agents include benzodiazepines, some tricyclic antidepressants, barbiturates, some anticonvulsants (valproate and carbamazepine), oral contraceptives, cocaine, and alcohol. Diagnostic testing focuses on identification of by-products of heme synthesis in the urine or measurement of PBG deaminase levels in the blood. Molecular testing may help to identify relatives of an affected patient who also are at risk for the disorder. Urine that is left standing may discolor, turning dark red or brown as a result of the presence of porphobilinogen and aminolevulinic acid. Treatment for AIP includes supportive care during attacks and the avoidance of offending agents. In addition, a high-carbohydrate diet, folic acid (a PBG diamine co-factor), intravenous heme, and the use of medications that suppress heme synthesis may be helpful.[95–98]

Autosomal Recessive Disorders

Homocystinuria

Classic homocystinuria is due to mutations of the *cystathionine β-synthase (CBS)* gene on chromosome 21q22.3 that results in decreased enzymatic activity of *CBS* and problems with conversion of homocystine to cystine and re-methylation of homocystine to methionine. Patients with preservation of some enzyme activity may respond to high dosages of pyridoxine (vitamin B_6), which acts as a co-factor for *CBS*. Deficiencies of other enzyme co-factors (e.g., B_{12} and folate) may also lead to symptoms. Patients with homocystinuria usually have unremarkable early histories, with development of symptoms in childhood. The patients tend to be tall and thin and are sometimes described as "marfanoid." They may have features of connective tissue disease, such as a pectus excavatum, lens dislocation, scoliosis, and a high-arched palate. Unlike patients with Marfan's syndrome, they may have restricted mobility of their joints. It is thought that high levels of homocystine may interfere with collagen cross-linking, which results in connective tissue symptoms. In addition, abnormalities in collagen can lead to disruptions of the vascular endothelium and thrombotic events with disabling or fatal consequences. High levels of homocystine or other factors are also thought to be neurotoxic and, when left untreated, lead to intellectual disability and learning disabilities. During the 1960s and 1970s, these patients were reported to have increased rates of schizophrenia, which was attributed to the hypothesized central role of methionine in both disorders. More recent studies have not supported an increased risk of schizophrenia or psychosis but have shown depression, obsessive–compulsive disorder, personality disorders, and other behavioral disturbances. Urinary nitroprusside testing for disulfides and measurement of high levels of homocystine and methionine (the precursor of homocystine) in the blood help make the diagnosis. Newborn screening for homocystinuria has been available in some states for more than 30 years. Molecular testing is also available to detect biallelic pathogenic variants in *CBS*. Treatment focuses on providing a diet low in methionine and supplementation with vitamin co-factors and cystine (which becomes an essential amino acid in these patients). Use of the supplement betaine also aids in lowering homocystine levels.[99,100]

Wilson's Disease

Wilson's disease is due to mutations in the *ATP7B* gene, located on chromosome 13q14.21, which lead to copper deposition in the CNS as a result of decreased levels of copper-transporting adenosine triphosphatase (ATPase). Signs and symptoms of liver dysfunction (e.g., jaundice, hepatomegaly, cirrhosis, hepatitis) may be present, along with abnormal liver function tests. Of particular importance to psychiatrists are changes in personality, mood lability (including pseudobulbar palsy), cognitive decline, and other behavioral changes that may be among the earliest symptoms of Wilson's disease.[101] A recent small study has also reported significantly higher rates of bipolar disorder and depression in Wilson's patients.[102] Neurologic symptoms are most often extrapyramidal in nature and can include tremor, dysarthria, muscular rigidity, parkinsonism, dyskinesia, dystonia, and chorea. Seizures may also occur. The hallmark of this disorder is the Kayser–Fleischer ring, a yellow-brown ring (a consequence of copper deposition in the cornea) that is visible on slit-lamp ophthalmologic examination. Accumulations of copper in other organ systems may result in a variety of complications, including arthritis, renal tubular dysfunction, and cardiomyopathy. Confirmatory diagnostic testing includes measurement of reduced bound copper and ceruloplasmin in the serum and increased copper excretion in the urine, as well as testing to detect *ATP7B* mutations. Copper deposits may be seen on head magnetic resonance imaging (MRI) or in the liver by way of a liver biopsy. Treatment, in the form of chelation of copper (with medications such as D-penicillamine), treatment with zinc and supplementation with antioxidants, is available. Avoidance of copper-rich foods, such as shellfish, liver, chocolate, and nuts, is recommended. Of note, patients with Wilson's disease may be overly sensitive to extra-pyramidal effects of antipsychotic medications.[103] Unfortunately, liver damage may progress to liver failure and necessitate liver transplantation in some patients.[104]

Metachromatic Leukodystrophy

Metachromatic leukodystrophy is a lysosomal storage disorder with deficiency of the enzyme arylsulfatase A and mutations in the *ARSA* gene located on chromosome 22q13.31. As a result, abnormal storage of galactosyl sulfatide (cerebroside sulfate) occurs in the white matter of the central and peripheral nervous systems. The disorder may occur in infancy, childhood, or adulthood. For the later-onset forms psychiatric symptoms may be an earlier manifestation of the disease, with a decline in cognition, personality changes, and psychotic features (including hallucinations and delusions). In some cases, psychosis may predate the onset of other symptoms by several years. Two adult-onset forms are associated with specific genetic changes, including homozygous *P426L* mutations and heterogeneous carriers of *I179S* mutations. Neurologic symptoms may include ataxia and walking difficulties, dysarthria and dysphagia, and pyramidal signs. Vision loss may also occur. Brain MRI may show periventricular changes; eventually white matter atrophy caused by loss of myelin may be noted. In this disorder, the relationship between myelination deficits and the psychosis may provide a better understanding of the role of connectivity in the development of schizophrenia. Diagnostic testing involves measurement of elevated urine sulfatides and decreased levels of arylsulfatase A in blood. Confirmatory molecular testing of the ARSA gene is available. No treatment is currently available, although bone marrow transplantation may delay the progression of symptoms and is most beneficial when done prior to symptom onset.[94,105–107]

Niemann–Pick Disease, Type C

Niemann–Pick disease, type C (NPC) is a condition that results in abnormal cholesterol esterification and lipid storage in lysosomes caused by mutations in the *NPC1* gene on chromosome 18q11–q12 or the *NPC2* gene on 14q24.3. The disorder may appear in childhood or adolescence (and rarely in adulthood) with early findings of ataxia, coordination problems, and dysarthria. Vertical supranuclear palsy is the hallmark of the disorder. Seizures and hepatosplenomegaly may be present. Psychiatric symptoms include progressive cognitive decline and dementia and may be presenting symptoms in late-onset disorders. In addition, several reports have documented the initial presentation of this disorder as psychosis or schizophrenia as well as bipolar disorder and OCD. Diagnosis is based on demonstration of characteristic pathologic findings in the skin or bone marrow; abnormal cholesterol esterification in fibroblasts; and molecular analysis of the *NPC1* gene, which is positive in 95% of cases. Of note is that panels testing blood and urine specimens for lysosomal storage diseases will be normal in NPC, so diagnostic suspicion must direct a more comprehensive work-up.[108–111]

GM2 Gangliosidosis (Tay–Sachs Disease, Late-onset Type)

Tay–Sachs disease is another lysosomal storage disease, with accumulation of GM2 gangliosides in neurons. Mutations in the *HEXA* gene on chromosome 15q23–q24, which encodes the alpha subunit of hexosaminidase A, lead to an enzyme deficiency. Most clinicians are familiar with the infantile-onset form of the disorder but may not be aware of the later-onset forms that can occur with preservation of some enzymatic activity. Patients may present with psychiatric symptoms of psychosis, mood lability, catatonia, and cognitive decline. Physical findings are those of progressive neurologic dysfunction and include early ataxia, coordination problems, dysarthria, and progressive neurologic dysfunction (e.g., with dystonia, spasticity, and seizures). Macular cherry-red spots, the hallmark of the early-onset form, are not present in the later-onset form. Diagnosis is based on analysis of enzyme levels in the blood or mutation analysis, which is especially helpful for prenatal genetic counseling. Tay–Sachs may occur in people of various ethnic and racial backgrounds, and prenatal screening is offered, especially to those of Ashkenazi Jewish descent, wherein the carrier rate is estimated to be 1:30, and to French Canadians, who have a carrier rate of 1:50. There is no treatment available for Tay–Sachs disease.[112,113]

X-linked Disorders

X-linked Adrenoleukodystrophy

X-linked adrenoleukodystrophy is also a disorder of abnormal storage but in the peroxisome instead of the lysosome. In this disorder, deficiency of lignoceroyl-CoA ligase results from mutations in the *ABCD1* gene on Xq28 and leads to accumulation of very long-chain fatty acids (VLCFAs) in the cerebral white matter and adrenal cortex. On account of its X-linked manner of inheritance, male subjects are described with the full syndrome. Female carriers, however, can also exhibit a spectrum of associated symptoms with varying degrees of severity, and they may be misdiagnosed with other disorders, including multiple sclerosis. Often, the first signs and symptoms of the disorder result in a diagnosis of ADHD for affected males. In the adult-onset form, high rates of mania and psychosis are reported. Other early signs may include difficulty with gait, handwriting, or speech. Progressive loss of motor skills, vision, and hearing, accompanied by continued decline in cognition, occurs over a period of months to years. Accumulation of VLCFAs in the adrenal cortex may cause elevation of adrenocorticotropic hormone and other findings associated with adrenal dysfunction. These adrenal abnormalities, brain MRI findings, and elevated levels of VLCFAs in the blood can lead to the diagnosis. Confirmatory molecular testing for mutations in the *ABCD1* gene is available. Treatment for adrenal dysfunction is recommended, but there is no treatment available for the neurologic sequelae of this disease, insofar as the use of Lorenzo's oil has not proven to be effective. Bone marrow transplantation has been proposed, but concerns about the high morbidity and mortality rate associated with the procedure have limited its use.[114–116]

Urea Cycle Defects—Ornithine Transcarbamylase Deficiency

Disorders of the urea cycle interfere with the normal urinary excretion of excess nitrogen via conversion to urea. Several enzymes make up the urea cycle, and deficiencies of these enzymes lead to variable failure to manage nitrogenous waste from protein. Ornithine transcarbamylase (OTC) deficiency is one of the more common urea cycle disorders, and it is inherited in an X-linked manner as a result of mutations in the *OTC* gene on Xp21.1. Although male subjects with this disorder usually present in the neonatal period with marked hyperammonemia and resultant sequelae, female carriers of the *OTC* gene may have a more variable course, owing to lyonization of X chromosomes. Their presentations may occur at any age, and female carriers range from being asymptomatic to being as severely affected as their male counterparts. Psychiatric symptoms in affected female carriers may include intermittent episodes of delirium, ataxia, lethargy, and confusion.[117–122] Patients may report a history of self-restriction of protein in the diet or severe decompensations with vomiting illnesses or fasting (which may result in an endogenous protein load via catabolism of muscle). During symptomatic episodes elevations of ammonia, urine orotic acid, and liver function, accompanied by a characteristic pattern of plasma amino acids, aid in diagnosis. Confirmatory molecular diagnostic testing by mutation analysis, or enzymatic assay of liver tissue, is available. Treatment is focused on maintaining a low intake of dietary protein and providing supplemental essential amino acids and urea cycle intermediates. Acutely, medications that allow alternate excretion of nitrogen compounds may be used for high ammonia levels; in some cases hemodialysis is required for rapid control of hyperammonemic episodes. Of note, the use of valproate has been reported to cause acute liver failure in patients with OTC and also to precipitate a hyperammonemic crisis in female carriers. It is thought that valproate inhibits urea synthesis and can lead to hyperammonemia.[123,124] Hyperammonemic crisis has also been observed in female carriers on a high-protein diet.

Lesch–Nyhan Syndrome

Lesch–Nyhan syndrome is a disorder of purine metabolism owing to deficiency of hypoxanthine-guanine phosphoribosyltransferase (HPRT), caused by mutations in the *HPRT1* gene at Xq26–27.2. Hyperuricemia and hyperuricuria occur and can result in deposition of urate crystals in the joints, kidneys, and bladder. Affected males exhibit hallmark behaviors of self-injury and self-mutilation (including head-banging and biting of lips and fingers). Mutilation may be severe enough to warrant removal of teeth or the use of restraints. Additional symptoms may include aggression, depression, anxiety, motor stereotypies, distractibility, and attentional deficits and seem to be more strongly related to deficiencies of guanine recycling. Intellectual disability may occur, although progressive loss of cognition does not. Diagnostic testing reveals increased uric acid production and excretion, decreased HPRT activity, and confirmatory molecular analysis of the *HPRT1* gene. Although allopurinol may control sequelae of high uric acid, it does not ameliorate the neurologic or psychiatric symptoms. There is some suggestion that dysfunction of dopamine metabolism may be related to the CNS pathology in this disorder.[125–128]

Mitochondrial Disorders

Disorders that involve dysfunction of the mitochondria are diverse and include disorders of fatty acid beta-oxidation or pyruvate metabolism and dysfunction of the Krebs cycle or oxidative phosphorylation by the electron transport chain. Commonly, they may be thought of as disorders of energy metabolism. Mitochondrial disorders are inherited from the mother, in the case of those coded for by genes located in the mitochondrial genome, or from either or both parents in those coded for by genes located in the nuclear genome. Mitochondrial syndromes may be characterized as specific disorders (e.g., mitochondrial encephalopathy with lactic acidosis and stroke-like episodes) or may involve dysfunction of multiple organ systems (e.g., cardiomyopathy, diabetes, hearing loss). Body tissues with high energy demands, including the brain, may be preferentially affected. Psychiatric symptoms and conditions in mitochondrial disorders are largely uncharacterized but may include depression, delirium, dementia, and psychosis. Additionally, current thinking about the role of inflammation in contributing to the development of psychiatric disorders may indicate a pathway where deficiencies in energy production can lead to symptoms. Mitochondrial dysfunction may be suggested by elevations of lactate or pyruvate or by presence of by-products of fatty acid oxidation or other mitochondrial pathways. Diagnosis by analysis of specific mutations is available for some disorders, whereas others require functional analysis of pathways using skin or muscle tissue. Dietary and vitamin supplementation, prevention of lactic acidosis with acute decompensations, and management of associated medical conditions are the mainstays of treatment for mitochondrial disorders.[129,130]

Teratogen Exposure

A variety of syndromes and characteristic features are associated with prenatal exposure to prescribed medications, alcohol and drugs of abuse, maternal illnesses (e.g., diabetes) and infectious agents, chemicals, radiation, and other toxins. Physical, cognitive, and psychiatric findings vary depending on the amount and timing of exposure. A detailed prenatal history should be obtained as part of a comprehensive evaluation of a patient.

Fetal Alcohol Spectrum Disorders

Alcohol is the major teratogen to which fetuses are exposed; it can result in a wide spectrum of cognitive, behavioral, and physical findings known as fetal alcohol spectrum disorder (FAS). The severity of symptoms appears to be dose related, although a critical threshold of alcohol intake has not been identified. High levels of blood alcohol (achieved by binge drinking) may result in more severe manifestations. Psychiatric symptoms and conditions include ADHD, depression, mood lability, anxiety, aggression, and oppositional defiant behaviors. Physical features include prenatal and postnatal growth deficiency and a characteristic facial appearance manifested by a small head, a flattened mid-face, the presence of epicanthal folds, a flat philtrum with a thin upper lip, and small jaw. Learning disabilities and cognitive limitations are common. Diagnosis rests on clinical features with recognition of characteristic findings in the context of a known history of prenatal alcohol exposure. There is a spectrum of features seen encompassing full fetal alcohol syndrome on the most severe end to partial FAS (with some of the features) and/or alcohol-related neurodevelopmental disorder (where there may be no outward physical features). Exposure to multiple drugs *in utero* should also be considered in all patients evaluated for FAS. No confirmatory laboratory or imaging tests are available, although recent MRI studies have documented structural abnormalities of the brain with absence or small size of the corpus callosum being reported in FAS patients.[131–134]

CONCLUSION

Because the selected genetic and metabolic syndromes described in this chapter are frequently associated with psychiatric symptoms, an awareness of these disorders is important for the general psychiatrist. Given the surge in recent psychiatric genetic technologies, we anticipate that an understanding of the underlying genetics of psychiatric disorders will become increasingly important in refinement of diagnostic and treatment criteria in the coming years.

REFERENCES

Access the reference list online at https://expertconsult.inkling.com/.

SUGGESTED READING

Gene Clinics, available at: http://www.Geneclinics.org

Online Mendelian Inheritance in Man (OMIM), available at: http://www.ncbi.nlm.nih.gov/omim/

POSSUM and software, available at: http://www.possum.net.au/

Coping With Illness and Psychotherapy of the Medically Ill

36

Steven C. Schlozman, M.D.
James E. Groves, M.D.
Anne F. Gross, M.D.

Management of psychiatric illness in medically ill individuals requires knowledge of medicine and psychiatry as well as specialized psychotherapeutic techniques. In inpatient settings, challenges to compassionate psychological care are abundant (e.g., decreasing length of stays, severe medical and surgical illnesses, prominent side effects of treatment, threats to privacy, and procedures and technology that limit a patient's ability to communicate). Nonetheless, consultation psychiatrists strive to improve the patient's ability to cope with trying circumstances that surround their illness and its treatment.

Illness is a stress that requires both patients and the systems that care for them to adapt (e.g., to ongoing pain, impaired cognition, loss of bodily function, threats to life, and disruptions in everyday function) via enhancements in coping strategies and interpersonal relationships. Problematic coping with illness can create serious problems for both patients and physicians. However, when addressing this phenomenon, it is important to recognize that few medical schools or residency programs train physicians in the management of interpersonal stress and discomfort (in patients and in themselves) that is engendered by medical illness. This absence stands in stark contrast to the way the art of medicine was conceptualized 100 years ago. Indeed, it is ironic, and yet understandable, that we experience a profound sense of impotence when a cure cannot be found, despite our increasing ability to heal the sick.[1,2]

Fortunately, the consultation–liaison (C-L) psychiatrist is ideally suited to assist both patients and physicians with the demands of caring for the medically ill. From a psychological standpoint, the psychiatrist appreciates the powerful emotions and defense mechanisms that swirl in and around the hospital bed. These observations are relevant in both the consultative setting and in the outpatient office. In fact, specific psychotherapeutic techniques (e.g., cognitive-behavioral therapy [CBT] and group therapy) have been developed for work with the medically ill. This chapter addresses the fundamentals of coping, the process of adaptation to illness, as well as the art of working psychotherapeutically with the medically ill.

WHAT EXACTLY IS COPING?

Coping is best defined as problem-solving behavior that is intended to bring about relief, reward, quiescence, and equilibrium. Nothing in this definition promises permanent resolution of problems. It does imply a combination of knowing what the problems are and how to go about embarking on a correct course that will improve function.[3,4]

In ordinary language, the term *coping* is used to mean only the outcome of managing a problem, and it overlooks the intermediate process of appraisal, performance, and correction that most problem-solving entails. Coping is not a simple judgment about how some difficulty was worked out. It is an extensive, recursive process of self-exploration, self-instruction, self-correction, self-rehearsal, and guidance gathered from outside sources.

At virtually every step of patient care, physicians and patients actively assess coping ability. Though this appraisal is not always conscious, the conclusions drawn about how a patient is processing his or her illness have a tremendous impact on therapeutic decisions, on psychological well-being, and indeed on the overall course of illness. However, accurate appraisal of coping skills is hampered by muddled definitions of coping, by competing methods of assessment, by a general lack of conscious consideration of how a patient copes, and by uncertainty about whether particular coping styles are effective.[3–6]

Early conceptualizations of coping centered around the Transactional Model for Stress Management were put forth first by Lazarus[7] and colleagues in the late 1960s. This conceptualization stressed the extent to which a patient interacts with his or her environment as a means of managing the stress of illness. These interactions involve appraisals of one's medical condition in the context of psychological and cultural overlays that vary from patient to patient. Although this definition of coping persists, it may be too broad to allow for standard assessments of patients. Thus, though multiple studies of patient coping exist, most clinicians favor a more open-ended approach to evaluation that considers the unique backgrounds that the patient and the doctor bring to the therapeutic setting.[6]

Coping with illness and its ramifications cannot help but be an inescapable part of medical practice. Therefore, the overall purpose of any intervention, physical or psychosocial, is to improve coping with potential problems beyond the limits of illness itself. Such interventions must take into account both the problems to be solved and the individuals most closely affected by the difficulties.

How anyone copes depends on the nature of a problem as well as on the mental, emotional, physical, and social resources one has available for the coping process. The hospital psychiatrist is in an advantageous position to evaluate how physical illness interferes with the patient's conduct of life and to see how psychosocial issues impede the course of illness and recovery. This is accomplished largely by knowing which psychosocial problems are pertinent, which physical symptoms are most distressing, and what interpersonal relations support or undermine coping.

Assessment of how anyone copes, especially in a clinical setting, requires an emphasis on the "here and now." Long-range forays into the past are relevant only if they illuminate the present predicament. In fact, more and more clinicians are adopting a focused and problem-solving approach to therapy with medically ill individuals. For example, supportive therapies for medically ill children and adults in both group and individual settings have reduced psychiatric morbidity, and have had measurable effects on the course of non-psychiatric illnesses.

WHO COPES WELL?

There are few paragons who cope exceedingly well with all problems. For virtually everyone, psychiatrists included, sickness imposes a personal and social burden, threat, and risk; these reactions are seldom precisely proportional to the actual dangers of the primary disease. Therefore, effective copers may be regarded as individuals with a special skill or with personal traits that enable them to master many difficulties. Characteristics of good copers are presented in Table 36-1. These characterizations are collective tendencies; they seldom typify any specific individual (except the heroic or the idealized). No one copes exceptionally well at all times, especially with problems that are associated with risk and that might well be overwhelming. However, effective copers appear able to choose the kind of situation in which they are most likely to prosper. In addition, effective copers often maintain enough confidence to feel resourceful enough to survive intact. Finally, it is our impression that those individuals who cope effectively do not pretend to have knowledge that they do not have; therefore, they feel comfortable turning to experts who they trust. The better we can pinpoint which traits a patient appears to lack, the better we can help a patient cope.

TABLE 36-1 Characteristics of Good Copers

1. They are optimistic about mastering problems and, despite setbacks, generally maintain a high level of morale.
2. They tend to be practical and to emphasize immediate problems, issues, and obstacles that must be conquered, even before visualizing a remote or ideal resolution.
3. They select from a wide range of potential strategies and tactics, and their policy is not to be at a loss for fallback methods. In this respect, they are resourceful.
4. They heed various possible outcomes and improve coping by being aware of consequences.
5. They are generally flexible and open to suggestions, but they do not give up the final say in decisions.
6. They are composed, although vigilant, in avoiding emotional extremes that could impair judgment.

WHO COPES POORLY?

Bad copers are not necessarily bad people, nor even incorrigibly ineffective people. In fact, it is too simplistic merely to indicate that bad copers have the opposite characteristics of effective copers. As was stressed earlier, each patient brings a unique set of cultural and psychological attributes that impacts the capacity to cope. Bad copers are those who have more problems in coping with unusual, intense, and unexpected difficulties because of a variety of traits. Table 36-2 lists some characteristics of poor copers.

Indeed, structured investigations into the psychiatric symptoms of the medically ill have often identified many of the attributes of those who do not cope well. Problems such as demoralization, anhedonia, anxiety, pain, and overwhelming grief all have been documented in medical patients with impaired coping.

WHAT INTERFERES WITH OUR ABILITY TO ADAPT TO ILLNESS?

Adaptation to medical illness is affected by individual factors, by intrahospital factors, and by extrahospital factors;[8] understanding all three is crucial to an assessment of how an individual will adapt to illness. Individual (intrapersonal) factors include psychiatric diagnoses (including, but not limited to, depression, anxiety, neurocognitive disorders, substance use disorders, post-traumatic stress disorder [PTSD], factitious disorders, somatic symptom and related disorders, and sleep–wake disorders; their developmental stage, their experience with trauma, and their understanding of the illness). In addition, personality style and personality disorders (including histrionic, obsessive, paranoid, narcissistic, and borderline personality disorders) affect how a person copes with receiving bad news, how they interact with medical staff, and how they communicate with others in their life.[8] Holland and colleagues[9] described the "Five Ds" when discussing what illness means to a patient (e.g., distance [the interruption of interpersonal relationships]; dependence [having to rely on others]; disability [inability

TABLE 36-2 Characteristics of Poor Copers

1. They tend to be excessive in self-expectation, rigid in outlook, inflexible in standards, and reluctant to compromise or to ask for help.
2. Their opinion of how people should behave is narrow and absolute; they allow little room for tolerance.
3. Although prone to firm adherence to preconceptions, they may show unexpected compliance or be suggestible on specious grounds, with little cause.
4. They are inclined to excessive denial and elaborate rationalization; in addition, they are unable to focus on salient problems.
5. Because they find it difficult to weigh feasible alternatives, they tend to be more passive than usual and they fail to initiate action on their own behalf.
6. Their rigidity occasionally lapses, and they subject themselves to impulsive judgments or atypical behavior that fails to be effective.

to achieve]; disfigurement; and death). Intrahospital factors include the characteristics of the illness (e.g., its time course, the intensity of pain, its impact on sleep, surgical interventions, and chemotherapy), whereas extrahospital variables (e.g., finances, housing, interpersonal relationships, and sociocultural/language barriers) are also key issues.[8]

THE ROLE OF RELIGION

The significance of religious or spiritual conviction in the medically ill deserves special mention. Virtually every C-L psychiatrist works with patients as they wrestle with existential issues (such as mortality, fate, justice, and fairness). Such ruminations cannot help but invoke religious considerations in both the patient and the physician; moreover, there is a growing appreciation in the medical literature for the important role that these considerations can play.

In some investigations, being at peace with oneself and with one's sense of a higher power was predictive of both physical and psychiatric recovery.[10,11] However, other studies have suggested that resentment toward God, fears of God's abandonment, and a willingness to invoke satanic motivation for medical illness were all predictive of worsening health and an increased risk of death.[12]

Because the C-L psychiatrist's role involves identification and strengthening of those attributes that are most likely to aid a patient's physical and emotional well-being, effective therapy for the medically ill involves exploration of the religious convictions of a patient; fostering those elements is most likely to be helpful. It is *never* the role of the physician to encourage religious conviction *de novo*. At the same time, ignoring religious content risks omitting an important element of the psychotherapeutic armamentarium.

THE MEDICAL PREDICAMENT—BRINGING IT ALL TOGETHER

Coping refers to how a patient responds and deals with problems within a complex of factors that relates to disease, sickness, and vulnerability. In approaching chronically ill patients, it is helpful to conceptualize *disease* as the categorical reason for being sick, *sickness* as the individual style of illness and patienthood, and *vulnerability* as the tendency to be distressed and to develop emotional difficulties in the course of trying to cope.

Given these definitions, the psychiatrist needs to first ask *why now*? What has preceded the request for consultation? How does the patient show his or her sense of futility and despair? How did the present trouble, both the medical and the corresponding coping challenges, come about? Was there a time when such problems could have been thwarted? It is also important to note that not infrequently the treatment team is even more exasperated than the patient. In these instances, one must guard against the assumption that it is only the patient who is troubled by the medical predicament.

In fact, if there is any doubt about the gap between how the staff and a patient differ in cultural bias and social expectations, one should listen to the bedside conversation. Good communication may not only reduce potential problems, but it actually helps patients to cope better. Good coping is a function of empathic connection and respect between the patient and the physician regarding the risks and points of tension related to treatment. The psychiatrist is not the sole vessel to hold professional concerns about coping, but has unique skills that are ideally suited to address the challenges of how patients cope. As already mentioned, much of chronic disease evokes existential issues (such as death, permanent disability, low self-esteem, dependence, and alienation); these are fundamentally psychiatric concerns.

Given all of this, it is important to remember that psychiatry does not arbitrarily introduce psychosocial problems. If, for example, a patient is found to have an unspoken, but vivid, fear of death or to be suffering from an unrecognized and unresolved bereavement, fear and grief are already there, not superfluous artifacts of the evaluation itself. Indeed, open discussion of these existential issues is likely to be therapeutic; active denial of their presence is potentially detrimental, because it risks empathic failure and the poor compliance that accompanies the course of patients who feel misunderstood or unheard.

Being sick is, of course, much easier for some patients than for others, and for certain patients, it is preferred over trying to make it in the outside world. There is too much anxiety, fear of failure, inadequacy, pathological shyness, expectation, frustration, and social hypochondriasis to make the struggle for holding one's own appealing. At key moments of life, sickness is a solution. Although healthy people are expected to tolerate defeat and to withstand disappointments, others legitimize their low self-esteem by a variety of excuses, denial, self-pity, and symptoms, long after other patients return to work. Such patients thrive in a complaining atmosphere and even blame their physicians. These are perverse forms of coping and they complicate the task of the hospital psychiatrist.

The clinician must also assess the motivation of staff and patients when a psychiatric intervention is requested. Additionally, clinicians need to be aware that the real question is not always the problem for which one is consulted. For example, the request for psychiatric consultation to treat depression and anxiety in a negativistic and passive–aggressive patient is inevitably more complicated than a simple recognition of certain key psychiatric symptoms. Those with primitive defenses can generate a profound sense of hopelessness and discomfort in their treaters. It is often an unspoken and unrecognized desire by physicians and ancillary staff that the psychiatrist shifts the focus of negativity and aggression onto himself or herself, and away from the remaining treatment team. If the consulting psychiatrist is not aware of these subtleties, the intent of the consultation will be misinterpreted and the psychiatrist's efforts will ultimately fall short.

COPING AND SOCIAL SUPPORT

Every person needs, or at least deserves, a measure of support, sustenance, security, and self-esteem, even if they are not patients at all, but human beings encountered at a critical time.

In assessing problems and needs, the psychiatrist can help by identifying potential pressure points (e.g., health and wellness, family responsibility, marital and sexual roles, jobs and money, community expectations and approval, religious and cultural demands, self-image and sense of inadequacy, and existential issues) where trouble might arise.

Social support is not a hodgepodge of interventions designed to cheer up or straighten out difficult patients. Self-image and self-esteem, for example, depend on the sense of confidence generated by various sources of social success and support. In a practical sense, social support reflects what society expects and therefore demands about health and conduct.

Social support is not a "sometime" thing, to be used only for the benefit of those too weak, needy, or troubled to get along by themselves. It requires a deliberate skill that professionals can cultivate, in recognizing, refining, and implementing what any vulnerable individual needs to feel better and to cope better. In this light, it is not an amorphous exercise in reassurance, but a combination of therapeutic gambits opportunistically activated to normalize a patient's attitude and behavior. Techniques of support range from concrete assistance to extended counseling.[13,14] Their aim is to help patients get along without professional support. Social support depends on an acceptable image of the patient, not one that invariably "pathologizes." If a clinician only corrects mistakes or points out what is wrong, bad, or inadequate, then insecurity increases and self-esteem inevitably suffers.

COURAGE TO COPE

Most psychiatric assessments and interventions tend to pathologize and to emphasize shortcomings, defects, and deviation from acceptable norms. Seldom does an examiner pay much attention to positive attributes (such as confidence, loyalty, intelligence, hope, dedication, and generosity). One of the commonly neglected virtues in clinical situations is that of courage.

Courage in a clinical sense should not be confused with "bravery under fire." The derring-do of heroes is seldom found among ordinary people, who usually have more than their share of anxiety and apprehension when facing unfamiliar, unknown, and threatening events. Threats are manifest on many levels of experience, ranging from actual injury to situations that signify, for example, failure, disgrace, humiliation, embarrassment. In a sense, threat is "negative support" because it may do or undo everything that positive support is supposed to strengthen. It pathologizes. The courage to cope is a real but seldom recognized element in the attributes that affect the coping process. Nevertheless, in coping well, the courage to cope means a wish to perform competently and to be valued as a significant person, even when threatened by risk and anonymity.

Hope, confidence, and morale go together and can be directly asked about because most patients know what these terms mean without translation. Naturally, few people readily admit their tendency to fail, shirk, or behave in unworthy ways. Nevertheless, a skillful interview gets behind denial, rationalization, posturing, and pretense without evoking another threat to security or self-esteem.

Courage requires an awareness of risk as well as a willingness to go it alone, despite a substantial degree of anxiety, tension, and worry about being able to withstand pressure and pain. Courage is always accompanied by vulnerability, but it engages itself in the courage to cope.

ASSESSMENT OF VULNERABILITY

Vulnerability is present in all humans, and it shows up at times of crisis, stress, calamity, and threat to well-being and identity.[15–21] How does a patient visualize threat? What is most feared, say, in approaching a surgical procedure, a diagnosis, anesthesia, possible invalidism, failure, pain, or abandonment (by one's physician or family)?

Coping and vulnerability have a loosely reciprocal relationship; the better one copes, the less distress he or she experiences as a function of acknowledged vulnerability. In general, a good deal of distress often derives directly from a sense of uncertainty about how well one will cope when called on to do so. This does not mean that those who deny or disavow problems and concerns are superlative copers. The reverse may be true. Courage to cope requires anxiety confronted and dealt with, not phlegmatic indifference to outcome.

Table 36-3 shows 13 common types of vulnerability. Table 36-4 describes how to find out about salient problems, the strategy used for coping, and the degree of the resolution attained.

Seven different existential states were identified by Griffith and Gaby[22] that can be regarded as moving toward (resilience), or away from (vulnerability), assertive coping techniques (Table 36-5). They argued that an essential job of the psychiatrist is to help patients sustain characteristics of resiliency and to combat vulnerability. Confusion, defined as "an inability to make sense of one's situation," can be seen in patients who have delirium or dementia or for whom a clear medical diagnosis does not exist. Asking "How do you make sense of your experience?" can be helpful in organization, planning, and judging, and can lead to improved coherence. Communion, defined as the "felt presence of a trustworthy person," versus isolation can be assessed by asking, "Who do you believe understands your situation?" Despair or hopelessness have been associated with poor coping. Questions that assess hope include "What sorts of things keep you from giving up?" Feeling meaningless can be detrimental to one's ability to fight illness; questions that enhance purpose include, "Who keeps you alive?" Agency, defined as "the sense that one can make meaningful choices and that one's actions matter," can combat helplessness by empowering patients to be heard by their doctors. Asking "What issues involved in your treatment concern you the most?" embraces a sense of agency and diminishes helplessness. Showing courage, as opposed to cowardice, in the face of fear, can be elicited by asking, "Have there been times when you wanted to give up but you didn't?" Finally, experiencing a sense of gratitude rather than a sense of resentment can help combat feelings of depression and anxiety. The clinician can ask, "What things in your life are you most grateful for?" or "Has your illness taught you anything meaningful?"[22] While speaking with patients, it is helpful to establish which of these areas of vulnerability can be improved upon. Vulnerability, except in extreme forms (such as depression, anger, and anxiety), is difficult to characterize exactly, so the astute clinician

TABLE 36-3 Vulnerability

Hopelessness:	Patient believes that all is lost; effort is futile; there is no chance at all; a passive surrender to the inevitable
Turmoil/ Perturbation:	Patient is tense, agitated, restless, hyperalert to potential risks, real and imagined
Frustration:	Patient is angry about an inability to progress, recover, or get satisfactory answers or relief
Despondency/ Depression:	Patient is dejected, withdrawn, apathetic, tearful, and often unable to interact verbally
Helplessness/ Powerlessness:	Patient complains of being too weak to struggle anymore; cannot initiate action or make decisions that stick
Anxiety/Fear:	Patient feels on the edge of dissolution, with dread and specific fears about impending doom and disaster
Exhaustion/ Apathy:	Patient feels too worn out and depleted to care; there is more indifference than sadness
Worthlessness/ Self-rebuke:	Patient feels persistent self-blame and no good; he or she finds numerous causes for weakness, failure, and incompetence
Painful Isolation/ Abandonment:	Patient is lonely and feels ignored and alienated from significant others
Denial/Avoidance:	Patient speaks or acts as if threatening aspects of illness are minimal, almost showing a jolly interpretation of related events, or else a serious disinclination to examine potential problems
Truculence/ Annoyance:	Patient is embittered and not openly angry; feels mistreated, victimized, and duped by forces or people
Repudiation of Significant Others:	Patient rejects or antagonizes significant others, including family, friends, and professional sources of support
Closed Time Perspective:	Patient may show any or all of these symptoms, but in addition foresees an exceedingly limited future

TABLE 36-4 How to Find Out How a Patient Copes

Problem:	*In your opinion, what has been the most difficult for you since your illness started? How has it troubled you?*
Strategy:	*What did you do (or are doing) about the problem?* Get more information (rational/ intellectual approach) Talk it over with others to relieve distress (share concern) Try to laugh it off; make light of it (reverse affect) Put it out of mind; try to forget (suppression/denial) Distract myself by doing other things (displacement/dissipation) Take a positive step based on a present understanding (confrontation) Accept, but change the meaning to something easier to deal with (redefinition) Submit, yield, and surrender to the inevitable (passivity/fatalism) Do something, anything, reckless or impractical (acting out) Look for feasible alternatives to negotiate (if *x*, then *y*) Drink, eat, take drugs, and so on, to reduce tension (tension reduction) Withdraw, get away, and seek isolation (stimulus reduction) Blame someone or something (projection/disowning/externalization) Go along with directives from authority figures (compliance) Blame self for faults; sacrifice or atone (undoing self-pity)
Resolution:	*How has it worked out so far?* Not at all Doubtful relief Limited relief, but better Much better; actual resolution

Adapted from Weisman AD: *The realization of death: a guide for the psychological autopsy*, New York, 1974, Jason Aronson Inc.

must depend on a telling episode or metaphor that typifies a total reaction.

HOW TO FIND OUT MORE ABOUT COPING

Thus far, we have discussed the following: salient characteristics of effective and less effective copers; methods by which deficits in patients can be identified and how clinicians can intervene; potential pressure points that alert clinicians to different psychosocial difficulties; types of emotional vulnerabilities; and a format for listing different coping strategies, along with questions about resolutions and increasing resiliency.

The assessment and identification of ways in which a patient copes or fails to cope with specific problems requires both a description by the patient and an interpretation by the psychiatrist. Even so, this may not be enough. Details of descriptive importance may not be explicit or forthcoming. In these situations, the clinician must take pains to elucidate the specifics of each situation. If not, the result is only a soft approximation that generalizes where it should be precise. Indeed, the clinician should ask again and again about a topic that is unclear and re-phrase, without yielding to clichés and general impressions.

TABLE 36-5 How to Assess Areas of Vulnerability Versus Resiliency

Confusion versus Coherence	How do you make sense out of your experience?
Isolation versus Communion	Who do you believe understands your situation?
Despair versus Hope	What sorts of things keep you from giving up?
Helplessness versus Agency	Who keeps you alive?
Meaninglessness versus Purpose	What issues about your treatment concern you the most?
Cowardice versus Courage	Have there been times when you wanted to give up but did not? What prevented you from giving up?
Resentment versus Gratitude	What things in life are you most grateful for? Has your illness taught you anything meaningful?

Adapted from Griffith J, Gaby L: Brief psychotherapy at the bedside: countering demoralization from medical illness, *Psychosomatics*. 2005 Mar-Apr; 46(2): 109–116.

Psychiatrists have been imbued with the value of so-called empathy and intuition. Although immediate insights and inferences can be pleasing to the examiner, sometimes these conclusions can be misleading and totally wrong. It is far more empathic to respect each patient's individuality and unique slant on the world by making sure that the examiner accurately describes in detail how problems are confronted. To draw a quick inference without being sure about a highly private state of mind is distinctly unempathic. As most other individuals, patients give themselves the benefit of the doubt and claim to resolve problems in a socially desirable and potentially effective way. It takes little experience to realize that disavowal of any problem through pleasant distortions is itself a coping strategy, not necessarily an accurate description of how one coped.

Patients who adamantly deny any difficulty tend to cope poorly. Sick patients have difficult lives, and the denial of adversity usually represents a relatively primitive defense that leaves such patients unprepared to accurately assess their options. Carefully timed and empathic discussion with patients about their current condition can help them address their treatment more effectively and avoid maladaptive approaches.

On the other hand, patients may attempt to disavow any role in their current illness. By seeking credit for having suffered so much, such patients reject any implication that they might have prevented, deflected, or corrected what has befallen them (see Table 36-4). Helping these patients does not necessarily require that they acknowledge their role in their particular predicament. Instead, the empathic listener identifies and provides comfort around the implicit fear that these patients harbor (i.e., that they somehow deserve their debilitation).

Suppression, isolation, and projection are common defenses. Effective copers seem to pinpoint problems clearly, whereas bad copers, as well as those with strong primitive defenses, seem to seek relief from further questions without attempting anything that suggests reflective analysis.

In learning how anyone copes, a measure of authentic skepticism is always appropriate, especially when it is combined with a willingness to accept correction later on. The balance between denial and affirmation is always uncertain. The key is to focus on points of ambiguity, anxiety, and ambivalence while tactfully preserving a patient's self-esteem. A tactful examiner might say, for example, "I'm really not clear about what exactly bothered you, and what you really did. …"

The purpose of focusing is to avoid premature formulations that gloss over points of ambiguity. An overly rigid format in approaching any evaluation risks overlooking individual tactics that deny, avoid, dissemble, and blame others for difficulties. Patients, too, can be rigid, discouraging alliance, rebuffing collaboration, and preventing an effective physician–patient relationship.

HOW TO BE A BETTER COPER

It is important to recognize that in evaluating how patients cope, examiners should learn about their own coping styles and cultivate characteristics of effective copers. It is not enough to mean well, to have a warm heart, or to have a head filled with scientific information. Coping well requires open-ended communication and self-awareness. A false objectivity obstructs appraisal; an exaggerated subjectivity only confuses what is being said about whom. Confidence in being able to cope can be enhanced only through repeated attempts at self-appraisal, self-instruction, and self-correction. Coping well with illness—with any problem—does not predict invariable success, but it does provide a foundation for becoming a better coper.

CASE 1

Ms. A, a 50-year-old woman was admitted to the inpatient cardiology service for chest pain; her medical history was notable for having had an internal cardioverter defibrillator (ICD) following a cardiac arrest 2 months earlier. Psychiatry was consulted to assess and manage her anxiety and her refusal of recommended cardiac procedures related to her having received multiple ICD discharges before her arrival at the hospital.

When the C-L psychiatrist interviewed Ms. A, she described feeling vulnerable and afraid of dying; discharges of her ICD filled her with anticipatory anxiety of additional shocks. She described having flashbacks of her cardiac arrest, as well as insomnia, irritability, and guilt (over having caused her health problems by drinking alcohol to excess). She refused psychotropic medications and said, "I am already on too many meds!"

The psychiatrist met with Ms. A several times over the next few days and taught her diaphragmatic breathing and progressive muscle relaxation. She reported that her anxiety diminished and she became more fully engaged in her care. She agreed to an outpatient referral for cognitive-behavioral therapy.

ADDITIONAL PSYCHOTHERAPEUTIC TECHNIQUES IN THE MEDICALLY ILL POPULATION

Cognitive-behavioral therapy (CBT) is a structured and often short-term psychotherapeutic modality that has been effective in the treatment of many psychiatric conditions (including anxiety, depression, PTSD, and suicidal crises); it is a technique that involves assessment of the relationship among a patient's cognitive process, emotions, and behaviors. Literature has shown its efficacy in reducing anxiety and depression associated with a host of medical conditions (including cancer, chronic pain, HIV infection, and patients requiring an implantable cardioverter defibrillator).

A recent Cochrane review analyzing psychological interventions for women with non-metastatic breast cancer found that CBT lessened depression, anxiety, and mood disorders when compared with controls, and that individual CBT improved quality of life. The review also found that group-based psychological interventions demonstrated a non-significant overall survival benefit.[23] The combination of CBT and hypnosis effectively decreased negative affect and improved positive affect in breast cancer patients receiving radiation therapy.[24] CBT changed maladaptive cognitions and behaviors in these patients while leading to more adaptive cognitive processes; hypnosis (involving direct suggestion of decreasing negative affect and increasing positive affect) also led to improvement. In HIV-infected individuals, rates of depression are high, and co-morbidity is associated with increased rates of risky behaviors, poorer disease outcome (e.g., with a decreased CD4 count, an increased viral load, an increased progression to AIDS, and an increased mortality rate), as well as poor treatment adherence. In a randomized clinical trial, CBT improved adherence and decreased depressive symptoms in a significant proportion of patients.[25] Multiple studies support the efficacy of CBT in those with chronic pain; this may result from altering perceived pain control, self-efficacy, and psychological distress (including depression and anxiety).[26] Patients requiring an ICD often suffer from significant psychological distress, including depression and anxiety, associated with receiving multiple shocks. A CBT intervention for patients recently receiving an ICD demonstrated improvement in symptoms of PTSD and reduced avoidance as well as fewer depressive symptoms in women.[27] Recently, Levin and colleagues[28,29] described how to conduct a cognitive therapy assessment in acute medical settings, and implement interventions that target hopelessness, anxiety, cognitive distortions, and suicidality.

As described earlier in the chapter, characteristics of people who cope well with medical illnesses have been identified. Positive emotional health (including well-being, positive affect, and resilience) is associated with improved health outcomes in diabetic patients.[30] In patients with cardiac disease, positive psychological attributes (including optimism) may be associated with improved cardiac outcomes via their impact on physiologic and behavioral mechanisms. DuBois et al.'s[31] review of positive psychology interventions in cardiac patients provides sample exercises.[31]

Meaning-centered group psychotherapy focuses on techniques to alleviate the loss of spiritual wellness and subsequent existential suffering that can occur as someone faces advanced cancer. A recent study by Breitbart and colleagues[32] found that meaning-centered group psychotherapy led to multiple beneficial outcomes, including improved quality of life, reduction in depression, and amelioration of physical distress in patients with advanced or terminal cancer. In general, group psychotherapeutic interventions remain a critical technique to offer to the medically ill.

REFERENCES

Access the reference list online at https://expertconsult.inkling.com/.

Electroconvulsive Therapy and Neurotherapeutics

37

Aura M. Hurtado-Puerto, M.D.
Carlos G. Fernandez-Robles, M.D.
Michael E. Henry, M.D.
Cristina Cusin, M.D.
Sheri Berg, M.D.
Joan A. Camprodon, M.D., M.P.H., Ph.D.

OVERVIEW

Treatment options in neuropsychiatry include psychotherapy, psychopharmacology, and neuromodulation. This chapter focuses on neuromodulation, a group of device-based interventions able to modulate pathologically altered brain regions and circuits using electromagnetic energy or surgical ablation. Neuromodulation therapies (also known as brain stimulation or somatic therapies) can be divided into three main groups: non-invasive, convulsive, and invasive. Non-invasive methods are applied transcranially, without the need for surgery or the induction of seizures. Transcranial magnetic stimulation (TMS) is the most paradigmatic modality. Convulsive methods apply higher-density electromagnetic charges with the goal of inducing a generalized seizure, under general anesthesia and with close medical monitoring. Electroconvulsive therapy (ECT) remains the oldest and most commonly used modality. Last, invasive neuromodulation requires surgery to implant stimulating electrodes—such as in vagus nerve stimulation (VNS) and deep brain stimulation (DBS)—or for the controlled ablation of specific limbic pathways. In this chapter, we will review these treatments from least to most invasive, describe these techniques, their indications, and their safety profile.

TRANSCRANIAL MAGNETIC STIMULATION

Transcranial magnetic stimulation (TMS) is a non-invasive and non-convulsive treatment able to modulate neural excitability and connectivity of cortical nodes and their networks by applying strong and rapidly changing electromagnetic pulses on the surface of the skull. Since its invention in 1985, TMS has developed as a useful technology with basic science and clinical applications, including diagnostic and therapeutic uses. Notably, in 2008, the FDA cleared the use of repetitive TMS (rTMS) using high-frequency stimulation to the left dorsolateral prefrontal cortex (DLPFC) for the treatment of major depressive disorder (MDD). Since that time, a total of four different TMS systems have been cleared by the FDA for the treatment of MDD.

Technique

TMS is a clinical application of Faraday's principle of electromagnetic induction. The basic equipment includes an electrical capacitor connected to a metallic coil encased in a protective plastic cover. The coil is placed on the surface of the skull and a powerful and rapidly changing electrical current is passed through it, generating a magnetic field that travels unimpeded through the soft tissue, bone, and cerebrospinal fluid (CSF) all the way to the cortex. The cortex, which is electrically conductive, acts as a pick-up coil and transforms the magnetic energy into a secondary electrical current, which in turn forces an action potential on neurons and a volley of activity through the axons to the synapse, leading to activation of the post-synaptic neuron and beyond.

TMS leads to circuit-wide modulation, and not just local stimulation.[1] The *direct* effects of TMS are restricted to the superficial cortical neurons: the magnetic field weakens as it travels away from the TMS coil, and its capacity to induce neuronal action potentials disappears approximately 3 centimeters from the skull surface. However, the effects on these cortical neurons spread to the post-synaptic neuron, and then to the next post-synaptic neuron, initiating a cycle that is able to modulate an entire circuit of interest, including deep cortical or subcortical nodes.[2] Thus, TMS allows for *indirect* trans-synaptic modulation of deep structures as long as the appropriate cortical target is selected.

The TMS parameter space includes anatomic variables (such as location and depth) and physiologic variables (such as stimulation frequency, pulse intensity, and duration). The anatomic target for stimulation is a window that provides modulatory access to a network of interest, and therefore has a critical impact on the effects of TMS, which are primarily determined by the functional anatomy and connectivity of the stimulated region. In the case of major depressive disorder (MDD), current guidelines set the DLPFC as the stimulation target,[3] a node that has been shown to exert top-down control over limbic structures (e.g., anterior cingulate cortex, hippocampal regions, and amygdala) and is pathologically altered in MDD.[4,5]

The depth of stimulation is proportional to the strength of the magnetic field, which decreases as it travels away from its source (the coil). Nevertheless, the primary factor affecting depth is the coil design. Different coil architectures are available, with two main types: the circular coil and the figure-of-8 coil, though the latter is most commonly used given its greater focality.[6,7]

Therapeutically, TMS is applied as a series of consecutive pulses, called repetitive TMS (rTMS) and can be delivered at various frequencies. *Low-frequency rTMS* (1 Hz) has similar effects to long-term depression (LTD), causing inhibition of the stimulated area. Conversely, *high-frequency rTMS* (>5 Hz, though typically 10–20 Hz) resembles long-term potentiation (LTP) producing local facilitation. Other complex stimulation patterns—such as theta burst stimulation—have been developed recently and promise to add greater efficiency, with much shorter stimulation time and longer after-effects.[8]

The stimulation intensity determines how much energy is applied with each individual TMS pulse. Intensity is generally individualized according to the patient's specific cortical excitability, assessed by the motor threshold, which can be determined by the clinician according to the protocols by Rossini and co-workers.[9] This individualization of TMS stimulation is important for both its efficacy and safety.

Duration of stimulation applies to each session and also to an entire course of treatment. For example, a typical antidepressant therapeutic session uses 3000 pulses over the course of 37 minutes, and the treatment course involves 36 sessions over the course of 9 weeks.

The latest guidelines for TMS antidepressant treatment suggest stimulating the left DLPFC at a high frequency (10 Hz), using 3000 pulses per session at 120% of the motor threshold intensity. The acute course involves 30 daily sessions (given Monday through Friday) over 6 weeks, followed by a taper period with 2 weekly sessions for an additional 3 weeks.[10]

Indications

TMS was approved in the United States in 2008, when the Food and Drug Administration (FDA) cleared high frequency repetitive TMS (rTMS) for "the treatment of [MDD] in adult patients who have failed to receive satisfactory improvement from prior antidepressant medication in the current episode".[11] In 2013, TMS H-coils—producing deeper stimulation—were approved for the same purpose. TMS is also used diagnostically for the assessment of pathologies affecting the motor system (such as brain or spinal cord injury or multiple sclerosis) and for the pre-surgical mapping of motor and language areas.

TMS is an effective primary or adjunctive treatment for depression. The pivotal trial that led to the FDA-clearance of therapeutic TMS[12] demonstrated the antidepressant efficacy of TMS monotherapy with response rates of 23.9% to 24.5% (compared with 12.3% to 15.1% for placebo) and remission rates of 14.2% to 17.4% (compared with 5.5% to 8.9% for placebo) after 6 weeks of treatment. After the taper period, the therapeutic outcomes continued to improve (27.7% response and 20.6% remission rate). An NIMH-funded multi-center trial reported similar results.[13]

Although large randomized controlled trials are crucial to identify the pure and true efficacy of a treatment, by design they generally recruit patients who do not reflect the standard clinic patient (who may have several psychiatric and medical comorbidities, varying degrees of severity, and treatment-resistance, and may be on several medications, including psychoactive agents). An open-label, naturalistic trial, sought to assess the antidepressant effectiveness of TMS in 339 typical clinical patients using the same FDA-approved protocols used in the pivotal trials. This study allowed patients to continue on their current psychiatric treatment (medication and therapy) while undergoing TMS. After the acute phase of treatment, the response rate was 41.5% to 58% and the remission rate was 26.5% to 37.1%.[14] A separate study assessed the duration of benefit in this same population at 1-year follow-up, and found that two-thirds of the responders/remitters maintained their designation and less than 30% of the initial responders/remitters relapsed.[15]

Safety

TMS has a remarkably benign profile. Absolute contraindications are limited to metallic implants in the area of stimulation (including brain stimulators, medication pumps, and cochlear implants) and cardiac pacemakers.[16] Noteworthy, TMS has been tested in patients with DBS and considered relatively safe, granted the DBS pulse generator is turned off; extreme caution is advised since data are limited.[17] As with any other therapy, the clinician should weigh the risk–benefit ratio carefully.

The main safety concern remains the potential for seizure induction when applying rTMS. Various reports have estimated the similar seizure risk: 20 seizures out of approximately 300,000 research and clinical sessions;[16] seven events out of 250,000 clinical sessions applied to 8000 patients since the FDA clearance in 2008 until 2012;[18] and six events in 5000 patients receiving stimulation with the deep H-coil.[19] The estimated risk was one event in 30,000 treatment sessions; this was commensurate with the seizure risk of most antidepressant medications. Seizures triggered by TMS can happen during—but not after—a treatment session. Consequently, although rTMS can initiate a seizure it cannot cause epilepsy. Therefore, patients should be screened for personal and familial history of epilepsy, as well as other factors that increase seizure risk (e.g., concomitant medications that lower seizure threshold, history of head injury or malformations), in order to evaluate the risk and benefit more accurately. If a patient is considered to benefit greatly from rTMS, while being at a moderate risk of seizure, this appraisal allows for the implementation of special safety measures around their stimulation sessions. Other more frequent and more benign side effects are headaches, facial or muscle twitching, vasovagal syncope, discomfort limited to the area of stimulation, anxiety, and tinnitus. To minimize the impact on hearing, patients should wear earplugs.[3,16]

ELECTROCONVULSIVE THERAPY

Electroconvulsive therapy (ECT) has been used to treat severe psychiatric illnesses for over 75 years. During this time, improvements in the equipment, and in dosing schedules, as well as the addition of general anesthesia have greatly increased its safety and have brought ECT into the modern era. Its continued use reflects the large number of affectively ill individuals who are unresponsive to drugs or are intolerant of their side effects.

Technique

The routine pre-ECT work-up should include taking a thorough medical history, performing a physical examination, and obtaining an electrocardiogram (ECG), and a comprehensive metabolic panel. Additional studies and consultations should be obtained as needed, based on co-morbid conditions.

The issue of whether to combine a psychotropic medication with ECT is a matter of much speculation. In general, a patient should be taken off medications that have not been beneficial, despite an adequate dosage and duration of therapy. Older case reports cautioned that patients undergoing ECT while taking lithium may be particularly prone to severe cognitive disturbance, a prolonged time to awakening or breathing, or prolonged or spontaneous seizures; however, more recent case series indicate that the combination may be used safely.[20,21] Nonetheless, when lithium and ECT are used in combination, the patient should be monitored for signs of confusion and targeted for lower lithium serum levels. Benzodiazepines, which are antagonistic to the ictal process, should also be decreased or discontinued whenever possible.[22] Second-generation antipsychotics and antihistaminic drugs can replace benzodiazepines as anxiolytic agents. Tricyclic antidepressants (TCAs) can create cardiovascular management problems and should be discontinued. Monoamine oxidase inhibitors (MAOIs) and ECT may be combined, while caution is advised to avoid toxic drug interactions.[23] In patients with a pre-existing seizure disorder, anticonvulsants should be maintained for patient safety and the elevated seizure threshold over-ridden with a higher-intensity stimulus and the use of bilateral electrode placement. Anticonvulsants used for mood stabilization or augmentation are generally discontinued, or tapered if discontinuation is not possible.

ECT should be performed in collaboration with an anesthesiologist familiar with the techniques and cardiovascular effects of ECT. The American Society of Anesthesiologists has endorsed the use of cardiac monitoring and pulse oximetry on all patients undergoing general anesthesia. General anesthesia is induced with barbiturates (methohexital) or other short-acting induction agents (e.g., propofol or ketamine). Paralysis is most commonly achieved with use of succinylcholine.

The choice of electrode placement in ECT remains controversial. Both right unilateral (RUL) and bilateral (BL) placements have advantages and disadvantages. RUL ECT causes less cognitive impairment than BL ECT, but it is less efficacious.[24,25] At the Massachusetts General Hospital, RUL ECT is used at the outset for most patients; the exceptions are patients with catatonia and treatment-resistant mania. Patients are switched to BL ECT when depressive symptoms prove refractory to 6 to 12 unilateral treatments. The factor most commonly associated with ineffective unilateral ECT is use of threshold stimulus intensity.[26] RUL stimuli should be 300% to 600% above the seizure threshold with the electrodes placed in the d'Elia position.[24,27]

Use of brief-pulse (0.5–1 ms) waveforms has become the standard practice in the United States. Although sine-wave stimuli were used previously, the brief-pulse waveform is more efficient and is associated with less post-treatment confusion and amnesia.[28] Ultra-brief pulse-width (0.3 ms) RUL ECT, is slightly less efficacious than brief-pulse ECT but it can greatly minimize cognitive side effects.[29]

The schedule of administration is usually three times a week, although new trends are favoring a twice-weekly schedule, as it appears to be as effective and to be associated with less memory impairment. The improvement, however, is slower with this approach, posing a challenge in inpatient settings. Once-a-week ECT administration has not provided additional advantages and it slows the antidepressant effect to a clinically unacceptable level.[30]

Generalization of the seizure to the entire brain is essential for efficacy. Most ECT instruments have a built-in, dual-channel EEG monitor that can measure electrical activity in the brain. No relationship has been detected between the clinical antidepressant response to ECT and the duration of the induced seizure or total seizure time during the course of treatment. After ECT, a nurse should monitor patients carefully; vital signs should be taken regularly and pulse oximetry monitored.

The average number of ECT procedures necessary to treat major depression is consistently reported to be between 6 and 12. The use of more than one seizure per session (multiple-monitored ECT) has shown minimal advantage over conventional ECT and has dramatically increased the occurrence of cognitive side effects.[31]

After successful treatment, the risk of relapse is greater than 50% at 6 months without the use of maintenance medication.[32] In general, maintenance ECT (i.e., one treatment per month, on average) has been an efficacious, safe, well-tolerated, and cost-effective intervention compared with maintenance pharmacotherapy alone, with its greatest impact consisting of reducing relapse, recurrence, and re-hospitalization in treatment-resistant patients.[33]

Indications

Although ECT may be used as a first-line treatment, it is usually used further down the treatment algorithm. The most common indication for ECT is a major depressive episode (in the context of unipolar or bipolar depression), but other indications include mania, psychosis, and catatonia. Within these diagnoses, the severity of the mood symptoms and the associated risk of suicide or violence, past psychotherapy, medication failures, history of prior response to ECT, and the patient's inability to tolerate further medication trials are important considerations in the decision to treat with ECT.

In depressed patients, longer depressive episodes, psychotic symptoms, and medication failure at baseline are robust predictors of lower response rate to ECT.[34] Nonetheless, most patients who receive ECT for depression are considered to be treatment-resistant. In practice, treatment resistance usually reflects a combination of medications tried and clinical acuity. Less acute, non-suicidal patients have more time to try several classes of antidepressant medications or non-invasive neuromodulation (i.e., TMS) before moving to ECT. Suicidal ideation is often an important consideration in the decision to use ECT and has been reported to respond to ECT 81% of the time.[35] Older, medically vulnerable patients with limited social supports may also need to move to ECT sooner to minimize morbidity and mortality.

Psychotic illness is another indication for ECT. Although it is not a routine treatment for schizophrenia, ECT alone and in combination with a neuroleptic, results in sustained improvement of symptoms in patients with chronic schizophrenia.[36] Evidence suggests that ECT may be an effective and safe clozapine-augmentation strategy in treatment-resistant schizophrenia.[37] Furthermore, in young adults with intractable first-episode schizophrenia and schizophreniform disorder, ECT was a highly efficacious treatment option.[38]

ECT has been known to cause and treat mania,[39,40] but drug treatment remains the first-line therapy. Nevertheless, in controlled trials, ECT has been at least as effective as lithium, and in acute mania, more than 50% of cases have remitted with it.[41] ECT is also an effective and safe treatment for those with mixed affective states.[42]

ECT has proven effective in the treatment of catatonia with reported response rates of 85% to 93%,[43,44] and should be considered in those patients who fail to achieve full resolution with medications. Of all patients who failed to respond to pharmacotherapy, 59% improved with ECT.[19] Characteristic features, such as waxy flexibility and *gegenhalten*, predict a faster response to ECT than other features, such as echophenomena.[45] ECT is considered a definitive treatment for excited catatonia and delirious mania, whereas available pharmacologic options are of limited efficacy.[46,47] The use of ECT can be life-saving in cases of malignant catatonia and neuroleptic malignant syndrome.[48] The timing of administration is crucial, as use of ECT within 3 days of the onset of symptoms has been associated with significantly higher survival rates.[49,50]

While initially most patients receive a medication trial regardless of their diagnosis, ECT is a primary treatment for mood-disordered patients who are severely malnourished, dehydrated, and exhausted, as well as those presenting with depression with psychotic features, as these patients do not improve with an antidepressant alone,[51] and the combination of an antidepressant and an antipsychotic medication may be difficult to tolerate. The reported response rate with ECT in psychotic depression is 80%.[52]

Several case series have documented the effectiveness of ECT in the treatment of behavioral disturbances, aggression, and pathologic yelling associated with severe dementia (refractory to medications).[53–55] Depressed patients with pre-existing dementia are likely to develop severe cognitive deficits after ECT; fortunately, most individuals return to their baseline level of cognition after treatment, especially when dementia pharmacotherapy is co-administered.[56]

Finally, ECT has been helpful alleviating motor symptoms of Parkinson's disease,[57–60] behavioral symptoms of Huntington's disease[61] and controlling intractable pain (secondary to neuropathic pain, fibromyalgia, and complex regional pain syndrome, among other syndromes) in patients with comorbid depression.[62–65]

Safety

ECT is generally considered a safe procedure. An examination of a national patient safety database, found only six events that were determined to be serious injuries associated with ECT in 73,440 treatments.[66] The largest study on mortality related to ECT in United States, reported only one death specifically linked to ECT and four additional deaths thought to be plausibly associated, in 49,048 ECT treatments.[67] A more recent review, found no causal association between ECT and death in 99,728 treatments.[68]

As ECT's technique and anesthesia monitoring have improved, factors that were formerly considered absolute contraindications have now become relative risk factors. The patient is best served by carefully weighing the risk of treatment against the morbidity or lethality of remaining depressed. The prevailing view is that there are no absolute contraindications to ECT; however, several conditions warrant careful work-up and management when ECT is considered.[69]

Cognitive

Current evidence indicates that ECT is neuroprotective and increases hippocampal and amygdalar gray matter volume.[70,71] There is no evidence for structural brain damage as a result of ECT.[72] Nonetheless, there are important effects on cognition. Post-treatment confusion and disorientation in the immediate period after ECT has been well-documented; bilateral electrode placement, high stimulus intensity, inadequate oxygenation and prolonged seizure activity are known risk factors; older patients and those with an underlying neurologic condition are at risk of longer and more severe episodes.[73] Between 5% and 12% of patients develop motor restlessness, disorientation, panic-like behavior, and combativeness, known as post-ictal agitation (PIA). A single 0.5-mg/kg IV propofol bolus administered after the end of the seizure reduced the incidence of PIAs significantly.[74]

Development of severe delirium after ECT is rare, and it requires discontinuation of treatment. Usually, substantial improvement occurs within 48 hours of the last treatment; if symptoms persist after cessation of treatment, a full neurologic work-up is indicated to rule out underlying causes other than ECT.

The most common cognitive side effect is anterograde amnesia (difficulty recalling new information); autobiographic memory and verbal and non-verbal recall impairments are also observed. Objective measures have found memory loss to be relatively short term (<6 months after treatment),[75] whereas subjective accounts differ markedly depending on the assessment method.[76] ECT predominantly affects memory of prior personal events that are near the treatment date, with BL ECT causing more memory disturbances than RUL ECT.[77] The least amount of memory deficit is seen with a unilateral ultra-brief pulse stimulus.[78]

Other CNS Adverse Effects

Intracranial pressure increases and the blood–brain barrier becomes more permeable during ECT. In years past, space-occupying brain lesions were considered an absolute contraindication to ECT; now the general consensus is that if a lesion is relatively small, solitary, and not associated with significant mass effect, edema, or increased intracranial pressure, ECT probably does not present a greater-than-usual risk of neurologic deterioration; however, larger or multiple masses (e.g., metastatic lesions), edema, increased intracranial pressure, or mass effect should be considered relative contraindications and measures should be taken to reduce edema and intracranial pressure if treatment is undertaken.[61] The most common intracranial risk factor is recent cerebral infarction. Retrospective reviews of ECT after recent cerebral infarction indicate that, when the treatment is properly performed, the complication rate is low.[79] The interval between infarction and treatment with ECT should be determined by the urgency and need for depression treatment.

Cardiovascular

The heart is physiologically stressed during ECT. Parasympathetic discharge immediately after electrical stimulation suppresses the heart rate followed by a sympathetic outflow, resulting from a rise in circulating catecholamine levels that peak about 3 minutes after the onset of seizure activity.[80]

After the seizure ends, the parasympathetic tone remains strong, often causing transient bradycardia, with a return to baseline function after 5 to 10 minutes. The cardiac conditions most commonly worsened by this autonomic stimulus are ischemic heart disease, congestive heart failure (CHF), hypertension, and cardiac arrhythmias. If properly managed, these conditions should not represent a significant increase in morbidity during ECT.

The contraindication of ECT within 6 months of a myocardial infarction is no longer absolute. A more rational approach involves careful balancing of the cardiac function and the risk of untreated depression.[81] Patients with compensated CHF generally tolerate ECT well, although temporary, non-life-threatening cardiac arrhythmias may occur.[82] In hypertensive patients, a retrospective study examining blood pressures before and after ECT concluded that ECT does not worsen blood pressure beyond the peri-treatment period.[83] For patients with coronary artery disease or hypertension, short-acting intravenous (IV) β-blockers effectively reduce stress on the heart. Esmolol or labetalol given IV immediately before the anesthetic induction is usually sufficient.[84] Nitroglycerine causes vasodilation, thus reducing cerebral blood flow and cardiac workload, and it is useful in patients with extremely high cardiovascular risk.[85]

Duration of the QTc in the baseline ECG appears to be a helpful predictor of arrhythmias during ECT.[86] Atrial fibrillation, with its attendant risk of embolic stroke, is another cardiac condition that must be stabilized prior to starting a course of ECT.[87] Adequate anticoagulation for at least 1 month should be sufficient to minimize the risk to acceptable levels. In the event of needing to treat the patient urgently, a transesophageal echocardiogram is required to adequately visualize the left atria. Patients with cardiac pacemakers are known to tolerate ECT uneventfully. Current guidelines advise that pacemakers should be reprogrammed to the asynchronous mode for ECT to protect against under- or over-sensing from electromagnetic interference.[88]

The current recommendation for patients with an automatic implantable cardioverter defibrillator is to turn it off during ECT, to carefully monitor the rhythm, and to have an external defibrillator available.[89] Cardiac arrest is a rare complication of ECT. Some patients have a period of asystole after the ECT stimulus that may last several seconds (and can be mistaken for a true arrest).[90] Patients who receive non-convulsive stimuli are especially at risk, because the intense parasympathetic outflow caused by the stimulus is not counteracted by the sympathetic outflow of the seizure itself, and severe bradycardia or arrest may ensue.

Respiratory

Despite the fact that anesthesia for ECT requires a brief period of ventilation, ECT is safe in patients with chronic obstructive pulmonary disease (COPD) and asthma;[62] recent guidelines recommend the administration of prescribed inhalers on the morning of the ECT treatment. However, caution is recommended in patients taking theophylline, because this drug has been associated with prolonged seizures and status epilepticus.[63]

Pregnancy

ECT is an effective treatment for severe mental illness during pregnancy and the risks to the fetus and to the mother from ECT are low.[64] Preparation for ECT during pregnancy should include a pelvic examination, discontinuation of non-essential anticholinergic medications, uterine tocodynamometry, IV hydration, and adequate antacid therapy. During ECT, elevation of the pregnant woman's right hip, external fetal cardiac monitoring, intubation, and avoidance of excessive hyperventilation are recommended.[65] The fetus may be protected from the physiologic stress of ECT by virtue of its lack of direct neuronal connection to the maternal diencephalon.

VAGUS NERVE STIMULATION

Vagus nerve stimulation (VNS) is a relatively low-risk surgical intervention that does not require craniotomy, but the implantation of a stimulating electrode around the left vagus nerve. VNS has FDA-approved indications for the treatment of epilepsy and MDD.

Technique

VNS is implanted using two incisions: at the cervical level, electrodes are placed around the left vagus nerve; in the left subclavicular space, a second incision allows for the subcutaneous implantation of an internal pulse generator (IPG). Subcutaneous tunneling enables the passage of wires connecting the stimulating electrodes with the IPG. The system can be turned on after a 2-week postoperative period with a wireless controller that communicates transcutaneously with the IPG.

The exact mechanism of action of VNS is not fully understood. Neuroanatomic and functional connectivity evidence may harbor clues to its mechanism of action. It is known that peripheral stimuli to the left vagus nerve (at the cervical level) primarily reach the brain, since 80% of the fibers of this nerve are afferent. Noteworthy, some efferent fibers in the *left* vagus nerve innervate the sinoatrial node in the heart and do not affect heart rate;[91] this contrasts with the innervation of the atrioventricular node by the *right* vagus nerve, which affects heart rate. Afferent fibers of the left vagus enter the brain and reach the *nucleus tractus solitarius* (NTS), which is known to relay signals to the parabrachial nucleus, periaqueductal gray, cerebellum, limbic and paralimbic regions, *locus coeruleus*, and dorsal raphe.[92] Nuclei in the two latter structures contain serotoninergic and noradrenergic neurons that project across the central nervous system. The parabrachial nucleus, in turn, has projections to the nucleus of the *stria terminalis*, amygdala, hypothalamus, and thalamus—known to be implicated in the pathophysiology of MDD. Successively, the thalamus has projections to various cortical structures including the insula, orbitofrontal, and prefrontal cortices.[92] Studies using functional neuroimaging demonstrate increased blood flow in patients receiving VNS in various regions shown to be hypoactive in depressed patients,[93,94] such as the left dorsolateral and ventrolateral prefrontal cortices.[95]

Stimulation parameters include: output current, pulse width (i.e., pulse duration), frequency, and duty cycle (stimulation generally follows an on/off pattern, e.g., 30 s/5 min). Clinical trials submitted to the FDA for approval of VNS in MDD used the following median parameters: 0.75 mA, 500 μs, 20 Hz, 30 s on and 5 min off (10% duty cycle), as described above.[96] In practice, current and duty cycle tend to be more aggressive; this has raised retrospective concern for trials using subtherapeutic parameters. Clinically, current can be as high as 3 mA and duty cycles should stay below 50% (i.e., 60 s on and 2 min off), as animal studies suggest the possibility of vagus nerve damage.

Management of VNS patients is generally ambulatory, requiring the use of a wireless controller that is placed over the IPG in the subclavicular region that allows transcutaneous changes of the stimulation parameters by clinicians. Patients have a different controller with limited capacities, generally just turning the system on/off, and sometimes the modulation of a given parameter within a narrow pre-specified range, and programmed by the treating clinician.

Indications

Approved in the USA, Europe, and Canada for the treatment of epilepsy, observations identified an antidepressant benefit in epilepsy patients independent of the anticonvulsive effects.[97,98] This led to a series of clinical trials in patients with MDD that eventually prompted the FDA approval of VNS for the treatment of MDD in 2005.

Controlled studies assessing the efficacy of VNS for treatment-resistant MDD have generally been designed with "treatment-as-usual" as a minimum control condition for all participants. Hence, none received a placebo intervention. Customarily, these designs protect patients by providing standard-of-care treatment, while yielding results with many covariates and possible confounders given the lack of a true placebo control. For example, upon the 1-year follow-up evaluation of 205 patients enrolled in an open-label VNS plus treatment-as-usual trial, 27.2% of patients responded and 15.8% met criteria for remission.[99] Most studies found that longer stimulation periods (1 year vs 3 months) increased response and remission rates. Moreover, response rates at this follow-up doubled those observed at 3 months, suggesting a long-term period may be required for optimal effects of this treatment.[99,100]

Safety

Side effects of VNS encompass standard risks of the surgical procedure in addition to stimulation-specific iatrogenesis. The most common side effect is voice alteration (54% to 60% of patients), associated with surgical manipulation of the left vagus nerve, which may affect the laryngeal and pharyngeal branches. Other side effects include neck pain, cough, dyspnea, and paresthesias.[99] Fortunately, these complications typically dissipate over time or by reducing the frequency or pulse width.

DEEP BRAIN STIMULATION

Deep brain stimulation (DBS) is a surgical neuromodulation treatment based on the stereotactic implantation of electrodes in deep neural structures. Current FDA-approved indications include movement disorders (e.g., Parkinson's disease, dystonia, essential tremor) and obsessive–compulsive disorder (OCD), although ongoing research is exploring additional indications. As with other psychiatric neurosurgical treatments, DBS candidates are evaluated by a multidisciplinary team to confirm the appropriate indication according to the stringent inclusion criteria of severity and treatment-resistance.

Technique

DBS technology consists of a battery-powered IPG, usually implanted in the subclavicular space; a pair of wires that travel subcutaneously via the neck, all the way to the skull surface and into the intracranial space via a burr hole; and the stimulating electrodes, which are stereotactically placed in a disease-relevant structure (different for each condition). The programing and control of the IPG are comparable with those described for VNS. Furthermore, most DBS systems have four contact electrodes whose polarity can be changed, allowing for greater flexibility.

OCD treatment involves the implantation of DBS electrodes in the ventral capsule/ventral striatum (VC/VS), while other conditions require implantation in alternative structures relevant to that disease process (e.g., the subthalamic nucleus for Parkinson's disease or the subgenual cingulate BA25 for MDD). Similar to the VNS controller management, clinicians can change the parameters of stimulation using a wireless programmer placed over the IPG, and patients have a controller as well, with limited control over the system (usually turning the stimulation on/off).

Indications

DBS is currently part of the standard of care for the treatment of movement disorders (such as Parkinson's disease, dystonia, or essential tremor). In 2009, the FDA cleared the use of DBS to the VC/VS for the treatment of refractory OCD, under a humanitarian device exemption. Results have not been conclusive for its application in other psychiatric conditions, but clinical trials are underway for conditions including MDD, Tourette's syndrome, addictions, and Alzheimer's disease.

A meta-analysis of 31 studies and 116 patients with OCD recently reported that 60% of patients responded to DBS treatment with >35% reduction in Yale–Brown Obsessive Compulsive Scale (Y-BOCS) and a Y-BOCS reduction of 45.1%.[101] No significant differences were identified between stimulation of the striatum (ventral capsule/ventral striatum, nucleus accumbens, anterior limb of the internal capsule, and ventral caudate nucleus) compared to the subthalamic nucleus. Positive predictors of response included older age-of-onset of symptoms and sexual or religious obsessions and compulsions.

Safety

DBS complications can be surgical or secondary to the maladaptive stimulation of brain structures. Side effects that are related to the surgical procedure itself (e.g., hemorrhage, infection, and seizures[102]) have an incidence between 1% and 4%. Those related to the stimulated regions (e.g., mania, hypomania, worsening of depressive symptoms, anxiety, difficulty concentrating and gustatory or olfactory disturbances)[102,103] can be reversed with readjustment of the stimulation parameters, contrasting with the irreversible effects of ablative procedures.

ABLATIVE LIMBIC SURGERY

These procedures are irreversible by nature and are the last resort for the most severe and treatment-resistant patients. Exploration of ablative surgeries became notorious in the 1940s, when frontal lobotomies were done empirically and often produced serious adverse events. Since then, techniques have evolved to be much less invasive and precise, leading to a dramatic decrease in adverse events.[104] These surgeries are indicated in patients with intractable mood disorders and OCD, with response rates between 30% and 70%.[105,106] Four procedures are commonly considered: anterior cingulotomy, anterior capsulotomy, subcaudate tractotomy, and limbic leucotomy (which is the combination of both cingulotomy and subcaudate tractotomy). Side effects are rare with rates comparable with DBS, and include infection, headache, seizures, bleeding, cognitive deficits, and nausea.[106,107]

CASE 1

Mr. V, a 48-year-old lawyer, with complaints of marked irritability, depressed mood, indecisiveness, distractibility, hyporexia, insomnia, and anhedonia for the past 8 months, was seen in the Emergency Department (ED). He reported spending long night hours working on cases without getting tired. In addition, he acknowledged a history of psychological and physical abuse by his father during childhood, who had an alcohol use disorder. He was diagnosed with post-traumatic stress disorder after his father physically assaulted him at the age of 15. After treatment, this was resolved. He described being taken to the hospital when he was 17 after he "woke up" on the floor of his kitchen while making lunch. Upon evaluation, a tilt-table test revealed an autonomic dysregulation, thus confirming the diagnosis of a vasovagal syncope—the possibility of a seizure was ruled out. During adulthood, he has been diagnosed with MDD on three separate occasions and received pharmacologic and psychotherapeutic treatment.

Upon initial evaluation by his psychiatrist for the current episode, she found him to have a markedly depressed mood without psychotic features, elation, or disturbances in thought process or language. After ruling out underlying organic disturbances, she started a fluoxetine trial at 20 mg, increasing the dose up to 60 mg with no improvement of Mr. V's symptoms. She then switched to paroxetine 20 mg, which produced sedation and the need for a brief medical leave. She started a trial with duloxetine, titrated up to 90 mg producing mild symptom improvement during 2 months. Mirtazapine was added and titrated up to 45 mg, with mild but incomplete improvement. Given the lack of appropriate response to medications, Mr. V was referred for a neurotherapeutic evaluation.

On interview, Mr. V was alert, oriented, and cooperative. His major concerns involved sadness, amotivation, anergia, dysexecutive syndromes, and fatigue. He endorsed occasional thoughts that he may be better off dead, but denied suicidal ideation, plan, or intent. Given his current symptoms of depression without psychosis or mania, lack of response to four medications of three different classes, and absence of seizures, cardiac pacemaker or metallic foreign bodies in the head and neck, a course of TMS was recommended.

REFERENCES

Access the reference list online at https://expertconsult.inkling.com/.

Psychopharmacology in the Medical Setting

38

Jonathan R. Stevens, M.D., M.P.H.
Theodore A. Stern, M.D.
Maurizio Fava, M.D.
Jerrold F. Rosenbaum, M.D.
Jonathan E. Alpert, M.D., Ph.D.

OVERVIEW

The mental health professional in the general medical setting faces many challenges posed by co-morbid medical disorders and concurrent medications that hinder the detection of psychiatric symptoms and alter the effectiveness, tolerability, and safety of psychiatric drug treatment. In today's complex medical environment, many patients receive a host of medications from different specialists.[1] As illustrated in the case study below, communication between specialties may not always occur, particularly when care is provided in different healthcare systems, using dissimilar information management platforms, or on an emergency basis. Clinicians with expertise in psychopharmacology are well versed in the contemporary literature on medications and their effects (and side effects), and effectively communicate this knowledge to medical colleagues, patients, and patients' families. Successful psychopharmacology in the medical setting is knowing where, when, and how to use medicines safely and to their maximum effect, as well as which medicines to use for which disorders, the doses necessary to provide relief of symptoms, when to change medicines, when to combine them, and when to stop them.

As a guide to making informed decisions about use of psychotropic medication in the medical setting, this chapter is broadly divided into three sections. The first section focuses on principles of psychopharmacologic practice. The second portion reviews the rapidly expanding knowledge base regarding pharmacokinetics and drug–drug interactions. The final segment reviews some of the important psychiatric uses of non-psychiatric medications in daily clinical practice. The aim of this chapter is to share what adept psychopharmacologists do to help patients find relief from their symptoms, avoid harm from potential drug–drug interactions and, ideally, achieve remission.

CASE 1

Mr. C, a 75-year-old with a long-standing history of schizophrenia, was well managed on clozapine (300 mg/day) for 3 years. His medical problems included hypertension, a dilated cardiomyopathy, and a history of ventricular tachycardia (VT) for which he received an automatic implanted cardioverter defibrillator (AICD).

Four months after placement of his AICD, he was noted to be hypoxic during a routine outpatient AICD interrogation. Mr. C was sent to the Emergency Department (ED), where a transthoracic echocardiogram revealed a large circumferential pericardial effusion, without tamponade. A subxiphoid pericardial window was created and his AICD generator lead was removed as the suspected cause of his hemopericardium (via perforation of the right ventricle).

Within 48 hours of this procedure, however, Mr. C developed VT (with rates up to 200 beats per minute); a "code" was called. He received magnesium and intravenous (IV) amiodarone (150 mg), which resulted in a return to normal sinus rhythm within 10 minutes. In light of his AICD-related complication, Mr. C was loaded on amiodarone instead of replacing his AICD. Mr. C remained hemodynamically stable and was discharged on a regimen of amiodarone (400 mg/day) and his pre-admission dose of clozapine.

Mr. C returned to his group home. However, 2 days later, he developed dry mouth, dizziness, blurred vision with dilated pupils, sedation, and confusion. A clozapine serum level revealed a concentration of 1580 ng/mL (his combined clozapine plus norclozapine level was 1786 ng/mL), which was significantly greater than his pre-hospital level (242 ng/mL). Staff at his group home confirmed that he had been adherent to his medication regimen. Mr. C's outpatient psychiatrist, suspicious that potent cytochrome P450 isoenzyme (CYP) inhibitors (e.g., amiodarone) could increase circulating levels of drugs with fairly narrow therapeutic indices (e.g., clozapine), halved the dose of clozapine (to 150 mg/day). Two weeks later, Mr. C's serum clozapine level decreased (to 355 ng/mL) and his mental status returned to baseline.

PRINCIPLES OF PSYCHOPHARMACOLOGIC PRACTICE

The complicated clinical and psychosocial contexts in which psychotropic medications are often administered in the general hospital call on a sound understanding of basic principles that underlie the practice of psychopharmacology.[2] If pharmacologic efforts fail to achieve their intended goals, a review of these principles often helps to uncover potential explanations and to re-direct treatment.

Initiating Treatment

The appropriate use of psychotropic medications starts with as precise a formulation of the diagnosis as possible. The use of an antidepressant alone for a depressed college student presenting to an Emergency Department (ED) might be appropriate if the diagnosis is of a major depressive episode; less pertinent if the diagnosis is of an adjustment disorder; and seriously inadequate and quite possibly harmful if the diagnosis is of a bipolar disorder or a substance use disorder. As a rule, the "ready, fire … aim" approach should be avoided and it is best to defer pharmacologic treatment until a good working diagnosis can be reached. The establishment of a psychiatric diagnosis, however, often requires longitudinal assessment of course and treatment response. Many symptoms of psychiatric disorders may be obscured by co-occurring medical conditions, substance use, or inaccurate patient reports. In acute clinical situations, however, it is often not possible to defer the implementation of psychotropic medications until a diagnosis is fully clarified. In this context, it is crucial to document probable and differential diagnosis, to outline the rationale for selecting a particular treatment over others, and to indicate the kind of information needed to achieve greater diagnostic certainty. When a disorder appears in a sub-syndromal form, such as minor depression, the rationale and goals for proceeding with psychopharmacologic treatment should be well defined.

The identification of target symptoms plays an integral role in establishing a pre-treatment baseline and in later efforts to monitor the success of treatment. These symptoms might include aggression, insomnia, anhedonia, delusions of reference, hallucinations, or the frequency and intensity of suicidal longings. The identification of target symptoms—particularly clusters of target symptoms—serves to focus attention on the symptoms revealing greatest danger, disability, and distress to the patient while also informing the patient about the core symptoms of his or her illness and the specific goals for which psychotropic medications have been recommended.

For some conditions, clinician-rated instruments, such as the Brief Psychiatric Rating Scale,[3] the Hamilton Rating Scale for Depression,[4] the Hamilton Rating Scale for Anxiety,[5] and the Young Mania Scale,[6] provide useful, well-studied templates for the serial assessment of relevant symptoms. In addition, the patient and family or other caregivers can be recruited in formal efforts to monitor progress. In the case of episodic or complex presentations, the use of daily mood charts, patient-rating scales such as the Quick Inventory for Depressive Symptomatology,[7] or sleep logs reveal temporal patterns[8] (e.g., rapid mood cycling) and associations (e.g., to menstrual cycle or medication changes) that are not apparent cross-sectionally during office or bedside visits.

Along with the assessment of target symptoms, evaluation of current levels of function and subsequent changes with treatment relevant to quality of life are an integral part of good psychopharmacologic practice. Thus, for an outpatient, the clinician might query about improvement in work or school function, family and other social relationships, and use of leisure time. For an inpatient, progress in the level of independence and reduction in the overall degree of anguish can help confirm the adequacy of treatment, because lack of improvement along these dimensions directs attention to residual symptoms or to problems not initially apparent.

Since the last edition of this handbook, the Global Assessment of Function scale and its single composite score that pertains to quality of life has fallen out of favor.[9] In its place, some clinicians use the Clinical Global Impression (CGI) scale.[10] This scale, widely used in clinical trials, rates severity of disease on a scale of 1 to 7 (from normal to most extreme) and improvement on a scale of 1 to 7 (from very much improved to very much worse) and provides a simple quantitative means to document overall treatment outcome. The *Diagnostic and Statistical Manual of Mental Disorders*, 5th edition (DSM-5) Disability Study Group recommends that practitioners use the World Health Organization Disability Assessment Schedule (WHODAS 2.0) to measure disability for routine clinical use.[11] The WHODAS 2.0 is applicable to patients with any health condition. WHODAS 2.0 evaluates the patient's ability to perform activities in six domains of functioning (e.g., self-care) and uses these to calculate a score representing global disability.[12]

The understanding that a patient's psychiatric condition is influenced by psychosocial factors does not imply that psychotropic medications should be withheld. A major depression evolving in the setting of a spouse's chronic illness or panic attacks emerging in the weeks following the break-up of a significant relationship may well be as severe and as responsive to pharmacologic treatment as the same disorders that developed in other patients without similar precipitants. Vague referrals to counseling do not constitute sufficient treatment under such circumstances and may be viewed by patients as dismissive. If psychotherapy is recommended and pharmacotherapy deferred, the referral to psychotherapy—whether, for example, to individual cognitive therapy, to couples therapy, or to a pain management group (i.e., behavioral treatment)—must be viewed with the same deliberateness as the prescription of medication, and it should include a plan for follow-up. If substantial progress is not made within a clinically appropriate time frame (e.g., no more than 8 to 12 weeks for a moderately severe episode of major depression), then the adequacy of the psychotherapy should be re-evaluated. Severity, chronicity, and risk of recurrence of symptoms are often more relevant in determining the need for pharmacotherapy of psychiatric conditions than the presence of aggravating life circumstances or a caricatured description of illness as chemical or reactive.

Reciprocally, the expanding range of safe and well-tolerated psychotropic agents, such as the selective serotonin re-uptake inhibitors (SSRIs) and other newer antidepressants, does not alter the imperative to explore the use of non-medication interventions whenever medications are considered. An assessment of a patient for psychiatric medications should include an equally careful evaluation for other targeted interventions instead of, or in addition to, pharmacotherapy or psychotherapy. Often uniquely helpful are judicious referrals to parenting classes; elder care; Alcoholics Anonymous, Narcotics Anonymous, and Al-Anon; vocational assessment and rehabilitation; support groups for persons who are bereaved, who are going through separation, and who have medical disorders (e.g., epilepsy, human immunodeficiency virus [HIV] infection); and psychiatric self-help groups, such as those sponsored by the Depression and Bipolar Support Alliance (DBSA).

Patient education and informed consent are important legal and ethical imperatives that are also critical to the success of a course of treatment with psychotropic medications. If the capacity of the patient to make his or her own decisions fluctuates or is questionable, the clinician should obtain the patient's permission to include family or other patient-appointed persons in important treatment decisions. When a patient clearly lacks the capacity to make such decisions, formal legal mechanisms for substituted judgment should be used. Such mechanisms, however, in no way diminish the importance of educating a patient about medications and target symptoms to the fullest extent possible. When one presents recommendations to a patient about medications, information about diagnosis, target symptoms, treatment options, and anticipated means of follow-up should be included, as well as the medication's name, class, and dosing instructions. Side effects that are common (e.g., dry mouth, nausea, tremor, drowsiness, sexual dysfunction, weight gain) should be reviewed together with side effects that are uncommon but require immediate attention, such as a dystonia on an antipsychotic, painful and prolonged erection on trazodone, or a rapidly progressing rash on lamotrigine. Patients should be specifically cautioned about the risks of abrupt discontinuation of a psychotropic drug. Dietary and drug restrictions must be clearly described and, particularly in the case of preventing a hypertensive crisis with monoamine oxidase inhibitors (MAOIs), should be provided in written form as well.

Prescribers have a duty to disclose to patients the information necessary for them to make informed decisions about treatment recommendations.[13] Some prescribers have mixed feelings about the disclosure of side effect information (particularly about serious adverse reactions) to patients. They argue that providing such information may result in unnecessary anxiety and perhaps non-adherence to the medication. The consequence of such an approach carries a violation to patient's civil rights, and bears serious liability and responsibility if an adverse effect occurs and the patient has not been informed. Downplaying potential adverse events inherent in a particular medicine to mislead patients to give consent, may set the ground for a malpractice lawsuit. In the context of urgent, life-threatening conditions (such as acute mania), counseling about some potential adverse effects, particularly those not anticipated in the foreseeable future (e.g., tardive dyskinesia or perinatal risks), can be deferred until greater clinical stability is achieved and the risks and benefits of longer-term treatment can be meaningfully addressed.

All too often omitted in discussions preceding the initiation of medications, are clear information about the anticipated time course of response (whether to anticipate improvement in hours or weeks), the anticipated length of treatment, and the ready availability of strategies to address side effects, or lack of efficacy. Psychopharmacology decisions possess great meaning to patients and the goal of treatment is not simply to recommend or prescribe "the right" medicine for a given diagnosis. Patients may view medicine as a magic cure, a method of mind control, a poisonous substance, or a gift (especially if the prescriber gives it as a sample). Exploring a patient's reluctance to initiate treatment might elicit a variety of concerns, including the fear that medication will be stigmatizing, might engender physical or psychological dependence, might be "mind-altering" or personality transforming, might mask a problem rather than treat it, might imply consignment to life-long treatment, or reflect a narrow therapeutic philosophy. The faithfulness of a patient to a recommended course of treatment is invariably strengthened by a physician's dedicated efforts to elicit and address misgivings and potential misunderstandings at the outset. Referral to relevant websites and written materials on diagnosis and treatment are usually welcomed by patients and family members as a source of more detailed information, particularly when longer-term treatment is anticipated.

Selecting and Administering Medication

For many common psychiatric disorders, there exist at least several agents within a single class that are known to have roughly equivalent efficacy. Decisions regarding choice of a particular medication for a patient should give considerable weight to previous treatment response and the current feasibility of the medication in terms of cost, tolerability, and complexity of dosing. Anticholinergic, hypotensive, and sedative effects of drugs must be considered carefully, particularly when prescribing medications to elderly patients or patients who are medically frail.

Knowledge of a patient's genetic background may help clinicians provide a personalized medicine strategy by predicting both drug response and risk for adverse events. Pharmacogenetics is becoming more impactful to clinical practice and promises improved accuracy when selecting a medicine for a specific individual. Within psychiatry, studies have found genetic variations associated with altered treatment response/efficacy and increased side effect risk. Genetic testing for such variations may help identify which patients are more or less likely to respond to psychotropics and which are likely to experience an increased side effect burden.[14] Large randomized controlled trials are needed to further substantiate the utility of genetic testing in psychiatry.

Once a drug is chosen, the goal should be to achieve a full trial with adequate dosages and an adequate duration of treatment. Inadequate dosing and duration count are among the principal factors in treatment failure for patients with accurate diagnoses. In the service of decisions regarding a patient's care weeks or months later, it is crucial to document whether a trial of medication succeeded, failed, or was abbreviated because of clinical deterioration, medication side effects, poor adherence to treatment, or drug abuse. Suffering is unnecessarily prolonged and resources are poorly used when medications that were previously ineffective have been tried again because of inadequate documentation of failure or when medications that could have been effective are avoided because previous trials of those medications had not been flagged as having been incomplete.

Medication dosages should be adjusted to determine the lowest effective dosage and the simplest regimen. There is significant variability among individual patients with respect to response, blood levels, the expression of side effects, and the development of toxicity, such that the recommended dosage ranges provide only a general guide. Documentation of a patient's response to a particular dosage becomes a meaningful reference point for future treatment. As a rule, elderly patients should be started on lower dosages than younger patients, and the interval between dosage changes should be longer because the time to achieve steady-state levels is often prolonged. In the elderly, often there is also prolonged storage of medication and active metabolites in body tissues. Nevertheless, the goal of reaching an effective dosage must be pursued with equal determination in the elderly as in younger patients.

For patients with chronic psychiatric conditions, exacerbation of symptoms might prompt increases in the dosages of medications or addition of other medications. So too, for patients presenting acutely with severe disorders, medication dosages may be titrated up more rapidly than usual or combined with other psychotropic medications at an early point such that the lowest effective dosage and simplest regimen is likely to be unclear. Under these circumstances, re-evaluation for cautious reduction of dosage when an appropriate interval of stability has followed should be routine. When a patient's care is likely to be transferred to another clinician or another setting, such as a chronic care facility or a community health center, it is essential that such a plan be communicated to the accepting clinical staff to avoid committing a patient to long-term treatment with dosages or regimens that are excessive.

The attentive management of side effects plays an important role in developing a therapeutic alliance and improving the quality of life for a patient who may be on psychopharmacologic treatment for months or years. Although some adverse events require immediate discontinuation of the drug (e.g., serotonin syndrome or neuroleptic malignant syndrome [NMS]), most can be addressed initially with a dosage reduction, modification in the timing or by dividing doses, taking the medication with or without food, a change in the preparation of medication (e.g., from valproic acid to divalproex sodium), or guidance about sleep hygiene, exercise, or diet (e.g., caffeine, fluids, or fiber). When such measures prove unhelpful in addressing a side effect that is causing distress or that poses a safety risk, other measures must be considered, such as prescribing benztropine for extrapyramidal symptoms (EPS) on high-potency antipsychotic medicine or bupropion for sexual dysfunction on SSRIs, or replacing the offending medication with a more tolerable agent. For side effects that are likely to be transient and not dangerous, a patient's understanding that a variety of straightforward strategies are available in the case of persistence or worsening may be enough to help the patient endure the side effects until they subside.

Sometimes the best recommendation for a psychopharmacologist to offer is to "stay the course" and to counsel against making a medicine change. Though difficult in practice, it is best to avoid responding to short-term crises with long-term changes in medication. The decision to discontinue a successful antidepressant and substitute another in the setting of despair and insomnia following a traumatic event, offers the patient the prospect of benefit from the new medication weeks hence, while currently depriving the patient of active treatment known to have been effective. Although it may seem tempting to respond proportionally to a patient's marked distress with a fundamental change in established treatment, exacerbations that are thought likely to be transient are most reasonably addressed with interventions that are short term and focused coupled with adequate follow-up.

Approach to Treatment Failure

Lack of improvement, clinical worsening, or the emergence of unexpected symptoms require a concerted re-evaluation of diagnosis, dosage, drugs, and disruptions. Some patients require higher-than-usual doses of medicine or augmentation strategies involving combined-medication regimens.

Diagnosis

Among at least one-third of patients with major psychiatric disorders, initial treatment fails to bring about significant improvement despite accurate diagnosis. Nevertheless, treatment failure should motivate a careful review of history, initial presentation, and symptoms that seem incongruous with the provisional diagnosis (e.g., confusion in a patient with a seemingly mild depression; olfactory hallucinations in a patient presenting with panic attacks). A patient with fatigue out of proportion to other depressive symptoms might have a primary sleep disorder, such as obstructive sleep apnea. A depressed and cachectic elderly patient who fails to improve despite a series of adequate courses of antidepressant might turn out to have a psychotic depression, early dementia, carcinoma, or a frontal lobe tumor. A patient with obsessive–compulsive disorder who appears increasingly bizarre and erratic on an SSRI might have an undiagnosed bipolar disorder exacerbated by the antidepressant.

Dosage

Apparent treatment refractoriness is often the result of prescribing subtherapeutic dosages or the patient's nonadherence, and when treatment fails, the onus is on the clinician to confirm the adequacy of the dosage. Whenever possible, blood levels of prescribed medications help establish whether a patient is taking the medications and, for medications with established dosage ranges (e.g., lithium, anticonvulsants, TCAs, and methylphenidate, but not generally antipsychotics, SSRIs, or newer antidepressants), whether the medication dosages are likely to be in a therapeutic range. When adequate dosages of a drug prescribed to a conscientious patient fail to achieve consistent plasma concentrations or clinical response, the clinician must consider factors that affect drug metabolism, such as cigarette smoking, chronic alcohol use, or use of concurrent medications that result in lower levels of the drug. Less commonly, patients experience clinical deterioration after changes in their prescription brand, such as when generic preparations are substituted for brand name medications, causing variation in the bioavailability of the active agent.

Drugs

Many patients compartmentalize their use of medications and forget to mention as-needed or over-the-counter (OTC) medications or treatments prescribed in different settings. When psychopharmacologic treatments fail, a careful re-evaluation of the patient's current non-psychiatric medication use is warranted. Thus, a patient whose panic disorder responds incompletely to full dosages of a high-potency benzodiazepine may be unaware that his or her condition is aggravated by use of a β-agonist inhaler, sympathomimetic decongestant, or consumption of highly caffeinated beverages. So, too, a patient with bipolar disorder, previously stabilized on lithium but now presenting with hypomania, might not have realized the importance of reporting the initiation of prednisone for a flare of inflammatory bowel disease.

Widely consumed herbal and other natural remedies marketed as dietary supplements (e.g., St. John's wort, steroid-type agents) can participate in clinically important drug interactions;[15,16] the possibility of such interactions may be easily missed, however, because the use of alternative and complementary therapies is typically reported by patients only on direct inquiry by their clinician. Details of alcohol, diet pill, and illicit drug use must be carefully elicited as factors that, when excessive, often masquerade as, and at the very least exacerbate, other psychiatric disorders and can jeopardize the safety and efficacy of pharmacotherapy.

Disruptions

Although psychosocial stressors are not an excuse for psychopharmacologic nihilism, neither can they be meaningfully ignored as potential impediments to treatment. Incomplete remission of depressive symptoms in a patient living with an alcoholic spouse or of a psychotic exacerbation in a patient with schizophrenia whose community residential treatment facility has closed, should be met both by aggressive efforts to ensure the adequacy of pharmacologic treatment and by equally determined efforts to develop a plan to address the environmental factors that appear to be compromising a patient's recovery.

Combined Therapy

In clinical practice, many patients—particularly the elderly, the medically ill, or the medically complex—receive multiple medications. Moreover, general medical co-morbidity is common among patients with psychiatric disorders, elevating the likelihood of complex medication regimens and polypharmacy.[17] As in other areas of medicine, polypharmacy has become an increasingly accepted approach in psychiatry for addressing difficult-to-treat disorders.[18] The term *polypharmacy* may carry a pejorative connotation suggesting a thoughtless, irrational, or non-evidence-based approach to the prescribing of medicine. Indeed, haphazard polypharmacy puts patients at risk due to an increased likelihood of adverse medication reactions and drug–drug interactions. In contrast, "rational" or "strategic" combined psychopharmacologic approaches can be used for the treatment of psychiatric or medical co-morbidity,[19] as augmentation for patients with an insufficient response to a single agent, and for the management of treatment-emergent adverse effects.[20] Examples of the rational use of combined treatment include the addition of a benzodiazepine to an SSRI to hasten treatment response in panic disorder, use of lithium and a stimulant medication to treat co-occurring bipolar disorder and attention-deficit/hyperactivity disorder (ADHD), or the addition of modafinil to mitigate the sedating effects of clozapine for a patient with schizophrenia.

Therefore, a patient's use of two or more psychotropic medications ought not be viewed reflexively as in need of dismantling. One patient might arrive at a precisely adjusted, albeit complicated, regimen through a series of careful trials guided by a single experienced clinician, whereas another may accumulate multiple medications in a haphazard fashion across diverse treaters and settings. For the former patient, even a modest dosage change can result in a severe relapse that threatens the patient's safety or livelihood, whereas for the latter, a directed plan to taper medications and perhaps even to "start from scratch" is likely to be most helpful.

Discontinuing Medications

The discontinuation of psychotropic drugs must be carried out with as much care as their initiation. For patients on complicated regimens of psychotropic medications, periodic review for dosage reduction and potential discontinuation must be standard. Because data providing guidelines for drug discontinuation are scarce, the process is often empirical. Successful discontinuation, therefore, relies heavily on a good knowledge of a patient's history, together with adequate follow-up.

Assessment of a patient for discontinuing a drug involves appreciating the short-term risks of rebound and withdrawal as well as the long-term risks of relapse and recurrence. Rebound effects are the transient return of symptoms for which a medication has been prescribed (e.g., insomnia or anxiety), and withdrawal effects are the development of new symptoms characteristic of abrupt cessation of the medication, such as muscle spasms, delirium, or seizures following discontinuation of high-dosage benzodiazepine; hot flashes, nausea, unusual shock-like sensations, or malaise following discontinuation of an antidepressant.[21]

To make sound decisions regarding the re-instatement of medications, it is essential to distinguish rebound and withdrawal effects from relapse. *Relapse* is typically a persistent rather than self-limited state associated with a more delayed onset, and the re-emergence of clinically significant symptoms of the underlying illness in the absence of (or sometimes despite the continuation of) active treatment. The return of daily panic attacks after a remission of several months and an exacerbation of psychosis requiring hospitalization after 2 years of exclusively outpatient treatment are examples of relapse.

For disorders that can occur episodically, such as major depression, the term *relapse* refers more precisely to the recrudescence of symptoms during an initial period of remission, whereas the additional term *recurrence* refers to return of symptoms following a defined period of full remission (at least 4 to 6 months) on or off continued treatment. In the case of recurrence, the re-appearing symptoms are conceptualized as denoting a new episode rather than a continuation of the one previously treated.

In parallel with the concepts of relapse and recurrence, continuation of treatment refers to the ongoing use of medication prescribed to consolidate a remission of symptoms brought about by an initial (acute) phase of treatment to prevent relapse. *Maintenance treatment* refers to a more extended course of medication thereafter aimed at preventing recurrences and is reserved for patients with an illness characterized by chronicity, past recurrences, or particular severity. For major depression, acute treatment is typically in the range of 6 to 12 weeks, whereas continuation treatment extends 4 to 6 months beyond that point, and maintenance treatment may extend a further 1 to 5 years or more depending on the clinical context. Although antidepressants appear to be more effective than placebo during long-term treatment, the number of controlled antidepressant trials focusing on treatment of depression beyond the first year remains limited.[22]

A taper of medications over 48 to 72 hours is typically adequate to minimize the risk of rebound or withdrawal. With respect to relapse or recurrence, however, patients at risk may well benefit from a more protracted, carefully monitored taper of medications. This allows rapid reinstatement of full-dosage treatment at the early signs of worsening to avert a more serious escalation. Analyses of discontinuation of lithium[23] and antipsychotic agents[24] suggest that a too-rapid cessation can, in fact, increase the risk of relapse when compared with a more gradual taper. Findings such as these suggest that for elective discontinuation of psychotropic medications, a taper lasting at least 2 to 4 weeks should be considered.

With patients for whom the consequences of relapse are likely to be severe (e.g., most patients with bipolar and psychotic disorders), an extended taper with dosage reductions of no more than 25% at intervals of no less than 4 to 6 weeks is likely to be a more prudent course. For patients who have anxiety disorders and are maintained on high-potency benzodiazepines, the introduction of a targeted course of therapy (e.g., a cognitive-behavioral panic disorder group) in preparation for a drug taper is likely to further reduce the risks of relapse.[25]

Far from being an afterthought, decisions regarding the timing and pace of drug discontinuation should be regarded as an integral part of psychopharmacologic management and remain an important topic for further study.

PHARMACOKINETICS

Pharmacokinetic processes refer to absorption, distribution, metabolism, and excretion, factors that determine plasma levels of a drug and the local availability of a drug to biologically active sites—in short, what the body does to the drug.[26] Pharmacokinetics also refers to the mathematical analysis of these processes. Advances in analytic chemistry and computer methods of pharmacokinetic modeling[27] and a growing understanding of the molecular pharmacology of the hepatic isoenzymes responsible for metabolizing most psychotropic medications have furnished increasingly sophisticated insights into the disposition and interaction of administered drugs.

Because the pharmacokinetics of a medication are subject to myriad influences, including age, genes, gender, diet, disease states, and concurrently administered drugs, a working knowledge of pharmacokinetic principles is of particular relevance to psychopharmacology in medical settings. Although pharmacokinetics refers to only one of the two broad mechanisms (the other being pharmacodynamics) by which drugs interact, pharmacokinetic interactions involve all classes of psychotropic and non-psychotropic medications.[28] An overview of pharmacokinetic processes is a helpful prelude to a discussion of specific drug–drug interactions by psychotropic class.

Absorption

Factors that influence drug absorption are generally of less importance in determining the pharmacokinetic properties of psychiatric medications than factors influencing subsequent drug disposition (e.g., drug metabolism). The term *absorption* refers to processes that generally pertain to orally (rather than parenterally) administered drugs, for which alterations in gastrointestinal (GI) drug absorption can affect the rate (time to reach maximum concentration) or the extent of absorption, or both. The extent or completeness of absorption, also known as the *fractional absorption*, is measured as the area under the curve (AUC) when plasma concentration is plotted against time. The bioavailability of an oral dose of drug refers, in turn, to the fractional absorption for orally compared with intravenously (IV) administered drug. If an agent is reported to have a 90% bioavailability (e.g., lorazepam), this indicates that the extent of absorption of an orally administered dose is nearly that of an IV-administered dose, although the rate of absorption may well be slower for the oral dose.

Because the upper part of the small intestine is the primary site of drug absorption through passive membrane diffusion and filtration and both passive and active transport processes, factors that speed gastric emptying (e.g., metoclopramide) or diminish intestinal motility (e.g., opioids or cannabis) can facilitate greater contact with, and absorption from, the mucosal surface into the systemic circulation, potentially increasing plasma drug concentrations. Conversely, bulk laxatives, such as psyllium, magnesium-based antacids, lactulose, kaolin-pectin, and cholestyramine, can bind to drugs, forming complexes that pass unabsorbed through the GI lumen.

Changes in gastric pH associated with food or other drugs alter the non-polar, un-ionized fraction of drug available for absorption. In the case of drugs that are very weak acids or bases, however, the extent of ionization is relatively invariant under physiologic conditions. Properties of the preparation administered (e.g., tablet, capsule, or liquid) can also influence the rate or extent of absorption and, for an increasing number of medications (e.g., bupropion, lithium, most stimulant medicines, quetiapine, and venlafaxine—to name a few), preparations intended for slow release are available.

The local action of enzymes in the GI tract (e.g., monoamine oxidase [MAO]; cytochrome P450, CYP3A4) may be responsible for metabolism of drug before absorption. This is of critical relevance to the emergence of hypertensive crises that occur when excessive quantities of the dietary pressor tyramine are systemically absorbed in the setting of irreversible inhibition of the MAO isoenzymes for which tyramine is a substrate.

Following gut absorption, but before entry into the systemic circulation, many psychotropic drugs are subject to first-pass liver metabolism. Therefore, conditions that affect hepatic metabolism of drug (e.g., primary liver disease) or conditions that impede portal circulation (e.g., congestive heart failure) are likely to increase the fraction of drug available for distribution for the majority of psychotropic drugs, thereby contributing to clinically significant increases in plasma levels of drug.

There has been increasing focus on the role of the drug transporter P-glycoprotein (Pgp) in drug absorption. While the tissue distribution of Pgp influences the effect of psychotropics and the interaction potential for drugs such as risperidone, nortriptyline, and citalopram at the interface between the blood and central nervous system (CNS), Pgp is also found in other areas of the body such as the intestines, which are a major site for drug absorption into the body.[29] The Pgps found in the gut have not been as extensively studied; however, it is well known that the expression of Pgp in other tissues can be induced and inhibited by other drugs. It is thought that some interactions, mainly seen with the antiepileptic drugs (AEDs), previously assumed to be a result of CYP450 alterations, instead may actually be mediated by the modulation of the Pgp activity at the point of drug absorption or distribution.[30] The capacity of St. John's wort to lower blood levels of several critical medications (e.g., cyclosporine, indinavir) is hypothesized to be related to an effect of the botanical agent on this transport system.

Distribution

Drugs distribute to tissues through the systemic circulation. The amount of drug ultimately reaching receptor sites in tissues is determined by a variety of factors, including the concentration of free (unbound) drug in plasma, regional blood flow, and physiochemical properties of drug (e.g., lipophilicity or structural characteristics). For entrance into the CNS, penetration across the blood–brain barrier is required. Fat-soluble drugs (e.g., benzodiazepines, antipsychotics, cyclic antidepressants) distribute more widely in the body than water-soluble drugs (e.g., lithium), which distribute through a smaller volume of distribution. Changes with age, typically including an increase in the ratio of body fat to lean body mass, therefore, result in a net greater volume of lipophilic drug distribution and potentially greater accumulation of drug in adipose tissue in older than in younger patients. A similar potential exists for female compared with male patients because of their generally higher ratio of adipose tissue to lean body mass.[27]

In general, psychotropic drugs have relatively high affinities for plasma proteins (some to albumin but others, such as antidepressants, to α_1-acid glycoproteins and lipoproteins). Most psychotropic drugs are more than 80% protein-bound. A drug is considered highly protein-bound if more than 90% exists in bound form in plasma. Fluoxetine, aripiprazole, and diazepam are examples of the many psychotropic drugs that are highly protein-bound. In contrast, venlafaxine, lithium, topiramate, zonisamide, gabapentin, pregabalin, levomilnacipran, and memantine are examples of drugs with minimal protein binding and therefore minimal risk of participating in drug–drug interactions related to protein binding.

A reversible equilibrium exists between bound and unbound drug. Only the unbound fraction exerts pharmacologic effects. Competition by two or more drugs for protein-binding sites often results in displacement of a previously bound drug, which, in the free state, becomes pharmacologically active. Similarly, reduced concentrations of plasma proteins in a severely malnourished patient or a patient with a disease that is associated with markedly lowered serum proteins (e.g., liver disease, the nephrotic syndrome) may be associated with an increase in the fraction of unbound drug potentially available for activity at relevant receptor sites. Under most circumstances, the net changes in plasma concentration of active drug are, in fact, quite small because the unbound drug is available for redistribution to other tissues and for metabolism and excretion, thereby offsetting the initial rise in plasma levels. It is important to be aware, however, that clinically significant consequences can develop when protein-binding interactions alter the unbound fraction of previously highly protein-bound drugs that have a low therapeutic index (e.g., warfarin). For these drugs, relatively small variations in plasma level may be associated with serious untoward effects.

Metabolism

Most drugs undergo several types of biotransformation, and many psychotropic drug interactions of clinical significance are based on interference with this process. *Metabolism* refers to the biotransformation of a drug to another form, a process that is usually enzyme-mediated and results in a metabolite that might or might not be pharmacologically active and might or might not be subject to further biotransformations before eventual excretion. A growing understanding of hepatic enzymes, and especially the rapidly emerging characterization of the CYP isoenzymes and other enzyme systems including the uridine-diphosphate glucuronosyltransferases (UGTs) and flavin-containing monooxygenases (FMOs),[31] has significantly advanced a rational understanding and prediction of drug interactions and individual variation in drug responses.

Phase I reactions include oxidation (e.g., hydroxylation, dealkylation), reduction (e.g., nitro reduction), and hydrolysis, metabolic reactions typically resulting in intermediate metabolites that are then subject to phase II reactions, including conjugation (e.g., glucuronide, sulfate) and acetylation. Phase II reactions typically yield highly polar, water-soluble metabolites suitable for renal excretion. Most psychotropic drugs undergo both phase I and phase II metabolic reactions. Notable exceptions are lithium and gabapentin, which are not subject to hepatic metabolism, and a subset of the benzodiazepines (lorazepam, oxazepam, temazepam), which undergo only phase II reactions and are therefore especially appropriate when benzodiazepines are used in the context of concurrent medications, advanced age, or disease states in which alterations of hepatic metabolism is likely to be substantial.

The synthesis or activity of hepatic microsomal enzymes is affected by metabolic inhibitors and inducers, as well as distinct genetic polymorphisms (stably inherited traits). Table 38-1 lists enzyme inducers and inhibitors common in clinical settings. These should serve as red flags that beckon further scrutiny for potential drug–drug interactions when they are found on a patient's medication list. In some circumstances an inhibitor (e.g., grapefruit juice) or an inducer (e.g., a cruciferous vegetable, such as Brussels sprouts) is a drug but it may be another ingested substance.

Inhibitors impede the metabolism of a concurrently administered drug, producing a rise in its plasma level,

TABLE 38-1 Commonly Used Drugs and Substances That Inhibit or Induce Hepatic Metabolism of Other Medications[18,26]

INHIBITORS	INDUCERS
Antifungals (ketoconazole, miconazole, itraconazole)	Barbiturates (e.g., phenobarbital, secobarbital)
Macrolide antibiotics (erythromycin, clarithromycin, triacetyloleandomycin)	Carbamazepine
	Oxcarbazepine
Fluoroquinolones (e.g., ciprofloxacin)	Phenytoin
	Rifampin
Isoniazid	Primidone
Antiretrovirals	Cigarettes
Antimalarials (chloroquine)	Ethanol (chronic)
Selective serotonin re-uptake inhibitors (fluoxetine, fluvoxamine, paroxetine, sertraline)	Cruciferous vegetables
	Charbroiled meats
Duloxetine	St. John's wort
Bupropion	Oral contraceptives
Nefazodone	Prednisone
β-Blockers (lipophilic) (e.g., propranolol, metoprolol, pindolol)	
Quinidine	
Valproate	
Cimetidine	
Calcium channel-blockers (e.g., diltiazem)	
Grapefruit juice	
Ethanol (acute)	

whereas inducers enhance the metabolism of another drug, resulting in a decline in its plasma levels. Although inhibition is usually immediate, induction, which requires enhanced synthesis of the metabolic enzyme, is typically a more gradual process. A fall in plasma levels of a substrate might not be apparent for days to weeks following introduction of the inducer. This is particularly important to keep in mind when a patient's care is being transferred to another setting where clinical deterioration may be the first sign that drug levels have declined. Reciprocally, an elevation in plasma drug concentrations could reflect the previous discontinuation of an inducing factor (e.g., cigarette smoking, carbamazepine) just as it could reflect the introduction of an inhibitor (e.g., fluoxetine, valproic acid).

Although the CYP isoenzymes represent only one of the numerous enzyme systems responsible for drug metabolism, they are responsible for metabolizing, at least in part, more than 80% of all prescribed drugs. The capacity of many of the SSRIs to inhibit CYP isoenzymes fueled great interest in the pattern of interaction of psychotropic and other drugs with these enzymes in the understanding and prediction of drug–drug interactions in psychopharmacology. The CYP isoenzymes represent a family of more than 30 related heme-containing enzymes, largely located in the endoplasmic reticulum of hepatocytes (but also present elsewhere, including gut and brain), which mediate oxidative metabolism of a wide variety of drugs as well as endogenous substances, including prostaglandins, fatty acids, and steroids. The majority of antidepressant and antipsychotic drugs are metabolized by or inhibited by one or more of these isoenzymes.[32] Table 38-2 summarizes the interactions of psychiatric and non-psychiatric drugs with a subset of isoenzymes that have been increasingly well characterized. In addition to the numerous publications in which these interactions are cited,[18,26,27] several relevant websites are regularly updated, including www.drug-interactions.com. The relevance of these and other interactions is highlighted in a later section of this chapter, in which clinically important drug–drug interactions are reviewed.

Within the group of CYP isoenzymes, there appears to be a polymodal distribution of metabolic activity in the population with respect to certain isoenzymes (including CYP2C19 and 2D6). Most people are normal (extensive) metabolizers with respect to the activity of these isoenzymes. A smaller number are poor metabolizers, with deficient activity of the isoenzyme. Probably very much smaller numbers are ultra-rapid metabolizers, who have more than normal activity of the enzyme, and intermediate metabolizers, who fall between extensive and poor metabolizers. Persons who are poor metabolizers with respect to a particular CYP isoenzyme are expected to have higher plasma concentrations of a drug that is metabolized by that isoenzyme, thereby potentially being more sensitive to or requiring lower dosages of that drug than a patient with normal activity of that enzyme. These patients might also have higher-than-usual plasma levels of metabolites of the drug that are produced through other metabolic pathways that are not altered by the polymorphism, thereby potentially incurring pharmacologic activity or adverse effects related to these alternative metabolites.

Studies on genetic polymorphisms affecting the CYP system suggest ethnic differences.[33] Approximately 15% to 20% of Asian Americans and African Americans appear to be poor metabolizers with respect to CYP 2C19 compared with 3% to 5% of whites. Conversely, the proportion of frankly poor metabolizers with respect to CYP 2D6 appears to be higher among white (approx. 5% to 10%) than among Asian and African Americans (approx. 1% to 3%). As our understanding of the clinical relevance of genetic polymorphisms in psychopharmacology expands, commercial genotyping tests for polymorphisms of potential relevance to drug metabolism will likely become commonplace. For the use of certain drugs, notably carbamazepine, the US Food and Drug Administration (FDA) recommends genotyping Asians for the *HLA B*1502* allele owing to data implicating the allele as a marker for carbamazepine-induced Stevens–Johnson syndrome and toxic epidermal necrolysis in Han Chinese.[34] Future study of genetic polymorphisms and their relevance to the prediction of drug response promises new ways to compensate for a gene defect (pharmacodynamic genetic variations) or to adjust medication dosage based on the rate at which a patient metabolizes medication (pharmacokinetic genetic variations).

Excretion

Because most antidepressant, anxiolytic, and antipsychotic medications are largely eliminated by hepatic metabolism, factors that affect renal excretion (glomerular filtration, tubular re-absorption, and active tubular secretion) are generally far less important to the pharmacokinetics of these drugs than to lithium, for which such factors can have

TABLE 38-2 Selected Cytochrome P450 Isoenzyme Substrates, Inhibitors, and Inducers[a,18,26]

ISOENZYME	SUBSTRATES	INHIBITORS	INDUCERS
1A2	Alosetron, asenapine, caffeine, clomipramine, clozapine, cyclobenzaprine, estradiol, fluvoxamine, mirtazapine, melatonin, olanzapine, propranolol, ramelteon, riluzole, ropinirole, tacrine, tizanidine, theophylline, zolmitriptan	Amiodarone, artemisinin, cimetidine, **ciprofloxacin**, fluoroquinolones, **fluvoxamine**, ginkgo, grapefruit juice, methoxsalen, mexiletine, oral contraceptives, tranylcypromine, vemurafenib, zileuton	**Carbamazepine**, charbroiled meats, cigarette smoking (tobacco), cruciferous vegetables, modafinil, montelukast, **primidone**, **rifampin**, ritonavir, St. John's wort
2B6	Bupropion, methadone, selegiline	Desipramine, doxorubicin, paroxetine, sertraline, sorafenib, thiotepa	**Carbamazepine**, dexamethasone, efavirenz, modafinil, nilotinib, **phenobarbital**, **phenytoin**, **primidone**, rifampin
2C9	Celecoxib, diclofenac, fluoxetine, meloxicam, piroxicam	Amiodarone, **delavirdine**, efavirenz, fluconazole, **gemfibrozil**, ketoconazole, leflunomide, miconazole, omeprazole, sorafenib	Carbamazepine, dexamethasone, griseofulvin, **phenytoin**, **primidone**, rifampin, **rifapentine**, **secobarbital**
2C19	Amitriptyline, carisoprodol, citalopram, clomipramine, diazepam, escitalopram, imipramine, venlafaxine	**Chloramphenicol**, **delavirdine**, esomeprazole, fluconazole, fluoxetine, **fluvoxamine**, **gemfibrozil**, modafinil, omeprazole, sertraline, **ticlopidine**, tranylcypromine, voriconazole	Aspirin, **carbamazepine**, norethindrone, **phenytoin**, prednisone, rifampin St. John's wort, vilazodone
2D6	Amitriptyline, amoxapine, amphetamine, aripiprazole, atomoxetine, brexpiprazole, β-blockers (lipophilic), chlorpromazine, clomipramine, clozapine, codeine, desipramine, dextromethorphan, diltiazem, donepezil, doxepin, duloxetine, encainide, escitalopram, flecainide, fluoxetine, fluvoxamine, haloperidol, hydroxycodone, iloperidone, imipramine, lidocaine, metoclopramide, mCPP, mexiletine, mirtazapine, nifedipine, nortriptyline, ondansetron, olanzapine, phenothiazines (e.g., thioridazine, perphenazine), propafenone, risperidone, tamoxifen, tramadol, trazodone, venlafaxine, vortioxetine	Amiodarone, antimalarials, **bupropion**, **chlorpromazine**, cimetidine, **cinacalcet**, citalopram, clomipramine, clozapine, **delavirdine**, desipramine, duloxetine, fluoxetine, haloperidol, ketoconazole, methadone, metoclopramide, paroxetine, phenothiazines, protease inhibitors (ritonavir), quinidine, sertraline, terbinafine, ticlopidine, tipranavir, tranylcypromine, yohimbine	Dexamethasone, glutethimide, rifampin
3A4, 3A5	Alfentanil, alprazolam, amiodarone, amprenavir, aripiprazole, armodafinil, bromocriptine, buspirone, Cafergot, calcium channel blockers, caffeine, carbamazepine, cisapride, clonazepam, clozapine, cyclosporine, dapsone, diazepam, disopyramide, efavirenz, estradiol, fentanyl, indinavir, HMG-CoA reductase inhibitors (lovastatin, simvastatin), lidocaine, loratadine, methadone, midazolam, mirtazapine, nimodipine, pimozide, prednisone, progesterone, propafenone, quetiapine, quinidine, ritonavir, sildenafil, tacrolimus, testosterone, triazolam, vilazodone, vinblastine, warfarin, zaleplon, ziprasidone, zolpidem, zonisamide	Antifungals, **boceprevir**, calcium channel blockers, **clarithromycin**, cimetidine, **conivaptan**, efavirenz, erythromycin, fluconazole, fluvoxamine, **grapefruit juice**, **indinavir**, **itraconazole**, **mibefradil**, **nefazodone**, **nelfinavir**, **ritonavir**, **saquinavir**, **telaprevir**, telithromycin, verapamil, **voriconazole**	Bosentan, **carbamazepine**, glucocorticoids, modafinil, oxcarbazepine, **phenobarbital**, **phenytoin**, **primidone**, pioglitazone, **rifampin**, **rifapentine**, ritonavir, **St. John's wort**, troglitazone

Bold indicates strong inhibitor/inducer.
[a]Drugs.com: *Drug interactions checker*. Retrieved from www.drugs.com/drug_interactions.php. Accessed August 12, 2016.
HMG-CoA, hydroxy-methylglutaryl co-enzyme A; mCPP, meta-chlorophenylpiperazine.

clinically significant consequences. Conditions resulting in sodium deficiency (e.g., dehydration, sodium restriction, use of thiazide diuretics) are likely to result in increased proximal tubular re-absorption of lithium, resulting in increased lithium levels and potential toxicity. Lithium levels and clinical status must be monitored especially closely in the setting of vomiting, diarrhea, excessive evaporative losses, or polyuria. Factors, such as aging, that are associated with reduced renal blood flow and glomerular filtration rate (GFR) also reduce lithium excretion. For this reason, as well as for their reduced volume of distribution for lithium because of the relative loss of total body water with aging, elderly, patients typically require lower lithium dosages than younger patients, and a low starting dosage (i.e., 150 to 300 mg/day) is often prudent. Apparently separate from pharmacokinetic effects, however, elderly patients may also be more sensitive to the neurotoxic effects of lithium even at low therapeutic levels. On the other hand, factors associated with an increased GFR, particularly pregnancy, can produce an increase in lithium clearance and a fall in lithium levels.

For other medications, renal excretion can sometimes be exploited in the treatment of a drug overdose. Acidification of the urine by ascorbic acid, ammonium chloride, or methenamine mandelate increases the rate of excretion of weak bases, such as the amphetamines and phencyclidine (PCP). Therefore, such measures may be important in the emergency management of a patient with severe phencyclidine or amphetamine intoxication. Conversely, alkalinization of the urine by administration of sodium bicarbonate or acetazolamide can hasten the excretion of weak acids including long-acting barbiturates, such as phenobarbital.

Mildly to moderately impaired renal function does not typically prompt routine changes in the dosage or dosing intervals of psychotropic medications other than lithium. In patients with severe impairment of kidney function, however, there may be accumulation of metabolites and, to a lesser extent, of the parent compound across repeated doses. An increase in the dosing interval and possible reduction in drug dosage should therefore be considered in this setting, particularly in the case of chronically administered agents with active metabolites.

Renal excretion is only one contribution to the *elimination half-life*, a pharmacokinetic construct that refers to the time required for the plasma concentration of a drug to be reduced by one half. The elimination phase (also referred to as the β-phase) reflects all processes that contribute to drug removal, including renal excretion, hepatic metabolism, and, to a much lesser extent, other factors (e.g., loss of drug in sweat or biliary secretions) potentially affecting drug clearance (the volume of blood or plasma cleared of drug per unit time). For the majority of drugs, whose elimination follows first-order kinetics (i.e., their rate of elimination is proportional to the amount of drug in the body rather than equal to a constant amount), steady-state drug levels are reached in four to five elimination half-lives, whereas, on discontinuation, almost all drug is out of the body within five half-lives.

For drugs that are administered for their single-dose effects (e.g., an as-needed benzodiazepine or antipsychotic) rather than for long-term effects of repeated administration (e.g., antidepressants), the duration of action of the drug depends not only on the elimination half-life but also often more critically on the initial phase of drug redistribution from the systemic circulation to other tissues, such as muscle and fat.

DRUG INTERACTIONS

The scientific literature on psychotropic drug–drug interactions has grown immensely since first reviewed in the *Massachusetts General Hospital Handbook of General Hospital Psychiatry* in 1978.[35] Despite impressive advances in clinical and molecular pharmacology, much of the literature on drug–drug interactions remains a patchwork of case reports, post-marketing analyses, extrapolation from animal and *in vitro* studies, and inferences based on what is known about other drugs with similar properties. Fortunately, well-designed studies of drug–drug interactions are an increasingly integral part of drug development.

Drug–drug interactions refer to alterations in drug levels or drug effects (or both) attributed to the administration of two or more prescribed, illicit, or OTC agents in close temporal proximity. Although many drug–drug interactions involve drugs administered within minutes to hours of each other, some drugs can participate in interactions days or even weeks after they are discontinued because of prolonged elimination half-lives (e.g., fluoxetine) or owing to their long-term impact on metabolic enzymes (e.g., carbamazepine). Some drug–drug interactions involving psychotropic medications are life-threatening, such as those involving the co-administration of MAOIs and drugs with potent serotoninergic (e.g., meperidine) or sympathomimetic (e.g., phenylpropanolamine) effects.[36] These combinations are therefore absolutely contraindicated.

However, most drug–drug interactions in psychopharmacology manifest in subtler ways, often leading to poor medication tolerability and compliance due to adverse events (e.g., orthostatic hypotension, sedation, irritability), diminished medication efficacy, or puzzling manifestations, such as altered mental status or unexpectedly high or low drug levels. Drug combinations that can produce these often less-catastrophic drug–drug interactions are usually not absolutely contraindicated. Some of these combinations may, indeed, be valuable in the treatment of some patients though wreaking havoc for other patients. The capacity to anticipate and to recognize both the major, but rare, and the subtler, but common, potential drug–drug interactions allows the practitioner to minimize the impact of these interactions as an obstacle to patient safety and to therapeutic success.

It is crucial to be familiar with the small number of drug–drug interactions in psychopharmacology that, though uncommon, are associated with potentially catastrophic consequences. These include drugs associated with ventricular arrhythmias, hypertensive crisis, serotonin syndrome, Stevens–Johnson syndrome, seizures, and severe bone marrow suppression. In addition, drug–drug interactions are important to consider when a patient's drugs include those with a low therapeutic index (e.g., lithium, digoxin, warfarin) or a narrow therapeutic window (e.g., indinavir, nortriptyline, cyclosporine), such that relatively small alterations in pharmacokinetic or pharmacodynamic behavior can jeopardize a patient's well-being. In addition, it is worthwhile to consider potential drug–drug interactions whenever evaluating a patient whose drug levels are unexpectedly variable or extreme or a patient with a confusing clinical picture (such as clinical deterioration) or with unexpected side effects. Finally, drug–drug interactions are likely to be clinically salient for a patient who is medically frail or elderly, owing to altered pharmacokinetics and vulnerability to side effects, as well as for a patient who is heavily using alcohol, cigarettes, or illicit drugs or who is being treated for a drug overdose.

Given the widespread use of combined pharmacotherapeutic regimens for many difficult-to-treat disorders, the vast literature of reported and potential drug–drug interactions, and the increasingly litigious society in which physicians practice, the physician today is faced with a dilemma when evaluating the potential significance of drug–drug interactions. Fortunately, an increasing range of resources are available, including e-prescribing software packages (often embedded within electronic health records), will automatically check for potential drug–drug interactions when a clinician prescribes medicine, as well as regularly updated websites (such as www.drug-interactions.com) that may detect and prevent potential interactions.

Numerous factors contribute to inter-individual variability in drug response. These factors include treatment adherence, age, gender, nutritional status, disease states, and genetic polymorphisms that can influence risk of adverse events and treatment resistance.[37] Drug–drug interactions are an additional factor that influences how patients react to drugs. The importance of these interactions depends heavily on the clinical context. In many cases, the practical impact of drug–drug interactions may be small compared with other factors that affect treatment response, drug levels, and toxicity. It is reasonable therefore to focus special attention on commonly used classes of drugs and the contexts in which drug–drug interactions are most likely to be clinically problematic.

Antipsychotic Drugs

Antipsychotic drugs, used in the treatment of schizophrenia, schizoaffective disorder, organic psychoses, mood disorders, and an increasingly broad range of other psychiatric conditions, include the phenothiazines (e.g., chlorpromazine, fluphenazine, perphenazine, thioridazine, trifluoperazine); butyrophenones (haloperidol); thioxanthenes (thiothixene); indolones (molindone); diphenylbutylpiperidines (pimozide); dibenzodiazepines (loxapine); and the second-generation, atypical agents (clozapine, risperidone, olanzapine, quetiapine, ziprasidone, aripiprazole, paliperidone, asenapine, lurasidone, iloperidone, brexpiprazole, and cariprazine). As a class, they are generally rapidly, if erratically, absorbed from the GI tract after oral administration (peak plasma concentrations ranging from 30 minutes to 6 hours). They are highly lipophilic and distribute rapidly to body tissues with a large apparent volume of distribution. Protein-binding in the circulation ranges from approximately 90% to 98%, except for molindone, paliperidone, and quetiapine, which are only moderately protein-bound.

The antipsychotics generally undergo substantial first-pass hepatic metabolism (primarily oxidation and conjugation reactions), reducing their systemic bioavailability when given orally compared with intramuscular (IM) administration, the fractional absorption of which nearly approximates that of IV administration. Most of the individual antipsychotics have several pharmacologically active metabolites (e.g., paliperidone is 9-hydroxyrisperidone, the primary active metabolite of risperidone).[38]

Because of their propensity to sequester in body compartments, the elimination half-life of antipsychotics is quite variable, ranging from approximately 6 to 90 hours. For some antipsychotics, elimination pharmacokinetics appears to be especially complex, and the disappearance of drug from the systemic circulation may take much longer, as it does for the newer agent, brexpiprazole, whose half-life can exceed 90 hours.[39]

The lower-potency antipsychotics (including chlorpromazine, clozapine, thioridazine, quetiapine) are generally the most sedating and have the greatest anticholinergic, antihistaminic, and α_1-adrenergic antagonistic effects, whereas the higher-potency antipsychotics (including aripiprazole, haloperidol, loxapine, and others) are comparatively more likely to be associated with an increased incidence of extrapyramidal symptoms (EPS), including akathisia, dystonia, and parkinsonism.

The atypical antipsychotics generally have multiple receptor affinities, including antagonism at dopamine D_1 to D_4 receptors, serotonin (5-HT) 5-HT_1 and 5-HT_2 receptors, α_1- and α_2-adrenergic receptors, histamine H_1 receptor, and cholinergic muscarinic receptors, with variations across agents. Thus, for example, clozapine and olanzapine have notably greater affinity at the muscarinic receptors than the other agents, and aripiprazole is actually a partial agonist at the D_2 receptor.

Although the more complex pharmacologic profile of second-generation, atypical agents, as well as the older low-potency antipsychotics, has generally been associated with a lower risk of EPS, the same broad range of receptor activity also poses greater risk of *pharmacodynamic interactions*. Pharmacodynamic interactions refer to the pharmacologic effects that result from interactions at the same or interrelated biologically active (receptor) sites.

Lower-potency drugs, as well as some atypical antipsychotics (e.g., asenapine, risperidone, quetiapine), can produce significant hypotension, especially when combined with vasodilator or antihypertensive drugs related to α_1-adrenergic blockade (Table 38-3).[40,41] Severe hypotension has been reported when chlorpromazine has been administered with the angiotensin-converting enzyme (ACE) inhibitor captopril. Hypotension can develop when epinephrine is administered with low-potency antipsychotics. In this setting, the α-adrenergic stimulant effect of epinephrine, resulting in vasodilation, is unopposed by its usual pressor effect because α_1-adrenergic receptors are occupied by the antipsychotic. A similar effect can result if a low-potency antipsychotic is administered to a patient with pheochromocytoma. Finally, hypotension can develop when low-potency antipsychotics are used in combination with a variety of anesthetics, such as halothane, enflurane, and isoflurane.

In addition, the low-potency antipsychotics have quinidine-like effects on cardiac conduction and can prolong Q-T and P-R intervals.[42] Ziprasidone may also cause Q-T prolongation, although clinically significant prolongation (QTc >500 ms) appears to be rare when administered to otherwise healthy subjects.[40] Significant depression of cardiac

TABLE 38-3 Selected Drug Interactions With Antipsychotic Medications[2,41,45]

DRUG	POTENTIAL INTERACTION
Antacids (aluminum- and magnesium-containing)	Interference with absorption of antipsychotic agents; fruit juice
Carbamazepine	Decreased antipsychotic drug plasma levels; additive risk of myelosuppression with clozapine
Cigarettes	Decreased antipsychotic drug plasma levels; reduced extrapyramidal symptoms
Rifampin	Decreased antipsychotic drug plasma levels; reduced extrapyramidal symptoms
TCAs	Increased TCA and antipsychotic drug plasma levels; hypotension, depression of cardiac conduction (with low-potency antipsychotics)
SSRIs	Increased SSRI and antipsychotic drug plasma levels; arrhythmia risk with thioridazine and pimozide
Bupropion, duloxetine	Increased antipsychotic drug plasma levels; arrhythmia risk with thioridazine
Fluvoxamine, nefazodone	Increased antipsychotic drug plasma levels, arrhythmia risk with pimozide; seizure risk with clozapine
β-Blockers (lipophilic)	Increased antipsychotic drug plasma levels; improved akathisia
Anticholinergic drugs	Additive anticholinergic toxicity; reduced extrapyramidal symptoms
Antihypertensive, vasodilator drugs	Hypotension (with low-potency antipsychotics and risperidone)
Guanethidine, clonidine	Blockade of antihypertensive effect
Epinephrine	Hypotension (with low-potency antipsychotics)
Class I antiarrhythmics	Depression of cardiac conduction; ventricular arrhythmias (with low-potency antipsychotics, ziprasidone)
Calcium channel blockers	Depression of cardiac conduction; ventricular arrhythmias (with pimozide)
Lithium	Idiosyncratic neurotoxicity

SSRI, selective serotonin re-uptake inhibitor; TCA, tricyclic antidepressant.

conduction, heart block, and life-threatening ventricular dysrhythmias can result from co-administering low-potency antipsychotics or ziprasidone with class I antiarrhythmics (e.g., quinidine, procainamide, disopyramide); it can also result from the TCAs, which have quinidine-like activity on cardiac conduction, and when administered in the context of other aggravating factors including hypokalemia, hypomagnesemia, bradycardia, or congenital prolongation of the QTc. Pimozide also can depress cardiac conduction as a result of its calcium channel-blocking action, and the combination of pimozide with other calcium channel blockers (e.g., nifedipine, diltiazem, verapamil) is contraindicated.

Another clinically significant pharmacodynamic interaction arises when low-potency antipsychotics, particularly clozapine or olanzapine, are administered with other drugs that have anticholinergic effects, including TCAs, benztropine, and diphenhydramine.[41] When these drugs are combined, there is a greater risk of urinary retention, constipation, blurred vision, impaired memory and concentration, and, in the setting of narrow-angle glaucoma, increased intraocular pressure. With intentional or inadvertent overdoses, a severe anticholinergic syndrome can develop, including delirium, paralytic ileus, tachycardia, and dysrhythmias. With lower affinity for muscarinic cholinergic receptors, the high-potency agents and non-anticholinergic atypical agents (e.g., risperidone, aripiprazole) are indicated when anticholinergic effects need to be minimized.

The sedative effects of low-potency agents and atypical antidepressants are also often additive to those of the sedative–hypnotic medications and alcohol. In patients for whom sedative effects may be especially dangerous, including the elderly, the cautious selection and dosing of antipsychotics should always take into account the overall burden of sedation from their concurrent medications. For these patients, starting with low and divided doses is often an appropriate first step.

Because dopamine receptor blockade is a property common to all antipsychotics, they are all likely to interfere, although with varying degrees, with the efficacy of levodopa in the treatment of Parkinson's disease. When antipsychotic treatment is necessary in this setting, the low-potency antipsychotics, clozapine and quetiapine, have been preferred.[43] Reciprocally, antipsychotics are likely to be less effective in the treatment of psychosis in the setting of levodopa, stimulant use, and direct agonists (e.g., ropinirole) that facilitate dopamine transmission. Nevertheless, these agents have been combined with antipsychotics, in cautious modestly successful efforts, to treat the negative symptoms of schizophrenia (including blunted affect, paucity of thought and speech, and social withdrawal).

Elevated prolactin is common in patients on antipsychotics, particularly the higher-potency agents (e.g., haloperidol, risperidone, paliperidone). It often manifests with irregular menses, galactorrhea, diminished libido, or hirsutism. Antipsychotic-induced prolactin elevations associated with clinical symptoms can be abated by reducing the dosage of the offending agent, switching to a prolactin-sparing agent (e.g., aripiprazole, brexpiprazole, clozapine, quetiapine, ziprasidone), adding adjunctive amantadine (200 to 300 mg/day) or a dopamine agonist, such as cabergoline (0.5 to 4 mg/week).[44] At present, the management of sustained asymptomatic hyperprolactinemia—which is far more clinically common—is less well defined.

The risk of agranulocytosis, which occurs rarely with the low-potency antipsychotics, is much higher with clozapine, with an incidence as high as 1% to 3%. For this reason, the combination of clozapine with other medications associated with a risk of myelosuppression (e.g., carbamazepine) should be avoided. Similarly, because clozapine lowers the seizure threshold to a greater extent than other antipsychotics, co-administration with other medications that significantly lower the seizure threshold (e.g., maprotiline) should be avoided or combined with an anticonvulsant should be avoided or combined with an anticonvulsant.

Pharmacokinetic drug interactions are quite common among the antipsychotic drugs. Plasma levels of the antipsychotic drugs, however, can vary as much as 10-fold to 20-fold between patients even on monotherapy, and, as a class, they have a relatively wide therapeutic index.[45] Therefore, factors that alter antipsychotic drug metabolism might not have apparent clinical consequences. Another exception has to do with patients who are maintained on antipsychotics carefully tapered to the lowest effective dosage. In these patients, a small decrease in antipsychotic levels, as can occur with the introduction of a metabolic inducer or an agent that interferes with absorption, can bring them below the threshold for efficacy.

Antipsychotic drug levels may be lowered by aluminum-containing or magnesium-containing antacids, which reduce their absorption and are best given separately. Mixing liquid preparations of phenothiazines with beverages, such as fruit juices, presents the risk of causing insoluble precipitates and inefficient GI absorption.

Carbamazepine, known to be a potent inducer of hepatic enzymes, has been associated with reduction of steady-state antipsychotic drug plasma levels by as much as 50%. This effect is especially important to bear in mind as a potential explanation when an antipsychotic-treated patient appears to deteriorate in the weeks following the introduction of carbamazepine. Oxcarbazepine can also induce antipsychotic drug metabolism, as can a variety of other anticonvulsants, including phenobarbital and phenytoin.

Cigarette smoking may also be associated with a reduction in antipsychotic drug levels through enzyme metabolism.[46] As inpatient units and community residential programs have widely become smoke-free, there are often substantial differences in smoking frequency between inpatient and outpatient settings. Among patients who smoke heavily, consideration should be given to the impact of these changes in smoking habits on antipsychotic dosage requirements, particularly for those taking olanzapine and clozapine.

SSRIs and other antidepressants with inhibitory effects on CYP isoenzymes can also produce an increase in the plasma levels of a concurrently administered antipsychotic agent (Table 38-3). Thus, increases in clozapine, olanzapine, haloperidol, and asenapine plasma levels can occur when these drugs are co-administered with fluvoxamine. Increases in risperidone, aripiprazole, iloperidone, and typical antipsychotic levels can follow initiation of fluoxetine, paroxetine, bupropion, duloxetine, and sertraline. Quetiapine and ziprasidone levels can rise following addition of nefazodone, fluvoxamine, or fluoxetine.

Phenothiazine drug levels may be increased when co-administered with propranolol, another inhibitor of hepatic microenzymes. Because propranolol is often an effective symptomatic treatment for antipsychotic-associated akathisia, the combined use of the β-blocker with an antipsychotic drug is common. When interactions present a problem, the use of a water-soluble β-blocker, such as atenolol, which is not likely to interfere with hepatic metabolism, provides a reasonable alternative.

Mood Stabilizers

Lithium

Lithium is absorbed completely from the GI tract; it achieves peak plasma concentrations after approximately 1.5 to 2 hours for standard preparations and 4 to 4.5 hours for slow-release preparations. It distributes throughout total body water and, in contrast to most psychotropic drugs, does not bind to plasma proteins and is not metabolized in the liver. It is filtered and re-absorbed by the kidneys, and 95% of it is excreted in the urine. Lithium elimination is highly dependent on total body sodium and fluid balance; it competes with sodium for re-absorption in the proximal tubules. To a lesser extent, lithium is re-absorbed also in the loop of Henle but, in contrast to sodium, is not re-absorbed in the distal tubules. Its elimination half-life is approximately 24 hours; clearance is generally 20% of creatinine clearance but is diminished in elderly patients and in patients with kidney disease. The risk of toxicity is increased in these patients as well as in patients with cardiovascular disease, dehydration, or hypokalemia. The most common drug–drug interactions involving lithium are pharmacokinetic.[47] Because lithium has a low therapeutic index, such interactions are likely to be clinically significant and potentially serious (Table 38-4).

Among the best-studied of these interactions are thiazide diuretics and drugs that are chemically distinct but share a similar mechanism of action (e.g., indapamide, metolazone, quinethazone). These agents decrease lithium clearance and thereby steeply increase the risk of lithium toxicity. Loop diuretics (e.g., furosemide) appear to interact to a lesser degree with lithium excretion, presumably because they block lithium re-absorption in the loop of Henle, potentially offsetting possible compensatory increases in re-absorption more proximally.[48] The potassium-sparing diuretics (e.g., amiloride, spironolactone, triamterene) also appear to be less likely to cause an increase in lithium levels, but close monitoring is indicated when these drugs are introduced.[49] The potential impact of thiazide diuretics on lithium levels does not contraindicate their combined use, which has been particularly valuable in the treatment of lithium-associated polyuria. Potassium-sparing diuretics have also been used for this purpose. When a thiazide diuretic is used, a lithium dosage reduction of 25% to 50% and close monitoring of lithium levels are required. Monitoring of serum electrolytes, particularly potassium, is also important when thiazides are introduced because hypokalemia enhances the toxicity of lithium. Although not contraindicated with lithium, ACE inhibitors (e.g., captopril) and angiotensin II receptor antagonists (e.g., losartan) can elevate lithium levels, and close monitoring of levels is required when these agents are introduced.[49]

A probable pharmacodynamic interaction exists between lithium and agents used clinically to produce neuromuscular blockade (e.g., succinylcholine, pancuronium, decamethonium) during anesthesia. Muscle paralysis can be significantly prolonged when these agents are administered to the lithium-treated patient.[50] Although the mechanism is unknown, the possible inhibition by lithium of acetylcholine

TABLE 38-4 Selected Drug Interactions With Lithium[2,49]

DRUG	POTENTIAL INTERACTION
Aminophylline, theophylline, acetazolamide, mannitol, sodium bicarbonate, sodium chloride load	Decreased lithium levels
Thiazide diuretics	Increased lithium levels; reduction of lithium-associated polyuria
Non-steroidal anti-inflammatory drugs, COX-2 inhibitors, tetracycline, spectinomycin, metronidazole, angiotensin II receptor antagonists, angiotensin-converting enzyme inhibitors	Increased lithium levels
Neuromuscular blocking drugs (succinylcholine, pancuronium, decamethonium)	Prolonged muscle paralysis
Anti-thyroid drugs (propylthiouracil, thioamide, methimazole)	Enhanced anti-thyroid efficacy
Antidepressants	Enhanced antidepressant efficacy
Calcium channel blockers (verapamil, diltiazem)	Idiosyncratic neurotoxicity
Antipsychotic drugs	Idiosyncratic neurotoxicity, neuroleptic malignant syndrome risk

COX-2, cyclo-oxygenase-2.

synthesis and release at the neuromuscular junction is a potential basis for synergism.

Lithium interferes with the production of thyroid hormones through several mechanisms, including interference with iodine uptake, tyrosine iodination, and release of triiodothyronine (T_3) and thyroxine (T_4). Lithium can therefore enhance the efficacy of anti-thyroid medications (e.g., propylthiouracil, thioamide, methimazole) and has also been used preoperatively to help prevent thyroid storm in the surgical treatment of Graves' disease.[51]

There have been isolated reports of various forms of neurotoxicity, which is usually, but not always, reversible, when lithium has been combined with SSRIs and other serotoninergic agents, calcium channel blockers, antipsychotics, and anticonvulsants (e.g., carbamazepine).[52] In some cases, features of the serotonin syndrome or NMS have been present.[53] Although it is worthwhile to bear this in mind when evaluating unexplained mental status changes in a lithium-treated patient, the combination of lithium with these classes of medication is neither contraindicated nor unusual.

Many of the non-steroidal anti-inflammatory drugs (NSAIDs) (including ibuprofen, indometacin, diclofenac, naproxen, mefenamic acid, ketoprofen, piroxicam) have been reported to increase serum lithium levels, potentially by as much as 50% to 60% when used at full prescription strength. This can occur by inhibition of renal clearance of lithium by interference with a prostaglandin-dependent mechanism in the renal tubule. The cyclooxygenase (COX)-2 inhibitors (e.g., celecoxib, rofecoxib), can also raise lithium levels. Limited data available suggest that sulindac,[54] phenylbutazone,[55] and aspirin[56] are less likely to affect lithium levels. A number of antimicrobials are associated with increased lithium levels, including tetracycline, metronidazole, and parenteral spectinomycin. In the event that these agents are required, close monitoring of lithium levels and potential dosage adjustment are recommended.

Conversely, a variety of agents can produce decreases in lithium levels, thereby increasing the risk of psychiatric symptom breakthrough and relapse. The methylxanthines (e.g., aminophylline, theophylline) can cause a significant decrease in lithium levels by increasing renal clearance; close blood level monitoring with co-administration is necessary. A reduction in lithium levels can also result from alkalinization of urine (e.g., with acetazolamide use or with sodium bicarbonate), osmotic diuretics (e.g., urea, mannitol), or from ingestion of a sodium chloride load, which also increases lithium excretion.

Valproic Acid

Valproic acid is a simple branched-chain carboxylic acid that, like several other anticonvulsants, has mood-stabilizing properties. Valproic acid is 80% to 95% protein-bound and is rapidly metabolized primarily by hepatic microsomal glucuronidation and oxidation. It has a short elimination half-life of approximately 8 hours.[54] Clearance is essentially unchanged in the elderly and in patients with kidney disease, whereas it is significantly reduced in patients with primary liver disease.

In contrast to some other major anticonvulsants (e.g., carbamazepine, phenobarbital), valproate does not induce hepatic microsomes. Rather, it tends to inhibit oxidation reactions, thereby potentially increasing levels of co-administered hepatically metabolized drugs, notably including lamotrigine, as well as some TCAs, such as clomipramine, amitriptyline, and nortriptyline (Table 38-5).[55,56] A complex pharmacokinetic interaction occurs when valproic acid and carbamazepine are administered concurrently. Valproic acid not only inhibits the metabolism of carbamazepine and its active metabolite, carbamazepine-10,11-epoxide (CBZ-E), but it also displaces both entities from protein-binding sites. Although the effect on plasma carbamazepine levels is variable, the levels of the unbound (active) epoxide metabolite are increased, with a concomitant increased risk of carbamazepine neurotoxicity. Conversely, co-administration with carbamazepine results in a decrease in plasma valproic acid levels. Nevertheless, the combination of valproate and carbamazepine has been used successfully in the treatment of patients with bipolar disorder who were only partially responsive to either drug alone.[57] Oral contraceptives as well as carbapenem antibiotics have also been associated with decreases in plasma valproic acid levels; enhanced monitoring of levels and valproate dose adjustments are recommended when these agents are used

Cimetidine, a potent inhibitor of hepatic microsomal enzymes, is associated with decreased clearance of valproic

TABLE 38-5 Selected Drug Interactions With Valproate and Carbamazepine

DRUG	INTERACTION WITH VALPROATE
Carbamazepine	Decreased valproate plasma levels; increased plasma levels of the epoxide metabolite of carbamazepine; variable effects on plasma levels of carbamazepine
Phenytoin	Decreased valproate plasma levels; variable effects on phenytoin plasma levels
Phenobarbital	Decreased valproate plasma levels; increased phenobarbital plasma levels
Oral contraceptives	Decreased valproate plasma levels
Carbapenem antibiotics	Decreased valproate plasma levels
Lamotrigine	Increased lamotrigine levels; hypersensitivity reaction
Aspirin	Increased unbound (active) fraction of valproate
Cimetidine	Increased valproate plasma levels
Fluoxetine	Same as above
Clonazepam	Rare absence seizures

DRUG	INTERACTION WITH CARBAMAZEPINE
Phenytoin	Decreased carbamazepine plasma levels
Phenobarbital	Same as above
Primidone	Same as above
Macrolide antibiotics	Increased carbamazepine plasma levels
Isoniazid	Same as above
Fluoxetine	Increased carbamazepine plasma levels
Danazol	Same as above
Verapamil	Same as above
Diltiazem	Same as above
Propoxyphene	Same as above
Oral contraceptives	Induction of metabolism by carbamazepine
Corticosteroids	Same as above
Thyroid hormones	Same as above
Warfarin	Same as above
Cyclosporine	Same as above
Phenytoin	Same as above
Ethosuximide	Same as above
Carbamazepine	Same as above
Valproate	Same as above
Lamotrigine	Same as above
Tetracycline	Same as above
Doxycycline	Same as above
Theophylline	Same as above
Methadone	Same as above
Benzodiazepines	Same as above
TCAs	Same as above
Antipsychotics	Same as above
Methylphenidate	Same as above
Modafinil	Same as above
Thiazide diuretics	Hyponatremia
Furosemide	Same as above

TCA, tricyclic antidepressants.

acid, resulting in increased levels. The dosage of valproic acid may need to be reduced in the patient starting cimetidine, but not other H_2-receptor antagonists.[58] Elevated levels of valproic acid have also been reported sporadically with fluoxetine and other SSRIs. Aspirin and other salicylates can displace protein binding of valproic acid,[59] thereby increasing the unbound (free) fraction, which can increase the risk of toxicity from valproate even though total serum levels are unchanged.

Lamotrigine

Lamotrigine is a phenyltriazine anticonvulsant that is moderately (50% to 60%) protein-bound and metabolized primarily by glucuronidation. Its most serious adverse effect is a life-threatening hypersensitivity reaction with rash, typically, but not always, occurring within the first 2 months of use.[60] The incidence among patients with bipolar disorder is estimated at 0.8 per 1000 among patients on lamotrigine monotherapy and 1.3 per 1000 among patients on lamotrigine in combination with other agents.

The risk of adverse effects including hypersensitivity reactions and tremor is increased when lamotrigine is combined with valproic acid. As much as a two-fold to three-fold increase in lamotrigine levels occurs when valproic acid is added, related to inhibition of glucuronidation of lamotrigine.[61] Accordingly, the *Physicians' Desk Reference* (PDR) provides guidelines for more gradual dosage titration of lamotrigine and lower target dosages when introduced in a patient already taking valproate. When valproate is added to lamotrigine, the dosage of lamotrigine should typically be reduced by one-half to two-thirds.

Conversely, lamotrigine levels can be decreased by as much as 50% when administered with metabolic inducers, particularly other anticonvulsants (including carbamazepine, primidone, and phenobarbital). Therefore, guidelines have been developed for dosing lamotrigine in the presence of these metabolic-inducing anticonvulsants. Similar-magnitude reductions in lamotrigine levels have been reported in patients on oral contraceptives, requiring an increase in the dosage of lamotrigine.[62] Lamotrigine levels and symptom status should be monitored closely when oral contraceptives or metabolic-inducing anticonvulsants are started.

Carbamazepine and Oxcarbazepine

Carbamazepine is an iminostilbene anticonvulsant structurally related to the TCA imipramine. Carbamazepine is slowly and inconsistently absorbed from the GI tract; peak serum concentrations are achieved approximately 4 to 8 hours after oral administration. It is only moderately (60% to 85%) protein-bound. Carbamazepine, a potent inducer of hepatic metabolism, can also induce its own metabolism, such that elimination half-life can fall from 18 to 55 hours to 5 to 20 hours over a matter of several weeks, generally reaching a plateau after 3 to 5 weeks.[2]

Most drug drug interactions with carbamazepine occur by pharmacokinetic mechanisms. Drugs whose metabolism is increased by carbamazepine include valproic acid, phenytoin, ethosuximide, lamotrigine, alprazolam, clonazepam, TCAs, antipsychotics, doxycycline, tetracycline, thyroid hormone, corticosteroids, oral contraceptives, methadone, theophylline, warfarin, and cyclosporine. The concurrent administration of carbamazepine with any of these drugs can cause significant reductions in plasma levels and can lead to therapeutic failure. Patients of child-bearing potential who are taking oral contraceptives must be advised to use an additional method of birth control.

Several drugs inhibit the metabolism of carbamazepine, including the macrolide antibiotics (e.g., erythromycin, clarithromycin, triacetyloleandomycin), isoniazid, fluoxetine, valproic acid, danazol, propoxyphene, and the calcium channel blockers verapamil and diltiazem. Because of its low therapeutic index, the risk of developing carbamazepine toxicity is significantly increased when these drugs are administered concurrently. Conversely, co-administration of phenytoin or phenobarbital, both microsomal enzyme inducers, can increase the metabolism of carbamazepine, potentially resulting in sub-therapeutic plasma levels. Carbamazepine has also been associated with bone marrow suppression, and its combination with other agents that interfere with blood cell production (including clozapine) should generally be avoided. The combination of carbamazepine with thiazide diuretics or furosemide has been associated with severe symptomatic hyponatremia,[63] suggesting the need for close monitoring of electrolytes when these medications are used concurrently.

Oxcarbazepine, a structural derivative of carbamazepine, appears to be a less-potent metabolic inducer than its parent compound, although it still can render certain important agents (particularly CYP3A4 substrates) less effective because of similar pharmacokinetic interactions.[2] Women of child-bearing potential should therefore receive guidance about supplementing oral contraceptives with a second effective form of birth control, as with carbamazepine. As with carbamazepine, oxcarbazepine is also associated with risk of hyponatremia.

Other Anticonvulsants

Other anticonvulsants have become available that, as with valproate, carbamazepine, and lamotrigine, are being explored in treating bipolar disorder and other psychiatric conditions. In contrast to older anticonvulsants with demonstrated effects on mood, much less is known about the potential pharmacokinetic interactions involving these newer agents, including topiramate, zonisamide, gabapentin, and pregabalin. At present, none of these anticonvulsants can be justified as a monotherapy for any phase of bipolar disorder, but they may have a role as an adjunct treatment in some bipolar patients.

Topiramate

Topiramate is a sulfamate-substituted monosaccharide, related to fructose, a rather unusual chemical structure for an anticonvulsant. Topiramate is used less commonly for its putative mood-stabilizing effects[64] than its weight-reducing effects[65] and utility in substance-abusing populations.[66,67]

Topiramate is quickly absorbed after oral use. Most of the drug (70%) is later excreted in the urine unchanged; therefore, it requires dosage reduction in the setting of renal insufficiency. The remainder is extensively metabolized by hydroxylation, hydrolysis, and glucuronidation. Topiramate inhibits carbonic anhydrase; therefore, the concomitant use of other carbonic anhydrase inhibitors (e.g. acetazolamide) can lead to an increased risk of forming kidney stones. Patients adhering to a ketogenic diet can also be prone to nephrolithiasis with topiramate treatment and should be instructed to stay well hydrated.[68]

In the presence of hepatic enzyme inducers (e.g., carbamazepine), the elimination of topiramate may be increased by up to 50%. Based on its properties as a weak inhibitor of CYP2C19 and an inducer of CYP3A4, topiramate can increase plasma levels of phenytoin but decrease plasma concentrations of estrogens in women taking oral contraceptives.[2]

Zonisamide

Zonisamide is a sulfonamide anticonvulsant used in patients with partial seizures.[69] As with topiramate, zonisamide is under investigation in psychiatry to facilitate weight loss in bipolar patients, and it might have fewer adverse cognitive effects. The FDA has warned that zonisamide can cause metabolic acidosis in some patients. As a result, patients should have their serum bicarbonate levels assessed before starting treatment and periodically during treatment with zonisamide, even in the absence of symptoms. Zonisamide is metabolized mostly by the CYP3A4 isoenzyme; its metabolism is inhibited by ketoconazole, cyclosporin, miconazole, fluconazole, and carbamazepine (in descending order).[70]

Gabapentin and Pregabalin

Gabapentin—used at present in psychiatry for patients with anxiety, mood instability, or pain—is not a salt, but it resembles lithium because it is not hepatically metabolized, is not appreciably protein-bound, and is excreted by the kidney largely as unchanged drug. As with lithium, therefore, it is essential to adjust the dosage according to changes in renal function.

As with gabapentin, pregabalin is rapidly absorbed when administered on an empty stomach, undergoes negligible metabolism in humans, has very low protein-binding, and is eliminated from the systemic circulation primarily by renal excretion unchanged. Studies have shown that pregabalin has a role in treating chronic pain disorders, such as fibromyalgia[71] and spinal cord injuries. Although *in vivo* studies have shown no significant pharmacokinetic interactions for pregabalin, it might have potential interactions with opioids (pregabalin is synergistic with opioids in lower dosages), benzodiazepines, barbiturates, alcohol, and other drugs that depress the CNS.

Antidepressants

The antidepressant drugs include the TCAs, the MAOIs, the SSRIs, the atypical agents (bupropion, trazodone, nefazodone, and mirtazapine), and the serotonin–norepinephrine re-uptake inhibitors (SNRIs) (venlafaxine, duloxetine, milnacipran, desvenlafaxine, and levomilnacipran).

Although the TCAs and MAOIs are used infrequently, they continue to serve a valuable role in the treatment of more severe, treatment-resistant depressive and anxiety disorders despite the wide range of drug–drug interactions they entail.

SSRIs and Other Newer Antidepressants

The SSRIs (e.g., fluoxetine, sertraline, paroxetine, fluvoxamine, citalopram, escitalopram, vilazodone, vortioxetine) share similar pharmacologic actions, including minimal anticholinergic, antihistaminic, and α_1-adrenergic blocking effects and potent pre-synaptic inhibition of serotonin re-uptake.[2] Vilazodone and vortioxetine act as serotonin re-uptake inhibitors and agonize/antagonize various serotonin receptors (i.e., vilazodone is a partial agonist at the 5-HT_{1A} receptor, vortioxetine acts as an agonist or antagonist at 5-HT_{1A}, 5-HT_{1B}, 5-HT_3, 5-HT_{1D}, and 5-HT_7). There are important pharmacokinetic differences that account for distinctions among them with respect to potential drug interactions (Table 38-6).

Nefazodone, similar to trazodone, is distinguished from classic SSRIs by its antagonism of the 5-HT_2 receptor and differs from trazodone in its lesser antagonism of the α_1-adrenergic receptor. Mirtazapine blocks the 5-HT_2 receptor, 5-HT_3 receptor, and the α_2 adrenergic receptors. Venlafaxine/desvenlafaxine, duloxetine, milnacipran/levomilnacipran similar to TCAs, inhibit serotonin and norepinephrine re-uptake, but, in contrast to TCAs, they are relatively devoid of post-synaptic anticholinergic, antihistaminic, and α_1-adrenergic activity. Milnacipran is FDA-approved only for fibromyalgia, while its enantiomer levomilnacipran is approved for major depressive disorder (MDD). While venlafaxine is predominantly serotoninergic at low to moderate dosages, duloxetine and, especially, milnacipran/levomilnacipran are potent inhibitors of both the norepinephrine and serotonin transporters across clinical dosage ranges.

Although not an approved antidepressant, the norepinephrine re-uptake inhibitor atomoxetine, indicated for the treatment of ADHD, might have a role in depression pharmacotherapy as a single agent or as adjunctive treatment. It is neither a significant inhibitor nor inducer of the CYP system, but owing to its adrenergic effects, the risk of palpitations or pressor effects is likely to be greater than with serotoninergic agents when combined with prescribed and OTC sympathomimetics, and its use with MAOIs is contraindicated.

All of the SSRIs (except for fluvoxamine [77%], citalopram [80%], and escitalopram [56%]) as well as nefazodone, are highly protein-bound (95% to 99%). Venlafaxine, desvenlafaxine, milnacipran, and levomilnacipran are minimally protein-bound (15% to 30%), whereas duloxetine is highly protein-bound (90%).[2] All of the antidepressants are hepatically metabolized, and all of them except paroxetine and duloxetine have active metabolites. The major metabolites of sertraline, citalopram, and desvenlafaxine, however, appear to be minimally active. Elimination half-lives range from 5 hours for venlafaxine and 11 hours for its metabolite, O-desmethylvenlafaxine, to 2 to 3 days for fluoxetine and 7 to 14 days for its metabolite, norfluoxetine. Nefazodone, similar to venlafaxine, has a short half-life (2 to 5 hours), with fluvoxamine, sertraline, paroxetine, citalopram, and escitalopram in the intermediate range of 15 to 35 hours.[2] Food can have variable effects on antidepressant bioavailability, including an increase for sertraline, a decrease for nefazodone, and no change for escitalopram.

The growing knowledge about the interaction of the newer antidepressants with the CYP isoenzymes has revealed differences among them in their pattern of enzyme inhibition

TABLE 38-6 Potential Drug Interactions With the Selective Serotonin Re-Uptake Inhibitors and Other Newer Antidepressants

DRUG	POTENTIAL INTERACTION
MAOIs	Serotonin syndrome
Secondary amine TCAs	Increased TCA levels when co-administered with fluoxetine, paroxetine, sertraline, bupropion, duloxetine
Tertiary amine TCAs	Increased TCA levels with fluvoxamine, paroxetine, sertraline, bupropion, duloxetine
Antipsychotics (typical) and risperidone, aripiprazole	Increased antipsychotic levels with fluoxetine, sertraline, paroxetine, bupropion, duloxetine
Thioridazine	Arrhythmia risk with CYP 2D6-inhibitory antidepressants
Pimozide	Arrhythmia risk with CYP 3A4-inhibitory antidepressants (nefazodone, fluvoxamine)
Clozapine and olanzapine	Increased antipsychotic levels with fluvoxamine
Diazepam	Increased benzodiazepine levels with fluoxetine, fluvoxamine, sertraline
Triazolobenzodiazepines (midazolam, alprazolam, triazolam)	Increased benzodiazepine levels with fluvoxamine, nefazodone, sertraline
Carbamazepine	Increased carbamazepine levels with fluoxetine, fluvoxamine, nefazodone
Theophylline	Increased theophylline levels with fluvoxamine
Type 1C antiarrhythmics (encainide, flecainide, propafenone)	Increased antiarrhythmic levels with fluoxetine, paroxetine, sertraline, bupropion, duloxetine
β-Blockers (lipophilic)	Increased β-blocker levels with fluoxetine, paroxetine, sertraline, bupropion, duloxetine
Calcium channel blockers	Increased levels with fluoxetine, fluvoxamine, nefazodone
Tizanidine	Increased tizanidine levels with fluvoxamine

CYP, cytochrome P450; MAOI, monoamine oxidase inhibitor; TCA, tricyclic antidepressant.

that are likely to be critical to the understanding and prediction of drug–drug interactions.

Cytochrome P450 2D6

Fluoxetine, norfluoxetine, paroxetine, bupropion, duloxetine,[72] sertraline (to a moderate degree), and citalopram and escitalopram (to a minimal degree)[26] all inhibit CYP2D6, which accounts for their potential inhibitory effect on TCA clearance and the metabolism of other CYP2D6 substrates. Other drugs metabolized by CYP2D6—and whose levels can rise in the setting of CYP2D6 inhibition—include the type 1C antiarrhythmics (e.g., encainide, flecainide, propafenone) as well as β-blockers (e.g., propranolol, timolol, metoprolol), antipsychotics (e.g., risperidone, haloperidol, aripiprazole, iloperidone, thioridazine, perphenazine), TCAs, and trazodone. CYP2D6 converts codeine and tramadol into their active form; hence the efficacy of these analgesics may be diminished when concurrently administered with a P450 2D6 inhibitor. So too, as P450 2D6 converts tamoxifen into its active N-desmethyl tamoxifen form for treatment of neoplasms, the use of inhibitors of 2D6 should be carefully re-evaluated during tamoxifen treatment.

These observations underscore the need to exercise care and to closely monitor when prescribing these SSRIs, bupropion, or duloxetine in the setting of complex medical regimens. Plasma TCA levels do not routinely include levels of active or potentially toxic metabolites, which may be altered by virtue of shunting to other metabolic routes when CYP2D6 is inhibited. Therefore, particularly in the case of patients at risk for conduction delay, electrocardiography and blood level monitoring are recommended when combining TCAs with SSRIs, duloxetine, or bupropion.

Cytochrome P450 3A4

Fluoxetine's major metabolite (norfluoxetine), fluvoxamine, nefazodone, and, to a lesser extent, sertraline, desmethylsertraline, citalopram, and escitalopram inhibit CYP3A4. All of these agents therefore have the potential for elevating levels of pimozide and cisapride (arrhythmia risks), methadone, oxycodone, fentanyl (respiratory depression risks), calcium channel blockers, the statins, carbamazepine, midazolam, and many other important and commonly prescribed substrates of this widely recruited CYP enzyme.

Cytochrome P450 2C

Serum concentrations of drugs metabolized by this sub-family may be increased by fluoxetine, sertraline, and fluvoxamine. Reported interactions include decreased clearance of diazepam on all three SSRIs, a small reduction in tolbutamide clearance on sertraline, and increased plasma phenytoin concentrations reflecting decreased clearance on fluoxetine. Warfarin is also metabolized by this sub-family, and levels may be increased by the inhibition of these enzymes. SSRIs can interact with warfarin by still other, probably pharmacodynamic mechanisms (such as depletion of platelet serotonin). Although the combination is common, increased monitoring is recommended when SSRIs are prescribed with warfarin.

Cytochrome P450 1A

Among the SSRIs, only fluvoxamine appears to be a potent inhibitor of CYP1A2. Accordingly, increased serum concentrations of theophylline, haloperidol, clozapine, olanzapine, and the tertiary amine TCAs including clomipramine, amitriptyline, and imipramine can occur.[26] Because theophylline and TCAs have a relatively narrow therapeutic index and because the degree of elevation of antipsychotic blood levels appears to be substantial (e.g., up to four-fold increases in haloperidol concentrations), additional monitoring and consideration of dosage reductions are necessary when fluvoxamine is co-administered with these agents.

Additional Interactions

Mirtazapine, although neither a potent inhibitor nor inducer of the CYP isoenzymes, has numerous pharmacodynamic effects including antagonism of the histamine, α_2-adrenergic, 5-HT_2 and 5-HT_3, and muscarinic receptors, creating the possibility of myriad pharmacodynamic interactions (including blockade of clonidine's antihypertensive activity).[73] It also has the possible benefit of attenuated nausea and sexual dysfunction that can occur with SSRIs.[74]

The serotonin syndrome is a potentially life-threatening condition characterized by confusion, diaphoresis, hyperthermia, hyperreflexia, muscle rigidity, tachycardia, hypotension, and coma.[75] Although this can arise whenever an SSRI is combined with a serotoninergic drug (e.g., L-tryptophan, clomipramine, venlafaxine) and drugs with serotoninergic properties (e.g., lithium, mirtazapine, dextromethorphan, tramadol, meperidine, pentazocine), the greatest known risk is associated with the co-administration of an SSRI with an MAOI; this is absolutely contraindicated. In view of the long elimination half-life of fluoxetine and norfluoxetine, at least 5 weeks must elapse after fluoxetine discontinuation before an MAOI can be safely introduced. With the other SSRIs, an interval of 2 weeks appears to be adequate.

The weak, reversible MAOI antimicrobial linezolid, used for treatment of multi-drug-resistant Gram-positive infections, has been implicated in a small number of post-marketing cases of serotonin syndrome in patients on serotoninergic antidepressants, typically patients on SSRIs, as well as other medications, including narcotics.[76] The co-administration of SSRIs with other serotoninergic agents is not contraindicated, but it should prompt immediate discontinuation in any patient on this combination of drugs who presents with mental status changes, fever, or hyperreflexia of unknown origin.

Tricyclic Antidepressants

TCAs are thought to exert their pharmacologic action by inhibiting the pre-synaptic neuronal re-uptake of norepinephrine and serotonin in the CNS with subsequent modulation of both pre-synaptic and post-synaptic α-adrenergic receptors. While clinically effective, TCAs have been replaced by SSRIs and newer antidepressants that cause fewer side effects. TCAs also have significant anticholinergic, antihistaminic, and α-adrenergic activity as well as quinidine-like effects on cardiac condition, and in these respects they resemble the low-potency antipsychotic drugs, which are structurally similar.[2]

TCAs are well absorbed from the GI tract and subject to significant first-pass liver metabolism before entry into the systemic circulation, where they are largely protein-bound, ranging from 85% (trimipramine) to 95% (amitriptyline). Peak plasma concentrations are reached approximately

2 to 6 hours after oral administration. They are highly lipophilic, with a large volume of distribution. TCAs are extensively metabolized by hepatic microsomal enzymes, and most have pharmacologically active metabolites.[77] Additive anticholinergic effects can occur when the TCAs are co-administered with other drugs possessing anticholinergic properties (e.g., low-potency antipsychotics, antiparkinsonian drugs), potentially resulting in an anticholinergic syndrome. SSRIs, SNRIs, atypical antidepressants, and MAOIs are relatively devoid of anticholinergic activity, although the MAOIs can indirectly potentiate the anticholinergic properties of atropine and scopolamine. Additive sedative effects are not uncommon when TCAs are combined with sedative–hypnotics, anxiolytics, or narcotics or alcohol (Table 38-7).

TCAs possess class 1A antiarrhythmic activity and can lead to depression of cardiac conduction, potentially resulting in heart block or ventricular arrhythmias when combined with quinidine-like agents (including quinidine, procainamide, and disopyramide as well as the low-potency antipsychotics).[78,79] The antiarrhythmics quinidine and propafenone, inhibitors of CYP2D6, can additionally produce clinically significant elevations of the TCAs, thus increasing the risk of cardiotoxicity through both pharmacodynamic and pharmacokinetic mechanisms.[80] The arrhythmogenic risks of a TCA are enhanced in a patient with underlying coronary or valvular heart disease, a patient with a recent myocardial infarction or hypokalemia, and in a patient receiving sympathomimetic amines, such as amphetamine stimulants.[81]

TCAs also interact with several antihypertensive drugs. TCAs can antagonize the antihypertensive effects of guanethidine, bethanidine, debrisoquine, or clonidine via interference with neuronal re-uptake by noradrenergic neurons. Conversely, TCAs can cause varying degrees of postural hypotension when co-administered with vasodilator drugs, antihypertensives, or low-potency neuroleptics.

Hypoglycemia has been observed with secondary and tertiary TCAs, particularly in the presence of sulfonylurea hypoglycemic agents,[2] suggesting the need for close monitoring.

Pharmacokinetic interactions involving the TCAs are often clinically important. The antipsychotic drugs (including haloperidol, chlorpromazine, thioridazine, and perphenazine) are known to increase TCA levels by 30% to 100%.[18] Cimetidine and methylphenidate can also raise tertiary TCA levels, as predicted by microsomal enzyme inhibition. The antifungals (e.g., ketoconazole), macrolide antibiotics (e.g., erythromycin), and calcium channel blockers (e.g., verapamil and diltiazem) as inhibitors of CYP3A4, can also impair the clearance of tertiary amine TCAs, thereby requiring a reduction in TCA dosage. SSRIs have been associated with clinically significant increases in TCA plasma levels, believed to be the result of inhibition primarily, but not exclusively, of CYP2D6.[18] Similar elevations of TCA levels would be expected with other potent CYP2D6 inhibitor antidepressants (e.g., duloxetine, bupropion). Inducers of CYP enzymes can increase the metabolism of TCAs. Thus, plasma levels of TCAs may be significantly reduced when carbamazepine, phenobarbital, rifampin, or isoniazid are co-administered or in the setting of chronic alcohol or cigarette use.

TABLE 38-7 Selected Drug Interactions With Tricyclic Antidepressants

DRUG	POTENTIAL INTERACTION
Carbamazepine Phenobarbital Rifampin Isoniazid	Decreased TCA plasma levels
Antipsychotics Methylphenidate SSRIs Quinidine Propafenone Antifungals Macrolide antibiotics Verapamil Diltiazem Cimetidine	Increased TCA plasma levels
Class I antiarrhythmics	Depression of cardiac conduction; ventricular arrhythmias
Guanethidine Clonidine	Interference with antihypertensive effect
Sympathomimetic amines (e.g., epinephrine)	Arrhythmias, hypertension (e.g., isoproterenol, epinephrine)
Antihypertensives Vasodilator drugs Low-potency antipsychotics	Hypotension
Anticholinergic drugs	Additive anticholinergic toxicity
MAOIs	Delirium, fever, convulsions
Sulfonylurea hypoglycemics	Hypoglycemia

MAOI, monoamine oxidase inhibitor; SSRI, selective serotonin re-uptake inhibitor; TCA, tricyclic antidepressant.

Monoamine Oxidase Inhibitors

Monoamine oxidase is an enzyme located primarily on the outer mitochondrial membrane and is responsible for intracellular catabolism of the monoamines. It is found in high concentrations in brain, liver, intestines, and lung. In pre-synaptic nerve terminals, MAO metabolizes cytoplasmic monoamines. In liver and gut, MAO catabolizes ingested bioactive amines, thus protecting against absorption into the systemic circulation of potentially vasoactive substances, particularly tyramine.

Two sub-types of MAO have been distinguished: intestinal MAO is predominantly MAO_A, whereas brain MAO is predominantly MAO_B. MAO_A preferentially metabolizes norepinephrine and serotonin. Phenylethylamine and benzylamine are the prototypic substrates for MAO_B. Both MAO sub-types metabolize dopamine and tyramine. Among the currently available MAOIs, phenelzine, tranylcypromine, and isocarboxazid are non-specific inhibitors of both MAO_A and MAO_B; selegiline is primarily an inhibitor of MAO_B, though it is a mixed MAO_A and MAO_B inhibitor at higher dosages.[36]

When patients are using MAOIs, dietary[82,83] and medication restrictions must be closely followed to avoid serious interactions. The MAOIs are, therefore, generally reserved for use in responsible or supervised patients when adequate trials of other classes of antidepressants have failed. That said, MAOIs have enjoyed renewed clinical interest, due in part to the approval of a transdermal form of selegiline for the treatment of depression. The two major types of MAOI drug–drug interaction are the serotonin syndrome and the hypertensive (also called *hyperadrenergic*) crisis.

Hypertensive Crisis

Hypertensive crisis is an emergency characterized by an abrupt elevation of blood pressure, severe headache, nausea, vomiting, and diaphoresis; intracranial hemorrhage or myocardial infarction can occur. Prompt intervention to reduce blood pressure with the α_1-adrenergic antagonist phentolamine or the combination of sodium nitroprusside and a β-blocker may be life-saving.[84] Potentially catastrophic hypertension appears to be due to release of bound intraneuronal stores of norepinephrine and dopamine by indirect vasopressor substances. The reaction can therefore be precipitated by the concurrent administration of vasopressor amines, stimulants, anorexiants, and many OTC cough and cold preparations; these include L-dopa, dopamine, amphetamine, methylphenidate, phenylpropanolamine, phentermine, mephentermine, metaraminol, ephedrine, and pseudoephedrine.[85] By contrast, direct sympathomimetic amines (e.g., norepinephrine, isoproterenol, epinephrine), which rely for their cardiovascular effects on direct stimulation of postsynaptic receptors, rather than on pre-synaptic release of stored catecholamines, appear to be somewhat safer when administered to patients on MAOIs (although they are also contraindicated).

Hypertensive crises may also be triggered by ingestion of naturally occurring sympathomimetic amines (particularly tyramine), which is present in various food products,[82,83] including aged cheeses (e.g., stilton, cheddar, blue cheese, or camembert, rather than cream cheese, ricotta cheese, or cottage cheese), yeast extracts, fava (broad) beans, over-ripe fruits (e.g., avocado), pickled herring, aged meats (e.g., salami, bologna, and many kinds of sausage), chicken liver, fermented bean curd, sauerkraut, many types of red wine and beer (particularly imported beer), and some white wines. Although gin, vodka, and whiskey appear to be free of tyramine, their use should be minimized during the course of MAOI treatment, as with other antidepressants, because of the risk of exaggerated side effects and reduced antidepressant efficacy. Other, less-stringent requirements include moderate intake of caffeine, chocolate, yogurt, and soy sauce. Because MAO activity can remain diminished for nearly 2 to 3 weeks following the discontinuation of MAOIs, a tyramine-free diet and appropriate medication restrictions should be continued for at least 14 days after an MAOI has been discontinued.[36]

The lowest dose available of transdermal selegiline (6 mg/24 h) has been shown to have minimal risks of hypertensive crisis on a normal diet and therefore does not require the same level of restriction. Based on the more limited data available for the doses of 9 mg and 12 mg/24 hours, food effects cannot be ruled out; therefore, the FDA advises that patients receiving these doses follow dietary modifications that include the avoidance of tyramine-rich food and beverages during treatment and for up to 2 weeks after therapy has been completed.[86] While the FDA recommendation for dietary modifications for the 9 mg and 12 mg doses are largely based on theoretical concerns, there are reports of adverse events with the selegiline transdermal system due to diet.[87] However, some authors[68] have used the 9 mg and 12 mg doses without a restricted diet and report no increases in blood pressure. The package insert also recommends following dietary modifications for two weeks after a dose reduction to 6 mg/24 hours. No dose adjustment is necessary for patients with mild-to-moderate renal or hepatic impairment.

Serotonin Syndrome

The serotonin syndrome the other major drug–drug interaction involving the MAOIs, occurs when MAOIs and serotoninergic agents are co-administered.[88] Potentially fatal reactions most closely resembling the serotonin syndrome can also occur with other drugs with less-selective serotoninergic activity, most notably meperidine and dextromethorphan, a widely available cough suppressant. Both of these medications, similar to the SSRIs, SNRIs, and clomipramine, are absolutely contraindicated when MAOIs are used. Other serotoninergic medications (e.g., buspirone and trazodone) are not contraindicated but should be used with care.

The 5-HT_1 agonist triptans, used in the treatment of migraine, have been implicated in serotonin syndrome when administered to patients on MAOIs. Other narcotic analgesics (e.g., propoxyphene, codeine, oxycodone, morphine, alfentanil, or morphine) appear to be safer alternatives to meperidine, but, in conjunction with MAOIs, their analgesic and CNS-depressant effects may be potentiated and rare serotonin syndrome-like presentations have been reported.[89] If opioid agents are necessary, they should be started at one-fifth to one-half of the standard dosages and gradually titrated upward, with monitoring for untoward hemodynamic or mental status changes.

St. John's Wort

Although the efficacy of St. John's wort for depression has not been well established, it has emerged as one of the most carefully studied herbal preparation when it comes to drug–drug interactions. Initial concerns about the generally weak, though potentially variable, MAOI activity of this botanical and the associated risk of serotonin syndrome when combined with serotoninergic agents have only been weakly borne out, with few cases of serotonin syndrome reported despite widespread concurrent use of St. John's wort with serotoninergic antidepressants. However, case reports and clinical trials indicate that some critical medications may be rendered less effective in some patients concurrently taking St. John's wort.[90,91] These medications include immunosuppressants (such as cyclosporine and tacrolimus), coumarin anticoagulants, antiretrovirals, theophylline, digoxin, amitriptyline, and oral contraceptives. Although the precise mechanisms and herbal constituents responsible for these effects remain to be elucidated, the primary focus has been on CYP3A4 and P-glycoprotein. A paucity of systematic information exists concerning potential drug interactions and adverse effects of other herbal products, including a possible risk of increased bleeding in patients on *Ginkgo biloba* and warfarin and of hepatotoxicity in patients on certain kava preparations.[92]

Psychostimulants and Modafinil

Psychostimulants

Psychostimulants have provided an often rapidly effective treatment of depressive symptoms among elderly and medically frail patients, including those with heart disease or HIV infection, who would be at particular risk from anticholinergic, hypotensive, sedative, or quinidine-like effects of the TCAs.[93–96] Although the broader range of options presented by the newer antidepressants has limited the need for stimulants in these settings, stimulants continue to be recruited as antidepressants and antidepressant adjuncts to the SSRIs, SNRIs, and bupropion in the management of treatment-refractory depression. In addition, the cautious combination of methylphenidate and dextroamphetamine with MAOIs has been found to be effective in a subset of treatment-refractory depressed patients[97,98] and in efforts to treat particularly severe postural hypotension from the MAOIs. In view of the high risk of hypertensive crises, the addition of stimulants to MAOIs for antidepressant augmentation should remain an option only in exceptional cases in which other options (e.g., ECT) have been carefully weighed.

Methylphenidate, one of the most commonly used stimulants in modern psychiatric practice, has low bioavailability (20% to 30%) in orally administered forms and undergoes extensive pre-systemic metabolism through hydrolysis or de-esterification with limited oxidation.[99,100] Carboxylesterase-1A1 (CES-1), located in the stomach and liver, is the primary enzyme involved with first-pass methylphenidate metabolism. Difference in an individual's hydrolyzing enzyme activity, linked to variants in human CES-1 gene,[101] can lead to wide variations in methylphenidate metabolism (and corresponding methylphenidate blood concentrations) in certain persons. A transdermal preparation of methylphenidate, which avoids much of the first-pass metabolism through CES-1, is also available.

In combination with other drugs, psychostimulants, such as methylphenidate, have been linked to increased plasma levels of TCAs and possibly other antidepressants; increased plasma levels of phenobarbital, primidone, and phenytoin; increased prothrombin time on anticoagulants; attenuation or reversal of the guanethidine antihypertensive effect; and increased pressor responses to vasopressor drugs. Methylphenidate has been implicated in putative drug interactions more often than dextroamphetamine or mixed amphetamine salts; however, decades of clinical experience with methylphenidate and other psychostimulants suggests these medicines are safe and effective for appropriately screened patients, including those on more-complex medical regimens.

Modafinil/Armodafinil

The relatively benign side-effect profile of modafinil (and its *R*-enantiomer, armodafinil), together with its stimulant-like properties but differing mechanism, have motivated efforts to define the potential role of this wakefulness-promoting agent currently approved for treatment of narcolepsy. Its success as a treatment for fatigue in neurologic conditions (e.g., multiple sclerosis)[102] suggests the possibility of usefulness as a treatment for drowsiness related to other causes, including medications (e.g., antipsychotic-induced sedation). In addition, it is used off-label, like the psychostimulants, for treating depression co-morbid with medical illness[103] and as an antidepressant adjunct in refractory depression.[104] Several studies have suggested efficacy for ADHD,[105–107] though the use of modafinil and armodafinil for this purpose remains an off-label practice.

Clinical and pre-clinical studies have suggested that modafinil and armodafinil may be less likely than methylphenidate or dextroamphetamine to generate euphoria;[108] nevertheless, they are Schedule IV medications and their abuse liability is not yet known to be less than the psychostimulants in real-world clinical settings. Modafinil and armodafinil interact with the CYP isoenzymes as a minimal to moderate inducer of 3A4 and as an inhibitor of the 2C isoforms.[109,110] Modafinil and armodafinil can thereby engage in drug–drug interactions with common substrates, including oral contraceptives (the levels of which can decrease) and β-blockers and warfarin (the levels of which can increase), which requires monitoring and patient education. It is important to advise use of a second non-hormonal form of contraception in modafinil and armodafinil-treated patients on oral contraceptives. Like St. John's wort, modafinil has also been implicated as a factor in lowered cyclosporine levels, presumably through P450 3A4 induction, and should be used with extreme care in patients on immunosuppressants that rely on this enzyme for metabolism.

Benzodiazepines

The benzodiazepines are a class of widely prescribed psychotropic drugs that have anxiolytic, sedative, muscle-relaxant, and anticonvulsant properties. Their rate of onset of action, duration of action, presence of active metabolites, and tendency to accumulate in the body vary considerably and can influence both side effects and the success of treatment. Most benzodiazepines are well absorbed on an empty stomach, with peak plasma levels achieved generally between 1 and 3 hours, although with more rapid onset of some (e.g., diazepam, clorazepate) than others (e.g., oxazepam).[2] Duration of action of a single dose of benzodiazepine generally depends more on distribution from systemic circulation to tissue than on subsequent elimination (e.g., more rapid for diazepam than lorazepam). With repeated doses, however, the volume of distribution is saturated, and elimination half-life becomes the more important parameter in determining duration of action (e.g., more rapid for lorazepam than diazepam). A benzodiazepine that is comparatively short-acting on acute administration can therefore become relatively long-acting on long-term dosing. Benzodiazepines are highly lipophilic and distribute readily to the CNS and to tissues. Plasma protein-binding ranges from approximately 70% (alprazolam) to 99% (diazepam).[2]

Of the benzodiazepines, only lorazepam, oxazepam, and temazepam are not subject to phase I metabolism. Because phase II metabolism (glucuronide conjugation) does not produce active metabolites and is less affected than phase I metabolism by primary liver disease, aging, and concurrently used inducers or inhibitors of hepatic microsomal enzymes, the 3-hydroxy substituted benzodiazepines are much preferred in older patients and patients with liver disease. Perhaps the most common and clinically significant interactions involving benzodiazepines are the additive

CNS depressant effects, which can occur when a benzodiazepine is administered concurrently with barbiturates, narcotics, or ethanol. These interactions can be serious because of their potential to cause excessive sedation, cognitive and psychomotor impairment, and, at higher dosages, potentially fatal respiratory depression. The specific benzodiazepine antagonist, flumazenil, may be used in the management of a severe benzodiazepine overdose.

Pharmacokinetic interactions include a decreased rate of absorption, but not extent of absorption, of benzodiazepines in the presence of antacids or food. This is more likely to be a factor in determining the subjective effects accompanying the onset of benzodiazepine action for single-dose rather than repeated-dose administration. Carbamazepine, phenobarbital, and rifampin can induce metabolism, lowering levels of benzodiazepines that are oxidatively metabolized. In contrast, potential inhibitors of CYP3A4 (including macrolide antibiotics, antifungals such as ketoconazole and itraconazole, nefazodone, fluvoxamine, cimetidine) have been associated with decreased clearance and therefore increased levels of the triazolobenzodiazepines. A similar reaction occurs with several non-benzodiazepine sedative–hypnotics (e.g., zolpidem, zaleplon, eszopiclone), which are also metabolized through this pathway. The metabolism of diazepam depends in part on CYP2C19. Decreased diazepam clearance has been reported with concurrent administration of a variety of agents including fluoxetine, sertraline, propranolol, metoprolol, omeprazole, disulfiram, low-dose estrogen-containing oral contraceptives, and isoniazid.[54]

PSYCHIATRIC USES OF NON-PSYCHIATRIC MEDICATIONS

In the general hospital, consideration of the psychiatric complications of non-psychiatric medications is an integral part of the evaluation of alterations in mood, behavior, or mental status. A selected array of non-psychiatric medications that are associated with neuropsychiatric symptoms are listed in the text in the differential diagnosis of mood changes, delirium, psychosis, and anxiety in the medical setting. Nevertheless, whether by extrapolation from known *in vitro* mechanisms or through serendipity, non-psychiatric drugs have also been found to be useful in the treatment of psychiatric illness. These include medications that ameliorate the side effects of psychotropic drugs, as well as the growing number of non-psychiatric medications studied for the treatment of mood, anxiety, psychotic, substance abuse, attentional, and tic disorders.

Medications for Psychotropic Drug Side Effects

The importance of attentive management of psychotropic drug side effects for alleviating the patient's suffering, for developing a therapeutic alliance, and for increasing the likelihood of the patient's adherence to necessary treatment continues to fuel the search for effective pharmacologic strategies when more conservative measures fail to reduce dangerous or difficult-to-tolerate side effects.[7] Anticholinergic agents (benztropine 1 to 2 mg twice a day; biperiden 1 to 3 mg twice a day; and trihexyphenidyl 1 to 3 mg twice a day) and, less often, anticholinergic antihistamines (diphenhydramine 25 to 50 mg twice a day) and amantadine (100 mg two to three times a day) are widely used for managing the parkinsonian side effects of antipsychotics. Benztropine (2 mg) and diphenhydramine (50 mg) are also used IM or IV for the acute management of dystonia. Anticholinergic side effects are not uncommon, however, and combination of these drugs with other highly anticholinergic agents (e.g., tertiary amine TCAs) invites the risk of frank toxicity. In this regard, IV physostigmine has been used in the emergency management of the anticholinergic syndrome, which includes delirium and tachyarrhythmias.

β-Blockers (including propranolol starting at 10 to 20 mg one to two times a day or the less centrally active atenolol [approx. 50 mg/day]) have been useful for akathisia from antipsychotics and antidepressants, for lithium-associated tremor, and, less commonly, for jitteriness on antidepressants. Although the risk of depression on β-blockers is likely to be quite small, it is still reasonable nevertheless to monitor for alterations in mood whenever moderate to high dosages of the more lipophilic CNS active agents are used (e.g., propranolol dosages >80 mg/day).[111,112]

Diuretics, including amiloride 5 to 10 mg one to three times a day and hydrochlorothiazide 50 to 100 mg/day, have been successful in treating disruptive polyuria on lithium, albeit potentially requiring reduction of lithium dosage and close monitoring of lithium levels and serum potassium. Anticholinergic side effects, including urinary retention, constipation, blurred vision, and dry mouth, may be treated with bethanechol 10 to 25 mg one to three times a day; dry mouth and blurred vision can also be treated with 1% pilocarpine ophthalmic solution. Excessive sweating on antidepressants is infrequently treated with the α_1-adrenergic agent terazosin (1 mg for every hour of sleep) and doxazosin (1 to 2 mg for every hour of sleep), as well as with anticholinergic agents, such as benztropine (0.5 to 1.0 once or twice daily) or glycopyrrolate (1 to 2 mg once daily to three times a day).

Pharmacologic attempts to reduce orthostatic hypotension on antidepressants have included caffeine or cautious introduction of T_3 (25 to 50 μg/day); T_4 (50 to 200 μg/day); the mineralocorticoid fludrocortisone (0.05 to 0.5 mg/day); salt tablets (600 to 1800 mg/day); methylphenidate, or dextroamphetamine (5 to 20 mg/day). These measures tend to be used after other measures have failed, including efforts to maximize hydration and to improve venous return from the lower extremities by calf muscle exercises or surgical support stockings.

Nausea or indigestion that is not responsive to change in dosing strategy or a change in preparation has been successfully treated with nizatidine (150 to 300 mg/day), famotidine (20 to 40 mg/day), or metoclopramide (5 to 10 mg one to two times a day). Metoclopramide, a cholinergic agonist and dopamine antagonist, has been associated rarely with extrapyramidal and dyskinetic effects, akathisia, and a case of mania, and because it increases gastric motility, it can potentially affect the absorption of co-administered medications. With respect to the H_2 antagonists, although all are capable of producing mood and cognitive changes, including delirium, cimetidine, which has been most closely associated with these effects, is also a potent inhibitor of CYP metabolism, rendering it least preferable among these agents for use in patients on multiple psychotropic medications. Similarly, omeprazole, an inhibitor of the gastric proton pump, appears to be an inducer of CYP1A2 and an inhibitor of CYP2C, and its potential impact on the metabolism of concurrent medications should therefore be considered when it is prescribed. Agents that block 5-HT_3 receptors also may be helpful in reducing nausea related to serotoninergic agents. Although ondansetron is an option, a less-expensive, albeit less-selective, alternative for appropriate candidates is mirtazapine.

Diarrhea not responsive to changes in preparation or dosing is often responsive to standard agents, such as loperamide or diphenoxylate. Acidophilus (1 capsule/meal) and cyproheptadine (2 to 4 mg one to three times a day) have also been used as anti-diarrheal strategies.

Weight gain on psychotropic medications is common, distressing, and associated with risk of diabetes and hyperlipidemia. In addition to behavioral strategies for weight reduction, attention has also been directed toward pharmacologic strategies. Metformin currently has one of the largest databases of studies showing its superiority to placebo.[113] Other classes of medicines may also be helpful, including the anticonvulsants topiramate[114] (25 to 100 mg one to three times a day) and zonisamide (up to 600 mg daily). The H_2 antagonists, including nizatidine[115] (up to 300 mg daily), have also showed promise in curbing weight gain, as have dopaminergic agents and bupropion.

Sexual dysfunction has proved to be a particularly common and troublesome side effect of antidepressants, especially the SSRIs, including diminished libido, erectile dysfunction, ejaculatory delay, and anorgasmia. As an alternative to switching medications (e.g., to bupropion, mirtazapine, vilazodone, vortioxetine), a variety of partly effective strategies have been marshaled for when dosage reductions or drug holidays[116] have not been feasible. These include sildenafil (25 to 100 mg/day);[55,117,118] yohimbine (2.5 mg as needed up to 5.4 mg three times a day),[74] potentially complicated by jitteriness, dizziness, or irritability; cyproheptadine (4 to 16 mg/day), with the potential, although apparently quite small, risk of interfering with efficacy of serotoninergic antidepressants; bethanechol (10 to 25 mg one to three times a day); and amantadine (100 mg two to three times a day). Psychotropic medications have also been used in an effort to treat sexual dysfunction, including bupropion (75 to 300 mg/day),[119] nefazodone (50 to 200 mg/day), trazodone (25 to 100 mg/day), and buspirone (5 to 20 mg two to three times a day), as have dopamine agonists, such as ropinirole.[120] Improvement may be limited not only by the lack of more effective pharmacologic strategies but also by the impact of depressive illness on sexual interest and by the influence of relevant psychosocial factors (e.g., marital conflict) that can accompany the depression.

α_1-Adrenergic Antagonists

Prazosin, the α_1-adrenergic receptor antagonist used for many years to treat hypertension, has been demonstrated (in several open-label trials, chart reviews, and an increasing number of placebo-controlled trials) to offer possible benefit at dosages of up to 10 mg at bedtime in the treatment of core symptoms of post-traumatic stress disorder (PTSD), particularly nightmares, insomnia, and hyperarousal.[121,122] Side effects include orthostatic blood pressure changes and dizziness, and particular caution does need to be observed when administered concurrently with other agents with α_1-adrenergic blocking properties, including low-potency antipsychotics.

α_2-Adrenergic Agonists

The antihypertensive clonidine is highly lipophilic and readily crosses the blood–brain barrier, where it stimulates α_2-adrenergic receptors, thereby inhibiting norepinephrine release. Diminution of norepinephrine results in decreases in peripheral resistance, renal vascular resistance, heart rate, and blood pressure. Clonidine is available as oral tablets or a transdermal patch. Oral clonidine is indicated for the treatment of hypertension in adults, but has a broad range of psychiatric uses, including ADHD, oppositional defiant disorder (ODD), PTSD, sleep disturbances, substance-induced withdrawal (particularly withdrawal from opioids),[123] Tourette's syndrome, chronic headaches, and hyperactive/impulsive behaviors in patients with autism spectrum disorders. Although generally more likely to cause sedation and hypotension than other treatments for akathisia (e.g., anticholinergic medications, β-blockers, and benzodiazepines), clonidine has also been used to reduce akathisia refractory to other agents.[124] The clinical literature involving psychiatric applications of transdermal clonidine is considerably smaller. Although controlled trials are generally lacking, guanfacine, another α_2-adrenergic receptor agonist antihypertensive drug, appears to be useful for many of the same indications as clonidine but with the potential advantages of a longer half-life and generally less sedation.[125,126]

β-Blockers

In addition to their role in the treatment of akathisia and tremor, the non-selective β-adrenergic receptor antagonists, which block the β_1-adrenergic receptors in heart and brain and β_2-adrenergic receptors in lung, blood vessels, and brain (including glial cells), have been among the first-line treatments for organically based aggressive behavior.[127,128] Anti-aggression β-blockers include the lipid-soluble agents propranolol, pindolol, and nebivolol, and the water-soluble agent nadolol.[129] It is unclear how β-blockers mediate psychoactive effects. Some studies report benefits with β-blockers that do not cross the blood–brain barrier, suggesting that both central and peripheral mechanisms are involved.

β-Blockers (e.g., propranolol 10 to 40 mg or the equivalent) have been used widely to reduce symptoms associated with performance anxiety[130] and are not uncommonly used for this purpose by musicians and public speakers. The β-blockers have had limited use for treatment of autonomic arousal associated with other anxiety states, including social phobia, PTSD, generalized anxiety disorder, and panic disorder.

The prescription of β-blockers is potentially hazardous in a variety of common clinical conditions, including bronchospastic pulmonary diseases, insulin-dependent diabetes, hyperthyroidism, significant peripheral vascular disease, and congestive heart failure. In addition, β-blockers entirely or primarily eliminated by liver (e.g., propranolol, metoprolol, and pindolol) may be inhibitors of, as well as substrates for, hepatic microsomal enzymes and are therefore more likely to be subject to pharmacokinetic drug interactions than β-blockers primarily cleared by kidney (e.g., atenolol, nadolol, and sotalol).[131]

REFERENCES

Access the reference list online at https://expertconsult.inkling.com/.

Psychopharmacologic Management of Children and Adolescents

39

Jonathan R. Stevens, M.D., M.P.H.
Amy F. Vyas, M.D.
Boris A. Lorberg, M.D.
Jefferson B. Prince, M.D.
Theodore A. Stern, M.D.

OVERVIEW

Similar to adults, hospitalized children can develop psychiatric illness as a result of psychosocial stresses of hospitalization (e.g., loss of control, threat of illness, separation from caregivers), effects of general medical conditions (e.g., infections), use of medications or substances (e.g., drug–drug interactions, drug withdrawal), and exacerbation of preexisting psychiatric vulnerabilities. The decision to use psychotropics in this population should be based on a careful diagnostic formulation and consideration of the limited database on the risks and benefits of using, as well as not using, psychotropics. Despite increasing research efforts, expanding clinical experience, and a continued rise in prescriptions for psychoactive medications to pediatric patients, a large gap remains between empirical support and clinical practice. Children represent a significant proportion of those affected with depression, schizophrenia, and bipolar disorder—medical conditions with a prominent global health burden—though their representation among clinical drug trials worldwide is less than 15%.[1] General guidelines for the use of psychoactive medications in children and adolescents are provided in Table 39-1; they are consistent with the American Academy of Child and Adolescent Psychiatry's (AACAP) policy statement on prescribing psychotropic medications for children and adolescents.[2]

ISSUES IN CLINICAL MANAGEMENT

The safe and effective use of psychotropics in pediatric patients rests on many of the same principles reviewed in Chapter 38. However, there are special factors to consider when prescribing or recommending psychiatric medications for youth.

The first of these issues is the off-label use of medications. The Food and Drug Administration (FDA) approves the use of medications in specified clinical situations. However, the FDA allows practitioners to use medications in clinical situations not included in the official labeling—that is, practitioners may use a medication for clinical situations other than the approved use or use it in age groups in which it has not been formally studied.[3] Medical advances are often made with use of drugs in conditions that are not yet approved by the FDA.

The second issue deals with obtaining consent to use medications. Except in emergency situations, consent must be obtained from the custodial parent or the legal guardian before any compounds can be used in pediatric patients. This consent process involves a discussion of the diagnosis being treated, the prognosis with or without treatment, the potential risks and benefits of the proposed intervention, and a discussion of treatment alternatives. The practitioner also needs to assess the reliability of the parents before initiation of outpatient treatment because it will be their responsibility to administer the drugs on an outpatient basis. If the parents cannot reliably administer the medication, this type of intervention may be precluded.

A third issue involves developmental factors. Both pharmacodynamic and pharmacokinetic factors may influence the safety, tolerability, and efficacy of medications in the pediatric population.[4] Pharmacodynamic factors, such as the ongoing development of neural networks, may affect the response to medications. Similarly, pharmacokinetic factors may influence the absorption, distribution, metabolism, and excretion of medications. Pediatric patients may require higher doses of medication to achieve the same benefit as adults, perhaps as a result of more extensive or rapid metabolism by the liver or increased renal excretion (owing to a higher glomerular filtration rate). Furthermore, the pharmacokinetics in children and adolescents may be different for short- and long-term exposures.

CASE 1

Jacob, a 15-year-old boy with attention deficit hyperactivity disorder (ADHD), presented to the Emergency Department (ED) in the early morning hours following an apparent intentional overdose of lisdexamfetamine (Vyvanse). Jacob's mother (his legal guardian) told ED staff that she was awakened when she heard "banging sounds" on the wall of an adjacent room. She found her son on the floor, unresponsive to commands, and observed his legs shaking violently, thereby hitting the wall. His mother found an empty bottle of lisdexamfetamine (prescribed by Jacob's pediatrician during the previous academic year when Jacob was failing academically) by his side. She stated that Jacob stopped taking this medicine months ago because "he didn't like the way it made him feel" in terms of suppressed appetite, emotional blunting, and difficulty sleeping. She suspected there were "about 20" 50 mg tablets unused, suggesting an ingestion of 1000 mg of the amphetamine-based stimulant.

On the ambulance ride to the ED, Jacob received lorazepam 5 mg intravenously (IV) for a suspected seizure. Jacob had no history of seizures and his general medical history was benign, aside from two concussions sustained while skateboarding. In the ED, Jacob was somnolent, but arousable. His vital signs showed mild hypertension and tachycardia; an electrocardiogram (ECG) suggested a possible left bundle branch block. He received activated charcoal (without gastric lavage or acidification of the urine) and was transferred to the intensive care unit (ICU) for additional monitoring.

Within hours of his transfer to the ICU, Jacob experienced waxing and waning periods of agitation and confusion. He yelled at "demons and devils" and believed that he was "in hell." He threatened to leave the hospital and tried to pull out his IV lines. ICU staff consulted the psychiatric consultation service, who, after reviewing cardiac monitoring data, recommended IV haloperidol 5 mg for Jacob. This intervention was rapidly effective and Jacob received only one additional dose of this medicine during his ICU stay.

Ultimately, Jacob transferred to an acute care pediatric psychiatric unit, where he was diagnosed with major depressive disorder (MDD), in addition to ADHD. His psychotic symptoms did not recur; therefore, his mental status changes in the ICU were attributed to an amphetamine (or other stimulant) intoxication delirium. After 2 weeks of inpatient psychiatric care, Jacob transitioned to residential level of care on liquid fluoxetine (after refusing to take any medicines in tablet form). He refused pharmacologic treatment for ADHD, though his mother had consented to re-start stimulant medicine.

Take home points

- It is important to tell parents to keep medications locked in a safe.
- Supra-therapeutic doses of stimulants can decrease seizure threshold.
- Haloperidol is an effective medication for managing pediatric delirium and severe agitation.

TABLE 39-1 General Guidelines for the Use of Psychoactive Medications in Children and Adolescents

1. The use of psychotropics should follow a careful evaluation of the child and the family (including psychiatric, medical, and social considerations).
2. Consideration should be given to the child's non-psychiatric disorders, and an exclusionary differential diagnosis should be considered, particularly in an acute medical setting.
3. Children who manifest transient symptoms related to an adjustment to a medical illness or to a loss should be considered for non-pharmacologic treatment; pharmacologic care should be reserved for severe or refractory cases.
4. Pharmacotherapy should be considered as part of a comprehensive treatment plan that includes individual and family psychotherapy, educational and behavioral interventions, and careful medical management; it should not be presented as an alternative to these interventions. However, pharmacotherapy should be considered as an initial treatment when it is known to be superior to other modalities.
5. If a patient has a psychiatric disorder that may respond to a psychotropic, the clinician should decide which psychotropic to use and take into consideration the age and weight of the child and the severity and nature of the clinical picture. The diagnosis and target symptoms should be defined before the initiation of pharmacotherapy.
6. The family and the child should be familiarized with the risks and benefits of this intervention, the availability of alternative treatments, the possible adverse effects, the potential for interactions with other medications, the realization that unforeseeable adverse events may arise, and the prognosis with or without treatment. Permission to use medications should be obtained from the custodial parent or from the patient's legal guardian.
7. Ongoing assessment of pharmacologic interventions is necessary. When a medication is thought to be either ineffective or inappropriate to the current clinical situation, it should be tapered and discontinued under careful clinical observation. Appropriate alternatives should be reviewed with the family before initiation.
8. Pediatricians, family practitioners, other medical staff, mental health professionals, and child psychiatrists should work collaboratively in the pharmacologic management of children.

MEDICAL PRECAUTIONS AND CONTRAINDICATIONS

In the presence of active pediatric illness, special precautions apply when using psychotropics. For example, in the presence of pre-existing cardiac disease that might impair cardiac conduction, tricyclic antidepressants (TCAs) either alone or in combination with antipsychotics should be used cautiously; a cardiac evaluation should be considered before initiating treatment.

Because non-selective β-blockers may cause severe bronchoconstriction and bradycardia, they are contraindicated in patients with asthma, congestive heart failure, sinus bradycardia, first-degree atrioventricular block, and Wolff–Parkinson–White syndrome. Similarly, β-Blockers should not be used in conjunction with α-adrenergic medications because of concerns over heart block. β-blockers can mask the symptoms of hypoglycemic crisis and thyrotoxicosis and therefore should be used with caution in patients with diabetes and hyperthyroidism.

Atypical antidepressants (e.g., bupropion), antipsychotics, and TCAs may lower the seizure threshold. *The Physicians'*

Desk Reference (PDR)[5] notes that stimulants are associated with seizures (as illustrated in the case study), though clinical experience and recent investigations show this is a rare occurrence at manufacturer-recommended dosage ranges. Patients with ADHD and an epileptiform EEG have an increased risk of seizures.[6] However, published guidelines for the evaluation of attention deficit/hyperactivity disorder (ADHD) do not recommend a baseline electroencephalogram (EEG) as part of the work-up, and recent data indicate that patients with ADHD and a normal EEG are at minimal risk for seizures.

Antidepressants, antipsychotics, and anti-anxiety agents can produce central nervous system (CNS) depression; therefore, these agents should be used with caution in patients with a chronic respiratory disease.

Known drug interactions should also be considered. Psychostimulants generally do not generate significant interactions with other agents, with the exception of monoamine oxidase inhibitors (MAOIs); however, many antidepressants, antipsychotics, and anticonvulsants can interact with a wide array of drugs (see Chapter 38). Psychotropics should be used with caution in pediatric patients with renal or hepatic dysfunction. In these patients psychotropics with specific metabolic pathways (i.e., renal or hepatic) should be selected or the dose decreased and serum levels closely monitored.

Clinicians are encouraged to access readily available databases to receive up-to-date information about their metabolism and interactions with other medications.

EMERGENCY INTERVENTIONS: TREATMENT OF ACUTE AGITATION OR AGGRESSION

Typically, the request for the emergency use of psychotropics deals with the initial management of acutely assaultive or self-injurious behaviors. Use of emergency psychotropics should be conducted in concert with behavioral interventions and aimed at addressing the crisis situation, its causes, and its psychosocial impact.[7] If reduced stimulation and general calming measures are ineffective, pharmacotherapy should be considered. Low doses of a short-acting benzodiazepine (e.g., lorazepam 0.5 to 1 mg) or a sedating antihistamine (e.g., diphenhydramine 25 to 50 mg) can be used to reduce acute anxiety, agitation, and insomnia with few side effects. These agents can be administered orally, intravenously (IV), or intramuscularly (IM). Behavioral disinhibition can occur among children and should be monitored. In severe or agitated psychotic states, low to medium doses of a sedating antipsychotic (e.g., chlorpromazine 25 to 150 mg, olanzapine 2.5 to 10 mg, or quetiapine 25 to 300 mg) may be very effective in reducing concomitant anxiety, agitation, or psychosis. For children with active hallucinations or severe disturbances of reality, a higher-potency antipsychotic (e.g., risperidone at 0.25 to 3 mg orally or haloperidol 2.5 to 10 mg orally, IV, or IM) may be necessary. Often a combination of a benzodiazepine and an antipsychotic may be necessary for severe agitation. Extra caution is advised when co-administering IM lorazepam and olanzapine due to elevated risk of cardiorespiratory depression. Medications used for crisis management should not be continued indefinitely, unless they are indicated for the treatment of a co-existing psychiatric disorder.

DELIRIUM

Delirium is a transient derangement of cerebral function with global impairment of cognition and attention. It is frequently accompanied by disturbances of the sleep–wake cycle and changes in psychomotor activity. Delirium may be an early warning of a deteriorating medical condition, a toxic insult, or a brain injury, and it may be accompanied by self-injurious behaviors, such as pulling out IV lines. In adolescents, clinicians should consider substance intoxication and drug interactions (between prescribed medications and illicit substances, such as marijuana) in the differential.

Treatment is usually directed at both the cause and the symptoms. Correction of metabolic abnormalities, removal of agents that may be exacerbating the symptoms, or treatment of the underlying injury or infection is generally followed by reversal in the delirium. After attempting to re-orient and decrease the sensory input, the practitioner may need to implement pharmacologic intervention. Generally, antipsychotics are useful if hallucinations or delusions are present, whereas anxiolytics (i.e., benzodiazepines) help reduce anxiety and apprehension. As mentioned previously, antihistamines (e.g., diphenhydramine 25 to 50 mg orally or IM every 6 to 8 hours) or benzodiazepines (e.g., lorazepam 0.5 to 2 mg orally, IM, sublingually [SL], or IV every 4 to 6 hours) are among the most benign choices for agitation and anxiety. In older children or adolescents who do not respond to these treatments or in those with psychosis, severe dyscontrol, or agitation, risperidone or haloperidol can be used, with the dose repeated every 6 hours if needed. Psychotropic medications should be withdrawn with resolution of the delirium.

CHILDHOOD ANXIETY DISORDERS

Children tend to be anxious when receiving care in any medical setting. When the level of anxiety impairs the child (or practitioner) and is unremitting, a child should be assessed for an anxiety disorder. Anxiety problems may also manifest in children as multiple somatic complaints, such as headaches and stomachaches. Childhood anxiety disorders are relatively common and tend to persist into adult life. The three most common childhood anxiety disorders seen in medical settings are separation anxiety disorder, generalized anxiety disorder (GAD) of childhood, and acute stress disorder. Other anxiety disorders, such as post-traumatic stress disorder (PTSD), obsessive–compulsive disorder (OCD), and tic disorders may be present in hospitalized children.

In separation anxiety disorder, the predominant disturbance is a developmentally inappropriate excessive anxiety on separation from familial surroundings. It is called *separation anxiety* because it is assumed that the main disturbance is the child's inability to separate from the parent or major attachment figures. When separation occurs or is anticipated, the child may experience severe anxiety to the point of panic. Although it may develop during the pre-school age, it more commonly appears in older children.

Similar to GAD in the adult patient, the essential feature of childhood GAD is excessive worry and fears that are not focused on a specific situation or a result of psychosocial stressors. Affected children may manifest an exaggerated or unrealistic response to the comments or criticisms of others.

Four medications have been approved for OCD treatment in children and adolescents; to date, only duloxetine (Cymbalta) is FDA-approved for non-OCD anxiety in pediatric patients. Duloxetine is approved for the treatment of GAD in patients aged 7 to 17 years, but is not routinely used clinically. A ten-week randomized controlled trial demonstrated duloxetine was superior to placebo as evidenced by changes from baseline Pediatric Anxiety Rating Scale scores.[8a] However, based on the efficacy and safety demonstrated in multiple randomized controlled trials (RCTs), the selective serotonin re-uptake inhibitors (SSRIs) fluoxetine, sertraline, and fluvoxamine appear to be the first-line medications for the treatment of separation anxiety disorder and GAD in children.[8b] The literature on benzodiazepines, tricyclic antidepressants (TCAs), buspirone, pregabalin, gabapentin, and β-blockers is mixed (at best). Acute stress disorder develops within 1 month of an acute traumatic event and lasts for a maximum of 1 month. It is manifest by anxiety, dissociative symptoms, persistent re-experiencing of the trauma, and avoidance of stimuli that evoke recollections of the trauma. The nature, severity, duration, and proximity to the trauma are factors that influence the development of acute stress disorder. In a number of patients, acute stress disorder may continue beyond 1 month and develop into PTSD. Effective management is focused on ensuring safety and reducing pain, anxiety, and fear. Recent investigations of children with burns suggest that aggressive management of pain with morphine may reduce and secondarily prevent PTSD.[9] Pediatric patients with PTSD are likely to have co-morbidity with other psychiatric disorders, a history of neglect or abuse, or both.[10]

In adults with PTSD, SSRIs have been shown to be useful in reducing symptoms of anxiety, depressed mood, rage, and obsessional thinking. In fact, both sertraline and paroxetine are approved for treatment of PTSD in adults and are often used in pediatric patients.[11] β-Blockers, in particular propranolol, have been studied as a means of reducing arousal symptoms of PTSD.[12] Similarly, α-adrenergic agents, such as prazosin, clonidine, and guanfacine, may similarly reduce nightmares, anxiety, hyperarousal, impulsivity and—in the case of clonidine and guanfacine—improve attention.[13]

In patients with dissociation, medications (such as the benzodiazepines or gabapentin) that enhance gamma-aminobutyric acid (GABA), may reduce the severity of anxiety. In patients with fear or terror, the short-term use of atypical antipsychotics in low doses may be useful. Long-term treatment of acute stress disorder and PTSD uses both pharmacologic and psychotherapeutic modalities.[14]

High-potency (e.g., clonazepam 0.25 to 1 mg three times per day) or medium-potency (e.g., lorazepam 0.25 to 1 mg three times per day) benzodiazepines can be effective for short-term relief of anxiety. A shorter-acting compound (e.g., lorazepam) can be very effective in managing more acute situations (e.g., anxious or agitated reactions to psychosocial crises). Doses of 0.5 to 1 mg of lorazepam given orally or SL are often effective. Lorazepam may be administered IM in an emergency. Use of short-acting benzodiazepines requires multiple daily doses. Long-term use should be avoided whenever possible.

In general, the clinical toxicity of benzodiazepines is low, but higher rates of disinhibition are observed in the pediatric population than in adults. Children who become disinhibited on high-potency benzodiazepines may respond more favorably to the mid- or low-potency agents (e.g., diazepam). The most commonly encountered short-term adverse effects of benzodiazepines are sedation, disinhibition, and depression.

When long-term treatment in older adolescents is warranted, long-acting benzodiazepines (such as clonazepam) may be preferable. For clonazepam an initial dose of 0.25 to 0.5 mg can be given at bedtime. The dose may be increased by 0.5 mg every 5 to 7 days depending on the clinical response and the side effects. Typically, doses between 0.25 and 2 mg per day are effective. Potential benefits of the longer-acting compounds are once-daily dosage and a decreased risk of withdrawal symptoms on discontinuation of treatment.

Buspirone is a non-benzodiazepine anxiolytic without anticonvulsant, sedative, or muscle-relaxant properties. Clinical experience with this drug suggests limited anti-anxiety efficacy in the acute setting, but greater utility in the chronic management of pediatric anxiety. The effective daily dose ranges from 0.3 to 0.6 mg/kg.

One controlled study with high-dose imipramine demonstrated efficacy under controlled conditions.[15] However, TCAs have had only limited usefulness for management of pediatric anxiety disorders given their narrow therapeutic window.

AKATHISIA

Akathisia is a movement disorder experienced as inability to sit still (the term is derived from the Greek and literally means "not to sit"). In children and adolescents, it is most often seen as a side effect of antipsychotics or antidepressants. Akathisia may be confused with ADHD or agitation. Historically, patients are free from akathisia before starting an antidepressant or antipsychotic or reducing an anticholinergic medication. As with adults, treatment of akathisia in the pediatric population involves reducing the dose of the offending medication to the lowest effective dose and then adding either β-blockers or benzodiazepines (0.5 to 1 mg three times per day of lorazepam). Although several β-blockers are likely to be effective, propranolol has good CNS penetration and is typically used. Propranolol should be initiated at 10 mg two times per day and the dose increased every several days to effect.

Studies in adults have demonstrated the efficacy of the potent selective β-1 blocking agent betaxolol in reducing akathisia.[16] Betaxolol has a long half-life (allowing once-daily dosing) and has minimal medication interactions. Betaxolol is generally started at 5 mg and can be titrated as tolerated to doses between 10 mg and 20 mg/day.

ATTENTION DEFICIT HYPERACTIVITY DISORDER

A common psychiatric condition, ADHD, is found in 3% to 10% of school-age children.[17] ADHD is characterized

TABLE 39-2 FDA-Approved Treatments for Attention Deficit Hyperactivity Disorder

GENERIC NAME	BRAND NAME	FORMULATIONS AND STRENGTHS	DURATION OF BEHAVIORAL EFFECT (h)	COMMENTS
Amphetamines				
D-amphetamine	Dexedrine	Tablets: 5, 10 mg	3–6	
	Dexedrine Spansule	Spansules: 5, 10, 15 mg		
	ProCentra	Oral solution: 5 mg/5 mL		
Mixed amphetamine/ dextroamphetamine	Adderall	Tablets: 5, 7.5, 10, 12.5, 15, 20, 30 mg	4–6	
	Adderall XR	Capsules: 5, 10, 15, 20, 25, 30 mg	8–10	Capsule with 1:1 ratio of IR to DR beads
	Evekeo	Tablets: 5, 10 mg	10	Racemic amphetamine sulfate, 1:1 D-amphetamine and L-amphetamine
	Dyanavel	Oral suspension: 2.5 mg/mL	8–13	Shake the bottle before administering the dose
Lisdexamfetamine dimesylate	Vyvanse	Capsules: 20, 30, 40, 50, 60, 70 mg	8–12	Inactive prodrug in which L-lysine is chemically bonded to D-amphetamine
Methylphenidates				
Methylphenidate	Ritalin	Tablets: 5, 10, 20 mg	3–4	
	Methylin	Tablets, chewable: 2.5, 5, 10 mg	3–4	
		Oral solution: 5 mg/5 mL, 10 mg/5 mL (500 mL)	3–4	
	Ritalin LA	Capsules: 10, 20, 30, 40 mg	8–9	Capsule with 1:1 ratio of IR beads to DR beads
	Metadate ER	Tablets: 10, 20 mg	5–8	
	Metadate CD	Capsules: 10, 20, 30 mg	8–9	Capsule with 3:7 ratio of IR beads to DR beads
	Concerta	Tablets: 18, 27, 36, 54 mg	8–12	Ascending profile, OROS technology
	Daytrana	Transdermal patch: 10, 15, 20, 30 mg/9 h	9	Delivery rate of 1.1, 1.6, 2.2, 3.3 mg/h for the patches, respectively, based on 9-h wear times in patients ages 6–12 years
	Quillivant XR	Oral suspension: 25 mg/ 5 mL	8–12	Shake the bottle before administering the dose
	QuilliChew ER	Chewable tablets: 20, 30, 40 mg	8	
	Aptensio XR	Capsules: 10, 15, 20, 30, 40, 50, 60 mg	9–12	May be swallowed or opened and contents mixed into food.
Dexmethylphenidate	Focalin	Tablets: 2.5, 5, 10 mg		*d-threo*-enantiomer of methylphenidate, twice as potent as racemic methylphenidate
	Focalin XR	Capsules: 5, 10, 20 mg		

by the classic triad of impaired attention, increased impulsivity, and excessive motor activity, although many children manifest only inattentiveness. With developmental variations, ADHD affects children of all ages (as early as age 3), and it persists into adulthood about half of the time.[18] Within the medical setting, ADHD needs to be differentiated from environmental stimulation, iatrogenic causes (e.g., use of β-agonists), or other psychiatric disorders (e.g., anxiety, depression, mania, or intoxication). Pharmacotherapy remains the cornerstone of ADHD treatment (Table 39-2).[19]

FDA-Approved Treatments for ADHD

Stimulants

Since the 1940s, stimulants have been used safely and effectively in the treatment of ADHD. There are three main stimulant families (Table 39-2): methylphenidate (MPH) (e.g., short-acting Ritalin and Metadate, long-acting Concerta and Metadate-CD), transdermal Daytrana, or liquid Quillivant XR), dextroamphetamine (DEX) (i.e., short-acting Dexedrine tablets, long-acting Dexedrine spansules, and Vyvanse), and a mixture of dextroamphetamine salts (DEX) plus mixed amphetamine salts (MAS) (i.e., short-acting Adderall, long-acting Adderall-XR, Evekeo, and liquid Dyanavel).

Stimulants increase intra-synaptic (extra-cellular) brain concentrations of dopamine; norepinephrine; and, to a lesser extent, serotonin (5-HT).[20] After oral administration, stimulants are rapidly absorbed and preferentially taken up into the CNS. Stimulants bind poorly to plasma proteins; this partially explains their relative paucity of drug–drug interactions. MPH is metabolized primarily by plasma-based esterases to ritalinic acid that is excreted in the urine. The amphetamines are 80% excreted in the urine unchanged; 20% undergo hepatic metabolism. Acidification of the urine may enhance excretion of the amphetamines. Of note, MPH is not usually detected on routine drug screening.

Methylphenidate

Originally formulated in 1954, methylphenidate was produced as an equal optical isomer mixture of *d,l-threo*-MPH and *d,l-erythro*-MPH. Because the *erythro* form of MPH was linked with cardiovascular (CV) side effects, MPH is now manufactured as an equal mixture of *d,l-threo*-MPH. Later studies found that the *d-threo*-MPH isomer was twice as active as the *l-threo* one. The *d-threo* isomer of MPH (*d-threo*-MPH or *dex*-MPH) is marketed as Focalin. With regard to conversion and potency, 10 mg of Ritalin is biologically equivalent to 5 mg of Focalin.

The time-to-peak plasma concentration with oral administration of immediate-release *d,l-threo*-MPH (e.g., generic MPH, Ritalin, Metadate, Methylin) is variable (1 to 2 hours); its half-life is 2 to 3 hours. Behavioral effects of immediate-release MPH peak 1 to 2 hours after administration and tend to dissipate in 3 to 5 hours. Although generic MPH has a similar pharmacokinetic profile to Ritalin, it is more rapidly absorbed and peaks sooner.

Novel methods of delivering MPH have become available; each is intended to extend the clinical effectiveness of stimulants. Although these medications all deliver a stimulant, their pharmacokinetic profiles differ. Concerta (OROS methylphenidate) uses the OROS technology to deliver a 50:50 racemic mixture of *d,l-threo*-MPH. An 18 mg caplet of Concerta delivers the equivalent of 15 mg MPH (5 mg MPH three times per day) providing 12-hour coverage. Initially, the 18 mg caplet provides 4 mg MPH and delivers the additional MPH in an ascending profile over 12 hours.[21] The recommended dose of Concerta is between 18 to 54 mg per day, although trials in adolescents studied doses up to 72 mg per day.[21] If Concerta is cut or crushed, its delivery system is compromised.

Metadate-CD (MPH-MR) capsules (10, 20, and 30 mg; may be sprinkled) contain *d,l-threo*-MPH with 30% of immediate-release beads and 70% of extended-release beads.[22] Metadate-CD delivers 30% or 6 mg of *d,l-threo*-MPH initially and is designed for 8-hour coverage.

Ritalin-LA (MPH-ERC) capsules (10, 20, 30, and 40 mg; may be sprinkled) deliver 50% of its *d,l-threo*-MPH initially and another bolus approximately 3 to 4 hours later, thereby providing approximately 8 hours of coverage.

The primarily active form of MPH is the *d-threo* isomer,[23] which has become available in both immediate-release tablets (Focalin 2.5, 5, and 10 mg) and extended-delivery capsules (Focalin XR 5, 10, 15, and 20 mg). The efficacy of D-MPH is well established in children, adolescents, and adults under double-blind conditions.[24,25] D-MPH is approved to treat ADHD in children, adolescents, and adults in doses of up to 20 mg per day and has been labeled to provide 12 hours of coverage. Although the research is not definitive, 10 mg of MPH appears to be approximately equivalent to 5 mg of D-MPH, and clinicians can reasonably use this estimate in clinical practice.

For patients who have difficulty tolerating an oral stimulant formulation or for patients who need flexibility in the duration of medication effect, the MPH Matrix Transdermal System (MTS; Daytrana; 10-, 15-, 20-, and 30-mg patches[26]) delivers MPH through the skin. The patches are applied once daily and are intended to be worn for 9 hours, although in clinical practice they can be worn for shorter or longer periods. The MTS usually takes effect within 2 hours and provides coverage for 3 hours after removal of the patch. Because the MPH is absorbed through the skin, it does not undergo first-pass metabolism in the liver; therefore, patients require lower doses with the patch compared with oral preparations (10 mg MTS is equivalent to 15 mg extended-release oral MPH).

For youth who have difficulties swallowing tablets or capsules, a long-acting liquid form of MPH may be useful. Extended-release liquid MPH (Quillivant XR) is supplied as a powder that is reconstituted with water by the pharmacist prior to dispensing. The resulting ER MPH suspension has a concentration of 25 mg/5 mL (5 mg/mL) and does not require refrigeration. It is composed of cationic polymer matrix particles that bind *d,l-threo*-methylphenidate racemic mixture via an ion exchange mechanism; it is a blend of uncoated and coated particles that is ~20% immediate-release (IR) and 80% ER methylphenidate.[27] The liquid has a fruit flavoring. At doses of 20 to 60 mg once daily, this preparation provides effective treatment of ADHD symptoms for up to 12 hours.[28] An extended-release chewable formulation of MPH (QuilliChew ER) is also offered in 20, 30, and 40 mg cherry-flavored chewable tablets, containing 30% immediate-release methylphenidate and 70% extended-release methylphenidate. This preparation provides therapeutic effect for about 8 hours.

Amphetamines

Mixed amphetamine salts (MAS; Adderall) are a racemic mixture of approximately 3:1 of D- to L-amphetamine.[5] The two isomers have different pharmacodynamic properties, and some patients with ADHD preferentially respond to one isomer over another. Data on children with ADHD suggest that, when compared with immediate-release MPH, the peak behavioral effects of Adderall occur later and are more sustained.[29]

The extended-delivery preparation of MAS is a capsule containing two types of Micotrol beads (MAS XR; Adderall XR). The beads are present in 50:50 ratios, with immediate-release beads designed to release MAS in a fashion similar to that of MAS tablets, and delayed-release beads designed to release MAS 4 hours after dosing.[5] A single dose of MAS-XR 20 mg is bioequivalent to 10 mg of an MAS tablet dosed twice per day. The efficacy of MAS XR is well established in youth with ADHD.[30]

Dextroamphetamine (DEX; Dexedrine) tablets contain only the *D*-isomer of amphetamine. DEX tablets achieve peak plasma levels 2 to 3 hours after oral administration and have a half-life of 4 to 6 hours. Behavioral effects of DEX tablets peak 1 to 2 hours after administration and last 4 to 5 hours. When DEX spansules are used, behavioral effects last 6 to 9 hours.

Lisdexamfetamine dimesylate (LDX; Vyvanse), is an amphetamine pro-drug in which L-lysine, a naturally occurring amino acid, is covalently linked to D-amphetamine. After oral administration, the pro-drug is hydrolyzed in the body to release D-amphetamine. Although lisdexamfetamine appears to have less abuse liability and overdose protection, it is a CII schedule drug. It is available in doses of 30, 50, and 70 mg that appear to be comparable with MAS XR doses of 10, 20, and 30 mg, respectively.[31]

Guidelines on the Use of Stimulants in Children

The AACAP guidelines on the use of stimulants in children and adolescents recommend starting with a longer-acting preparation in most cases. Clinicians can initiate therapy at 18 mg Concerta or 20 mg Metadate-CD or Ritalin-LA for MPH products or 5 to 10 mg Adderall-XR or Dexedrine spansules. However, in the hospital setting, clinicians may prefer short-acting stimulants, starting with lower doses (2.5 to 5 mg/day for children and adolescents, 5 to 10 mg/day for adults), given in the morning with food. The dose is titrated upward every 3 to 5 days until a beneficial effect is noted or adverse effects emerge. Typically, the half-life of the short-acting stimulants necessitates at least twice-daily dosing, with the addition of similar or smaller afternoon doses, based on breakthrough symptoms. Although the PDR lists maximum dosages for amphetamine products at 40 mg per day and 60 mg per day for MPH, patients often benefit from suggested daily doses that range from 0.3 to 1.5 mg/kg per day for amphetamine products and from 0.5 to 2 mg/kg per day for MPH products. Thus, an older adolescent may need immediate-release MPH up to 30 mg three to four times daily or amphetamine 15 to 20 mg three to four times a day.

Numerous short-term (<12 weeks) clinical trials show that approximately 70% of patients with ADHD respond to stimulants. A positive dose–response relationship of stimulants is present for both hyperactivity and inattention. Longer-term trials have demonstrated the tolerability and continued efficacy of stimulants in patients treated continuously over 2 years.

Despite the vast literature and excellent safety profile of stimulants, studies indicate that approximately one-third of children and adolescents with ADHD either do not respond or manifest intolerable adverse effects; these outcomes necessitate alternative treatments. Fortunately, ATMX and other off-label treatments (including antidepressants, antihypertensives, and wakefulness medicines) are available.

Side Effects of Stimulants

Although generally well-tolerated, stimulants can cause clinically significant side effects (e.g., anorexia, nausea, insomnia, nightmares, headaches, dizziness, dry mouth, anxiety, irritability, dysphoria, rebound phenomena). Rates and types of stimulant-induced side effects appear to be similar in all ADHD patients, regardless of age. In patients with a current co-morbid mood or anxiety disorder, clinicians should consider whether a presenting complaint reflects the co-morbid disorder, a side effect of the treatment, or an exacerbation of the co-morbidity. Moreover, although stimulants can cause these side effects, many ADHD patients experience these problems before treatment; therefore, it is important for clinicians to document these symptoms at baseline.[32] Although tolerance to the effects of stimulants has been debated, data from the NIMH Multimodal Treatment of ADHD study demonstrated the persistence of stimulant-associated medication effects. Strategies to manage common stimulant-related side effects are listed in Table 39-3.

Medication Interactions With Stimulants

The interactions of stimulants with other prescription and OTC medications are generally mild and not a major source of concern.[20] Co-administration of stimulants with MAOIs is the only true contraindication to their use: it may result in a potentially life-threatening hypertensive crisis. Concomitant use of sympathomimetic agents (e.g., pseudoephedrine or caffeine) may potentiate the effects of both substances and exacerbate sleep difficulties. Stimulants are associated with small increases in heart rate and blood pressure

TABLE 39-3 Strategies to Address Stimulant Side Effects[33]

FREQUENCY OF SIDE EFFECT	STIMULANT SIDE EFFECT	SUGGESTED INTERVENTIONS
Common	Decreased appetite	Dose after meals. Encourage frequent snacks. Drug holidays. Decrease dose.
	Behavioral rebound	Try a sustained-release stimulant. Add reduced dose in late afternoon.
	Irritability/dysphoria	Try another stimulant medication. Consider co-existing conditions (e.g., depression) or medications (e.g., antidepressants).
	Sleep problems	Institute a bedtime routine. Reduce or eliminate afternoon dose. Reduce overall dose. Restrict or eliminate caffeine.
	Edginess	Change preparation, change class of stimulant. Consider adding low-dose beta blocker.
	Dry mouth	Proactive dental hygiene, encourage sips of water through the day, use of biotene or equivalent, avoid sugared candies.
Rare	Exacerbation of tics	Observe. Try another stimulant or class of ADHD medications (e.g., alpha-adrenergic drugs).
	Psychosis/euphoria/mania/depression	Stop treatment with stimulants. Refer to mental health specialist.

that are usually insignificant. Although data on the co-administration of stimulants with TCAs suggest little interaction between these compounds,[34] careful monitoring is warranted when prescribing stimulants with either TCAs or anticonvulsants because of potential cardiovascular (CV) and CNS effects. For complex patients or those with co-morbidities, using stimulants in combination with a variety of other psychotropics is common in clinical practice and appears to be well tolerated and effective.

Atomoxetine

A highly selective norepinephrine re-uptake inhibitor, ATMX (Strattera) increases intra-synaptic norepinephrine. ATMX was initially developed as an antidepressant but became FDA-approved as a non-stimulant (hence, not a controlled agent) for the treatment of ADHD.

In the initial trials, ATMX was dosed twice a day (up to 2 mg/kg per day). Later studies demonstrated its efficacy and tolerability when dosed once a day,[35] with its best tolerability occurring when dosed in the evening.[36] ATMX should be initiated at 0.5 mg/kg per day; after several days, it can be increased to 1.2 mg/kg per day. Current guidelines recommend a maximum once-daily dose of 1.4 mg/kg per day. It may take up to 10 weeks to see the full benefits of ATMX treatment (although some patients achieve an early response).[37]

Although generally well-tolerated, the most common side effects in children and adolescents taking ATMX include dyspepsia, dizziness, and reduced appetite. In older adolescents, ATMX may be associated with dry mouth, insomnia, nausea, decreased appetite, constipation, decreased libido, dizziness, and sweating.[38] When patients experience nausea, the dose of ATMX should be divided and administered with food. Sedation is often transient, but it may be helped by either administering the dose at night or dividing the dose. If mood swings occur, patients should be evaluated and their diagnosis reassessed.

The impact of ATMX on the CV system appears to be minimal.[39] ATMX was associated with a mean increase in the heart rate of 6 beats per minute and an increase in both the systolic and diastolic blood pressure of 1.5 mmHg. Extensive ECG monitoring indicates that ATMX has no apparent effect on QTc intervals, and ECG monitoring aside from routine medical care is not indicated.

Based on an FDA public health advisory, the manufacturer added a black box warning regarding the development of suicidal ideation in patients treated with ATMX. As with the SSRIs, there was a slight increase in suicidal thinking in controlled trials of ATMX. Parents should monitor for any such occurrences and for unexpected changes in mood or behavior.

ATMX is metabolized primarily in the liver to 4-hydroxyatomoxetine by the cytochrome CYP P450 2D6 enzyme, and it is primarily excreted in the urine.[40] ATMX does not appear to inhibit 2D6. Although patients identified as poor metabolizers (i.e., having low 2D6 activity) appear to tolerate ATMX, they seem to have more side effects; a reduction in the dose may be necessary. Therefore, in patients who are also on strong 2D6 inhibitors (e.g., fluoxetine, paroxetine, and quinidine), it may be necessary to reduce the dose of ATMX. Use of ATMX is contraindicated with MAOIs.

Alternative (Non-FDA-Approved) Treatments for ADHD

Bupropion Hydrochloride (Wellbutrin, Zyban)

Bupropion hydrochloride (Wellbutrin, Zyban) is a unicyclic aminoketone (unrelated to other antidepressants) that modulates both norepinephrine and dopamine. Bupropion is approved for the treatment of depression and as an aid for smoking cessation in adults, and it has improved ADHD symptoms in children, adolescents,[41] and adults.[42] Although helpful, the magnitude of bupropion's effect is less than that seen with stimulant medicines and more similar to ATMX. Bupropion can be particularly useful in patients with ADHD and co-morbid conditions (e.g., ADHD and nicotine dependence,[43] substance use[44] and mood disorders, substance abuse and conduct disorder, depression,[41] and bipolar disorder [BPD]).[45] In light of the high rates of marijuana use in patients with ADHD, it is important for clinicians to note that adolescents treated with bupropion may experience increased irritability during marijuana withdrawal.[46]

Bupropion appears to be more stimulating than other antidepressants, and it may cause irritability, exacerbate tics, and induce seizures (more often than do other antidepressants). Seizures appear to be dose-related (above 450 mg/day) and are more likely to occur in patients with bulimia or a seizure disorder.

Treatment should be initiated at 37.5 mg per day of the immediate-release (IR, TID dosing), 100 mg sustained-release (SR, BID dosing), or 150 mg extended-release (XL, once-daily dosing) and titrated gradually as indicated. Although dosage guidelines are not available for children, in one study, doses of 3 to 6 mg/kg per day were given. As in adults, no single dose of the IR preparation should exceed 150 mg, SR 200 mg, or XL 450 mg.

Tricyclic Antidepressants

Although controlled trials in ADHD youth[47] and adults demonstrate the efficacy of TCAs, their effects are less robust than are those of stimulants. On the other hand, possible advantages of TCAs over stimulants include once-daily dosing, the option of monitoring plasma drug levels, and a negligible abuse liability. TCAs may be particularly useful in patients with co-morbid anxiety; ODD;[48] tics;[49] and, theoretically, depression (in adults). However, given concerns about potential cardiotoxicity and the availability of ATMX, use of the TCAs has been significantly curtailed. Desipramine (DMI) and nortriptyline are associated with lower risks of adverse effects (e.g., sedation, dry mouth, and impairment in cognition) than imipramine and other tertiary amine TCAs and therefore may be better tolerated.

α-Adrenergic Agonists

Clonidine

Clonidine is an imidazoline derivative with α-adrenergic agonist properties; it has been primarily used in the treatment of hypertension. At low doses, it appears to stimulate inhibitory, pre-synaptic adrenergic autoreceptors in the CNS.[50] Clonidine has achieved an increasing prominence in pediatric psychopharmacology because of its wide range of uses and relative safety. Although clonidine ameliorates symptoms of ADHD, its overall effect is less than the stimulants[51] and likely smaller than ATMX, TCAs, and bupropion. Clonidine appears particularly helpful in patients with ADHD and co-morbid conduct disorder or ODD, tic disorders, and ADHD-associated sleep disturbances. In addition, clonidine has been increasingly reported to be useful in developmentally disordered patients to control aggression toward self and others.[52]

Clonidine is a relatively short-acting compound with a plasma half-life ranging from approximately 5.5 hours (in children) to 8.5 hours (in adults). Usual dose ranges from 3 to 10 μg/kg per day given generally in divided doses, once, twice, three, or four times per day. A longer-acting preparation (Kapvay) or transdermal therapeutic system (clonidine TTS) may simplify clonidine dosing. Therapy is usually initiated at the lowest manufactured dose of half (0.05 mg) of a 0.1-mg tablet, depending on the size of the child (approx. 1 to 2 μg/kg per day) and increased depending on the clinical response and adverse effects. The initial dosage can more easily be given before bedtime because nocturnal sedation will not adversely affect daytime function.

The most common short-term adverse effect of clonidine is sedation, which tends to subside with continued treatment. It can also produce hypotension, dry mouth, vivid dreams, depression, and confusion. Except in overdose, clonidine is not known to be associated with long-term serious adverse effects. Because abrupt withdrawal of clonidine has been associated with rebound hypertension, slow tapering is advised. In addition, extreme caution should be exercised with the co-administration of clonidine with β-blockers or calcium channel-blockers because adverse reactions, including complete heart block, have been reported.[53] After reports of several sudden deaths related to clonidine use, concerns about the safety of co-administration of clonidine with stimulants were raised.[54] However, these cases were thoroughly examined, and no causative link between use of the combination and sudden death was found. Accumulating evidence suggests that combining clonidine with stimulants may be a successful strategy in reducing ADHD in children and adolescents who experience a partial response to stimulants alone.[55] Current guidelines are to monitor blood pressure when initiating and tapering clonidine, but ECG monitoring is not usually necessary.

Guanfacine (Tenex)

The clonidine-like but more selective, α_2-adrenergic agonist compound, guanfacine (Tenex, Intuniv), has been used as an alternative to clonidine for the same indications.[56,57] Possible advantages of guanfacine over clonidine include less sedation and a longer duration of action. When compared with clonidine, guanfacine may be more useful in improving the cognitive (inattention) symptoms of ADHD (and less effective in reducing the behavioral symptoms of impulsivity, aggressiveness, and hyperactivity). Trials of children with ADHD and co-morbid tic disorder treated with guanfacine (in doses ranging from 0.5 mg twice per day to 1 mg three times per day) showed reduction in both tics and ADHD. Controlled data also demonstrated the benefit of guanfacine in reducing tic severity and ADHD symptomology.[58]

Guanfacine treatment is associated with minor, clinically insignificant decreases in blood pressure and pulse rate. The adverse effects of guanfacine include sedation, irritability, and depression. Several cases of apparent guanfacine-induced mania have been reported, but the impact of guanfacine on mood disorders remains unclear. The guanfacine extended-release formulation (Intuniv) at doses of 2, 3, and 4 mg per day shows greater efficacy than placebo and favorable tolerability in children 6 to 17 years of age with ADHD.[56]

Novel Treatments for ADHD

Modafinil/Armodafinil

Modafinil and its stereo-isomer, armodafinil, are novel stimulants that are distinct from amphetamine. They are approved for the treatment of narcolepsy, shift-work sleep disorder, and obstructive sleep apnea with residual excessive sleepiness. Unlike the broad brain area activation observed with amphetamine, modafinil/armodafinil appears to activate specific hypothalamic regions.[57] Although initial trials in adults were negative, in controlled pediatric trials, modafinil demonstrated efficacy in the treatment of ADHD.[59,60] Nonetheless, the FDA voted that modafinil is "not approvable" for pediatric ADHD owing to possible Stevens–Johnson syndrome in pediatric patients. Therefore, use of modafinil or armodafinil should include patient/guardian education about the risk of developing a serious and potential life-threatening dermatologic reaction. It may be reasonable to consider combining modafinil with stimulants,[61] but clinicians should be aware of the potential to exacerbate mania.[62]

MOOD DISORDERS

Depression

Children and adolescents may develop a variety of depressive disorders (including major depressive disorder [MDD]; persistent depressive disorder or mood disturbances that are primary or associated with medical conditions; substance use or abuse; and as a result of psychosocial problems). In the medical setting, clinicians are challenged to differentiate transient symptoms of depression from true depressive disorders. Children often manifest worry, hopelessness, and sadness as primary symptoms related to their own illness, whereas adolescents typically display anxiety, anger, or withdrawal. If the symptoms are episodic and associated with limited impairment, they are generally considered an adjustment disorder with depressed or anxious mood. These patients usually respond to reassurance, environmental intervention, or interpersonal or cognitive-behavioral therapy (CBT). In the outpatient medical setting, children and adolescents with depression may present for evaluation for medical symptoms of unclear etiology. During routine examination these patients may appear sad, withdrawn, apathetic, anxious, angry, or irritable. Although many families seek care from PCPs for depression, most family physicians and pediatricians believe they are inadequately trained to screen for, evaluate, and manage pediatric depression.[63]

Severe presentations of depression (i.e., MDD) are a common mental health problem in adolescents worldwide, with an estimated 1-year prevalence of 4% to 5% in mid- to late-adolescence.[64,65] The prevalence of MDD increases with advancing age. Epidemiologic studies from community and clinical samples estimate that the prevalence of MDD is approximately 0.3% in pre-schoolers, 2% in children, and between 1.5% and 9% in adolescents. By the end of adolescence, the cumulative incidence of MDD is estimated at 20%.[66] Although the gender ratio appears equal in children with MDD, by the age of 14, girls appear twice as likely to experience depression as boys.[67] However, additional data suggest that boys and girls who develop depression during prepubescence experience similar symptoms, rates of recovery, relapse, and co-morbidity.[68] Depressive disorders in older children and adolescents commonly co-occur with anxiety, ADHD, and conduct and substance use disorders.[69] The challenge to the clinician is to recognize the developmental progression of co-morbidity. Children initially may be evaluated and treated for ADHD, only to develop depression several years later during their treatment for ADHD.

Suicidal ideation, threats, and behaviors are commonly seen among children and adolescents with psychiatric disorders. These behaviors are of great concern to clinicians who need to ensure the safety of patients within the medical setting and identify patients at increased risk for self-injurious behaviors. Depression in adolescents is a major risk factor for suicide, the second-to-third leading cause of death in this age group,[8] with more than half of adolescent suicide victims reported to have a depressive disorder at the time of their death.[70]

Pharmacotherapy of Depression

Unfortunately, the pharmacotherapy of youth with depression is less straightforward than it is with adults. Unlike in adults, TCAs are not an effective treatment for adolescents with depression. Fluoxetine, a selective serotonin re-uptake inhibitor (SSRI), seems effective in meta-analyses,[71] and randomized, controlled trials (RCTs).[72–74] Escitalopram, another SSRI, is FDA-approved for the treatment of adolescent depression, though evidence is inconsistent for other antidepressants. Even in the best circumstances, antidepressants are only moderately effective in adolescents with depression.[72]

Update on Antidepressant-Associated Suicidality

Against this backdrop, the FDA warning of potentially increased suicidal thinking and behavior in children and adolescents taking an SSRI has added complexity to an already challenging treatment situation. Clinicians who recommend or prescribe antidepressants to pediatric populations must be aware of this important clinical issue.

In 2004, the FDA issued a black box warning describing the probable risk of increased suicidality in children and adolescents and suggested close monitoring for side effects and response in youth. The following year, antidepressant manufacturers were required to include a black box warning on antidepressant product labels.[75] Then, in 2007, the FDA updated the warning on antidepressants to include young adults (aged 18 to 24) during initial antidepressant treatment.

The FDA's black box labeling of antidepressant medications for the pediatric population has had far-reaching consequences. In the United States, prior to 2005, the rate of diagnosed new episodes of pediatric depression increased consistently between 1999 and 2004. In 2005, however, the rate decreased sharply and returned to 1999 rates.[76–78] Strikingly, as depression diagnoses decreased, overall estimates of depressive symptomatology actually increased, suggesting clinician resistance to providing a new depression diagnosis to clinically depressed youth.[79] Some authors[80] reported a 47% reduction in the use of antidepressants in the United States from 2002 to 2006 among patients aged 5 to 21 years, who had not previously been exposed to antidepressants. Interestingly, antidepressant rates remained the same in this age group for those who had been previously exposed to treatment.[80]

Perhaps the most notable change in prescribing practice was noted in non-psychiatrists. Among providers, 3.9% of family medicine practitioners, and 11.5% of pediatricians, but only 0.8% of psychiatrists, reported that they no longer treated young patients with antidepressants.[80] Researchers[81] found a decrease in the use of all SSRIs in the pediatric population after the FDA issued its 2004 advisory; others[82] showed that fluoxetine prescriptions increased for those newly prescribed an antidepressant following the regulatory action. Moreover, after the FDA's warnings, prescribing clinicians reported that 14% to 22% of guardians and 9% of pediatric patients refused treatment with antidepressants.[81,83] The FDA recommended that patients meet with a physician weekly for the first 4 weeks of medication initiation, bi-weekly for a month, and after 12 weeks of treatment.[84] Despite this recommendation, a study showed that the frequency of follow-up appointments showed little to no change following the FDA's guidelines.[85]

The most serious and unintended effect of FDA advisories may have been on pediatric suicides. Gibbons and coworkers[86] provided a comparative study of suicide prevalence rates in the pediatric populations in the United States and the Netherlands, pre- and post-regulatory agency warnings. This study showed that, after 2003, antidepressant prescription rates in the United States decreased for all groups under age 60. The magnitude of the decrease in prescription rates was inversely proportional to age; the decrease in the two youngest age groups (up to age 14) was approximately 20% and 30% overall for new prescriptions.[87] The decrease in SSRI prescription rates in youth occurred at a time when the suicide rate *increased* by 14% from 2003 to 2004 among children and adolescents.[87]

Suicidal risk in relation to antidepressant use remains controversial.[87,88] Several studies, including a meta-analysis, suggest a significant association with such risk,[88] especially in young people. Individuals younger than 25 years of age treated with antidepressants are more likely than older adults to develop thoughts about suicide. However, a large meta-analysis[89] showed that the benefits of such treatments still outweighed the risks (numbers needed-to-treat 10, vs numbers needed-to-harm 143). It remains unknown whether the suicidality risk attributable to antidepressants extends to longer-term use (i.e., beyond several months). However, there is substantial evidence from placebo-controlled maintenance trials in adults with depression that the use of antidepressants can delay the recurrence of depression.

With the mixed evidence and because untreated depression in adolescents is itself so strongly associated with the risk of suicide, suicidal risk should be monitored in this clinical group, irrespective of treatment choice. In the current environment, it is prudent to inform patients and parents of this risk and urge close observation for clinical worsening, suicidality, and unusual changes in behavior, especially during the initial 1 to 2 months of a course of drug therapy or whenever the dose is changed.

Pharmacokinetics of Antidepressants in Children and Adolescents

Although the main pharmacodynamic effects of SSRIs are similar, the SSRIs are structurally dissimilar to one another and vary in their pharmacokinetics and drug interactions. The SSRIs inhibit specific hepatic isoenzymes and thereby increase the serum levels of other compounds. In the medical setting, treatment with antidepressants may produce clinically significant medication interactions. Parents and clinicians should be aware that SSRIs may interact with antibiotics, for example, especially macrolide derivatives currently used for pediatric patients. Clinicians need access to updated databases on medication interactions and current references.

Fluoxetine is a racemic mixture that is metabolized to its active metabolite, norfluoxetine. Both fluoxetine and norfluoxetine are substrates of CYP2C9, 2C19, 3A4, and 2D6. Both fluoxetine and norfluoxetine are potent inhibitors of 2D6 and therefore may increase the levels of medications that are metabolized through 2D6 (e.g., certain antidepressants, antipsychotics, analgesics, calcium channel blockers, β-blockers, dextromethorphan, and ATMX). In the pediatric population, mean steady states of fluoxetine and norfluoxetine occur, on average, within 4 weeks, although high between-patient variability was observed. Furthermore, on average, children accumulated higher amounts of fluoxetine (two-fold) and norfluoxetine (1.7-fold) compared with adolescents. Accumulation of fluoxetine and norfluoxetine in adolescents was similar to the profile for adult patients. The clinical implications of this finding are that most children should be started on fluoxetine 10 mg/day.

Sertraline, which is produced as the S-enantiomer and metabolized to its active metabolite desmethylsertraline, is a substrate of 2B6, 2C9, 2C19, 2D6, and 3A4. Both sertraline and desmethylsertraline are modest inhibitors of 2C9, 2C19, and 3A4. Case reports have shown that sertraline increases the concentration of phenytoin, pimozide, warfarin, cyclosporine, and diazepam. Sertraline is known to inhibit glucuronidation, and it has been reported to cause toxic levels of lamotrigine. Levels of sertraline may be reduced by adjunctive analgesic agents, such as carbamazepine and phenytoin.[89] In one study, the mean steady-state half-life of sertraline 50 mg per day was significantly shorter than the single-dose half-life (15.3 ± 3.5 hours vs 26.7 ± 5.2 hours; $p<0.001$) and the mean steady-state half-life of 100 to 150 mg/day of sertraline (20.4 ± 3.4 hours).[90] Therefore, adolescents may need doses greater than 50 mg/day to achieve a therapeutic response for depression. Similarly, treatment with sertraline 200 mg/day, the T_{max} (14.6 ± 16.1 vs 10.8 ± 8 hours) and half-lives of sertraline (26.2 ± 8.4 vs 27.1 ± 8.2 hours) and its main metabolite desmethylsertraline (78.5 ± 50.6 vs 75.4 ± 37.1 hours) were similar in children and adolescents, respectively. Overall results suggest linear pharmacokinetics of sertraline in pediatric patients across the dose range of 50 to 200 mg/day, and the authors concluded that sertraline can be safely used within the adult dosage schedule.

Citalopram (CIT), a racemic mixture of R- and S-citalopram (S-CIT), is demethylated via 2C19, 2D6, and 3A4. It is a mild inhibitor of 2D6, but in general it has few medication interactions. Reis and co-workers,[91] using data from two trials, studied the pharmacokinetics of CIT in 44 patients younger than 21 years of age who were treated naturalistically with a mean dose of CIT 30 mg/day. As in adults, large inter-individual variability in levels of serum CIT and its main metabolite desmethylcitalopram (DCIT) and didesmethylcitalopram (DDCIT) were observed in these adolescents. The mean serum half-life of CIT was 36 hours. These authors found that the pharmacokinetics of CIT was influenced by gender, smoking status, the menstrual period, and treatment with oral contraceptives. The active enantiomer S-CIT is available as Lexapro. As with CIT, it has few medication interactions.

Though the role of fluvoxamine and paroxetine in treatment of child and adolescent depression is presently limited, it should be noted that fluvoxamine is a substrate of 2D6 and 1A2, has no significant metabolites, and is described as a pan-inhibitor because it is a potent inhibitor of 2B6, 2C9, and 3A4 and a mild inhibitor of 2D6. When adding any medication to fluvoxamine, clinicians should be cautious. Paroxetine is an S-enantiomer that is a substrate of 2D6 and, to a lesser degree, 3A4. Paroxetine has no significant metabolites, is a potent inhibitor of 2B6 and 2D6, and is a mild inhibitor of 1A2, 2C9, 2C19, and 3A4. Co-administration of paroxetine with substrates of 2D6 (e.g., antidepressants, antipsychotics, analgesics, calcium channel blockers, β-blockers, antiarrhythmics), or 2B6 (e.g., bupropion, nicotine, sertraline, diazepam, tamoxifen) is likely to increase levels of the substrate.[89]

The profiles of the pK for novel antidepressants have been reported as well. Bupropion is mainly metabolized by 2B6 to its main metabolite hydroxybupropion. Bupropion acts as a modest inhibitor of 2D6. Although smoking does not affect the pK profile, co-administration with paroxetine, sertraline, or other 2B6 inhibitors may cause interactions.

Clinical Use of SSRIs

Selection of an SSRI should take into consideration tolerability (e.g., side-effect profile), anticipated medication interactions, half-life (e.g., potential for bipolar switching), and adherence. SSRIs should be initiated at low doses (e.g., 5 to 10 mg fluoxetine; 12.5 to 25 mg sertraline; 5 to 10 mg citalopram; 2.5 to 5 mg escitalopram; 5 to 10 mg paroxetine; 12.5 to 25 mg fluvoxamine; and 18.75 to 37.5 mg venlafaxine) and titrated upward slowly.[92] As with fluoxetine, sertraline, paroxetine, and citalopram, escitalopram is now available as an elixir. Once an antidepressant response is obtained, patients and their families often benefit from encouraging adherence to prevent relapse; however, the ideal length of treatment in pediatric patients requires further study. After treatment is completed (typically 6 to 12 months after remission), the SSRIs should be tapered slowly, to prevent both a discontinuation syndrome and recurrence of symptoms. Patients and their families need education regarding the monitoring of future depressive episodes. However, only 60% of adolescents with depression will show an adequate clinical response to an initial treatment trial with an SSRI.

Side Effects and Complications

In general, SSRIs are well-tolerated and have fewer side effects than TCAs, especially when taken in overdose. Common adverse effects of SSRIs include manic activation, agitation, gastrointestinal symptoms, irritability, insomnia, sexual dysfunction, and weight loss. Whereas paroxetine, fluoxetine, citalopram, and sertraline may be associated with agitation and increased energy, fluvoxamine appears to generate sedation and is useful in children with sleep difficulties associated with mood symptoms. Given the lack of CV effects of SSRIs, monitoring of vital signs and the ECG does not appear necessary unless there is an additional medical concern.[93,94] Similarly, no specific blood monitoring appears necessary in children receiving SSRIs.

Activation, which is distinguished from a change in mood or impulse control, may be related to either akathisia, hyperactivity, or disinhibition; it usually responds to lowering of the dose. Signs of mania (which may include impulse dyscontrol, mood swings, grandiosity, hypersexuality, and aggression) may be observed and accompany bipolar switching. Treatment of mania relies on pharmacologic approaches. Celebration may occur in SSRI-treated anxious children who experience relief of their anxiety; they may seem impulsive or uninhibited. Adolescents prescribed SSRIs may also experience sexual side effects, although reports of these side effects are minimal in controlled studies in this population.

As in adults, children may experience a discontinuation syndrome as they are tapered off SSRIs or if they miss scheduled doses. Typically, this syndrome occurs among those taking SSRIs with shorter half-lives (e.g., paroxetine or venlafaxine), although it can occur with any antidepressant. As in adults, the discontinuation syndrome is typically characterized by physical symptoms (e.g., nausea, gastrointestinal disturbance, diarrhea, dizziness, insomnia, lightheadedness, headache, shakiness, and sensations of a mild electrical shock), cognitive symptoms (e.g., confusion, poor memory, cloudiness, and forgetfulness), and emotional symptoms (e.g., increased crying, mood lability, and anxiety).[95] Patients and parents should be educated about the discontinuation syndrome, and steps should be taken to prevent its occurrence (including the use of SSRIs when necessary, encouraging adherence, tapering SSRIs gradually, and ensuring that the manufacturer of the medication stays the same throughout treatment if a patient is taking a generic preparation). When patients experience a discontinuation syndrome, re-introducing the medication usually provides relief, although some patients may need to be switched to an SSRI with a longer half-life.

Bipolar Disorder

Pediatric bipolar disorder (BPD) is a relatively recent phenomenon in the modern child psychiatry landscape. Moreover, many children and adolescents with BPD seek medical attention in Emergency Departments (EDs) or develop severe symptoms (e.g., unremitting temper tantrums) during medical hospitalizations. Pre-pubertal mania is usually co morbid with ADHD, and these patients typically present with extreme hyperactivity, impulsivity, and aggression.[96,97] Children with BPD commonly present with extreme irritability or an explosive mood associated with poor psychosocial function. These children often over-react to minor environmental stressors (mood reactivity). Additional symptoms consistent with mania include grandiosity, unmodulated high energy, decreased need for sleep, over-talkativeness, increased goal-directed and pleasurable activity (e.g., social, work, school, and sexual), and poor judgment (e.g., seeking out reckless activities). Although the juvenile symptom complex of mania should be differentiated from ADHD, conduct disorder, depression, trauma, substance use and abuse, and psychotic disorders, these disorders commonly co-occur with childhood mania.[98]

Pharmacotherapy

Until recently, lithium was the only FDA-approved drug for the treatment of BPD in children 12 years of age and older. In 2007, the FDA approved the use of risperidone (Risperdal) for acute treatment of manic or mixed episodes of bipolar I disorder in children 10 to 17 years of age. In 2008, the FDA approved aripiprazole (Abilify) for acute treatment of manic or mixed episodes associated with BPD (type I) in pediatric patients between the ages of 10 and 17. In 2009, the FDA approved olanzapine (Zyprexa) for acute treatment of manic or mixed episodes associated with bipolar I disorder in adolescents aged 13 to 17 years of age, and then quetiapine (Seroquel) for treatment of manic or mixed episodes of BPD in patients aged 10 to 17 years old. In 2015, the FDA approved asenapine (Saphris) for acute management of manic or mixed episodes of BPD in children between 10 and 17 years old.

Unfortunately, early-onset BPD appears less responsive to lithium.[99] Therefore, children and adolescents with BPD are often treated with combinations of lithium, anticonvulsants, and atypical antipsychotic mood stabilizers.[100] If the patient does not respond to an adequate trial (in dose and time) of a single agent or cannot tolerate the medication, subsequent trials with alternative medication(s) are recommended. In manic or mixed presentations, with psychotic symptoms, additional antipsychotic treatment is recommended. In BPD with prominent symptoms of depression, combined treatment with a mood stabilizer and an antidepressant is indicated. Clinicians must be wary of the potential destabilizing effects of SSRIs in the treatment of bipolar depression in children and adolescents. Recent data indicate that the management of BPD with or without co-morbid disorders (depression and ADHD) may require treatment that combines several therapeutic agents.

Lithium

The use of lithium carbonate in BPD and treatment-resistant unipolar depression appears helpful; surprisingly, it has not been studied under controlled conditions. The usual starting dose of lithium ranges from 150 to 300 mg/day in divided doses, two or three times per day. Weller and co-workers[101] published dosage guidelines for lithium in children 6 to 12 years of age, suggesting the initial total daily doses (administered three times per day) of 600 mg/day for patients weighing <25 kg; 900 mg/day for patients weighing 25 to 40 kg; 1200 mg/day for patients weighing 40 to 50 kg; and

1500 mg/day for patients weighing 50 to 60 kg. Unfortunately, there is no known therapeutic serum lithium level in children. Based on the adult literature, serum levels of 0.8 to 1.5 mEq/L for acute episodes and levels of 0.4 to 0.8 mEq/L for maintenance therapy are suggested.

Common short-term adverse effects of lithium include gastrointestinal symptoms (e.g., nausea, vomiting), renal symptoms (e.g., polyuria, polydipsia), and CNS symptoms (e.g., tremor, sleepiness, memory impairment). Short-term adverse effects associated with the use of lithium are generally dose-related. The incidence of toxicity increases directly with increased serum levels, and symptoms respond favorably to dose reduction. The chronic administration of lithium may be associated with metabolic (e.g., substantial weight gain and decreased calcium metabolism), endocrine (e.g., decreased thyroid functioning), dermatologic (e.g., acne), cardiac, and renal dysfunction. Thus, it is necessary for children to be screened for renal function (e.g., blood urea nitrogen, creatinine), thyroid function (e.g., thyroid-stimulating hormone), ECG, and calcium level before lithium treatment is started and that these tests be repeated every 6 months. Female patients should undergo a pregnancy test and be educated about the dangers of lithium exposure during pregnancy. Particular caution should be exercised when lithium is used in patients with neurologic, renal, or CV disorders.

Carbamazepine

Carbamazepine, approved for treatment of pediatric seizures (e.g., psychomotor, grand mal) and trigeminal neuralgia, is structurally related to the TCAs. Carbamazepine is not FDA-approved for the treatment of pediatric mania; however, anecdotal reports and some studies support its consideration.[102,103]

Carbamazepine induces its own metabolism, which is usually complete after 3 to 5 weeks on the medication. Carbamazepine has many medication interactions (see Table 38-5), induces the metabolism of substrates of 3A4 (e.g., haloperidol, phenytoin), and may reduce levels of valproic acid and increase lithium levels by reducing lithium clearance. Inhibitors of 3A4 (e.g., erythromycin) may increase levels of carbamazepine. The plasma half-life after chronic administration is between 13 and 17 hours. The therapeutic plasma concentration is variably reported as 4 to 12 μg/mL, and recommended daily doses in children range from 10 to 20 mg/kg, administered twice per day. Because the relationship between the dose and the plasma level is variable and uncertain with marked inter-individual variability, plasma level monitoring is recommended. Common short-term side effects include dizziness, drowsiness, nausea, vomiting, and blurred vision. Idiosyncratic reactions (e.g., bone marrow suppression, liver toxicity, and skin disorders, including Stevens–Johnson syndrome), have been reported but are rare. However, given the seriousness of these reactions, careful monitoring of blood counts and liver and renal function is warranted initially and during treatment.

Oxcarbazepine

Oxcarbazepine (Trileptal) appears to have fewer reports of medication interactions and adverse effects (e.g., less effect on bone marrow and skin). However, minimal data are currently available regarding its efficacy in pediatric BPD. Clinicians who prescribe it should monitor for hyponatremia and be aware that it can induce the metabolism of ethinyl estradiol.

Valproic Acid

Valproic acid (VPA) is an FDA-approved anticonvulsant for the acute and maintenance treatment of BPD in adults; by extension, it may be useful in the treatment of juvenile BPD. However, the evidence for VPA in childhood BPD has been mixed at best.

VPA is primarily metabolized by the liver; it has a plasma half-life of 8 to 16 hours and a therapeutic plasma concentration of 50 to 100 μg/ml. Recommended initial daily doses are 15 mg/kg per day that are gradually increased to a maximum of 60 mg/kg per day, administered three times a day. Common short-term side effects include sedation, thinning of hair, anorexia, nausea, and vomiting. Idiosyncratic reactions (e.g., bone marrow suppression and liver toxicity) have been reported but appear to be rare. Asymptomatic elevations of serum glutamic oxaloacetic transaminase usually resolve spontaneously. Although fatalities resulting from hepatic dysfunction have been reported in children younger than 10 years of age with monotherapy, these have occurred primarily in children younger than 2. The risk of serious hepatic involvement is increased by concomitant use of other anti-seizure medications and may be dose-related. Careful monitoring of blood counts and liver and renal function are warranted initially and during treatment. Hyperammonemia has been reported, and depending on clinical impression, monitoring ammonia levels may be appropriate.

Atypical Antipsychotics

The atypical antipsychotic medications (especially clozapine [Clozaril], olanzapine [Zyprexa], quetiapine [Seroquel], risperidone [Risperdal], ziprasidone [Geodon], and aripiprazole [Abilify]) are a principal strategy in the pharmacologic management of pediatric BPD. These medications differ from "typical" antipsychotics (e.g., chlorpromazine, haloperidol) in their receptor profile (D_2 blockade and the fact that they affect multiple other receptors, including serotonin), reduced likelihood of causing EPS, reduced likelihood of causing hyperprolactinemia (the exception is risperidone), and a greater benefit on the negative symptoms of psychosis and on cognition. Whenever these medications are used, patients and families should be informed about the potential for side effects, including EPS, akathisia, neuroleptic malignant syndrome, tardive dyskinesia (TD), and dystonias. Although the risk of developing TD is lower with the atypical medications, the rate of occurrence is unknown. Patients treated with antipsychotic medications should be monitored regularly with the Abnormal Involuntary Movement Scale (AIMS) examination.

Risperidone

Risperidone is FDA-approved for the treatment of pediatric mania. Risperidone is usually started at 0.25 mg once or twice per day and titrated up to 3 to 4 mg/day in most pediatric patients, although it appears to retain its atypical properties in doses up to 6 mg/day. Its common adverse effects include weight gain, sedation, drooling, and elevation of prolactin levels. Although EPS is not common, clinicians should be aware of this possibility and recognize it when it occurs. As for adults, children and adolescents with EPS can be treated with oral or IM diphenhydramine or benztropine. Although pK studies in children are lacking, data in adults indicate that risperidone reaches peak concentrations within 1 hour, is metabolized through CYP 2D6, and has a half-life of 3 hours in extensive metabolizers and 17 hours in poor metabolizers.[104] There are case reports of hepatotoxicity, tachycardia, prolongation of the QTc interval, and stroke (in elderly patients).

Aripiprazole

Aripiprazole (Abilify) was FDA-approved for manic and mixed states in pediatric BPD I in 2008. Aripiprazole appears to have mixed agonist–antagonist properties and is described as a "dopamine/serotonin stabilizer." It has a long half-life and does not appear to cause significant interactions with other medications that are metabolized through the P450 system. It can cause akathisia. It is usually started at 2.5 to 5 mg/day and is titrated to 10 to 15 mg/day (up to 30 mg/day in adult trials).

Olanzapine

Olanzapine is currently FDA-approved for acute treatment of BPD in adolescents aged 13 to 17 years old. In adults on atypical antipsychotics, hyperglycemia, new-onset diabetes, and diabetic ketoacidosis (50% occurred in those without weight gain) have been observed during treatment.[105,106] Olanzapine is available in injectable, tablet, and oral disintegrating tablet (Zydis) forms. Olanzapine is typically initiated at 2.5 to 5 mg and can be titrated up to 20 mg. Olanzapine is metabolized by way of glucuronidation (primary) and oxidation via CYP1A2.[89]

Quetiapine

Quetiapine has been FDA-approved for use of acute treatment of manic or mixed episodes of bipolar disorder in pediatric patients aged 10 to 17. Quetiapine is typically started at 25 mg twice daily, with a target dose of 400 to 600 mg/day. The pK of quetiapine has not been formally studied in children and adolescents. Data from adult studies indicate that quetiapine is readily absorbed from the GI tract and reaches peak concentrations 1.5 hours after ingestion. It is metabolized primarily in the liver by CYP 3A4 and does not appear to be affected by gender, smoking, or race. Occurrence of EPS appears low, but quetiapine can cause dizziness, sedation, and weight gain.

Ziprasidone

The atypical antipsychotic ziprasidone (Geodon) may also be used in the treatment of pediatric BPD, though the FDA has not granted approval. Ziprasidone may increase QTc intervals; thus, before using it a baseline ECG and family history of cardiac problems (especially early-onset arrhythmia) should be obtained. Although ziprasidone is primarily metabolized through aldehyde oxidase, it is also metabolized in part via CYP3A4. Co-administration of ziprasidone with medications that may also lengthen the QTc interval (e.g., thioridazine, pimozide, droperidol, class IA and III antiarrhythmics) is not recommended. In children and adolescents, ziprasidone is started at 10 to 20 mg/day or twice per day and can be increased upward to 40 to 60 mg twice per day.

Asenapine

Asenapine (Saphris) is an atypical antipsychotic currently approved for treatment of manic or mixed episodes of BPD in pediatric patients aged 10 to 17 years. Asenapine has an unusual pharmacologic profile, in that it antagonizes a combination of dopamine, serotonin, norepinephrine, and histamine receptors.[107] Asenapine is available in a cherry-flavored sublingual formula that requires the patient refrain from eating or drinking within 10 minutes of administration. Recommended dosing for asenapine begins at 2.5 mg twice daily and can be increased up to 10 mg twice daily. Sedation is the most common side effect in youth, though weight gain, dysgeusia, oral parasthesia, and dizziness have also been reported.

Alternative Anticonvulsants

Gabapentin (Neurontin) is approved as an adjunct therapy for seizures. It is not significantly metabolized in humans and has few medication interactions.[108] Trials with gabapentin for BPD in adults have been negative; however, it has reduced anxiety.

Lamotrigine (Lamictal) is an anticonvulsant approved in the maintenance treatment of BPD type I in adults. Lamotrigine's labeling contains a boxed warning that serious rashes, including Stevens–Johnson syndrome, occur in approximately 1% of patients younger than 16 years of age. The risk for rash seems to increase if lamotrigine is increased too quickly, the initial dose is greater than recommended, or it is administered with VPA.

Topiramate (Topamax) is an anti-epileptic that has shown variable utility in treatment of BPD in adults. Topiramate has a half-life of approximately 24 hours, is excreted unchanged in the urine, and inhibits carbonic anhydrase as well as CYP2C19.

DEVELOPMENTAL DISORDERS

The term *developmental disorders* includes intellectual disability, autism spectrum disorders, and specific developmental disorders previously called *learning disabilities* (e.g., non-verbal learning disability). The term intellectual disability has replaced the term mental retardation in DSM-5; severity levels are now classified by adaptive functioning rather than by IQ, and the IQ criteria based on approximate rather than absolute cutoffs (e.g., 65 to 75 rather than 70). At any given time, approximately 1% to 3% of the population meet the diagnostic criteria for intellectual disability.[109] Autism spectrum disorder symptoms develop prior to the age of three and typically involve unusually restricted behaviors with impaired development of social skills (e.g., reciprocal interactions), communication skills (e.g., idiosyncratic language), and sensory–motor skills (e.g., hyporeactivity and hyper-reactivity to sensory stimulation). Individuals with developmental disorders are at an increased risk of seizure disorders, hearing loss, and other medical co-morbidities.

Intellectual Disability

In general, the treatment of specific developmental disorders is largely remedial and supportive. Although psychotropics can temporarily control behavioral and psychiatric complications in some children with developmental disorders, they have not been shown to affect the cardinal symptoms and the basic course of the underlying disorders.

If the child with a developmental disorder also meets diagnostic criteria for ADHD or a mood disorder, the guidelines described for the treatment of these disorders are applicable. For example, stimulants appear generally well tolerated and effective in reducing symptoms of hyperactivity and impulsivity in patients with intellectual disability.[110]

Autism Spectrum Disorders

Children with autism spectrum disorders often have aggressive, hyperactive, repetitive, and self-injurious behaviors that may respond to pharmacologic treatment. Risperidone and aripiprazole are FDA-approved for the symptomatic treatment of irritability (including aggression, deliberate self-injury, and temper tantrums) in children and adolescents with autism. Several RCTs with these two agents have demonstrated moderate and clinically significant benefits in behavioral control, including disruptive and repetitive behaviors, hyperactivity, and self-injury.[111–113] Social and language impairments were only slightly modified by treatment, although results differed among studies. Moreover, open trials with a variety of atypical antipsychotics, including olanzapine[114] and ziprasidone[115] have similarly shown promise in modulating maladaptive behaviors in patients with developmental delay.

A number of alternative pharmacologic agents, in addition to antipsychotics, may be employed for complications or co-morbidities of developmental disorders. Considering the relatively low toxicologic profile of these drugs compared with the antipsychotics, they are the preferred treatment for the management of these children. β-Blockers (e.g., propranolol) may improve self-regulation in patients with developmental disorders and thus reduce agitation, aggression, and self-abusive behaviors.[116] Propranolol is usually given in divided doses throughout the day. Treatment is typically initiated at 10 mg twice per day and increased as clinically indicated to a dose range of 2 to 8 mg/kg per day. Short-term adverse effects of β-blockers are usually not serious and generally abate when the drug is decreased or stopped. Nausea, vomiting, constipation, and mild diarrhea have been reported. Psychiatric side effects appear to be relatively infrequent but can occur; symptoms include vivid dreams, depression, and hallucinations. Because abrupt cessation of this drug may be associated with rebound hypertension, a gradual taper is recommended. In a similar manner, clonidine,[117] lofexidine,[118] and buspirone[119] have been used to diminish aggression in patients with developmental disorders.

For children with prominent obsessive behavior, rigidity, or compulsive rituals, SSRIs may be helpful. In many cases, the full antidepressant dosage (discussed later) is necessary; however, children should be started with the lowest possible dose to prevent adverse effects, such as disinhibition or agitation. Controlled trials in adults treated with fluoxetine[120] and fluvoxamine[121] have shown positive results. However, studies in children have been less robust. Benzodiazepine use in youth with autism spectrum disorders is commonly associated with the adverse effect of disinhibition, and may result in restlessness and more disturbed behavior.

Several RCTs have supported the appropriateness of stimulant use in children with autism spectrum disorders. A preponderance of the evidence suggests that symptoms of ADHD are common in those with autism spectrum disorders and that MPH is an empirically supported treatment to target ADHD symptoms in PDD. However, tolerability remains a problem, and caregivers should be cautioned to be watchful for potential adverse effects. With the increasing recognition of autism spectrum disorders in young children, further studies are needed to clarify the roles of AMPH and non-stimulant medications in the treatment of ADHD symptoms in children with PDD.

PSYCHOTIC DISORDERS

The term *psychosis* is generally used to describe the abnormal behaviors of children with grossly impaired reality testing. The diagnosis of psychosis requires the presence of either delusions (false implausible beliefs) or hallucinations (false perceptions that may be visual, auditory, or tactile). Often, psychosis in children is seen with MDD, BPD, or severe dissociative states, such as PTSD. Psychotic disorders in children, as in adults, can be functional or organic. Functional psychotic syndromes include schizophrenia and related disorders and the psychotic forms of mood disorders. Psychosis can develop secondary to CNS lesions as a consequence of medical illness, trauma, or drug use. Children may manifest psychosis for a substantial amount of time without indicating its presence to parents or caregivers. Therefore, all children with major mood disorders or those who have manifested abnormal or bizarre behaviors should be queried for the presence of psychosis.

Currently, the atypical antipsychotics are first-line agents in the pharmacotherapy of psychosis in children and adolescents. Aripiprazole, olanzapine, quetiapine, and risperidone are FDA-approved to treat chronic psychosis (e.g., schizophrenia) in youth aged 13 and older.

In clinical practice, atypical antipsychotics are initiated at low doses and gradually titrated up to achieve efficacy. Risperidone, for example, may be started at 0.25 mg twice a day and can be increased every day or two under the close observation of the medical setting. In patients treated over the long term with risperidone, clinicians should monitor weight, vital signs, and laboratory results (e.g., triglyceride, cholesterol, prolactin).[122,123] Olanzapine and quetiapine are generally more sedating and are initiated at 2.5 to 5 mg/day and 25 to 50 mg/day, respectively.[124]

If trials with two or three atypical antipsychotics are ineffective, a trial with a typical agent (e.g., chlorpromazine, haloperidol) should be considered. The usual oral dosage of antipsychotics ranges between 3 and 6 mg/kg per day for the low-potency phenothiazines (e.g., chlorpromazine) and between 0.1 and 0.5 (up to 1) mg/kg per day for the high-potency antipsychotics (e.g., haloperidol). Antipsychotic medications have a relatively long half-life and therefore should not be administered more than twice daily.

Common short-term adverse effects of antipsychotics are drowsiness, increased appetite, and weight gain (Table 39-4). Anticholinergic effects (e.g., dry mouth, nasal congestion, blurred vision) are more commonly seen with the low-potency phenothiazines. Short-term adverse effects

TABLE 39-4 Side-Effect Risk Profiles of Common Second-Generation Antipsychotic Medications Used in Children and Adolescents[125,126]

SECOND GENERATION ANTIPSYCHOTICS (BRAND NAME)	ANTICHOLINERGIC	DIABETES	HYPERLIPIDEMIA	HYPER-PROLACTINEMIA	HYPOTENSION	SEDATION	TARDIVE DYSKINESIA	WEIGHT GAIN
Aripiprazole (Abilify)	0	+	+	0	+	+	+	+
Asenapine (Saphris)	0	+	+	+	0	+	+	+
Clozapine (Clozaril)	+++	+++	++/+++	0	+++	+++	0	+++
Iloperidone (Fanapt)	0	+	+	+	+	+	+	+
Lurasidone (Latuda)	0	+	+	+	0	+	+	+
Olanzapine (Zyprexa)	++	+++	++/+++	+/++	+	+/++	+	+++
Paliperidone (Invega)	0	+	+/++	++	+	+	+	++
Quetiapine (Seroquel)	0/+	++	+/++	0	++	++	0	++
Risperidone (Risperdal)	0	+	+/++	++	++	+	+	++
Ziprasidone (Geodon)	0	+	+	0	+	+	+	+

0, low risk; +, mild risk; ++, moderate risk; +++, high risk.

of antipsychotics are generally managed with adjustments of the dose and the timing of administration. Excessive sedation can be avoided by using less sedating agents and prescribing most of the daily dose at nighttime. Drowsiness should not be confused with impaired cognition; it can usually be corrected by adjusting the dose and the timing of administration. In fact, there is no evidence that antipsychotics adversely affect cognition when used in low doses. Anticholinergic adverse effects can be minimized by choosing a medium- or high-potency compound.

Acute dystonia, akathisia (motor restlessness), parkinsonism (bradykinesia, tremor, and lack of facial expressions), and other EPSs are more commonly seen with the high-potency compounds (butyrophenones and thioxanthenes) and have been reported to occur in up to 75% of children receiving these agents. The extent to which antiparkinsonian agents (e.g., anticholinergic drugs, benztropine, trihexyphenidyl, antihistamines, the anti-viral agent amantadine) should be used prophylactically when antipsychotics are introduced is controversial. Whenever possible, antiparkinsonian agents should be used only when EPS emerge. Akathisia may be particularly problematic in young patients because it is often under-recognized.

A benign withdrawal dyskinesia and a syndrome of deteriorating behavior have been associated with the abrupt cessation of these drugs. As in adults, the long-term administration of antipsychotic drugs may be associated with tardive dyskinesia (TD). Although children appear generally less vulnerable than adults to developing TD, there is an emerging consensus that this potentially worrisome adverse effect may affect children and adolescents in 10% to 15% of cases.[127] Prevention (appropriate use for a clear indication, clear target symptoms, periodic drug discontinuation to assess the need for drug use) and early detection (with regular monitoring) are the only effective treatments for TD.

Little is known about the potentially lethal neuroleptic malignant syndrome in juveniles; however, preliminary evidence indicates that its presentation is similar to that in adults. This syndrome may be difficult to distinguish from primary CNS pathology; concurrent infection; or other, more benign side effects of antipsychotics that include EPS or anticholinergic toxicity. Treatment appears similar to those strategies used in adults.

In patients who do not respond to trials with either first-line atypical or typical antipsychotics or who experience significant dyskinesia from these medications, consideration should be given to a trial with clozapine (Clozaril).[128] In the United States and Europe, there has been considerable experience with clozapine in adolescents. Established dose parameters are not yet available; however, in one open study of clozapine for schizophrenic youths, doses from 125 to 825 mg/day (mean = 375 mg/day) for up to 6 weeks were necessary for effectiveness.[129] Although remarkably effective in chronic treatment-resistant schizophrenia and affective psychosis, clinicians should be mindful of clozapine's dose-related risk of seizures and an increased risk of leukopenia and agranulocytosis in adolescents.

COMBINED AGENTS

Increasingly, multiple agents have been used in both clinical practice and research settings for the treatment of child and adolescent psychiatric disorders. This need has arisen out of an emerging awareness of the high rates of co-morbidity described in clinical and epidemiologic studies of juvenile psychiatric disorders. Previously, the law of parsimony dictated a single cause for each symptom complex; this led to the use of large doses of individual agents for a given disorder, often resulting in intolerable adverse effects. In contrast, the use of combined pharmacotherapy has permitted more targeted treatment and greater efficacy, often achieved with lower doses and fewer adverse effects.

Fluoxetine and MPH, for instance, have been described as useful in the management of children with depression and ADHD.[130] In addition, controlled investigations of single agents have produced inconclusive findings in many disorders. Enhanced response rates have been reported when traditional agents are combined. For example, improved anti-ADHD efficacy has been shown with the combination of stimulants and antihypertensives such as clonidine or guanfacine.

On the other hand, growing use of combined pharmacotherapy in children has drawn intense attention from the media and regulatory agencies.[131,132] On balance, rational use of combined psychotropics may produce significant benefits in the hands of experienced clinicians. It has become imperative for future research to provide clinicians with the evidence base for combined-agent pharmacotherapy.

REFERENCES

Access the reference list online at https://expertconsult.inkling.com/.

Mind–Body Medicine

Micaela B. Owusu, M.D., M.Sc.
Deanna C. Chaukos, M.D.
Elyse R. Park, Ph.D., M.P.H.
Gregory L. Fricchione, M.D.

40

OVERVIEW

The National Center for Complementary and Integrative Health defines Mind–Body Medicine as an approach that "focuses on the interactions among the brain, mind, body, and behavior, and on the powerful ways in which emotional, mental, social, spiritual, and behavioral factors can directly affect health."[1] Mind–Body Medicine may also be conceptualized as the scientifically based dimension of what was once named "Complementary and Alternative Medicine" (CAM). In 2012, approximately 45% of Americans were using CAM therapies and spending US$30.2 billion in out-of-pocket expenses to pay for them.[2,3] Mind–body therapies accounted for 17% of this CAM usage.[4] Mind–Body Medicine uses the evidence-based effects of thoughts, beliefs, emotions, and behaviors to positively influence health.

The field of medicine may be thought of as having three component areas: medications, procedures, and self-care.[5] This has been called the "Three-Legged Stool" model. In this schema, Mind–Body Medicine may be conceptualized as the self-care leg, comprised of information derived from the subspecialty of Psychosomatic Medicine. To promote healing, it employs an array of heterogeneous, researched techniques, including meditation, biofeedback, autogenic training, hypnosis, yoga, tai chi, qi gong, and autogenic training (Table 40-1). In this chapter, we will point out the common elements of these techniques and the core elements of the mind–body approach, which can all elicit the relaxation response (RR). The focus on a repetitive activity (such as breathing, or a phrase, word, or prayer) and disruption of the train of everyday thoughts and concerns are the two main features of eliciting the RR; a physiologic state of decreased stress characterized by diminished heart rate, blood pressure, respiratory rate, and oxygen consumption, along with peripheral vasodilatation.[5]

Mind–Body Medicine is often seen as a philosophical concept of healing and health, as well as a group of techniques. Many of these techniques originated in ancient Eastern cultural traditions and may have a religious foundation based on a particular conceptualization of human life. However, even though some people attain benefits from the religious aspects, they are not essential for their therapeutic effect. Throughout this chapter, we describe how recent research is providing evidence for the effectiveness of these treatments, establishing their scientific value and facilitating their integration into mainstream medicine.

Mind–Body Medicine approaches are mainly complementary to current allopathic therapies, but for some conditions, they may also be efficacious when used alone. Within this framework, Mind–Body Medicine takes center stage as it stresses a multi-system integrative model.

STRESS PHYSIOLOGY

All mind–body strategies utilize focus and a non-judgmental stance to quiet the mind and body. In other words, these techniques modulate the physiologic stress response. Later in this chapter, we discuss various hypotheses that link stress physiology to the efficacy of mind–body techniques. Preliminary research illustrates that diverse mind–body techniques have the effect of dampening the stress response; thus, it has been hypothesized that the downstream effects of chronic stress (and the associated morbidity) may also be alleviated by mind–body strategies. Here, we discuss the broad physiologic impact of chronic stress.

Definition of Stress and Distress

Being alive involves *stress* as a stimulus; stress requires biological, psychological, and social adaptations. *Eustress* can be thought of as the normal physiologic workings of the living organism. *Pathogenic stress* or *distress* occurs when homeostasis is threatened or perceived to be so in the setting of overwhelming or sustained external and internal stressors.[6] Alterations in the environment may provoke a physiologic *stress response* mediated by several interconnected physiologic networks constituting the *stress system*, composed of elements of the central nervous system (CNS), the hypothalamus–pituitary–adrenal (HPA) axis, and the immune system. Stressors, the stress response, and the stress system are the three key elements in this process.

Distress is accompanied by overactivity of the stress response system mediated primarily by hypothalamic corticotrophin releasing hormone (CRH) and locus coeruleus-derived norepinephrine (NE). Walter Cannon, in the early 1900s, did groundbreaking work on one axis of the stress response system, the autonomic nervous system (ANS).[7] He focused on a particular branch of ANS, the sympathetic nervous system (SNS) and its connection to "*the flight–fight response*." Hans Selye, another 20th century stress researcher, focused on the HPA axis.[8]

TABLE 40-1 Description of Common Mind–Body Therapies

MIND–BODY THERAPY	DESCRIPTION
Autogenic training	Uses visualization and affirmation techniques to perform manualized self-relaxation
Biofeedback	Use of quantitative sensory modalities (such as heart rate monitoring) to learn to control physiologic processes
Hypnosis	Use of suggestion in a relaxed state of consciousness to elicit behavioral change
Meditation	One of many practices that focuses attention on a bodily sensation, thought, object, or word to promote observation with a stance of non-judgment
Progressive muscle relaxation	Serial contraction and relaxation of muscle groups, often in conjunction with guided imagery and breathing
Tai chi	Derived from martial arts, this practice focuses energy on precise choreographed physical movements that are perfected over years of practice
Qi gong	A moving meditation and health practice focused on internal organ energy derived from Traditional Chinese Medicine
Yoga	One of multiple styles of meditative movement practices based in Indian philosophy utilizing postures, breathing, and relaxation

Data from National Center for Complementary and Integrative Health (NCCIH): Complementary, alternative, or integrative health: what's in a name? Bethesda, 2016, NCCIH. Available from: https://nccih.nih.gov/health/integrative-health and Bertlsch SM, Wee CC, Phillips RS, et al: Alternative mind–body therapies used by adults with medical conditions. *J Psychosom Res*. 2009; 66: 511–519.

Autonomic Nervous System

The CNS and the peripheral ANS have opposing sympathetic (SNS) and parasympathetic (PNS) components. While the SNS promotes the stress response, the PNS can dampen this effect and restore balance in the autonomic system. With practice, engaging in mind–body techniques facilitates a switch from SNS to PNS. These interconnected systems maintain homeostasis by modulating different bodily functions and controlling the administration, distribution, and use of energy. In this way, the brain adapts the level of functioning of different organs to global bodily demands, autoregulated by negative feedback and feed-forward mechanisms. The SNS dominant stress response is adaptive in the short term to mediate a fight-or-flight behavior. However, *distress* occurs when the SNS is overactivated by either chronic or acutely overwhelming stressors that make restoration of homeostasis through balance with the PNS difficult. When this occurs persistently, chronic sympathetic activation (i.e., distress) may lead to chronic diseases in organ systems that are sensitive to prolonged alterations in autonomic control—the cardiovascular, respiratory, gastrointestinal, renal, endocrine, and immune systems, among others.[9]

Activation of the stress response via the SNS stimulates metabolism, cardiac output (through increased heart rate), vascular tone, respiration (through increased breathing rate and oxygen consumption), muscle contraction, increased beta and reduced alpha brain wave activity. Simultaneously, the stress response suppresses the PNS resulting in reduced activity of the excretory, gastrointestinal, and reproductive systems.[10] The neurobiologic pathways for this stress response are detailed below.

The stress response is elicited by efferent pathways from the central nucleus of the amygdala (which stimulates the parabrachial nucleus to increase respiration), the dorsomedial nucleus of the vagus nerve (that suppresses the PNS), and the lateral hypothalamus (which activates the SNS). Through reciprocal neuronal pathways connecting the amygdala to the medial prefrontal cortex (PFC), the specific emotional experience of stress will differ, but is typically associated with fear. During panic attacks, for example, the fear is of imminent death; in social phobia, the fear is of embarrassment; in post-traumatic stress disorder (PTSD), the traumatic memory is remembered or re-experienced; in obsessive–compulsive disorder (OCD), obsessional ideas recur and intrude; and in generalized anxiety disorder, anxiety is ever present and non-specific.

Hypothalamic–Pituitary–Adrenal Axis

Activation of the HPA axis results in secretion of glucocorticoids, hormones that act at many levels to modulate the body's energy resources and restore the body to homeostasis after acute disruption.[11] The medial parvocellular division of the paraventricular hypothalamic nucleus (PVN) houses neurons that release the CRH required for adrenocorticotrophin hormone (ACTH) secretion from the pituitary through stimulation of G-protein-coupled receptors.[12] ACTH moves through the systemic circulation arriving at the adrenal cortex where it promotes synthesis and secretion of the corticosteroid cortisol. The early pathway hypothalamic CRH neurons are regulated by bottom-up direct somatic, visceral, and humoral excitatory sensory afferents that provide a reflexive stress response. Simultaneously, the hypothalamus receives anticipatory voluntary top-down stress signals from paralimbic medial PFC and limbic forebrain structures, a set of structures related to the control of emotional responses, behavior, and long-term memory. When integrated, these two pathways (bottom-up and top-down) modulate the HPA axis through tuning of the PVN CRH output.

The HPA output hormone, cortisol, circulates to stimulate hepatic glycogenolysis, proteolysis, and lipolysis, mediates vasoconstriction, suppresses innate immunity, reproductive function, and bone and muscle growth, and inhibits mood leading to depression. In the short term, these mechanisms are adaptive to mobilize resources for the fight-or-flight response. However, when prolonged, this profile becomes pathologic.

Appraisal

Cognitive and emotional appraisal of whether a situation constitutes a stressor is accomplished by the brain.[13] A stressor is most distressing when it is perceived as such. While certain experiences are universally threatening, there is individualized variability among appraisals of particular threats. Depending on one's appraisal, the physiologic mediators of the stress response may or may not emerge.[14]

The PFC regions cooperate to help us plan for the future and manage higher-order decision-making. When we are not stressed, the PFC and its extensive connections orchestrate behavior, thought, and emotion in a reasonable, goal-directed and regulated way. This situation potentiates a top-down guidance of attention and thought (via dorsolateral PFC), error monitoring, and reality testing (via dorsomedial PFC), inhibition of inappropriate actions (via inferior PFC) and regulation of emotions (via ventromedial PFC).[15] When we are distressed, on the other hand, the amygdala stimulates the bottom-up stress response pathways in the HPA axis and the brainstem with outpourings of cortisol, NE, and dopamine.[16,17]

The neurochemical environment of highly elevated cortisol and NE may impair PFC top-down regulation and strengthen amygdala-driven bottom-up dynamics. Stress-induced catecholamine excess impairs PFC higher-order control enabling supremacy of the activated amygdala fear-conditioning, sensory hypervigilance, and habituated motor responses.[15]

Immune System

The immune system also plays an important role in the stress response. The immune system evolved in association with enormous microbial threat. Specifically, cell-mediated innate immunity evolved to have a high sensitivity at the expense of a low specificity to any and all perceived threats. The result is a highly reactive immune system that is easily triggered into a persistently activated state that may contribute to excessive metabolic wear and tear.[18] We become susceptible to this activation when our psychosocial stressors stimulate our macrophages into an immune response not only in the periphery, but also in the brain in a process termed *neurogenic neuroinflammation*.[19]

As depicted above, stress stimuli result in release of catecholamines and glucocorticoids. NE and epinephrine directly stimulate beta-adrenergic receptors on macrophages resulting in activation of transcription factor NF-κB. Under normal circumstances, cortisol binds glucocorticoid receptors on the macrophage surface to inhibit the NF-κB system. However, under conditions of chronic stress, functional resistance of monocyte-macrophages to cortisol negative feedback permits continuation of NF-κB signaling resulting in continued pro-inflammatory cytokine release.[20] These immune cell-derived pro-inflammatory signals from the catecholamine cascade consequently outweigh the anti-inflammatory effects of the glucocorticoids.

NF-κB is a bridge between stress and oxidative cellular activation through its stimulatory effects on the secretion of pro-inflammatory cytokines from immune cells (IL-1, IL-6, TNF-α).[21,22] This cascade promotes downstream cellular oxidative stress and alterations in neurotransmitter metabolism, neuroendocrine action, and neuroplasticity.[23,24] Pro-inflammatory immune cell product TNF-α, for example, can have direct toxic effects on oligodendrocytes resulting in apoptosis and neuronal demyelination.

These aspects of the immune response's physiology have relevance in the genesis or progression of multiple diseases in high stress situations. Empirically, distress has been related to proneness to viral infections, progression from HIV to AIDS, flares of multiple sclerosis, lupus, arthritis, and risk of developing coronary heart disease and Alzheimer's disease.[25–30]

Specificity of the Stress Response

From an evolutionary developmental perspective, the stress response is an adaptive phenomenon. However, it is a biological reflection of early stages in our species' development, and thus, it is not always well suited to deal with the specific types of chronic daily stressors we face in modern life. To understand how the stress response, which was evolutionarily designed to help us survive, can also hurt us, we will employ two opposing concepts: allostasis and allostatic load.

ALLOSTASIS, ALLOSTATIC LOADING, AND NF-κB

Allostasis is a stress-specific term meaning the ability to achieve stability through change.[31] It refers to the biologic mechanisms that protect the body from internal and external stress thereby maintaining internal homeostasis. But sometimes, the stress system cannot maintain the internal balance for various reasons.

In the presence of chronic stress, the persistent overactivation of allostatic systems can lead to a variety of diseases. This long-term effect of the physiologic response to stress has been called *allostatic loading*—the metabolic wear and tear on the organism at the cellular level that occurs as the price for maintaining allostasis.[32] It is the brain's stress response system, consisting of the amygdala, lateral hypothalamus-driven SNS, the HPA axis, and the medial basal hypothalamus-related inflammatory response, that serve as conduits to the body's end organs of what the brain mesocorticolimbic system processes as a challenge or a threat.

There are four proposed mechanisms associated with allostatic load:[33] (1) frequent stress or multiple stressors; (2) prolonged exposure to stress and the consequent lack of adaptation; (3) inability to shut off allostatic responses or delayed shutdown once a stressor is terminated; and, (4) inadequate (insufficient) response. These burdens lead to an over-activation of other systems in order to compensate for failed allostasis.

Mind–body therapies, such as meditation, may reduce allostatic loading via epigenetic pathways of gene expression. The genes of interest are involved in oxidative metabolism, apoptosis, activation of NF-κB, and ribosomal functioning. In one study, the cross-sectional peripheral blood mononuclear cell gene expression profile of experienced meditators (M group) was compared with the gene expression profile taken at two times in novices who had never learned the core meditative RR practice. Results showed that certain gene expression profiles in the M group and 8 weeks post-RR training novice group differed significantly from the pre-training novice group.[34] The transcriptome changes seen with RR practice relate to more efficient mitochondrial metabolism with improvement in insulin function, cell aging, and reduction in NF-κB immune activation. These effects may relate to the known physiologic results of RR elicitation, which include reduction in blood pressure and oxygen consumption.

When stress is removed, proinflammatory transcription factor NF-κB usually downregulates within 60 minutes. Some individuals are unable to downregulate this quickly, suggesting a variability in stress perception that can be translated into prolonged NF-κB activation. This differential response to stress stimuli may be a product of genomic activation differences. The group of individuals who are unable to downregulate NF-κB quickly, may theoretically benefit most from RR training.

In another example of how mind–body therapies reduce oxidative stress, they have been shown to improve telomerase activity and protect against telomere shortening. Stress and aging, in contrast, hasten telomere shortening.[35]

Mind–Body Medicine offers interventions to reduce stress (allostatic load) and enhance resiliency, thereby promoting health and preventing illness.

RESILIENCY

Resiliency is a term that comes to us from structural engineering and refers to the ability to rebound from a stressor. Resiliency reflects good adjustment across different domains in the face of significant adversity. It consists of five major capacities: (1) the capacity to experience reward and motivation nested in dispositional optimism and high positive emotionality; (2) the capacity to circumscribe fear responsiveness so that one can continue to be effective through active coping strategies despite fear; (3) the capacity to use adaptive social behaviors to secure support through bonding and teamwork and to provide support through altruism; (4) the ability to use cognitive skills to re-interpret the meaning of negative stimuli in a more positive light; and (5) the integration of a sense of purpose in life along with a moral compass, meaning, and spiritual connectedness.[36]

There are increasing studies identifying biochemical correlates of resiliency, typically attributable to HPA axis pathways. For example, single nucleotide polymorphisms (SNPs) of the CRH type 1 receptor gene may moderate the effects of child maltreatment on susceptibility to depression in adulthood.[37] Additionally, four SNPs of FKBP5 (a gene that codes for a protein involved in glucocorticoid receptor sensitivity) have been found to modulate the association of child abuse with the risk of PTSD in adulthood.[38] Polymorphisms of the catecholamine transport enzyme COMT alter levels of circulating catecholamines in response to stress, resulting in altered resilience to anxiety and negative mood states.[39] There are also epigenetic mechanisms of resiliency in which the environment can change chromatin structure through methylation or acetylation of histones or direct methylation of DNA.

THE MIND–BODY MEDICINE HYPOTHESES

Four hypotheses of Mind–Body Medicine emerge based on the science summarized above.[40] The first hypothesis is that the mind and body are a unity. Every external and internal experience produced is the result of and results in biological reactions in the brain. These biologic reactions change the ecology of the brain and this transduction of experience unifies what we consider to be *mind* activity and *body* function.

The second hypothesis is that psychosocial stress gets transduced into cellular stress. This cellular stress is mitochondrial oxidative stress, and every cell receives psychosocial stress in this physiologic way via the stress response systems.

The third hypothesis is that this cellular oxidative stress is what uncovers disease vulnerability. This is essentially a non-specificity stress diathesis model. For example, if both of my parents died of coronary artery disease, it is a good bet that I have genetic vulnerability to coronary artery disease. I may not manifest that vulnerability if I can build my cardiovascular resiliency by holding my psychosocial stress, and by extension, my cellular oxidative stress, in check. Our genetic endowment is not completely writing the script for us, and this fact is revolutionizing the field of Psychosomatic Medicine. The environment is having its say in terms of which genes are activated or inactivated through epigenetic transcriptomic effect.

This leads to the fourth hypothesis, the *Mind–Body Medicine Equation*.[41] Building on the earlier work of medical sociologist George Albee,[42] it is a very simple and heuristic model of disease vulnerability. Consider a division equation with the numerator as stress and the denominator as resiliency. The quotient approximates one's allostatic loading and provides a metric of one's vulnerability to illness in the future (Figure 40-1). If you flip the numerator to resiliency and the denominator to stress, this inverse quotient depicts propensity to health.

In clinical practice, for example, if one cares for patients with systemic lupus erythematosus, if you stratify the patient cohort by level of social support when you populate the variables in the equation, there will be variability in the denominator (resiliency). This care provider may then hypothesize that individuals with low social supports will have increased propensities for lupus flares. There are many examples of this relationship in the research literature from rheumatologic to cardiac to gastrointestinal diseases.

Because of this relationship, doctors and nurses should be mindful of this equation when they evaluate patients and create treatment plans. This is particularly critical in the field of Psychosomatic Medicine, where patients may struggle

$$\frac{\text{Stress+Genetic Vulnerabilities}}{\text{Resiliency+Genetic Endowments}} = \frac{\text{Oxidative Stress}}{\text{Antioxidation}} = \text{Propensity to Disease}$$

Figure 40-1 Mind–Body Medicine equation. *(From Fricchione, Gregory L., M.D. Compassion and Healing in Medicine and Society: On the Nature and Use of Attachment Solutions to Separation Challenges. pp. 440. © 2011 Johns Hopkins University Press. Reprinted with permission of Johns Hopkins University Press.)*

with physical, cognitive, and emotional ramifications of illness. There should be some ability in the clinical encounter to get an objective feel for the level of patient stress and the level of patient resiliency.[41]

So what is an example of a comprehensive mind–body strategy available to relieve stress and enhance resilience? The Benson–Henry Institute for Mind–Body Medicine (BHI) at the Massachusetts General Hospital, uses the Stress Management and Resiliency Training (SMART)-Relaxation Response Resiliency Program (3RP), which combines integrative medicine consultations with management of stress-related conditions (see a mind–body clinical case, Case 1).[41]

CASE 1

Mr. B, a 35-year-old man was admitted to inpatient medicine for the fourth time in the past year with a subacute flare of ulcerative colitis. His primary inpatient treatment team noticed his progressive increases in anxiety and irritability with each admission. He was short-tempered with staff and fewer of his family members remained at his bedside. His outpatient gastroenterologist noted that he frequently felt afraid about his future health status, frustration at not being able to participate in activities that he enjoyed (such as meals with friends), and increasing difficulties keeping up at his fast-paced job. He complained of chronic abdominal pain with notable worsening during moments of anxiety, anger, and sadness. His psychiatric review of systems was notable for diminished sleep due to worries about his work, but he had no other psychological or neurovegetative signs of depression. There was no concern about a history of mania or psychosis. Psychiatry consultation was requested to assist with inpatient management and aftercare planning for his emotional, behavioral, and physical symptoms.

The consultant provided a 20-minute instruction on how Mr. B could practice eliciting the relaxation response through focused breathing, directed attention and mindfulness, and non-judgmental observation of his thoughts. He recommended using the technique daily. Throughout his 3-week hospitalization, the consultant provided supplementary guided imagery meditations to assist Mr. B envision a life with less pain. Intermittently, Mr. B required use of trazodone for sleep.

In conjunction with the acute anti-inflammatory medications offered by the primary team, Mr. B reported that use of these mind–body therapies significantly increased his self-efficacy and remarkably reduced the intensity of his pain, though it still arose intermittently. He was discharged after 3 weeks with less irritability. He accepted a referral to the local mind–body center where he engaged in an 8-week group program to develop these self-healing skills and receive psychiatric follow-up. His outpatient gastroenterologist continued to see him regularly, but noted that his flares became less frequent and Mr. B appeared to be coping well with his chronic illness.

The SMART-3RP program is designed to target five resiliency capacities, intervening in one's ability to: (1) adapt to stress and circumscribe fear responses by eliciting the RR and participating in lifestyle behaviors that buffer against the stress response and promote the RR; (2) engage sources of social support and increase opportunities to be pro-social; (3) generate cognitive habits of adaptive thinking to counter negative, stress-activating thoughts; (4) experience appreciation of life and its joys and cultivate optimism and positive thinking in daily pursuits; and (5) engage in meaningful social, empathic, and altruistic activities that foster a sense of spiritual connectedness. Specifically, this treatment intervenes on three core components: (1) promoting the relaxation response; (2) decreasing the stress response; and (3) promoting growth enhancement.

Patients referred to SMART-3RP group interventions first learn RR with a component of mindfulness and yoga to enhance the subsequent didactic component. Cognitive behavioral skills are then taught in the group setting with the goal of breaking the negative thinking traps and catastrophizing that can lead to pathogenic stress. Also in the group setting, social support is an important component, as is encouragement of pro-social behavior. Optimism and belief in conscious positive expectation are important parts of the positive psychology aspect of our approach, as is accenting meaning, purpose, gratitude, and life enjoyment.[42] Spirituality, basically defined as a sense of connectedness to something greater than ourselves, is also addressed in the SMART-3RP. In addition, exercise and nutrition education are important factors. The SMART-3RP is designed to reduce stress and enhance resiliency, thereby increasing the denominator of the above mind–body equation and thus reducing propensity to disease. Results show that the SMART-3RP reduces the frequency of 12 out of 23 somatic symptoms on the Medical Symptom Checklist, significantly decreases frequency and intensity of psychological symptoms on the Symptom Checklist-90-Revised, and increases health-promoting lifestyle behaviors on the Health Promoting Lifestyle Profile-II.[43] In patients with functional bowel disorders, the SMART-3RP reduced symptomatology, while also changing peripheral blood mononuclear cell gene expression to result in a reduction in the NF-κB pathway.[44] BHI investigators have assessed the feasibility and acceptability of the 3RP with pilot trials among medical patients and clinical providers. Pilot trials have shown that the 3RP treatment is efficacious among participants, with reported post-treatment improvements in mood and positive affect, stress coping, and life/work satisfaction, and resiliency.

In a preliminary study, exposure to the SMART-3RP reduced billable encounters and associated services in a hospital-insured employee pool suggesting that the program may contribute to reductions in healthcare utilization.[45]

USE AND EFFICACY OF MIND–BODY TECHNIQUES

A significant interest in Mind–Body Medicine among the general population has been documented in national surveys in the United States.[46] Mind–body therapies were most frequently used for different chronic conditions, such as anxiety, depression, chronic pain, insomnia, gastrointestinal disorders, and fatigue, for which currently available therapies are not entirely satisfactory. In fact, anxiety and pain have been proposed as the symptoms that best predict the public's search for alternative therapies.[47] However, the main reason why people use these kinds of interventions is not dissatisfaction with conventional medicine, but because they have found these interventions to be more congruent with their own values, beliefs, and philosophical orientations toward health and life.[48]

The RR-based approaches have been shown to be beneficial in many disorders.[49] However, not all studies are reliable, and caution must be used. Many studies have methodologic problems, and statistical significance is not synonymous with efficacy. With these caveats in mind, Astin and colleagues noted there is strong to moderate evidence based on meta-analyses of mind–body intervention efficacy in the following medical conditions: cardiovascular disease, cancer treatment tolerance, incontinence, surgical outcomes, insomnia, chronic low back pain, arthritis self-care, and hypertension.[50] Mind–body interventions have also been shown to be effective for depression and anxiety symptoms[51,52] and are regularly incorporated into some of today's most popular manualized psychotherapies. Many other disorders are also likely to respond to mind–body interventions, but sufficient studies have either not been done or are too numerous to describe here.

Because they promote self-care, mind–body interventions also appear to be cost-effective. It has been documented that these approaches reduce ambulatory visits, post-surgical days in the hospital, unnecessary procedures and medical costs.[53,54] As part of the cost-effectiveness analysis, mind–body interventions also improve patient satisfaction, sense of control, and quality of life.[55] It should also be stressed that mind–body interventions, in most cases, are to be used as complementary therapies in combination with conventional medical treatments and procedures.[51] Further research is needed to define the role of Mind–Body Medicine in primary prevention (stop disease before it occurs) as well as in secondary (slow disease progression) and tertiary prevention (decrease impact of chronic disease), considering that stress plays a role in the onset of many diseases and in their exacerbations.[52] This is particularly important since the major healthcare challenge facing the 21st century world is chronic non-communicable diseases, of which neuropsychiatric disorders, are included.[53]

CONCLUSIONS

The heuristic Mind–Body Medicine Equation can be derived from the research described above. In this equation, the propensity to disease is defined by a relationship between the stress burden and genetic vulnerability as numerator and the personal resources which help us to cope with stressors (resiliency) and genetic endowment as denominator. Mind–Body Medicine lowers the numerator and increases the denominator through enhanced self-management skills, such as the ability to elicit the relaxation response, cognitive skills, social support, prosocial behavior, positive psychology, and spiritual beliefs. Gene expression changes, induced epigenetically, may form the links within the denominator between genes and resiliency and within the numerator between genes and stress. Thus, Mind–Body Medicine interventions are effective and critical in buffering against stress and in building resiliency.[41]

Mind–Body Medicine is an important bridge between clinical medicine and public health. All physicians should evaluate stress and resiliency in their patients and consider use of mind–body approaches for treatment and prevention to promote mental and physical health. Additionally, since patients rely on their professional and lay caregivers, who likely fall prey to stress themselves, Mind–Body Medicine approaches can benefit all individuals engaged in health care.

REFERENCES

Access the reference list online at https://expertconsult.inkling.com/.

Chronic Disease and Unhealthy Habits: Behavioral Management

41

Elizabeth Pegg Frates, M.D.
Elyse R. Park, Ph.D., M.P.H.
A. Eden Evins, M.D., M.P.H.
Gregory L. Fricchione, M.D.

OVERVIEW

Lifestyle choices are associated with the development of chronic non-communicable diseases (NCDs). Centuries ago, Hippocrates emphasized the power of exercise and nutrition; he noted, "If we could give every individual the right amount of nourishment and exercise, not too little and not too much, we would have found the safest way to health." Over the past few decades, a bevy of research papers have supported this ancient wisdom. Among these was a 1993 study on the identification of non-genetic factors that contribute to death in the United States.[1] McGinnis and Foege[1] examined the literature from 1977 to 1993 and determined that 19% of all deaths were attributable to tobacco use, 14% were attributable to poor diet and physical inactivity, and 5% were attributable to alcohol consumption. Eleven years later, Mokdad and colleagues[2] reported on statistics from the United States population from the year 2000. They pointed out that the main chronic diseases causing death in the United States were cardiac disease, cancer, stroke, and chronic respiratory disease. In addition, they highlighted the root causes of those diseases and thus, the actual causes of death; among these were behaviors (e.g., tobacco use, accounting for approximately 19% of deaths; poor diet and physical inactivity, accounting for approximately 17% of deaths; and alcohol consumption, accounting for approximately 4% of deaths).[2] These studies and others helped to connect addictions and lifestyle choices to the development of NCDs. To address these notable behaviors, *Healthy People 2020* created goals to: increase the proportion of adults who meet current National Guidelines physical activity guidelines for aerobic physical activity and for muscle-strengthening activity; decrease smoking prevalence of adults to 12%; enhance restorative sleep (70.8% of adults get sufficient sleep, defined as ≥8 hours for those aged 18 to 21 years and ≥7 hours for those aged 22 years and older, on average, during a 24-hour period); increase the proportion of adults who are at a healthy weight to 33.9% thereby decreasing the proportion of adults who are obese to 30.5%.[3]

According to the American Psychological Association's *Stress in America 2015 Survey*, stress also contributes to unhealthy behaviors. Among Americans who have tried to make a lifestyle change in the past 5 years, many are still trying to lose weight (58%), reduce stress (53%), eat a healthier diet (49%), get more sleep (47%), and exercise more (45%).[4]

The NCDs (cardiovascular diseases, chronic respiratory diseases, cancer, diabetes, arthritis and neuropsychiatric diseases) take an enormous toll, not only in terms of mortality but also in terms of disability and the ballooning of healthcare costs. For this reason, the NCDs represent the most important global health challenge of the 21st century.[5] Lifestyle is crucial in the etiology of NCDs, and healthcare providers need to work with patients to reduce these important risk factors.[5]

The idea that Americans have some control over their chances of acquiring a chronic condition is becoming more mainstream. The five healthy habits index is commonly used in research. These five habits include: not smoking; maintaining a body mass index (BMI) <25; eating a healthy diet with high intake of fiber, low levels of refined carbohydrates, a high ratio of polyunsaturated fat compared with saturated fat, and low intake of trans fats; drinking alcohol in moderation (two drinks or less a day for men and one drink or less a day for women); and exercising regularly (at least 20 minutes 3 times a week of aerobic exercise).[6] Gradually, the public awareness of these healthy indices has increased. Unfortunately, over the past 20 years, changes in adherence rates to healthy habits in the United States has not changed for the better.[7] For example: obesity levels in the United States rose from 28% to 36%; the percentage of people engaging in regular physical activity dropped from 53% to 43%; the percentage of people eating ≥5 servings of fruits and vegetables in a day decreased from 42% to 26%; adherence to all five healthy indices went down from 15.2% to 8.5%; and, adherence rates to healthy habits were not more likely in people with chronic disease (e.g., cardiac disease, high blood pressure, high cholesterol, and diabetes).

Increased awareness of healthy habits does not necessarily translate into increased adoption of healthy lifestyles. As Sir Francis Bacon stated in the 17th century, "Knowledge is power." However, knowledge alone is not powerful enough to instill lasting behavior change.

HEALTHY HABITS AND DISEASE PREVENTION AND MANAGEMENT

Lifestyle intervention studies have demonstrated that adopting healthy lifestyles reduces morbidity and mortality of disease. Without question, obesity is a growing health concern. Therefore, losing weight and maintaining a healthy weight at or below a BMI of 25, is a goal for many people in the United States. However, simply adding healthy habits, even if they do not alter someone's weight or BMI, is also beneficial. Matheson and colleagues[8] examined healthy habits (e.g., being a non-smoker, consuming greater than five servings of fruit and vegetables a day, engaging in physical activity more than 12 times a month, and drinking alcohol in moderation) in people in different weight categories (normal weight, overweight, and obese). Their results demonstrated that adding healthy behaviors to people's lifestyles resulted in a significant decrease in mortality, regardless of baseline BMI. This was especially beneficial for those who were obese.[8]

Research has shown that practicing healthy habits can reduce mortality and help people prevent chronic disease. For example, Ford and colleagues[9] found that by adhering to four healthy lifestyle factors: never smoking, maintaining a BMI <30, being physically active for ≥3.5 hours per week, and adhering to a healthy diet (high intake of fruits, vegetables, whole-grain bread, and low meat consumption) approximately 80% of chronic diseases could be prevented. Several years later, Akesson and colleagues[10] in Sweden, conducted a population-based prospective cohort study in Swedish men who were followed for 11 years. They concluded that by not smoking; by consuming only moderate amounts of alcohol; by following a healthy diet; by walking/bicycling for longer than 40 minutes each day; by exercising for at least 1 hour a week; and by maintaining a waist circumference <95 cm, 79% of myocardial infarctions could be avoided.

Collectively, current interventions target multiple risk factors (MRFs)—as a lifestyle change—rather than individual behaviors. Indeed, in 1982, the Multiple Risk Factor Intervention Trial, a randomized trial of a multi-factor intervention program on mortality from coronary heart disease (CHD) among high-risk men, consisted of treatment for hypertension, counseling for cigarette smoking, and dietary advice for lowering blood cholesterol levels.[11]

Lifestyle medicine is the burgeoning area of medicine that encourages and prescribes healthy habits (e.g., regular exercise, healthy eating patterns, and stress management to treat, reverse, and prevent disease). A landmark study published in the *New England Journal of Medicine* randomized overweight, pre-diabetic patients into three groups: placebo, metformin, and a lifestyle intervention. The lifestyle intervention targeted losing 7% of body weight by following a diet low in calories and low in fat, as well as aiming to accumulate 150 minutes of physical activity in a week. A 16-hour curriculum covering diet, exercise, and behavior modification was also part of the lifestyle intervention. These sessions, taught by case managers, were flexible and individualized. The participants also had monthly individual group sessions that reinforced the lessons. Subjects were followed for 4 years and then evaluated to see how many of the subjects, who were all pre-diabetic, went on to develop diabetes. Compared with the placebo group, the cumulative incidence of diabetes in the metformin group was 31% less, and the cumulative incidence of diabetes in the lifestyle intervention group was 58% less than the placebo group. The lifestyle medicine intervention was more effective in helping pre-diabetic patients avoid the diagnosis of diabetes than both the placebo and the metformin group.[12]

Our lifestyles affect our ability to manage, treat, and prevent disease through different mechanisms. One of those involves gene expression changes. Ornish and colleagues[13] demonstrated that a 3-month intensive lifestyle intervention with a focus on exercise, stress management, and nutrition could modulate gene expression in patients with prostate cancer. This epigenetics research encourages healthcare practitioners to prioritize counseling patients on behavior change.

The effect of one component alone, specifically exercise, on health has been the subject of much research. A recent meta-analysis that examined the efficacy of exercise, compared with drug interventions, on the mortality rate of people suffering from specific chronic disease (including heart disease, chronic heart failure, stroke, and diabetes), revealed that in many cases, exercise can be as effective as medicine.[14] Investigating the effects of exercise on mood and anxiety has also become a topic of interest in the medical literature. Several studies support the use of exercise as an adjunct treatment for depression and anxiety.[15–20] In one study, researchers demonstrated that state anxiety was reduced after even one 50-minute session of aerobic or resistance training exercise at a level of 70% to 80% of maximum heart rate, in subjects with elevated anxiety levels.[21] These studies did not recommend using exercise instead of medicine, but rather in conjunction with medications. Exercise can be prescribed in a safe and effective way.[22] Moreover, providers who exercise are more likely to counsel their patients on exercise, and specifically, providers counsel patients on exercises that they themselves perform, such as aerobic training or strength training.[23]

The evidence shows that adopting healthy lifestyles helps patients prevent and manage chronic disease. However, starting on, counseling in, and sustaining healthy habits is a challenge for patients and for clinicians. Specific skills and tools (such as the use of the Transtheoretical Model of Change, the 5As, motivational interviewing, positive psychology, appreciative inquiry, and goal setting) can be developed by practitioners to empower patients to adopt healthy lifestyles. There is a five-step cycle that incorporates all of these strategies and techniques and serves as a guide for providers counseling patients on lifestyle changes.

Patients often need support when seeking to stop an unhealthy behavior and start a new health-promoting behavior.

TRANSTHEORETICAL MODEL OF CHANGE

The Transtheoretical Model of Change was developed by James Prochaska, PhD, after working for 20 years with patients who suffer from addictions. It is useful, not only as a tool for treating addictions, often in conjunction with medication, but for increasing exercise, adopting a healthy diet, and changing other behaviors. This model separates patients into categories of readiness for change, including pre-contemplation (not willing or wanting to change), contemplation (considering changing), preparation (getting ready to make a change), action, and maintenance.[24] Recognizing the stage of change that a patient is in is the first step. Then, counseling follows according to their stage of change. This model allows providers to tailor their counseling to the needs of the patient based on their stage of change.

Pre-contemplation

Those individuals who are pre-contemplative, say they cannot and are not ready to change. By raising their awareness of the importance of the problem, providers increase the chances that their patients will address the issue. For example, if an obese patient is eating "fast foods," reporting that he has no time to cook, no money to buy healthy foods, and states that since he has never been successful at losing weight he will not even try, then asking the patient about his understanding of the risks of being obese is a good place to start. "What is your understanding about the risks of being obese?" is an open ended question that will allow a patient to share his knowledge and beliefs. Building on his response to this question, other risks can be added. This will raise his awareness. Sharing the story of a patient who lost weight and kept it off might be another effective strategy for someone who is pre-contemplative. In this stage, the goal is for him/her to consider learning more about his/her behavior and the effects of their behavior.

For patients who are not motivated to change, the "5 Rs" can be used:

- Relevance—Make it relevant to the patient's current health and health goals;
- Risks—Elicit the patient's perceptions of short- and long-term health risks of their behavior (e.g., obesity's impact on shortness of breath, long-term cardiac risk);
- Rewards—Encourage the patient to think about possible rewards for future changes in health behavior;
- Roadblocks—Identify barriers to making a behavior change (e.g., other smokers at work, friends who drink excessively); and,
- Repetition—Repeat these discussions each time you see the patient.

Contemplation

Contemplators say they may or might change. For contemplators, using experiential techniques, including raising awareness and dramatic relief, is effective. In this stage, a provider can also use self-re-evaluation by encouraging the patient to identify with a healthy role model. In addition, the use of imagery is helpful for contemplators. In so doing, the patient can begin to create a vision of who they might become. Asking the patient to consider what life would be like if they were enjoying healthy meals throughout the day and avoiding fast foods is one way to encourage the use of imagery. This allows the patient to ponder the possibilities of changing behavior and then to put those possibilities in their own words. By reviewing and emphasizing the pros of change and the cons of staying the same, the patient will start to realize the importance of change and the possible rewards that will come with change. When treating a contemplator, the goal is for him/her to think deeply about the reasons/causes that underlie their behaviors and consider evaluating different options.

Preparation

People who are in the preparation phase about their potential plans for modifying the target behavior have already convinced themselves that change is worth the effort. The focus is on making a commitment to change, using social support from family and friends, and finding healthy substitutes that can be used in place of the unhealthy habit. For a patient looking to lose weight by consuming less fast food, the healthcare provider might brainstorm about quick healthy meals, starting with breakfast, to help the person in preparation move to action. Identifying a friend, co-worker, neighbor, or family member who can be a buddy in the process or a supporter will help the patient make progress. Creating a start date, or for smoking—a "quit date"—and making it public (e.g., by writing it down, posting it on social media, or sharing it with the healthcare provider, friends, or family) will help the person in preparation get ready for action. Making this commitment is called self-liberation. When treating someone in preparation, the goal is action, specifically, creating a plan to change behaviors and initiating medication if that is part of the plan.

Action

When treating someone in preparation, the goal is one of action, specifically, carrying out action-oriented plans. The people in the action phase have been practicing the new healthy behavior for at least a month, but less than 6 months, and they still need behavioral counseling and may still need medication treatment. Encouraging healthy substitutions and fostering relationships with people who support the healthy behavior pattern are also important. In addition to these strategies, focusing on the types of rewards the patient is experiencing and receiving from the newly adopted healthy behavior is key. Checking labs and pointing out a change in cholesterol or glucose control can serve to encourage the patient to sustain the behavior. If the patient has experienced positive changes in BMI or in body composition, these can act as powerful rewards. The patient may notice improved mood or decreased stress. It is important to ask the patient what they noticed since adopting the healthy habit.

Maintenance

People in the maintenance phase have been practicing the healthy habit for over 6 months, but they also need ongoing encouragement and support and may continue medication to sustain this behavior. Using similar techniques to those in the action phase will work. Those patients in maintenance often respond well to the idea of becoming a mentor to someone who is new to the process of change. This can be a useful way for them to stay on track and to help another person who is struggling with a similar issue.

BEHAVIOR MODIFICATION COUNSELING: THE "5 As"

The 5 As of behavior change counseling are: Assess, Advise, Agree, Assist, and Arrange. Following the 5 As of behavior change counseling is useful as it helps to engage the patient, to put a plan in motion, and to track progress with the plan.[25]

Assess

First, assess the patient's risk factors, signs and symptoms, social history, past medical history, lab results, physical exam, exercise history, dietary patterns, stress levels, sleep quality and quantity, substance use, and level of social connection. Assessing the patient's current level of interest in change and stage of change according to the Transtheoretical Model of Change is also part of the assessment phase of counseling.

Advise

After asking questions and gathering information during the initial assessment phase of the counseling, the provider moves to the second A: advising. The provider can then target the information on behavior change to address the patient's current disease state, risk factors, and unhealthy behaviors. Meeting the patient's stage of change and tailoring the advice to the stage will save time and increase the chances that the advice is heard, understood, and followed. An understanding of the Transtheoretical Model of Change is essential for behavior change counseling, especially when crafting advice that will be accepted and utilized by the patient.

Agree

After crafting advice that targets the patient's stage of change, disease state, symptoms, complaints, needs, desires, and hopes for the future, the next step is to check in with the patient. The third A stands for agree. It is important to acknowledge that the patient's autonomy and agreement with the plans for the change process. Instead of just telling the patient what to do without asking for feedback, this strategy ensures that the patient is in agreement with the plan. If the patient does not agree, a dialogue about the best way forward will unfold. This step creates a partnership between the patient and the provider.

Assist

Assist is the fourth A. In this phase, the provider assists the patient in making the change plan a reality. This could involve writing prescriptions for exercise or a healthy eating pattern, encouraging participation in a stress management program, or requesting a referral to a nutritionist, sleep lab, or physical therapist. The provider works closely with the patient to find support systems and community resources near the patient's home that can assist the patient in following through with the plan and achieving the stated goals.

Arrange

The fifth and final A represents arranging follow-up. This last phase is critical because it puts accountability into the change plan. The patient knows that there will be another visit in which the provider will follow-up on the topics and strategies discussed in the session. The provider needs to ask about the plan, which has been recorded in the medical record, during the follow-up visit. Focusing on all five steps of behavioral change counseling helps providers cultivate a supportive environment and conduct sessions that foster movement toward the targeted healthy behaviors.

A FIVE-STEP CYCLE FOR COACHING PATIENTS TO ADOPT HEALTHY HABITS

The collaboration embodied in the "5 As" of behavior change counseling helps propel patients forward on their behavior change journeys.[26] With collaboration, the expertise of the provider in disease management, health goals, behavior change, and national guidelines are combined with the expert knowledge of that patient in his or her own life: needs, desires, fears, desires, past successes, strengths, weaknesses, previous failed attempts to change, and potential supportive friends and family that might help the patient achieve his or her goals. Both the provider and the patient provide essential information in the partnership. The provider refrains from telling the patient exactly what to do and realizes that the patient can have his or her own effective solutions to problems that arise during the process of behavioral change. Threatening, convincing, arguing, demanding, and cajoling are all ineffective tactics when counseling patients on behavior change. An example of a threat is: "If you don't exercise regularly, you will keep gaining weight and suffer a heart attack." A more collaborative approach to motivate someone to begin an exercise program is to ask, "How would your life be different if you were exercising regularly?" Eliciting information from patients and building on their statements helps them feel heard, understood, and validated

When collaborating with a patient to help start a new healthy behavior, there is a five-step cycle that can help providers conduct coaching conversations that are motivating, inspiring, and in line with the 5 As of behavioral counseling.[27] The five steps are: (1) express empathy; (2) align motivation; (3) build confidence and self-efficacy; (4) co-create SMART goals; and, (5) set accountability. Then, the cycle starts again with expressing empathy. The five-step cycle of collaboration is compatible with the 5 As. They are used in concert (Figure 41-1).

Expressing empathy is the first step of the five-step cycle. Research shows that physicians who score highly on the Jefferson Scale of Empathy have patients with lower levels of LDL cholesterol and hemoglobin A_{1C}.[28] Making sure to be fully present and mindful during the behavior change counseling session is critical. This might require a provider to elicit his or her own relaxation response by taking a few deep breaths before the session, or by entering a mindful state through opening awareness in a non-judgmental way and finding a sense of calm prior to the session. With an open and quiet mind, the provider is able to listen fully to the patient's story and to provide useful, individualized advice after thoughtful questioning. Fully understanding the patient's situation is important to increase the patient's trust in the provider. After listening carefully to the sentences, words, tone of voice, body language, cadence, and facial expressions of the patient, the provider can respond with reflections that demonstrate to the patient that he or she was listening, that he or she followed the patient's story and train of thought, and that he or she understood the patient's emotional state. As Theodore Roosevelt said, "No one cares what you have to say until they know how much you care."

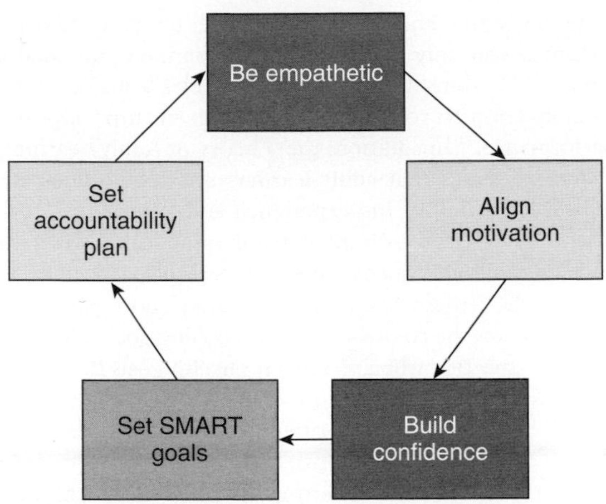

Figure 41-1. Five-step cycle as a coaching model. *(From Frates EP, Moore MA, Lopez CN, et al. Coaching for behavior change in physiatry.* Am J Phys Med Rehabil. *2011;90(12):1074–1082. Reprinted with permission.)*

This first step of expressing empathy is the basis for creating a meaningful connection and for forming a therapeutic partnership for behavioral change.

The second step is to align motivation. In this step, the provider uses motivational interviewing (MI) to help a patient discover and declare his or her own motivation for change.[29] Step 1 of the cycle emphasizes empathy and fully understanding the patient while taking a non-judgmental approach. In Step 2, the patient is encouraged to express their own *change talk*. Change talk is language that provides the pros for change, the cons for remaining the same, the desire for change, the ability to change, the reasons for change, and the need for change. One of the main goals of MI is to evoke change talk.

Through MI, a clinician can elicit a patient's reasons for change. The clinician's role is then, through questioning and listening, to illustrate the discrepancy between a patient's current behavior and his/her health goals. MI is influenced by the Stage of Change Theory, Rogerian Patient-centered Therapy, and cognitive-behavioral therapy (CBT). Yet, distinct from CBT, MI conceptualizes motivation as a constantly changing state. Distinct from Rogerian therapy in its patient-centered approach, it differs, in that it is directive. MI is also goal-directed, through negotiations between the clinician and the patient. During times of elevated motivation, CBT skills may be integrated with MI, to apply action goals, such as cutting back on the number of cigarettes per day, or to target barriers to achieving smoking cessation goals, such as using stress management practices to alleviate stress-related smoking triggers.

Underlying MI are the beliefs that motivation is a fluctuating state, in which ambivalence is a welcome and important part of change, and every patient has a potential for change. MI goals include: (1) building a patient's intrinsic motivation to change (e.g., beginning with an exercise routine or quitting smoking), and (2) resolving ambivalence about change (e.g., creating and amplifying the discrepancy between the patient's current behavior and their expressed goals). For example, a patient says that they want to get 8 hours of sleep a night, to feel well rested, but starting the next day consistently goes to bed 6 hours before their alarm will ring. Lastly, four MI principles are: (1) express empathy (through skillful reflective listening); (2) develop discrepancy (ask evocative questions to enable the patients to express reasons for change); (3) roll with resistance (avoid arguing for change); (4) support self-efficacy (the patient's belief, perceived confidence in his/her ability to change). A 2010 meta-analysis of 14 studies that compared MI with brief advice and usual care for smoking cessation concluded that MI yielded an increase in quitting[30] (RR = 1.27; CI = 1.14–1.42).

Some basic skills used in MI, can be recalled through the mnemonic "OARS": asking Open-ended questions, stating Affirmations, using Reflections, and giving Summaries. MI involves establishing a connection and exploring the patients feelings, beliefs (e.g., hopelessness), and values (e.g., importance of longevity) to help them work through ambivalence or ever-changing motivations. This includes addressing his/her reasons for their behaviors; the relation of behaviors to his/her values and goals; and build his/her confidence.[29] Another technique used in MI is to elicit-provide-elicit. The provider elicits what information the patient would like to hear or what topics interest them. In this way, the provider checks in with the patient on how much the patient already knows; this diminishes wasting time by supplying the patient with information that he or she already has. With this method, the provider provides that requested information. After imparting knowledge, the provider asks what the patient learned. This ensures a collaborative relationship in which the patient is an active member. It also makes sure that the provider was successful in explaining the concepts, and checks in on what the patient was able to comprehend and recall. MI is an effective skill that can empower patients. It helps patients align their own motivation for change. MI has been studied in weight loss and stroke, and has shown promise in many other areas (including HIV care, dental outcomes, alcohol use, tobacco use, and physical inactivity).[31–33]

Step 3 builds confidence and self-efficacy. Confidence is the feeling of strength that comes from a belief in one's abilities. Self-efficacy is the belief that one can complete a task successfully. In general, being confident and believing in one's self will help patients persist in their process of behavioral change. Feeling assured that one can do a certain activity or conquer a specific challenge (such as taking a walk at lunch time), is more specific and requires focused work on that particular task. To build self-efficacy, the patient needs to feel comfortable with the difficulty of the specific activity and to feel strong enough, mentally and physically, to meet that challenge. By practicing, patients build self-efficacy. By recalling times when they performed the target activity in the past, the patient can also build self-efficacy. This step invites the provider to use positive psychology, a strengths-based approach, and appreciative inquiry to help the patient move forward on their behavior change journey. Seligman,[34] considered one of the founders of the field of positive psychology, promotes the process of bringing out the patient's individual strengths. By identifying his or her strengths, the patient acknowledges the power inside him or her, and this helps to build confidence.[34] Finding ways to use these signature strengths in the pursuit of health goals and in the behavior change process can be an effective and rewarding technique to propel patients forward.

By asking questions that elicit a positive emotion, the provider is setting the stage for creative thinking and brainstorming that are both important in a behavior change counseling session. Positive emotions include love, joy, gratitude, serenity, interest, hope, pride, amusement, inspiration, and awe.[35] Frederickson's[36] broaden-and-build model highlights the fact that positive emotions can help people stimulate new ideas, gain new perspective, as well as appreciate the broad picture in a situation. Thus, positive emotions can help people build enduring personal resources.[36] Asking a question that explores a positive experience, such as "What was the highlight of your week?" "When was a time that you reached a goal? Tell me about that," or "What is going really well in your life right now?" will serve to bring out the positive core, and corresponding emotions, in a person.

Accentuating the positive core is a key concept in Appreciative Inquiry (AI), an interviewing style that uses positive experiences in the present to create positive experiences in the future. In this method of interviewing, the idea is that appreciating and acknowledging the positive aspects of a person, situation, or organization brings forward more positive experiences.[37] This work has been used in the healthcare setting, and on an organizational and individual level with success. With AI, the provider works to build confidence by defining the focus or goal in the behavior change process, then discovering the best of what is, after that, dreaming about what might be, then designing a plan for the future, and finally, experiencing destiny by learning from and adjusting to what unfolds. The goal is to define, discover, dream, design, and deliver. A study using AI with dementia patients demonstrated positive results[38] and a recent review of the medical literature revealed that AI was effective in multiple domains, including care of patients with dementia, elderly patients at the time of discharge from the hospital, and use within medical practices.[39] Building confidence and self-efficacy is an important step in the cycle and there are many different ways to accomplish this.

Step 4 is to co-create SMART goals. SMART goals are specific, measurable, action-oriented, realistic, and time-sensitive.

S = Specific: Goals should be straightforward and emphasize what you want to happen. Specific is the "What, Why, and How" of the SMART model.

M = Measurable: Goals with measurable outcomes should be selected, so that you can see the results of change. How will you know when you reach your goal?

A = Action-oriented: Identify action goals and specify what you will do.

R = Realistic: The goal needs to be something you can strive toward and achieve.

T = Time-sensitive: Set a time frame for the goal—initially very short term (i.e., this week).

Co-creation is used here to remind the provider to make sure the patient agrees with the goal. A provider can check to see if a goal is SMART by asking five questions: Is this a goal that is detailed and explicitly stated? How will the patient measure the outcome of the goal? Will the patient be doing something in particular to achieve the goal? How likely is it that the patient can reach the goal in the stated time frame? What is the timeline for meeting the goal? To answer these questions, the provider must be connecting, communicating, and collaborating with the patient, as the patient is the only one who can determine if the goal is realistic. Working toward a goal provides a major source of motivation to reach the goal, which in turn, improves performance.[40] In addition, the Theory of Adult Learning, *andragogy*, states that adult learners are autonomous and self-directed, full of life experience and knowledge, goal-oriented, relevancy-oriented, and practical.[41] Keeping andragogy in mind when co-creating goals helps the provider to treat the patient like an adult learner and a partner. It also facilitates the co-creation of compelling goals. Research demonstrates that when patients set health goals that match their life goals, they are more likely to reach their health goals.[42] Setting goals helps patients to focus on the behavior change process and to prioritize it.

Step 5 in the cycle is setting accountability. This step ensures that patients are working on their goals. In the 5 As, this is consistent with the fifth A, for arranging follow-up. The patient needs to feel that this is important enough to the provider that he or she will check in on the goals the next time they meet. Prior to the next follow-up visit, a provider can check in by e-mail, by phone, or by postcard. This can be accomplished with the help of administrative staff at the office. Helping the patient identify a buddy for the behavior change will allow for accountability between visits. A family member or friend can serve as the behavior-change buddy. If the buddy has similar goals and can take walks with the patient or start consuming more vegetables at the same time as the patient, it adds another level of importance to the goals for the patient and the buddy. Using a tracking system, such as a pedometer or wearable device, can be a useful method of providing feedback and thus setting accountability. A written log can be as effective as a method that uses the latest technology. The method must match the patient preferences. Thus, setting accountability is an important part of the five-step cycle.

After setting accountability, the cycle starts again with empathy. Empathy propels the cycle forward. When the patient returns for the follow-up visit, the provider needs to be open, non-judgmental, and supportive, regardless of the success or lack of success the patient experienced. If there was failure, then the goal is to learn from the failure and move forward. Approaching the process with a growth mindset allows patients to take risks, try new things, and challenge themselves without the fear of shame, blame, and guilt, which often comes with failure. With a growth mindset, failures or mis-steps are opportunities to learn and grow.[43] Each week, there are usually moments of success or positivity and asking about these in the follow-up appointment is important. "What went well this week?" is a great way to start a follow-up session. The patients usually report on their failures right away and often neglect the small successes. Expressing empathy after listening to the successes and setbacks that the patient experienced when trying to achieve the goal is a priority for follow-up sessions with a patient seeking to change a behavior. Empathy is key when counseling on behavior change.

Behavior change is not a quick fix, and it is not easy. It takes collaboration, connection, time, patience, understanding, and an organized approach that will help patients stay engaged in their behavior change plan.

CASE 1

Mrs. M, a 57-year-old, overweight female with a history of depression was recently informed by her primary care doctor that she is pre-diabetic. She is divorced and has two adult children in college. Mrs. M quit smoking 15 years ago. Over the past 10 years, her weight has been increasing, although she occasionally goes on a diet and loses 15 pounds but regains the weight within 3 months. She comes to the office today because she is anxious about her new diagnosis of pre-diabetes. Since she watched her uncle suffer with diabetes for years, she is afraid of having her lower leg amputated like her uncle did.

After listening attentively, the provider expressed empathy by reflecting on what she heard. "It sounds like you are anxious because you are afraid that the diagnosis of pre-diabetes means you are on your way to a below-the-knee amputation, and with that, your life will change dramatically." After that, the patient nods her head sheepishly. Then, the provider asks her an open-ended question, "What could you do to control your blood sugars?" She answers by reporting, "My primary care doctor said that if I lose weight I could reverse the pre-diabetes and avoid the diagnosis of diabetes altogether, but I have tried to lose weight for 10 years, and I am afraid that I will never succeed." The provider notes that the patient is in the contemplative stage of change. She keeps listening attentively, and the patient continues, "If I could stick with eating more vegetables and fewer sweets and if I could find an exercise that I like, I might be able to lose weight and keep it off." Then, the provider uses another reflection. "If you can eat healthy foods in healthy portions and start exercising regularly, then you might be able to control your weight and stop worrying about getting an amputation, which is pretty powerful motivation to stick with a healthy lifestyle." Mrs. M. then reflects and says, "I have never had such a powerful motivator before. I really don't want an amputation. I wish I could find a plan that worked for me to lose weight. I want to do it. I just don't think I can." By reminding Mrs. M that she successfully quit smoking, the provider points out that the patient has been successful with behavior change in the past. She admits that it took several attempts for her to be successful at quitting smoking and it was not until she had a powerful motivator, which was her teenager starting to smoke her cigarettes, that she was able to quit. She says that the fear of amputation is equally as powerful so she thinks this time maybe she can be successful with her weight loss attempts. The provider reviews the past successes and failures of the weight loss attempts and highlights the importance of learning from the failed attempts. The provider also asks if she wants to hear about research on pre-diabetes and lifestyle interventions. Because the patient expresses an interest, the provider shares some data and statistics with her. After checking in with the patient to see how much of the discussion resonated with the patient, the provider learns that the patient is very interested in exercise, specifically. She had used walking with friends to help her quit smoking. With that cue, the provider asks if the patient wants to learn about some research on exercise and its ability to reduce anxiety levels. The patient is eager to hear about that topic and is able to demonstrate a clear understanding of how exercise could help her blood glucose as well as help reduce her anxiety level, which was the reason for her visit.

Together, the patient and provider create a SMART goal for the week. Originally, Mrs. M says she wants to walk for 1 hour for 7 days this coming week, because she read that people need to be active for 60 minutes each day to lose weight. The provider asks her how realistic this goal is, given her work schedule. Then, the patient remembers that she stopped walking because her old sneakers were bothering her bunions and her feet were hurting with each step. So, they co-created a SMART goal for this week, which is for Mrs. M. to buy sneakers that fit her feet and feel good when she walks. After purchasing appropriate sneakers, Mrs. B is to walk for one 20-minute session on Wednesday, which is her day off. They set accountability by making the follow-up appointment. At the end of the appointment, Mrs. M says her anxiety seems better already, since she has a doable plan to control her weight, and she is hopeful that she will be successful this time.

At the follow-up visit, Mrs. M proudly wears her new sneakers, and the provider congratulates her on making the time to go to the store and buy the sneakers. Although she was only able to walk for 10 minutes, because she said it started to rain, the provider recognizes her effort to meet her goal and reinforces the fact that walking for 10 minutes is better than not walking at all. She asks Mrs. M how it felt when she was walking, and Mrs. M reports that she liked walking outside and being in nature on a trail near her house.

Mrs. M gradually increases her walking to 5 days a week for 1 hour each session. She starts noticing that her clothes are feeling baggy. Also, she starts changing her diet to add more vegetables, to cut down on desserts and to monitor the glycemic index of her foods. After 3 months, she has lost 15 pounds and she slowly continues to lose weight. She takes a cooking class at the local community center and starts eating healthy meals at home, while enjoying the preparation and creation of delicious food, following a Mediterranean dietary pattern of eating, with plenty of vegetables, nuts, seeds, healthy protein, and whole grains. After a year, her blood sugars are consistently in the normal range, and her BMI is normal.

SMOKING PREVALENCE AND CHARACTERISTICS OF SMOKERS

In 2012, 18.1% of adults in the United States were current smokers.[44] The prevalence of smoking differs by gender and race/ethnicity and even by socioeconomic status; specifically, individuals who have lower incomes and fewer years of education and those with a mental illness have the highest rates of smoking. Individuals who smoke have higher rates of depression and mental illness; 36.5% across psychiatric disorders,[45] and smoking rates are estimated at 53% among individuals with serious mental illness. While counseling is effective, first-line medications in conjunction with counseling can increase abstinence rates by 200–300% over counseling alone.[46] In considering smoking patterns, the issue of electronic cigarettes (known as e-cigs) is also important. E-cigs are electronic devices that deliver a nicotine vapor. Rates of e-cig use are increasing; the most common reasons for use of e-cigs are to try to cut down/quit smoking or for use in places where combustible cigarettes are not allowed. The value of e-cigs as a significant harm reduction or to help smokers stop smoking is unknown.[47]

Quitting Cigarette Smoking

Most smokers begin by the age of 18, and the majority of smokers want to quit. Each year, two-thirds of adult smokers try to quit,[48] but only 6% will become non-smokers, if unassisted.[49] Quitting is indeed a process. There are many different ways that a smoker can engage in quitting; individuals can quit by going "cold turkey" or by cutting back and tapering. Smokers cut back/taper by smoking only in certain places (e.g., no smoking in the car, or in certain rooms in the home), only during certain times (e.g., only after work hours), or only a certain number of cigarettes smoked by day. Many individuals find it helpful to record one's smoking, to better understand his/her smoking habits and associated patterns, and to set up a cutting back/tapering schedule. Daily monitoring of one's cigarette intake can be a great tool to facilitate a quit. Negative emotions (e.g., depression, anxiety, stress) complicate smoking cessation attempts. Individuals often use smoking to help regulate these emotions; in turn, quitting attempts, in particular, withdrawal symptoms, can exacerbate these negative emotions. However smoking cessation has been shown in many studies to improve anxiety, depression, negative affect, and stress.[50]

Smoking Cessation Behavioral Treatments

The United States Public Health Service guidelines, recommend that all smokers receive a brief clinician-delivered model, the 5 As: Ask, Advise, Assess, Assist, and Arrange follow-up.[51] The 5 As increase the likelihood of smoking cessation. Studies report that clinician-delivered rates of assist (recommending and/or providing counseling or prescriptions) are low, which is unfortunate because these are the most impactful for patients.[52–55]

Smokers may obtain treatment in individual or group settings and treatment can be delivered via an in-person counselor, or with other modalities, as stand-alone or adjunctive treatment, including telephone-based counseling, text messaging, web-based programs, and phone apps. Here, we discuss CBT and mindfulness approaches to smoking cessation.

Cognitive-Behavioral Therapy Approaches

Cognitive-behavioral treatments focus on building an awareness of and adaptation for negative thinking patterns and associated emotions and behaviors. CBT strategies for cessation include:

- Tracking daily intake
- Identification and management of triggers, including withdrawal symptoms. A simple strategy for this is ACE, Avoid, Change and Escape, in anticipating or coping with a trigger. Avoid: "How can you avoid triggers?"; Change: "What can you do to change a situation to lessen your chances of being around smoking?;" Escape: "How do you get away from a situation in which you are being exposed to smoking?"
- Social support (enhancing one's emotional and smoking-specific support)
- Emotional regulation (focusing on the role of mood changes, in relation to smoking and quitting attempts)
- Stress management and relaxation training (using strategies such as meditation and deep breathing)
- Environmental modification (creating smoke-free environments or decreasing exposure to smokers and cigarette smoking)
- Coping with cravings. Many smokers experience physical and psychological urges to smoke, in particular in the earlier stages of quitting. Stress management and mind–body strategies—such as diaphragmatic breathing, guided imagery, body scanning, yoga progressive muscle relaxation, brief meditation, or mindful walking—can be used to deal with these urges. The "4 Ds" can also be helpful to remember and use: Delay—take a moment; Drink (water); Distraction—focus on or do something else; and Deep—breathing.

Mind-Body Approaches or Mindfulness

Mindfulness involves purposeful attention, and non-judgmental awareness of present experiences.[56] Mindfulness exercises (mindful meditation, body scan, mindful walking) can increase awareness and acceptance of smoking cues, which, in turn, helps smokers tolerate smoking triggers and choose behaviors/responses other than smoking as a response to smoking cues. Focusing on this experience, a smoker may learn that an urge became fleeting. Mindfulness programs help smokers use mindfulness skills to manage negative emotions and thoughts about cues and have been found to be efficacious to help smokers quit.[57,58]

Smoking Cessation Medications

The most effective way to quit smoking is to combine counseling treatment with FDA-approved smoking cessation medications. A careful psychiatric and medical intake, as well as a review of previous medication use, will determine the most effective medication and dose. Smoking cessation medications can be used for smokers with varying levels of quit motivation[59] during the process of quitting. Specifically, using this combination of evidence-based behavioral treatment and medication approximately doubles abstinence rates.[60] Currently, there are eight first-line medications for smoking cessation. Five are types of nicotine therapy (patch, lozenge, gum, inhaler, and spray), bupropion (Zyban, Wellbutrin), and varenicline. Nicotine-replacement therapy (NRT) involves using "clean" nicotine substitutes that target withdrawal symptoms. Bupropion SR (Zyban, Wellbutrin SR) is an antidepressant that inhibits re-uptake of dopamine and norepinephrine, reducing cravings for tobacco. Varenicline (Chantix) is a non-nicotine medication that interferes with nicotine receptors; it has both agonist and antagonist function—blocking pleasure in conjunction with withdrawal symptoms. In 2009, the FDA published a public health advisory on the neuropsychiatric side effects of varenicline and bupropion but recent research suggests that these fears may have been over-stated prompting an upcoming FDA review.[46] A recent Cochrane Database review found that varenicline and combination NRT were superior to mono NRT or bupropion.[61] In the largest smoking cessation study to date, with over 8000 smokers randomized, and first head-to-head comparison of all first-line smoking cessation aids in smokers with and without mental illness, varenicline, bupropion, and nicotine patch were each more effective than placebo, with varenicline more effective than bupropion, and NRT, and none had greater neuropsychiatric safety signal than placebo in either cohort. Quitting rates are consistently significantly higher for smokers who use varenicline than for other monotherapies.[46,62–65]

REFERENCES

Access the reference list online at https://expertconsult.inkling.com/.

Complementary Medicine and Natural Medications

42

Felicia A. Smith, M.D.
David Mischoulon, M.D., Ph.D.

OVERVIEW

Complementary and alternative medical (CAM) therapies constitute a diverse spectrum of practices and beliefs in current medical practice. The National Institutes of Health has defined CAM as "healthcare practices outside the realm of conventional medicine, which are yet to be validated using scientific methods."[1] The term *natural medications* refers to medications derived from natural products that are not approved by the U.S. Food and Drug Administration (FDA) for their proposed indication.[2] Natural medications under the category of CAM may include hormones, vitamins, plants, herbs, fatty acids, amino acid derivatives, and homeopathic preparations, among others. Although natural medications have been used for thousands of years, their use in the United States has increased dramatically over the past two decades.[3,4] The consultation psychiatrist must therefore be informed about these medications to provide comprehensive patient care. This chapter provides an overview of the use of natural medications in psychiatry. Issues pertaining to general safety and effectiveness are discussed first, followed by a more specific look at some of the remedies used for mood disorders, anxiety and sleep disorders, menstrual disorders, and dementia. The final section is devoted to a description of two non-medication alternative therapies: acupuncture and hypnosis.

EFFICACY AND SAFETY

Despite the increase in both government and industry sponsorship of clinical research involving natural medications, data regarding efficacy and safety are still limited.[5] Moreover, the safety and efficacy of combining natural medications with more conventional medications remains unclear.[5] This situation is very important to the consultation psychiatrist because of the prevalence of polypharmacy often seen in inpatient medical settings. It is also noteworthy that patients frequently do not disclose use of CAM therapies to their physician,[4] thereby making it essential to ask patients specific questions about use of prescribed and over-the-counter medications. Finally, preparations of natural medications often vary in purity, quality, potency, efficacy, and side effects. The remainder of this chapter outlines what is currently known in this regard for a few such natural medications.

MOOD DISORDERS

Omega-3 fatty acids, St. John's wort (SJW), *S*-adenosyl-methionine (SAMe), folic acid, vitamin B_{12}, and inositol have all been used for mood disorders. Here we describe the efficacy, possible mechanisms of action, dosing, adverse effects, and drug interactions of each of these medications. Because of the nature of consultation psychiatry, a particular emphasis is placed on the interface between their psychiatric and other medical uses, as well as on drug interactions.

Omega-3 fatty acids are polyunsaturated lipids derived from fish oil that have been shown to have benefits in a variety of health domains including rheumatoid arthritis, Crohn's disease, ulcerative colitis, psoriasis, and systemic lupus erythematosus.[6] Cardioprotective effects have been demonstrated, as have several neuropsychiatric benefits. Eicosapentaenoic acid (EPA) and docosahexaenoic acid (DHA) are thought to be psychotropically active omega-3 fatty acids.[2] Lower rates of depression and bipolar disorder have been detected in countries where more fish is consumed, suggesting that omega-3 fatty acids may play a protective role in these disorders.[7] Omega-3 fatty acids also may have a role in the treatment of both bipolar disorder and unipolar depression. About 30, mostly positive, studies on patients with unipolar depression have been reported.[8] Although efficacy studies in bipolar illness have been more mixed,[9–12] most of the benefit in bipolar illness may be related to alleviating or preventing depression rather than mania.[13] In fact, there have been reports of cycling in bipolar patients who take omega-3 preparations without concomitant mood stabilizers,[14] so caution is warranted when treating bipolar patients. Recent evidence suggests that overweight patients with elevated serum inflammatory biomarkers may be especially responsive to EPA.[15] Similarly, the omega-3s may prevent depression in individuals taking interferon therapy for hepatitis.[16] Mixed results have been shown in the areas of postpartum depression[17–20] and schizophrenia.[21–23]

Although their mechanism of action is not completely clear, omega-3 fatty acids may function in the same way as mood stabilizers, by inhibiting G-protein signal transduction via reduced hydrolysis of phosphatidylinositol and other membrane phospholipids.[24] Other proposed mechanisms include neuronal membrane stabilization and anti-inflammatory effects.[24] Commercially available preparations of omega-3 fatty acids vary in composition, and recent evidence suggests that the optimal ratio of EPA to DHA is approximately 3 : 2 or at least 60% EPA.[25] Psychotropically active dosages are generally thought to be in the range of 1 to 2 g/day, with the major side effect being dosage-related gastrointestinal (GI) distress.[8] There is a theoretical risk of increased bleeding, particularly at doses >3 g/day, so concomitant use of high-dose NSAIDs or anticoagulants is not recommended,[8] though recent evidence suggests that these concerns may have been exaggerated.[26] In sum, the use of omega-3 fatty acids is promising, particularly given the range of potential benefits and the relatively low toxicity seen thus far. However, larger studies are still needed.

St. John's wort (*Hypericum perforatum* L.) has generally been shown to be more effective than placebo in the treatment of mild to moderate depression,[14,27] and as effective as low-dose tricyclic antidepressants (TCAs) (e.g., imipramine 75 mg, maprotiline 75 mg, or amitriptyline 75 mg).[2,14,27] Data comparing SJW and selective serotonin re-uptake inhibitors (SSRIs) are more mixed,[27] though some believe that depression severity may have contributed to some negative studies.[2,5,14] Although hypericin is thought to be the main antidepressant ingredient in SJW, polycyclic phenols, pseudohypericin, and hyperforin are also thought to be active ingredients. Possible mechanisms of action include the inhibition of cytokines, a decrease in serotonin receptor density, a decrease in re-uptake of neurotransmitters, and monoamine oxidase inhibitor (MAOI) activity.[2,5] SJW should not be combined with SSRIs because it has mild MAOI activity and there is a risk of serotonin syndrome, but no special diet is required for the patient on SJW.[14] The metabolism of SJW is thought to be hepatic. Suggested dosages range from 900 to 1800 mg three times per day depending on the preparation, and adverse effects include dry mouth, dizziness, constipation, and phototoxicity. A switch to mania in patients with bipolar disorder may also occur.[14,28] Finally, a number of drug–drug interactions with SJW are particularly noteworthy for the consultation psychiatrist. Because hyperforin induces cytochrome P450 (CYP) 3A4 expression, therapeutic activity of the following medications may be reduced: warfarin, cyclosporine, oral contraceptives, theophylline, digoxin, and indinavir.[2,5,14] Transplant rejections have been reported as a result of interactions between SJW and cyclosporine;[14] therefore, transplant recipients should not use SJW. Individuals with human immunodeficiency virus infection and on protease inhibitors should also avoid SJW because of drug interactions. In conclusion, SJW appears to be better than placebo and equivalent to low-dose TCAs for the treatment of mild depression. It may also perform comparably with SSRIs, but more data are needed. It may not be as effective for more severe forms of depression. Care should be taken because of the drug–drug interactions mentioned earlier.

In dosages of up to 3200 mg/day, SAMe has been shown to elevate mood in depressed patients. Meta-analyses and comprehensive reviews support antidepressant efficacy of SAMe when compared with placebo and TCAs.[29–32] However, many studies have used IM and IV preparations, as well as oral SAMe; early oral preparations of SAMe were unstable and rapid decomposition may have resulted in less robust efficacy findings.[29] Recent comparisons with SSRIs have suggested similar efficacy, but have been limited by high placebo response rates.[32] Current oral preparations, although tosylated for improved shelf life, may nonetheless require high dosages for adequate bioavailability—in some instances, as much as 2000 to 3000 mg/day; the medication is relatively expensive, and the out-of-pocket cost may be prohibitive to some.[14,29,30]

S-adenosyl-methionine is the principal methyl donor in the one-carbon cycle, and SAMe levels depend on availability of the vitamins folate and B_{12}. SAMe donates methyl groups to hormones, neurotransmitters, nucleic acids, proteins, and phospholipids. Thus, SAMe has been proposed to work as an antidepressant by providing methyl groups in the reactions that result in the synthesis of acetylcholine, serotonin, and dopamine.[33] Potential adverse effects are relatively minor and include anxiety, agitation, a switch to mania, insomnia, dry mouth, bowel changes, and anorexia.[29,30,33] Sweating, dizziness, palpitations, and headaches have also been reported.[29,30,33] At least one case has been reported of suspected serotonin syndrome when SAMe was combined with clomipramine in an elderly woman.[34] No significant drug–drug interactions have been reported, and there is no apparent hepatotoxicity.[29,30,33] SAMe, therefore, is a natural medication that shows promise as an antidepressant. It appears to be relatively safe and is without significant interactions thus far, making it a particularly good candidate for augmentation therapy. One open study and one controlled study have demonstrated benefit from open SAMe augmentation in SSRI partial responders.[35,36] Recent evidence also suggests a gender-related effect favoring men, with regard to alleviation of depression and sexual dysfunction.[37] Further study, particularly comparisons against newer antidepressants, will help clarify issues of efficacy and safety.

Folate and B_{12} vitamins obtained in the diet, play important roles in the synthesis of central nervous system (CNS) neurotransmitters (e.g., serotonin, dopamine, and norepinephrine). Sequelae of folate and vitamin B_{12} deficiencies include a variety of neuropsychiatric and general medical conditions (e.g., macrocytic anemia, neuropathy, cognitive dysfunction or dementia, and depression). Folate deficiency may result from inadequate dietary intake, malabsorption, inborn errors of metabolism, or an increased demand (e.g., as seen with pregnancy, infancy, bacterial overgrowth, and rapid cellular turnover).[33,38]

Certain drugs may also cause folate deficiency. These include anticonvulsants, oral contraceptives, sulfasalazine, methotrexate, triamterene, trimethoprim, pyrimethamine, and alcohol.[39] Vitamin B_{12} deficiency states may also result from inadequate dietary intake, malabsorption, impaired utilization, and interactions with other drugs. Included in such drugs are colchicine, H_2 blockers, metformin, nicotine, oral contraceptive pills, cholestyramine, K-Dur, and zidovudine.[39] Folate deficiency may also hinder antidepressant response,[40] and folate supplementation may be a beneficial adjunct to SSRI-refractory depression.[41] Vitamin B_{12} deficiency, in turn, may cause an earlier age of onset of depression.[2] The recommended daily dosage of vitamin B_{12} is 6 μg, and that of folate is 400 μg. Because both vitamins are involved in the synthesis of CNS neurotransmitters, adequate levels provide optimal neurotransmitter synthesis that may aid in reversing depression. Finally, folate may mask vitamin B_{12} deficiency by correcting macrocytic anemia while neuropathy continues, so vitamin B_{12} levels should be routinely measured when high dosages of folate are given. Folate may also reduce the efficacy of phenytoin, methotrexate, and phenobarbital.[42] In summary, correction of folate and B_{12} deficiencies may improve depression or augment other antidepressant therapy. The prescription form of 5-methyltetrahydrofolate (5-MTHF; Deplin) may present a desirable treatment option for depressed patients; 5-MTHF is thought to penetrate the blood–brain barrier more readily than other folate forms, and it may, in theory, deliver more of the active product to its site of action.[38] 5-MTHF may also bypass genetic anomalies in the enzyme methylene tetrahydrofolate reductase (MTHFR), which can prevent the adequate conversion of other folate forms into 5-MTHF. A recent double-blind randomized controlled trial (RCT) of Deplin augmentation for SSRI non-responders suggested benefit with 15 mg/day of Deplin added to the baseline antidepressant.[43] Deplin is FDA-approved for treatment or prevention of vitamin deficiencies, and requires a prescription. There are preparations, such as Cerefolin and Cerefolin-NAC, that contain additional nutrients (vitamins B_2, B_6, B_{12}, and N-acetylcysteine), and may have benefits in dementia, but rigorous evidence is still lacking. Psychiatrists should be mindful of potential deficiency states (as outlined here) and should check serum levels in patients (such as elderly patients, the medically ill, alcoholics, or those who have not responded to antidepressant treatment) at risk for deficiencies.

Inositol, a natural isomer of glucose, is present in common foods. It has been found in small studies to be effective in the treatment of depression, panic disorder, obsessive–compulsive disorder (OCD), bulimia, binge-eating disorder, and possibly bipolar depression.[44–48] Recent work supports efficacy in pediatric bipolar disorder when combined with omega-3 fatty acids.[49] Effective dosages range from 12 to 18 g/day. Negative monotherapy trials with inositol have been run with patients with schizophrenia, dementia, attention deficit hyperactivity disorder, premenstrual dysphoric disorder, autism, and electroconvulsive therapy-induced cognitive impairment.[5,50] Augmentation studies of inositol with SSRIs in patients with depression and OCD have been mostly negative.[51–53] One crossover comparison of inositol against fluvoxamine for panic disorder suggested similar efficacy for both agents.[46] Inositol is a polyol precursor in brain second-messenger systems that may reverse desensitization of serotonin receptors.[2,5] Mild adverse effects include GI upset, headache, dizziness, sedation, and insomnia. There is no apparent toxicity or known drug interactions at this time.[2,5] Treatment with inositol for the indications mentioned here currently appears safe and remains promising.

ANXIOLYTICS AND HYPNOTICS

Three natural agents are often used for their anxiolytic and hypnotic properties: valerian, melatonin, and kava. Valerian (*Valeriana officinalis*) is a sedating plant extract that has been used for over 2000 years. It is thought to promote natural sleep after several weeks of use by decreasing sleep latency and by improving overall sleep quality. The effects on slow-wave sleep increase with time. Valerian is thought to work by decreasing gamma-aminobutyric acid (GABA) breakdown.[2,5] Sedative effects are dosage-related, with usual dosages in the range of 450 to 600 mg about 2 hours before bedtime. Dependence has not been an issue, nor has daytime drowsiness. Adverse effects, thought to be uncommon, include blurry vision, GI symptoms, headache, and dystonia. Meta-analyses have questioned valerian's hypnotic efficacy; some studies may have been limited by the powerful and distinctive smell of valerian, which renders double-blinding more difficult.[54] Because of potential hepatotoxicity, valerian should be avoided in patients with liver dysfunction. Major drug interactions have not been reported. Although valerian has been used as a hypnotic for many years (in pediatric and elderly populations as well as adults) with relatively few reported adverse effects, more trials are needed to further quantify its efficacy and safety.

Melatonin is a hormone made in the pineal gland that has gained popularity for its use by travelers to avoid jet lag. It is derived from serotonin and is thought to play a role in the organization of circadian rhythms via interaction with the suprachiasmatic nucleus.[55] Melatonin generally facilitates falling asleep within 1 hour, no matter what time of day it is taken. Optimal dosages, although this is controversial, are thought to be in the range of 0.25 to 0.30 mg/day. Some preparations, however, contain as much as 5 mg of melatonin.[2,5] There are prolonged-release forms of melatonin that may provide more sustained sleep. Daytime sleepiness and confusion have been noted with high dosages. Other reported adverse effects include decreased sex drive, retinal damage, hypothermia, and fertility problems. Moreover, melatonin is contraindicated in pregnancy and in immunocompromised patients.[2,5] There are few reports of drug–drug interactions. In conclusion, melatonin is a promising and relatively safe hypnotic, probably best used in people with insomnia secondary to circadian disturbances, and potentially useful in children with sleep difficulties. Caution should be taken in patients at risk, as noted.

Kava (*Piper methysticum*) is derived from a root originating in the Polynesian Islands. Although it is believed to have a mild anxiolytic effect, study results have been mixed. The mechanism of action is attributed to kavapyrones, which are central muscle relaxants involved in GABA receptor binding and norepinephrine uptake inhibition.[2,5] The suggested dosage is 60 to 120 mg/day, with GI upset, headaches, and dizziness being the major adverse effects. Toxic reactions, however, have been seen at high dosages or with prolonged use and include ataxia, hair loss, respiratory problems, yellowing of the skin, and vision problems. Even more worrisome are reports of severe, sometimes fatal, hepatotoxicity, including some requiring liver transplantation.[2,5] For this reason, kava has been banned in certain parts of the world. Recent investigations suggest that the toxicity may have been due to molds developing as a result of a long time interval between harvest and preparation.[56] Although kava appears to be somewhat efficacious in the treatment of mild anxiety, current concerns about safety make cautious use essential. It should be used only under a physician's supervision, preferably for no longer than 3 months (with monitoring of liver function tests), and should be avoided by people who are taking other potentially hepatotoxic drugs or who have a history of recent alcohol abuse or liver disease of any sort.

PREMENSTRUAL AND MENOPAUSAL SYMPTOMS

Black cohosh (*Cimicifuga racemosa*) at a dosage of 40 mg/day has been shown to reduce physical and psychological menopausal symptoms.[57] Active ingredients are thought to be triterpenoids, isoflavones, and aglycones, which may participate in suppression of luteinizing hormone in the pituitary gland.[2,5] Mild side effects include headache, dizziness, GI upset, and weight gain. In the past few years, a few reports have emerged of possible liver toxicity, convulsions, and cardiovascular problems, although some have argued that these toxicities could not be conclusively linked to black cohosh.[58] Black cohosh is not recommended for individuals who are pregnant or who have heart disease or hypertension. More data are needed to further specify beneficial effects as well as safety profiles.

COGNITION AND DEMENTIA

Ginkgo biloba comes from the seed of the ginkgo tree and has been a part of Chinese medicine for thousands of years. It has generally been used for the treatment of impaired cognition and affective symptoms in dementing illnesses; however, a possible new role has emerged in the management of antidepressant-induced sexual dysfunction.[59] Diminished memory and abstract thinking are target symptoms when used for individuals with dementia. Studies have shown modest but significant improvements, with a dosage of 120 mg/day, in both cognitive performance and social function.[60] Progression of disease may be delayed by 6 to 12 months. Further evidence suggests greater improvement for those with mild dementia and stabilization at most with more severe disease.[61] *Ginkgo biloba* has been proposed to enhance learning capacity, as evidenced by one study of healthy young volunteers who made significant improvements in speed of information processing, executive processing, and working memory when on the medication.[62] The body of evidence as a whole has been mixed,[63–65] however, and a recent systematic review suggests a lack of convincing evidence for acute or long-term benefits in young and healthy people.[66] The active components of ginkgo, flavonoids and terpene lactones, stimulate nerve cells that are still functional,[2,5] which seems to provide protection from pathologic effects such as hypoxia, ischemia, seizures, and peripheral damage. Because ginkgo has been shown to inhibit platelet-activating factor, it should be avoided in those at high risk of bleeding. Other side effects include headache, GI distress, seizures in epileptics, and dizziness. The suggested dosage of *Ginkgo biloba* is 120 to 240 mg/day with at least an 8-week course of treatment. However, full benefit may not be seen for a year. Comparisons between ginkgo and FDA-approved nootropics, based on a few meta-analyses[67] and one head-to-head study of ginkgo versus donepezil in patients with Alzheimer's disease,[68] suggest better tolerability for ginkgo, but somewhat more modest efficacy than cholinesterase inhibitors. *Ginkgo* can also be combined safely and effectively with cholinesterase inhibitors with apparent potentiation between the two medications.[69,70] In conclusion, *Ginkgo biloba* appears to be a safe and efficacious cognition-enhancing medication. It may also have a role in reducing antidepressant-induced sexual dysfunction, although this evidence is mixed and must be regarded as preliminary.[71] Further studies are needed to fully understand its complete and long-term effects.

Dehydroepiandrosterone (DHEA) is an androgenic hormone synthesized primarily in the adrenal glands, which is converted to testosterone and estrogen.[72] Although study results have been somewhat mixed, DHEA is thought to play a role in enhancing memory and in improving depressive symptoms.[72–75] Mechanisms of action may include modulation of *N*-methyl-D-aspartate receptors and $GABA_A$ receptor antagonism.[72] Synthetic DHEA is available in an oral formulation and as an intra-oral spray, with dosages ranging from 5 to 100 mg/day. As in many other natural remedies, strength and purity are not regulated. In women, there is a risk for weight gain, hirsutism, menstrual irregularity, voice changes, and headache. Men may experience gynecomastia and prostatic hypertrophy, and the effects on hormone-sensitive tumors are not known.[72] Although early data are promising for DHEA, larger studies must be undertaken to clarify risks versus benefits before it may be safely recommended.

NON-MEDICATION THERAPIES

Acupuncture has been used in Eastern countries for several millennia for the treatment of neuropsychiatric disorders, especially pain. Acupuncture is quite safe, with no major adverse events reported in a recent review of over 65,000 treatments.[76] Although some data support its use to treat a wide range of psychiatric disorders, including schizophrenia, bipolar disorder, substance abuse, and mood and anxiety disorders, the lack of an ideal placebo has been a major barrier in establishing its efficacy in Western studies. However, recent findings in the arena of functional neuroimaging may provide a deeper understanding of the role of acupuncture in mediating pain perception.[77] Further study will help elucidate potential neuropsychiatric benefits of this ancient Eastern treatment.

Hypnosis can be defined as "an event or ritual between a hypnotist and an hypnotic subject in which both agree to use suggestion to bring about a change in perception or behavior."[78] Hypnosis is thought to depend on the dissociative and imaginative abilities of the subject, on the motivation of the subject, and on the relationship between the hypnotist and the subject.[78] Mechanisms are unclear, but levels to which a patient can be hypnotized tend to fall on a bell-shaped curve. Although hypnosis may be used for a wide variety of medical and psychiatric conditions, the following disorders often respond better than others: anxiety, pain, asthma, phobias, nausea, vomiting, and bulimia.[78] Contraindications include unwillingness to be hypnotized, a history of paranoia, and an inexperienced hypnotist. Clinicians should exercise caution in patients with post-traumatic stress disorder or dissociative disorders, as hypnosis may precipitate intrusive (or false) memories in a patient who is not ready to confront them.[79] Because hypnosis may be employed at the bedside, it is particularly attractive to the consultation psychiatrist. Finally, hypnosis is a powerful tool when administered by properly trained individuals, and it may be used alone or as an adjunct in the treatment of a wide array of medical disorders.

CONCLUSION

The spectrum of CAM therapies is quite diverse in current medical practice and is gaining significant popularity in the United States. Historical lack of scientific research in this area has contributed to deficiencies in knowledge with respect to safety and efficacy of many of the natural remedies on the market today. A recent surge in funding by government and industry sources should help in this regard. Current knowledge about a few such therapies is addressed in this chapter, including proposed treatments for mood disorders, anxiety and sleep disorders, menstrual disorders, and dementia. Many of these therapies may prove to be a valuable addition to the armamentarium of treatments available to psychiatrists in the future. A particular emphasis was placed on potential adverse effects and drug–drug interactions, given the nature of consultation psychiatry. A general knowledge of these therapies and routine questioning about their use is an essential part of comprehensive care by the consultation psychiatrist.

CASE 1

Mr. A, a 40-year-old librarian with no significant medical history, presented to the Emergency Department (ED) with a chief complaint of a "panic attack." He had been in his usual state of health until a few hours earlier. His only significant health issue was a diagnosis of major depression made a year earlier, for which he was taking fluoxetine, 20 mg daily.

During the interview, Mr. A reported that he was feeling restless and agitated, had a headache that would not go away, despite taking acetaminophen, was nauseated and shivering with goose bumps, and could feel his heart "beating out of my chest." On physical exam, he was noted to have dilated pupils, tachycardia, mildly elevated blood pressure, and profuse sweating.

Upon further questioning, Mr. A noted that he had just started taking St. John's wort (SJW), which he had bought in a health food store upon a friend's recommendation. He felt the fluoxetine had not been working very well lately and he had been getting more depressed, so he decided to combine the two drugs.

The ED physician investigated whether there might have been an interaction between the two drugs and found that serotonin syndrome could occur with the combination of selective serotonin re-uptake inhibitors (SSRIs) and SJW, due to SJW's monoamine oxidase inhibitor (MAOI) activity. Mr. A was diagnosed with serotonin syndrome secondary to a drug–drug interaction. He was started on intravenous (IV) fluids and kept overnight for observation. By the next morning, he had stabilized and was discharged home with instructions to not take SJW again while he was on fluoxetine or any other SSRI. Mr. A agreed to follow-up with his regular psychiatrist as soon as possible.

REFERENCES

Access the reference list online at https://expertconsult.inkling.com/.

Difficult Patients

Franklin King IV, M.D.
James E. Groves, M.D.

43

OVERVIEW

The medical equivalent of war is the care of the difficult patient. Doctors soldier steadily on through all kinds of clinical chores, arduous schedules, and "administrivia," but when they get to the types of patients variously called "obnoxious,"[1] "needy," "crocky,"[2] "malignant," and even "hateful,"[3] they fight the worst battles of their careers, become prone to clinical blunders, mess up their personal lives, violate boundaries, and get sued. The good news is that—almost without exception—the "difficult patient" situation makes the consulting psychiatrist more useful to treating physician and patient alike than in any other medical encounter. Harrowing though such situations may temporarily be, it is just this kind of consultation that earns the trust and respect of the physician consultee and generates more consultation requests later on (and, really, there are few better ways for a psychiatrist starting out to build a practice than by becoming a specialist on the care of the difficult patient). Before turning to management strategies, it is worth reviewing the presentations of difficult patients.

CASE 1

Ms. A, a 38-year-old woman with a history reported in the chart as being significant for obesity, lower back pain, systemic lupus erythematosus, chronic tinnitus, fibromyalgia, and bipolar disorder, was admitted to the hospital for fever and cough. Pneumonia was initially diagnosed, and her medical symptoms had been improving with antibiotics. However, care had been increasingly complicated by her escalating demands and seemingly endless physical complaints: she had been complaining of back pain, "because of my lupus flare" (despite any objective evidence of autoimmune exacerbation), with repeated requests for oxycodone as the only medication that will help; urinary symptoms, despite a normal exam and laboratory findings; and insomnia and anxiety. In addition, Ms. A continued to leave the hospital to smoke cigarettes and at times, went off the unit for hours at a time, and lashed out at the physician team when they told her that she needed to be present for morning rounds. Conflict broke out among staff; some nurses had excellent rapport with her and viewed her as a sympathetic character, who was at the mercy of a cold and indifferent attending physician and senior resident, as well as their apparently heartless colleagues on the night shift—who just didn't seem to understand how much Ms. A was suffering. On his first nightfloat shift on this service, the junior resident prescribed lorazepam for insomnia, despite the daytime team's instructions to withhold benzodiazepines. This error was corrected the following night, but the next morning, Ms. A told the junior resident, "I need to sleep because of my bipolar. If you don't give me my lorazepam, I'm gonna kill myself". An argument ensued between the patient and the junior resident, which escalated and resulted in a loud verbal conflict between the resident, the nurse, and the charge nurse. By the time the consultant received the consult request (delivered in an indignant, angry tone by the rotating subintern), the entire staff was in an uproar.

TYPES OF DIFFICULT PATIENTS

Delirious patients may be assaultive. Guilty, bereaved spouses can be litigious. Temporal lobe epileptic patients are often clingy and viscous. Manic patients are emotional cyclones. Celebrities at times generate anxiety in their caregivers. Patients with schizophrenia can be non-compliant. Anyone when ill can regress and become angry, dependent, and hypochondriacal—yet none of these difficult situations necessarily produces "difficult patient" scenarios.

Difficult patients are almost always persons with personality disorders, or at least those who, in the face of medical illness, severe psychosocial stress, alcohol and substance use disorders (SUDs), regressively display the maladaptive traits so characteristic of the personality-disordered patient. This highlights the importance of differentiating state versus trait: true personality disorders lie closer to trait because they are relatively durable over time, while SUDs and eating disorders lie closer to state because change, when it occurs, can be dramatic. In the *Diagnostic and Statistical Manual of Mental Disorders*, 5th edition (DSM-5),[4] personality disorders are defined by clusters of traits, while SUDs are associated with maladaptive behaviors that the substance gives rise to. However, the consultant will do well to remember that patients encountered on inpatient units are often at their worst—and as personality disorders are diagnosed based on traits observed over time, the patient with "borderline traits" may not meet criteria for the actual *personality disorder* despite seeming to exhibit evidence during an acute medical illness. Despite their reputation of being intractable and chronic conditions, even the stability of full-fledged personality disorders over time has come under scrutiny in recent years, as prognosis, change, and recovery now appear perhaps more favorable for some disorders than previously thought.[5–7]

Not all patients with personality disorders are difficult patients or necessitate psychiatric consultation. Looking at pure types through the lens of DSM-5, those not necessarily belonging to the difficult patient paradigm are paranoid, schizoid, and schizotypal personality disorders (cluster A), and avoidant, dependent, and obsessive–compulsive personality disorders (cluster C), which do not necessarily belong to the difficult patient paradigm. Patients with a paranoid personality disorder deserve brief mention, however, as the nearly boundless suspiciousness, hostility towards others, and extreme employment of projection often render them problematic to the primary clinical team when they must—always reluctantly—seek medical care.[8]

Nonetheless, although some of these may be difficult patients, it is really when we look into Cluster B disorders that a pit of despair opens: antisocial, borderline, and narcissistic (for the sake of this discussion, histrionic patients are grouped with borderline patients because, as difficult patients, they are almost indistinguishable). With these three diagnoses, comprising the dramatic-emotional-erratic cluster, there is almost a complete overlap between difficult patients and personality disorders. DSM-5 defines them as the following:

- Antisocial personality disorder involves a pattern of disregard for, and violation of, the rights of others.
- Borderline personality disorder is characterized by a pattern of instability in interpersonal relationships, poor self-image, labile and dysphoric affects, and marked impulsivity.
- Narcissistic personality disorder is embodied by a pattern of grandiosity, a need for admiration, and a lack of empathy.

The key word here is *pattern*. Personality traits lead to personality disorder when they are "inflexible and pervasive across a broad range of personal and social situations," leading to significant distress or impairment in multiple domains of functioning.[4] These traits are enduring for most of the life span, and deviate markedly from the expectations of the patient's culture. Finally, they do not result from another mental or physical disorder, such as depression or head trauma.

Antisocial and Narcissistic Personality Disorders

Patients with antisocial personality disorder display the defining trait of disregard for the rights of others. The disorder satisfies the general criteria for the other personality disorders and consistently manifests at least three of the following traits:[4] rule-breaking; deceitfulness (e.g., lying, conning others); impulsivity or poor planning (resulting in a parasitic lifestyle that is sustained by manipulating others); aggressiveness (with repeated assaults and fights); irresponsibility (failing to sustain a job or uphold financial obligations); and a lack of conscience, remorse or empathy.

Narcissistic personality disorder[4] defines itself in the grandiosity and lack of empathy shown by at least five of the following traits: arrogance; a preoccupation with fantasies of power, beauty, love, brilliance, or money; convictions of "specialness"; a hunger for admiration; entitlement; exploitation and manipulativeness; stunted empathy (an inability to "feel into" the other person); envy; and displays of contemptuousness.

Antisocial personality disorder and narcissistic personality disorder are similar in terms of selfishness but different in terms of social destructiveness. One could think of the difference as that between criminality and shabby ethics. Whether these two entities differ more in degree or in kind is a question perhaps better left to religion or philosophy, yet in psychiatry one view has been that the personality disorders have similar ego defects (except in degree) and similar underlying psychic organizations[9–11] or even a common *borderline personality organization*.[12] If it is true that a change in social context (e.g., incarceration) brings out borderline personality in persons who otherwise look antisocial, as some have claimed,[13] there may be some utility to the notion of a core personality disorder called *borderline with several variant presentations*. At any rate, the management strategies discussed subsequently work for borderline and for other personality disorders alike, given a rigorous application and a sufficiently strong social structure.

The concept of an underlying or core borderline personality organization is a metaphor that has considerable utility in the discussion of the difficult patient. In the medical setting, antisocial and narcissistic patients are difficult only when they are acting like borderlines. The idea is that the underlying good–bad split or fragmented borderline personality organization is held together by the self-promoting program of the antisocial person and the grandiosity of the narcissist. Antisocial and narcissistic patients who believe their physicians' interests parallel their own are unctuous and un-difficult ("prison sincerity"). When the psychopathy and grandiosity are punctured by illness or injury and thwarted by medical treatment, the underlying fragmented, rageful, splitting, attacking borderline comes out. In the discussion that follows, therefore, *borderline personality* is the referent paradigm of difficulty, to be discussed more at length and used interchangeably with *difficult patient*.

Borderline Personality Disorder

"Borderline personality" was originally named[14] because it seemed to psychoanalysts to lie between the psychoses and the neuroses. Borderline patients are dreaded for their impulsivity, swings from love to hate, and maddening irrationality. They split the world into exaggerated dichotomies of good and evil. An interpersonal middle ground does not exist. These patients, by some combination of innate rage and inept parenting, cannot find a moderate position in any aspect of mental life.[15]

Borderline patients have a multi-faceted personality disorder that goes beyond the repeated self-injurious behavior once referred to as the "behavioral specialty" of the disorder,[16] with characteristics grouped into four broad domains of affective, interpersonal, behavioral, and cognitive features.[17] Symptoms range from bordering on psychosis, in which the patient is chaotic or irrational, to bordering on neurosis, in which the patient desperately clings to others to feel real—reflective of historical assumptions that the disorder represented a "border" state between psychosis and neurosis. The borderline patient exhibits five or more of the following traits: frantic efforts to avoid or prevent (usually perceived) abandonment, a pattern of intense interpersonal relationships characterized by unstable alternations between idealization and devaluation; unstable sense of self or identity; impulsive behaviors that may be self-damaging; recurrent suicidal ideation, attempts, threats, or self-mutilation; marked mood reactivity and affective instability; inappropriate, intense anger and poor self-control of anger; chronic feelings of emptiness, and transient paranoid ideation and dissociative symptoms.[4]

In the past, borderline personality was sometimes held to be a sub-set of biological depressive illness or a variant of traditional diagnoses, such as hysteria, sociopathy, or alcoholism. This is likely reflective of the high rates of co-morbid psychiatric disorders found in this population: one of the more rigorously conducted studies to date followed 290 borderline personality patients, and found that even at 6-year follow-up, 75% of these patients surveyed met criteria for a mood disorder (61% for major depression), 35% for post-traumatic stress disorder (PTSD), 34% for an eating disorder, 29% for panic disorder, and 19% for a substance use disorder (SUD).[18] More striking is the fact that this represented a decline from initial surveys, and that even in patients whose borderline personality remitted, psychiatric co-morbidity remained high. Rates of remission of symptoms of both borderline personality and affective disorders have similarly been shown to reciprocally delay the time to recovery of each other, suggesting an interplay of related, but separate, etiologies.[19] Unfortunately, borderline personality disorder remains both underdiagnosed[20] as well as misdiagnosed (often as bipolar disorder).[21] The consultant would therefore do well to thoroughly review the diagnostic criteria and differential diagnosis of this disorder.

Regardless of sub-type or co-morbid diagnosis, however, borderline patients can abruptly flee treatment or develop psychotic transference and delusions about their caregivers.[22–24] Short, circumscribed episodes of delusional thinking in unstructured situations and when under stress are almost pathognomonic.[24–26] Borderlines display a signature trait, poor observing ego,[27] which is a dense denial of vital aspects of reality and irrationality to a degree that almost has to be seen to be believed. Although the relation of borderline personality to schizophrenia was long debated, it is likely that if there is a "border" with a biological illness, it is closer to affective illness without being completely tangential to it.[28]

Heredity plays a crucial role in the cause of borderline personality, with 42% to 68% of the variance found to be associated with genetic factors.[29] Innate intolerance to anxiety and a constitutional tendency toward rage have long been accepted even by psychoanalytic theorists regarding borderline personality.[30] Individual features of borderline personality disorder have also been found to run in families.[31] Many studies have examined the co-aggregation of borderline personality and other psychiatric disorders in families; however, a recent review found that while evidence was suggestive of a familial relationship of borderline personality with major depressive disorder (MDD) and SUDs, conclusions are limited by methodologic problems in most studies and more evidence is needed.[32]

Psychologically based theories also focus on the family of origin.[33] Psychoanalysts view borderline personality as arising from failure by the patient's mother to foster coherent differentiation between self and object in the first 18 months of life,[34,35] leading to the development of pathologic ego defenses. The patient does not learn to tolerate negative affect associated with separation;[36,37] this continues the child's clinging into adulthood, as if others were desperately needed parts of the self.[12,38,39] The borderline's adult relationships are called *transitional* after the transitional object.[40–42] The patient's mother (possibly borderline herself[43]) apparently feared fusion with (and destruction of or by) the child. She could not let the child separate because of her own fears of being alone. On rapprochement, she tended to reject the child for "deserting" her.[40–46] She mostly saw the child as her own transitional object and—used as the imaginary playmate of the mother—the child never grew into an emotionally separate human being.

In borderline personality, the boundaries between the self and others are blurred, so that closeness seems to threaten fusion. Sexuality and dependency are confused with aggression. Needs are experienced as rage. Long-term relationships disintegrate because of an inability to find optimal interpersonal distance. Because of inadequate ego mechanisms of defense, there is little ability to master painful feelings or to channel needs or aggression into creative outlets. Ambivalence is poorly tolerated. Impulse control is dismal. The patient has a fragmented mental picture of the self and views others as all bad and simultaneously all potent, a chaotic mixture of shameful and grandiose images.[15]

In addition to the literature on inadequate parenting, borderline personality is linked with parental neglect and abuse, particularly severe or sexual abuse.[47,48] The analytically based theory put forth is that the child victim of sexual abuse (especially of chronic abuse[49]) used dissociation[50] as a defense against massive psychic trauma, and the dissociation became habitual, undermining ego integration. This association with abuse is seen as variously explaining phenomena ranging from a propensity toward dissociative psychotic-like episodes, rage, sexual disorders, psychotic–erotic transferences in psychotherapy, and self-mutilation. The literature on abuse has the important effect of spotlighting the relationship between borderline phenomena and dissociation, something the older literature under-emphasized. Although the exact role that abuse plays in the development of borderline personality is still being worked out, it is clear that a significant number of borderline patients, when asked to give a history of such abuse, do so; this has to be taken into account in management.[51,52]

Borderline personality occurs in perhaps 2% of the population.[53] Despite its small size, the borderline cohort stands out in the general hospital because of its florid presentation, notoriety for frequent utilization of both psychiatric and medical services, and because of the feelings of anger and helplessness stirred up in the caregivers.[54–56]

These patients often make themselves medical outcasts because they ruthlessly destroy the care they crave. However, because of this, the diagnosis of borderline personality has unfortunately attracted a considerable amount of bad press, both within the lay public, the medical community at large,

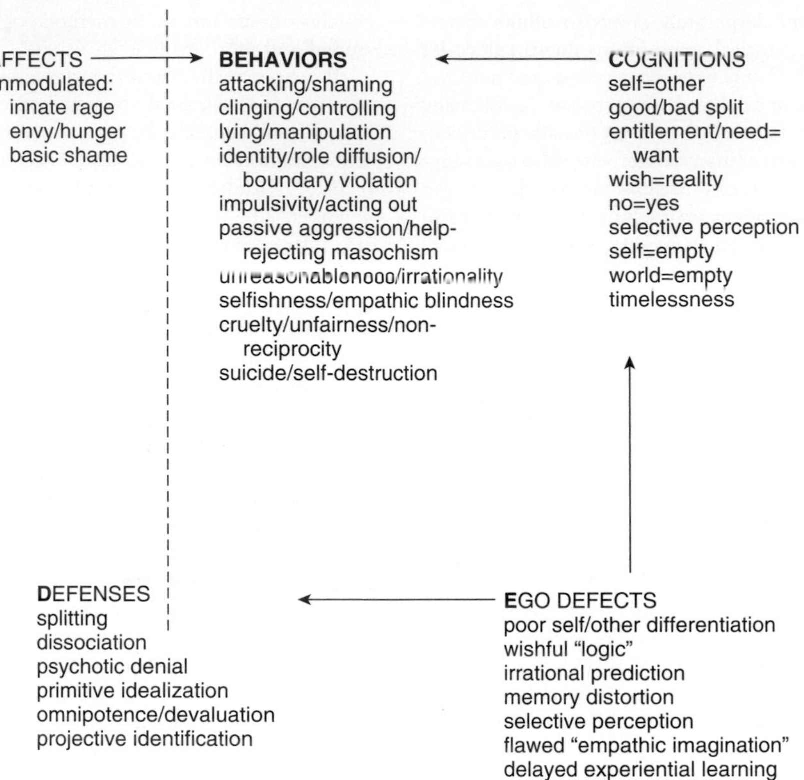

Figure 43-1. The difficult patient's types of problem behavior.

and even among psychiatrists and other mental health clinicians.[57–60] This fact begs the question of how this affects psychiatric, medical, and nursing care, as clinicians who seek to avoid the difficult patient may overlook important clinical signs and under-diagnose disease, in an unconscious effort to limit patient interaction. Medical co-morbidity in borderline patients is significant, at least partly due its association with obesity;[61,62] a 10-year longitudinal study found that compared ever-recovered to never-recovered borderline patients, the latter had significantly higher rates of chronic health conditions—notably obesity, diabetes, urinary incontinence, and osteoarthritis—as well as poorly defined illnesses, such as chronic fatigue syndrome and fibromyalgia.[63] They also had higher rates of poor health-related life-style choices, financial burdens related to medical illness, and higher rates of utilization of costly medical services. Appropriate medical care is thus sorely lacking in this population, shunned as it is by the medical community—and thus adroit management of the inpatient medical team is of paramount importance in effecting sound patient care, as is discussed later in the chapter.

DIFFICULT BEHAVIOR AND THE CONSULTEE

The previous discussion about the DSM-5 diagnoses of difficult patients must be leavened with a simple fact: it is not the diagnosis of these patients that makes them difficult for the consultee—it is their behavior. The relationship of the behavior to other aspects of mental life is schematized in Figure 43-1.

Such patients have abnormally intense affects, poorer-than-average neutralizers of affect, or both. In any case, raw rage, naked dependency, and ontologic shame are present and are often found on the surface. The cognitive structures that ordinarily temper intense affects are distorted and primitive. The ego weakness of the patient is shown by the absence of higher-level defenses and by the primitive nature of the ones that are present.[64]

Under pressure of intense affect (rage, terror, shame), the patient uses dissociation to a greater or lesser extent and enters the dream-like state that persons ordinarily enter only in extreme emergencies. In this dissociated state (which is probably present much of the time to some degree), the patient is distracted, numb, and difficult to reach. The pervasiveness of dissociation is one feature of borderline personality that is insufficiently discussed in the literature; however, it can contribute drastically to the pathologic cognitions of borderline patients and place a distorting lens of unreality between them and the real world.

Besides dissociation, the borderline patient uses denial of major aspects of reality to cope. This mythification of the external, threatening world is displayed in defenses called *primitive idealization*, *omnipotence*, and *devaluation*. As the names imply, these are metaphors for the dreamy, wishful, mythified world the difficult patient inhabits, a world of black and white and good and evil. These maladaptive defenses may be all too visible in the medical setting, but even more troubling are two others with which such patients unsuccessfully try to manage their extreme negative affects: splitting and projective identification.[64]

Splitting is by definition a rigid separation of positive and negative thoughts or feelings. Normal persons are ambivalent and can experience two contradictory feeling states at one time; the borderline personality characteristically shifts back and forth, entirely unaware of one feeling state while in another. Sometimes one state is rigidly held while its opposite is projected onto the environment. Splitting may protect the patient from the anxiety of reconciling contradictory extremes (at the expense of the already unstable personality). In social systems,[65–69] borderline patients can split the staff into warring "good" and "bad" factions that unwittingly act out the patient's internal world.

Projective identification[70–74] is said to consist of taking an unwanted aspect of the self, such as cruelty or envy, and wholly ascribing it to ("projecting it into") another. The patient then unconsciously pressures that person to own the projected attribute. Unaware that a self-fulfilling prophecy is being set-up, the recipient complies with the projection and acts it out. These two mechanisms can complement each other, with projective identification being used to "confirm" one side of a polarized, split view of the world.[15]

Although the long-term psychotherapy of the borderline patient can involve therapeutic undoing of these defenses,[12,75] it is inadvisable—even dangerous—to confront such defenses in brief encounters in the medical setting. It is crucial, however, to be aware of their presence. For example, awareness of borderline splitting prepares the consultant to deal with the division of the medical staff into "good ones" and "bad ones." Recognition of the patient's primitive idealization, of a physician for instance, can help the consultant prepare for the furious devaluing that is to follow.

Helping the Consultee

The medical setting is a social system with its own history, boundaries, hierarchy, customs, and taboos. The introduction of a difficult patient into this culture sometimes places such stress on the system as to cause malfunctions in caregiving or outright extrusion of the patient, a situation that active psychiatric consultation can prevent. Difficult patients are exquisitely vulnerable to caregivers' ordinary imperfections in communication and consistency, and they are often remarkably attuned to their caregivers' normal negative feelings of anxiety, shame, anger, and depression. Such patients are especially vulnerable to feelings of rejection by caregivers, and their shaky defenses are even more compromised than usual by the stresses of illness and treatment.

After initial diagnosis and treatment of the patient, the consultant's next priority should be to gauge the amount of distress the staff is under. A psychologically naive medical staff can regress to a helpless or vengeful position in response to the patient's ingratitude, intractability, impulsivity, manipulativeness, dependency, entitlement, and rage. Regression in any social system can emerge as disagreement among staff; it can take the form of inappropriate confrontation of the patient, or it can manifest itself as a deterioration in the patient's behavior.[15] Regression seems to occur when there exists a large disparity between what is expected and what is found.[76] Troublesome dissonance of this sort between patient and staff generally occurs in any or all of three dimensions: perception of reality, values governing control and aggression, and rules about interpersonal closeness (Table 43-1).

The earliest clue to the nature of the dissonance lies in the consultation request.[77] Its tone, covert messages, intensity, timing, and route by which it reaches the consultant all can reflect the dissonance between patient and staff expectations. Consultation is sought when the patient is out of touch with the staff's reality. In this case, dissonance can range from mild (when the patient is from a different culture) to severe (when the patient is psychotic). When the patient is docile, the request is matter-of-fact; when the patient manifests grotesquely sexual or aggressive behavior, the consultant might receive a shrill, disorganized call for help.

TABLE 43-1 Consultation Management of Staff and Difficult Patient Dissonance in the Medical Setting

TYPE OF DISSONANCE: CONSULTATION REQUEST	PATIENT'S PROBLEM BEHAVIORS	CONSULTANT'S WORK WITH THE CONSULTEE	CONSULTANT'S WORK WITH THE PATIENT
Dissonant reality: vague, confusing request for help; puzzled tone	Inappropriate to realities of illness or hospital; denial and demandingness	Explains patient's reality to staff; models "reality testing"	Diagnosis of any cognitive disorders; gives medication and reality-testing request
Aggressive dissonance: request to control or remove patient; fearful or angry tone	Menacing, self-destructive, or suicidal	Recommends social, chemical, or physical restraints necessary for safety	Evaluates potential violence; searches for source of patient's panic
Staff and patient dissonance regarding interpersonal distance: request consultant to take over care of patient; depressed, guilty tone to consultation request	Dependent Rejecting	Gives permission to say "no" to patient's unrealistic, excessive demands Diminishes guilt and depression by stating impossibility of entirely satisfying patient	Clarifies for patient that some, but not all, needs can be realistically met Allows patient some distance; repeatedly appeals to patient's "entitlement" and autonomous side
	Manipulative (dependent and rejecting)	Serves as forum for hatred toward patient; voices hateful feelings but behaves non-sadistically	Bargains; sets firm, non-interpretive limits on manipulation; clarifies patient's self-interest

Consultation is sought when the patient's aggression violates staff expectations. The staff expects to be in control of the patient, who is expected to be grateful, compliant, and non-destructive. Dissonance in this dimension can range from mild, when the patient sulks, to severe, when the patient is violent or self-destructive. The tone of such a consultation request ranges from irritation to anger or outright fear, depending on the kind of aggression the patient displays.

Consultation is sought when the patient's need for closeness is different from what the staff deems appropriate. The staff expects the patient to be involved with the caregivers but to keep a certain distance. When the patient asks for repeated reassurances or when the patient makes inexhaustible or contradictory demands, a depressed, guilty request often ensues. Arrogant, peremptory consultation requests often herald a hostile, dependent, manipulative patient; depressed, tired requests can foretell an empty, clinging patient.

The primitive defenses[78] of the difficult patient can stimulate staff disagreement (Table 43-2). To cope with deep feelings of self-loathing, the patient might see the staff as loathsome—otherwise why would they care (projective identification)? Or the patient may see the staff as magically all good, to keep all the badness in the world away (primitive idealization). To make sense of a world in which people are both good and bad, such a patient might choose some people on the staff to be "all good" and some to be "all bad" (splitting). This "explains" for the patient "why" things always go wrong: the patient is caught between good and bad forces outside the self and therefore they are not the fault of the self. When the patient views the staff through the defense of splitting, the staff might eventually behave as if it were so. The patient will tell an "all good" staff member what terrible things an "all bad" staff member has done, said, or thought and then swear the "good" one to secrecy. As less and less communication takes place and the patient escalates demands, the "good" staff and "bad" staff begin to disagree about the care of the patient because the borderline patient may be "good" with "good" staff and vice versa. The remedy for this depends on re-establishing open staff communication, even if it is hostile, to enable staff to get a well-rounded view of the patient. Firm, non-punitive limit setting[65,67] (Table 43-3) is crucial for inpatient treatment because it must be made clear that the patient cannot destroy the caregiving system or be destroyed by it, no matter how intense the wishes or fears may be.

It is a natural human instinct to confront such patients angrily, but caregivers should exercise precautions during confrontations. Avoiding a confrontation of narcissistic entitlement is as important as it is difficult.[79] Such patients exude an offensive sense of deservedness that is always tempting for an overworked staff to confront angrily and suddenly. Often the difficult patient has only this sense of entitlement to keep a fragmented personality together during the stresses of hospitalization. Entitlement for the narcissist is what hope and faith are to normal persons. Preserving it requires a deliberate effort. Taken together, what Tables 43-2 and 43-3 show is that such behavior of the difficult patient (e.g., manipulativeness and entitled demanding)—obnoxious though they may be—sometimes function as defenses at a relatively high level for that patient. Stripping them away makes the patient fall back on even lower-level defenses, such as psychotic denial and dissociation, or—worse—to be defenseless, panic, or explode.

Setting limits, avoiding confrontation, and avoiding overstimulation of the desire for closeness and rage are difficult to arrange in the fast-paced medical milieu.[79] Prevention of staff splitting is especially difficult because of the various sub-cultures in medicine. If, for instance, the patient chooses the nurses to be "all bad" and the physicians to be "all good,"

TABLE 43-2 Manifestations of Primitive Ego Defenses: the Difficult Patient in the Medical Setting
Splitting: Keeping completely apart two opposite ideas and their associated feelings. Staff are divided into "good ones" and "bad ones," reflecting the patient's incapacity to achieve ambivalence enough to see that caregivers have human limits, with "good" and "bad" qualities at the same time.
Projective identification: The tendency to see some staff as "bad" as the patient feels. This gets translated into behavior based on the following kind of "logic": "I'm bad and you take care of me, which means you're as rotten as I am, otherwise you wouldn't care for me." This perception is so powerfully held that the staff receiving it tend to act it out unconsciously.
Primitive denial: The alternating expungement from consciousness of first one and then another perception of opposite quality (in which it is called *splitting*) or a wish so powerful that it obliterates crucial aspects of reality contradicting that wish. For instance, fear might cause the patient to deny a serious condition and flee the hospital where it could be treated.
Primitive idealization: The tendency to see some staff as totally "good" to protect the patient from "bad" staff or from the patient's medical condition.
Omnipotence and devaluation: A shift (splitting) between the need to establish a relationship with a magical, powerful staff (primitive idealization) versus the conviction of omnipotence in the self that makes all others impotent by comparison (primitive idealization of the self). Omnipotent caregivers are supposed to deliver to the patient perfect care to protect against disease, and when this does not happen, the staff is seen as impotent and hateful. (Splitting makes the perception shift dramatically, whereas projective identification causes the staff to buy into the patient's primitive projections, making them come true).

Adapted from Groves JE: Management of the borderline patient on a medical or surgical ward: the psychiatric consultant's role, *Int J Psychiatry Med* 1975; 6: 337–348.

TABLE 43-3 Rules for Confronting the Difficult Patient
Acknowledge the real stresses in the patient's situation.
Avoid breaking down needed defenses.
Avoid overstimulating the patient's wish for closeness.
Avoid overstimulating the patient's rage.
Avoid confronting narcissistic entitlement.

Adapted from Adler G, Buie DH: The misuses of confrontation with borderline patients, *Int J Psychoanal Psychother* 1972; 1: 109–120.

the nurses may displace anger to the physicians but be unable to express it directly because of role-induced sanctions, and the physicians may see the nurses as incompetent and unable to comprehend their treatment plan for the patient. Such situations are fertile ground for the splitter and require concerted effort toward open communication.

Pathologic dependency manifests in one of its extremes as manipulativeness: an intense, covert, contradictory, self-defeating attempt to get needs met.[3,78] It is the behavioral manifestation of a need by the patient to get close but at the same time, maintain a safe distance from sources of emotional support. Some patients feel so empty that, paradoxically, getting their needs met threatens them with engulfment; they are so famished that closeness can actually make them feel merged with someone else and therefore not really alive. Such patients seem to have a deathly fear of what they most crave.

In limit-setting confrontations with manipulative and entitled patients, the consultant might have to model for the staff firmness, repetition, and an appeal to the patient's sense of entitlement (rather than an assault on it): "You deserve the best medical care we can give, and that's why we're recommending X, Y, and Z." The consultant has to keep uppermost in mind the appeal to the entitlement and not get drawn into logical or illogical arguments. Moreover, it is important to avoid interpreting the resistance to cooperation as a fear of dependency, a tactic that would at best leave the patient somewhat bewildered. Repetition is crucial. Encounters to engage compliance often have to be repeated two or three times at varying intervals before the patient agrees, for instance, to take medication.

Dependent, manipulative patients stir up sadism in the caregivers, which inhibits the setting of effective limits. The consultant supports the staff's self-esteem and performance by reinforcing strengths rather than by pointing out weaknesses, by teaching, by lending a conceptual framework to mitigate anxiety, by modeling interactions, and, most of all, by matter-of-factly stating that such patients stir up hatred even in the best of caregivers. Whenever the staff brings even a hint of negative reference to the patient, the consultant can say something like, "Yeah, these patients are manipulative and irritating as hell!" or, "Everybody hates this kind of patient." This personalization, juxtaposed with the consultant's own non-sadistic behavior toward the patient, legitimizes hostility toward the patient, but shares it among staff rather than inflicting it on the patient.

In general, the earlier in the hospitalization the consultant is called, the more overt is the reason for the consultation and the more effective will be the intervention because the difficult patient has had less time to project into the staff the intense, seemingly inborn shame such patients possess in great abundance. Late in the hospitalization, the consultant may be urgently called in to see the patient for vague reasons and arrive to find the situation in a shambles, the patient in restraints, the staff ashamed and in bitter conflict—and nobody either willing or able to say what has been going on.

Consultant's Role

The consultant's role in the management of the difficult patient consists of a specialized type of consultee-oriented approach, in which countertransference hatred and fear are drawn away from the patient and strategically metabolized within the relationship between staff and consultant. The consultant should actively promote a behavioral management practicum[78] placed in the medical chart for reference and as a symbol of the psychiatrist's helping presence. This "recipe" discusses communicating clearly with the patient and among staff; understanding the patient's need for constant interaction with personnel; dealing with entitlement without confronting needed defenses; and setting firm limits on dependency, manipulativeness, rage, and self-destructive behavior.

Generally, the consultant's approach should first lead directly to the consultee. The request should be elicited in person or at least on the phone because the written record never reveals all of the problems in the management of the difficult patient. Then the consultant goes to the nursing staff to get a history of the patient's responses to hospital routine. Next, the consultant reads the chart and compares medication orders with records of medication actually administered. The consultant will have generated some hypotheses and is now ready to test them in the examination of the patient. As the consultant proceeds through these steps, an orderly plan emerges (Table 43-4).

One helpful approach is the consultee-oriented model of consultation,[80] which involves thinking of the patient and staff as a single entity and dealing as much as possible with the strong, healthy part. The entity consists of two parts. One part, the difficult patient, has problems with object relations, pathologic behavior exacerbated under stress, and several self-defeating and infuriating defenses, especially splitting. To prevent being split, the consultant should try to deal mainly with the healthy part, the staff. Because the

TABLE 43-4 Order of Priorities for the Difficult-Patient Consultation in the Medical Setting

1. Rapidly evaluate the most pressing psychiatric problems, beginning with physical or social restraints if the patient appears about to lose control of violent or self-destructive impulses.
2. Create a differential diagnosis of the difficult patient, with an explicit biopsychosocial formulation of the predominant conflicts and stressors.
3. Identify dissonance between staff and patient and formulate a plan of action to reduce it (Table 43-1).
4. Provide treatment recommendations—psychological and pharmacologic (Table 43-1), short-term and long-term—taking into account the ongoing medical regimen and implicitly addressing dissonance between staff and patient while explicitly addressing the patient's conflicts.
5. Educate the consultee and staff to reduce dissonance and to lend a conceptual framework for dealing with future difficult patients.
6. Actively participate without grandstanding or actually taking over the total psychological care of the patient.
7. Follow-up and be involved in disposition planning for the medical and psychiatric needs of the patient.

Adapted from personal communications with Hackett TP, Weisman AD, Cassem NH, Alonso AW, Stewart TW, Nobel K, Renner JA, Surman OS, and many others.

staff is often closely linked in an unwilling, hateful, and guilty alliance with the patient and its collective self-esteem is already damaged by encounters with the patient, the consultant should not damage it further by interpreting the staff's pathology.

The attempt to ally with staff rather than the patient is destined to encounter several kinds of resistance at the outset. First, the patient is eager to engage the consultant to find out whether the consultant is "all good" or "all bad." Second, the staff, needing distance from its sense of failure, wants the consultant to take over the care of the patient completely. Third, neither the staff nor the patient has the energy to understand what is going on; they are in pain and want relief now, preferably by removal of the patient.

The alliance with the staff depends to a large extent on previous experience with the consultant, how long it takes to answer the consultation request, and how much sense the advice makes. The alliance with the difficult patient is dramatically less important in terms of outcome than the alliance with the staff. Such patients are incapable of forming a real alliance, and their "alliances" are mostly primitive idealization. Ideally, the patient should be seen only briefly if there are enough data from other sources, and the staff is told that the consultant will work mainly with staff and see the patient infrequently.

Visiting the patient should be reserved in the early stages for the specific purpose of the consultant's alliance with the staff. Following the initial patient interview, the consultant goes to see the patient when a magical gesture of "taking over" is needed to comfort a desperate staff, when staff members feel that the consultant does not know how much they are suffering, and when the staff needs a specific model for carrying out recommendations on limit-setting or reality testing.

The consultation note, by its tone, specific information, and description of the patient in a way the staff can immediately recognize, remains in a medical record day and night as a tangible symbol of the consultant's helping presence. It outlines the request, history, mental status at the hour of the examination, and the psychiatric history. It is explicit about medications, and the potential for suicide and for violence. It includes specific, concrete management recommendations.

CASE 2

This was the conclusion of a consultation note for a difficult patient who had been spitting into her central line.

Impression: Ms. B is thought to have borderline personality disorder, a chronic, severe personality disorder, meaning that her moods can fluctuate rapidly and severely and she has only marginal social adjustment. These chronic traits have likely worsened as a result of the stress of her current medical condition.

Recommendations: Have brief, daily staff conferences to compare notes and reach a consensus about her surgical treatment plan. Try to have the same staff members work with Ms. B each day; bear in mind that she tends to panic at each change of shift. Set firm limits on her multiple and contradictory demands. She is quick to rage when her demands are not met and may threaten suicide. Do not imply that Ms. B does not deserve the things she demands, but rather say over and over again that you understand what she is asking, but because you feel she deserves the best possible care, you are going to continue to recommend the course dictated by your experience and judgment. If she continues spitting into her central line, assure her that physical restraint will ensue. Initiate suicide precautions (and search her luggage). Medication recommendations are delineated as shown below.

The consultant addresses dissonance arising from the patient's version of reality; tendency to act out; and demandingness, neediness, and rage. The consultant gives a mandate for open communication and daily staff conferences to prevent staff splitting and to provide a supportive environment. Firm limits, without challenging the patient's sense of entitlement, are set forth explicitly. The task now becomes one of seeing that recommendations are effected. There is nothing more frustrating than laboring to devise a treatment plan only to find that it is not carried out. When this happens, the consultant often finds that the source of resistance is still-unresolved dissonance between staff and patient (Table 43-1).

Nowhere in the previous discussion is the unconscious motivation of the patient or of the staff brought to the attention of either. This is what is meant by *non-interpretive intervention*. Psychoanalytic interpretations foster a temporary regression and have no place in the consultation with the disruptive medical–surgical patient.[78] Instead, the consultant analyzes and reduces dissonance by speaking of its behavioral roots and consequences while resisting the temptation to illuminate interesting unconscious processes.

Medication

The psychopharmacologic management of borderline personality disorder (the referent paradigm for difficult patients) is complex: despite the high exposure of this group to psychiatric polypharmacy,[18,81,82] robust evidence supporting the use of medications remains limited, and, as of 2016, there remains no FDA-approved medication for the treatment of borderline personality. However, the general consensus among experts is that, although the role of medications in the long-term care of borderline personality remains to be determined and should never be the sole or first-line treatment modality, medications—especially for short-term use—nonetheless can be helpful in reducing specific symptoms within borderline personality.[83–86] It is important to add that medications may also serve as transitional objects and vehicles for the patient's projection,[86,87] especially during times of dysregulation such as may occur during admission to a general hospital. Thus, the inexperienced clinician may be easily deceived into attributing changes in symptoms to pharmacologic interventions—and fall into the trap of "symptom chasing" while ignoring the often context-specific manifestation of borderline personality symptoms (e.g., rapid improvement of "depression" upon hospital admission or "relapse" of self-injurious behavior prior to or just after discharge). When prescribing medications, the consultant would do well to not "over-sell" the role of medications to the patient and consultee, but to also provide the hopeful attitude that medications can indeed play a role—albeit a partial one—in improvement of specific symptoms.[86]

Reflecting the variability in presentation of borderline personality and other cluster B personality disorders, four clusters of personality disorder symptoms—difficulty with cognition or perceptual organization, impulsive and aggressive behavior, mood instability and dysphoria, and suppression of anxiety—have been proposed as targets for pharmacotherapy.[88] The symptoms within each cluster might have a common neurobiological substrate that can serve as a rationale for treatment selection.

The impulsive–aggressive dimension and the mood-instability dimension are the two most relevant to cluster B personality disorders and, hence, the difficult patient. Anger, aggression, and behavioral disinhibition constitute primary impairments in the former domain. While selective serotonin reuptake inhibitors (SSRIs) were previously thought to be helpful based on earlier studies,[89] subsequent meta-analyses have not found evidence to support their use outside of treatment of comorbid depression and anxiety.[83–85] In small clinical trials, efficacy has been found for the mood-stabilizing agents lamotrigine[90] and valproate[91] in improving impulsive or aggressive behavior. Topiramate[92–94] and aripiprazole[95] were also found to reduce anger, but a subsequent meta-analysis questioned the design and funding of these trials.[85] Haloperidol may be useful in controlling agitation, although this effect could be nonspecific.[85] Quetiapine has more recently emerged as effective in reducing aggression.[96]

The mood-instability dimension consists of mood dysregulation, dysphoria, emotional lability, and depression. These likely have broad neurotransmitter underpinnings, possibly related to dysfunction in serotonergic, cholinergic, or noradrenergic systems. For affective instability, antipsychotics (haloperidol, aripiprazole, and olanzapine) and mood stabilizers (valproate, topiramate, and lamotrigine)[87,97] have shown some efficacy in smaller trials, most of which unfortunately have significant limitations.[87] The clinician who suspects major depression in the borderline patient, however, should note that depressive symptoms in borderline personality often resolve on their own, and should ensure that the borderline personality itself is being treated first.[19] Treatment of depression in borderline personality (via both pharmacologic as well as somatic therapies) seems to show a slower and less complete treatment response to both pharmacologic as well as somatic therapies than in patients with major depression without comorbid borderline personality,[98,99] and personality disorder may also predict accelerated rates of relapse.[100]

Atypical antipsychotics may have a nonspecific effect in reducing the outward expressions of intense emotions, such as rage, as well as reducing anxiety and alleviating cognitive-perceptual states (such as dissociative symptoms and brief episodes of paranoia).[87] Quetiapine has shown the most promise recently, as a randomized, placebo-controlled trial found superiority over placebo of low-dose extended-release quetiapine in reducing global borderline personality symptoms. Interestingly, the efficacy was similar for the 150-mg and 300-mg groups, but the 300-mg group suffered more adverse events.[101]

Regarding difficult patients with other personality disorders, a symptom-based approach, like that described above for borderline personality, may prove useful. Pharmacotherapy is not recommended for the treatment of other cluster B personality disorders (i.e., narcissistic personality disorder [NPD]; and antisocial personality disorder [APD]).[102]

Miscellaneous medications, ranging from methylphenidate to levodopa, have been reported to help difficult patients,[15] and there seem to exist single case reports touting almost any conceivable drug.[103] Given the present state of knowledge, it seems appropriate for the consultant to remember that mind and body are not separate, and that many seemingly insoluble problems respond to a search for, and aggressive treatment of, comorbid psychiatric conditions, especially affective and SUDs. Common and uncommon medical conditions may mimic personality disorders (e.g., three random instances in the literature are narcolepsy, Wolfram's syndrome, and Addison's disease[104–106]). Also, over the life-time of any given patient, the relationship with a supportive physician is as healing as any drug.

PSYCHIATRIST'S WORK WITH THE PATIENT

Although design and promotion of the behavior management protocol and consultation with the staff are the initial work of the consultant, the psychiatrist performs the following tasks with the patient directly:

- The psychiatric mental status examination, differential diagnosis, and formulation (including the use of observations of transference and countertransference)
- Assessment of suicide potential
- Assessment of present need for control of violence (as opposed to making a prediction of dangerousness)
- Assessment of, and recommendations around, co-morbid psychiatric disorders and maladaptive behaviors
- Rarely a highly focused, brief (one- or two-session) tactical psychotherapeutic intervention.

Differential Diagnosis

If the consulting psychiatrist does not provide them, there will not be a good mental status examination, psychiatric history, or biopsychosocial formulation in the medical record. However skilled or willing other specialists may be, only the psychiatrist has an understanding of the minute-to-minute fluctuations of transference and countertransference that occur early, even in a single interview (countertransference is so important as to be almost a diagnostic discriminator of borderline personality).[107] Also, there is a kind of rigor and discipline that the experienced psycho-diagnostician brings to these situations: no one else in the medical setting is, for instance, going to perform a Mini-Mental State Examination, ask about earliest memories, a history of sexual abuse, the content of dreams and fantasies, sexual worries, religious and spiritual concerns, disordered thoughts, and suicidal ideation—all in one interview—and then put them together into a differential diagnosis and formulation.

Differential diagnosis is crucial because comorbidity is almost a hallmark of the difficult patient, and it is surprising (if not impossible) to encounter a cluster B patient who does not also have at least one of the following diagnoses: another personality disorder, substance abuse disorders, affective disorders, anxiety disorders (especially panic and phobias), eating disorders, obsessive–compulsive disorder, PTSD, adult attention deficit/hyperactivity disorder, impulse control disorders, or other disorders.

Suicide Assessment

Patients with borderline personality disorder are at increased risk for suicide; specific risk factors described within this population include higher levels of impulsivity, hostility, low levels of harm-avoidance and high levels of novelty-seeking, comorbid substance and affective disorders, personal connection to suicide (family member, caregiver), and poor psychosocial functioning.[108,109] Suicide risk assessment is discussed in detail in Chapter 44. However, it bears mentioning here, given that difficult patients on the inpatient medical unit—due to the interplay of personality factors, active psychiatric comorbidity, and, often, psychological stress and regression in the face of acute medical illness—are often at increased risk of suicide. For the difficult patient, in addition to the usual risk factors, recent worsening in the medical condition along with perceived rejection by caregivers[110] adds considerably to the risk of suicide. Suicides and suicide attempts in medical and surgical settings correlate highly with primary psychiatric disorders, but hopelessness related to severe medical illness and anger over the loss of social supports have also been found to be significant.[110,111] Many suicide attempts occur in a clinical setting, in which the patient's experience is of being abandoned: during failing treatment, at times of imminent discharge, in conjunction with disputes with the staff, or during staff holidays. Negative countertransference itself may also be a poor predictor.[112] That the characteristics and demographics of suicides in non-psychiatric medical settings differ from those of patients in psychiatric settings,[113] coupled with the fact that personality-disordered patients may at their most vulnerable during a medical admission, underscores the fact that a detailed and thorough consideration of the suicide risk is warranted for every difficult patient the consultant encounters.

Assessment of Potential for Violence

Problems arising when the patient has difficulty controlling aggression are helped when the consultant defines for the staff the range of responses, from supporting the sulking patient or even giving in to a mildly over-controlling patient, to absolute limits on violence. The medical staff fear over-reacting, and the consultant reduces anxiety by defining the management of varying degrees of aggression. Disruptions are mostly born of self-protective or fearful impulses in the confused or delirious patient. Rarely, however, a patient becomes dangerous. In those instances, the most common warning is fear; someone becomes scared of the patient. Staff almost never fear delirious behavior, controllable anger, or senile pique, but they do tend to become wary, then edgy, then frightened. This intuition in the caregivers is often the only warning the consultant gets before an explosion. Ominous signs in the patient are rapidly increasing demandingness; more frequent and intense anger, especially with abusive language; and mounting agitation and paranoia. The general feeling in the medical setting of an implacable crescendo of menace surrounding the patient is another ominous sign.

Before any decision about physical restraint of the patient is made, hospital security guards should be standing by on the ward. This is a first step in the decision-making process. Security can always be dismissed with thanks after standing by, but to delay summoning help until after such a decision is made risks panicking the patient, who may have an uncanny ability to sense an impending confrontation.

Such ideas refer to control of violent behavior in the immediate situation. Occasionally, however, the consultant is asked about the long-range "dangerousness" of the patient. This is an opinion that involves extrapolating from present behavior in a known, observed situation to a guess about the patient's interaction with a different milieu, one that might contain drugs, weapons, and situations beyond the psychiatrist's ken. Medicine is about healing, not social control. Dangerous persons (e.g., the person with an antisocial personality who commits rape) may in some sense be "difficult patients," but in these situations, they are not patients at all, but criminals.

Psychiatric opinions outside the medical purview violate an important boundary and feed the fallacy that all bad behavior is somehow psychiatric and that mentally ill persons have no personal responsibility for their behavior. What the psychiatrist can do, however, is document medical history from the consenting patient about drugs, access to weapons, felony convictions, and the like. Surprisingly often, such a patient discloses useful information in the context of a skillfully elicited childhood history of enuresis, fire-setting, and cruelty to animals. ("Were you ever accused of setting fires? Did anybody ever say you were mean to the neighbor's pets?") Such patients can be oddly eager to resurrect old denials and often are still indignant about them. They then sometimes go on to give themselves away and provide information needed to protect caregivers and other patients in the medical setting.

Substance Abuse

Substance use is one area in which the consultant can be most useful to patients with primitive personality problems. Substance use is such an issue for a significant proportion of difficult patients that excess alcohol can be thought of as a personality disorder in a bottle. A significant number of borderline patients—one-fifth in one study—abuse substances.[18] Of these, perhaps up to a fourth have such a good response to abstinence that they no longer meet diagnostic criteria for the disorder,[114] and the absence of an active substance use disorder (SUD) has been found to be the strongest single predictor of remission of borderline personality symptoms over time.[18]

Readers are referred to Chapters 14 and 15 for further information on the diagnosis and management of alcohol and SUDs. However, it is important to note that personality-disorder patients can benefit from 12-step recovery programs, given that they have two ingredients known to help primitive character pathology: an emphasis on taking responsibility for oneself (as opposed to cultivating the victim role) and a highly structured series of steps and methods. Moreover, there is commonality between a central tenet of one of the most successful treatments for borderline personality, dialectical-behavioral therapy (DBT)—that of embracing both acceptance and change—and one of the philosophical underpinnings of 12-step programs, embodied in the Serenity Prayer.[115] DBT itself can also be helpful for SUDs in patients with borderline personality.[116] Not least in importance, there are myriads of such groups meeting at almost any hour of the day or night in every location in the urban United States.

Not surprisingly, it requires great skill to persuade a difficult patient to identify with one of the 12-step programs. First, there is almost always dense denial of the abuse problem, along with a need to see the self as powerless and victimized. Splitting patients and narcissists see themselves as "better than" persons in Alcoholics Anonymous, for example, and are so vulnerable to shame that they hesitate to take on another attribute they see as shameful. Also, the general culture outside such programs has little real information about what they can accomplish, so the patient is not only ashamed, but also usually ignorant of these resources.

There is an art to getting a difficult patient to consider that a problem with addiction, codependency, or the like may be the root of much of the suffering the patient endures. Practicing this art involves accumulating knowledge about such programs and having familiarity with some persons helped by them. It involves the ability to discern when the patient might be receptive, first to acknowledging an addictive problem and second to considering such a program. It involves knowing how to elicit information in a non-shaming way ("Do you find yourself drinking more than you really want to be drinking?"), presenting the condition as a disease and "not the person's fault," and introducing the ideas gradually in a non-threatening way. ("Did your mom ever turn to Al-Anon for help with your father's drinking?" "Did you ever get help from the Adult Children of Alcoholics program or something like that?")

No difficult patient is ever educated easily, and it usually requires multiple inputs from numerous sources over many months even to begin to get some of these options accepted by the patient. The consulting psychiatrist is ideal to introduce such ideas and, given the relapse rate of difficult patients, might get another opportunity with the same patient in the future. The consultant can at least start the educational process without making the patient feel ashamed.

Brief Tactical Psychotherapy

Psychotherapy is a risky proposition, and the consultant is wise to resist the temptation to do much on the medical-surgical unit. Rarely, however, the crisis of an illness provides a unique chance for insight and growth for the patient with a primitive personality. This lucid interval is incidentally produced when an illness and treatment cut through the veils of dissociation surrounding such patients, their maladaptive projective defenses, and their habitual externalization of responsibility. In this context, sometimes the patient asks not only the superficial "Why me?," but also the deeper question, "Who am I that this is happening to?" In a certain sense, catastrophe throws the primitive individual into a developmental crisis, in which there may be the potential for recouping a bit of the developmental lack of progress in the first 2 years of life—the maturation from the paranoid position to the depressive position—along with a capacity for grieving and developing empathy for others that such maturational steps entail.

A study of changes in pathologic narcissism in a cohort of subjects followed for several years[117] found that the majority of them had improved significantly and that the improvement related to life achievements, new durable relationships, and disillusionment. These subjects displayed decreased grandiosity and deeper empathy for others as evidenced by better relationships. The disillusionment related to these improvements, moreover, had occurred at a critical juncture in the person's development and was of a certain type—challenging but not devastating. Rather than questioning the construct validity of narcissistic personality disorder (as was done in the study), the findings plausibly support the idea that certain painful, constructive real-life experiences help people change their primitive pathology. (That brief therapeutic interventions can further this process, even in primitive patients, is shown in some of the therapies detailed by Malan, Budman, Strupp, Bloom, Horowitz, and especially Winnicott.)[118]

This is the rationale for a certain brief, tactical intervention by the psychiatric consultant who encounters the difficult patient during a medical or surgical crisis: how to keep the disillusionment from being completely devastating and help the patient make sense of it in terms of personal identity. (As Figure 43-1 shows, a vague sense of personal identity underlies much of the pathology of the difficult patient.) The patient is in a process of trying to adapt to the illness or injury, to work through it, to grieve losses, and to contain fears. In this context, the psychiatrist's aim is not merely to help further this grieving or adjusting process, but to accomplish a deeper, more lasting goal: using the illness or injury process as a template or map for other life changes, using the crisis of the moment to help the patient learn new ways of thinking about the self, and coping with rage, terror, and shame.

The tactical brief therapy of the difficult patient falls into two types of maneuvers: *containment* and *intervention*. Containment involves control of uncontrolled affect, distorted cognition, and destructive behavior. Intervention consists of correcting the misdirection of the patient's trajectory, previously determined by pathologic affect, distorted cognition, and self-defeating behavior. Containment and intervention roughly correspond to the two parts of traditional psychotherapy: the frame (scheduling, vacations, fee, phone calls, limits on acting out, confidentiality) and the content (symptoms, history, development, associations, discourse, dreams, fantasies, defenses, adaptation, transference, countertransference, and other non-framework components of therapy). This "moment" of brief tactical psychotherapy assumes the patient in the medical situation is temporarily contained and already in a dialogue with the psychiatrist about the illness or injury that brought the patient to this place at this time.

The therapist's first task—and therapist is what the consultant becomes at this moment—is to listen to see whether the patient is asking for intervention. The patient signals such readiness not only by addressing the impact of the illness or injury but also by mentioning the overall meaning of the patient's life, the patient's "story," the over-arching narrative that helps any human being make sense of the world. If the tactical intervention is to be helpful, the patient must be the one to push for it. The therapist's experience at this point is of being passively drawn into the patient's turbulent material, yet actively steering the discussion away from affects too intense on the one side and cognitions that are psychotically distorted on the other.

Up to this point, the therapist's job has been careful listening and containment. If the patient is ready, the patient will introduce these two themes: the overall story of the patient's life and its meaning, and the meaning of the illness or injury that is serving as the focus of the tactical psychotherapeutic moment. The patient will tend to see the medical crisis as thematically pertinent to the meaningful life story—for instance, just another in a long series of persecutions, a punishment for something bad the patient has done or is. The life story is generally a standard narrative of a search for perfect safety and love, a quest for power so the patient will never again be scared; there are seldom any major surprises at this point.

The therapist's first active step in the tactical intervention occurs now: labeling the life story; labeling the symbolic, adding metaphoric meaning of the illness or injury; and labeling the pain that is at the interface of the two. This is almost like offering a "title" for the story. ("All your life you've been a survivor; now you wonder if you can survive this terror.") The idea here is that, to survive, individuals have to construct a meaningful narrative of the crisis. Under pressure of converting experience into symbols and then into meaning, the primitive person may be forced to construct a more realistic life narrative (and hence a more coherent sense of personal identity).

If the patient continues to be receptive to tactical intervention, two things happen at this point: first, production of deeper material in symbolic form (mention of a fantasy or recurrent dream, some external, cultural symbol or icon, a movie or a television character) and, second, a rather pointed question for the therapist about what to do (an acceptance by the patient of the therapist as a relatively separate, helpful person). This turning point requires careful listening because the key organizing theme of the patient's life (as the patient sees it) is presented in this one moment of symbol formation along with the rather concrete question that follows directly after.

Here the therapist does not answer the patient's question about what to do with the illness assaulting the meaning in the patient's life. The therapist labels the assault, points out the crisis in meaning, and thematically throws the question back to the patient. ("In a way you're asking how to cope with this thing, but in a deeper way you're saying that you're Scarlett O'Hara, since you just mentioned her. How would Scarlett handle what you're going through?")

What the patient says next reveals whether the tactical linking of the two meanings and two stories seemed useful to the patient. If so, the patient produces more details of the life story, again asking the therapist what to do about the illness or injury. Again the therapist throws responsibility back to the patient, labeling meaningfulness issues and the importance of the illness or injury to it. ("You just mentioned losing your husband—like Scarlett O'Hara—and now you're asking how to cope with your boyfriend's reaction to your mastectomy. Scarlett fell back on Tara and her own resources. What resources do you have to draw on?")

This working-through cycle of question and deflection continues as long as the therapist has time and the patient has the strength to bear the rage, terror, or shame of the moment. Usually the patient soon fatigues and moves the subject back to some specific entitled demand, such as getting more pain medication. This signals that the therapy part of the encounter is now over and that the consultant is once again back to management of the difficult patient.

Although the brief tactical psychotherapy just described is probably the most useful first-line approach for the inpatient consultant, other psychotherapeutic methods have been designed for the treatment of borderline personality disorder and can be applied to other difficult patients as well. Dialectical-behavioral therapy (DBT),[119] transference-focused psychotherapy (TFP),[120] mentalization-based therapy (MBT),[121] and schema-focused therapy (SFT)[122] each are highly operationalized treatments and have a somewhat different theoretical perspective; all have shown efficacy in randomized, controlled trials for improving outcomes for those with borderline personality disorder.[123–126]

Although full implementation of these therapies is obviously not possible during a few consultation visits, familiarity with the theory and techniques they rely upon can enhance the consultant's ability to make sense of, and employ a therapeutic tool, in diverse situations.[127] Indeed, as these very different forms of therapy have been found to produce similar results,[128] a set of common factors for any successful therapy of borderline patients has been proposed.[129]

Table 43-5 summarizes these treatments and provides examples of how they can be adapted to encounters with the difficult patient.

TERMINATION

Preparation of the difficult patient for discharge from the hospital is fraught with hazards. The patient not only might intensify disruptive behavior to prolong the hospital stay but also might simultaneously try to leave prematurely. The patient might secretly infect dressings or IV lines with saliva or feces and develop a fever while threatening to leave the hospital against medical advice. Or the patient might increase suicidal gestures, such as wrist slashing, to manipulate (get close to/stay distant from) the staff. Firm limits on sabotage and elopement should be discussed with the staff. Around termination, they should be more observant of the patient and more visible and firm. A specific discharge date should be firmly adhered to,[130] despite a predictable worsening in the patient's psychological status.

After the patient has left, it is preferable for the consultant to touch base with the staff and the consultee once more to review the treatment and to share some of the consultant's own feelings. In this way, the consultant not only "terminates" with the staff but also paves the way for future work with the next difficult patient who comes to the general hospital.

TABLE 43-5 Psychotherapies for Borderline Personality Disorder and Their Relevance to the Difficult Patient

THERAPY	DEVELOPER	RELEVANT THEORY*	RELEVANT TECHNIQUES	EXAMPLE WITH THE DIFFICULT PATIENT
Dialectical behavioral therapy	Marsha Linehan	The patient is more emotionally vulnerable and reactive and is therefore ill-suited to a normal social environment	Acknowledge and validate the patient's difference while also encouraging change	*Consultant*: "This ward is a difficult place for you. Everyone's too busy to give you the help you need, and this illness is one of the most distressing things that's ever happened to you. Your rage and fear make sense. That being said, the doctors and nurses here really are trying their best. They're at least meeting you a third of the way. Do you think you could cut them a little more slack? Do you want me to communicate anything to them for you?"
Transference-focused psychotherapy	Otto Kernberg, John Clarkin	The patient is frozen in a state of immature emotional development where self is split into multiple negative and positive parts experienced successively in time, each infused with maladaptively powerful affects. Personality therefore lacks consistency and cohesion	Interpret the patient's successive self-states to enhance the patient's awareness of the multiple roles she or he plays, which fosters a more integrated self	*Consultant*: "You say the doctors here are the best ever, but the nurses are all bitches. And at first you told me I understood you like no one else. But now that I'm trying to enforce the rules to protect your safety, you're ready to throw me on the trash heap. So it's almost like I experienced two different people: first you were so warm and tender and the next minute you were like a warrior ready to cleave me in two. Aside from letting you take off your heart monitor leads, which you know is too dangerous right now, how can we help you feel better heard and cared for?"
Mentalization-based therapy	Peter Fonagy, Anthony Bateman	The patient cannot make sense of the actions of self and others on the basis of intentional mental states, such as desires, feelings, and beliefs	Point out the patient's actions to help the patient draw a link between actions and what the patient is thinking and feeling; identify the patient's reactions to the therapist's words or actions and help them guess what you're feeling and thinking	*Consultant*: "Can you tell me what you were feeling and thinking while you were cutting yourself with that razor you brought in? Were you scared? Were you angry because we did something wrong?" *Patient*: "I told you to get the f*** out of here!!" *Consultant*: "I'm concerned about you and terrified when you scream like that. I know that scares other staff too. We'll need those restraints to keep you safe until we can understand you better and help you cope with this more safely."

Table continued on next page

TABLE 43-5 Psychotherapies for Borderline Personality Disorder and Their Relevance to the Difficult Patient—cont'd

THERAPY	DEVELOPER	RELEVANT THEORY*	RELEVANT TECHNIQUES	EXAMPLE WITH THE DIFFICULT PATIENT
Schema-focused therapy	Jeffrey Young; influenced by the work of Aaron Beck	The patient's inner world is characterized by five modes, or aspects of self, that interact in destructive ways: the abandoned and abused child, the angry and impulsive child, the detached protector, the punitive parent, and the healthy adult	Develop the "healthy adult" by "limited reparenting," emotion-focused work (e.g., imagery and dialogues), cognitive restructuring and education, and breaking behavioral patterns	*Patient*: "I don't take my heart pills or my insulin usually for the simple reason that I'm a drop out and a druggie and what's the point of someone like me continuing to take up space on this earth." *Consultant*: (who has already established that the patient is not depressed but rather personality-disordered) "Multiple times already I've heard you be extremely hard on yourself. It would be useful to give that particular voice of yours a name. How about 'My Abusive Step-father?' When you hear yourself talking like that, try to remember that name. With outpatient therapy, you can learn how to tell that part of yourself to leave the rest of you alone and gradually he'll go away for good."

Note: The patient = the borderline personality-disordered or difficult patient.

*With minor differences in emphasis all of these theories assume the same etiologic factors: innate temperamental difficulties, or an abusive or neglectful (or poorly matched in terms of temperament) relationship with a caregiver in early life.

REFERENCES

Access the reference list online at https://expertconsult.inkling.com/.

Care of the Suicidal Patient

44

Rebecca Weintraub Brendel, M.D., J.D.
Katherine A. Koh, M.D., M.Sc.
Roy H. Perlis, M.D., M.Sc.
Theodore A. Stern, M.D.

OVERVIEW

Suicide, or intentional self-harm with the intent of causing death, is the 11th leading cause of death in the United States, accounting for more than 40,000 deaths each year.[1] Non-lethal self-inflicted injuries are even more prevalent, accounting for nearly 800,000 Emergency Department (ED) visits per year[2] and reflecting the high ratio of suicide attempts to completed suicides. Psychiatric disorders, as the most powerful risk factor for both completed and attempted suicide, are associated with more than 90% of completed suicides[3,4] and with the majority of attempted suicides.[5–7] In addition, medical illness, especially chronic illness, is also associated with an increased risk of suicide.[8]

Psychosomatic medicine psychiatrists must be familiar with the evaluation and treatment of patients who contemplate, threaten, or attempt suicide, not only because of the risk of suicide associated with psychiatric and medical illness, but also because they are likely to be asked to evaluate patients who are medically or surgically hospitalized following a suicide attempt. Although guided by knowledge of epidemiologic risk factors for suicide (Table 44-1), the clinician must rely on a detailed examination and on clinical judgment in the evaluation of current suicide risk.

EPIDEMIOLOGY AND RISK FACTORS

Epidemiology

Suicide accounts for 1.6% of the total number of deaths in the United States each year.[1] Although no nationwide data on annual attempted suicides are available, research indicates that for every completed suicide, approximately 10 to 40 attempts are made;[9,10] of note, some individuals make more than one unsuccessful attempt. Each year, EDs treat nearly 800,000 self-inflicted injuries or suicide attempters.[2] These visits represent approximately 1.9% of all annual ED visits.[2] Recent trends suggest that after a period of decline in suicide rates in the United States from 1986 to 1999, suicide rates have increased almost steadily between 1999 and 2014, with greater annual percentage increases after 2006.[10] Use of firearms is the most common method of committing suicide for both men and women in the United States, accounting for between 50% and 60% of annual suicides.[11] Suffocation, including hanging, is the second most common cause of suicide overall in the United States, and the second most common cause in men, accounting for approximately 11,400 suicide deaths per year.[1] Poisoning, including drug ingestion, is the third most common cause of completed suicide in the United States and the second most common cause in women, accounting for approximately 6800 deaths per year.[1] However, between 1999 and 2014, the percentages of suicides involving firearms and poisoning declined, while suicides involving suffocation increased.[10] Historically, drug ingestion has accounted for the majority of unsuccessful suicide attempts.[12–14]

Suicide rates differ by age, gender, and race. Rates generally increase with age; people older than 65 years are 1.5 times more likely to commit suicide than are younger individuals, whereas white men over age 85 years have an even higher rate of suicide.[15–18] The number of suicides in the elderly is disproportionately high; the elderly appear to make more serious attempts on their lives and are less apt to survive when medical complications from an attempt ensue—one out of four attempts in this group results in a completed suicide.[16,17,19] Although the elderly have the highest suicide rates, suicide in young adults (between the ages of 15 and 24) rose three-fold between 1950 and 1990, becoming the third leading cause of death following unintentional injuries and homicide.[11,20,21] From 1990 to 2003, the suicide rate declined in the 10- to 24-year-old age group.[21,22] However, in 2004, for the first time in a decade and a half, the suicide rate in this age group increased by 8%.[22] In addition, hanging/suffocation became the most common method of suicide among girls in this age group.[22] Since 2008, the rate of suicide in this population has continued to increase.[18] In females, the largest percentage increase in suicide rates between 1999–2014 was in the 10 to 14 age group, increasing by 200%.[10]

Men are more likely to complete suicide than are women, although women are more likely to attempt suicide than are men. Four times more men than women complete suicide,[9,11,18] although women are three to four times more likely than men to attempt suicide.[9,23] The reasons for these disparities have not been established clearly. Whites and Native Americans attempt and commit suicide more than non-whites.[5,9,11,21] African Americans and Hispanics have approximately half the suicide rate of whites.[9,18,24,25]

TABLE 44-1 Risk Factors for Suicide

Psychiatric illness
- Major depression
- Bipolar disorder
- Alcoholism and drug dependence
- Schizophrenia
- Character disorders
- Organic brain syndrome
- Panic disorder

Race
Marital status (widowed, divorced, or separated)
Living alone
Recent personal loss
Unemployment
Financial/legal difficulties
Co-morbid medical illness (having chronic illness, pain, or terminal illness)
History of suicide attempts or threats
Male gender
Advancing age
Family history of suicide
Recent hospital discharge
Firearms in the household
Hopelessness

TABLE 44-2 Percentage of Suicides With a Given Psychiatric Disorder

CONDITION	PERCENTAGE OF SUICIDES
Affective illness	50
Drug or alcohol abuse	25
Schizophrenia	10
Character disorders	5
Secondary depression	5
Organic brain syndromes	2
None apparent	2

Psychiatric Risk Factors

Psychiatric illness is the most powerful risk factor for both completed and attempted suicide. Psychiatric disorders are associated with more than 90% of completed suicides[3,4,25,26] and with the vast majority of attempted suicides.[5–7] Mood disorders, including major depressive disorder (MDD) and bipolar disorder, are responsible for approximately 50% of completed suicides, alcohol and drug abuse for 25%, psychosis for 10%, and personality disorders for 5% (Table 44-2).[27,28]

Up to 15% of patients with MDD or bipolar disorder complete suicide, almost always during depressive episodes;[29] this represents a suicide risk 30 times greater than that of the general population.[30,31] True life-time risk may be somewhat lower, because these estimates (and those for the other diagnoses discussed later) typically are derived from hospitalized patient samples.[27] The risk appears to be greater early in the course of a life-time disorder, early on in a depressive episode,[32] in the first week following psychiatric hospitalization,[33] in the first month following hospital discharge,[33] and in the early stages of recovery.[33] The risk may[34] or may not[35] be elevated by co-morbid psychosis. A 10-year follow-up study of almost 1000 patients found that those who committed suicide within the first year of follow-up were more likely to be suffering from global insomnia, severe anhedonia, impaired concentration, psychomotor agitation, alcohol abuse, anxiety, and panic attacks, whereas those who committed suicide after the first year of follow-up were more likely to be suffering from suicidal ideation, severe hopelessness, and a history of suicide attempts.[34] A study of 667 patients with MDD found that patients who reported prior suicide attempts had more current general medical conditions, more current alcohol or other substance abuse, more work hours missed in the past week than non-attempters, and also reported more current suicidal ideation.[36]

Approximately 15% to 25% of patients with alcohol or drug dependence complete suicide,[32,37] of which up to 84% suffer from both alcohol and drug dependence.[37] The suicide risk appears to be greatest approximately 9 years after the commencement of alcohol and drug addiction.[3,38] The majority of patients with alcohol dependence who commit suicide suffer from co-morbid depressive disorders,[32,39,40] and as many as one-third have experienced the recent loss of a close relationship through separation or death.[41]

Nearly 20% of people who complete suicide are legally intoxicated at the time of their death.[42] Alcohol and drug abuse are associated with more pervasive suicidal ideation, more serious suicidal intent, more lethal suicide attempts, and a greater number of suicide attempts.[43] Use of alcohol and drugs may impair judgment and foster impulsivity.[33,44]

Approximately 10% of patients with schizophrenia complete suicide, mostly during periods of improvement after relapse or during periods of depression.[40,45,46] The risk for suicide appears to be greater among young men who are newly diagnosed,[46–48] who have a chronic course and numerous exacerbations, who are discharged from hospitals with significant psychopathology and functional impairment, and who have a realistic awareness and fear of further mental decline.[40,48] The risk may also be increased with akathisia and with abrupt discontinuation of neuroleptics.[32] Patients who experience hallucinations (that instruct them to harm themselves) in association with schizophrenia, mania, or depression with psychotic features are probably at greater risk for self-harm, and they should be protected.[49]

Between 4% and 10% of patients with borderline personality disorder and 5% of patients with antisocial personality disorder commit suicide.[50] The risk appears to be greater for those with co-morbid unipolar depression or alcohol abuse.[51,52] Patients with personality disorders often make impulsive suicidal gestures or attempts; these attempts may become more lethal if they are not taken seriously. Even manipulative gestures can turn fatal.[49] A prospective cohort study of 7968 patients examined suicide rates up to 4 years after a deliberate self-harm episode and found an approximately 30-fold increase in risk of suicide compared to the general population.[53]

As many as 15% to 20% of patients with anxiety disorders complete suicide,[54] and up to 20% of patients with panic disorder attempt suicide.[55] Although the risk of suicide in patients with anxiety and panic disorders may be elevated secondary to co-morbid conditions (e.g., MDD and alcohol or drug abuse), the suicide risk remains almost as high as that of major depression, even after co-existing conditions are taken into account.[56] The risk for suicide attempts may be elevated for women with an early onset and with co-morbid alcohol or drug abuse.[55] Patients with obsessive–compulsive disorder (OCD) have also been found to be at high risk for suicidal behavior, with a history of suicide attempt reported in 27% of subjects in one study.[57]

The first prospective study of body dysmorphic disorder (BDD) found that patients with BDD have rates of suicidal ideation that are approximately 10 to 25 times higher than those in the general population and that their suicide attempt rate was 3 to 12 times higher. The completed suicide rate of patients with BDD is still being studied.[58]

One study of 754 inpatients and 1100 patients assessed following discharge from a psychiatric inpatient unit found that nearly a quarter of the inpatient suicides occurred within the first 7 days of admission—the majority died by hanging. Post-discharge suicide was most frequent in the first 2 weeks after leaving the hospital, with the highest number of deaths occurring on the first day following discharge.[59]

Medical Risk Factors

Medical illness, especially of a severe or chronic nature, is associated with an increased risk of suicide and is thus considered a risk factor for completed suicide (even though there is most likely a multi-factorial relationship between medical illness and suicide).[8,60,61] Medical disorders are associated with as many as 35% to 40% of suicides[62] and with as many as 70% of suicides in those older than 60 years.[63] Acquired immunodeficiency syndrome (AIDS), cancer, head trauma, epilepsy, multiple sclerosis, Huntington's chorea, organic brain syndromes, spinal cord injuries, hypertension, cardiopulmonary disease, peptic ulcer disease, chronic renal failure, Cushing's disease, rheumatoid arthritis, and porphyria have each been reported to increase the risk of suicide. Notably, however, few investigations concerning the increased risk for suicide in these populations have controlled for the effects of age, gender, race, psychiatric disorders, other medical disorders, or use of medications. There have also been few studies of patients who commit suicide on general hospital medical or surgical units. A review of these rare cases suggests that agitation and a readily available lethal means of suicide are potent risk factors (as are past psychiatric illness, substance abuse, suicidal ideation, and depression).[64]

Patients with AIDS appear to have a suicide risk that is greater than that of the general population, and estimates of the increased risk range from 7 to 66 times greater than the general population.[27,65,66] While some studies suggest that the risk of suicide in human immunodeficiency virus (HIV) infection has increased approximately seven-fold,[8,65] others suggest that HIV-positive individuals do not have a significantly increased risk of death from suicide.[67] Testing for antibodies associated with HIV infection has resulted in an immediate and substantial decrease in suicidal ideation in those who turned out to be seronegative; no increase in suicidal ideation was detected in those who were seropositive.[68] Sexual orientation among men, in and of itself, has not been identified as an independent risk factor for completed suicide.[69] Recent studies suggest that gay, lesbian, and bisexual individuals have a higher life-time prevalence of suicide attempts than heterosexual individuals.[70] Cancer patients have a suicide rate that is almost twice as great as that found in the general population, and the risk appears to be higher in the first 5 years after diagnosis.[65,71,72] A large retrospective cohort study of patients diagnosed with cancer in the United States from 1973 to 2002 found that suicide rates varied among patients with cancers of different anatomic sites, with the highest risks observed in the following order: the lung and bronchus, stomach, oral cavity and pharynx, and larynx.[72] Head and neck malignancies have been associated with a risk of suicide 11 times greater than that of the general population (possibly due to increased rates of tobacco and alcohol use and the resultant facial disfigurement and loss of voice).[65] In men, gastrointestinal cancers are associated with a greater risk of suicide.[58] Other factors that may place cancer patients at greater risk include poor prognosis, poor pain control, fatigue, depression, hopelessness, delirium, disinhibition, prior suicide attempts, recent losses, and a paucity of social supports.[73,74]

As with cancer patients, individuals with head trauma, multiple sclerosis, and peptic ulcer disease have approximately twice the risk of suicide as those in the general population.[65,75,76] In patients with head injuries, the risk appears to be greater in those who suffer severe injuries and in those who develop dementia, psychosis, character changes, or epilepsy.[75–77] In patients with multiple sclerosis, the risk may be higher for those diagnosed before age 40 years and within the first 5 years after a diagnosis has been made.[78] In patients with peptic ulcer disease, the increased risk is thought to be due to co-morbid psychiatric and substance use (especially alcohol) disorders.[65,77]

Between the increased risk of suicide of approximately two-fold for cancer, head trauma, multiple sclerosis, and peptic ulcer disease, and the increased risk in HIV-infected/AIDS patients (estimated to be at least nearly seven-fold), there are a number of medical illnesses associated with intermediate increases in suicide risk. These illnesses and conditions include epilepsy, systemic lupus erythematosus, spinal cord injuries, Huntington's disease, organic brain syndromes, and chronic renal disease. Patients with end-stage renal failure treated with hemodialysis may have the highest risk of all subgroups.[65,79] As many as 5% of patients with chronic renal failure on hemodialysis die from suicide; those who travel to medical centers for dialysis have a higher suicide rate than those who are dialyzed at home. The risk for suicide among these patients may be as high as 400 times that of the general population.[80]

Patients with epilepsy are five times more likely than those in the general population to complete or to attempt suicide.[65,81–83] Sufferers of temporal lobe epilepsy, with concomitant psychosis or personality changes, may also be at greater risk.[65,81,82,84]

Delirious and confused patients may suffer from agitation and destructive impulses and be unable to protect themselves from harm.[73] In victims of spinal cord injury, the risk is actually greater for those with less severe injuries.[85,86]

Hypertensive patients[77] and those with cardiopulmonary disease[49] may also have a higher risk for suicide than those in the general population. Although previous reports suggested that β-blockers could contribute to increased risk by promoting depression,[77] recent studies suggest that β-blockers do not increase the risk of developing depression.[87] Patients with diabetes have more hopelessness and thoughts of suicide than internal medicine outpatients, although fatal and non-fatal suicidal behavior has not been well-studied in this population.[88] Finally, an association between suicide and very low cholesterol levels has been reported, but the connection is still under investigation.[27]

Suicidal ideation in pregnancy has been associated with unplanned pregnancy, current major depression, and a co-morbid anxiety disorder.[89] Completed suicide and suicide attempts are less frequent during pregnancy and the post-partum period than they are in the general population of women. However, suicides account for almost 20% of post-partum deaths.[90]

Surgical procedures have also been associated with a higher risk of suicide. Six epidemiologic studies have concluded that the suicide rate in women who received cosmetic breast implants was approximately twice the expected rate based on estimates in the general population.[91–96]

Bariatric surgery is associated with an increased risk of death from non-disease-related causes, including suicide, compared with other severely obese individuals and the general population.[97] More research is necessary to determine whether these high rates of suicide are due to pre-existing psychiatric illness in cohorts of surgery patients or to the post-surgical complications of the surgery or its impact on quality of life.[98]

Suicide has been distinguished from life-ending acts and end-of-life decisions in the literature, based on patients with chronic kidney disease and dialysis.[99] Discussion of physician-assisted suicide is addressed in the end-of-life chapter. Among patients with advanced AIDS, the desire for hastened death has been found to be 4.6% to 8.3%, significantly lower than the rate found in studies of patients with advanced or terminal cancer.[100]

Familial and Genetic Risk Factors

A family history of suicide, a family history of psychiatric illness, and a tumultuous early family environment have each been found to have an important impact on the risk for suicide.[11,62] As many as 7% to 14% of persons who attempt suicide have a family history of suicide.[101] A family history of suicide confers approximately a two-fold increase in the risk for suicide after family psychiatric history is controlled for.[102] This increased suicide risk may be mediated through a shared genetic predisposition for suicide, psychiatric disorders, or impulsive behavior,[32,47,103] or through a shared family environment in which modeling and imitation are prominent.[104]

Genetic factors are supported by evidence that monozygotic twins have a higher concordance rate for suicide and suicide attempts than do dizygotic twins, and by evidence that biological parents of adoptees who commit suicide have a higher rate of suicide than do biological parents of non-suicidal adoptees.[103,105] However, little is known about the specific genetic factors that confer this risk. Studies have largely focused on serotonin neurotransmission, including genetic mutations in the rate-limiting enzyme in serotonin synthesis, L-tryptophan hydroxylase, serotonin receptors, and the serotonin transporter; however, this investigation is still preliminary.[102,106–108] Overall, it is estimated that one-third to one-half the risk of suicide is genetically mediated.[102]

Numerous familial environmental factors may also contribute to suicide risk. A tumultuous early family environment (including early parental death, parental separation, frequent moves, and emotional, physical, or sexual abuse) increases the risk for suicide.[109] A meta-analysis suggested that suicide attempts were twice as likely to occur in adults who suffered childhood sexual abuse compared with adults who were not abused.[109] A child's risk of future suicide attempts or completion may also be increased through modeling of suicidal behavior in important family members.

Social Risk Factors

Widowed, divorced, or separated adults are at greater risk for suicide than are single adults, who are at greater risk than married adults.[110,111] Married adults with young children appear to carry the lowest risk.[33,49,62] Living alone substantially increases the risk for suicide, especially among adults who are widowed, divorced, or separated.[33] Social isolation from family, relatives, friends, neighbors, and co-workers also increases the chance of suicide.[47,62] Conversely, the presence of social supports is protective against suicide.[102]

Significant personal losses (including diminution of self-esteem or status[62,63]) and conflicts also place individuals, particularly young adults and adolescents, at greater risk for suicide.[3,112] Bereavement following the death of a loved one increases the risk for suicide over the next 4 or 5 years, particularly among people with a psychiatric history (including suicide attempts) and in those who receive little family support.[32,113] Unemployment, which may produce or exacerbate psychiatric illness or may result from psychiatric illness,[32] increases the likelihood of suicide and accounts for as many as one-third to one-half of completed suicides.[42,62] This risk may be particularly elevated among men.[35] Financial and legal difficulties also increase the risk for suicide.[33,114]

The annual number of suicides among soldiers on active duty in the Army, Army Reserve, and Army National Guard has reached a 28-year high, having risen steadily between the years 2004 and 2008.[115] The wars in Afghanistan and Iraq have been associated with the highest suicide rates in the United States military personnel since tracking began in 1980.[116] One study of suicide risk among veterans of Operations Iraqi Freedom and Enduring Freedom showed that the overall risk was not significantly elevated compared to that in the general population, but suicide risk was increased for former active-duty veterans and for veterans diagnosed with a selected mental disorder.[117] However, a study of patients in the Veterans Health Administration in fiscal year 2001 found that the suicide rates were significantly higher than in the general population.[118]

The presence of one or more firearms in the home appears to increase the risk of suicide independently for both genders and all age groups, even when other risk factors, such as depression and alcohol abuse, are taken into account.[6,112,119] For example, adolescents with a gun in the household have suicide rates between 4 and 10 times higher than other adolescents.[120]

Past and Present Suicidality

A history of suicide attempts is one of the most powerful risk factors for completed and attempted suicide.[121] As many as 10% to 20% of people with prior suicide attempts complete suicide.[122] The risk for completed suicide following an attempted suicide is almost 100 times that of the general population in the year following the attempt; it then declines but remains elevated throughout the next 8 years.[32] People with prior suicide attempts are also at greater risk for subsequent attempts and have been found to account for approximately 50% of serious overdoses.[123] The clinical use of past suicide attempts as a predictive risk factor may be limited in the elderly because the elderly make fewer attempts for each completed suicide.[62]

The lethality of past suicide attempts slightly increases the risk for completed suicide,[32] especially among women with psychiatric illness.[39] The dangerousness of an attempt, however, may be more predictive of the risk for suicide in those individuals with significant intent to suicide and a realization of the potential lethality of their actions.[124]

The communication of present suicidal ideation and intent must be carefully evaluated as a risk factor for completed and attempted suicide. As many as 80% of people who complete suicide communicate their intent either directly or indirectly.[62] Death or suicide may be discussed, new wills or life insurance policies may be written, valued possessions may be given away, or uncharacteristic and destructive behaviors may arise.[62]

People who intend to commit suicide may, however, be less likely to communicate their intent to their healthcare providers than they are to close family and friends.[45] Although 50% of people who commit suicide have consulted a physician in the month before their death, only 60% of them communicated some degree of suicidal ideation or intent to their physician.[45] In a study of 571 cases of completed suicide who had met with their healthcare professional within 4 weeks of their suicide,[125] only 22% discussed their suicidal intent. Many investigators believe that ideation and intent may be more readily discussed with psychiatrists than with other physicians.[125,126]

Hopelessness, or negative expectations about the future, is a stronger predictor of suicide than is depression or suicidal ideation,[127,128] and may be both a short-term and long-term predictor of completed suicide in patients with major depression.[45]

Contact With Physicians

Nearly half of the people who commit suicide have had contact with their primary care provider (PCP) within 1 month of committing suicide.[33,45,129] Approximately three-quarters of people who commit suicide have seen a PCP in the year before the suicide.[129] Many of these individuals have sought treatment from their PCP for somatic rather than for psychiatric complaints.[130] Rates of psychiatric encounters in the period before completed suicides are lower than those for primary care contacts.[129] In the month before a completed suicide, approximately one-fifth of suicide-completers obtained mental health services, and in the year before a completed suicide, approximately one in three suicide completers had contact with a mental health professional.[129]

PATHOPHYSIOLOGY

Suicide is a behavioral outcome with a large number of contributing factors, rather than a disease entity in itself. Therefore, in order to understand the pathophysiology of suicidality, it is necessary to examine the differences between individuals with a given set of predisposing factors who do not attempt or complete suicide and those who do. Research has focused on a wide array of neurobiologic and psychological topics in an attempt to better understand the pathophysiology of suicide. Neurobiologic inquiries have included neurotransmitter analyses, genetic studies, neuroendocrine studies, biological markers, and imaging studies.[8]

Of all the neurotransmitters, the relationship of serotonin to suicidality has been most widely studied.[8] Specifically, an association between reduced serotonergic activity, as indicated by lower levels of cerebrospinal fluid (CSF) 5-hydroxyindoleacetic acid (5-HIAA), and serotonin dysfunction and suicidality has emerged since the 1970s.[102,131–142] This finding is independent of underlying psychiatric diagnoses.[132,133] Changes in norepinephrine transmission in suicide have also been investigated, but although there may be some association between a decreased number of noradrenergic neurons and suicidality,[143] overall, CSF studies have shown no significant difference in norepinephrine metabolites in those with suicidal behavior.[102,143] Data regarding the role of dopamine in suicide are inconclusive.[102,142,144,145] Lastly, heightened hypothalamic–pituitary–adrenal (HPA) axis activity has been implicated in the pathophysiology of suicide, although not all studies of the relationship between the HPA axis abnormalities and suicidal behavior have reached the same conclusions.[8,30,102,133,142]

Psychological aspects of suicide typically focus on psychodynamic and cognitive perspectives, and they have contributed to a vast literature on the topic. Suicide can be conceptualized as anger turned on oneself or anger toward others directed at the self.[146–148] Suicide has also been seen as being motivated by three driving forces: the wish to die, the wish to kill, and the wish to be killed.[148] Deficits in ego function have also been postulated to predispose to suicide,[146] as have poor object relations.[148] Hopelessness is a central psychological correlate of suicide, and extensive study on it has suggested that hopelessness may be the best overall predictor of suicide.[102] Shame, worthlessness, poor self-esteem, early traumatic relationships, and intense psychological pain are also key concepts in the understanding of suicide.[148,149] In addition, poor coping skills, antisocial traits, hostility, dependency or over-dependency, self-consciousness, and high intro-punitiveness have also been associated with suicide.[148,150] Finally, research has postulated correlations between observed neuroanatomic, neurotransmitter, and neuroendocrine findings in suicide and attendant cognitive traits of loser status, no escape, and no rescue as central to understanding suicidal behavior.[133]

CLINICAL FEATURES AND DIAGNOSIS

The patient at risk for suicide varies along a continuum (from an individual with private thoughts of wanting to be dead or to commit suicide, to a gravely ill individual who requires emergent medical attention as the result of a self-inflicted injury aimed to end his or her life). There is no characteristic presentation for a suicidal patient. As a result, suicide risk must be assessed in all patients, and it depends on a thorough clinical assessment; the patient who has contemplated, threatened, or attempted suicide requires special consideration. The thoughts and feelings of the individual must be elicited and placed in the context of known risk factors for suicide.

Although useful as a guide to populations who may be more likely to commit or to attempt suicide, risk factors alone are neither sensitive nor specific in the prediction of suicide. Their pervasive prevalence in comparison with the relatively low incidence of suicide in the general population may also lead to high false-positive rates. A multiple logistic regression model that used risk factors (e.g., age, gender, psychiatric diagnoses, medical diagnoses, marital status, family psychiatric history, prior suicide attempts, and suicidal ideation) failed to identify any of the 46 patients who committed suicide over a 14-year period from a group of 1906 people with mood disorders.[151] Similarly, a multiple regression analysis aimed at predicting risk classification by treatment disposition of individuals after a suicide attempt had only slightly more than a two-thirds concordance with the decisions made by the treating clinician.[152]

An evaluation for suicide risk is indicated for all patients who have made a suicide attempt, who have voiced suicidal ideation or intent, who have admitted suicidal ideation or intent on questioning, or whose actions have suggested suicidal intent despite their protests to the contrary. All suicide attempts and thoughts of suicide should be taken seriously, regardless of whether the actions or thoughts appear manipulative in nature. The work group on suicidal behaviors of the American Psychiatric Association outlined the four critical features of a comprehensive assessment of patients with suicidal behaviors in its 2003 practice guideline: a thorough psychiatric evaluation, specific inquiry about suicidality, establishment of a multi-axial diagnosis, and estimation of suicide risk.[148] The key facets of each of these components are detailed in Table 44-3.

The Joint Commission Sentinel Event Alert was established in 2016 to assist healthcare organizations in better identifying and treating individuals with suicidal ideation, given the increasing rates of suicide in the United States. A large number of patients at risk for suicide do not receive outpatient mental health treatment in a timely manner following discharge from EDs and inpatient psychiatric settings.[153] The risk of suicide is three times as likely during the first week after discharge from a psychiatric facility[154] and remains high within the first year[155] and over the first 4 years[156] after discharge.[157]

The Joint Commission Sentinel Event Alert provides guidance on strategies for detecting suicidal ideation, taking immediate action, planning aftercare, educating, and documenting. In terms of detection, it recommends screening all patients for suicide using a brief, standardized, evidence-based screening tool in non-acute or acute care settings. In terms of taking immediate action, it recommends keeping high-risk patients under one-to-one observation and creating physically safe healthcare environments; for lower-risk patients making appointments for outpatient behavioral health (as opposed to asking them to make it themselves); and for every patient providing information on suicide prevention help lines, identifying coping strategies, and encouraging restriction of access to lethal means. In terms of after-care planning, it recommends developing treatment plans that directly target suicidality, such as evidence-based clinical approaches including CBT for Suicide Prevention (CBT-SP), the Collaborative Assessment and Management of Suicide (CAMS), and Dialectical Behavioral Therapy (DBT). In terms of education and documentation, it recommends educating all staff about how to identify and respond to patients with suicidal ideation systematically, as well as providing careful documentation of decisions regarding the care and referral of patients at risk for suicide.

The approach to the patient at risk for suicide should be non-judgmental, supportive, and empathic. The initial establishment of rapport may include an introduction, an effort to create some degree of privacy in the interview setting, and an attempt to maximize the physical comfort of the patient during the interview.[49] The patient who senses interest, concern, and compassion is more likely to trust the examiner and to provide a detailed and accurate history. Often ambivalent about their thoughts and plans, suicidal patients may derive significant relief and benefit from a thoughtful and caring evaluation.[47,49]

The patient should be questioned about suicidal ideation and intent in an open and direct manner. Patients with thoughts of and plans for suicide are often relieved when they find someone with whom they can speak about the unspeakable. Patients without suicidal ideation do not have the thoughts planted in their mind and do not develop a greater risk for suicide.[47,49,158] General questions concerning thoughts about suicide can be introduced in a gradual manner while obtaining the history of present illness. Questions such as: "Has it ever seemed like things just aren't worth it?"[49] or "Have you had thoughts that life is not worth living?"[47] may lead to a further discussion of depression and hopelessness. "Have you gotten so depressed that you've considered killing yourself?"[49] or "Have you had thoughts of killing yourself?"[46] may open the door to a further evaluation of suicidal thoughts and plans.

Specific questions concerning potential suicide plans and preparations must follow any admission of suicidal ideation or intent. The patient should be asked when, where, and

TABLE 44-3 Components of the Suicide Evaluation

Conduct a thorough psychiatric examination
- Establish initial rapport
- Combine open-ended and direct questions
- Gather data from family, friends, and co-workers
- Conduct a mental status examination

Suicide assessment
- Ask specifically about thoughts of suicide and plans to commit suicide
- Examine the details of the suicide plan
- Determine the risk/rescue ratio
- Assess the level of planning and preparation
- Evaluate the degree of hopelessness
- Identify precipitants

Establish a psychiatric and/or medical diagnosis
- Obtain history
- Use data from a psychiatric examination
- Incorporate data from prior or current treaters

Estimate suicide risk
- Evaluate risk factors
- Evaluate available social supports

how an attempt would be made, and any potential means should be evaluated for feasibility and lethality. An organized and detailed plan involving an accessible and lethal method may place the patient at higher risk for suicide.[42] The seriousness of the wish or the intent to die must also be assessed. The patient who has begun to carry out the initial steps of a suicide plan, who wishes to be dead, and who has no hopes or plans for the future may be at greater risk. The last-mentioned domain (plans for the future) may be assessed by asking questions such as, "What do you see yourself doing 5 years from now?" or "What things are you still looking forward to doing or seeing?"[49]

Many clinicians have addressed the issues of lethality and intent by means of the risk/rescue ratio.[159] The greater the relative risk or lethality and the lesser the likelihood of rescue of a planned attempt, the more serious is the potential for a completed suicide. Although often useful, the risk/rescue ratio cannot be applied as a simple formula; instead, one must examine and interpret the particular beliefs of a given patient. For example, a patient may plan an attempt with a low risk of potential harm but may sincerely wish to die and believe that the plan will be fatal; the patient may thus have a higher risk for suicide. Conversely a patient may plan an attempt that carries a high probability of death, such as with an acetaminophen overdose, but may have little desire to die and little understanding of the severity of the attempt; the patient may thus have a lower risk.[42,148]

The clinician must attempt to identify any possible precipitants for the present crisis in an effort to understand why the patient is suicidal. The patient who must face the same problems and stressors following the evaluation or who cannot or will not discuss potential precipitants may be at greater risk for suicide.[42] The clinician must also assess the social support in place for a given patient. A lack of outpatient care providers, family, or friends may elevate a patient's risk.[47,62]

The examiner who interviews a patient after a suicide attempt needs to evaluate the details, seriousness, risk/rescue ratio, and precipitants of the attempt. The patient who carries out a detailed plan, who perceives the attempt as lethal, who thinks that death will be certain, who is disappointed to be alive, and who must face unchanged stressors will be at a continued high risk for suicide. The patient who makes a calculated, pre-meditated attempt may also be at a higher risk for a repeat attempt than the patient who makes a hasty, impulsive attempt (out of anger, a desire for revenge, or a desire for attention), or the patient who is intoxicated.[49]

A thorough psychiatric, medical, social, and family history of the patient who may be at risk for suicide should be completed to evaluate the presence and significance of potential risk factors. Particular attention should be paid to the presence of MDD, alcohol or drug abuse, psychotic disorders, personality disorders, and anxiety disorders. The presence of multiple significant risk factors may confer an additive risk.

A careful mental status examination allows the clinician to detect psychiatric difficulties and to assess cognitive capacities. Important aspects to evaluate in the examination include level of consciousness, appearance, behavior, attention, mood, affect, language, orientation, memory, thought form, thought content, perception, insight, and judgment.[159,160] A psychiatric review of systems aids in the detection of psychiatric disease.

The clinician should interview the family and friends of the patient at risk to corroborate gathered information and to obtain new and pertinent data. The family may provide information that a patient is hesitant to provide and that may be essential to his or her care.[42,47,49] A patient who refuses to discuss an attempt or who insists that the entire event was a mistake may speak in an open and honest manner only when confronted with reports from his or her family. The evaluation of suicidal risk and the protection of the patient at risk are emergent procedures, which may take precedence over the desire of the patient for privacy and the maintenance of confidentiality in the physician–patient relationship. Concern over a life-or-death situation may obviate obtaining formal consent from the patient before speaking to family and friends.[49]

TREATMENT OF SUICIDE RISK

The treatment of suicide risk begins with stabilization of medical sequelae of suicidal behaviors. Attention to current or potential medical conditions must be prompt, and medical evaluations must be complete. The severity of the psychiatric presentation should not distract a clinician from his or her obligation to provide good medical care.[42] Once the patient is medically stable, or if the patient is suicidal but has not acted on suicidal impulses, the focus of treatment can shift to initiation of treatment for the underlying causes of the desire for death. Components of the treatment of suicide risk include providing a safe environment for the patient, determining an appropriate treatment setting, developing a treatment plan that involves appropriate somatic and psychotherapeutic interventions, and reassessing safety, suicide risk, psychiatric status, and treatment response in an ongoing fashion (Table 44-4).[148]

Throughout the evaluation and treatment of the suicidal patient, safety must be ensured until the patient is no longer at imminent risk for suicide. Appropriate intervention and the passage of time may aid in the resolution of suicidal ideation and intent.[42,49] A patient who is at potential risk for suicide and who threatens to leave before an adequate evaluation is completed must be detained, in accordance with statutes in most states that permit the detention of individuals deemed dangerous to themselves or others.[161] Patients who attempt to leave nonetheless should be contained by locked environments or restraints.[42]

Potential means for self-harm should be removed from the reach of a patient at risk. Sharp objects (such as scissors, sutures, needles, glass bottles, and metal eating utensils)

TABLE 44-4 Treatment of Suicide Risk
Stabilize the medical situation
Create a safe environment
• Remove potential means for self-harm
• Provide frequent supervision
• Use restraints as needed
• Detain involuntarily if necessary
Identify and treat underlying mental illness
Identify and modify other contributing factors

should be removed from the immediate area. Other items to limit access to include extra sheets or towels, pajamas with ties, belts, plastic bags, headphones, electrical cords, telemetry wires, batteries, hospital gloves, or IV bags and tubing when not in use. Open windows, stairwells, and structures to which a noose could be attached must be blocked. Medications or other dangerous substances that patients may have in their possession must be secured by staff in a location out of the patient's access.[42] Appropriate supervision and restraint must be provided at all times for a patient at risk for suicide. Frequent supervision, constant one-to-one supervision, physical restraints, and medications may be used alone or in combination in an effort to protect a patient at risk. The least restrictive means that ensures the safety of the patient should be used. For patients who are hospitalized, off-floor tests should be carefully considered and, if needed, patients should be accompanied by staff. If possible, suicidal patients' rooms should not be near exits. It is also important that all items brought by visitors be carefully checked to ensure no dangerous materials were acquired.[157]

A decision about the appropriate level of care and treatment setting for the suicidal patient is critical. The patient's safety is paramount, and decisions about level of care—from discharge home with outpatient follow-up to involuntary hospitalization—should be based on risk determinations and methods most likely to protect the patient from self-harm, even when the patient disagrees. Those who are at high risk for suicide, or who cannot control their suicidal urges, should be admitted to a locked psychiatric facility. A patient who is at high risk but who refuses hospitalization should be committed involuntarily.

A patient who requires psychiatric hospitalization should be informed of the disposition decision in a clear, direct manner. Possible transfers should proceed as quickly and efficiently as possible because a patient may become quite tense and ambivalent about the decision to hospitalize. Those who agree to voluntary hospitalization and who cooperate with caregivers may have the highest likelihood of successful treatment.[49] A 3-year study of patients at a university ED in Zurich found that older patients were more likely to be hospitalized after a suicide attempt and that nearly half of patients admitted for psychiatric treatment were voluntary.[152] In a regression analysis of the same sample, more aggressive methods of suicide attempt (defined as not overdose or cutting), a history of previous inpatient treatment, and a current diagnosis of psychosis or schizophrenia were associated with inpatient admission.[152]

The clinician should always take a conservative approach to the treatment of suicidal risk and the maintenance of patient safety, and err, if necessary, on the side of excess restraint or hospitalization. From a forensic standpoint, the clinician sued for battery secondary to the use of restraints or to involuntary commitment would be easier to defend than the clinician sued for negligence secondary to a completed suicide. Acting in accordance with good clinical judgment in the best interest of the patient brings little danger of liability.[49] Adequate documentation should include the thought processes behind decisions to supervise, restrain, discharge, or hospitalize.[49]

Although managed care may place pressure on a clinician to avoid hospitalization through the use of less costly alternatives, there is no substitute for sound clinical judgment. In particular, safety contracts or suicide prevention contracts, while intended to manage risk, are generally over-valued and of limited utility.[162] Specifically, suicide contracts depend on the subjective beliefs of the psychiatrist and the patient and not on objective data; they have never been shown to be clinically efficacious.[162] In addition, many suicide attempters and completers had suicide contracts in place at the time of the suicidal act.[163,164] Finally, a suicide contract is not a legal contract and it has limited utility, if any, if litigation should ensue from a completed suicide.[165,166]

Somatic therapies to target underlying psychiatric illness are a mainstay of the management of the suicidal patient. However, though psychiatric illness is a significant risk factor for suicide and treatment of underlying psychopathology is associated with decreased suicide risk, with few exceptions psychiatric medications have not independently been associated with a decrease in suicide. The two notable exceptions are long-term treatment with lithium (in affective illness)[167,168] and clozapine (in schizophrenia).[169,170]

Because depression is the psychiatric diagnosis most associated with suicide, psychopharmacologic treatment of depression is a central facet of management of suicide risk. However, antidepressants have not been shown to decrease suicide risk.[171] Although one recent study found a higher rate of suicide after discontinuation of antidepressants compared with ongoing antidepressant treatment, the study was small and further investigation is required.[172]

Controversy regarding the relationship of selective serotonin re-uptake inhibitor (SSRI) antidepressants and suicide has now spanned more than a decade. In the early 1990s, reports of a possible increase in suicidal ideation and suicidal behavior in both adults and children on SSRIs emerged.[173,174] In 2004, the Food and Drug Administration (FDA) issued a black box warning for all antidepressants related to the risk of suicide in pediatric patients.[175] In 2007, the FDA proposed that makers of all antidepressants update the existing black box warning to include warnings of increased suicidal ideation and behavior for adults ages 18 to 24 years during the first 2 months of treatment.[176] Nonetheless, controversy about SSRIs and suicide persists in both adults and children. For example, in 2004, before the FDA advisory opinion, the American College of Neuropsychopharmacology's Task Force on SSRIs and Suicidal Behavior in Youth failed to find an association between SSRIs and increased suicidality in children; this was confirmed and extended in their final report.[177,178] Another study also showed an improvement in depression and a reduction in suicidal thinking when fluoxetine was combined with cognitive-behavioral therapy (CBT), compared with placebo and CBT.[179]

The controversy has extended to the issue of whether the publicity surrounding the black box warning has had a significant effect in decreasing physician prescription of antidepressants for children and adolescents[180] and whether there are spillover effects on community treatment for adults with depression. One study found a spillover effect into community treatment for adults with depression, including a lower rate of diagnosis of depression than would have been expected by historical trends and a reduction in antidepressant prescription rates for adults with depression.[181] However, others have argued that the black box warnings had modest and targeted effects limited to the pediatric population.[182] One study that examined the United States data on prescription rates for SSRIs from 2003 to 2005 in children and adolescents found an association between decreased prescription rates and increases in suicide rates in children and adolescents.[183] However, making such an association has been heavily cautioned against and contested.[184] A meta-analysis of randomized controlled trials (RCTs) emphasized that the risks of suicidal ideation and suicidal attempts must be weighed in the context of the benefits of antidepressants for pediatric MDD, OCD, and non-OCD anxiety disorders.[185]

In adults, there has been similar controversy about a possible relationship among use of SSRIs and increased suicidality and self-harm. Multiple large studies that assessed the risk of suicide and self-harm have been completed; they largely concluded that SSRIs were not associated with a greater risk of suicide or violence.[186–189] However, debate has continued.[190] Three papers published in the *British Medical Journal* reached varying conclusions and raised some questions about the data used in a previous analysis.[191–193] One analysis of 477 RCTs of more than 40,000 patients found no evidence that SSRIs increased the risk of suicide, but found weak evidence of an increased risk of self-harm.[191] A second review of RCTs with a total of 87,650 patients reached the opposite conclusion, finding an association between suicide attempts and the use of SSRIs.[192]

A case–control study of 146,095 individuals with a first prescription for depression found no greater risk of suicide or non-fatal self-harm in adults prescribed SSRIs as opposed to those prescribed tricyclic antidepressants (TCAs), although there was some weak evidence for increased non-fatal self-harm with use of SSRIs in patients under age 18 years.[193] A case–control study of Medicaid beneficiaries aged 19 to 64 years who had been hospitalized for depression found no association for suicide and suicide attempts with antidepressant drug use.[194] An observational study of over 225,000 United States veterans with a new diagnosis of depression found patients who received monotherapy with SSRI had approximately one-third the risk of suicide attempts compared to those who received no medication.[195] A study of 1,264,686 people over 66 years of age, which matched 1138 suicide cases with four comparison subjects for each case, found that the use of SSRIs compared with other antidepressants was associated with an increased risk of completed suicide only for the first month of use.[196]

What is clear from a review of the data on SSRIs, is that more study is needed. Because SSRIs are prescribed for treatment of an underlying illness characterized by anxiety, agitation, and suicidality, it is difficult to separate out drug effect from illness effect. Whether the medication might affect the patient's threshold for reporting ideation, rather than the actual occurrence of suicidal ideation itself, has also been raised.[197] Notwithstanding the continuing controversy, SSRIs do have the obvious advantage over TCAs and monoamine oxidase inhibitor (MAOI) antidepressants of being relatively safe in overdose.

Finally, because pharmacotherapy for depression typically requires several weeks for onset of efficacy, electroconvulsive therapy (ECT) may be indicated in cases in which suicide risk remains high or antidepressants are contraindicated.[198] ECT is associated with a decrease in short-term suicidal ideation.[147] Its use is best established for depression, and it may also be recommended for pregnant patients and for patients who have not responded to pharmacologic interventions.[147]

Psychotherapeutic interventions are widely used to manage suicide risk, although few studies have addressed psychotherapy outcomes in the reduction of suicidality. Nonetheless, clinical practice and consensus supports the use of psychotherapy and other psychosocial interventions, despite the need for further study. There is emerging evidence of the efficacy of multiple psychotherapeutic modalities in the treatment of depression, borderline personality disorder, and suicide risk *per se*, including psychodynamic psychotherapy, CBT, dialectical behavioral therapy, and interpersonal psychotherapy.

CASE 1

Ms. C, a 45-year-old woman with a history of MDD and opiate dependence, was brought to the Emergency Department after jumping off a bridge in a suicide attempt. She was profoundly depressed, anhedonic, and hopeless, with persistent suicidal ideation. She appeared very depressed, made little eye contact, and was reluctant to engage in conversation. In the hospital, she met regularly with physical therapy and occupational therapy and was encouraged to attend groups. Ms. C was maintained on fluoxetine (20 mg/day) which she had been taking at home, but the dose was increased to 30 mg/day. Due to her high risk for suicide and lithium's link with decreased suicidal ideation, she was started on lithium (300 mg BID) for adjunctive treatment of depression. She was given quetiapine for anxiety and melatonin (5 mg PO Q 6PM) for sleep.

After a week in the hospital, she reported improvements in mood, energy, and sleep. She met frequently with psychiatric staff and began to open up about her life stressors, including conflict with her boyfriend and difficulty with employment. Her affect brightened, and she expressed her love of working with horses and engaging with her faith. By the time of discharge she expressed significant improvement in her mood, gratitude for the hospitalization, and her plans to spend more time with her family, her horses, and to engage with her faith.

Her symptoms of depressed mood, anhedonia, poor concentration, hopelessness, and suicidal ideation were consistent with a major depressive episode. Though she reported that she had been thinking about suicide for 6 months, she described her decision to jump on that particular day as impulsive. She endorsed no manic symptoms to suggest bipolar disorder and no psychosis. Though she had a history of substance use, she had not used drugs on the day of her suicide attempt. Since she sustained an orbital bone fracture, a brain injury was a possibility, although head imaging did not reveal any pathology. Thus, Ms. C appeared to be experiencing depression in the setting of stressors (e.g., conflict with her boyfriend and lack of employment), and her suicide attempt appeared to be in the setting of inadequately treated disease, stress, and overwhelmed coping skills. Her risk factors for suicide included depressed mood, relationship stress, lack of stable employment, and lack of outpatient treaters.

Upon discharge, she was able to identify ways she would increase her social support, engage in activities more meaningful to her, create day structure, and begin with an outpatient treater. She also identified her antidepressant augmentation as very helpful to her. It seems that the combination of the contained environment of the hospital, a supportive treatment team, increasing her antidepressant, adding an augmenting agent with known anti-suicide effects, and using a multidisciplinary approach that also included psychology, PT, and OT services was what allowed this patient to improve and develop a plan for a more meaningful life moving forward.

DIFFICULTIES IN THE ASSESSMENT OF SUICIDE RISK

Clinicians may encounter obstacles with certain patients, or within themselves, during the evaluation of suicide risk. They must be adept in the examination of patients who are intoxicated, who threaten, or who are uncooperative, and they must be aware of personal feelings and attitudes (e.g., anxiety, anger, denial, depression, helplessness, indifference, rejection, intellectualization, or over-identification) to allow for better assessment and management of the patient at risk. A survey study found that only 25% of patients who had self-disclosed suicidal ideation on a computer survey had suicidal ideation or other mental health issues documented in the chart; a majority of these patients were discharged to their home.[199]

A patient who is intoxicated may voice suicidal ideation or intent but retract such statements (frequently) when sober. A brief initial evaluation while the patient is intoxicated, and when his or her psychological defenses are impaired, may reveal the depth of suicidal ideation or the reasons behind a suicide attempt.[49] A more thorough final examination when the patient is sober must also be completed and documented.[42,49]

A patient who threatens should be evaluated in the presence of security officers and should be placed in restraints as necessary to protect both the individual and the staff.[49] Those who are uncooperative, may refuse to answer questions despite all attempts to establish rapport and to create a supportive and empathic connection. Stating "I'd like to figure out how to be of help, but I can't do that without some information from you" in a calm but firm manner might be helpful. Patients should be informed that safety precautions will not be discontinued until the evaluation can be completed and that they will not be able to sign out against medical advice. Their capacity to refuse medical treatments should be carefully questioned.[49] A patient who refuses to cooperate until restraints are removed should be reminded of the importance of the evaluation and should be enlisted to cooperate with the goal of removing the restraints. Statements such as "We both agree that the restraints should come off if you don't need them. I am very concerned about your safety, and I need you to answer some questions before I can decide if it's safe to remove the restraints," might be helpful.[49]

A clinician may experience personal feelings and attitudes toward a patient at risk for suicide, which must be recognized and which must not be allowed to interfere with appropriate patient care.[146] Clinicians may feel anxious because of the awareness that an error in judgment might have fatal consequences. They may feel angry at a patient with a history of multiple gestures or at a patient who has used trivial methods, often resulting in poor evaluations and punitive interventions. Angry examiners may inappropriately transfer a patient with a low risk for suicide to a psychiatric facility or may discharge a patient with a high risk to home.[49] Attitudes of ED staff toward patients who have attempted suicide may vary based on gender, age, and hospital site.[200]

Some clinicians are prone to experience denial as they evaluate and treat patients at risk for suicide. They may conspire with the patient or family in the stance that voiced suicidal ideation was "just talk" or that an attempt was "just an accident." Others may practice intellectualization and choose to believe that suicide is "an act of free will" and that patients should have the personal and legal right to kill themselves.[42]

Clinicians commonly over-identify with patients with whom they share personal characteristics. The thought, "I would never commit suicide" may become translated into the thought, "This patient would never commit suicide," and serious risk may be missed.[49] The examiner may try to assure patients that they will be fine or may try to convince them that they do not feel suicidal. Patients may thus be unable to express themselves fully and may not receive proper evaluation and treatment.

A clinician who performs evaluations for patients who have made suicide attempts and who have been admitted to general hospital floors has to be aware of his or her own reactions to the patient, as well as to those of the staff. In addition, medical and surgical staff often develop strong feelings toward patients who have attempted suicide, and at times they wish that these patients were dead. The clinician must diffuse such charged situations, perhaps by holding group meetings for those involved to make them more aware of their negative feelings so that they are not acted out.[201] Such intervention may prevent mismanagement and premature discharge. Institutions should be aware of the need for guidelines for and management of immediate, short-term and long-term responses in the event of an in-hospital suicide.[202]

REFERENCES

Access the reference list online at https://expertconsult.inkling.com/.

45

Emergency Psychiatry

Abigail L. Donovan, M.D.
Laura M. Prager, M.D.
Suzanne A. Bird, M.D.

INTRODUCTION

Over the past 20 years, emergency psychiatry has developed into an independent subspecialty practice within psychiatry. Although formal board certification requirements are lacking, all accredited US psychiatric residency-training programs follow minimum training guidelines for emergency psychiatry.[1] The emergence of emergency psychiatry as a specialized practice parallels the recent dramatic increase in patient volume in emergency care settings. In 2001, there were over 2 million visits to US Emergency Departments (EDs) for mental health-related chief complaints, accounting for more than 6% of all ED visits, and representing an increase in the percentage of all visits by 28% over the previous decade.[2] By 2007, 8% of all ED visits were related to mental health complaints.[3]

Psychiatric emergencies encompass a range of clinical presentations and diagnoses. Typically, patients seek treatment in a state of crisis, unable to be contained by local support systems. Crises may be understood and addressed from a variety of perspectives, including medical, psychological, interpersonal, and social. Symptoms often consist of an overwhelming mental state that puts the patient or others at risk. Patients may have suicidal or homicidal ideation, overwhelming depression or anxiety, psychosis, mania, or acute cognitive or behavioral changes; these presentations may occur in the context of active substance use. Emergency services are also used for non-emergent conditions.[2] Increasing numbers of patients seek treatment at EDs for non-urgent conditions, in order to secure outpatient referrals due to a general scarcity of community-based outpatient resources, or an inability to navigate the complex mental healthcare system. This volume increase, coupled with the dearth of available outpatient services, the limited number of inpatient psychiatric beds, and the demands of insurance companies for prior authorization for care, has led to longer lengths of stay for many psychiatric patients in the ED, especially for, among others, those who demonstrate acute safety issues (suicidal or homicidal ideation), are hostile and aggressive, have significant but not necessarily active co-morbid medical issues, or are uninsured.[4]

The scope of emergency psychiatry includes core skills for psychiatric practice, as well as more specialized skill sets. In addition to the evaluation and treatment of acute psychiatric conditions, practitioners of emergency psychiatry must evaluate and manage suicidal behavior, homicidal (or violent) behavior, agitation, delirium, and substance intoxication or withdrawal states. Because clinical practice lies at the interface of medicine and psychiatry, emergency psychiatrists must also be skilled in the assessment and treatment of medical conditions that involve psychiatric symptoms.

This chapter provides a foundation for the clinical aspects of psychiatric emergency care. First, we review the psychiatric emergency evaluation, and then address special topics including common emergency psychiatric presentations, management of acute substance intoxication and withdrawal, management of agitation, the emergency treatment of children who present with acute psychiatric crises, and legal issues in emergency psychiatry.

DEMOGRAPHICS

As of 1991, the United States had approximately 3000 dedicated psychiatric emergency services (PESs).[5] By 2007, roughly 86% of general hospitals provided some type of emergency psychiatric care, with 45% having either a psychiatric emergency service or an in-house consultation service and 41% contracting with an outside source for emergency psychiatric care.[6] Approximately 29% of the patients treated are diagnosed with psychosis, 25% with substance abuse, 23% with major depression, 13% with bipolar disorder, and 22% with personality disorders;[7] co-morbidity is common. Approximately one-third to one-half of patients voice suicidal ideation.[5]

Though patients may self-refer to a PES, many are referred by family, friends, primary care providers, medical specialists, community mental health providers, and employees of local, state, and public agencies. Multiple high-profile school shootings have prompted schools in the United States to refer students to PESs for emergency risk assessments.[8] Police officers and representatives of the legal system can also be a source of referrals, as there is often overlap between the mentally ill and/or active substance users and the legal system. Patients with acute psychiatric illnesses, e.g., delirium or paranoia that manifests as hostility or aggression, are sometimes taken into custody for their own safety or for the safety of others. Such patients require emergency psychiatric assessment to determine if their behavior is primarily due to an acute psychiatric illness and if they require mental health services.[9]

TYPES OF DELIVERY MODELS

Delivery of emergency psychiatric services within a general hospital typically falls into one of two models. In the first, the PES exists as an independent service, either co-located with a general emergency department or located separately in a stand-alone facility nearby. In the second model, the PES functions as a consultation service that provides recommendations to primary emergency medical services. Some institutions utilize hybrid models; the type of service offered within a specific hospital is usually determined by the volume of patients and available financial and staff resources.[10]

Delivery of emergency psychiatric care through an independent service offers several benefits. The first is safety: a PES that is separated from the chaos of a busy ED offers a secure environment, in which providers can assess patients within a less-stimulating environment while also limiting access to dangerous objects. Such a unit allows the staff to observe the patients, formulate an initial diagnosis, and initiate psychiatric treatment rapidly. The unit may also have security staff who are trained to understand mental health issues, and can help maintain a safe environment for patients and staff. Many units also have specialized rooms for restraint and seclusion.[10] In addition, an independent PES is more likely to have individual rooms for private interviews, thus protecting patients' privacy and allowing them to maintain their dignity.

Another benefit of a dedicated psychiatric unit is the opportunity to staff the unit with specialized personnel with training in emergency psychiatric care.[5,10] An interdisciplinary staff of psychiatrists, nurses, social workers, and case managers can enhance the care of psychiatric patients, by coordinating medical evaluations with ED colleagues, initiating psychopharmacologic treatment, focusing on therapeutic patient interactions, and using their specialized knowledge of psychiatric services to facilitate appropriate disposition. Psychiatric staff also manage the milieu in an emergency unit, provide individual support to patients, and recognize when situations require immediate intervention.

Some PESs also have access to "crisis beds" that are able to provide 24- to 72-hour observation. The ability to observe a patient whose mental state may change significantly after the initiation of antipsychotics or with a period of sobriety may decrease the need for inpatient hospitalization.[5,10,11]

THE PSYCHIATRIC INTERVIEW

The psychiatric emergency evaluation is a concise, focused evaluation with the goals of diagnostic assessment, management of acute symptoms, and disposition to the appropriate level of care. Just as a medical ED visit involves an initial triage (a brief evaluation of the severity of the problem), many emergency psychiatry models also depend on an initial assessment of the dangerousness of the psychiatric complaint, as well as the overall medical stability of the patient. This initial determination of acuity should screen for active medical issues, including those that may cause a change in mental status or psychiatric symptomatology.

Many patients are willing to participate in a psychiatric evaluation, but some are not. Most states have legislation that allows for holding individuals against their will if there is evidence of inability to care for self, or dangerousness to self or others due to mental illness. In the PES, if patients meet these criteria, they may be held involuntarily for further evaluation.

The cornerstone of the initial psychiatric evaluation is a careful history that focuses on the temporal relationship between the acute symptoms that led to the emergency visit, associated signs and symptoms, and possible precipitants. In addition, important aspects of the evaluation also include information regarding significant medical history, psychiatric diagnoses and treatments, current and past medications, allergies and adverse reactions to medications, patterns of substance use, family history, and psychosocial history. Specific history of prior suicide attempts or violent behavior should always be included in an emergency assessment. Table 45-1 describes components of the evaluation, and Table 45-2 describes the special features of a substance use evaluation.

It is important to consider all of the information that could be included in an evaluation and then to focus on areas that are most relevant to the patient at hand. The interview should be a fact-gathering mission, and the elements of the history should both tell a story about the current symptoms and provide support for the ultimate disposition. For example, though the developmental history may not be an important part of the evaluation for an otherwise healthy-appearing adult patient with depression, it is very important in the assessment of a young patient with obvious cognitive deficits.

TABLE 45-1 The Emergency Psychiatric Interview and Evaluation

- Chief complaint
- History of present illness, with a focus on symptoms and the context for these symptoms
- Safety evaluation, with assessment of suicidal and homicidal ideation, plan or intent, and any associated risk factors as well as gross changes in ability to care for self
- Active and past medical history
- Psychiatric history, particularly symptoms or events similar to the current presentation; include diagnoses, current treaters, previous hospitalizations, suicide attempts and violent behavior
- Allergies and adverse reactions to medications
- Current medications, including an assessment of treatment compliance
- Social history, particularly how it contributes to the context for the emergency visit
- History of trauma
- Substance use history
- Legal history
- Access to firearms
- Family psychiatric history, including a family history of suicide
- Mental status examination
- Review of medical symptoms, particularly any medical symptoms that may account for the patient's presentation
- Vital signs
- Physical examination, if indicated
- Laboratory studies and other tests, if indicated
- Assessment, including a summary statement, a statement about the patient's level of safety, and a rationale for disposition recommendations
- Diagnoses
- Plan for immediate management and disposition recommendations
- Documentation of any significant interventions (e.g., medication administration) and the outcome.

TABLE 45-2 The Substance Use Disorder Interview

For each substance used, assess the following:

- Age of first use
- Recent pattern of use and duration
- Method of use (e.g., drinking, smoking, intranasal, IV)
- Time of last use and amount used
- Medical sequelae of use (including accidents, overdoses, infections)
- Social sequelae (relationship problems, school or work absences, legal problems)
- Longest period of sobriety
- Previous treatment (detoxification programs, outpatient programs, partial hospitalization)
- Method of maintaining sobriety
- Participation in self-help programs (e.g., Alcoholics Anonymous, Narcotics Anonymous)
- Risk for withdrawal syndrome
- Patient's motivation to cut down or stop substance use
- Patient's need for assistance meeting goals to cut down or stop substance use

The emergency evaluation always includes an assessment of the patient's living situation and social supports, as well as a brief understanding of how s/he spends the day (e.g., at work, at school, or in a therapeutic program). This assessment defines the patient's baseline level of function. In addition, in many countries, including the United States, a review of the patient's health insurance is necessary because it often dictates the types of treatment programs that are available for disposition.

Often, PES presentations are complicated, and patients may be unable, or unwilling, to provide an accurate history. Therefore, it is important to collect information from multiple sources including, but not limited to, outside medical records, family, friends, treaters, police, emergency personnel, pharmacies, or statewide prescription monitoring programs. Ideally, patients will give consent for collateral sources to be contacted. If a patient declines to give this permission, the importance of the type of information sought must be balanced against a violation of the patient's wishes and a potential violation of confidentiality. In addition, clinicians should be mindful about only gathering, and not releasing, information, particularly without patient consent. When data can be obtained and corroborated from various sources, psychiatrists are able to make better informed risk assessments and disposition decisions.

THE MEDICAL EVALUATION

The purpose of the medical evaluation, often called "medical clearance," is to determine that there is no identifiable medical cause contributing to the patient's psychiatric presentation that requires acute medical intervention, and that the patient is medically stable enough to receive care in their intended disposition setting.[12] Consideration of medical etiologies and co-morbidities is important because many psychiatric hospitals have limited resources to manage medical conditions. The ED medical evaluation may be the most comprehensive that the patient receives, particularly because many psychiatric patients do not have regular contact with primary care physicians. A missed medical diagnosis because of an assumed psychiatric diagnosis could result in dire consequences. Yet, there is no standard process for medical clearance in the ED, and the need for routine laboratory and other diagnostic testing remains controversial.[12]

TABLE 45-3 Tests to Consider in the Medical Evaluation of Patients With Psychiatric Symptoms

- Complete blood count ([CBC] to monitor for infection, blood loss)
- Electrolytes, blood urea nitrogen (BUN), creatinine (metabolic changes, hyponatremia or hypernatremia, abnormal kidney function, dehydration)
- Glucose (hypoglycemia or hyperglycemia)
- Liver function tests and ammonia (e.g., liver dysfunction due to hepatitis or alcohol abuse)
- Pregnancy test
- Serum toxicology screen (ingestion, intoxication, poisoning)
- Medication levels (ingestion of medications, e.g., lithium and tricyclic antidepressants)
- Urine toxicology screen (to identify or confirm substance abuse)
- Calcium, magnesium, and phosphorus (hypoparathyroidism or hyperparathyroidism, eating disorders, poor nutrition)
- Folate (alcohol dependence, poor nutrition, depression)
- Vitamin B_{12} (megaloblastic anemia, dementia)
- Thyroid-stimulating hormone; this result may not be available immediately, but it may be available during an extended observation period (hypothyroidism or hyperthyroidism)

The following tests and imaging studies may also be considered in the medical work-up:

- Computed tomography (CT) (acute hemorrhage or trauma)
- Magnetic resonance imaging (MRI) (higher resolution than CT for potential brain masses or lesions, posterior fossa pathology, or when radiation exposure is contraindicated)
- Electrocardiogram (EKG)
- Electroencephalogram (seizure, changes due to ingestion of medications, dementia)
- Lumbar puncture (infection, hemorrhage)

Adapted from Smith FA, Alpay M, Park L: Laboratory tests and diagnostic procedures. In: Stern TA, Herman JB, Gorrindo TL, editors. *Psychiatry update and board preparation. 3rd edition*. New York: McGraw-Hill; 2012.

Non-geriatric patients with presentations consistent with their prior psychiatric histories, without significant medical conditions or active physical complaints, may be sufficiently evaluated by history, review of systems, physical examination, and vital signs, without additional laboratory testing. Elderly patients or those with known medical problems, new-onset psychiatric symptoms, or a change in previous psychiatric symptoms, will benefit from additional medical testing, including labs or even diagnostic imaging.[12–14] Practitioners should be vigilant of factors (e.g., homelessness or substance use) which may put patients at risk for additional medical conditions. The medical tests to consider are listed in Table 45-3.

One retrospective study demonstrated that, among patients with a known psychiatric history and no medical complaints (38%), screening laboratories and radiographic results yielded no additional information; those patients could have been referred for psychiatric evaluation with the history, physical examination, and stable vital signs alone. Among the patients deemed to require further medical evaluation (62%), all had either reported medical complaints or their medical histories suggested that further evaluation would be necessary.[15] Another study demonstrated that two-thirds of ED patients with new-onset psychiatric symptoms had an organic cause.[16] These studies suggest that careful screening is important among patients with new-onset symptoms, but additional medical tests may be of little benefit among patients with known psychiatric disorders and without physical complaints or active medical issues.

THE SAFETY EVALUATION

The safety evaluation is a mandatory component of every emergency evaluation and it assesses the imminent likelihood that an individual will attempt to harm oneself or someone else. Suicide is the eighth leading cause of death in the United States, and more than 90% of patients who commit suicide have at least one psychiatric diagnosis.[17] Patients 15 to 24 years of age and those over 60 are at the highest risk for suicide. The safety evaluation is a key factor in determining the overall plan for disposition.

The psychiatrist must ask about thoughts, plans, and intent of suicide and homicide. These questions should be followed by more specific questions about access to lethal means, particularly firearms. If a patient has a plan or intent to commit suicide, the potential lethality of the plan, as well as the patient's perception of the risk, must be assessed. A medically low-risk plan may still coincide with a strong intent to die if the patient believes that the lethality is high. Similarly, the possibility that the patient could have been rescued if s/he had attempted the plan should be evaluated; an impulsive ingestion of pills in front of a family member conveys less risk than a similar attempt in a remote location. If a patient has attempted suicide previously, details of that attempt may facilitate an understanding of the current risk. In addition, the clinician should assess other risk factors for suicide, which include the presence and severity of a major mental illness, substance use, impulsivity, family history of suicide, recent loss (social, occupational, or financial), and medical illness, including chronic pain.

The assessment of risk for violence is similar. Every patient should be asked about thoughts to harm others, as well as potential plans and intent. Observation of the patient's mental status, behavior, and impulsivity during the interview provides important information. Because previous violence is the strongest predictor of future violence, it is important to explore prior episodes of violence, triggers for those events, and the role of substance use. Questions about legal issues related to violence are also appropriate. In addition, any intended target(s) of future violence should be identified, if possible. If there is a likelihood of violence directed toward a specific person, there may be a duty to protect the identified target, potentially through containment and treatment of the patient or through warning the identified target. As jurisdictions differ in their approach to these duties, consultations with hospital legal counsel can be helpful when discharge is considered for a potentially violent patient.

Whenever possible, the safety evaluation should include contact with others who know the patient. Although civil commitment laws differ between states, most states have provisions for the containment of a patient who is deemed at acute risk for harm to self or others. In cases where the patient has expressed suicidal or homicidal ideation, which then resolves during the course of the assessment, a clear plan must be created for steps that the patient should take if these thoughts return. Most often, these involve contact with family members and treaters, and a return to a psychiatric evaluation center or ED.

PSYCHIATRIC SYMPTOMS AND PRESENTATIONS

Diagnosis using *Diagnostic and Statistical Manual of Mental Disorders*, 5th edition (DSM-5)[18] criteria can be difficult in the PES because patients are seen at a single point in time, often in crisis, whereas definitive diagnosis frequently requires a longitudinal assessment of symptoms. Nevertheless, consideration of the major diagnostic syndromes (e.g., mood disorders, psychosis, anxiety disorders, substance use disorders, and a change in mental status caused by a medical etiology, such as delirium) should be part of the emergency assessment. The following pages will outline some common psychiatric presentations.

Depression

Depression is a common reason for seeking treatment at a PES. The severity of depression may vary from mild to extremely severe; it may occur with or without psychosis or suicidal thinking. Anxiety or anger attacks are often co-morbid with depression, and a history of mania or mixed episodes must be assessed in every depressed patient to screen for bipolar disorder. Potential effects on mood from substance use as well as other medical conditions, especially hypothyroidism and chronic pain, must be considered. While the severity of symptoms, functional level, available treatment, and social supports may contribute to a disposition determination, the assessment of safety is critical to treatment planning.

Mania

Manic patients can often be disruptive and provocative, with pressured speech, grandiosity, irritability, and flight of ideas. Such patients may be dressed or behave in an odd or seductive manner and may have impulsively traveled long distances. In mania with psychosis, paranoid thoughts and delusions or hallucinations often arise, leading to a lack of insight. It is important to assess for medical causes of mania, including acute intoxication, steroid use, or hyperthyroidism. Judgment is often significantly impaired during manic episodes and patients' safety and ability to care for themselves must be carefully assessed.

Anxiety

Although symptoms of anxiety may reflect a primary anxiety disorder, anxiety in the ED patient often heralds other disorders. Patients with psychosis may first describe anxiety about people trying to harm them; patients with depression may have anxiety about financial or relationship difficulties. Psychomotor agitation, fidgeting, and pacing co-occur with anxiety but may also correlate with psychosis, alcohol withdrawal, or cocaine intoxication. Medical problems (e.g., hyperthyroidism) and medication side effects (e.g., akathisia) may also present with anxiety. Chest pain and shortness of breath resulting from a panic attack are also common ED presentations that require thorough medical evaluation in concert with a psychiatric evaluation.

Psychosis

Patients with psychosis suffer from disorganized thinking, hallucinations, delusions, or other forms of disordered thought (e.g., ideas of reference, thought broadcasting, or thought insertion). Patients with psychosis vary greatly in the severity of their symptoms; they may be affected by paranoia that has undermined their work or relationships or suffer from delusions or aggressive behavior. Because some patients have lost touch with reality and may be at risk for agitation or dangerousness, careful attention to the safety of staff and other patients must be maintained.

Medical causes for psychosis must be ruled out, particularly among patients without a prior history of psychosis or whose age falls outside the usual range for the onset of psychosis (late teens to mid-20s). Seizure disorders, delirium, metabolic changes, infections, ingestion, stimulant intoxication, and withdrawal from alcohol or benzodiazepines should be considered in the differential for new-onset psychosis. Among the elderly with new-onset hallucinations, delirium and dementia should be strongly considered.

Personality Disorders

Patients with personality disorders presenting to the ED often require a significant amount of time and emotional energy. Such patients may request special services or favors that are outside of the normal routine of the unit. They may file complaints or even threaten to kill themselves or others if the clinician is unwilling to provide the desired treatment. These threats often are statements of desperation, though each statement must be evaluated in the context of a patient's history and current situation.

Problems often occur because of splits between staff members who disagree about how the patient should be managed. A critical aspect of treatment for these patients is for the PES team to provide consistent, clear boundaries regarding the scope of care available, the role of individual staff members, and the goal of the emergency intervention. Outside contacts who know the patient may be able to provide insight for the purposes of the safety assessment.

Catatonia

Patients with catatonia typically require coordinated care between emergency medicine and emergency psychiatry clinicians, and rapid diagnosis and treatment is critical. Catatonia can be due to a number of underlying organic (e.g., seizures, infections, neoplasms, metabolic derangements, etc.) and psychiatric (e.g., mood disorders, schizophrenia) etiologies, and full work-up of all potential etiologies is required. While the underlying disorder will require treatment, treatment of the catatonia itself should be initiated rapidly, typically with parenteral benzodiazepines. Antipsychotic medication should be avoided in catatonic patients until after the catatonia has been lysed. Malignant catatonia is characterized by the triad of mental status change, rigidity and fever, and carries increased morbidity and mortality. A full discussion of catatonia can be found in Chapter 23.

Trauma

Patients presenting to the PES frequently have a history of trauma, even if it is not a presenting chief complaint. All patients should be asked whether they have been a victim of violence or trauma; if they have symptoms of post-traumatic stress disorder (PTSD); and whether they are safe in their current living environment. Patients need not describe explicit details about past traumas. Clinicians should also be mindful of the potential for patients being unintentionally re-traumatized during their ED visit. The sights and sounds of the busy and acute ED can be overwhelming and triggering for patients with a trauma history. In addition, patients who have previously had negative interactions with the mental health field (including civil commitments or physical restraints) may also find the psychiatric evaluation process itself to be potentially re-traumatizing. Awareness of these vulnerabilities can influence where a patient waits in the ED and how the clinician may approach the assessment.

Intoxication or Withdrawal

Patients with substance intoxication or withdrawal often come to the attention of emergency personnel because of acute medical symptoms (e.g., unconsciousness, difficulty breathing, confusion). However, they may also present requesting referral for detoxification services or other substance use disorder (SUD) treatment. SUDs are frequently co-morbid with other psychiatric conditions. The following will outline commonly seen SUDs in the PES and key concepts in their assessment.

Alcohol

Alcohol intoxication can cause disorientation, ataxia, and slurring of speech; when toxic blood alcohol levels (BALs) are present, respiratory depression, coma, and death may follow. Chronic alcohol use leads to tolerance and a higher BAL without severe symptoms. For alcohol intoxication, treatment typically consists of observation, maintenance of the airway, and administration of IV fluids. Patients who are acutely intoxicated from alcohol may also be agitated and aggressive, requiring restraints and medication for their own and others' safety. Although evidence-based protocols are lacking, consensus guidelines suggest the use of first-generation antipsychotic medication (e.g., haloperidol) when necessary.[19]

Alcohol withdrawal is medically dangerous and can be life-threatening. Alcohol withdrawal can lead to anxiety, irritability, tremor, autonomic instability (elevated blood pressure, pulse, and temperature), and sometimes seizures. Patients with chronic alcohol use can be in withdrawal, despite the presence of alcohol in their blood because of a relatively lower concentration of alcohol, compared with their usual (intoxicated) state. Treatment of alcohol withdrawal generally involves use of oral or IV benzodiazepines (initially titrated to normalize vital signs and then tapered over several days) and fluid repletion. A high-potency antipsychotic (e.g., haloperidol) can decrease psychomotor agitation associated with withdrawal. Prophylactic treatment with benzodiazepines for patients at high risk of alcohol withdrawal is beneficial in the ED, unless patients are likely to be discharged shortly, with a high likelihood of resuming alcohol consumption. All patients with alcohol use disorders, regardless of withdrawal status, should be given prophylactic thiamine (to prevent Wernicke's encephalopathy), folic acid, and multi-vitamins.

In more severe cases, alcohol withdrawal can lead to delirium tremens, which consists of a change in mental status, disorientation, visual or tactile hallucinations, and severe autonomic instability. Delirium tremens is a medical emergency with a mortality rate of 5% to 10%; it requires immediate medical care and treatment with IV benzodiazepines, sometimes parenteral antipsychotic agents, thiamine, and fluids.[20]

Benzodiazepines and Barbiturates

Intoxication with benzodiazepines and barbiturates appears similar to alcohol intoxication; it involves the presence of slurred speech, confusion, ataxia, and respiratory depression. Withdrawal is also potentially life-threatening; management is similar to that of alcohol withdrawal, including use of oral or IV benzodiazepines or barbiturates.

Opiates

Opiate intoxication is characterized by drowsiness, decreased heart rate, and pupillary constriction. The greatest risk of opiate overdose is respiratory depression. Frequently, accidental overdoses occur when patients either miscalculate their dose after a period of abstinence (because of decreased tolerance) or when the drug is more potent than expected. Opiate intoxication can be treated emergently with naloxone, an opioid antagonist, although drowsiness and respiratory depression may return as the naloxone wears off. In addition, naloxone will cause an acute and uncomfortable withdrawal syndrome that often leads to agitation on awakening.

Opiate withdrawal is not typically life-threatening. Early symptoms include anxiety, yawning, diaphoresis, rhinorrhea, dilated pupils, abdominal and leg cramping, and chills. Elevated blood pressure, pulse, and temperature, as well as nausea and vomiting, will follow. A urine drug screen can usually confirm recent opiate use although toxic screens vary in which agents can be detected. In the emergency setting, withdrawal management is typically limited to symptomatic treatment with clonidine for autonomic instability (monitor for hypotension), dicyclomine for abdominal cramps, and quinine sulfate for leg cramps (limit to once per day due to cardiovascular or renal toxicity). Optimally, the patient can be referred to a licensed detoxification facility or outpatient buprenorphine provider for post-ED treatment.

Cocaine

Patients with cocaine use disorders often present to the ED suffering from medical complaints (e.g., chest pain), mood, anxiety, or psychotic symptoms. The symptoms and signs of cocaine intoxication include euphoria and grandiosity, irritability or agitation, insomnia, dilated pupils, and psychomotor restlessness (e.g., pacing, hand wringing, or choreiform-like movements). Patients may have elevated blood pressure and temperature, tachycardia, palpitations, chest pain, and shortness of breath. An oral benzodiazepine is often indicated for the discomfort of acute cocaine intoxication although some patients experience hallucinations, paranoia, or agitation requiring antipsychotic medication. With very high doses of cocaine, patients can experience decreased responsiveness, seizures, and severe autonomic changes followed by coma and risk of cardiac arrest or ventricular fibrillation; treatment is supportive. Serum toxicology screens for cocaine, if available, may confirm very recent use of cocaine (within hours), whereas urine toxicology may confirm use up to 24 hours previously.

Although there is no clearly described withdrawal syndrome for cocaine, patients often experience a very strong urge to sleep once cocaine has left their system. They also describe feeling weak and tired, often depressed and with persistent cravings for days to weeks after use has ended.

Crystal Methamphetamine

Intoxication with crystal methamphetamine and other amphetamines may be recognized by mood lability or irritability, psychomotor agitation, confusion, and sweating. More severe cases may include paranoia, hallucinations, seizures, cardiac toxicity, and fever. Treatment is supportive but agitation can be extreme and often requires parenteral medication with both benzodiazepines and antipsychotics.[21] Withdrawal leads to agitation, irritability, sleep disturbance, and depressed mood.

Phencyclidine

Phencyclidine (PCP; also known as "angel dust") intoxication is characterized by agitation, paranoia, hallucinations, and violent or bizarre behavior. Intoxication can cause nystagmus, ataxia, and slurred speech; at higher doses, it may lead to seizures, hypertensive crisis, coma, and death. Treatment is supportive and should include management in a contained setting (because of the risk of violence). Benzodiazepines are generally considered first-line medication as first-generation antipsychotics may be associated with a lowered seizure threshold. PCP-induced psychosis can last from days to weeks; these patients may require hospitalization if symptoms do not improve within several hours.[21] There is no withdrawal syndrome from PCP.

Marijuana

Marijuana is a common drug of abuse. Symptoms of intoxication include relaxed or elevated mood, alteration in the perception of time, tachycardia, and conjunctival injection.[21] Patients may report paranoia or hallucinations, although in these cases, it is important to assess for other illicit drugs and for underlying psychiatric disorders, as marijuana can both cause a substance-induced psychosis and increase psychotic symptoms in patients with pre-existing psychotic disorders.

Substance Intoxication and the Safety Assessment

Even beyond these signs and symptoms, substance intoxication can impact the overall psychiatric assessment, especially the safety assessment. It is not unusual for patients to present with intoxication and reporting suicidality or other safety concerns. While an assessment upon initial presentation is important, a full safety assessment cannot be complete until the patient has been re-evaluated when clinically sober. Some patients may no longer feel suicidal when sober, and may be appropriate for less restrictive levels of care. All patients should be educated that ongoing substance use is a risk factor for impulsive behavior, suicide, and violence to others. Regardless of expressed safety concerns, no patient should be discharged from the ED while acutely impaired from intoxication. These patients frequently present management challenges to ED and mental health providers alike.

Change in Mental Status

When evaluating a patient with a mental status change, the emergency psychiatrist must identify the underlying etiology. In general, mental status changes result from delirium (due to an organic cause), dementia, or psychiatric conditions. Because psychiatric conditions are often diagnoses of exclusion, delirium and dementia must be ruled out. The Folstein Mini-Mental State Examination[22] can be useful to screen for cognitive changes. Dementia, a chronic and progressive condition characterized by memory and other cognitive impairments, may underlie more acute presentations of psychosis or agitation, particularly in older patients. Dementia is discussed elsewhere in this textbook (see Chapter 11).

Delirium, as defined by DSM-5,[18] is a fluctuating disturbance in attention, awareness, and cognition that is caused by a variety of medical conditions, substance intoxication or withdrawal, toxic exposure, or a combination of multiple etiologies. (For a more complete discussion of the causes and of delirium, see Chapter 10.) Delirium, also known as acute confusional state or encephalopathy, typically has an acute onset (over hours to days), a fluctuating course, and is reversible. Disturbance in consciousness, reduced awareness of the environment, attentional difficulties, disorientation, and an inability to think or speak coherently are common symptoms. Psychomotor agitation is also common, though psychomotor retardation is possible. Symptoms typically associated with psychiatric diagnoses (e.g., auditory and visual hallucinations, acute changes in mood, psychotic or disorganized thoughts) may also be seen in delirious states.

Delirium may be due to serious or life-threatening conditions. These conditions include Wernicke's encephalopathy, hypoxia, hypoglycemia, hypertensive encephalopathy, intracerebral hemorrhage, meningitis/encephalitis, poisoning (exogenous or iatrogenic), and seizures. Their assessment and treatment are outlined in Table 45-4. Other conditions (including subdural hematoma, septicemia, subacute bacterial endocarditis, hepatic or renal failure, thyrotoxicosis or myxedema, delirium tremens, anticholinergic toxicity, and complex partial status epilepticus) may require acute intervention.[23] Treatment of delirium optimally involves immediate treatment of the underlying etiology; however, patients who are delirious and presenting with confusion and/or agitation may benefit from symptomatic treatment.

MANAGEMENT OF ACUTE SYMPTOMS

After ruling out contributory medical causes and identifying a working psychiatric diagnosis, the PES's primary goal is to manage acute crises. Interventions chosen will depend on the patient's needs, the severity of illness, and the resources available. For some patients, the intervention may be speaking to an understanding clinician, who can form an alliance, demonstrate empathy, and provide reassurance. Other patients require IM medication or restraint for agitation. Between those extremes are various therapeutic interventions designed to manage the acuity of the patient's situation, provide education about mental illness and treatment, and help the patient and family members make informed decisions about treatment. The types of interventions include environmental, psychological, and

TABLE 45-4 Potentially Life-Threatening Causes of Delirium

CONDITION	DIAGNOSTICS	TREATMENT
Wernicke's encephalopathy	Clinical triad: change in mental status, gait instability, ophthalmoplegia	Thiamine 500 mg IM (may see improvement over the course of hours)
Hypoxia	Oxygen saturation/ABGs	Treat etiology, give oxygen
Hypoglycemia	Blood glucose	PO/IV administration of glucose, dextrose, sucrose, or fructose
Hypertensive encephalopathy	Blood pressure	Antihypertensive medication
Hyperthermia/hypothermia	Temperature	Cooling or warming interventions
Infectious process (e.g., sepsis, bacteremia, subacute bacterial endocarditis)	Infectious disease work-up	Treat infectious agent or site
Intracerebral hemorrhage	MRI/CT	Per hemorrhage type or location
Meningitis/encephalitis	LP, MRI	Antibiotic medication, immunotherapy
Metabolic (e.g., chemical derangements, renal failure, hepatic failure, thyroid dysfunction)	Laboratory investigations	Per derangement
Poisoning/toxic reaction (e.g., environmental exposures, medications, alcohol, illicit substances)	Toxicology panel	Per toxin
Status epilepticus	EEG	Anticonvulsants and/or IV benzodiazepines

ABGs, Arterial blood gases; CT, computed tomography; EEG, electroencephalogram; IM, intramuscular; IV, intravenous; LP, lumbar puncture; MRI, magnetic resonance imaging; PO, oral (*per os*).

pharmacologic. Patients with agitation may also require physical interventions (seclusion and restraint—the options of last resort).

Environmental Intervention

Although resources and space may be limited, environmental interventions can be critical for patients in crisis. The environment determines if the patient will sit, stand, or lie on a stretcher; if s/he will wear street clothes or a hospital gown; and if the clinician will be alone with the patient or be accompanied by family members or other emergency staff. If possible, the interview should occur in a quiet, clean setting, where the patient and clinician can both sit comfortably and not be overheard by others (unless safety concerns necessitate the presence of additional staff or security). Attention to the patient's basic needs (e.g., offering a blanket or something to drink or eat) may assist in forming an alliance.

Psychological Intervention

Forming an alliance during a brief interview in an emergency setting can be a challenge. EDs and PESs are often busy, with long waits for evaluation and treatment; PES clinicians are often pulled in different directions. A sympathetic comment after a patient has experienced an extended wait can facilitate an alliance.

The psychiatric clinician should allow patients a few minutes at the beginning of the interview to describe their situation. Beginning the interview with several open-ended questions will help the patient feel heard and allow a brief assessment of the patient's mental status. Because of time constraints, the PES evaluation often involves more closed-ended screening questions (to rule out major symptoms or diagnoses) than occur in other psychiatric arenas. Empathic comments demonstrate concern and allow the clinician to interject with appropriate questions to guide the interview.

In the PES, the psychological intervention is often pragmatic. It may consist of formation of an empathic connection and education about psychiatric symptoms, treatments, or the mental health system. The clinician may help the patient gain insight into the problem at hand and brainstorm about alternative solutions. Collaboration between the patient and the clinician may lead to a mutually agreeable treatment plan. The psychiatrist may offer reassurance that the patient is not alone and that help is available. The simple act of validating a patient's feelings of being overwhelmed can often be a therapeutic intervention. The patient's and the family's unstated wishes or concerns should be identified and managed.

The patient should be encouraged to identify coping skills that have been helpful at other times. Though the patient should be allowed to describe difficult feelings and release tension, there should be an expectation that the patient behave within the boundaries of what is safe and appropriate in that environment. When a patient is too ill to maintain these boundaries, referral to a higher level of care is typically indicated.

Another key to providing therapeutic care in the emergency setting is understanding potential countertransference reactions. Amid the stress of overcrowded and chaotic EDs and PESs, staff members at every level can become cynical and resentful. Although these reactions are understandable, clinicians must prevent these frustrations from influencing the treatment of patients. Acting on counter-transference reactions can lead to unprofessional behavior, compromising clinical care and safety. For many years at the Massachusetts General Hospital, psychiatric residents have participated in a weekly supervision session that focuses on recognizing countertransference reactions and enhancing resilience after long nights in the PES.[24] Awareness of stress levels and scheduled breaks (to eat meals and relax during long shifts) are necessary for the provision of good care.

Pharmacologic Intervention

The power of medication should not be underestimated in a psychiatric emergency. For some patients, particularly those who are psychotic or acutely agitated, administering medication may be the primary intervention. Medication can decrease anxiety and paranoia, improve disorganization, help a manic patient to sleep, or decrease symptoms of withdrawal. Patients who are initially overwhelmed may be able to participate in an interview and treatment planning after taking medication. Medication should be considered early and often in the process of an evaluation. If the patient uses a medication at home for similar symptoms or has tried a medication before, the same medication can be offered to minimize potential new side effects. If the patient has not tried medications, consideration of the symptoms, differential diagnosis, intended means of administration of the medication, and potential side effects can guide the choice.

Management of Agitation

In the PES, evaluation and treatment may be complicated by *agitation*, defined as the physical manifestation of internal distress. Agitation may be a sign of psychiatric illness, psychological distress, substance intoxication or withdrawal, or an underlying medical illness. Early signs include pacing, tapping of the fingers and feet, sighing, moaning, fidgeting, staring intensely, and appearing distracted by internal stimuli. Physical signs (e.g., elevations in blood pressure, pulse, or respiratory rate) may be noted. Pressured or loud speech, invasion of others' personal space, clenching of the jaw, or tension of other muscles often indicates escalating agitation. Agitation can herald a psychiatric emergency; it can jeopardize the safety of the patient and others.

Agitation is best managed by attempting to prevent or treat it as early as possible (see Case 1).

CASE 1

Mr. R, a 52-year-old man with a long history of schizophrenia was diagnosed in his early 20s after he became acutely paranoid, and violently assaulted a stranger who he believed was going to harm him. He had previously had multiple prior hospitalizations, and currently lived at a shelter supported by the state Department of Mental Health.

Over the past week, he stopped taking his psychiatric medications, which include haloperidol and lorazepam.

He had become progressively more paranoid and disorganized. Police were called to his shelter after he threatened to harm several staff members, and he was brought to the local ED.

Upon arrival in the ED, he was extremely agitated. He was quickly escorted to a private room in the PES, where a psychiatrist, psychiatric nurse, and security staff immediately attempted verbal de-escalation. Mr. R was quite upset that he could not smoke, but he did accept a nicotine patch. He was also offered, and accepted, haloperidol 5 mg and lorazepam 2 mg PO. He was also given a dinner tray, at which point he asked to be left alone to eat. After 1 hour, he was much calmer and able to participate in a complete psychiatric assessment.

To the extent possible, the agitated patient should be enlisted in this task (i.e., to monitor his/her internal state, report increases in anxiety or distress, and consider safe and effective means to reduce distress). Staff members should be well trained in verbal de-escalation. Key components of verbal de-escalation include empathic listening to the patient's concerns, validation of the patient's position, respectfully stating expectations for behavior, and offering choices where possible.[25] Staff should maintain an open, neutral stance, and speak calmly, in concise and simple language.

Modulation of the environment is another important initial step. When possible, patients should be moved to a quiet, private room, in order to decrease environmental stimulation. The room should have adequate space for the patient and staff, including security staff, to interact safely. Paranoid or previously traumatized patients may be particularly sensitive to personal space. The environment should be safe and free of anything that could be used to harm oneself or others.[25] Attention should be paid to the patient's physical comfort; offers of food, drink or a warm blanket can sometimes diffuse tension.

Pharmacologic interventions are critical for the management of agitation. Medication should be offered early and often to any patient at risk for agitation. The goal of using medication is to calm patients so they can participate in the assessment and treatment planning.[19] Potential medication options include benzodiazepines (particularly lorazepam: 0.5 to 2 mg PO or IM; a benzodiazepine should always be the first choice if alcohol withdrawal is suspected); second-generation antipsychotics (e.g., risperidone: 1 to 2 mg in oral tablet, liquid, or rapidly dissolving form; or olanzapine, 5 to 10 mg in oral tablet, rapidly dissolving, or parenteral form; the parenteral form should not be administered with benzodiazepines due to cardiorespiratory risks;[26] quetiapine: 25–100 mg in oral tablet form); and first-generation antipsychotics (e.g., haloperidol: 5 mg in oral or parenteral form). Oral medications should generally be offered first if the patient is willing, although very distressed patients will sometimes accept IM medication voluntarily for faster onset of action. IM medications are usually needed to treat severe agitation in an unwilling patient. A commonly used combination for severe agitation, optimally administered IM, is haloperidol 5 mg, lorazepam 2 mg, and diphenhydramine 50 mg (for prophylaxis of dystonia). Table 45-5 lists a range of medications that are used for adult patients in the PES. Elderly patients, children, patients with developmental or intellectual disabilities, and patients with a history of head injuries can be particularly sensitive to anticholinergic side effects or can experience paradoxical reactions to medications such as benzodiazepines. Review of prior medication responses is particularly helpful in these populations and smaller initial doses of medication should be used, with increases made slowly.

TABLE 45-5 Medications Frequently Used in the Psychiatric Emergency Service for Adult Patients

MEDICATION	STARTING DOSE[a]	FORMULATION AVAILABLE
Benzodiazepines		
Chlordiazepoxide (Librium)	25–50 mg	PO/IM/IV
Clonazepam (Klonopin)	0.5 mg	PO
Diazepam (Valium)	5–10 mg	PO/IM/IV (oral solution available)
Lorazepam (Ativan)	0.5–1 mg	PO/IM/IV (oral solution available)
Oxazepam (Serax)	15–30 mg	PO
First-Generation Antipsychotics		
Chlorpromazine (Thorazine)	25–50 mg	PO/IM (oral solution available)
Fluphenazine (Prolixin)	5–10 mg	PO/IM (oral solution available)
Haloperidol (Haldol)	5–10 mg	PO/IM/IV (oral solution available)
Perphenazine (Trilafon)	4–8 mg	PO (oral solution available)
Second-Generation Antipsychotics		
Olanzapine (Zyprexa)	5–10 mg	PO/IM[b]
Quetiapine (Seroquel)	25–50 mg	PO
Risperidone (Risperdal)	1–2 mg	PO[b] (oral solution available)
Other Agents		
Benztropine (Cogentin)	0.5–1 mg	PO/IM/IV
Clonidine (Catapres)	0.1 mg	PO
Diphenhydramine (Benadryl)	25–50 mg	PO/IM/IV (oral solution available)
Hydroxyzine (Vistaril)	25–50 mg	PO/IM
Propranolol (Inderal)	20 mg	PO (oral solution available)
Trazodone (Desyrel)	25–50 mg	PO

IM, Intramuscular; IV, intravenous; PO, oral (*per os*).

[a]Starting doses are for healthy adult patients. Consider lower doses in patients who are elderly, children or adolescents, developmentally or intellectually disabled, or have a history of head injury.

[b]Also available in an orally disintegrating tablet.

Restraint and Seclusion

Agitated or violent behavior should be managed with the least restrictive means possible; restraint (any method or device that immobilizes or restricts the patient's movement) and seclusion (involuntary confinement of a patient alone in a room or area) are interventions of last resort when patients are at imminent risk of harming themselves or others. These interventions can be associated with physical and psychological injuries to both patients and providers;[27] however, if verbal, environmental, and pharmacologic interventions are not successful, seclusion or restraint may be necessary to protect the safety of the patient and others. In such cases, the least restrictive intervention should be used; if patient safety permits, seclusion is preferable. For patients who remain at serious risk for harm, physical restraint may be the last resort to maintain their safety and the safety of those around them. A restraint represents a true psychiatric emergency, and all members of the multidisciplinary team should be involved in the management of the patient and the decision to use restraints, although the ultimate responsibility lies with the physician.

Patients in seclusion or restraint require regular monitoring of their medical and behavioral status. National regulations limit the amount of time a patient may remain in restraint; however, attempts should always be made to remove the restraints as soon as possible. Almost every patient who requires restraint or seclusion can benefit from medication to decrease the symptoms that led to agitation. In addition, after the restraint episode, patients (and staff) may benefit from a therapeutic debriefing in order to process the event and to allow the patient and staff to discuss how to avoid similar future events.

Disposition

The goals of the PES evaluation are to provide a therapeutic intervention, to arrive at a diagnostic and risk assessment, and to determine the most appropriate after-care, or disposition, for the patient. The acuity of the patient's symptoms, the safety assessment, the psychosocial support system, and the availability of services must all be weighed to determine the appropriate level of care. Optimally, the patient, family, and outpatient treaters should all participate in the disposition determination although patients with acute risk and/or with impaired judgment may require referral for involuntary hospitalization. Levels of care, ranging from most to least restrictive, include locked inpatient psychiatric units, unlocked crisis stabilization units, residential treatment services, detoxification units, partial hospitalization programs, and outpatient programs. The PES clinician must have a thorough knowledge of local mental health resources and the resources to access them. The availability of outpatient treatment varies greatly by location. Some PESs offer prescriptions for medications on discharge and even provide follow-up, while patients are awaiting referral to outpatient treatment. Other programs may have access to urgent appointments or an outpatient program with a short waiting list. Patients faced with significant social adversity, such as homelessness, may also benefit from referral to appropriate social service agencies.

EMERGENCY ASSESSMENT OF CHILDREN

Demographics

There are very few studies of emergency psychiatric presentations among children. It is estimated that between 1.6% and 3.3% of ED visits in patients younger than 19 are related to mental health conditions.[28,29] Adolescents between 13 and 17 years of age account for more than two-thirds of the visits, and suicide attempts account for 13% of the visits.[28] The most common diagnoses include substance-related disorders (24%), anxiety disorders (16%), and attention deficit and disruptive disorders (11%).[28] Frequent precipitants for ED visits include family crises (e.g., death, divorce, financial stress, domestic abuse), disturbed or truncated peer relationships, and recent change of school.[30–32]

Basic Principles

Few child psychiatric emergencies are life-threatening; all result from the complex interaction of psychosocial, biological, and systems issues.

The primary goal is the safety of the child, and this principle must guide all plans for treatment or disposition. The clinician must always consider the possibility of abuse or neglect as the precipitant for the visit to the ED.

The evaluation itself is based on a developmental approach. The clinician must choose age-appropriate techniques with which to conduct the examination, and the assessment must be based on a solid understanding of normative behavior within each developmental stage.

The emergency psychiatric assessment of a child is often more complicated and time-consuming than the evaluation of an adult. The clinician must be familiar with resources for children and families within the community mental health system. Thorough evaluation often requires phone calls to outside providers including, among others, pediatricians, school administrators, guidance counselors, and outpatient mental health professionals.

The Evaluation

The initial step in the assessment of a child in the PES is identification of the child's legal guardian(s). In routine cases, the legal guardians are the biological parents who accompany the child to the hospital. In complex cases, the child's legal guardian may be court-ordered to be only one parent, another relative, a foster parent, or a representative of the state agency responsible for the care and protection of children. Custody can be split into several parts, and one guardian can have legal (or decision-making) custody, while another guardian retains physical custody. Sometimes a child remains in the home of the biological parent, but a state agency assumes responsibility for decisions regarding medical care. The clinician should never assume that the adult who accompanies the child is the legal guardian or that a friend or neighbor can offer consent for the assessment. Except in very rare, extenuating circumstances, the legal guardian must come to the PES and participate in the evaluation because that person will be a key factor in disposition.

The clinician should base the method of assessment on the age of the child, although the interview may also include many standard elements of the psychiatric history as listed in Table 45-1. The *style* and *process* of the interview and mental status examination depend on the age of the child.

Pre-schoolers (1 to 5 years), many of whom may be preverbal, are generally unable to provide a coherent narrative of the events leading up to the ED visit. The clinician must interview the parent or guardian to obtain the details of the history but should also pay close attention to the interaction between the child and the caregiver, as well as to the child's hygiene. Mental status assessment should focus on the child's appearance, behavior, level of agitation, mood, affect, and ability to take direction and accept reassurance from the caregiver. Common precipitants for ED visits in this age group include impulsive or dangerous behaviors (e.g., running away from home or from a caregiver in a public place, fire-setting, or hitting a younger sibling).

Latency-age children (5 to 11 years) can often provide a clear description of the precipitating event but usually lack the ability to place that event within a larger context. It is often helpful to interview the parent or caregiver before meeting with the child. The mental status assessment includes observations of the child's interaction with the caregiver, attention to speech and language, and direct questions about mood, affect, and risk for self-injurious behavior. Children who are younger than 6 years of age might retain their magical thinking and thus not yet be able to distinguish fantasy from reality. The retention of magical thinking can make assessment of suicidality (i.e., the wish to die) difficult, as children who are not yet able to distinguish fantasy from reality because of developmental stage or developmental delay, may not recognize that death is a one-way street but instead imagine it as a place to which one can go and return.

Adolescents (12 to 18 years) should be interviewed alone before the clinician speaks with caregivers. This approach reinforces and supports the adolescent's desire for autonomy. Mental status assessment involves assessment of mood, affect, thought process and content, cognition, insight, and judgment, as well as suicidal and homicidal ideation.

Finally, the evaluation must include an assessment of the social situation. Being familiar with the local communities and school systems will help the clinician better understand the social context of the PES visit. An inner-city school with few resources is very different from a wealthy suburban school with counselors and school nurses who can identify new problems and monitor medications; knowing these details will help the clinician make appropriate decisions about the treatment plan. It is also important to know the types of treatments that the child has accessed before. A child whose severe depression has failed to improve after several medication trials and participation in months of residential treatment programs, is very different from one who seeks treatment for the first time.

As with adult patients, the options available for disposition vary widely by location and accessible resources through the hospital and community programs. The clinician must have an accurate working knowledge of these resources and how to access them in order to facilitate appropriate disposition planning.

Management

The agitated or aggressive child requires rapid diagnostic assessment and management. The differential diagnosis should focus first on organic (medical) causes of the behavior, including elevated lead levels (particularly for children under 5 years), seizure disorders, metabolic abnormalities, medication (prescription or over-the-counter) ingestion or overdose, substance intoxication or withdrawal, hypoxia, and infection.

If an organic etiology is suspected, vital signs and laboratory studies should be obtained immediately. Laboratory studies might include a complete blood count (CBC), serum electrolytes (including blood glucose), serum and urine toxic screens[33] and, in young women, a pregnancy test. It is usually helpful to decrease stimulation by placing the child in a private room, sometimes with one family member who can be soothing and reassuring. With very young children, it can be helpful to offer food and drink.

At times, it is necessary to administer medications to control agitated or acutely intoxicated children, particularly if they are in danger of harming themselves or others. It is best to ask the parent or guardian which medications the child usually takes and administer either an additional dose of a standing medication or an existing as-needed medication. Administration of an oral medication is always preferable to an IM injection, but it is not always possible if the child is unable to respond to verbal direction or limit-setting. If the child has never tried to swallow a pill before, oral medications that come in liquid formulations are best.

The choice of medication and route of administration depend on the severity of the agitation and the age of the child. Medications to consider include diphenhydramine (1.25 mg/kg per dose PO or IM if the child has no history of paradoxical excitation); clonidine (at a dose of 0.05 to 0.1 mg PO); a second-generation antipsychotic (e.g., risperidone: 0.5 to 1 mg in oral tablet, liquid, or rapidly dissolving form; or olanzapine: 2.5 to 5 mg in oral tablet, rapidly dissolving form or IM preparation); benzodiazepines (particularly lorazepam: 0.5 to 1 mg PO or IM can be helpful but can also cause paradoxical excitation and disinhibition); and for an older, acutely agitated adolescent, it is appropriate to use a high-potency antipsychotic (e.g., haloperidol) combined with a benzodiazepine and an anticholinergic agent (diphenhydramine or benztropine).

Physical restraints are sometimes necessary and should be placed only by trained security personnel according to guidelines established by the appropriate state and federal agencies. Family members should leave the room during any form of restraint and be debriefed later about the course of events and reasons for particular interventions.

LEGAL RESPONSIBILITIES OF THE EMERGENCY PSYCHIATRIST

The emergency psychiatrist is responsible for knowing the legal regulations and local standards of care related to capacity evaluations, confidentiality, release of information, civil commitment, and mandatory reporting. Although specific standards may differ, the following information may assist with understanding these general responsibilities. In all cases, careful documentation of decision-making is important. In complex cases, consultation with a forensic psychiatrist or legal counsel trained in mental health law may be helpful.

Capacity Evaluation

Capacity refers to the patient's ability to make an informed decision about a recommended medical procedure or treatment. While any physician can determine capacity, psychiatrists may be called upon to assist in challenging cases, especially when ED patients are refusing recommended treatment for acute medical problems. The determination of capacity is not based on legally determined criteria but rather on widely accepted clinical standards.[34] In addition, a capacity evaluation applies to a single decision at one moment in time; when in question, the patient's ability to make global medical decisions is determined through a court-based competency hearing, which is outside the purview of the hospital psychiatrist. A patient is presumed to have capacity to make medical decisions until proven otherwise. The key capacity evaluation components include: the assessment of whether the patient can express a choice that is stable over time, understand the relevant information, appreciate the consequences of their decision, and manipulate all of the data in a logical fashion. Furthermore, capacity exists on a sliding scale that incorporates a risk:benefit analysis of the particular treatment in question; a patient may have capacity to decline a treatment with low benefit and high risks and at the same time not have the capacity to decline a treatment with high benefit and low risks. In many cases, the psychiatrist will find that the patient's ability to make a clear and rational decision depends on an opportunity to learn more about the specific medical procedure. If the psychiatrist can coordinate further communication between the medical or surgical team and the patient, the capacity evaluation may become unnecessary.

Confidentiality and Release of Information

The care of psychiatric patients requires a strong commitment to confidentiality; in the emergency setting, all attempts are made to gain permission for any collateral contact. However, for patients who present a risk of harm to themselves or others, it is sometimes necessary to consult with treaters or family members without the patient's consent. It is important to document why the contact was made and to focus the contact on gaining information that will assist in the safety assessment. While the clinician may receive information necessary to assess the patient's safety, the clinician should limit the confidential information given to the other party.

Another situation in which a breach in confidentiality may be justified is when a clinician learns that a patient is at imminent risk to harm another individual. The standards for the clinician's duty to protect the potential victim are different in every state, but most are based on the original Tarasoff case in California in 1976.[35] Consultation with legal counsel is also recommended in situations involving duty to warn.

Civil Commitment

Civil commitment refers to the state's ability to hospitalize an individual involuntarily because of risk of harm or grave disability due to mental illness.[35] The commitment regulations and processes vary by state. Most regulations incorporate risk of harm to self, risk of harm to others, and inability to care for self, all owing to psychiatric pathology, as the basis for civil commitment. The safety evaluation described in this chapter provides the clinician with a basic outline of a risk assessment, which may lead to civil commitment. Hospital commitments by psychiatrists in the ED are generally for short periods of several days; more prolonged involuntary hospitalizations are typically a court ordered decision.

Mandatory Reporting

Most states have regulations regarding mandatory reporting for suspected abuse or neglect of children,[36] elders,[37] and individuals with physical or mental disabilities. In most cases, mandatory reporters are obligated to report situations in which they suspect abuse or neglect, whether or not they have clear evidence; they are protected against claims of a breach of confidentiality under these conditions.[35] Mental health clinicians should be aware of whether they are considered mandatory reporters in their state and how to contact the appropriate agencies.

CONCLUSION

Emergency psychiatry is a growing sub-specialty within psychiatry, driven in part by rapidly increasing rates of ED visits related to mental health and substance use disorders. The role of the emergency clinician is complex, and includes rapid assessment, stabilization, and treatment planning for these complicated and acute patients. These clinicians must be expert not only in a variety of acute psychiatric presentations, addictions and substance-induced conditions, but also in medical illnesses with psychiatric symptoms, management of agitation, local treatment resources, and legal issues in psychiatric care.

REFERENCES

Access the reference list online at https://expertconsult.inkling.com/.

46

Care at the End of Life

M. Cornelia Cremens, M.D., M.P.H.
Ellen M. Robinson, R.N., Ph.D.
Keri O. Brenner, M.D., M.P.A.
Thomas H. McCoy, M.D.
Rebecca Weintraub Brendel, M.D., J.D.

With more than 2.6 million deaths each year in the United States,[1] providing both competent and compassionate care for patients at the end of life is a crucial task for physicians. The Institute of Medicine identified end-of-life care as one of the priority areas for improvement of quality of care, and it specifically identified pain control in advanced cancer and care of patients with advanced organ failure as areas of focus.[2] In addition, professional organizations, including the American College of Physicians, issued guidelines for improving end-of-life care, including recommendations for clinicians to regularly assess patients for pain, dyspnea, and depression.[3,4]

Caring for patients at the end of life occurs amid an often complex background of medical, psychiatric, ethical, and legal concerns. Psychiatric issues (such as depression, anxiety, delirium, substance dependence, and coping difficulties) are common conditions encountered in the treatment of dying medically ill patients. This chapter provides an overview of the central principles of care, diagnosis, and treatment of patients at the end of life from the psychiatric perspective. It also examines current concepts in ethics and legal precedents that surround this evolving area of medicine, where advances in medical technology and practice have extended the human life span and led to the emergence of both opportunities and conflicts at the end of life.

GOALS OF TREATMENT

Psychiatrists face multiple challenges when caring for a dying patient, encompassing issues of diagnosis and treatment as well as larger ethical and legal considerations. Psychiatrists may be uniquely effective in helping a dying patient by ensuring optimization of palliative care and by assisting the patient and the family in the dying process. An important first step in the treatment of the dying patient is for the psychiatrist and the patient to define treatment goals. According to Saunders,[5] the primary aim of care is to help patients "feel like themselves" for as long as possible. Care at the end of life also offers an important opportunity, according to Kübler-Ross, to address and complete "unfinished business."[6] Common themes in this category include reconciliation with estranged friends or family, resolution of conflicts with loved ones, and the pursuit of remaining hopes. Additionally, according to Kübler-Ross,[6] patients who are dying go through a transformational process (which includes stages of denial, anger, bargaining, guilt/depression, and eventual acceptance). These stages may occur in a unique order, may occur simultaneously, and may last variable amounts of time. Psychiatrists and other physicians may assist the dying patient in the transition through these often difficult stages toward acceptance.

Hackett and Weisman[7] also developed five goals for "appropriate death" that may focus therapeutic efforts for the treatment of a dying patient. These goals include freedom from pain, optimal function within the constraints of disability, satisfaction of remaining wishes, recognition and resolution of residual conflict, and yielding of control to trusted individuals. Perhaps the most important principle in the treatment of the dying patient is that the treatment be individualized. That is, within these general goals and paradigms, each patient's unique characteristics will necessitate careful tailoring of clinical interventions. This case-by-case approach can be accomplished only by getting to know the patient, by responding to his or her needs and interests, by proceeding at his or her pace, and by allowing him or her to shape the manner in which those in attendance behave. There is no one best way to die. Everyone dies, but the goal for everyone is to have a good life to the end. In that vein a good death often means respecting the patient's wishes while caring for the patient, family and caregivers.

The recent surge of discussions regarding end-of-life care comes at a time with a burgeoning aging population who are concerned about their preferences being respected and are encouraged to make their preferences known. Gawande[8] cited that palliative care and documented end-of-life wishes established early in the course of life, illness, and impending death are essential. The Conversation Project began in 2010 to help provide an avenue to discuss death and end of life issues in open conversations with family and friends to talk about their wishes for end of life care and not fear talking about death (see: theconversationproject.org).[9]

Hospice provides an important function for the dying patient by incorporating spiritual and family support, pain management, respite services, and a multidisciplinary approach to medical and nursing care. When St. Christopher's Hospice opened in 1967 with Saunders as medical director, it was dedicated to enabling a patient, according to Saunders: "to live to the limit of his or her potential in physical strength, mental and emotional capacity, and social relationships."[5] Saunders viewed hospices as the "alternative to the negative and socially dangerous suggestion that a patient with an incurable disease likely to cause suffering should have the legal option of actively hastened death, that is, euthanasia."[5]

Currently, hospices provide home nursing, family support, spiritual counseling, pain treatment, medication, medical care, and some inpatient care for the terminally ill. In 1994,[8] this numbered approximately 340,000 dying persons, and by 2014, approximately 1.6–1.7 million patients received hospice services.[8] A decade ago, the average patient was enrolled roughly 1 month before his or her death, and the vast majority of patients had cancer.[9–11] According to 2014 data, cancer diagnoses now accounts for less than 50% of hospice admissions, and growth in these admissions has been attributable to dementia, stroke or coma, and lung diseases.[8] The average length of hospice enrollment in 2013 was 72.6 days, with a median length of service of 18.5 days.[5] Women were found to use hospice services more than men, whites more than blacks, and, overall, close to one in four older Americans used this service.[8] Higher hospice utilization rates were found for diseases that impose higher burden on caregivers or diseases with more prognostic accuracy.[8] The three causes of death with highest hospice utilization rates were malignancies, dementia, and heart disease.[8] Medicare pays for the vast majority of hospice services; in 2013 more than 87.2% of hospice patients received services through their Medicare benefits.[8] To qualify for hospice benefits, potential recipients of hospice care must, with their physician and the hospice medical director, determine the benefits provided by their Medicare plan, as there are many options with newer Medicare HMO and PPO plans.[12]

THE ROLE OF THE PSYCHIATRIST

Psychiatrists can play a crucial role in the effective management of patients at the end of life because of their abilities to appreciate the medical aspects of disease, to understand the highly subjective and individual factors that contribute to the personal significance of illness, to understand personality styles and traits, and to engage with patients to modulate maladaptive responses to illness.[13,14] To this end, the psychiatrist may serve many functions, including facilitating medical treatment; augmenting communication between the patient, the family, and the caregivers; and modeling those qualities that may be helpful for the patient. Above all, the psychiatrist's primary goals are the diagnosis and management of psychiatric symptoms and illnesses. As for all other patients, a consideration of all factors that contribute to psychiatric suffering including biological illnesses, psychological style, psychosocial factors and functional capacity, is essential. Studies indicate that psychiatric morbidity in the setting of terminal illness is very high.[15] The most common issues that lead to psychiatric interventions for the dying patient include major depression, anxiety, personality disorders, delirium and other organic brain syndromes, refractory pain, substance abuse, and difficulties surrounding bereavement.[16,17]

Depression

The more seriously ill a person becomes, the more likely the person is to develop major depression.[18] The prevalence rates of clinically significant depression in the terminally ill range from 20% to 50%.[15,19] Studies of terminally ill cancer patients have suggested rates of adjustment disorders of from 9% to 35% and rates of major depression from 8% to 26%.[20–26] Depression has also been associated with poor quality of life in amyotrophic lateral sclerosis.[27,28] Careful vigilance for depression is necessary, as both symptoms of depression and the impact of depression on other aspects of the patient's life and medical care are challenging. For example, Weisman formulated the wish to die as an existential signal of the person's conviction "that his potential for being someone who matters has been exhausted" (AD Weisman, personal communication). Ganzini and colleagues[29] documented that severely depressed patients made more restricted advance directives when depressed, and they changed them after their depression remitted. At Memorial Sloan-Kettering Cancer Center, Breitbart and Holland[30] studied terminally ill patients with cancer and acquired immunodeficiency syndrome (AIDS) who had suicidal ideation and compared them to similar patients *without* suicidal ideation. The primary difference was the presence of depression in the patients with suicidal thoughts.[30] Thus, aggressive treatment of depression is a cornerstone of care, as it dramatically decreases suffering and improves quality of life. In terms of specific treatments, psychiatrists may consider the use of rapidly acting treatments that target specific symptoms. In addition to antidepressants, stimulants are another useful class of agents; their advantages include the rapid onset of improved mood and the potentiation of co-administered narcotics (with less accompanying sedation). Suicidal ideation, if it appears, should not be thought of as an "understandable" response but rather as a condition that warrants immediate investigation and treatment.[17]

Desire to Hasten Death

It is also important to differentiate suicidal ideation from a stated desire to hasten death. In one study, suicide was distinguished from life-ending acts and end-of-life decisions in the literature based on patients with chronic kidney disease and dialysis.[31] The desire to hasten death has been identified consistently among a minority of terminally ill patients.[32–35] Among patients with advanced AIDS, 4.6% to 8.3% have expressed a desire for hastened death, a rate significantly lower than the rate found in studies of patients with advanced or terminal cancer.[36] Although the desire to hasten death is frequently associated with depression, other factors (such as pain, existential concerns, loss of function, and social circumstances) also play critical roles.[32,37–43] The psychiatric consultant needs to listen carefully to the patient who desires hastened death, to treat any underlying psychiatric or physical problem, and to take steps to lessen distress.[40,44]

Anxiety

Anxiety frequently occurs at the end of life and requires psychiatric attention.[17,19] Impending death can generate severe anxiety not only in those who face death themselves but also in their family members, friends, and caregivers. The patient who experiences anxiety surrounding death may not necessarily be able to articulate his or her fears, although anxiety may be related to prior losses or experiences that involve the death of others. Common fears associated with death include helplessness or loss of control, ideas of guilt and punishment, physical pain or injury, and abandonment.[16–18,45,46] The psychiatrist can address these fears and explore issues of isolation, abandonment, and suffering. Appropriate attention should be directed toward psychopharmacologic management of anxiety symptoms.

Personality Considerations

The terminally ill patient with a personality disorder (such as narcissistic or borderline personality disorder) or other coping difficulties can present a particular challenge for care providers. For the patient, help is hard if not impossible to accept and trust, which can interfere with his or her ability to take the comfort that is offered.[13,16,17] Much of the situation is out of his or her immediate control; this elicits regression and the use of more primitive defenses (such as splitting). This may manifest as poor communication with treaters, inadequate pain control, and difficulty in the resolution of interpersonal conflicts.[17] Psychiatrists may find it useful to call on psychodynamic diagnostic and treatment skills to assist such a person in accepting palliative care.[17] Treaters can help to transform the negative countertransference (on the part of caretakers) into an understanding of how best to help the patient undergo the dying process.[16,17] Working closely with family and friends of the patient, as well as the medical team, is important in these situations.[16,17]

Delirium and Cognitive Changes

As terminal illness progresses, medical complications (such as delirium and other cognitive changes) can occur.[47–51] These complications can manifest as confusion, psychosis, agitation, or a multitude of other symptoms and can be caused by the medical illness, its treatment, or both. Palliative care interventions should also be considered earlier in the course of deterioration from dementia, and goals of care for patients with dementia should include quality of life, dignity, and comfort.[47,52] Effective management of changes in affect, behavior, and cognition resulting from delirium or dementia is critical, as it can indicate worsening of medical illness and can greatly affect the quality of time spent with friends, family, and caretakers.[16,17,53]

Pain

Pain management can be a complex challenge requiring extensive expertise. Freedom from pain is basic to every care plan, and it should be achievable in most cases,[16] but management of breakthrough pain requires detailed assessments and management.[54–56] For a multitude of reasons, pain is often undertreated by medical staff.[57–61] Pain management may be particularly challenging for a patient with a history of substance dependence; patients with a history of addiction are more likely to receive inadequate pain management than patients without a history of substance abuse or dependence.[14,62,63] The reasons for this can include concerns about higher-than-expected (and escalating) dosages of opiates, potential misuse or diversion, and fears of legal consequences of prescribing narcotics to a patient with substance dependence.[62,64] Evidence of abuse may include unexpectedly positive results on toxicology screens, frequent requests for higher dosages, recurrent reports of lost prescriptions, and multiple visits to various providers or Emergency Departments for prescription refills.[65]

Physicians who prescribe to such patients may have divergent opinions about the treatment of substance dependence in the terminally ill. Some physicians feel that carefully monitoring a terminally ill patient on an opiate or actively treating the patient's substance dependence deprives the patient; however, optimal relief of suffering mandates acknowledgment and treatment of active substance abuse issues.[66] The goal of care requires the physician to separate the management of the patient's pain from the management of addiction, and to treat both.[14,67] Careful monitoring of a patient's narcotic use, use of a multidisciplinary team, encouragement of substance abuse treatment, limitation of prescribing power to a single provider, and use of screening tests (e.g., urine toxicology) may all be useful in the management of the terminally ill person with substance dependence.[68] Complementary therapies as part of end-of-life care for improvement of quality of life or moderation of pain distress are also being studied.[69]

Psychosocial Considerations

Optimal end-of-life care includes an understanding of the major areas of psychosocial concern (such as family, work, religion, faith, ethnicity, and culture). The presence of the family is crucial to help a patient resolve longstanding conflicts (if possible) and to provide a context for honoring and remembering the patient.[16] Psychiatrists can aid the family by encouraging the sharing of feelings among family members and by helping to create specific plans for the family (such as the compilation of commemorative items).[17] At the same time, an understanding of the complexities of family interactions (both positive and negative) helps prevent harm to a potentially fragile family system. For example, a recent randomized clinical trial of family-focused grief therapy found that it could help prevent pathologic grief in family members; however, it also had the potential to increase conflict in families where the level of hostility was high.[70]

As with family relationships, a sense of vocational identity can help create meaning for a patient at the end of life.[16] For some, work can be critical for self-esteem. As a patient can begin to feel less valuable when work ceases or retirement arrives, the presence of former and current colleagues can be quite supportive.

Similarly, thoughtful discussion about a patient's beliefs and faith can provide an opportunity for a patient to further his or her sense of meaning and thoughts about an afterlife.[17] Many patients are grateful for the chance to express thoughts about their faith. The patient's own clergyperson, if available, can often provide valuable information and insights about the patient and family and help smooth the course before death. Writers such as Allport[71] and Feifel[72] have contrasted an extrinsic religious orientation (in which religion is mainly a means to social status, security, or relief from guilt) with an intrinsic religious orientation (in which the values appear to be internalized and subscribed to as ends in themselves). Experimental work[73] and clinical experience[16] indicate that an extrinsic value system, without internalization, seems to offer less assistance in coping with a fatal illness than an intrinsic religious commitment (that can offer considerable stability and strength).

Last, patients from underserved communities or minority populations in the United States may have needs that are not served by the current health care system. Unfortunately, the same institutional, cultural, and individual factors that generate disparities in care for minority populations in general also affect care at the end of life.[74] These factors include lack of access to care, under-treatment of pain, and mistrust of the healthcare system.[74–76] Furthermore, important differences between ethnic groups and cultures can be found at all segments of end-of-life care. For example, several studies have shown that African-American patients, as well as older individuals from other ethnic backgrounds (such as Latino, Asian, or Native American), are somewhat less likely to have arranged for an advance directive as compared with Caucasian patients.[77] There are also important differences in terms of preferences for life-sustaining treatment. For example, in a study involving multiple ethnic groups, African-Americans had the highest rate of preferring life-sustaining treatment, and European-Americans had the lowest rates.[78] Multiple other studies have demonstrated a preference by African-Americans to choose more life-sustaining treatment and cardiopulmonary resuscitation in the face of terminal illness.[74,79–82]

Additionally, culture may influence the decision-making process.[83] For example, family-centered (rather than individual) decision-making is common in certain ethnic groups in the United States, which challenges the traditional Western model of the importance of individual autonomy. Studies have found a higher use of family-centered decision-making among Latino and Asian groups in the United States, which may include the decision to disclose (or not to disclose) the diagnosis of a terminal illness to an individual patient.[77] Thus, attention to cultural competency by psychiatrists plays a significant role in mediating end-of-life care for patients from all ethnicities and cultures.

CHALLENGES FOR CARE PROVIDERS

The emotional intensity associated with providing empathy and support for the dying patient during a time of need may challenge and tire caregivers (such as family and professional staff). A critical skill in end-of-life care is being able to hold end-of-life discussions[84] and to listen to the patient and families, asking open-ended questions.[85–88] End-of-life discussions with physicians have been associated with fewer aggressive interventions, which, in turn, is associated with improved quality of life and caregiver bereavement adjustment.[89] Structured, proactive, multidisciplinary communication systems that include an ethics consultation and palliative care teams have also been shown to improve communication during critical care and end-of-life care for patients and their families.[90–94] Barriers to patient–physician communication about end-of-life care include physicians' own perception that the patient is not ill enough or is not ready to have the conversation.[95] Special considerations should be given to pediatric populations.[96]

Caregivers may also experience helplessness and despair in the face of their powerlessness over a patient's approaching death.[97] If left unaddressed, these feelings in caregivers can cause the caregiver to avoid the patient, to retreat, or even to convey to him or her how burdensome he or she is to caregivers. This could be devastating to the helpless patient who looks to the caregiver for hope. Hence, among the greatest psychological requirements for caregivers is to learn to live with negative feelings and to resist the urge to avoid the patient actions that convey to the patient that he or she no longer matters. Certain traits make these empathic difficulties hazardous for some caregivers. Dependent persons who expect patients to appreciate, to thank, to love, and to nurture them are unconsciously prone to exhaust themselves regularly because they "can never do enough." This creates a pattern that may be sustainable for a patient with the capacity to nurture the caregiver, but it could have a disastrous outcome if the patient is depleted or intractably hostile. The harder the caregiver strives, the less rewarding the work becomes. Exhaustion and demoralization follow. Some caregivers want to please every physician they consult, and they come to a similar state of exhaustion because many of these patients cannot improve.

CASE 1

Ms. W, a 48-year-old woman with chronic paranoid schizophrenia struggled for years, often refusing psychiatric medications that were of benefit and resisting medical care for chronic kidney disease. Although she has an extensive group of professionals caring for her, her delusions and paranoia influenced her judgment and prevented her from accepting care. She has a legal guardian and lived in a psychiatric supported group home for many years.

Ms. W was admitted to an inpatient psychiatry service due to the increasingly severe psychotic symptoms and worsening kidney failure for which she historically and currently refused hemodialysis (HD). The decision to forego dialysis, even in the light of rising levels of potassium, was respected, as this had been her decision for many years according to those who had cared for her. Ms. W lived with persistent delusions that made HD untenable; it was a way of not interacting with the healthcare system.

Facing a life-threatening situation, both the decision to forego dialysis and not to offer resuscitation (CPR) was the immediate decision regarding her end-of-life decisions. Not to provide life-sustaining treatment to Ms. W became an ethical dilemma, weighing the tenet of "do not harm" or malfeasance with treatment of a life-threatening situation.

An ethics consult was requested to examine the risks, to interview the stakeholders, and to assess the suffering that HD would inflict on her. A clear mechanism existed to impose dialysis on Ms. W, through her guardian, could be justified. The opinion of the consultants was this would be a violation of the patient's personhood, dignity, and right to self-determination in her life's framework leading to irreparable harm to the patient.

The inpatient team, family, guardian, and outpatient caregivers were consulted and the decision to forego HD was established in light of the patient's years of refusing treatment and weighing the risks of harm and suffering. In the event that the kidney failure led to a life-threatening situation the decision to not offer CPR, in a patient who would not receive dialysis, would be unsuccessful and it would inflict pain and suffering at the end of her life.

ETHICS AND END-OF-LIFE CARE

Principles

End-of-life care carries, inherently, a host of ethical questions that the psychiatrist is likely to encounter. A brief discussion of principles is not intended to supplant the need for concrete individualized judgments for every patient. Principles provide anchor points from which clinical reasoning can proceed—specifically, when limitation of life-supporting treatment is proposed.

The primary obligation of the physician to the patient in traditional medical ethics has been expressed in both positive and negative terms. The negative goal, always referred to first, is not to harm the patient (*primum non nocere*). The positive obligation is to restore health, to relieve suffering, or both. Our contemporary dilemma, as Slater[98] has pointed out, arose because we now have many situations in which these two aims come into conflict (i.e., the more aggressive the efforts to reverse an incurable illness, the more suffering is inflicted on the patient).

A related problem is the difficulty in distinguishing treatments administered to relieve pain and suffering from those intended to hasten death.[99] The principle of double effect is commonly used to allow the administration of narcotics and sedatives with the intent to relieve suffering of dying patients, even though such administration may hasten death, but it is a principle that remains widely debated.[100–102]

Second, modern medicine respects patients' right to autonomy. This principle guarantees any competent patient the right to refuse any treatment, even a lifesaving one. This was the emphasis of the medical ethics of the 1970s and 1980s and it focused on refusing life-prolonging treatment, such as mechanical ventilation, and more recently, nutrition and hydration. Honoring such refusals presupposes that the patient is competent. It is important to remember that competent patients may make decisions that providers may view as irrational.[103] However, a patient cannot insist that the physician provides treatment that is considered futile.[104–108] Defining futility continues to be a goal of medical ethics as a balance is forged between the autonomy interest of patients to opt for aggressive treatment and concern by physicians that there is a duty not to offer or provide treatments that are ineffective.[109–111]

Another area of debate concerns the right for terminally ill patients with cancer to have access to investigational drugs.[112] A case was brought against the U.S. Food and Drug Administration (FDA) by an alliance named after Abigail Burroughs, a young woman who had been diagnosed with squamous-cell carcinoma of the head and neck at age 19 and had unsuccessfully attempted to obtain investigational drugs on a compassionate-use basis. In 2006, the U.S. Court of Appeals for the District of Columbia Circuit initially held that patients with cancer have a constitutional right of access to investigational cancer drugs.[113] On a re-hearing, however, the Court of Appeals reversed the decision and found that there is no fundamental right of access to experimental drugs for the terminally ill. Recent reports from the FDA outline the expanded access or compassionate use that outlines expanded access to investigational drugs for treatment and charging for the investigational drugs; this went into effect in 2012.

Limitation of Life-Sustaining Treatment

One salient concept for psychiatrists to understand is the limitation of life-sustaining treatment. Whenever the risks or burdens of a treatment appear to outweigh the benefits, use of that treatment should be questioned by both physician and patient. Limitation of life-prolonging treatment is generally reserved for three categories of patients. First, patients who have an irreversible illness, who are moribund, and who need to be protected from needlessly burdensome treatments may refuse life-sustaining treatment. This is widely accepted for patients who will die with or without treatment (such as the patient with advanced metastatic cancer). Second, because of the right to refuse treatment, competent patients who are not moribund but who have an irreversible illness have also been allowed to have life-sustaining treatments stopped. Last, competent patients with a reversible illness have the right to refuse any treatment, including life-saving treatments.

However, complications emerge when a patient is unable to make or voice a decision regarding his or her wishes. In these situations, the state has a recognized legal interest in preserving life, and it may be difficult to ascertain whether the patient had a countervailing autonomy interest. One historic example is the case of Karen Ann Quinlan, a 21-year-old woman who, in 1976, fell into an irreversible coma while at a party. This case became a legal battle between the right of Quinlan's mother (who, as her guardian, wished to withdraw life-sustaining treatment from her daughter and allow her daughter to die with dignity) and the state's interest in preserving life. In the end, the Supreme Court of New Jersey decided that, if it was believed, to a reasonable degree, that the coma was irreversible, life-sustaining treatment (e.g., with a respirator) could be removed.[114] Now, 40 years later, the standard medical recommendation in the case of irreversible coma is to stop all treatment (including nutrition and hydration). This judgment is made on the principle of the inevitability of death and the futility of any treatments to prevent it.

For patients in a persistent vegetative state (a state in which patients have a functioning brainstem but total loss of cortical function), a complicated scenario emerges.[115,116] The many clinical dilemmas in this condition are perhaps best exemplified by the Nancy Cruzan case in 1990. Seven years after the automobile accident that left her in a persistent vegetative state, Nancy Cruzan's feeding tube was removed. She died 12 days later. Her parents' request that the tube be removed initiated a journey that took them through the state and federal court system, up to the U.S. Supreme Court. The U.S. Supreme Court's decision[117,118] affirmed that competent patients have the right to refuse treatment, that foregoing nutrition and hydration is no different from foregoing other medical treatment (such as artificial ventilation or pressor agents), but that Missouri (and other states) could require "clear and convincing evidence" that the patient, while still competent, had rejected the idea of life-sustaining treatment under such circumstances. That is, the autonomy interest of the patient in a persistent vegetative state had to be weighed against the state's interest in protecting life. However, according to the U.S. Supreme Court, while Missouri could require clear and convincing evidence of a patient's wishes when that patient was previously competent, states could also adopt less rigorous standards.

The complicated scenario of the persistent vegetative state was more recently revisited in the Theresa Schiavo case of 2004.[119] In this case, Theresa Schiavo was determined to be in a persistent vegetative state, and her husband, who was her guardian, wished to withdraw life-sustaining nutrition and hydration from her, in accordance with what he believed her wishes would have been. However, her parents opposed removal of the life-sustaining measures. Although the Florida Supreme Court's decision upheld the decision to have her feeding tube removed, it did not re-visit or alter the legal rights of patients, in that it rested on a narrow legal analysis of the proper powers of each branch of the state government. Nonetheless, the case revived public debate about withdrawal of care at the end of life. After the case, many states began debating the amount of proof required to establish that an incompetent patient, when competent, would have opted to have his or her life-sustaining care withdrawn, and clinicians have had to re-visit the guidelines for the appropriate use of artificial nutrition and hydration.[120]

As a whole, the legal cases regarding end-of-life decision-making explicitly give patients the right to exercise their autonomy regarding what care they receive. For competent patients, these wishes may be expressed at the time that they are making decisions regarding end-of-life care through the use of advance directives that take effect in the event of future incapacity to make or express decisions about their care. These directives may be instructional, may appoint a surrogate decision-maker, or both. Instructional directives placing limits on life-sustaining treatment, however, may be difficult to interpret on clinical grounds. For example, requests (such as the desire that "no extraordinary means" be taken to preserve life) may be difficult to interpret in actual clinical settings. Advance directives that appoint a surrogate decision-maker with whom the patient has discussed his or her wishes may be a more flexible way to enact a patient's wishes. Specifically, a surrogate decision-maker can use his or her knowledge of the patient's prior expressed wishes in combination with the actual clinical scenario in order to more reliably lead to the outcome that the patient would have wanted, if competent.

Physician-Assisted Suicide

Although patients have broad rights of autonomy in expressing their wishes for end-of-life care, there are limits on a patient's ability to control his or her death. A patient may express the wish to have a physician end his or her life (euthanasia). One study of terminally ill cancer patients found that attitudes toward euthanasia and assisted suicide were determined by psychosocial traits and beliefs, including religious beliefs and perceptions of the amount of burden on families, rather than symptom intensity or disease severity.[121] Euthanasia, even when requested by the patient, is illegal in all 50 states and all US districts and territories, but is legal in the Netherlands, Belgium, Colombia, and Luxembourg. Physicians are prohibited from administering life-ending medication or directly causing death through affirmative action throughout the United States.

Unlike euthanasia, the practice of physician-assisted suicide, which allows physicians to help patients acquire the means to end their lives but does not permit the physician to actually administer those means, has begun to gain acceptance in the United States. Specifically, physician-assisted suicide is legal in the state of Oregon and has survived numerous legal challenges in the U.S. Supreme Court. Most recently, in 2006, the Supreme Court in *Gonzales v. Oregon* held that the U.S. Attorney General did not have the authority under federal law to prohibit doctors from prescribing regulated drugs for use in physician-assisted suicide in the setting of state law authorizing the practice.[122]

Under the Oregon Death with Dignity Act (DWDA),[123] physicians in Oregon are permitted to write prescriptions for lethal doses of medications to patients who request to die and meet the other requirements of the state law. Overall, the practice has contributed to a small proportion of deaths in Oregon (0.01%): from 1998 to 2009, there were 460 deaths by ingestion in Oregon.[124] The specific prevalence of psychiatric symptoms in individuals requesting physician-assisted suicide has not been extensively characterized. One study of 58 Oregon residents who had requested aid in dying from a physician or had contacted an aid-in-dying advocacy organization found that 15 participants met criteria for depression and 13 for anxiety.[125] Three of the 18 participants in the study who received a prescription for a lethal drug under the DWDA met criteria for depression.

Although Oregon has legalized the practice, organized medicine (and psychiatry) oppose the practice. Nonetheless, a second state, Washington, in 2008, passed an initiative for the Washington Death with Dignity Act[126] modeled on the Oregon DWDA, as have Vermont, Montana, and California. The debate[127–129] over physician-assisted suicide continues as other states consider passing laws that authorize it.

CONCLUSION

The aim of end-of-life care is to maximize the quality of life and to minimize the suffering of patients who are terminally ill. For many patients, the end of life marks an important opportunity to reflect, reconcile, and pursue remaining hopes. The psychiatrist can play an important role in the diagnosis and treatment of psychiatric illness in this setting, as well as in facilitating treatment, enhancing communication, and modeling caregiver qualities for families. From a psychiatric perspective, major depression and anxiety are commonly seen; suicidality should not be considered "understandable" or "normal" in this setting. Delirium, pain, and difficulties with coping are also common reasons for consultation requests. As in all other forms of psychiatric evaluation and treatment, it is crucial to consider any medical contribution to psychiatric symptoms. Aggressive treatment of depression, anxiety, and other psychiatric symptoms is a crucial part of holistic management. Additionally, psychosocial factors may play an important (and, at times, complicating) role in the care of these patients. Psychiatrists also should be aware of, and prepared to manage, many of the complex ethical and legal issues that arise in the care of these patients. Physicians have clear obligations in caring for their patients, and patients have rights to autonomy in their decision-making. Doctors often avoid frank conversations with patients regarding end-of-life decisions so as not to be perceived as having given up hope. The diagnosis, options for treatment in line with goals of care, and prognosis are best presented openly in an effort to guide the patients, family, and friends on a path to a peaceful, comfortable death with pain well controlled. Then, the conversations can continue with regard to acceptance, sadness, and an opportunity to say goodbye.

Sound clinical and ethical practice requires that the physician assist the terminally ill patient in the complex and often simultaneous processes of grieving and celebrating, reconciling conflicts and completing unfinished business, achieving last hopes and accepting that some goals are unrealized, while alleviating suffering and maximizing autonomy and personhood until death.

REFERENCES

Access the reference list online at https://expertconsult.inkling.com/.

REFERENCES

Pediatric Consultation

47

Kenny A. Lin, M.D.
Eric P. Hazen, M.D.
Annah N. Abrams, M.D.

OVERVIEW

Pediatric psychiatry consults are requested to address a diverse set of issues and needs. Similar to the work involving adult psychiatric consultations, the child psychiatrist evaluates the patient, acts as a liaison to the medical and nursing staff, manages the psychiatric needs and demands of patients and their families, and helps treatment teams unite around common goals of quality care. Additionally, the pediatric consultant incorporates child development into the formulation, works closely with parents, and also interacts with schools and social service agencies. This chapter reviews the pediatric consultation process and highlights its main differences from adult consultations. It focuses on important developmental and family-oriented concepts, common reasons for pediatric consultation, managing concerns about child maltreatment, psychological issues related to chronic medical illness in both patients and their parents, ethical issues, and future directions in the field.

Child psychiatric consultation has been utilized more as the clinical need has become more recognized and resources have grown. In 1985, Fritz and Bergman[1] surveyed more than 1000 members of the American Academy of Pediatrics and found that roughly two-thirds of pediatricians who have had an interaction with a psychiatrist remembered the consultation as necessary and helpful. However, half of the pediatricians rarely consulted a psychiatrist due to many factors, including lack of availability and family reluctance to engage with psychiatry. A 1993 study of pediatricians by Burket and Hodgin[2] found that more than half of the pediatric staff stated they rarely or never referred to child psychiatry, yet these same pediatricians estimated that more than 30% of their patients had emotional problems. Shaw and colleagues showed in 2006 and again in 2016, that pediatric psychiatry clinical needs have increased, with corresponding increases in consultation requests in outpatient, inpatient, and emergency room settings.[3,4] However, though the overall perceptions of child psychiatry consultation being helpful for pediatric staff and patients have remained consistent or even improved, funding issues continue to impact many consultation programs throughout the country.[4]

Early identification of children in need of consultation remains crucial. Bujoreanu and co-workers found that earlier psychiatric consultation during an admission led to shorter hospital stays and to lower hospital charges.[5] One strategy to ensure early identification is to implement routine, automatic psychiatric consultations for specific diagnoses (such as cancer, diabetes, cystic fibrosis, and failure to thrive), as well as for protracted or frequent hospital stays, nonadherence, and psychosocial dysfunction. Screening tools, such as the Pediatric Symptom Checklist (PSC)[6] or the Psychosocial Assessment Tool (PAT2.0),[7] may also help identify high-risk patients.

The consultant needs to be attuned not only to the needs of the child and the family, but also to the dynamics of the pediatric unit.[8,9] Assessment of how the child's situation is experienced by the pediatric team requires an awareness of the patient mix on the unit, recent deaths or other traumas, and attitudes toward certain diseases and presentations that may evoke strong emotions among staff (e.g., irritation when caring for a patient whose problems are perceived as "self-induced," such as with an eating disorder or intentional overdose). At times, the consultant may identify a psychologically vulnerable team member who needs referral for additional support.

Once consultation has been initiated, pediatricians highly value accessibility, timeliness in completing the consultation, close follow-up, and liaison work.[2] The consultant needs to make assessments and specific treatment plans in a timely fashion, to facilitate rapid high-quality communication between members of the healthcare delivery team, and to create seamless transitions from inpatient to outpatient care (involving follow-up and specific recommendations). These goals are facilitated by creation of relationships between the consultant and the pediatricians, interaction with community resources, and appreciation of the medical challenges from within the child's developmental frame of reference.[10,11]

CASE 1

An 11-year-old boy with autism spectrum disorder (ASD) was brought to the hospital by his parents due to a significant behavioral change and agitation over the previous 3 days. He was unable to communicate verbally and was dependent on his parents for toileting and other self-care needs. He was admitted to the pediatrics service for a medical work-up to determine if there was an organic etiology for his behavioral change. Child psychiatry was consulted to help with management of his agitation.

In the hospital, he continued to be quite agitated. He repeatedly tried to walk out his room, thrashed around in his bed, made loud yelling noises, and intermittently grabbed at members of the medical team. Hospital staff expressed frustration over not knowing how best to calm him, especially when his parents were asleep or away from the bedside. His parents were understandably fatigued, stressed, and frustrated. Staff wanted more guidance from the family regarding what triggered agitation and how best to soothe him, whereas his parents were looking to the staff for answers as to why their son was agitated and expected the staff to provide the answers. As a result, his parents expressed significant anger towards the staff. One of the child psychiatry consultant's roles was to help validate the parent's concerns, while also supporting the staff and helping them understand the reasons behind the parents' behaviors.

The consulting child psychiatrist helped develop a behavioral plan to manage the patient's challenging behaviors. This was done in collaboration with the family, occupational therapy, nursing staff, child life specialists, and the medical team. A developmental framework for this boy was particularly important, given his degree of developmental delay. History from the parents revealed that he very much liked having a stuffed dog toy in his bed, preferred specific clothing, and enjoyed certain cartoons that were usually watched by younger children, on an electronic tablet. He routinely listened to music at night before going to sleep. Occupational therapy brought a large exercise ball for him to bounce on, as well as other soft toys to squeeze. A customized behavioral plan was printed out and placed on the front of his chart, alerting any rounding or visiting medical staff. This included potential triggers to avoid (such as having many strangers in the room at once) and effective behavioral techniques for calming him (such as playing soothing music or using sensory toys, e.g., a squeeze ball). Recommendations for possible medications to be used in the event of severe agitation were also made.

Medical work-up revealed severe constipation that likely caused his abdominal pain and contributed to his agitation. This was treated effectively by the pediatrics team. He received rewards, such as extra time watching a preferred cartoon, offered for cooperation with his treatment regimen. As his constipation resolved, his agitation improved. The consulting child psychiatrist communicated with the patient's outpatient psychiatrist to coordinate care and assure appropriate follow-up.

THE PEDIATRIC CONSULTATION PROCESS

Initial Steps

The first step in any consultation is to understand the consultation questions (e.g., "Who initiated the consultation?" "What concerns underlie the question?" "What feedback does the consulting person need to be satisfied, and within what time frame?"). It can also be helpful to ask whether the patient and family have been notified about the consult. Once the questions are clarified, the consultant must gather the necessary history, including data provided by members of the medical team, the hospital record, observations from staff, and collateral information from social agencies or non-parent caretakers involved in a child's care, when appropriate.

Some pediatricians are especially sensitive to psychological concerns and have known the patient and family for several years. In university-affiliated hospitals, the consultant often deals with less experienced house staff on monthly rotating schedules and discussion with the referring physician is shifted toward teaching. A crucial function of ongoing consultation is the trusting relationship that should develop between the pediatrician, unit personnel, and the consultant. This trust creates an atmosphere in which the psychological needs of children are recognized, and the consultant's recommendations are carried out, even when this may take additional time and effort.

In the review of the medical record, it is especially important to note the observations of the nurses and child-life specialists. These individuals often have a wealth of information from sustained contact with the child and the family. They frequently have had considerable experience with other children of a similar age and with the same diagnosis, and thus, can sense how this child is coping as compared with a relevant peer group. The nurse usually takes a self-care and daily habit history on admission that emphasizes the child's pre-morbid level of functioning. The nurse may also record the most careful observations of the child's level of anxiety, state of aggression, and temperamental characteristics.[12–14] The role of the child-life specialist, trained in development, is to help children cope with the stress of hospitalization by organizing individual and group activities and providing coping strategies for challenges such as blood draws or other medical procedures. The child-life specialist often has the opportunity to observe children interact with peers and to use special hospital play materials.[15] Furthermore, many pediatric inpatient services have a social worker who reviews all or some of the admissions; this expanded social history may be helpful before the consultant meets the family and child. Staff input is a critical adjunct to the consultant's impression, which is usually based on only one or two interviews.

Interview Techniques for Child Psychiatric Consultation

The child and family should be prepared for the consultation. The referring physician should discuss the reasons for the referral with both the child and the parents so that the child feels included and does not feel that information is being withheld.

The interview of young children (younger than 3 years) requires largely indirect expressions of feelings and concerns via play and observation rather than by direct questioning. The consultant's interactive style should be active, interested, and playful. Toys could include finger puppets, stuffed animals, and dolls. First, one should carry out an unstructured observation, after which a gross developmental assessment is conducted. For children younger than 3 years of age, observations of the parent–child dyad are crucial. One should note: "What is the eye contact like between parent and child?" "Does the parent respond to cues in the child and vice versa?" "Are the parent and child "in sync"?" "Does the child look to the parent for reassurance and comfort?" "What is the child's temperament like, and how does the parent handle frustration?" "How do the child and parent handle separation?" "How does the child respond to strangers?" Stranger anxiety in the very young is expected, and the lack of any stranger anxiety may be a sign of attachment difficulties.

The 3- to 6-year-old child may still require that a parent be present throughout the interview. That request should be respected, although at some point in the interview an attempt should be made to have the parent leave the room. Developmental assessment, including language, social interaction, and gross and fine motor coordination, is a mandatory part of the interview. Drawings become a more important tool for some children to express troublesome thoughts and feelings. The psychiatrist should not expect to complete the evaluation in one visit. It may take several sessions, and the sessions may be short because of the child's fatigue or because other tests have been scheduled. The consultant may need to arrange visits to coincide with appropriate times for observing key behaviors, such as around meal times or dressing changes.

The latency-age child (age 7 to 12) can be a more verbal participant in the interview. The child should be questioned about current and previous school attendance, school behavior, school performance, after-school activities, friends, health (including mental health) of family members, family problems, and interaction of family members in response to traumatic events. The mental status examination should initially focus on the manner of relating. The child may be active and verbal or shy and inhibited. The consultant's approach should be flexible, depending on the child's interactive style. The active verbal child can be approached in the more traditional interview. The shy child may be engaged through drawings or games, such as checkers or video games. These activities can prove helpful in facilitating an alliance and in demonstrating organic deficits. The first few sessions may be necessary for the child to develop trust in the consultant and recognize that he will not be performing invasive or painful procedures. Many helpful observations of the child can occur in this initial phase, including assessment of pain, anorexia, and insomnia, assessment of coping strategies, and supportive comments about ways to deal with symptoms and difficult feelings.

Interviewing an adolescent (ages 13 to 18) can be more challenging with regard to building an alliance. In general, it is best to allow some time to interview adolescents without the parents or guardians present in order to provide a space to discuss uncomfortable or sensitive topics and to ensure that their voices are heard. Some adolescents may be reluctant to talk while others may express their emotions more intensely. Some adolescents may give an incomplete or distorted history, making collateral information from other family members essential. In general, it is helpful to approach the adolescent in a patient, easy-going manner. The consultant can build an alliance by providing a structure to the encounter, such as: informing the patient how long the interview might be, providing a thorough explanation and reason for referral, clarifying the limits and expectations of the interview, addressing confidentiality and its limits, and presenting the consultant as someone on the medical team here to help figure out more ways to help the patient. With the frame set, adolescents are able to feel more in control of the encounter, which may facilitate their engagement in the interview. The consultant should also clarify with the patient what he or she understands about the patient's medical condition, and allow the patient to provide an explanation from his or her point of view.

Some adolescents may be reluctant to engage or shrug their shoulders in response to questions. It is important to recognize that their silence may represent anxiety and vulnerability, rather than disinterest. It may be helpful to initiate the conversation with some safe topics, such as a sporting event, television show, or question about a photo or other belonging in the hospital room. Making empathic statements that address common expected issues, such as anxiety and the shocking novelty of being sick in the hospital, may also help facilitate more sharing.

The role of the family interview as the initial interview for the assessment of a child is somewhat controversial. Many clinicians believe that a family evaluation is essential to understanding a child, but that the timing of the family assessment may vary. A family evaluation is necessary in certain disorders, specifically somatic symptom and related disorders, feeding and eating disorders,[16] school phobia, and recurrent abdominal pain, in which family interaction may precipitate or maintain the symptoms.[17] In the pediatric intensive care unit, family evaluation sessions are routinely conducted when: the response to the child's hospitalization is inappropriate (either excessive or severely constricted); there is a history of psychiatric illness in family members; there is a question of maltreatment; or there is a question of whether the family is able to comprehend the clinical information adequately.[9] For other families, the assessments are less urgent.

Liaison With the Medical Team

Working With Clinical Staff

Child psychiatric consultation usually involves contact with more individuals than the patient and the referring physician. Parents are inherently a part of treatment as they give critical information and need to be actively involved in implementation of recommendations. During a hospitalization, nurses may assume some parental roles while the pediatric unit is the child's temporary home. Child and family behaviors have an impact on other patients and staff, and are likely to evoke intense feelings. Because many pediatric units encourage parental visitation and rooming-in, the potential impact of a distraught or disturbed parent on the entire floor is substantial. Lastly, patients with chronic illness may return repeatedly to the same floor over a 5- to 10-year period. Thus, many children become well known, and the depth of the staff's involvement grows over the years. Child psychiatric consultation includes an essential liaison role that is relevant to patient and family care, to inter-staff tensions, and to individual staff stress.

The model of primary nursing encourages continuity of care as one or two nurses are assigned to the child during the hospitalization, and often for repeated admissions as well. This practice is beneficial for the child's sense of trust, makes the nurse's role more personally satisfying, and can add a needed perspective if too many sub-specialists forget the child's needs. Unavoidably, primary nurses often become intensely involved in the child's personal and family life; thus, they have critical information and share the stress of the child's illness. The child psychiatrist can provide suggestions and supervision for dealing with difficult families or crises, review when psychiatric referral is indicated, and help in understanding the painful issues of chronic disease, suicide, and terminal illness.

For house staff, a common stressor is being relatively inexperienced and yet forced to deal with complex medical and psychological circumstances. This source of stress is clearest in the intensive care unit, where frustration mounts rapidly as children do not respond to treatment and can suffer life-long physical and neurologic damage. The consequences of multiple stressors (frustration with the patient's course, lack of sleep, and feeling incompetent) may lead to depression, substance abuse, or bitter tensions among house staff or nurses.

Part of the child psychiatrist's liaison function is to attend rounds, be aware of difficult clinical and family situations, get to know nurses and house staff through teaching and informal discussion concerning patients, and be aware of the early signs of behavior that are destructive to patient care and staff. With sufficient credibility, the child psychiatric consultant can organize family or multidisciplinary staff meetings that have a beneficial impact on the unit's functioning, and can relieve family or staff suffering.

Developmental and Family-Centered Approach to Consultation

In assessing a hospitalized child, the consultant must appreciate how the child's current presentation is understood in the context of his or her previous level of functioning and behavior, as well as in relation to other children in the same developmental phase. The consultant uses a developmental perspective, informed by collateral data regarding temperament, pre-morbid personality, and the family's functioning to evaluate the child's behavior, emotional state, and defensive style.

Knowledge of defense mechanisms provides insight into how children and their families cope with illness and hospitalization. In general, greater maturity of a child's defensive style helps when coping with anxiety; however, defensive patterns are complex. Defenses (including denial, isolation of affect, and intellectualization) help with modulation of anxiety.[10] For example, a teenager with cystic fibrosis may use isolation of affect and intellectualization when discussing what is needed for lung transplantation. An example of effective denial is the 10-year-old child with terminal cancer who is invested in completing his schoolwork and getting promoted to the 5th grade; this can maintain a sense of hope and future orientation, which can preserve day-to-day functioning. Use of an array of defenses that permits adherence with one's health care and facilitates investment in age-appropriate activities should be supported. Denial, when used by a withdrawn child, can mask psychopathology and prevent referral.[18]

Infancy

For the hospitalized infant, the key developmental challenge is to maintain the quality of the attachment between parent and child. The parental component of attachment begins while anticipating the infant's birth or adoption. An infant is a parent's most personal product, embodying the hopes that the child will ultimately possess the strengths and values the parent most values in himself or herself, and the wish that the child will have capacities that offset the parent's self-perceived deficiencies. No infant can meet all of the parents' conscious and unconscious expectations, yet most infants are accepted and loved when they enter the world. Parents adapt to the reality of the infant and embark on the life-long process of attachment that enables child and parent to weather the stresses and strains of caretaking and growing up while remaining committed and connected.

Parents with affective illness (including post-partum depression), anxiety disorders, psychotic disorders, character pathology, or intense guilt may have difficulty achieving the attunement that is necessary for attachment. The psychiatric consultant may be called on to differentiate between depression, character pathology, or anxious adjustment in the setting of inadequate parental attachment. Infants with medical conditions that interfere with feeding, limit access to holding and soothing, affect appearance, or cause irritability, present special challenges to the process of attachment. Ill infants require parents to be more mature because the unexpected circumstances may leave a parent feeling incompetent or unloved by the newborn. The medical staff can play a crucial role in successfully supporting new parents through this difficult early phase.

Infants and toddlers are largely non-verbal, and rely on a small, consistent number of caretakers who know them well enough to be attuned to their non-verbal communications. Therefore, the infant's experience of the stress of hospitalization is exacerbated by separations from the mother or primary caretaker. Bowlby's classic work on attachment[19] described the three phases of separation anxiety seen in infants:

1. *Protest*: The infant acutely, vigorously, loudly, and thrashingly attempts to prevent departure of the mother or rapidly attempts to recapture her. In the older child, this phase may appear as clinging, nagging, or bargaining as a parent is about to leave.
2. *Despair*: The infant is less active, may cry in a monotone with less vigor, begins to withdraw, and appears hopeless. Sometimes the withdrawal phase is mistakenly seen as a good adjustment because the infant is quieter.
3. *Detachment*: The infant seems more alert and accepting of nursing care. These new attachments are superficial, however, and the infant concomitantly shows a loss of affect or positive feeling when the mother appears. With chronic disease that requires numerous prolonged hospitalizations, the infant or young child may make many brief, inconsistent attachments and suffer numerous losses if the primary caretaker is regularly absent and many different surrogate caretakers interact with the infant. Spitz[20] referred to the overwhelmed infant's state as *hospitalism*.

Antecedents of Bowlby's more pronounced phases of separation occurring over minutes when a mother is unresponsive to her infant's attempts at relating have been found. In response to these findings of short-term and long-term consequences of maternal separations, hospitals encourage mothers to stay overnight with children and to participate in their child's care. In addition, nursing departments have instituted a primary nursing model to limit the number of nurses who care for each child.

Pre-School Age

Medical conditions in the pre-school phase (ages 3 to 6 years) are affected by three important aspects of the child's emotional and cognitive development: egocentricity, magical thinking, and body image anxiety. Egocentricity is the child's perception that all life events revolve around him or her. The child cannot imagine that others see the world from a vantage point different from his or her own. Magical thinking is the creative weaving of reality and fantasy to explain how things occur in the world. The combination of egocentricity and magical thinking may lead the pre-school-aged child to imagine that medical conditions are punishment for the child's own bad thoughts or deeds. For example, a 4-year-old with leukemia reported he got his "bad cells" from eating too many cookies. The young child needs ongoing support from family and medical staff to understand that the medical condition is not punishment or secondary to some unrelated experience. Without this support, the child's anxiety is likely to be much greater and be expressed as inhibition and withdrawal, or as behavioral outbursts. One understanding of the cause of body image anxiety comes from the pre-schooler's cognitive development, which leads the child to envision the body as a shell (skin) filled with blood, food, and stool, which could ooze out of any hole in the skin. This concept of the body being like a tire or water balloon that can be punctured with dire results may explain the preoccupation with bandages at this age, as well as fear of needle sticks and surgical procedures that seem to exceed what can be explained by painful experiences alone.

Some regression is to be expected in the stressed pre-schooler.[18] This may take the form of enuresis in a previously toilet-trained child, increased dependence on parents for help with dressing or eating, and episodes of unwillingness to use words to express wishes or use of baby talk. Each of these regressed behaviors serves to engage parents and nursing staff in a style of caretaking that may be more commonly associated with a baby or toddler.

Treatment approaches can assist the pre-schooler with adjustment to medical illnesses and interventions and can minimize regression. Pain should be controlled or eliminated whenever possible, even when it is not the fastest way to proceed. Procedures should be explained in simple terms to the child. The child needs to hear in the most basic terms what will be done, why it is needed, and what parts will be uncomfortable or painful. They will want to know where their parents will be before, during, and after the procedure. Interventions should be performed in designated locations, such as treatment rooms, and there should be safety zones, usually the child's hospital room and the playroom, in which no procedures are done. It is crucial for children of all ages to have safe places within the hospital setting, so that they are not on "high alert" at all times. Similarly, warning children about impending procedures may lead to protest acutely, but over time allows children to relax and not be constantly anticipating an unpleasant "surprise attack."

School Age

School age (6 to 12 years), also referred to as latency, is characterized by a host of new and developing skills in many arenas—academic, athletic, and artistic. The world outside the family becomes more important with the advent of best friends and status in friendship or interest groups. In the context of medical illness, the age-appropriate investment in mastery of skills may lead to improved coping with a better understanding of medical illnesses (although still rudimentary), pride in learning to anticipate regular treatments, medications, and procedures, better capacity to verbalize needs, and establishment of relationships with nursing staff and physicians. Children with pre-morbid competencies may weather the stress of illness somewhat better than their less capable peers. The stress of medical conditions, however, routinely leads to regression in all age-groups, so the improved coping skills of latency may not be observed in the hospital setting. Regression is common early in a chronic illness, with the potential for developing better coping after there has been time for adjustment. The level of function fluctuates according to the individual stressors (e.g., mood, malaise, pain, procedures, and prognostic changes) and family function. Offering age-appropriate activities (such as board games, video games, computers, puzzles, arts and crafts), and school tutors, helps children to function closer to their pre-morbid level and serves as a counterweight to the regressive pull of dependency, helplessness, and loss of control that often accompanies hospitalization. Later in a chronic illness, flexible denial can be a healthy component of coping. Flexible denial denotes the child's ability to suppress thoughts about the illness and invest in an array of activities, without abandoning the appropriate measures necessary for treatment of the illness.

It is common for latency-age and older children to have distorted or magical notions of the cause of the illness, which are typical of the thinking of younger children. It is helpful to invite all questions—by saying things like "I like to hear what children wonder about" or "There is no such thing as a silly question"—and invite fantasies about the medical condition by direct questions such as "What do you think might have caused your cancer?" Some children may be uncomfortable expressing themselves in a direct dialogue but may be willing to draw a picture of their cancer or to write a story about a child with an illness. Any outlet for expression can be helpful to elucidate the fears that underlie the child's anxiety.

In chronic illness, the latency-age years offer a less conflicted opportunity to foster positive health-related behaviors. The child should be able to give a simple, accurate explanation of the illness. The child should be learning the names of medications, their purpose, and when they are to be taken. At this age, a partially independent relationship between the child and the treating physician can be developed. Psychiatric intervention is warranted if the child is resistant to learning about the illness, if the child is regressed, if parents are noted to be intrusive or over-involved in the health care regimen, or if non-adherence to the medical treatment plan has become a means of fighting between child and parent. Allowing these patterns to proceed into adolescence will likely increase the risk of dysfunction and make intervention more difficult.

Adolescence

The adolescent, similar to an adult, enters the medical setting with the capacity to understand the meaning of an illness, including its possible ramifications. Developmentally, adolescents venture out with a more independent posture and leave behind the intense dependency on parents that is seen in younger children. This brings with it a particular sensitivity and vulnerability. The multiple demands of hospitalization (including deciphering the meaning of diagnoses and treatments while bearing the physical discomfort, limitations, pain, impact on appearance, and fears about the present and future) may overwhelm the adolescent's ability to exercise newly acquired independence in a developmentally appropriate way. The physical limitations imposed by illness may put adolescents at risk for major depression, especially when the illness interferes with activities that are key to the adolescent's emerging self-image.[21]

The assault on the teenager's autonomy may be particularly difficult to bear because it coincides with the strong developmental pull to individuate from parents and to establish an independent identity. Often the illness occurs at a time when other tensions between the adolescent and parent make relying on the parents uncomfortable or unacceptable. Faced with this emotionally complex dilemma, some teens become sullen, aggressive, non-adherent, or withdrawn, whereas others are able to negotiate the discomfort of returning to a more dependent, supportive relationship with parents.

Interview styles should respect the adolescent's wish for autonomy. One should engage the adolescent first before looking to the parents for their input. Adolescents should also be offered private time to share information that may not be easily shared in the company of parents. Sexual experiences or concerns and worries about parental coping or even death may not be voiced without privacy. The risks and benefits of treatments need to be presented to the adolescent with the recognition that his or her adherence is central to the success or failure of any treatment plan.

Family-Centered Care

In recent years, the concept of "family-centered care" has emerged as a care philosophy that highly values effective collaboration among patients, families, and healthcare providers, and promotes principles and practices that improve this collaboration.[22] It can be helpful to use this term when communicating with pediatric healthcare providers, who may be less accustomed than child psychiatrists to thinking about the family in a systemic manner, in order to share a common language about the need to include families in psychiatric assessments and treatment planning.

The child cannot be understood separately from the family. Serious or chronic illness in a child is a family crisis. The parents must cope with the uncertainty and the highs and lows associated with hospitalization. Abnormal laboratory results, adverse reactions, life-threatening crises, limitations on the child's future, and the specter of death suddenly become their reality. They observe their child in distress and they often feel fundamentally unable to protect the child. The hospital environment brings with it a host of medical professionals with as many personalities as there are consultants and caregivers; often, each seems to hold a crucial piece of the puzzle. Small nuances in the presentation of data or differing styles of optimism or pessimism among staff may radically shift the family's mood. There is rarely much privacy and sometimes none at all, whether in a shared room or in an intensive care unit.

Parental anxiety negatively affects the child's capacity to cope; to expect a parent to be other than anxious is unthinkable.[23,24] Parents are the child's most trusted and valuable resource; therefore, strategies to support the parents are crucial. Most parents evoke staff empathy and appreciate the skill and compassion of the treatment team. Certain parents are particularly challenging to support because of a particular combination of personality characteristics and coping style. Their distress, often fueled by a sense of helplessness, may be expressed either as devaluing staff or as apparent insensitivity to the sick child's needs. The consultant helps the team of caregivers understand the psychological meaning of the parents' troubling behavior so that they can continue to provide optimal care.[22,25]

Siblings are often the forgotten sufferers in the context of chronic or life-threatening illness.[26,27] They not only have worries about the sick sibling, but often they also lose the support of their parents. The parents may be physically absent, spending time at the hospital with the ill child and attempting to meet at least minimal work demands to support the family financially. They are often emotionally absent, depressed, or drained by the emotional demands of the sick child. Many parents feel angry at the well siblings for making any demands and for not selflessly understanding the seriousness of the ill child's predicament. This compounds the well siblings' guilt at the expectable feelings of resentment and jealousy toward the ill child who is receiving so much attention and so many gifts. If the illness results in death, the feelings of guilt and responsibility may become overwhelming.

Family interviews may aid in the assessment of the physically ill child and help the consultant target areas in the family system that may benefit from support. Families of ill children need to express their feelings about hospitalization and to obtain emotional support. Siblings often have distorted concepts of the child's illness that need to be corrected. A carefully planned family meeting can begin to clarify distortions, reduce family turmoil, improve coping skills, and dispel conflict between family and staff. During the meeting, the staff or the psychiatrist should evaluate the family's psychological state, including an assessment of coping mechanisms, anxiety level, available support, and ability to comprehend information.

REASONS FOR CONSULTATION REQUESTS

The child psychiatry consult practice pattern study by Shaw and associates[4] listed the most common reasons for consultation requests as: (1) suicide assessment (78.5% of survey responders indicated this as a common consult question); (2) differential diagnosis for medically unexplained symptoms (72.3%); (3) adjustment to illness, including depression and anxiety (58.5% and 55.4%, respectively); (4) psychotropic medication evaluation (49.2%); (5) delirium (29.2%); (6) treatment non-adherence (24.6%); and (7) management of psychiatric patients boarding on medical floors (23.1%).[4] The common reasons for child psychiatric consultation have remained consistent over time with the only addition being management of psychiatric patients boarding on medical floors that had not previously been listed. Consultants can also be called on to address behavioral difficulties that contribute to hospitalization, behavioral difficulties during hospitalization that compromise optimal medical care, child maltreatment in the form of physical or sexual abuse or medical neglect, and children and families who must cope with life-threatening or chronic illness.[4]

Primary Psychiatric Illnesses

Depression

Depression is a common disorder in hospitalized children. It may be a secondary response to acute or chronic illness, or it may be the primary diagnosis and present with somatic symptoms or behavioral problems. One of the obstacles to making the diagnosis of depression in the hospitalized child is the misconception that the child's dysphoric mood is appropriate to the stress of the situation and therefore does not deserve to be called depression. On the contrary, stress increases the likelihood that depression will occur; it does not invalidate the diagnosis.

Depression may be used to refer to a mood, symptom, or a syndrome. As a syndrome, depression in childhood is characterized by a persistent mood disorder and/or dysfunctional behavior, and, in older children, by self-deprecatory ideation. These symptoms or behaviors should represent a significant change in the child's pre-morbid function and not be a long-standing temperamental trait. The *Diagnostic and Statistical Manual of Mental Disorders*, 5th edition[28] (DSM-5), characterizes a major depressive episode as 2 weeks or more of persistent depressed or irritable mood and/or loss of interest in all or almost all activities, along with at least four additional associated symptoms.

Although the criteria are the same for children and adults, there are some clinical differences in how the symptoms manifest. For children younger than 6 years of age, the hallmarks of depression can include poor appetite or failure to grow and gain weight appropriately, disturbance of sleep, hypoactivity, and indifference to the surroundings and to primary caretakers.[29] Pre-pubertal children with an episode of major depression can present with separation anxiety, somatic complaints, irritability, or behavior problems.[30] These children may not give an accurate self-assessment of sustained mood, so dysphoria must be observed by caretakers over a prolonged period. Making the diagnosis of depression can be difficult in children who are sick because many of the symptoms they exhibit (e.g., decreased energy or loss of appetite) may be attributed to their medical illness.[31] Also, children who are sick can use denial as a coping mechanism and under-report their symptoms.[32]

Treatment of depression often involves psychotherapy, as well as child-life and recreational therapy, to support the child and family; sometimes therapy is used in conjunction with antidepressant medications. In a 2015 review and meta-analysis, Varigonda and colleagues[33] found that selective serotonin re-uptake inhibitor (SSRI) treatment gains for pediatric depression were greatest early in treatment, and overall the SSRI effect was smaller in children and adolescents compared to adults. Historically, there has been significant attention to the question of whether antidepressant treatment increases the likelihood of suicidal ideation in children and adolescents. In October 2004, the Food and Drug Administration (FDA) issued a "black-box warning" related to this concern, although, since then, there has been significant controversy in the research literature about the need for and impact of this warning.[34] Regardless, this concern should be addressed in discussions with patients and families as part of the discussion about the risks and benefits of pharmacotherapy. (See Chapter 39 for further discussion of the use of psychopharmacologic agents in children.)

Suicide

Suicide is the second leading cause of death among adolescents and young adults aged 10–25 years in the United States, accounting for nearly 17% of all deaths in this age group; furthermore, the frequency of suicide in this age group appears to be on the rise.[29] Suffocation is the most common means of completed suicide for children ages 10–14 years (52.9% of completed suicides), followed by use of firearms (40.9%).[29] For those between the ages of 15 and 24, the most common means switches to firearms (44.7% of completed suicides), followed by suffocation (39.6%).[29] In most cases, children who have made a suicide attempt must remain in the hospital or another secure facility until a thorough evaluation is completed and appropriate disposition is decided. This may occur via admission to the pediatric service, in conjunction with crisis intervention services in the Emergency Department, or in some cases by transfer directly to a psychiatric facility.

During the assessment of a potentially suicidal child, one should:

1. Gather details of the suicide attempt, including access to potentially lethal means (e.g., firearms, pills, a rope).
2. Assess the risk of an attempt—What did the child imagine would happen? What was the likelihood of rescue?
3. Determine the child's mind-set at the time of the attempt—Was there a clear precipitant? Was it an impulsive or a planned act? What prompted the attempt on that specific day?
4. Obtain a history of any suicide attempts in the patient, family members, or peers.
5. Pursue the child's understanding of death and fantasy of what his or her death would elicit in the family or other significant person (such as a boyfriend or girlfriend).
6. Ask about the child's feelings of remorse about the attempt or regrets about having survived.
7. Assess whether the child expresses feelings of hopelessness, helplessness, or despair.
8. Assess whether sexual orientation and/or gender identity are relevant issues, including familial or peer rejection, societal discrimination, bullying, or abuse.[35,36]
9. Assess how their racial or ethnic identity fits into the context of their community, and the extent of marginalization and vulnerability as a result of their minority status.
10. Assess whether the child is lonely or emotionally disconnected from others.
11. Determine whether the child used drugs or alcohol at the time of the attempt.
12. Determine whether the child is depressed, manic, or psychotic.

13. Determine whether the child identifies with someone who has committed suicide.
14. Assess the probability of physical or sexual maltreatment.
15. Conduct a family interview. Determine whether the parents are sad and frightened by the attempt or angry at the child for being manipulative.
16. Learn about therapeutic interventions that have been tried in the past. What is in place currently, and how good has adherence been with outpatient treatment?

Family issues (including a family history of depression, whether a family is modeling suicide, intra-familial tension, and real or imagined rejection of the suicidal child by the parents) should be assessed. If maltreatment is suspected, the appropriate child protective services agency must be contacted.

The consultant is initially asked to decide on the appropriate safety management for the suicidal child. This may include one or more of the following: one-to-one supervision, restrictions on movements around the unit or hospital, restrictions on access to potentially harmful objects, such as sharp objects or ligature (which may require a search of the belongings to which the patient has access in the hospital), strategies for managing potential agitation, and the presence of or separation from the parents. Ultimately the consultant needs to perform a thorough risk assessment and determine whether the child or adolescent should be hospitalized psychiatrically or managed as an outpatient (while either living at home or in another setting). Indications for psychiatric hospitalization may include: serious risk of death through suicide; little wish to be rescued; psychosis, identification with someone who has committed suicide; co-morbid drug or alcohol abuse; intense feelings of hopelessness and helplessness; intense anger or severe depression; lack of support systems; history of inability to use help; and vulnerability to further losses. Appropriate outpatient or day treatment will be required if the patient is not transferred to a psychiatric facility. In this case it is important to educate and engage the patient and his or her family in safety planning. This includes developing a plan for dealing with a crisis (such as contact information for treaters and access to hotlines), directing attention to limiting availability of lethal means of suicide, such as guns and medications (including over-the-counter medications such as acetaminophen), and emphasizing the need for vigilance about likely environmental contributors to suicidal behavior (such as substances and psychosocial stress).

Feeding and Eating Disorders

Anorexia nervosa (AN) is an illness characterized by significantly low weight in the context of a fear for gaining weight and/or a distorted perception of the thin body as fat. Amenorrhea is also a symptom of AN in post-menarche females, however, it is no longer a criteria for diagnosis in the DSM-5.[28] Onset of AN is typically in mid-to-late adolescence (14–18 years) and it is predominantly seen in females;[28] it may be associated with a stressful life event. Hospitalization of afflicted children is usually associated with severe weight loss, cardiovascular abnormalities (usually bradycardia), hypothermia, or electrolyte imbalance. The last-mentioned feature may reflect binging or purging, which can include vomiting or abuse of laxatives or diuretics. The goal of pediatric hospitalization is medical stabilization; additional interventions in the hospital are nutritional assessment and treatment, psychological assessment of the child and family, and recommendations for appropriate levels of psychiatric intervention after medical stabilization.[37] The assessment as to whether or not medical stabilization must be followed by intensive day or inpatient psychiatric treatment includes determination of the adolescent's recognition that he or she has a problem with eating behavior and self-image, the adolescent's motivation to participate in treatment (e.g., is he or she in denial about the eating disorder and resistant to eating the adequate nutrition presented in the hospital diet), and the parents' ability to support the adolescent and the need for psychotherapy (e.g., are they angry, intrusive, or controlling of the teen, or do they want to deny that the eating disorder is a problem?).

The DSM-5 introduced a new diagnosis related to disordered eating, Avoidant/Restrictive Food Intake Disorder (ARFID).[28] ARFID is characterized by an eating or feeding disturbance that leads to significant weight loss, nutritional deficiency, dependence on enteral feeding or oral nutritional supplements, and/or a significant impact to psychosocial functioning. Unlike AN, ARFID is not associated with body image distortion. Clinically, ARFID is seen in children who have a fear of aversive consequences (e.g., choking, vomiting), lack of interest in food or eating, or severe food selectivity due to sensory sensitivities. It is important to note that ARFID is intended to describe patients who are malnourished and medically fragile, not children who are simply "picky eaters" but otherwise healthy and medically stable.

The consultant will be called upon to assist with the assessment and management of a child with eating issues as well as to give recommendations about disposition once the patient is medically stable. Placement is based on whether the child or adolescent can live at home safely while consuming adequate calories and attending outpatient treatment appointments (e.g., psychotherapy, nutrition, and pediatric visits) versus the need for a more intensive and structured program (such as a day treatment or residential eating disorder unit). Often, the consultant, in conjunction with the social worker, spends a significant amount of time helping the parents accept the plan for psychotherapeutic treatment, especially if the team recommends that the patient not return home.

Somatic Symptom and Related Disorders

Some patients present to their pediatrician with intense somatic complaints (e.g., headaches, abdominal pain, constipation, dysmenorrhea, fatigue). In general, when cases are referred for psychiatric consultation, the pediatrician suspects that the intensity or the nature of the complaints is more likely to be an expression of emotional factors than medical conditions. Somatic symptoms and related disorders, as described in DSM-5, refer to a clustering of physical symptoms suggestive of a medical condition, but the severity of the symptoms or the level of functional impairment is not fully explained by the medical condition.[28] Although the DSM-5 lists specific disorders, including somatic symptom disorder, illness anxiety disorder, and conversion disorder (functional neurologic symptom disorder), the criteria for these conditions were established for adults. Often, children do not meet full criteria for these specific diagnoses. Recurrent somatic complaints are common in the pediatric population and are a frequent reason for psychiatric consultation. There also may be developmental considerations, with pre-pubertal children most often presenting with recurrent abdominal pain or headache and older children presenting with other pain and neurologic symptoms.[38]

The pediatrician's assessment, that symptoms are emotional in origin, is often at odds with the patient's and the parents' assessment. In psychosomatic illness, the child and family may be highly invested in a medical cause to explain the somatic complaints. They are not reassured by routine medical work-ups and they may pressure the physician to continue to search for a medical cause. Although the families of somatizing children have been found to have higher rates of anxiety and depression and to be more dysfunctional than other families,[39] they are typically resistant to undergoing psychiatric assessment. Parents may view any suggestion of the important role of psychological factors as an insult and as an indication that the clinician does not believe that the symptoms are real. These families prefer to have the child x-rayed and endoscoped for abdominal pain, rather than to discuss stressors, such as the child's increasing difficulty at school, the death of a grandparent, or parental discord. Often the child and parents focus on minimally abnormal test results and pressure the physician to pursue these findings. They may connect a series of irrelevant bits of data to create a medical theory that is not endorsed by the pediatrician. Commonly, families seek multiple specialists in an attempt to find someone who will support their medical theory. Unfortunately, if the parents search long enough, they will find either a specialist who will ignore the psychological factors and validate the parents' perspective or a more junior clinician who lacks the clinical experience to stop the "rule-out approach." If the psychological issues are not attended to, the condition is likely to become chronic and result in significant morbidity.

The presenting somatic symptoms serve as a solution, albeit a maladaptive one, to an emotional dilemma. For example, it may be easier for a child to get his recently divorced mother to focus on his needs by vomiting and by complaining of relentless abdominal pain than by articulating his deep sadness at his father's absence. Moreover, it may be easier for the mother to champion the cause of discovering a medical cause for her child's vomiting than to support and acknowledge the child's level of distress about the divorce.

The psychiatric consultant is well positioned to advocate for a balance of attention to medical and psychological factors in the consideration of somatization. This includes keeping in mind that it is not necessary to make the entire diagnosis the first day, week, or month, despite the wishes of the family. Restraint is called for in the pursuit of equivocal organic findings, without sacrificing a complete and appropriate medical work-up. It is often helpful to minimize the importance of a final diagnosis and instead to focus on reducing dysfunction.

Campo and Fritz[40] have proposed a method for assessing and managing pediatric somatization that includes the key elements in the assessment: acknowledgment of patient suffering and family concerns, exploration of prior assessment and treatment experiences, investigation of patient and family fears provoked by the symptoms, maintenance of alertness to the possibility that unrecognized physical disease and communications are at play, avoidance of unnecessary tests and procedures, avoidance of diagnosis by exclusion, and exploration of symptom timing, context, and characteristics. Mainstays of management include honesty, reassurance, emphasis of the rehabilitative approach (as opposed to the curative approach) to symptoms, consideration of family and group interventions in addition to individual management, and consolidation of care.

Therapeutic interventions for the somatizing patient include a medical–psychiatric team approach that emphasizes a consistent relationship between the clinicians, the child, and family. It is important to foster the continued presence of the pediatrician, because there may be a tendency for the pediatrician to withdraw after psychiatric referral has been made. If the family believes the presence of the psychiatrist leads to diminished access to the pediatrician, there may be escalating anxiety about physical symptoms, and it becomes difficult for the psychiatrist to maintain the critical alliance with the family. Pediatric re-examination without re-testing helps calm the family's medical anxiety and reduces the likelihood of continued doctor-shopping. Ongoing psychoeducation from team members can help the family re-frame the medical symptoms and enhance communication with caregivers. Inpatient pediatric rehabilitation sometimes may be necessary to address the physical components of the presentation and allow the child to regain strength and function in a supportive environment.

Often the child and family need different forms of psychotherapy to allow the child to let go of somatic symptoms and to move on to a healthy role. The child's medical symptoms frequently serve to stabilize the family system; therefore, family therapy may be required to change patterns of interactions. Couples therapy may also be used to help parents strengthen their adult relationship, so the child's illness is not needed to hold the couple together or to distract them from their discord. A child's individual therapy helps to build self-esteem, and allows the child to engage in developmentally appropriate activities that can increase his or her sense of agency or mastery, which leads to greater confidence and less need to rely on the sick role. Co-morbid psychiatric disorders in the child or family members must also be identified and treated appropriately, with the use of pharmacological agents as needed.

Psychiatric Factors That Affect Medical Illness

Medical illness and psychiatric illness are frequently co-morbid. Studies have shown higher rates of mental health problems in youth with a variety of chronic medical illness,[40,41] such as asthma,[42–44] diabetes,[45,46] epilepsy,[47–49] and inflammatory bowel disease.[50–53] In addition to the impact of illness-related symptoms and impairments on psychological function, complex interactions can arise between psychiatric factors and the symptoms, severity, complications, and even treatment of a medical illness.

In patients with type I diabetes, depression is associated with poorer glycemic control,[54] retinopathy,[55] and need for hospitalization.[56,57] Moreover, previous research had suggested type I diabetes was associated with significantly worse psychosocial and mental health issues. However, a 2014 Norwegian study suggests that adolescents with type I diabetes do not have significantly higher psychiatric co-morbidities, perhaps due to improvement in medical technology.[58]

For children with asthma, maternal anxiety and depression have both been associated with an increased risk of children developing asthma,[41] and 5-year-old children with more severe and persistent asthma were more likely to have anxiety, affective, somatic, and oppositional behavioral issues from ages 5 to 17.[42] In adolescents with asthma, there is an association between the severity of anxiety and depressive disorders and asthma symptom burden.[59]

Children with epilepsy have high rates of psychiatric co-morbidity, including anxiety disorders, affective disorders, and ADHD, with estimates ranging from 37% to 77%.[47,48] Children with symptomatic epilepsy and severe epilepsy syndromes also have high rates of global developmental delay and autism spectrum disorder; furthermore, the co-occurrence of intellectual disability in children with epilepsy predicts increased behavioral problems.[48,60]

In children and adolescents with inflammatory bowel disease, depression, and anxiety have been well documented as common co-morbidities.[51–53] Both disease-related inflammation and steroid treatment have been thought to affect the presence and expression of psychiatric symptoms, posing additional challenges to the detection and treatment of psychiatric illness.[51,52] Cognitive-behavioral therapy (CBT) has been proposed as a potential intervention to help target depression and to reduce gastrointestinal symptoms.[61]

Patients and families who have experienced stressful fear and helplessness in the course of life-threatening pediatric illness and treatment may develop post-traumatic symptoms of intrusive thoughts, hyperarousal, and avoidance.[62] Future medical care can then be complicated by post-traumatic symptoms that have been triggered by the medical setting.

Pediatricians rely on parental report in young children and self-report in older children to assess the need for intervention in many chronic conditions. When anxiety, dysphoria, emotional lability, or apathy are present, this increased distress often leads to a greater degree of medical interventions. In a study of asthmatics, steroid prescription was correlated with patients' expressed anxiety about an exacerbation and not with the degree of change on pulmonary function tests.[63] Follow-up studies have categorized this expressed anxiety as "dysfunctional breathing," and cautioned medical providers to distinguish between the two.[64,65] Apathy or dysphoria in a patient with severe lung disease (e.g., cystic fibrosis), can lead to less therapeutic coughing and to significant pulmonary compromise. Apathy as a result of frustration or helplessness in a child undergoing rehabilitation after a cerebrovascular accident (CVA) or car accident may interfere with physical therapy. Motivation is often a function of mood, and it is an essential feature of the sense of mastery and agency that we associate with striving toward maximal health. To help children become invested in their own best level of function, it is necessary to understand the emotional issues that impede the health-seeking process.

To understand the psychiatric factors involved in coping one should:

1. Ask the child what aspects of the illness and treatments are most difficult or frightening for him or her.
2. Invite the child to describe his or her own treatment goals and any disappointments experienced while reaching those goals.
3. Pursue the child's experience of how the illness and treatment affect his or her life outside of the hospital.
4. Learn whether the child feels that someone understands what it is like to be him or her.
5. Find out whether there is someone the child is particularly disappointed in for not understanding. Has the child felt deceived by anyone?
6. Determine whether the child knows someone with this condition, and how that person's condition has evolved and why.
7. Know the condition and its evolution.
8. Learn about what is the worst thing that could happen from the patient's point of view.

The goals of the physicians are sometimes at odds with the goals of the child. For example, a teenage girl who suffered a stroke but did not want to walk "like an old lady" with a cane, was sullen in rehabilitation because she did not want to give up her crutches. The many disappointments during hospitalization and unexpected re-hospitalizations are compounded when a patient feels that his opinion was not sought or her best efforts still resulted in setbacks, and can lead to anger, frustration, mistrust, anxiety, or apathy.[66,67] Engaging the child in voicing his or her experience may be therapeutic in itself. There may be ways of altering the hospital protocols to suit the child or adapting the child's treatment program to accommodate home-life priorities. The consultant is asked to assist the child during the hospital stay and to determine whether outpatient psychotherapy is warranted. Knowing how time is spent outside of the hospital and what the content of the frustrations covers informs this decision. Psychopharmacologic interventions may also be helpful, depending on the symptoms and the psychiatric diagnoses.

Behavioral Factors That Affect Health Outcomes

Accidents and non-adherence are the two major categories of behavioral difficulties that lead to the hospitalization of children. Accidents are a leading cause of pediatric Emergency Department (ED) visits and childhood deaths. It is not uncommon to find multiple accident-related ED visits for the same child; therefore, identifying the accident-prone child and gaining a better understanding of the causes of accidents may serve to prevent future and possibly more disabling injuries. Medical non-adherence is pervasive, but it runs along a spectrum from being benign to life-threatening. As a result, there are many cases of non-adherence (such as an incomplete course of antibiotics for an ear infection) that go undetected; other cases of non-adherence can lead to death (such as a diabetic teen who skips his or her insulin and embarks on a drinking binge).

Accidents

Unintentional injury remains the number one cause of death across all children and young adults.[29] All children experience accidents, but they are more likely to occur in children who are reckless, active, impulsive, or inadequately supervised. Predisposing conditions include ADHD, fetal alcohol syndrome, and lead exposure. Adolescents tend to view themselves as invulnerable and therefore may be prone to greater risk-taking and to accidents. It is necessary to gather the following information about the child's behavior before the accident:

1. Has the child had behavioral difficulty in school, at home, or with peers?
2. Has there been a change in the child's mood?
3. Is there evidence of a thought disorder?
4. Have there been problems leading to legal interventions?
5. Are these worrisome behaviors new or are they longstanding?

Supervision, particularly in younger children, plays a significant role in maintenance of child safety. When a child presents with an accidental injury, an assessment must be made as to whether the supervision has been adequate for the child's age; this usually involves an assessment of the parents or other caretakers. It is necessary to entertain the possibility that an accidental injury could be the result of maltreatment, a suicide attempt, or an act of intentional self-injury. These causes should be part of the clinician's routine consideration for an injured child.

Non-Adherence

Non-adherence may be secondary to an inadequate understanding of, or capacity to implement, the intended medical regimen. Often non-adherence is not an active decision to defy treatment recommendations. Instead, it may result from the patient being overwhelmed by a medical regimen or being tired of the chronicity of one. Some children leave the hospital on numerous medications that are to be administered several times each day. It is crucial for the pediatrician to review the medications with the family before planned discharge. Simplifying medication regimens as much as possible and having honest dialogues with parents and children about what is realistic at home is recommended. Highlighting critical medications and the consequences of not taking them engages the child and family as educated and informed collaborators in the child's health care.

Patients and families who are refractory to simple educational interventions to improve adherence may benefit from a more intensive intervention to address the issue, and the medical team may seek the consultant's input. Kahana et al.'s[68] meta-analysis evaluated how effective psychological interventions were in promoting adherence in pediatric chronic illness. They concluded that adherence was most likely to be improved by interventions that emphasized applied behavioral methods (such as problem-solving or parent training), or multi-component interventions, usually incorporating combined behavioral and educational treatments; however, education-only interventions did not lead to improved adherence.[68] As one might expect, these psychological interventions led to brief improvements and over time the effects were lost; this suggests that adherence-focused interventions likely need ongoing recurrent attention.[68]

With the advent of computer and digital technology, there are new methods for evaluating adherence as well as providing interventions. For example, electronic monitoring has been used to help track and categorize non-adherence patterns in pediatric cancer.[69] Other technologies such as MPEG audio layer-3 players, text messaging, computer or Internet-based systems, video games, and smart phone applications have been studied as intervention possibilities in asthma and diabetes management.[70–72] In a review by Baptist and colleagues,[70] computer-based interventions (e.g., interactive games, videos) were found to help increase asthma knowledge; unfortunately, this did not directly lead to improvements in healthcare utilization or other outcome measures. As mobile and digital technology become more developed, accessible, and even wearable, more research will be needed as to how they can be used for evaluation and intervention of adherence issues.

There can be many socioeconomic, emotional, and psychodynamic issues that lead children or parents to actively or passively disregard medical recommendation. For example, socioeconomic factors, such as low maternal education, low income, and households where mothers are not full-time caregivers have been associated with decreased adherence in the pediatric cancer population.[73] Denial on the part of either the child or the parent may result in non-adherence. In this scenario, the child or caretaker has the conscious or unconscious notion that if the prescribed medication or prescribed restrictions are ignored, it is as if the illness does not exist. The clinician may hear from the child, "Taking my pills makes me feel like I am sick," or from the parent, "I cannot make myself bring him in for his doctor's appointments because sitting in the clinic reminds me he has a bad liver." Suppression of thoughts about illness can be a healthy defense, allowing medically ill children and their families to cope with the stress of the illness, but denial leading to non-adherence is maladaptive and warrants psychotherapeutic intervention to minimize serious medical consequences.

Sometimes, non-adherence is an expression of anger, be it the child's anger at the parent or the child or family's anger at the physician, or at the illness itself. When the child is angry at the parents, non-adherence is guaranteed to elicit parental distress, which can be emotionally satisfying for the child. Psychologically absent in this schema is the child's awareness that he or she is actually harming him- or herself. The consultant can assist in altering the medical relationship, from a physician-to-parent-to-child relationship toward a more direct relationship between physician and child. By diminishing the parent's role in the communication of the healthcare regimen and of policing adherence, to the extent possible depending on the child's age, the pediatrician has the opportunity to build an alliance with the child that fosters a wish to please and thus to enhance adherence.

Psychotherapy serves the function of allying with the healthy part of the child and helping the child or adolescent appreciate that this style of acting-out anger and frustration with parents is self-injurious. Similarly, when the anger being acted-out is against the illness or the physician, the psychotherapeutic goal is to ally with the healthy part of the child, helping the child articulate the frustration with words rather than by acting them out in a self-destructive way. The consultant is called on to assess what aspect of this goal can be achieved during the hospital stay and when outpatient psychotherapy is warranted. The non-adherent child may be resistant to the idea of outpatient psychotherapy. Hospitalization offers the consultant a valuable opportunity for alliance-building by letting the child experience how talking (therapy) can be helpful.

Behavioral Difficulties During Hospitalization

Some children are referred for psychiatric consultation for the management of specific behavioral symptoms that interfere with medical care or with their own safety and the safety and comfort of other patients and medical staff. Their symptoms may include excessive activity, agitation, verbal or physical threats to staff and other children, and temper tantrums. Assessment should include medical, developmental, and social history from the child and family, a neurologic examination, nursing and child-life observations, and school reports, as needed.

Psychopharmacologic interventions may also be appropriate. The child with generalized anxiety or separation anxiety may benefit from a trial of a long-acting benzodiazepine (e.g., clonazepam) and/or an antidepressant.[74] Children with anxiety in association with particular procedures may benefit from pre-medication with shorter-acting benzodiazepines (e.g., lorazepam). Anticipatory anxiety can be managed with behavioral interventions (e.g., relaxation and visualization techniques, breathing exercises, child-directed distraction, nurse-led distraction, combined cognitive-behavioral interventions), as well as with psychotropics.[74,75] When ADHD is diagnosed, the child may respond quite dramatically to the addition of stimulant medication. Occasionally an underlying psychosis may be discerned, and the appropriate antipsychotic agent should be instituted. Agitation associated with delirium may require the use of antipsychotics to maintain a child's safety and to help clear the delirium until the underlying cause can be addressed.

Behavioral plans, especially for younger children, may be instrumental in establishing good behavior. The guiding principle underlying behavioral plans is to identify the key behaviors that are most problematic and provide incentives for the child to behave in positive ways. In younger children, sticker charts for swallowing pills and allowing blood drawing without a temper tantrum, are examples of common behavioral interventions. Younger children may receive stickers as the full reward, or after receiving a pre-determined number of stickers, a child may earn a toy. Older children may work toward special privileges (such as a trip to the gift shop, time outside with the child-life specialist, or a favorite meal brought in from outside the hospital). Other incentives (such as tickets to a hockey game), may be provided by the family. In addition to behavioral plans, children benefit from having a schedule for the day. An unstructured day increases uncertainty, boredom, and anxiety. Scheduling activity times, meal times, rest times, and procedure times can be helpful in providing the child with an increased sense of control over the hospital milieu.

Behavioral plans can be especially helpful for children with autism spectrum disorder (ASD), who are medically hospitalized. At baseline, children with ASD have high rates of social anxiety and sensory difficulties and often rely on familiar routines for comfort. In the hospital, their usual routines are disrupted and many new people and interventions are introduced, which may be overwhelming. Most children with ASD have communication impairments that can interfere with their ability to express their distress or to understand the need for certain medical interventions. Behavioral outbursts, including aggression or self-injury, and anxiety are not uncommon in the hospital setting and can cause significant distress for the patient, family, other patients, and staff.

Patients with ASD can benefit from specific, individualized behavioral plans that are developed collaboratively with the family and are easily accessible for staff; for example, posted on the patient's door. Parents can provide information to the team about preferred methods of communication, known triggers, individual signs of distress or escalation, and soothing strategies that work. Occupational therapy (OT) can be helpful in providing sensory-based interventions to help reduce agitation and distress. Use of visually oriented materials, such as story boards or visual schedules, can facilitate communication and help the patient understand what is happening and prepare for procedures or other interventions. Coordination and communication with outpatient providers is helpful, as they have a longer-standing history and relationship with the patient and family. Ideally an effective behavioral plan will decrease behavioral outbursts, provide uniform care, and avoid use of unnecessary medications or use of restraints.

Parental interactions often play a major role in the child's behavior in the hospital. Some behavioral outbursts may reflect the child's anxious response to the parent's escalating anxiety and inability to help the child feel safer in the hospital setting. Some parents may find it difficult to set limits on the child, in light of the sadness the parent feels at the child's medical condition. The child's behavior may represent an unconscious need to re-engage the parent in what had been the usual style of parenting. A parent's lack of limit-setting often feels to the child like emotional abandonment. In conjunction with the social worker doing family work or parent guidance, the consultant needs to help the parent feel competent to be an active parent again.

Children with behavioral difficulties invariably arouse negative feelings in the staff. There may be disagreements between staff members about how best to respond to particular behaviors, and the inconsistencies may foster further behavioral disturbances. Team meetings to develop a consistent plan and to facilitate good communication are essential. These team meetings are a good opportunity for the consultant to share his or her understanding of the psychological meaning of the behavior in a way that helps the staff feel more empathic with the child and the family.

CHILD MALTREATMENT

Child maltreatment is defined as any act or series of acts of commission or omission by a parent or other caregiver that results in harm, potential for harm, or threat of harm to a child.[76] Acts of commission constitute child abuse, in the form of physical abuse, sexual abuse, or psychological abuse. Acts of omission constitute child neglect, including a failure to provide (physical neglect, emotional neglect, medical neglect, or educational neglect) or a failure to supervise (inadequate supervision or exposure to violent environments).[76] In general, data collected from agencies such as the National Child Abuse and Neglect Data System (NCANDS), Administration for Children and Families, and Centers for Disease Control, all overseen by the US Department of Health and Human Services, have shown a trend from 1990 to 2013 toward a significant decline in the rate of overall child maltreatment. Neglect remains the most common form of maltreatment and continues to gradually increase in proportion to other maltreatment types.[77–80] Child maltreatment rates are higher among younger children, particularly highest from ages less than 1 to 11.[78]

Since the etiologic contributions to child maltreatment are diverse, a developmental-ecological perspective has been advocated in understanding the determinants of maltreatment, in which parenting behaviors are understood to be influenced by factors across multiple levels, including parental characteristics, the characteristics of the child, and the broader context.[81–83] Maltreatment may occur in the setting of multi-generational inadequate parenting, parental stress, substance abuse, and multiple family stressors (including domestic violence, a disrupted family unit, and cognitively limited or psychiatrically ill parents).[83] Low family income[84] is a risk factor, particularly among single-parent families,[85] as well as having a child with a disability.[86] Risk factors notwithstanding, maltreatment occurs in all socioeconomic and demographic environments, demanding constant vigilance in those who work with children.

The consequences of child maltreatment, including mental health problems, can be far-reaching.[81,87,88] Psychiatry may be consulted in cases where maltreatment is suspected. In some healthcare settings, a specialized child protection team may also be available to provide consultation and coordinate care. All physicians are mandated reporters of maltreatment, but only a suspicion is required; it is not necessary to prove maltreatment to file with the appropriate state child welfare agency.

Physical Abuse and Neglect

Physical abuse is defined as the intentional use of physical force against a child that results in, or has the potential to result in, physical injury.[76] Acts constituting physical abuse can include hitting, kicking, punching, beating, stabbing, biting, pushing, shoving, throwing, pulling, dragging, dropping, shaking, strangling/choking, smothering, burning, scalding, and poisoning.[76] The incidence of child physical abuse, based on data gathered by the US Department of Health and Services, has decreased from 3.4 per 1000 in 1990 to 1.1 per 1000 in 2007; however it then rose to 1.8 per 1000 in 2008 and remained relatively the same throughout to 1.7 per 1000 in 2013.[77,78,89] Children with disabilities have been shown to be at increased risk for violence,[86] and having emotional, psychological, or learning disability is associated with more abuse.[90]

Neglect, by comparison, is the failure by a caregiver to meet a child's basic physical, emotional, medical, or educational needs.[76] These children may present with failure to thrive or other consequences of inadequate nutrition, the occurrence of preventable accidents, dermatologic conditions related to poor hygiene, lack of routine and specialized medical appointments, and school absences. The incidence of neglect maltreatment was 7.3 per 1000 in 2000, which fell to 6.1 per 1000 in 2007, peaked to 8.1 per 1000 in 2009, and fell back to 7.3 per 1000 in 2013.[78] The overall proportion of how much neglect accounts for all maltreatment causes continues to rise, from 49% in 1990, to 60% in the early 2000s, to 75% in 2014.[77,78]

Abuse and neglect must be suspected before they can be diagnosed. Certain types and locations of injuries are suspicious. Bruises that resemble finger or hand prints, and those that appear on body surfaces that normally do not bear the brunt of an accidental fall (such as welts on the back as opposed to anterior shin bruises), should raise suspicion. Multiple bruises in various stages of healing are suggestive of abuse that has been ongoing. Clinicians should be suspicious when bruises, broken bones, and accidents have occurred that are inconsistent with the caretaker's explanation, when the caretaker admits and then recants culpability, or admits having observed the abuse being perpetrated and then recants the story. The caretaker may blame the injury on the child, suggesting it was self-inflicted or blame a sibling for an injury that appears beyond the developmental capability of the child. There may have been an inexplicable delay in seeking medical attention, or the person bringing the child for medical assistance may be vague or report having not been with the child during the injury and not knowing how it happened.

When physical maltreatment is suspected, the child at risk should be kept in a safe facility until the child welfare agency has determined the safety of the child's disposition. A full physical examination should be performed and well documented, checking the whole child for evidence of bruising or injury in various stages of healing. This is important both to ensure the child's safety and because there may be subsequent legal proceedings. A radiological bone series may be indicated to look for evidence of old and new fractures. A retinal examination should be performed for evidence of traumatic shaking of a young child. Siblings of a child suspected of having been abused must be assessed immediately because they are also at high risk for abuse.

Sexual Abuse

Sexual abuse is defined as any completed or attempted sexual act, sexual contact with, or exploitation (i.e., non-contact sexual interaction) of a child by a caregiver.[76] This involves the exposure of a child to a sexual experience that is inappropriate for his or her emotional and developmental level and that is coercive in nature.[91] As with physical abuse, reported rates of sexual abuse have declined since the 1990s, with an incident of 1.2 per 1000 in 1990 to a slow graduated decrease of 0.8 per 1000 in 2013.[78–80] However, it also important to note that sexual abuse is significantly under-reported due to reasons like shame and fear, and also from many methodological difficulties with estimating the prevalence of sexual abuse; for example, differences in definitions and screening tools.[92] Incest is present when sexual contact occurs between a child and a family member, including step-family members or members of a surrogate (foster) family. The highest reported rates of sexual abuse in 2007 (35.2% of sexual abuse reports) occur in the 12 to 15 age range.[93] Sexual abuse tends to be so disturbing and so emotionally intense a topic that there is risk of medical professionals abandoning a logical approach to assessment.

It has been proposed in the literature that, although there are no universal screening standards for sexual abuse, it is important to be aware of potential signs and symptoms of sexual abuse.[92] Reported symptoms may include nightmares, difficulty sleeping alone, sudden or worsening fear of the dark, bedwetting in otherwise toilet-trained child, anger outbursts, irritability, sadness and physical symptoms, such as headaches and stomach aches.[92] Observable signs may include caregiver separation anxiety, refusal to get undressed, unwillingness to be examined, using sexual language, sharing sexual knowledge that is not age appropriate, or being engaged in inappropriate sexual behaviors.[92]

In cases where there is unmistakable traumatic injury, sexually transmitted infection, or testimony that sexual abuse has occurred in the context of no physical evidence, assessment and documentation of the sexual abuse and disclosure must be approached with the assumption that legal proceedings are likely to follow. In these cases, there is ample information to make mandated reporting of the suspicion of abuse a requirement. The fewest number of people should question the child to minimize further trauma to the child and to decrease distortions. Ideally a single interview of the child should be conducted by a mental health professional with expertise in child sexual abuse and the appropriate police agency representative. The child psychiatry consultant's role is to support the child on the pediatric unit, without being involved in the sexual abuse examination.

Providers may also face scenarios where there are physical or behavioral symptoms suggestive of sexual abuse but there is no disclosure or implication of a perpetrator. In such cases, the child may present with medical symptoms, such as a urinary tract infection or vaginitis, or behavioral changes, such as sleep problems or depression.[91] These findings may arouse suspicion and should be followed up with a psychological assessment by the designated professional with expertise in child sexual abuse. Such an individual may assess a pre-schooler through play therapy, looking for themes of abuse in the fantasy play. During the play, the young child may reveal new information about sexual experiences. In the latency-aged child, additional information may be gleaned from the child's drawings, especially self-portraits or pictures of the family. Children and teenagers may be invited to disclose sexual abuse to the evaluator with questions such as, "Has anyone touched you in ways that made you feel uncomfortable or scared?" A follow-up question might be, "Would you tell me if they had?" and "Who could you tell, if someone was touching you or making you uncomfortable?" It is helpful to learn who a child feels he or she can talk to and to add new choices to the list, such as the pediatrician or school teacher as well as the consultant or another counselor. Even if a child is not yet ready to disclose, one hopes that it is therapeutic to assist a child in conceptualizing a plan for disclosing when he or she does feel ready.

In any case in which abuse is entertained, a family assessment is essential. There is no single personality profile of a sexual abuse perpetrator. Perpetrators may come from within the family or the community. The task of the psychiatric consultant is to explore sensitively the meaning of general symptoms that may be indicative of sexual abuse without suggesting that non-specific symptoms are pathognomonic of sexual abuse.

Medical Child Abuse

Medical child abuse is a caregiver pathology where as a result of the caregiver's reports of fabricated symptoms, the child can be a victim of physical abuse, psychological maltreatment, multiple unnecessary procedures, and potentially harmful medical care.[94,95] It was previously referred to as Münchausen syndrome by proxy and was first described as a pair of case reports in 1977.[96] It carries a DSM-5 diagnosis as "factitious disorder by proxy" and has similar names such as "pediatric symptom falsification" and "caregiver fabricated illness" in the pediatrics literature.[28,94,95] Though rare overall, one common presentation in which a parent, usually a mother,[96] consciously distorts her description of her child's symptoms or does things to the child to fabricate a picture of medical illness; she then seeks hospitalizations and medical interventions for the child. One American Academy of Pediatrics review reported that the most common presentations included bleeding, seizures, central nervous system depression, apnea, diarrhea, vomiting, fever, and rash; anorexia and feeding issues were reported as second most common.[95] The parent may also starve a child due to inaccurate beliefs of multiple allergies,[94] or cause life-threatening illness by injecting the child with medication, blood, or feces to ensure that a medical work-up continues.

Some of the individuals with this syndrome have had medical training in a health-related profession, such as nursing,[97,98] and they use their medical knowledge to create "illness" in their child. The mother is usually at the infant or young child's bedside. She tries to establish friendships with the nursing staff and is content as long as continued hospitalization and medical procedures are being scheduled and performed. She may become angry and agitated if she receives a report that her child is well and should be discharged home. Often she appears earnest and less anxious when serious diagnoses of the child are being entertained. If discharged, she may return within hours or days to the ED with an escalation of symptoms. The psychological understanding of this syndrome is that the mother needs the child to be sick to maintain her role as a "nurturant" mother in the protected, supported environment of the pediatric ward. She may gain a "curious sense of purpose and safety in the midst of the disasters which [she herself has] created."[97] She perceives the nurses to be her friends and the male physicians as caretaking men in her life. She lacks the empathy to be troubled by the pain and suffering she is inflicting on her child.

Medical child abuse is a difficult diagnosis to make without observing the caregiver doing something to the child. It may be suspected when a child's medical condition does not follow the expected course and the symptoms are persistently inconsistent. The symptoms may be observed only by the caregiver or may occur in conjunction with the caregiver's presence, and may be consistent with an intentional action. Undertaking the investigation of this diagnosis, and seeking concrete evidence of risk to the child at the hands of a parent may require input from hospital legal counsel and administration.

The American Academy of Pediatrics (AAP) Committee on Child Abuse and Neglect published an approach to recognizing and addressing medical child abuse.[94] They suggest that before making a diagnosis of medical child abuse, the physician must ask: (1) Are the history, signs, and symptoms of disease credible? (2) Is the child receiving unnecessary and harmful or potentially harmful medical care? (3) And if so, who is instigating the evaluations and treatment? They propose that medical child abuse is when medical care is harming the child as a result of the caregiver who is driving it.[94] The diagnosis is a pediatric diagnosis focused on what is happening to the child, and does not factor in the caregiver's motivations.[94]

It is crucial to protect the child's safety if this diagnosis is suspected. The reporters of this syndrome have described high mortality rates and significant morbidity.[94,99,100] The AAP suggests following these clinical principles in medical child abuse cases: (1) consult a pediatrician with child abuse experience; (2) carefully review records from all sources and have all involved physicians collaborate closely; (3) work with a multi-disciplinary child protection team; (4) allow treatment to occur at the least restrictive setting possible, but if necessary, do not hesitate to involve social agencies; and (5) involve the whole family in treatment.[94] The hospital legal department and child protective services should be notified of this diagnosis to protect the best interest of the child. If the parent thinks that she is being suspected of having hurt her child she may become angry and leave against medical advice (sometimes going straight to another hospital under the same or an assumed name). Perpetrators of medical child abuse are difficult to treat due to their psychological difficulties, persistent denial, and capacity for deception; recidivism is common.[101]

LIVING WITH CHRONIC ILLNESS

The vast majority of children with chronic illnesses cope well. They are not defined by their illnesses but rather by their individual strengths, personalities, and age-appropriate developmental issues. However, children with chronic illnesses are more likely than their peers to have a psychiatric disorder.[39,101] There is no one personality that coincides with a particular illness, but each chronic illness, such as asthma, diabetes, rheumatoid arthritis, cystic fibrosis, and sickle cell anemia, presents with particular challenges. These challenges present in terms of coping with: (1) the symptoms, such as pain or shortness of breath; (2) the timing of diagnosis, at birth, childhood, or adolescence; and (3) the requisite healthcare regimen, such as inhalers, IV antibiotics, or dietary restrictions. The meaning of the illness to the patient evolves according to relevant developmental issues throughout the individual's life. The consultant's task is to understand the meaning of the illness to the individual patient and family at this moment in development. The earlier section on development provides some general principles for understanding the effect of chronic illness throughout childhood, but the consultant must assess the unique experience of a particular child and family.[102–105]

The consultant needs to ask many questions to elucidate the patient's subjective experience of living with the chronic illness. Diagnostic instruments used in physically healthy children may not be useful in children with chronic illnesses. Some useful questions include what the worst or hardest thing is about the illness and if there is anything good about the illness. Similarly, what is the child's personal experience of the healthcare regimen? How has the child's experience of the disease changed as the child has grown older, or what events in the future are of concern? What are the child's peer relationships like, and how, if at all, does the illness affect these relationships? Who does the child tell about his or her illness, and when does the child do so in the course of the relationship? How does the child explain the illness to others, and how can he or she explain it to the consultant? What is the child's perception of the parental concerns about the illness? What are the areas of conflict between parent and child and between child and pediatrician or sub-specialist?

Chronic illness requires adjustment on the part of the child, the family, and sometimes the school. The child's personal strengths, such as music, sports, or academics, are assets in maintaining self-esteem and building important peer supports. Some children enjoy peer group opportunities, such as specialized camps for children who share a particular illness. Temperament and interpersonal capacities are also factors in the ease of a child's adjustment. Parental attitude toward the illness is crucial in setting the stage for the child's attitude. This may raise difficulties, because feeling worried, burdened, and isolated is a common experience among parents of children with chronic illness.[105] Excessive parental anxiety, anger, sadness, and guilt, however, are likely to impede the child's adjustment.[105,106]

The extent to which an illness interferes with age-appropriate activities, especially school, is an important factor in adjustment. Multiple hospitalizations are associated with greater emotional morbidity than is seen in an individual hospital stay.[107] Structuring the admissions to provide the child with protected times and protected places for play and dialogue, appropriate to the child's age, decreases the stress of the hospital environment. In-hospital tutoring for prolonged hospital stays and continued contact with friends in person, by phone, or online, can assist the child's comfort in returning to school.

CARE AT THE END OF LIFE

In recent years, the emerging subspecialty of pediatric palliative care has helped focus the attention of clinicians who participate in end-of-life care on the complex challenges to providing the best possible care to these children and their families.[108–110] In some treatment settings, there may be specialized clinical services dedicated to pediatric palliative care, and the psychiatric consultant may work closely with these services to address psychosocial needs.[111] In circumstances where these services are not available, the psychiatric consultant may be called upon to aid the patient, family, and medical team in a variety of ways.

A request for consultation may stem from issues related to problem-solving and decision-making in the context of life-limiting illness.[112] This may include initiating a dialogue between the medical team and the patient and family of the patient with life-threatening illness, clarifying the goals and hopes of treatment, and assisting in the evaluation of pros and cons related to specific treatments or treatment settings, including end-of-life care outside of the hospital[113] and planning for the location of death.[114] Because these issues may be frequently accompanied by emotional distress on the part of patients, families, and caregivers, psychiatric expertise may be sought. The psychiatric consultant may help to facilitate affectively intense discussions, and to help anticipate and interpret the reactions of children to issues around death and dying in the relevant developmental context.

In children, a mature conception of death can be viewed in components which may not be acquired simultaneously.[115] Key components include, in approximate order of typical acquisition,[116] concepts of universality, irreversibility, nonfunctionality (i.e., that the functions of life cease with death),[117] and causality. It should not be assumed that children either do not understand the concept of death or are too fragile to talk about it. The child's parents and the medical team may need education about whether and how to talk with the child about death and to involve the child in the plan of care.[118–120]

In addition, helping the seriously ill child to communicate his or her many small preferences, from being called a nickname rather than a formal name to whether or not to wake him or her for optional events or social activities, can create a greater sense of agency and help stave off the destructive force of helplessness. Facilitating peer interactions in the hospital playroom for the child and encouraging both formal and informal support groups for children and their parents can be invaluable. Many parents and children feel that the enormity of the child's illness has so changed their lives that old friends feel inadequate. The worries of the well world can feel alienating and out of touch with the child and the family's new reality. This experience can be isolating. Sharing pleasures and frustrations with other families facing cancer, a terminal neurologic syndrome, or a metabolic disease can be an antidote to the isolation. Many family friendships that begin on the ward survive long after a child dies.

Adolescents may desire to be more involved in their end-of-life planning, and consultants can be helpful in facilitating discussions in a developmentally appropriate manner. Wiener et al. highlighted how adolescents at the end of life really value providing their input and thoughts on: (1) what medical treatment they want or do not want; (2) how they would like to be cared for; (3) information for their family and friends to know; and (4) how they would like to be remembered.[121] The authors took these findings and created a new clinical tool, Voicing My CHOICES, which encompasses the above principles and can be a useful way of introducing and discussing these topics with adolescent and young-adult patients.

The consultant may also have a role in helping with the treatment of symptoms at the end of life, which may be under-recognized or under-treated. Studies of children who died of cancer have found that symptoms of pain, fatigue, and dyspnea occur in large numbers of patients, result in significant suffering, and persist despite attempts to treat.[122–125] In children with life-limiting illness of all kinds, the consultant may have a role in assisting with treatment of pain,[126–128] fatigue, dyspnea,[129] agitation,[130] anxiety, delirium, and depression.[131] Although the psychopharmacologic treatment of seriously ill or dying children is complicated, compassion dictates considering the use of psychiatric medications in this population if they may help relieve suffering.[132]

Families also need varying amounts of assistance to cope with the impending loss of a child, ranging from sympathy for their grief to guidance with how to make end-of-life decisions that reflect their values, preserve dignity, and minimize suffering. In a retrospective study of parents who lost children to cancer, the presence of unrelieved pain and a difficult moment of death were the most significant factors still affecting parents 4 to 9 years after the loss.[133] The same study also demonstrated that most parents had worked through their grief "a lot," and that factors which were associated with working through grief were sharing their problems with others during the child's illness, having access to psychological support during the last month of the child's life, and counseling being offered by healthcare staff within the last month of life.[134] Those parents who reported that they had not worked through their grief reported more physical and psychological health problems, increased sick leave, and increased utilization of healthcare services.[135] Parents who felt that health care given to their children was inadequate, that anxiety or pain had gone unrelieved, or that the parents' own needs (such as support and communication) were not met reported more feelings of guilt in the year following the death of the child.[136] Although support for grieving families at their time of loss can be beneficial, it is important to remember that grieving for the death of a child is a life-long process and community resources for bereaved families may help to work through grief and find meaning in a tremendous loss.

The child's care team may also struggle with the loss of a patient. Commonly, feelings of sadness and helplessness can surface, and it may feel difficult to maintain empathy for patients and families whose circumstances appear trivial by comparison or whose disorders seem "less real" or self-inflicted. Even when these factors are not present, continuous compassion directed at those in crisis can create emotional exhaustion that is termed "compassion fatigue."[137] The intensity of relationships formed in the course of providing care to children at the end of life may contribute to this phenomenon. The consultant may assist by educating members of the team about this phenomenon and dispelling stigma, and helping develop personal, professional, and organizational strategies to prevent and manage compassion fatigue.[138]

SUPPORT FOR PARENTS WITH SERIOUS ILLNESS

The Parenting at a Challenging Time (PACT) Model

Millions of children in the United States grow up in families in which a parent is medically ill. The psychiatric consultant may be asked to help facilitate communication about how parental illness can affect children, provide specific parent guidance, and share relevant community resources. Table 47-1 shows brief examples of parenting tips, with relevance to the child's developmental stage. Table 47-2 provides a list of various resources parents could access to help with their own coping, their family's coping, events, and other relevant resources. There is real clinical need for consultation in this capacity, as seen at the Massachusetts General Hospital, Parenting at a Challenging Time program. More clinical attention to and research about these issues is needed.

ETHICAL ISSUES

The psychiatric consultant faces many challenging ethical issues in the hospital. The consultant may be involved in helping children and families come to terms with psychologically complex decisions, such as pursuing continued

TABLE 47-1 Key Points and Parenting Tips by Developmental Stage

DEVELOPMENTAL STAGE	KEY POINTS	PARENTING TIPS
Infancy (birth to 2.5 years)	Concern with attachment and self-regulation	Maintain familiar routines Keep number of caretakers to a minimum
Pre-school years (ages 3 to 6 years)	Egocentricity + magical thinking = "I am to blame" Death is temporary and reversible	Maintain routines and loving limit-setting Repeatedly remind the child that the illness is not his or her fault
Latency (ages 7 to 12 years)	Mastery of skills Rules and fairness; simple cause-and-effect logic Peer-focused and image-conscious Intellectualization of death	Protect family time by limiting visitors and turning off the phone at meal times Set regular times for the child to show the ill parent the accomplishments of the week; attend to the details
Adolescence (ages 13 to 18 years)	Abstract thinking and behavior are not on the same plane Separation is developmental task but complicated by vulnerability of parent	Be cautious about assigning teens a parenting role with younger siblings Support relationships with trustworthy non-parental adults Foster safe independent behavior
Young adults (19 to 23 years)	Living away from home Serious relationship formation Longer time frame with regard to decision-making	Provide enough information to allow for decision-making Encourage balance between pursuing new life experiences and putting these on hold to spend precious time with the ill parent

TABLE 47-2 Resources for Patients

Resources for Cancer Patients

People Living With Cancer, From the American Society For Clinical Oncology (ASCO)

Offers educational information for patients and families (www.plwc.org)

American Psychosocial Oncology Society (APOS)

Provides a free help line to connect patients and families with local counseling services, as well as webcasts for professionals on topics such as "Cancer 101 for Mental Health Professionals" and "Psychosocial Aspects of Cancer Survivorship" (co-sponsored by the Lance Armstrong Foundation) (www.apos-society.org)

American Cancer Society (ACS)

Provides information on talking to children about cancer, as well as numerous other cancer-related topics (www.cancer.org)

The Wellness Community

A national, nonprofit organization that provides free online and in-person support and information to people living with cancer and their families (www.thewellnesscommunity.org)

Living Beyond Breast Cancer

A national education and support organization with the goal of improving quality of life and helping patients take an active role in ongoing recovery or management of the disease (www.lbbc.org)

Young Survival Coalition

Through action, advocacy, and awareness, this nonprofit seeks to educate the medical, research, breast cancer, and legislative communities and to persuade them to address breast cancer in women 40 and younger—and serves as a point of contact for young women living with breast cancer (www.youngsurvival.org)

Breast Cancer.org

Offers medical information about current treatments and research in breast cancer care and survivorship (www.breastcancer.org)

Hurricane Voices Breast Cancer Foundation

Among other breast cancer-related resources, this organization offers a family reading list of books and stories for children of all ages dealing with cancer, in particular with breast cancer (www.hurricanevoices.org)

CancerCare

The mission of this national nonprofit resource is to provide free professional help to people with all cancers through counseling, education, information, and referral and direct financial assistance. They offer online, telephone, and face-to-face support groups to those affected by cancer (www.cancercare.org)

Livestrong Foundation

Livestrong offers information and services to cancer survivors and the professionals who care for them (www.livestrong.org)

The Life Institute

This organization's online publication "Conversations from the Heart" provides an annotated list of resources for parents and professionals who want to learn more about how to have developmentally appropriate conversations with children about serious illness and death (www.thelifeinstitute.org)

Resources for Other Illnesses

American Heart Association (www.americanheart.org)
American Diabetes Association (www.diabetes.org)
ALS Association (www.alsa.org)
Brain Injury Association of America (www.biausa.org)
Colitis Foundation (www.colitisfoundation.org)
Cystic Fibrosis Foundation (www.cff.org/home)
Epilepsy Foundation (www.epilepsyfoundation.org)
National Multiple Sclerosis Society (www.nmss.org)
National Neurofibromatosis Foundation (www.nf.org)
Pulmonary Fibrosis Foundation (www.pulmonaryfibrosis.org)

aggressive treatments or assenting to "do not resuscitate" orders. Staff and families need help assessing the extent to which a child at a particular developmental level can understand and be included in such decision-making.

Confidentiality is complex in the hospital setting. The consultant must be clear about with whom information gathered in the consult will be shared and what the limits of confidentiality are. What cannot be kept confidential may be clear, such as suicidal ideation, but what can be confidential, such as a child's worry about a parent's sadness or a parent's trauma history, may be less apparent. The medical record is open to the full medical and support staff, and some personal information may be disclosed that is not relevant to the child's medical care.

FUTURE CONSIDERATIONS

The long-term benefits of psychiatric intervention must be assessed through outcome studies examining the impact of consultation on the quality of life of patients and families, on health outcomes, and the cost of care. Professionals who work with children are called on to advocate for the special needs of the young because they are not yet able to do so for themselves. Interventions that improve the psychological well-being of children maximize their productivity long into the future, and interventions that support families strengthen the community. As managed care, critical pathways, and advances in care decrease lengths of stay, increasingly consultation work will bridge to or be centered in outpatient settings and schools.[139] Being accessible, responsive, and communicative with primary care pediatricians will continue to be essential in the future. Sustained improvement in pediatric mental health services will require continuing and expanding collaboration between medical and child and adolescent psychiatric providers.

Efforts to reduce the distance between pediatrics and child psychiatry have led to more integration of behavioral care within the pediatric medical home, whether it is through an on-site embedded psychiatrist or other accessible consultation such as phone consultation. For primary care settings, the Bureau of Child and Maternal Health of the Public Health Service and the American Academy of Pediatrics have collaborated on projects that emphasize the psychosocial needs of children. *Bright Futures* integrates psychosocial issues into every recommended primary care visit.[140] Many pediatric practices are assessing mental health needs by using screening tools such as a Pediatric Symptom Checklist.[141] Some sub-specialty clinics, including those treating cystic fibrosis, cancer, diabetes, and endocrine disorders, have become more open to consultation at the time of medical diagnosis, at key points in the illness, and for non-adherence. In pediatric oncology, this has led to the development of psychosocial standards of care.[142] More work is needed to develop psychosocial standards of care for other illnesses. Research is needed to evaluate how integration and early involvement of psychiatry can save costs, reduce medical burden, and lead to better outcomes overall.

New technologies, such as telepsychiatry or e-mail consultation via electronic medical records systems (e.g., quick access to "curbside" questions or triaging appropriate referrals), are offering creative ways to offer pediatric psychiatric consultation to areas with little or no child psychiatry presence. This is a burgeoning area and more research is needed to explore its impact on cost-effectiveness, public health, and clinical outcomes.

REFERENCES

Access the reference list online at https://expertconsult.inkling.com/.

Care of the Geriatric Patient

48

M. Cornelia Cremens, M.D., M.P.H.
James M. Wilkins, M.D., D.Phil.
Ilse R. Wiechers, M.D., M.P.P., M.H.S.

OVERVIEW

The United States population over the age of 65 years has been increasing dramatically, reflecting improvements in health, nutrition, and medical care for the elderly. Illness (both medical and psychiatric) increases with advancing age in part due to stressful life events, the burden of co-morbid conditions, and combinations of medications used.[1] Roughly 40% to 60% of those hospitalized with medical and surgical illnesses are over the age of 65 years; such problems place them at greater risk for functional decline.[2] In addition, a reduction in hepatic, renal, and gastric function further impairs the elderly's ability to metabolize drugs.[3] By the year 2030, one in five Americans will be older than 65 years. Thus, psychiatric consultation to this group of patients is becoming ever more necessary while providing both complicated challenges and rewards.

CONSULTATION WITH GERIATRIC PATIENTS

Depression

Mood disorders associated with later life are a major public health problem. Depression is prevalent, unrelenting, immobilizing, and frequently fatal, especially in those with co-morbid medical illness.[4,5] In the United States, depression in the elderly accounts for higher rates of suicide than any other condition. Moreover, rates of suicide are higher in later life than they are in any other age group.[6] More than 90% of older individuals who commit suicide have a risk factor for suicide (e.g., depression or other mental disorders; a personal or family history of substance abuse disorder; stressful life events; a prior suicide attempt or a family history of an attempt; family violence, including physical or sexual abuse; firearms in the home, which is the method used in more than half of suicides; incarceration; or exposure to the suicidal behavior of others, e.g., family members, peers, or media figures).[7] In addition to having a higher prevalence of depression, older persons are more socially isolated and they use highly lethal methods more frequently. Suicide occurs early (often during the first 6 months) in the illness, but it can occur at any time, often in combination with other mental disorders.

Approximately 50% of those with neurologic diseases, cardiac diseases, or cancer, have depressive symptoms. The risk for depression in the post-stroke period is also high, with 25% to 50% developing depression within 2 years after a stroke.[8] Alzheimer's disease (AD) carries an increased risk of depression (found in 20% to 30% either before or at the time of diagnosis), and delusions are also prominent in depression associated with dementia.[9] Recent research confirms the association of depression with the increased risk of developing late-onset AD.[10] Fifty percent of patients with Parkinson's disease develop depression or have a history of depression with anxiety, dysthymia, or frontal lobe dysfunction.[11] Use of medications for medical problems often generates adverse effects and complicates the diagnosis of depression; moreover, medical illness may mimic depression and depression may mimic medical illness. In short, the elderly are at greater risk for depression due to the prevalence of these illnesses and their downstream sequelae.

Despite the fact that depression is a mood disorder comprising far-ranging symptoms (involving disordered sleep, diminished interests, guilt and ruminations, decreased energy or fatigue, impaired concentration, disturbed appetite, and suicidal thoughts or attempts), clinicians find that somatic complaints, rather than depressed mood, are often the reason for referral of the elderly and the medically ill.[12] These physical complaints lie on a continuum and can mimic medical problems (e.g., chest pain, headache, joint pain, nausea, dizziness, and weakness). Teasing out the symptoms of medical or surgical problems from the symptoms of depression can be a daunting task in the hospitalized patient. Physicians often misdiagnose or undertreat depression in the medically ill due to an overlap of these symptoms. The Geriatric Depression Scale (Table 48-1)[13] is a helpful tool in this regard; often the information provided by caregivers is crucial because elders may not be forthcoming with their symptoms.[14] The criteria for diagnosing depression at this time are the same as they are in the general population.

Substantial progress has been made in the treatment of elderly individuals with mood disorders, especially major depression.[15] Once the diagnosis has been established, prescription of an appropriate medication is part of the art of geriatric psychiatry. Since most of the antidepressants are equally effective for depression (Table 48-2), knowledge of how an antidepressant may alter the metabolism and therapeutic drug levels of other medications is crucial. For example, one may wish to start with an antidepressant agent with less cytochrome P450 drug interactions (e.g., citalopram). One needs to review the side effects of the

TABLE 48-1 Geriatric Depression Scale

Choose the best answer for how you felt this past week:

1. Are you basically satisfied with your life?
2. Have you dropped many of your activities and interests?
3. Do you feel that your life is empty?
4. Do you often get bored?
5. Are you hopeful about the future?
6. Are you bothered by thoughts you can't get out of your head?
7. Are you in good spirits most of the time?
8. Are you afraid that something bad is going to happen to you?
9. Do you feel happy most of the time?
10. Do you often feel helpless?
11. Do you often get restless and fidgety?
12. Do you prefer to stay at home, rather than going out and doing new things?
13. Do you frequently worry about the future?
14. Do you feel you have more problems with memory than most?
15. Do you think it is wonderful to be alive now?
16. Do you often feel downhearted and blue?
17. Do you feel pretty worthless the way you are now?
18. Do you worry a lot about the past?
19. Do you find life very exciting?
20. Is it hard for you to get started on new projects?
21. Do you feel full of energy?
22. Do you feel that your situation is hopeless?
23. Do you think that most people are better off than you are?
24. Do you frequently get upset over little things?
25. Do you frequently feel like crying?
26. Do you have trouble concentrating?
27. Do you enjoy getting up in the morning?
28. Do you prefer to avoid social gatherings?
29. Is it easy for you to make decisions?
30. Is your mind as clear as it used to be?

Answers and Scoring

1. No	6. Yes	11. Yes	16. Yes	21. No	26. Yes
2. Yes	7. No	12. Yes	17. Yes	22. Yes	27. No
3. Yes	8. Yes	13. Yes	18. Yes	23. Yes	28. Yes
4. Yes	9. No	14. Yes	19. No	24. Yes	29. No
5. No	10. Yes	15. No	20. Yes	25. Yes	30. No

This is the original scoring for the scale: one point for each of the correct answers as shown above.

Normal—0–9; mild depressives—10–19; severe depressives—20–30.

Adapted from Yesavage JA, Brink TL, Rose TL, et al: Development and validation of a geriatric depression rating scale: a preliminary report, *J Psychiatr Res* 1983; 17: 37–49.

antidepressant and then tailor its use to the patient's symptoms. For example, if a depressed patient is sleeping poorly and losing weight, one should select a sedating agent that is associated with weight gain. Drugs with anticholinergic effects and undue sedation should be avoided to reduce complications (e.g., falls, confusion, poor compliance). Moreover, since depression can complicate one's recovery from the medical or surgical problems, treatment should be swift and aggressive. Often, stimulants are used alone or in conjunction with a traditional antidepressant, such as a selective serotonin reuptake inhibitor (SSRI).[16] Electro-convulsive therapy (ECT) should be considered (and discussed with the patient and his or her family members) if a patient is not responsive to medications.[17]

Bipolar Disorder

Patients over the age of 65 years with bipolar disorder (BPD) may not have developed their affective illness early in life;[18] for many the illness began in middle age or later life, often in association with co-morbid neurologic insults.[19] Those patients with co-morbid neurologic diseases have a significantly later age-of-onset of their affective illness and are less likely to have a family history of a mood disorder. Snowdon[20] reported that 25% of patients whose mania arose after the age of 50 had a history of a neurologic disease and had significantly fewer genetic (familial) risk factors. A number of biological risk factors (including genetic factors and medical illnesses, particularly vascular conditions) have been identified for BPD in the elderly.[21]

Symptoms of mania or hypomania are manifested differently in the elderly, with more anger, irritability, aggression, delusions, and paranoia. In addition, less grandiosity and euphoria appear, episodes of mania are longer, and cycling may be more rapid. Treatment response is inconsistent, although lithium, anticonvulsants (e.g., divalproex sodium, carbamazepine, and lamotrigine), atypical antipsychotics (e.g., olanzapine, quetiapine, and risperidone), and antidepressants have all been beneficial in the treatment of elderly patients with BPD. Moreover, the differential diagnosis of secondary mania warrants special consideration.[22] Many of those with dementia or delirium present with mania secondary to their underlying illness. Although the treatment of secondary affective symptoms is similar to those of primary affective illness, an accurate diagnosis is important.

Delirium and Dementia

The discussions of consultation involving individuals with delirium or dementia are handled separately in chapters elsewhere in this book (see Chapters 10 and 11). However, they also warrant discussion in this chapter, given that the prevalence of dementia increases as age advances (3% to 12% of patients over the age of 65 years, and 25% to 46% of those over the age of 85 years have dementia)[23] and patients with mild dementia are at greater risk for developing delirium (leading to serious behavioral problems) during a hospitalization.[24] Dementia and delirium are often confused in the geriatric population; when consultants are asked to assess a patient for one condition, they often find the other.

The elderly are more vulnerable to delirium because of the numbers of medical problems encountered, changes in brain function, brain disorders (such as dementia), reduced hepatic metabolism of medications, and multi-sensory dysfunction. The elderly are at the highest risk for delirium, as are those with brain damage (including dementia and strokes), cardiac surgery, burns, substance withdrawal, and autoimmune diseases.[25–28] The morbidity and mortality of elderly patients with delirium is high; 15% to 26% die, often as a result of the problem responsible for the delirium.[28]

TABLE 48.2 Treatments Recommended for Depression in the Elderly

DRUGS	DOSE RANGE (mg/day)	COMMENTS
Tricyclic Antidepressants		
Nortriptyline	10–150	Reliable blood levels, minimal orthostasis
Desipramine	10–250	Mildly anticholinergic
Monoamine Oxidase Inhibitors		
Tranylcypromine	10–30	Orthostasis (may be delayed), pedal edema, weakly anticholinergic, dietary restrictions
Stimulants		
Dextroamphetamine	2.5–40	Agitation, mild tachycardia
Methylphenidate	2.5–60	
Modafinil	50–200	
Selective Serotonin Re-Uptake Inhibitors		
Fluoxetine	5–60	Akathisia, headache, agitation, GI complaints, diarrhea/constipation
Sertraline	25–200	
Paroxetine	5–40	
Fluvoxamine	25–300	
Citalopram	10–40	
Escitalopram	2.5–20	
Serotonin–Norepinephrine Re-Uptake Inhibitors (SNRI)		
Venlafaxine	25–300	Increased systolic blood pressure (SBP), confusion, lightheadedness
Duloxetine	20–60	Diarrhea
Other antidepressants		
Mirtazapine	15–45	Sedation, weight gain
Trazodone	25–250	Sedation, orthostasis, incontinence, hallucinations, priapism
Bupropion	75–450	Seizures, less mania/cycling headache, nausea

Performing a comprehensive medical evaluation (e.g., with assessment of oxygenation and infections, such as urinary tract infections) with an examination of the patient (including a careful neurologic assessment, even if it has been done by another physician), review of medications, and review of medication compliance, are keys to uncovering the etiology of the delirium and directing appropriate management. Medications with anticholinergic effects are often responsible for cognitive dysfunction and should be avoided. Diphenhydramine, a medication commonly given to elderly patients for sleep, can be problematic because of its strong anticholinergic properties.

Agitation and behavioral symptoms occur frequently in geriatric patients with dementia and delirium. First-line treatment for behavioral and psychological symptoms of dementia involves use of non-pharmacologic strategies that manipulate environmental and behavioral features (such as regularly scheduled routines for meals, sleep, and bathing). For geriatric patients with delirium, whenever possible, a family member or a familiar person should stay with the patient to re-orient them; this may minimize the need for medications or restraints. However, in those with delirium, both restraint and medication may be necessary. Restraints may also be required as a reminder not to get out of bed without supervision, because falls and subsequent hip fractures are common in the confused elderly. Hip fractures are associated with delirium and a poor prognosis for the elderly; they may never return to independent function following a hip fracture.[29] On the other hand, the risks associated with use of restraints are also greater among the elderly. Whenever possible, other ways to prevent falls should be entertained. Memory impairment in those with delirium persists in half of afflicted patients and becomes permanent.[30] Nursing home patients and patients with dementia are also at greater risk of delirium due to their impaired status.

Low doses of antipsychotics, either typical or atypical agents, are generally adequate to treat delirium in the elderly. One should increase the dose slowly, so as not to give more than is needed. Table 48-3 lists the types and doses of antipsychotics frequently used in the elderly. When patients are agitated and fail to cooperate with care or are unable to take oral medications, then IV haloperidol is often used to sedate and to reduce psychotic symptoms of delirium.[31,32] Elderly patients are initially started on lower doses (e.g., 0.5 to 2.0 mg of IV haloperidol). To adequately treat the delirium, the dose will need to be titrated.[30] While IV haloperidol can cause cardiac problems (with QTc widening and torsades de pointes), the etiology of polymorphic ventricular tachycardia is often difficult to determine.[33]

Atypical antipsychotics have been successfully used for treatment of delirium and agitation in the elderly and in those who are critically ill.[34,35] Again, doses must be titrated slowly to minimize adverse effects. Patients are maintained on the optimal dose until their symptoms resolve. Symptoms of delirium in the elderly can last up to 6 to 12 months, and it may be necessary to discharge a patient home on an antipsychotic medication. Patients with underlying dementia are at greater risk for developing delirium; the impact of cholinesterase inhibitors has been studied in this population.[36,37]

TABLE 48.3 Antipsychotics Commonly Used in the Elderly

AGENT/DOSE (mg)	SEDATION	ANTICHOLINERGIC	EXTRAPYRAMIDAL	COMMENTS
Low Potency				
Thioridazine (Mellaril) 10–50	High	High	Low	Significant hypotension
Intermediate Potency				
Perphenazine (Trilafon) 0.5–5	Medium	Medium	Medium	
High Potency				
Haloperidol (Haldol) 0.25–2	Low	Low	High	
Thiothixene (Navane) 0.5–4	Low	Low	High	
Fluphenazine (Prolixin) 0.5–2	Low	Low	High	
Atypical Antipsychotics				
Clozapine (Clozaril) 12.5–100	High	High	Very low	White blood cell (WBC) count each week Excessive drooling Hypotension
Risperidone (Risperdal) 0.25–3	Low	Low	Low	More EPS than initially reported
Olanzapine (Zyprexa) 2.5–10.0	Moderate	Medium	Low	
Quetiapine (Seroquel) 12.5–200	High	Low	Low	
Ziprasidone (Geodon) 20–120	Moderate	Low	Low	
Aripiprazole (Abilify) 5–20	Low	Low	Moderate	

In April 2005, FDA notified healthcare professionals that patients with dementia-related psychosis treated with atypical antipsychotic drugs are at an increased risk of death. Since issuing that notification, FDA has reviewed additional information that indicates the risk is also associated with conventional antipsychotics.

Antipsychotics are not indicated for the treatment of dementia-related psychosis.

Psychosis

Psychosis (manifested by hallucinations, delusions, disorganized speech, or disorganized or catatonic behavior) in the elderly has multiple etiologies. New-onset psychosis in the elderly should be rigorously worked-up for possible organic causes, such as trauma (e.g., concussion, subdural hematoma, intraparenchymal hemorrhage); organ failure (e.g., hepatic encephalopathy, hypertensive encephalopathy, electrolyte abnormalities, stroke, and seizures); drugs and toxins, infections (e.g., pneumonia, urinary tract infections); and substrate deficiencies (e.g., hypoxia, hypoglycemia, vitamin B_{12} or folate deficiencies). Once organic causes have been ruled out, the remaining differential diagnosis of psychosis in the elderly includes: various types of dementias (e.g., AD, Lewy body dementia, vascular dementia, frontal lobe dementia/Pick's disease, Parkinson's disease), all of which can manifest with symptoms of psychosis at any point during the illness; delirium; delusional disorders; BPD; schizoaffective disorder; schizophrenia (either early-onset or late-onset); and major depression with psychotic features.

Psychosis is most commonly associated with schizophrenia and delusional disorders, but in the elderly, delirium and psychosis are more commonly associated with dementia and have behavioral complications that accompany these diagnoses. Psychosis in dementia is often manifested by one of three general categories (i.e., delusions, hallucinations, and misconceptions). Delusions often include the themes of stolen items, infidelity, imposters, disorientation, a lack of familiarity with ordinary items, and fear of being alone or abandoned. Hallucinations may relate to sensory losses and to the usual sensory domains (e.g., visual, auditory, tactile). Frequent misconceptions include the misperceptions of objects, not recognizing oneself, and believing that television scenes are real here-and-now events. Symptoms of psychosis are distressing to family members and to caregivers. They can become dangerous if the individual is frightened or energized by them.

Although schizophrenia usually begins before the age of 30 years, late-onset schizophrenia is not rare. More than 20% of cases are diagnosed after the age of 40 years, and at least 0.1% of the population over age 65 years has a diagnosis of schizophrenia that started late in life, with a prognosis that may be made worse by delay and avoidance of treatment.[38] Aggressive treatment of symptoms and supportive care for patients with this diagnosis is imperative. Schizophrenia remains plastic into later life, with more prominent negative symptoms than positive symptoms. Numerous confounding factors (including cognitive decline, dementia, depression, medical co-morbidity, and use of medications for medical conditions) occur with aging. Further complications from treatment of psychosis include drug-induced side effects. In the elderly these side effects are often dramatic. Drugs with anticholinergic, orthostatic, sedative, and extrapyramidal symptoms (EPS) are relatively commonplace.[39] The elderly are more susceptible to tardive dyskinesia than are other age groups. The conventional antipsychotics have more adverse side effects than atypical agents, and higher-potency agents may be more useful than lower-potency ones. Atypical antipsychotics are often used in the elderly because of their sedative properties and their lack of EPS (when used at lower doses).[32,33] Atypical agents also reduce aggression associated with dementia.[40,41] However, they should be used with care, because there is a risk of adverse cerebrovascular events in patients with dementia.[42] The risk of death in patients taking typical antipsychotics is comparable with, or higher than, the rates in patients taking atypical antipsychotics.[43–45]

Dose equivalents of the atypical antipsychotics have been problematic, but a recent report by Woods[41] (using 100 mg/day of chlorpromazine as the standard), compared 2 mg/day for risperidone, 5 mg/day for olanzapine, 75 mg/day for quetiapine, 60 mg/day for ziprasidone, and 7.5 mg/day for aripiprazole, and outlined a more useful schedule. The caveat "start low and titrate up slowly" remains the gold standard; adding more medication is less harmful than is giving a large bolus of a drug with a long half-life. In certain instances, when agitation without psychosis is the primary problem, other medications to reduce anger (e.g., SSRIs, or other antidepressants that may cause sedation) are more apt to induce calm.[40,46]

Substance Abuse and Withdrawal

Patients of all ages should be asked about their use of alcohol and illicit substances. Alcoholism in the elderly is common; however, it often goes unreported by patients and is overlooked by physicians.[47,48] Alcohol-related problems in the elderly are a growing public health concern. A life-long pattern of daily drinking, even in small amounts, is problematic. The National Institute on Alcohol Abuse deems one drink (12 oz beer, 1.5 oz spirits, or 5 oz wine) per day to be the maximum intake considered to be moderate alcohol use for men and women 65 years of age or older.[49,50] The prevalence of alcoholism in the elderly is about 10% to 18% and is the second most frequent reason for admission to an inpatient psychiatric facility.[50] As with those in the general population, the risk of suicide in the elderly who abuse alcohol is staggering; it is second only to major depression.[51]

Older individuals with alcoholism often refuse treatment due to perceived negative stigma and significant denial of the problem.[49] Screening tools have not been of significant benefit, but as in all aspects of geriatric care, use of the team approach to diagnosis and treatment is essential.[52] Symptoms of problem drinking include insomnia, memory loss, confusion, anxiety, and depression, as well as somatic complaints that may mimic medical illness, further delaying accurate diagnosis.

Alcohol withdrawal is characterized by two or more of the following signs and symptoms: autonomic hyperactivity; tremor; insomnia; nausea or vomiting; transient visual, tactile, or auditory hallucinations or illusions; psychomotor agitation; anxiety; or tonic–clonic seizures.[47] With the loss of lean body mass associated with aging, the volume of distribution for alcohol is reduced; this results in an increased peak ethanol concentration after any amount of alcohol is consumed.[3]

Co-morbid illnesses, both psychiatric and medical, confound accurate diagnosis of both alcoholism and medical presentations.[48] Patients seen in consultation often are admitted for infection, trauma, cardiac disease, gastrointestinal disorders, renal diseases, and pulmonary conditions. Treatment of withdrawal in the elderly is more complex and requires close monitoring. Shorter-acting benzodiazepines (e.g., lorazepam) are the medications of choice, and one should begin with low doses and increase them slowly, so as to avoid oversedation. In some older patients, larger doses and longer-acting benzodiazepines (e.g., diazepam or chlordiazepoxide) are indicated, especially with those who have a history of seizures or *delirium tremens* (DTs). Often in those with chronic alcoholism who have a history of DTs or seizures, the gold standard remains chlordiazepoxide because its long-acting metabolites provide a slow taper and reduce the risk of seizures. Most important, aggressive treatment of symptoms limits the possibility of complications due to withdrawal or the development of DTs.

Anxiety

Recently, anxiety in the elderly (generally associated with normal aging and with medical, financial, and health-related hardships) has been recognized more often than it had been in the past. However, anxiety is not a direct consequence of normal aging, and the symptoms of anxiety should not be ignored. Beekman and associates[53] noted that loss of control and vulnerability to stress were the strongest risk factors for anxiety in later life. Both of these risk factors were common among elderly hospitalized patients. Anxiety co-exists with many other psychiatric diagnoses (such as depression, BPD, alcoholism, and dementia). Diagnostic challenges often arise when anxiety (e.g., worry, fear, apprehension, concern, foreboding) as well as somatic complaints (such as tachycardia, sweating, abdominal distress, dizziness, vertigo) develop in the context of a medical illness (e.g., diabetes with hypoglycemia, hyperthyroidism, or cardiac disease with hypoxia), because it can be manifest by similar symptoms.[54] Worries, fears, and concerns are often related to finances, dependency issues, loneliness, and memory loss. Manifestations of medical illness can mimic psychiatric symptoms; certain substances or medications (e.g., caffeine, stimulants, ephedrine, bronchodilators) produce anxiety-like symptoms. Withdrawal from a prescribed or an illicit drug can precipitate severe anxiety and panic; life-threatening withdrawal can result from sudden abstinence from alcohol, benzodiazepines, or barbiturates.

Fortunately, anxiety can be effectively managed in the elderly by use of medications, therapy, or a combination of the two.[54] In the general hospital, the treatment for anxiety involves use of benzodiazepines. However, because some older patients develop significant side effects (such as confusion, falls, oversedation, and paradoxical agitation) from benzodiazepines[55] they should be used cautiously (while observing for exacerbation of other problems, such as sleep apnea). Other agents (including selected antidepressants, such as trazodone and mirtazapine) can be used as well.

CASE 1

Mr. A, a 95-year-old man with dementia, depression, complicated grief, and anxiety was referred by his physician for treatment with psychotropics.

Mr. A and his family reported that his depressive symptoms appeared shortly after the death of his wife of more than 70 years; she had suffered from Alzheimer's disease (AD) for the past 10 years. After her death her caregiver remained to care for Mr. A, due to his decline in both activities of daily living (ADLs) and his instrumental activities of daily living (IADLs). Mr. A developed difficulty sleeping, lost weight, had a paucity of interests, experienced thoughts of death, and wished he was dead, although he had no thoughts of suicide ("I would never do that"). He was increasingly frail, had difficulty walking, fell frequently (with possible loss of consciousness) for several years. Evaluation by the Neurology Service on several occasions (due to recurrent falls and memory loss) led to a diagnosis of a mixed dementia, both vascular and AD. After his evaluation for memory loss, Mr. A was started on donepezil.

Mr. A's past medical history included a bilateral hip replacement and a right knee replacement, surgery for a multi-nodular thyroid, a history of stroke (with minimal loss of function), impaired hearing and vision, hypertension, benign prostatic hypertrophy, a TURP, several squamous cell cancers, non-sustained ventricular tachycardia, vaso-vagal syncope, orthostatic hypotension, falls (leading to a fractured spine, posterior C spine fusion), and back pain.

Over his life-time Mr. A was very active in his community, church, family, business, and philanthropic endeavors. He developed post-traumatic stress disorder (with nightmares and flashbacks of fighting the enemy) in the Second World War. His large extended family was supportive and available; nevertheless, Mr. A was not as engaged as he had been when his wife was alive. Mr. A sobbed when he spoke of his wife and their life together. With intense sadness and longing he sought comfort from his nocturnal caregivers.

Due to his difficulty sleeping and nighttime agitation with delusions, Mr. A was prescribed quetiapine and then mirtazapine; both caused daytime sedation and were discontinued. A selective serotonin re-uptake inhibitor and supportive therapy (to address his grief, depression, anxiety, and loneliness) was initiated.

SPECIAL CONSIDERATIONS IN THE GERIATRIC POPULATION

Pharmacotherapy

Polypharmacy, treatment with many medicines for the same condition, is extremely common in the elderly.[56] Older patients are at higher risk for polypharmacy because of the increased rates of chronic and co-morbid medical illness in this age group. Thus, concurrent use of multiple drugs does not necessarily connote inappropriate prescribing; it may in fact be sensible. Regardless, polypharmacy puts the elderly at increased risk for multiple adverse outcomes, including adverse drug reactions, falls, hospitalizations, nursing home placement, malnutrition, pneumonia, and death.[57–59]

The four key concepts relevant to polypharmacy in the elderly are the "prescribing cascade," the effects of aging, altered pharmacokinetics and pharmacodynamics, and multiple co-morbidities.[3] The "prescribing cascade" begins when an adverse drug reaction is misinterpreted as a new medical condition, for which another drug is then prescribed, placing the patient at risk of developing additional adverse effects relating to this potentially unnecessary treatment.[60] Age-related changes may exacerbate medication side effects in the elderly. Of particular concern are side effects, such as orthostatic hypotension, anticholinergic reactions, parkinsonism, sedation, and cardiac conduction disturbances. Changes in metabolism, distribution, and excretion that occur with aging result in longer half-lives, increased or decreased drug effects, and increased occurrence of drug toxicity. All of these issues need to be taken into consideration with the increased medical co-morbidities in the older population, which at times, necessitates the use of multiple medications.

One of the primary goals of the consultant is to prevent polypharmacy and its associated negative outcomes. One of the first and most critical steps of any geriatric psychiatry consultation should be a careful and detailed review of current medications and all recent medication changes, including both psychotropic and non-psychotropic agents as well as over-the-counter medications. A new medication should be added only when there is a clear indication for its use; one should consider non-pharmacologic treatments when appropriate. When starting new medications, one should start with low doses and slowly titrate them to achieve a therapeutic response. Many clinicians will stop titration too soon, thus giving the patient an inadequate trial of a medication; this is also a negative outcome. Hence, remember the adage "start low, go slow, but go all the way."

Healthcare Decision-Making

Consultants are often called to make determinations about the ability of elderly patients to make decisions regarding their health care. It is sometimes assumed that the elderly, regardless of the level of the cognitive impairment, cannot make such decisions. Although the details regarding capacity evaluations are dealt with elsewhere (see Chapter 51), it is worth noting the unique issues that surround surrogate decision-makers and the geriatric population.

As a rule, one should not assume that patients with cognitive impairment are unable to make their own healthcare decisions. Each case should be considered individually, taking into consideration the level of impairment, the medical decision being considered, and the risks of treatment versus non-treatment. As a result of the Patient Self-Determination Act of 1990, Medicare and Medicaid providers are required to educate all adult patients upon hospital admission about their right to participate in and to direct their own health care decisions, the right to accept or refuse treatment, and the right to prepare an advance directive. Geriatric patients should be encouraged to have conversations with family, friends, and caregivers about their wishes related to these issues, and should have surrogate healthcare decision-makers in place even if they are in the best of health. End-of-life conversations are important elements of care for older adults (see Chapter 46).

Emergency Department Care

Emergency Department (ED) visits are especially problematic for the elderly (who often manifest atypical presentations of illness); when the elderly are evaluated by someone with geriatric expertise, outcomes are improved. EDs are chaotic, even more so for elderly patients with cognitive or functional impairment. In such settings, the elderly often have extended waits, as those with more dramatic presentations are tended to; when this occurs, their symptoms may progress to a point where the physiologic reserves become exhausted. Although timely and accurate diagnosis is crucial, the diagnoses of delirium, depression, and dementia are frequently missed. One should remember that two-thirds of all cases of delirium in this age group occur in those with dementia.

Physicians in the ED may not have access to the patient's history; as a result they often attribute the presenting complaints to chronic problems or to symptoms of aging. Acute symptoms that bring an elderly patient to the ED are not a direct result of normal aging, even though physiologic functions and reserves diminish with aging; a rapid decline is not typical of the aging process and it requires immediate attention. Communication with third parties (e.g., caregivers, family members, primary care physicians, or nurses) is essential, because the elderly often deny or minimize their symptoms or situation. The elderly can be at risk for abuse or neglect, and be embarrassed or ashamed about their situation. The hurried, chaotic, and noisy ED environment exacerbates impairments in communication (that arise secondary to hearing loss, poor vision, and cognitive impairment).[61] Implementation of simple and compassionate interventions (such as providing warm blankets, keeping patients informed, re-orienting them, hydrating and feeding them, as well as attending to the needs of caregivers) improves care. Caregivers of elderly ED patients should also be mindful of the propensity for skin breakdown (when lying for protracted periods on hard surfaces). Psychiatric consultants with expertise in geriatrics can facilitate shorter stays and prevent iatrogenic complications. Education of ED staff with regard to the care of older patients in the acute setting (including management of end-of-life issues[62]) is still sorely needed.

It is also worth mentioning the medication reconciliation initiative outlined in the July 2006, Institute of Medicine (IOM) Report on Preventing Medication Errors.[63] This effort encourages development of a partnership between patients and their healthcare providers. It involves creation of a medication list (including new ones and those to be discontinued) that is provided to and discussed with older outpatients and their family members or caregiver. The IOM report found that a simple review of a patient's medications can eliminate numerous errors that increase the cost of care and improve communication with other healthcare providers. Use of electronic prescriptions (a recommendation of the IOM) is aimed at eliminating prescription errors and enhancing communication among providers about medications. According to a study cited in the IOM report, the annual cost of avoidable medication errors in Medicare enrollees (≥65 years) was over US$887 million. Over and above the monetary issue is the impact on pain and suffering, the need for family or caregiver assistance, and the loss of earnings. Ensuring medication reconciliation (with clear and concise instructions about the medications, their indications and side effects, and their various names and acronyms), at the time of hospital (or ED) discharge can lead to improved adherence and to fewer adverse drug reactions.

Elder Abuse

Each year, thousands of elderly are abused, neglected, and exploited by family members, caregivers, and others. Many of the victims are frail and vulnerable; they are unable to help themselves and they depend on those who abuse them to assist them with their basic needs. The psychiatric consultant often identifies these issues that may result in non-compliance with medications or with medical care. These issues may have contributed to the hospital admission and to ongoing medical or psychiatric problems.[53] All 50 states have reporting systems and toll-free hotlines to report concerns anonymously. Adult protective services (APS) agencies investigate the reports of suspected elder abuse and determine if abuse or neglect exists. Types of abuse are physical, sexual, psychological, financial, exploitative, and negligent.[64] More than a half million cases were reported to the APS in 1996 during a national incidence study done through the Administration on Aging. The cohort at greatest risk were those 80 years of age and older. In 90% of the cases the perpetrator was a family member; in two-thirds they were either adult children or spouses.[65]

The warning signs of abuse may be subtle, and the patient may not be willing to cooperate or agree to go forward with an investigation. Family or caregivers may be overwhelmed, depressed, or physically unable to continue to care for the elderly patient; the APS can guide them to appropriate services.

Families and Caregivers

Families and caregivers are often an integral part of the evaluation of the elderly. The consultant should begin by gathering information directly from the patient. However, when the patient is unable to provide information (e.g., because of altered mental status or cognitive impairment), gathering further collateral information is essential. Caregivers often serve as a crucial source of information regarding medication regimens and the patient's baseline in terms of both cognitive and functional status.

Dementia often causes tremendous suffering for patients, their families, and society. Patients are forced to become more dependent and to lose their independence in basic caring for themselves, which complicates other co-morbid conditions. An important part of any evaluation is the assessment of the health and well-being of the caregivers, family members, or employees of the patient, because they are at risk for developing anxiety and depression.[66,67] Caring for the caregiver is as important as caring for the patient.[68] The inordinate stress and burden can place the caregiver at risk for both medical and psychiatric crisis.

Loneliness has a significant impact on the older adult and the caregiver.[69] Serious poor health outcomes stem from loneliness such as reduced mobility, increased frailty, poor compliance with medications, depression, anxiety, and increased morbidity and mortality. Engaging older adults in activities they may enjoy as well as prior activities that gave them pleasure (e.g., music, singing, reading, walking). In Britain, it has become a national public health problem, with funding and programs designed to alleviate loneliness. Although not only an issue for older adults, older adults are more often isolated by retirement, loss of a spouse, and illness that may limit mobility.[70]

REFERENCES

 Access the reference list online at https://expertconsult.inkling.com/.

Psychiatric Illness During Pregnancy and the Postpartum Period

49

Charlotte Hogan, M.D.
Betty Wang, M.D.
Marlene P. Freeman, M.D.
Ruta Nonacs, M.D., Ph.D.
Lee S. Cohen, M.D.

OVERVIEW

Psychiatric consultation to obstetric patients typically involves evaluating and treating an array of psychopathology. Once thought to be a time of emotional well-being for women,[1] studies now suggest that pregnancy does not protect women from the emergence or persistence of psychiatric disorders.[2–4] Because many psychiatric conditions are chronic or recurrent and have high prevalence rates in women during the reproductive years, many women will become pregnant while receiving psychiatric treatment. Given the possibility of unplanned pregnancies, women of reproductive age should know the risks and benefits of their medications, even if they are not planning to become pregnant.

Optimally, a woman and her psychiatrist should plan ahead for a pregnancy and assess the risks and benefits of treatment before conception. Ideally, this planning helps avoid abrupt cessation of medications because of fear of exposing the fetus to medication, which is important because rapid discontinuation of medication increases the risk of relapse of mood episodes during pregnancy.[5,6] Medications with relatively benign reproductive safety profiles should be used as first-line agents in women of reproductive potential. The risks of untreated psychiatric disorders during pregnancy include pre-term delivery, low birth weight, poor nutrition, inadequate weight gain, poor prenatal care, inability to care for oneself, substance use (such as cigarettes or alcohol), and termination of the pregnancy.[7,8] In addition, untreated psychiatric disorders during pregnancy have been associated with altered developmental trajectories in infancy and childhood.[9] Depression during pregnancy is also a strong predictor of postpartum depression,[10] a condition that can have dire consequences for the mother, the baby, and the entire family. Therefore, it is critical to sustain maternal emotional well-being during pregnancy.

Pregnancy is an emotionally laden experience that evokes a spectrum of normal reactions, including heightened anxiety and increased mood reactivity. Psychiatric evaluation of pregnant women requires careful assessment of symptoms (such as anxiety or depression) and decisions about the nature of those symptoms, including normative or pathologic, manifestation of a new-onset psychiatric disorder, and exacerbation of a previously diagnosed or undiagnosed psychiatric disorder. Unfortunately, screening for psychiatric disorders during pregnancy or the puerperium has historically been uncommon. Recently, the American College of Obstetricians and Gynecologists (ACOG) and the U.S. Preventive Services Task Force (USPSTF) released formal recommendations calling for depression screening of all pregnant and postpartum women, with emphasis that adequate systems must ensure treatment and follow-up after screening.[11] Even when depressed pregnant women are identified, however, definitive treatment is often lacking[12] and patients are often untreated or incompletely treated.[13] Screening for depression during pregnancy followed by thoughtful treatment can minimize maternal morbidity as well as the potential impact of an untreated psychiatric disorder on infant development and family functioning.

Treatment of psychiatric disorders during pregnancy involves a thoughtful weighing of the risks and benefits of proposed interventions (e.g., pharmacologic treatment) against risks associated with untreated psychiatric disorders. In contrast to many other clinical conditions, treatment of psychiatric disorders during pregnancy is typically reserved for situations in which the disorder interferes in a significant fashion with maternal and fetal well-being; the threshold for treating psychiatric disorders during pregnancy tends to be higher than with other conditions. Women with similar illness histories often make very different decisions about their care in collaboration with their physicians during pregnancy.

DIAGNOSIS AND TREATMENT OF MOOD DISORDERS DURING PREGNANCY

Although some historical reports describe pregnancy as a time of emotional well-being that confers "protection" against psychiatric disorders,[14] more recent studies suggest rates of major and minor depression in gravid women (approximating 10% to 15%) that are similar in prevalence to non-gravid women.[15] Women with a history of major depression appear to be at particularly high risk for recurrence of depression during pregnancy, especially when antidepressants have been discontinued.[4]

Making the diagnosis of depression during pregnancy can be difficult because disturbances in sleep and appetite, symptoms of fatigue, and changes in libido do not always indicate an evolving affective disorder. Clinical features that can support the diagnosis of major depressive disorder (MDD) include anhedonia, feelings of guilt and hopelessness, poor self-esteem, and thoughts of suicide. In addition, symptoms that interfere with function signal a psychiatric condition that warrants treatment. Suicidal ideation is not uncommon during pregnancy, however risk of clear-cut, self-injurious or suicidal behavior appears to be relatively low in women who develop depression during pregnancy.[16]

Treatment for depression during pregnancy is determined by the severity of the underlying disorder, by a history of treatment responses, and by individual patient preferences. Neurovegetative symptoms that interfere with maternal well-being require treatment. Women with mild to moderate depressive symptoms may benefit from non-pharmacologic treatments that include supportive psychotherapy,[17] cognitive-behavioral therapy (CBT),[18] or interpersonal therapy (IPT),[19] all of which have been shown to ameliorate depressive symptoms during pregnancy.

Antidepressants

Antidepressant use has grown increasingly common, with a study from the Centers for Disease Control and Prevention (CDC) reporting that more than 15% of reproductive-aged women filled a prescription for an antidepressant medication during the years 2008–2013.[20] Although data accumulated over the last 30 years have suggested that some antidepressants have favorable risk–benefit profiles during pregnancy,[21,22] information regarding the full spectrum and relative severity of risks of prenatal exposure to all psychotropic medications is still incomplete. Importantly, the risks of medication use must be balanced in each individual against the risks associated with untreated psychiatric disorders that might adversely affect the mother and the fetus.

As is the case with other medications, four types of risk are typically cited with respect to potential use of antidepressants during pregnancy: risk of pregnancy loss or miscarriage, risk of organ malformation or teratogenesis, risk of neonatal toxicity or withdrawal syndromes during the acute neonatal period, and risk of long-term neuro-behavioral sequelae. In the past, a system established by the U.S. Food and Drug Administration (FDA) that classified medications into five risk categories: A, B, C, D, and X, was used to inform physicians and patients about the reproductive safety of various prescription medications. In this system, medications in category A were designated safe for use during pregnancy, whereas category X drugs were contraindicated, because of known risks to the fetus that outweighed any benefit to the patient. This system of classification had noteworthy limitations. First, categorization was often ambiguous and could lead to unwarranted conclusions. Second, the categorization was often assigned on the basis of only a small amount of animal data when human data were sparse or absent. Third, when larger and more rigorous studies became available on the reproductive safety profile of a medication, the category was rarely altered. And finally, the categorization system failed to take into account the risks of the untreated maternal psychiatric disorder for the woman and her fetus. For these reasons, in June 2015 the FDA replaced this system with the Pregnancy and Lactation Labeling Rule (PLLR), which requires descriptive safety information regarding pregnancy and lactation in the drug label. This includes a risk summary, clinical considerations, and data subsections for use in pregnancy, lactation, and treatment of patients with reproductive potential.[23] The letter classification system is now abolished and replaced by these more nuanced descriptions.

Randomized, placebo-controlled studies that examine the effects of medication use on pregnant populations are lacking and are largely considered unethical. Therefore, much of the data related to the profile of reproductive safety for a medication is derived from retrospective studies and case reports. Studies that have evaluated the reproductive safety of antidepressants have used a more rigorous prospective design,[24] or they have relied on large administrative databases or multi-center birth-defect surveillance programs.[25] The following paragraphs will provide an overview of currently available data on antidepressant use during pregnancy with regards to risk of pregnancy loss or miscarriage, risk of organ malformation or teratogenesis, risk of neonatal toxicity or withdrawal syndromes during the acute neonatal period, and risk of long-term neuro-behavioral sequelae.

Studies have not demonstrated a statistically increased risk of spontaneous miscarriage following prenatal exposure to antidepressants.[26] When compared with women with depression, women on antidepressants do not experience a higher rate of miscarriage.[27]

Regarding teratogenic risk, selective serotonin re-uptake inhibitors (SSRIs) have been studied extensively for safety during pregnancy. Large studies are reassuring; as a group of medicines, SSRIs are not major teratogens and do not increase risk of congenital malformation.[5,28] Initially, some reports suggested that first-trimester exposure to paroxetine was an exception to this finding, and reported that paroxetine was associated with an increased risk of cardiac defects (including atrial and ventricular septal defects).[29] More recent assessment of the data, including independent, peer-reviewed, comprehensive meta-analyses of studies assessing paroxetine exposure during the first trimester[30] failed to demonstrate the increased teratogenicity of paroxetine. Therefore, like other SSRIs, paroxetine may still be considered a first-line agent for women who have responded well to it before pregnancy. Tricyclic antidepressants (TCAs) have also been shown in the pooled available data to be safe for use during pregnancy with regards to risk of congenital malformations.[31]

Bupropion may be an attractive option for women who have not responded well to SSRIs or TCAs. Most data thus far have not indicated an increased risk of malformations associated with bupropion use during pregnancy.[32] However, one recent study suggested the possibility of an increased risk of cardiovascular malformations.[33] Bupropion deserves special consideration if a woman is attempting to abstain from smoking during pregnancy, as it helps with smoking cessation, and cigarettes are teratogenic. Bupropion may also be useful in treating attention deficit disorder, given that the reproductive safety profile of stimulants is more concerning than that of bupropion.[34]

Serotonin–norepinephrine re-uptake inhibitors (SNRIs), including venlafaxine and duloxetine, have been less well studied than other classes of antidepressant medications during pregnancy, but emerging data are reassuring that first-trimester exposure to these medications is not associated with a clinically important increase in risk of major congenital malformations.[35] Mirtazapine has not been thoroughly studied for safety during pregnancy. Case studies thus far have not identified any clear signal of increased risk of malformations,[36] so preliminary data are reassuring, but large definitive trials are necessary to assess risks that might be rare and thus only observable with adequate sample sizes.

Despite the growing literature that supports the relative safety of fetal exposure to SSRIs, multiple reports[37,38] have described adverse perinatal outcomes including decreased gestational age at delivery, low birth weight, and poor neonatal adaptation. However, others[39,40] have not noted these associations. Particular concern has been raised regarding the potential effects of late-pregnancy exposure to SSRIs; some newborns who were exposed to SSRIs exhibit a transient period (limited to several days following delivery) of jitteriness, tachypnea, and tremulousness.[41] In general, this neonatal adaption syndrome is a mild and benign syndrome not requiring any specific medical intervention.

Conflicting reports have also raised a question about whether SSRI use in later pregnancy is associated with a serious but rare developmental lung condition, persistent pulmonary hypertension of the newborn (PPHN). Chambers and colleagues raised this concern when they found an increased risk of PPHN with SSRI use in a nested case–controlled study. They reported the risk of PPHN with exposure to SSRIs after 20 weeks at about 1%.[42] Other research has been reassuring, with multiple large studies showing that the risk is much lower than initially estimated, or even that there is no association between SSRI use and PPHN at all.[43,44] Most recently, from a large Medicaid database of 3.8 million pregnancy outcomes, researchers demonstrated that the risk of PPHN was 0.3% for women who were treated with SSRIs, compared to 0.2% among those who were not.[45] Readers must be mindful that PPHN is correlated with multiple risk factors, including cesarean section, race, body mass index, and other factors not associated with SSRI use.[45]

Compared with the considerable data on risk of congenital malformations with prenatal antidepressant exposure, reproductive safety data regarding the long-term effects of prenatal antidepressant exposure on the developing fetal brain are more limited. In children exposed to fluoxetine, TCAs, venlafaxine, or no medication, no differences have been detected in behavioral or cognitive development (in terms of intelligence quotient, language, temperament, behavior, reactivity, mood, distractibility, and activity level)[46,47] among groups when followed through early childhood. Some recent studies have reported that rates of anxiety, autism spectrum disorder, and attention deficit disorder are more common in antidepressant-exposed children;[48] however, these studies do not account for the fact that maternal psychiatric illness itself is a known risk factor for these conditions.[49,50] That the higher prevalence of these disorders is more likely due to genes and maternal illness rather than to the medication exposure is supported by studies that have controlled for confounding factors, such as maternal psychiatric diagnosis and exposure to other medications.[51,52] While the data available are mostly reassuring, further investigation into the long-term neuro-behavioral effects of prenatal exposure to antidepressants is warranted.

Pharmacologic Treatment of Depression: Clinical Guidelines

Over the past several decades, as the pharmacologic treatment of depression has become more common, increased attention has been directed to the question of how to best manage women who suffer from depression throughout reproductive events. Clinical lore has suggested that women enjoyed positive mood during pregnancy, but more-recent data demonstrate that many women face substantial risk for recurrence or the new onset of depression during pregnancy. There is also a greater appreciation that depression poses risks for fetal and neonatal well-being that need to be taken into account during the risk–benefit decision-making process.

The majority of women who suffer from depression during pregnancy do not receive adequate treatment, despite the prevalence and consequences of untreated illness.[53] Despite the growing number of reviews on the subject, management of prenatal depression is still largely guided by experience, with few definitive data and no controlled treatment studies to inform management. The best treatment algorithms depend on the severity of the disorder, the patient's psychiatric history, her current symptoms, her attitude toward the use of psychiatric medications during pregnancy, and, ultimately, the patient's wishes. Clinicians must work collaboratively with the patient to arrive at the safest treatment plan based on currently available information.

In patients with less-severe depression, discontinuation of pharmacologic therapy during pregnancy should be considered. Though data on the use of IPT or CBT to facilitate antidepressant discontinuation before conception are not available, it makes sense to pursue such treatment for women on maintenance antidepressant therapy who are planning to become pregnant. These treatment modalities have been shown to reduce depressive symptoms during pregnancy.[18,54] Close monitoring of affective status is essential throughout pregnancy for women with a history of a mood disorder, regardless of whether medication is continued or discontinued. Psychiatrically ill women are at high risk for relapse during pregnancy, and early detection and treatment of recurrent illness can significantly reduce the morbidity associated with having prenatal affective illness.

Many women who discontinue antidepressants during pregnancy experience recurrent depressive symptoms.[55,56] In one study, women who discontinued their medications were five times more likely to relapse (with a rate of relapse of 68%)[4] as compared with women who maintained their antidepressants across pregnancy. Thus, women with recurrent or refractory depressive illness may decide (in collaboration with their clinician) that the safest option is to continue pharmacologic treatment during pregnancy to minimize the risk of recurrent illness. In this setting, the clinician should attempt to select medications during pregnancy that have a well-characterized reproductive safety profile that might obviate switching to one with a better reproductive safety profile.

In an ideal world, switching would occur before pregnancy and allow time for stabilization on a new medication. For example, one might switch from duloxetine, a medication for which there are sparse data on reproductive safety, to an agent such as fluoxetine or citalopram. In other situations, one may decide to use a medication for which information regarding reproductive safety is sparse, for example, a woman with refractory depression who has responded only to one particular antidepressant for which specific data on reproductive safety are limited (e.g., mirtazapine). She may choose to continue this medication during pregnancy rather than risk potential relapse associated with discontinuing the antidepressant or switching to another antidepressant for which the patient has no history of response.

Even if a woman continues taking an antidepressant during pregnancy, relapse can occur. Cohen and colleagues[4] reported that 26% of women who continued antidepressants had a relapse of MDD during pregnancy. Therefore, careful monitoring is required even if maintenance medications are continued. Only a small amount of information is available on the pharmacokinetic profile of SSRIs and newer antidepressants across pregnancy,[57,58] and some women experience lower serum medication levels in late pregnancy. Therefore, some women can require higher doses of medication as pregnancy progresses to maintain therapeutic benefits; this supports a need for frequent assessment. Older reports demonstrated that women might also have lower serum levels of TCAs in the third trimester.[59]

Women might also experience the new onset of depressive symptoms during pregnancy. For women who present with minor depressive symptoms, non-pharmacologic treatment strategies should be explored first. IPT or CBT may be beneficial for reducing the severity of depressive symptoms and can limit or obviate the need for medications. In general, pharmacologic treatment is pursued when non-pharmacologic strategies have failed or when it is felt that the risks associated with psychiatric illness during pregnancy outweigh the risks of fetal exposure to a particular medication.

In situations in which pharmacologic treatment is more clearly indicated, the clinician should select medications with the safest reproductive profile. SSRIs, with extensive data that support their reproductive safety, can be considered as first-line choices. Among the SSRIs, paroxetine is the most controversial (given reports regarding cardiovascular malformations with first-trimester exposure). However, as state previously, more comprehensive studies did not support this risk. Nevertheless, many women and their obstetric healthcare providers might remain apprehensive about use of paroxetine in pregnancy. The TCAs and bupropion have also been relatively well characterized and can be considered reasonable treatment options during pregnancy. Among the TCAs, desipramine and nortriptyline are preferred because they are less anticholinergic and less likely to exacerbate orthostatic hypotension during pregnancy.

When prescribing medications during pregnancy, an attempt should be made to simplify the medication regimen. For instance, one may select a more sedating antidepressant for a woman who presents with depression and a sleep disturbance instead of using a more activating antidepressant in combination with trazodone or a benzodiazepine.

In addition, the clinician must use an adequate dosage of medication to achieve or maintain remission. Often, the dosage of a medication is reduced during pregnancy in an attempt to limit risk to the fetus. However, this type of modification in treatment might instead place the woman at greater risk for recurrent illness. During pregnancy, changes in plasma volume and increases in hepatic metabolism and renal clearance can significantly affect drug levels.[60,61] Several investigators have described a reduction (up to 65%) in serum levels of TCAs during pregnancy.[61] Sub-therapeutic levels may be associated with depressive relapse; therefore, an increase in daily antidepressant dosage may be required to obtain remission.

With multiple studies supporting the finding of transient neonatal jitteriness, tremulousness, and tachypnea associated with peripartum use of SSRIs,[62] some physicians have suggested discontinuing antidepressants just before delivery to minimize the risk of neonatal toxicity. Another potential rationale for discontinuing antidepressants before delivery is derived from the assumption this would attenuate the risk of PPHN that has been associated with third-trimester exposure to SSRIs. However, the recommendation is not data-driven and such a practice can actually carry significant risk because it withdraws treatment from a patient precisely as she is about to enter the postpartum period, a time of heightened risk for affective illness. In consideration of the well-characterized risks to the baby and to siblings in the family of a woman with maternal depression, treatment goals should include having a woman approach the postpartum period in remission from depression. The strategy of discontinuing medication before delivery, however, would increase the risk of a woman's entering the postpartum period with depression, and recovery could require substantial time.

Severely depressed patients who are acutely suicidal or psychotic require hospitalization and treatment; electroconvulsive therapy (ECT) is often selected as the treatment of choice. Reviews of ECT during pregnancy note the efficacy and safety of this procedure.[63] In a review of the 339 cases of ECT during pregnancy published since 1941, only 11 of the 25 fetal or neonatal complications, including two deaths, were likely the result of ECT.[65] Given its relative safety, ECT may also be considered an alternative to conventional pharmacotherapy for women who wish to avoid extended exposure to psychotropics during pregnancy or for women who fail to respond to standard antidepressants.

BIPOLAR DISORDER

CASE 1

Ms. A, a 31-year-old professional with past psychiatric history of bipolar disorder type I, presents for consultation regarding pregnancy planning. She and her husband would like to conceive in the near future, and she seeks guidance on the safety of pregnancy given her psychiatric history and her medication regimen.

On interview, Ms. A is alert and engaged, presenting with stable euthymic mood. She describes having had two prior manic episodes for which she was psychiatrically hospitalized. Since starting lithium monotherapy 3 years ago, her mood has remained stable.

After gathering a complete psychiatric, medical, gynecologic, family, and social history, the consulting psychiatrist engages Ms. A in a careful discussion of the risks of mood disturbance during and after pregnancy, in addition to a discussion of the risks and benefits of various psychiatric treatment options during and after pregnancy. Based on this discussion, Ms. A decides to plan for a pregnancy while continuing lithium monotherapy during pregnancy and the postpartum period. She and her psychiatrist make a plan for close follow-up and monitoring.

Historically, women with bipolar disorder (BPD) have been counseled to defer pregnancy (given an apparent need for pharmacologic therapy with mood stabilizers) or to terminate pregnancies following prenatal exposure to drugs such as lithium or valproic acid. However, more recent and comprehensive data suggest that women can select treatment strategies that allow pregnancy with both the mother's and baby's safety in mind.

The risk of lithium exposure during pregnancy has been re-assessed and is considered far safer than it was decades ago. Concerns regarding fetal exposure to lithium, for example, have typically been based on early reports of higher rates of cardiovascular malformations (e.g., Ebstein's anomaly) following prenatal exposure to this drug.[64] While still thought to increase the risk of this rare condition, data suggest that the absolute risk of cardiovascular malformations following prenatal exposure to lithium is actually quite low. In the general population, Ebstein's anomaly occurs in 1/20,000 live births; with first-trimester lithium exposure, the risk is estimated as being at most 1/1000.[65] Prenatal screening with a high-resolution ultrasound and fetal echocardiography is recommended at about 16 to 18 weeks of gestation to screen for cardiac anomalies. Nonetheless, a woman with BPD is faced with a decision regarding use of lithium during pregnancy; it is appropriate to counsel such a patient about the very small risk of organ dysgenesis associated with prenatal exposure to this medicine.

Lamotrigine is another mood stabilizer that is an option for pregnant women who have BPD and who demonstrate a clear need for prophylaxis with a mood stabilizer. Well studied by several pregnancy registries, lamotrigine does not appear to increase the risk of major congenital malformations above that of the general population. Although early data caused concern for an increased risk of oral clefts following lamotrigine exposure, larger registries have not observed this association.[66,67]

Compared with lithium and lamotrigine, prenatal exposure to some anticonvulsants is associated with a far greater risk of organ malformation. A strong association between prenatal exposure to some mood stabilizers, including valproic acid and carbamazepine, and neural tube defects (3% to 8%) has been observed.[68,69] Fetal exposure to anticonvulsants has been associated not only with relatively high rates of neural tube defects, such as spina bifida, but also with multiple other anomalies including mid-face hypoplasia, congenital heart disease, cleft lip or palate (or both), growth retardation, and microcephaly. Factors that can increase the risk for teratogenesis include high maternal serum anticonvulsant levels and exposure to more than one anticonvulsant. This finding of dose-dependent risk for teratogenesis is at variance with that for some other psychotropics (e.g., antidepressants). Thus, when using anticonvulsants during pregnancy, the lowest effective dose should be used, anticonvulsant levels should be monitored closely, and the dosage should be adjusted appropriately. In addition, valproic acid has been associated with serious neuro-cognitive developmental anomalies, including lower IQ and impaired cognition across several domains in children who were exposed *in utero*.[70] Valproic acid exposure before birth also appears to increase risks of autism and attention deficit disorders later in childhood.[71,72] Ideally, women of reproductive age should avoid treatment with valproate, and it should not be considered a first-line therapy in women with reproductive potential. Information about the reproductive safety of newer anticonvulsants sometimes used to treat BPD, including gabapentin, oxcarbazepine, and topiramate, remains sparse.[73,74]

Prenatal screening for congenital malformations following anticonvulsant exposure (including cardiac anomalies) with fetal ultrasound at 18 to 22 weeks' gestation is recommended. The possibility of fetal neural tube defects should be evaluated with maternal serum alpha-fetoprotein (MSAFP) and ultrasonography. In addition, 4 mg a day of folic acid before conception and in the first trimester for women receiving anticonvulsants is often recommended. However, the supplemental use of folic acid to attenuate the risk of neural tube defects in the setting of anticonvulsant exposure has not been systematically evaluated.

Whereas use of mood stabilizers (including lithium and some anticonvulsants) has become the mainstay of treatment for managing both acute mania and the maintenance phase of BPD, the majority of patients with BPD are not treated with monotherapy. Rather, use of adjunctive conventional and newer antipsychotics has become common clinical practice for many patients with BPD. With growing data supporting the use of atypical antipsychotics as monotherapy in the treatment of BPD, patients and clinicians are seeking information regarding the reproductive safety of these agents.

To date, abundant data exist that support the reproductive safety of typical antipsychotics, and no definitive association between typical antipsychotic administration during pregnancy and risk of congenital malformations has been identified.[75] Recently, atypical antipsychotics have been the subject of increasing research regarding reproductive safety. Several large studies have released data that are largely reassuring regarding the safety of atypical antipsychotic exposure during pregnancy, with most showing either minimal or no increase in risk of major congenital malformations following atypical antipsychotic exposure.[76–78] More data are required to definitively understand these risks, and newer atypical antipsychotics (such as ziprasidone and lurasidone) are under-represented in these studies, limiting understanding of risks associated with their use during pregnancy. An atypical antipsychotic may be the optimal treatment for a pregnant woman with BPD who has responded to the medication in the past.

Patients with a history of a single episode of mania and prompt full recovery, followed by sustained well-being, may tolerate discontinuation of a mood stabilizer before an attempt to conceive.[79] Unfortunately, even among women with a history of prolonged well-being and sustained euthymia, discontinuation of prophylaxis for mania may be associated with subsequent relapse. In one study, the risk of recurrence of a mood episode during pregnancy in women who discontinued their mood stabilizer during pregnancy was 71%.[6]

For women with BPD and a history of multiple and frequent recurrences of mania or bipolar depression, several options can be considered. Some patients may choose to discontinue a mood stabilizer before conception as outlined earlier. An alternative strategy for this high-risk group is to continue treatment until pregnancy is verified and then taper off the mood stabilizer. Because the utero-placental circulation is not established until approximately 2 weeks following conception, the risk of fetal exposure is minimal. Home pregnancy tests are reliable and can document pregnancy as early as 10 days following conception, and with a home ovulation predictor kit, a patient may be able to time her treatment discontinuation accurately. This strategy minimizes fetal exposure to drugs and extends the protective treatment up to the time of conception, which may be particularly prudent for older patients because the time required for them to conceive may be longer than for younger patients. However, a significant potential problem with this strategy is that it can lead to relatively abrupt discontinuation of treatment, thereby placing the patient at increased risk for relapse. This strategy would require close clinical follow-up, so that patients could be monitored for early signs of relapse, and medications may be re-introduced as needed.

Another problem with the strategy of discontinuing mood stabilizers when the patient is being treated with valproic acid is that the teratogenic effect of valproic acid occurs early in gestation (between weeks 4 and 5), often before the patient even knows she is pregnant. In such a scenario, any potential teratogenic insult from valproic acid may have already occurred by the time the patient actually documents the pregnancy.

For women who tolerate discontinuation of maintenance treatment, the decision of when to resume treatment is a matter for clinical judgment. Some patients and clinicians prefer to await the initial appearance of symptoms before re-starting medication; others prefer to limit their risk of a major recurrence by re-starting treatment after the first trimester of pregnancy. Preliminary data suggest that pregnant women with BPD who remain well throughout pregnancy might have a lower risk for postpartum relapse than those who become ill during pregnancy.[79]

For women with particularly severe forms of BPD, such as with multiple severe episodes, and especially with psychosis and prominent thoughts of suicide, maintenance treatment with a mood stabilizer before and during pregnancy is strongly recommended. If the patient decides to attempt conception, accepting the relatively small absolute increase in teratogenic risk with first-trimester exposure to lithium or lamotrigine with or without an antipsychotic, for example, may be justified because such patients are at highest risk for clinical deterioration if pharmacologic treatment is withdrawn. Many patients who are treated with sodium valproate or other newer anticonvulsants, such as gabapentin, for which there are particularly sparse reproductive safety data, never received a lithium trial before pregnancy. For such patients, a lithium trial before pregnancy may be a reasonable option.

Even if all psychotropics have been safely discontinued, pregnancy in a woman with BPD should be considered a high-risk pregnancy, because the risk of major psychiatric illness during pregnancy is increased in the absence of treatment with a mood-stabilizing medication, and it is even higher in the postpartum period. Extreme vigilance is required for early detection of an impending relapse of illness, and rapid intervention can significantly reduce morbidity and improve overall prognosis. Therefore, close monitoring with assessment of mood, sleep, and other symptoms is urged throughout pregnancy and the immediate postpartum period.

Although the impact of pregnancy on the natural course of BPD is not well described, studies suggest that any "protective" effects of pregnancy on risk for recurrence of mania or depression in women with BPD are limited, and the risk for relapse and chronicity following discontinuation of mood stabilizers is high.[80] Given these data, clinicians and women with BPD who are either pregnant or who wish to conceive must carefully weigh the risks and benefits of medication against the risks of symptom relapse and the consequences this has for both mother and fetus.

PSYCHOTIC DISORDERS

Acute psychosis during pregnancy is an obstetric and psychiatric emergency. Similar to other psychiatric symptoms of new onset, first onset of psychosis during pregnancy requires a systematic evaluation. Psychosis during pregnancy can inhibit a woman's ability to obtain appropriate and necessary prenatal care or to cooperate with caregivers during delivery.[81]

Treatment of psychosis during pregnancy may include use of either typical or atypical antipsychotics. With regard to typical antipsychotics, high-potency neuroleptics, such as haloperidol or thiothixene, are preferred because lower-potency antipsychotics have some historical data for possible increased risk of congenital malformations associated with prenatal exposure.[82] However, their use is not absolutely contraindicated. Atypical antipsychotics have recently been the subject of several large studies regarding reproductive safety data.[76–78] These are largely reassuring, and to date do not identify any significant or consistent risk of major malformation with atypical antipsychotic exposure during pregnancy. More data are required in order to definitively understand risk, in addition to studies that include newer atypical antipsychotics, such as ziprasidone and lurasidone, but it appears that atypical antipsychotics are also a safe option for treating psychosis during pregnancy.

Psychiatric consultation may be requested to consider treatment options for mild or intermittent symptoms of psychosis or for pregnant women with chronic mental illness, such as schizophrenia, who have discontinued therapy with neuroleptics. Although as-needed neuroleptics are appropriate for treating milder symptoms of psychosis, introduction or re-introduction of maintenance antipsychotics should be considered in women with schizophrenia who have new-onset illness or a recurrent disorder. This approach can potentially limit overall exposure to these drugs by reducing the need for treatment with higher doses of drug during relapse. Patients with florid psychosis during labor and delivery might benefit from intravenous haloperidol, which can facilitate the patient's cooperation with the obstetrician, thereby enhancing the overall safety of the delivery.[83]

Decisions regarding the use of these agents and other psychotropics must be made on a case-by-case basis. Patients taking an antipsychotic drug may choose to discontinue their medication or switch to a better-characterized medication if they are taking a newer atypical antipsychotic. However, many women do not respond as well to the typical agents or have such severe illness that making any change in their regimen can place them at significant risk. Thus, women and their clinicians often choose to use whichever antipsychotic agent during pregnancy sustains function and prevents symptom relapse, while acknowledging that information regarding their reproductive safety remains incomplete.

ANXIETY DISORDERS

Although modest to moderate levels of anxiety during pregnancy are common, pathologic anxiety (including panic attacks) has been associated with a variety of poor obstetric outcomes, including increased rates of premature labor, low Apgar scores, and placental abruption.[84] Anxiety disorders are prevalent during pregnancy, however specific prevalence estimates vary widely.[85] For women with pre-pregnancy diagnoses, there is considerable variability in reported illness course, especially for obsessive–compulsive disorder (OCD) and panic disorder, with some studies suggesting improvement during pregnancy and others reporting worsening of symptoms.

Consultation requests regarding appropriate management of anxiety symptoms during pregnancy are common. The use of non-pharmacologic treatment, such as CBT and other types of psychotherapy, may be of great value in attenuating symptoms of anxiety, and for most patients it should be part of the treatment plan.[86] For some patients, psychotherapy may be sufficient to manage anxiety disorders during pregnancy.

For other patients, especially those who experience panic attacks associated with new-onset or recurrent panic disorder or those with severe generalized anxiety, pharmacologic intervention may be necessary. Many patients respond well to antidepressants, whose risks and safety profiles were discussed earlier. Concerns regarding a potential association between first-trimester exposure to benzodiazepines, and increased risk for oral clefts have been noted in some studies (risk for oral clefts was approximately 0.6% following first-trimester exposure),[87] while other more recent studies have not supported this association.[88] Pooled data analysis does not suggest an increase in risk of congenital malformations with benzodiazepine use during pregnancy.[89,90] Benzodiazepines, when used judiciously, may be a reasonable option for treating anxiety symptoms during pregnancy.

For patients with panic disorder who wish to conceive and do not want to remain on anxiolytic medication, a slow taper of the medication is recommended. Adjunctive CBT can help patients discontinue anti-panic agents and can increase the time to a relapse.[91] Some patients conceive inadvertently on anxiolytics and present for emergent consultation. Abrupt discontinuation of anxiolytic maintenance medication is not recommended given the risk for rebound panic symptoms or a potentially serious withdrawal syndrome. However, a gradual taper of a benzodiazepine (over more than 2 weeks) with adjunctive CBT may be pursued in an effort to minimize fetal exposure to medication.

If the taper of a medication is unsuccessful or if symptoms recur during pregnancy, reinstitution of pharmacotherapy may be considered. For patients with severe panic disorder, maintenance medication may be a clinical necessity. TCAs or SSRIs, perhaps in addition to benzodiazepines, are reasonable options for managing panic disorder during pregnancy. Although some patients choose to avoid first-trimester exposure to benzodiazepines (given historical data suggesting risk for cleft lip and palate), benzodiazepines may be used without significant risk during the second and third trimesters and can offer some advantage over antidepressant treatment because they may be used on an as-needed basis. Pharmacotherapy of severe anxiety during pregnancy includes treatment with benzodiazepines, TCAs, SSRIs, or SNRIs in addition to CBT.

With respect to the peripartum use of benzodiazepines, reports of hypotonia, neonatal apnea, neonatal withdrawal syndromes, and temperature dysregulation[92,93] have prompted recommendations to taper and discontinue benzodiazepines at the time of parturition. The rationale for this course is suspect for several reasons. First, given data that suggest a risk of puerperal worsening of anxiety disorders in women with a history of panic disorder and OCD,[94,95] discontinuation of a drug at, or about the time of, delivery places a woman at risk for postpartum worsening of these disorders. Second, data describe the use of clonazepam during labor and delivery at doses of 0.5 to 3.5 mg/day in a group of women with panic disorder without evidence of perinatal sequelae.[96]

ELECTROCONVULSIVE THERAPY

Consideration of the use of ECT during pregnancy typically generates anxiety among clinicians and patients. However, its safety record has been well documented since the 1940s,[97] particularly when instituted in collaboration with a multidisciplinary treatment team, including an anesthesiologist, a psychiatrist, and an obstetrician.[98] Requests for psychiatric consultation for pregnant patients who require ECT tend to be emergent and dramatic. For example, expeditious treatment is imperative in instances of mania during pregnancy or psychotic depression with suicidal thoughts and disorganized thinking. Such clinical situations are associated with a danger of impulsivity or self-harm. A limited course of treatment may be sufficient, followed by institution of treatment with one or a combination of agents (such as antidepressants, neuroleptics, benzodiazepines, or mood stabilizers). An additional option to consider for treatment-resistant depression (or for a pregnant woman with depression who does not want to take medications) would be transcranial magnetic stimulation (TMS), which appears to be safe during pregnancy and may be less likely than ECT to cause side effects. At least one study has demonstrated efficacy of TMS for treatment of depression during pregnancy,[99] but no studies have assessed its effectiveness in treating severe depression, and it is not clear how TMS compares to antidepressants for treatment of depression during pregnancy. For severe depression during pregnancy, pharmacotherapy and/or ECT remain the preferred treatment.

ECT during pregnancy tends to be under-used because of concerns the treatment will harm the fetus. Despite one report of placental abruption associated with the use of ECT during pregnancy,[100] considerable experience supports its safe use in severely ill gravid women. Thus, it becomes the task of the psychiatric consultant to facilitate the most clinically appropriate intervention in the face of partially informed concerns or objections.

BREAST-FEEDING AND PSYCHOTROPIC DRUG USE

The emotional and medical benefits of breast-feeding to mother and infant are clear. However, for some women, establishing breast-feeding can be difficult and can contribute to extreme sleep deprivation that can worsen the postpartum course of illness. It is important to consider the benefits and risks of breast-feeding given each woman's situation.

Given the prevalence of psychiatric illness during the postpartum period, a significant number of women might require pharmacologic treatment while nursing. Appropriate concern is raised, however, regarding the safety of psychotropic drug use in women who choose to breast-feed while using these medications. Efforts to quantify psychotropic drugs and their metabolites in the breast milk of mothers have been reported. The serum of infants can also be assayed to assess more accurately actual neonatal exposure to medications. The data indicate that all psychotropic drugs, including antidepressants, antipsychotic agents, lithium carbonate, and benzodiazepines, are secreted into breast milk. However, concentrations of these agents in breast milk vary considerably.

The amount of medication to which an infant is exposed depends on several factors:[101] the maternal dosage of medication, the frequency of dosing, and the rate of maternal drug metabolism. Typically, peak concentrations in the breast milk are attained approximately 6 to 8 hours after the medication is ingested. Thus, the frequency of feedings and the timing of the feedings can influence the amount of drug to which the nursing infant is exposed. By restricting breast-feeding to times during which breast milk drug concentrations would be at their lowest (either shortly before or immediately after dosing medication) exposure may be reduced; however, this approach might not be practical for newborns, who typically feed every 2 to 3 hours.

The nursing infant's chances of experiencing toxicity depend not only on the amount of medication ingested but also on how well the ingested medication is metabolized. Most psychotropics are metabolized by the liver. During the first few weeks of a full-term infant's life, there is a lower capacity for hepatic drug metabolism, which is about one-third to one-fifth of the adult's capacity. Over the next few months, the capacity for hepatic metabolism increases significantly and by about 2 to 3 months of age, it surpasses that of adults. In premature infants or in infants with signs of compromised hepatic metabolism (e.g., hyperbilirubinemia), breast-feeding typically is deferred because these infants are less able to metabolize drugs and are thus more likely to experience toxicity.

Since 1998, data have accumulated regarding the use of various psychotropics during breast-feeding.[101–103] The available data, particularly on the TCAs and SSRIs during breast-feeding, have been encouraging and suggest that the amounts of drug to which the nursing infant is exposed are low and that significant complications related to neonatal exposure to psychotropic drugs in breast milk are rare.[104–107] Typically very low or nearly undetectable levels of drug have been detected in the infant's serum; exposure to an SSRI during nursing does not appear to result in clinically significant blockade of serotonin (5-HT) re-uptake in infants.[108] Although less information is available on other antidepressants, serious adverse events related to exposure to these medications have not been reported.

Anxiety is prevalent during the postpartum period, and anxiolytics often are used in this setting. Data regarding the use of benzodiazepines while nursing indicate that amounts of medication to which the nursing infant is exposed are generally low.[109] Risk of adverse events in nursing infants exposed to benzodiazepines is very low; rare reports of sedation, particularly in infants exposed to other sedating drugs in addition to benzodiazepines, lead to a recommendation to monitor for sedation.[110] Benzodiazepines should be considered a reasonable treatment option for breast-feeding women with anxiety.

For women with BPD, breast-feeding can pose more significant challenges. First, on-demand breast-feeding can significantly disrupt the mother's sleep and thus can increase her vulnerability to relapse during the acute postpartum period. Second, there have been reports of toxicity in nursing infants related to exposure to some mood stabilizers in breast milk. Lithium is excreted at high levels in the mother's milk, and infants' serum levels are relatively high, about one-fourth that of the mother's serum levels,[111] thereby increasing the risk of neonatal toxicity (which includes cyanosis, hypotonia, and hypothermia). Although breast-feeding typically is avoided in women taking lithium, the lowest possible effective dosage should be used and both maternal and infant serum lithium levels should be followed in mothers who do breast-feed. In collaboration with the pediatrician, the child should be monitored closely for signs of lithium toxicity, and levels of lithium, thyroid-stimulating hormone (TSH), blood urea nitrogen (BUN), and creatinine should be monitored every 6 to 8 weeks while the child is nursing.

Several studies have suggested that lamotrigine reaches infants through breast milk in relatively high doses, ranging from 20% to 50% of the mother's serum concentrations;[112] this may be explained by poor neonatal metabolism of lamotrigine. In addition, maternal serum levels of lamotrigine increase significantly after delivery unless the dose is adjusted, contributing to high levels found in nursing infants. However, only one case of an adverse event related to this exposure has ever been reported (apnea in an infant breast-fed by a lamotrigine-toxic mother).[113] One worry shared by clinicians and new mothers is the risk for Stevens–Johnson syndrome, a severe, potentially life-threatening rash, most commonly resulting from a hypersensitivity reaction to a medication, that occurs in about 0.1% of patients who have BPD and are treated with lamotrigine.[114] Thus far, there have been no reports of Stevens–Johnson syndrome in infants exposed to lamotrigine. In fact, it appears that cases of drug-induced Stevens–Johnson syndrome are extremely rare in newborns. A single case report described a neonate who developed the syndrome after exposure to phenobarbital.[115]

Similarly, concerns have arisen regarding the use of carbamazepine and valproic acid. Both of these mood stabilizers have been associated in adults with abnormalities in liver function and with fatal hepatotoxicity. Hepatic dysfunction associated with carbamazepine exposure in breast milk has been reported several times.[116,117] The risk for hepatotoxicity appears to be greatest in children younger than 2 years; thus, nursing infants exposed to these agents may be particularly vulnerable to adverse events. Although the American Academy of Pediatrics has deemed carbamazepine and valproic acid to be appropriate for use in breast-feeding mothers, few studies have assessed the impact of these agents on fetal well-being, particularly in mothers who are not taking it for treatment of epilepsy. In women who choose to use valproic acid or carbamazepine while nursing, monitoring of drug levels and liver function testing is recommended. In this setting, ongoing collaboration with the child's pediatrician is crucial.

Consultation about the safety of breast-feeding among women treated with psychotropics should include a discussion of the known benefits of breast-feeding to mother and infant and the possibility that exposure to medications in the breast milk can occur. Although routine assay of infants' serum drug levels was recommended in earlier treatment guidelines, this procedure is probably not warranted; in most instances, infants have low or non-detectable serum drug levels and serious adverse side effects are uncommon. This testing is indicated, however, if neonatal toxicity related to drug exposure is suspected. Infant serum monitoring is also indicated when the mother is nursing while taking lithium, valproic acid, or carbamazepine.

PSYCHIATRIC CONSULTATION AND POSTPARTUM PSYCHIATRIC ILLNESS

The postpartum period is considered a time of risk for the development of affective illness. Research has identified sub-groups of women at particular risk for postpartum worsening of mood. At highest risk are women with a history of postpartum psychosis; up to 70% of women who have had one episode of puerperal psychosis experience another episode following a subsequent pregnancy.[118] Similarly, women with a history of postpartum depression are at significant risk, with rates of postpartum recurrence as high as 50%.[119] Women with BPD also appear to be particularly vulnerable during the postpartum period, with rates of postpartum relapse greater than 30%, and significantly higher for cases in which mood-stabilizing medication was not maintained throughout pregnancy.[120] In all women (with or without a history of MDD) the emergence of depressive symptoms during pregnancy significantly increases the likelihood of postpartum depression.[121]

Depression

Diagnosis

During the postpartum period, about 85% of women experience some mood disturbance. For most women the symptoms are mild; however, 10% to 15% of women experience clinically significant symptoms. Postpartum depressive disorders typically are divided into three categories: postpartum blues, non-psychotic major depression, and puerperal psychosis. Because these three diagnostic sub-types overlap significantly, it is not clear if they actually represent three distinct disorders. It may be more useful to conceptualize these sub-types as existing along a continuum, in which postpartum blues is the mildest and postpartum psychosis the most severe form of puerperal psychiatric illness.

Postpartum blues does not indicate psychopathology; it is common and occurs in approximately 50% to 85% of women following delivery.[122] Symptoms, including reactivity of mood, tearfulness, and irritability are, by definition, time-limited and typically remit by the 10th postpartum day. Because postpartum blues is associated with no significant impairment of function and is time-limited, no specific treatment is indicated. Symptoms that persist beyond 2 weeks require further evaluation and suggest an evolving depressive disorder. In women with a history of recurrent mood disorder, the blues may herald the onset of postpartum MDD.

Several studies describe a prevalence of postpartum MDD of between 10% and 15%.[122] The signs and symptoms of postpartum depression usually appear over the first 2 to 3 months following delivery and are indistinguishable from the characteristics of MDD that occur at other times in a woman's life. The presenting symptoms of postpartum depression often include depressed mood, irritability, and loss of interest in usual activities. Insomnia, fatigue, and loss of appetite are frequently described. Postpartum depressive symptoms also co-mingle with anxiety and obsessional symptoms, and women might present with generalized anxiety, panic attacks, or obsessive–compulsive symptoms.[123,124]

Although it is sometimes difficult to diagnose depression in the acute puerperium given the normal occurrence of symptoms suggestive of depression (e.g., sleep and appetite disturbance, low libido), it is an error to dismiss neurovegetative symptoms (such as severe decreased energy, profound anhedonia, and guilty ruminations) as normal features of the puerperium. In its most severe form, postpartum depression can result in profound dysfunction. Risk factors for postpartum depression include prenatal depression, prenatal anxiety, and a history of depression.

Treatment

A wealth of literature on this topic indicates that postpartum depression, especially when left untreated, may have a significant impact on the child's well-being and development. In addition, the syndrome demands aggressive treatment to avoid the sequelae of an untreated mood disorder, such as chronic depression and recurrent disease. Treatment should be guided by the type and severity of the symptoms and by the degree of functional impairment. However, before initiating psychiatric treatment, medical causes for mood disturbances (e.g., thyroid dysfunction, anemia) must be excluded. Initial evaluation should include a thorough history, physical examination, and routine laboratory tests.

Non-pharmacologic therapies are useful in the treatment of postpartum depression, and several studies examining efficacy of various psychotherapy modalities have yielded encouraging results. CBT specifically has been demonstrated in several studies as an effective treatment for postpartum depression,[125] and comparable in at least one study to treatment with fluoxetine.[126] IPT has also been shown to be effective for treating women with mild to moderate postpartum depression.[127]

These non-pharmacologic interventions may be particularly attractive to patients who are reluctant to use psychotropic medications (e.g., women who are breastfeeding) or for patients with milder forms of depressive illness. Further investigation is required to determine the efficacy of these treatments in women who suffer from more severe forms of postpartum mood disturbances. Women with more severe postpartum depression will likely have the best clinical response to a combination of pharmacologic treatment and non-pharmacologic therapies.

To date, only a few studies have systematically assessed the pharmacologic treatment of postpartum depression. Conventional antidepressants (e.g., fluoxetine, sertraline, venlafaxine) have shown efficacy in the treatment of postpartum depression.[128,129] In all of these studies, standard antidepressant doses were effective and well tolerated. The choice of an antidepressant should be guided by the patient's prior response to antidepressants and a given medication's side-effect profile. SSRIs are ideal first-line agents because they are anxiolytic, non-sedating, and well tolerated; bupropion is another good option. TCAs are sometimes used, and because they tend to be more sedating, they may be more appropriate for women who have prominent sleep disturbances. Given the prevalence of anxiety in women with postpartum depression, adjunctive use of a benzodiazepine (e.g., clonazepam or lorazepam) may be very helpful.

Some investigators have also explored the role of hormone manipulation in women who suffer from postpartum depression. The postpartum period is associated with rapid shifts in the reproductive hormonal environment, most notably a dramatic fall in estrogen and progesterone levels, and postpartum mood disturbance has been attributed to a deficiency (or change in the levels) in these gonadal steroids. Although early reports suggested that progesterone may be helpful,[130] no systematically derived data exist to support its use in this setting. A few small studies have described the benefit of exogenous estrogen therapy, either alone or in conjunction with an antidepressant in women with postpartum depression.[131,132] Although these studies suggest a possible role for estrogen in the treatment of women with postpartum depression, these treatments remain experimental. Estrogen delivered during the acute postpartum period is not without risk and has been associated with changes in breast-milk production and more significant thromboembolic events. Antidepressants are safe, well tolerated, and highly effective; they remain the clear first choice for women with postpartum depression.

In cases of severe postpartum depression, inpatient hospitalization may be required, particularly for patients who are at risk for suicide. In Great Britain, innovative treatment programs involving joint hospitalization of the mother and the baby have been successful; however, mother-and-infant units are much less common in the United States. Women with severe postpartum illness should be considered candidates for ECT. The option should be considered early in treatment because it is safe and highly effective. In choosing any treatment strategy, it is important to consider the impact of prolonged hospitalization or treatment of the mother on the infant's development and attachment.

Panic Attacks and Obsessive–Compulsive Disorder

Symptoms of postpartum generalized anxiety, panic attacks, and OCD are often included in the description of postpartum mood disturbance, and the relationship between postpartum depression and these anxiety symptoms is not fully understood. Co-morbid anxiety symptoms are particularly prominent in postpartum depression compared to non-postpartum MDD; one study demonstrated that 57% of women with postpartum-onset major depression reported obsessional thoughts compared of 36% of women with non-postpartum major depression, and that in the postpartum women obsessional thoughts were more frequent and more aggressive in nature.[133] Postpartum OCD has also been described in the absence of co-morbid postpartum MDD. Symptoms often include intrusive obsessional thoughts to harm the newborn in the absence of psychosis. Treatment with anti-obsessional agents, such as fluoxetine or clomipramine, in addition to CBT, has been effective.[134] Several investigators have also described postpartum worsening of panic disorder in women with pregravid histories of this anxiety disorder but with an absence of co-morbid depressive illness.[135]

Psychosis

Postpartum psychosis is a psychiatric emergency. The clinical picture is most often consistent with mania or a mixed state consistent with an episode of BPD[136] and can include symptoms of restlessness, agitation, sleep disturbance, paranoia, delusions, disorganized thinking, impulsivity, and behaviors that place mother and infant at risk. The typical onset is within the first 2 weeks after delivery, and symptoms can appear as early as the first 72 hours after delivery.

Although investigators have debated whether postpartum psychosis is a discrete diagnostic entity or a manifestation of BPD, treatment should follow the same algorithm to treat acute manic psychosis, including hospitalization and potential use of mood stabilizers, antipsychotics, benzodiazepines, and ECT (antidepressants should generally be avoided).

Prevention

It is difficult to reliably predict which women will experience a postpartum mood disturbance, but it is possible to identify certain sub-groups of women (e.g., women with a history of mood disorder) who are more vulnerable to postpartum affective illness. Several investigators have explored the potential efficacy of prophylactic interventions in these women at risk.

For women with a history of postpartum depression, Wisner and colleagues[137] have demonstrated in a double-blind, placebo-controlled study that there is a beneficial effect (lower rates of recurrent postpartum depression) from administering a prophylactic SSRI after delivery. Several studies demonstrate that women with a history of BPD or puerperal psychosis benefit from prophylactic treatment with lithium, instituted either before delivery (at 36 weeks of gestation) or no later than the first 48 hours following delivery.[138] Prophylactic lithium appears to significantly reduce relapse rates and diminish the severity and duration of puerperal illness.

Other studies have demonstrated the efficacy of non-pharmacologic interventions in women at risk of postpartum mood disturbance. These include interventions ranging from targeted psychotherapy, to coaching on infant behavioral interventions with the goal of reducing infant fussing and promoting sleep.[139]

In summary, postpartum depressive illness may be conceptualized along a continuum, in which some women are at lower risk for puerperal illness and others are at higher risk. Although a less aggressive, wait-and-see approach is appropriate for women with no history of postpartum psychiatric illness, women with BPD or a history of postpartum psychiatric illness deserve not only close monitoring but also specific prophylactic measures. All women should be screened for mood disturbance in the postpartum period, and referred for appropriate follow-up and treatment when indicated.

PERINATAL PSYCHIATRY: FROM SCREENING TO TREATMENT

Clinicians who manage the care of female psychiatric patients before, during, and after pregnancy may be called on to evaluate women who experience a broad spectrum of difficulties. Symptoms may be mild, although the consultant is typically requested when symptoms become severe. It is not uncommon for women to present weeks or even months after the onset of psychiatric symptoms. Many women and their healthcare providers mistakenly believe that even serious mood symptoms are normal postpartum reactions, and many women may be afraid or embarrassed to disclose that they are suffering from depression. Psychiatric disorders may emerge anew during pregnancy, although more often clinical presentations represent persistence or exacerbation of an existing illness. Physicians therefore should screen more aggressively for psychiatric disorders either before conception or during pregnancy, integrating questions about psychiatric symptoms and treatment into the obstetric history. Identification of at-risk women allows the most thoughtful, acute treatment before, during, and after pregnancy and signals the opportunity to institute prophylactic strategies that prevent psychiatric disturbances in women during the childbearing years.

Even among women with identified psychiatric illness during pregnancy, definitive treatment is often lacking or incomplete. The extent to which women suffering from postpartum psychiatric illness are under-treated as a group is also very well described. Perhaps one of the reasons for failure to treat women who have psychiatric disorders during pregnancy is the concern regarding fetal exposure to psychotropics. Many clinicians can conceptualize the need to weigh relative risks of fetal exposure on the one hand versus the risk of withholding treatment on the other. However, given the inability to absolutely quantify these risks, clinicians often defer treatment entirely and consequently put patients at risk for the sequelae of untreated maternal psychiatric illness. Clinicians should realize that the process of managing psychiatric illness during pregnancy and the puerperium is not a process like threading a needle; it is not clear-cut, and much treatment described in the literature is not evidence-based. However, thoughtful decisions can still be made with these patients as clinicians review available information with them and as clinician and patient realize that no decision is risk-free and no decision is perfect.

REFERENCES

Access the reference list online at https://expertconsult.inkling.com/.

Culture and Psychiatry

50

Justin A. Chen, M.D., M.P.H.
Michelle P. Durham, M.D., M.P.H., F.A.P.A.
Andrea Madu, B.A.
Nhi-Ha Trinh, M.D., M.P.H.
Gregory L. Fricchione, M.D.
David C. Henderson, M.D.

OVERVIEW

Race, ethnicity, and culture may all exert a tremendous impact on medical diagnosis, treatment, and outcomes. This is especially true in psychiatry, given the prominent role that culture plays in patients' interpretation and management of symptoms that fall within the affective, behavioral, and cognitive domains. Behaviors that appear bizarre in one cultural context may be perfectly acceptable in another. Although an in-depth understanding of every culture is impossible, familiarity with some basic principles will help minimize cultural clashes and reduce the risk of compromised medical care.

Understanding a patient's culture will aid in the delivery of high-quality care. However, a little knowledge can also be a dangerous thing. Variability among individuals is inevitable; a particular patient may not fit into a clinician's preconceived notion of his or her culture. Thus, the clinician must probe for clues regarding the patient's background, while remaining flexible enough to recognize when a patient's behaviors and clinical presentation do not necessarily match what is expected. The clinician should be aware of his or her own feelings, biases, and preconceptions about other cultures. In addition, the consulting psychiatrist must assess the impact of the hospital environment, the attitudes of the medical and ancillary care teams, and the patient's experience within the healthcare system. Mistrust of the healthcare system is common and may influence a patient's behavior, level of cooperation, and adherence to treatment. Furthermore, disparities in healthcare delivery have been well documented and are influenced by factors such as gender, race, ethnicity, and culture.

The role of culture in health care has become a topic of increasing importance due to rapid demographic changes in the United States. Although the US population already exhibits tremendous racial and ethnic diversity, projections expect this pattern to become further magnified in the coming decades. By 2044, non-Hispanic whites will be the minority race in the United States, and by 2060, nearly one in five of the nation's total population is projected to be foreign-born.[1] Most racial and ethnic groups are projected to experience growth between 2014 and 2060, with the largest rates of growth projected for Hispanics, Asians, and non-Hispanics of two or more races.[1]

CULTURE AND PSYCHIATRY

Culture is the collected body of beliefs, customs, and behaviors that a group (or people) acquire socially and transmit from one generation to another through symbols, shared meanings, teachings, and life experiences. It provides the tools by which members of a given society adapt to their physical environment, their social environment, and one another. It organizes groups with ready-made solutions to common problems and challenges.

Physical culture—as exemplified by art, literature, architecture, tools, machines, food, clothing, and means of transportation—can be observed directly through the five senses, and through items collected in a museum or recorded on film. Ideological culture refers to aspects of culture that must be observed indirectly, usually through specific behaviors and customs. These include beliefs and values, the reasons for considering some things sacred and other things ordinary, the characteristics and events of which a society is proud or ashamed, and the sentiments that underlie patriotism or chauvinism. Religion, philosophy, psychology, literature, and the meanings that people give to symbols are all part of the ideological aspect of culture. The physical level of culture yields more easily to change and to adaptation than does the ideological level, but without some understanding of the ideological aspect of culture, it is difficult to understand the meaning of a group purely at the physical level.

Each society establishes its own criteria regarding which forms of behavior are acceptable or abnormal, and which represent a medical problem. Learning more about an individual's culture and/or working with bilingual and bicultural interpreters can help to clarify normal and abnormal behaviors. It is also important to recognize that an individual may be influenced by multiple cultures or subcultures. The consulting psychiatrist must often employ the skills of a detective to verify whether a patient's statements or beliefs are appropriate to his or her environment, heritage, and culture.

Cultural Differences in Illness Presentation

Cultural differences in the presentation of psychiatric illnesses abound. For example, a woman originally from South Korea may present with chief complaints of dizziness, fatigue, and back pain, while she ignores other neurovegetative symptoms of depression, and is unable to describe feelings of dysphoria. American mental healthcare providers are generally unfamiliar with various Indo-Chinese cultural syndromes and culturally specific meanings attributed to certain symptoms.[2,3] For example, the Laotian way of describing feeling "tense" is feeling "like a balloon blown up until it is about to burst." Westermeyer,[4] in a case–controlled study in Laos, documented the general inability of Western psychiatrists to recognize the Laotian symptoms of depression. On the other hand, common American expressions, such as "feeling blue," cannot be readily translated into many other languages. A Cambodian clinician will ask Cambodian patients if they "feel blue" by using Khmer terms, which literally translate as "heavy, overcast, gloomy."

Similarly, the phenomenology of panic disorder may vary among minority groups within the United States. Compared with their Caucasian peers, for example, African Americans with panic disorder report more intense fears of dying or going crazy, as well as higher levels of numbing and tingling in their extremities, and exhibit higher rates of co-morbid post-traumatic stress disorder (PTSD) and depression. African Americans also use somewhat different coping strategies (e.g., religious practice and "counting one's blessings"), and endorse less self-blame. Cambodian populations may understand panic-like symptoms as *khyâl cap* (literally, "wind attacks") caused by *khyâl*, a wind-like substance, rising up in the body and causing a range of serious effects, including compressing the lungs or entering the cranium.[5]

Accurate evaluation of the meaning and significance of seemingly bizarre beliefs, hallucinations, and psychotic-like symptoms among diverse populations remains a clinical challenge. For example, a Puerto Rican woman who acknowledges hearing the voices of her ancestors may not be psychotic, as this phenomenon is relatively common among Caribbean Latinos in the absence of a thought disorder.[6] In many traditional, non-Western societies, spirits of the deceased are regarded as capable of interacting with, and possessing, those still alive. It may be difficult for the clinician to determine whether symptoms are bizarre enough to yield a diagnosis of a primary psychotic disorder without an adequate understanding of a patient's sociocultural and religious background. On the other hand, caution must be taken not to assume that bizarre symptoms are culturally appropriate when in fact they are a manifestation of psychiatric illness. A culture may interpret abnormal behavior as relating to some kind of voodoo or anger and therefore regard the symptoms as normal even though they are in fact consistent with a primary psychotic disorder. The use of bilingual and bicultural interpreters, along with the search for information from other sources (e.g., family, community leaders, religious officials) and attention to other more objective features of psychiatric illness (e.g., poor self-care, deterioration of personal and professional relationships) may help determine whether an individual's behavior is culturally acceptable or evidence of a psychiatric illness.

Western clinicians who search only for physiologic explanations for somatic complaints such as back pain, tinnitus, headaches, palpitations, and dizziness may miss depression or anxiety. Afflicted patients are often prescribed meclizine for dizziness and analgesics for pain by their primary care providers, when an antidepressant or anxiolytic would have been most appropriate. The appropriate diagnosis and treatment will only be elucidated if sufficient time and attention are spent understanding the cultural factors affecting an individual's distress, a process that is described further in the following section.

Cultural Assessment for Clinicians

The *Diagnostic and Statistical Manual of Mental Disorders*, 5th edition (DSM-5)[7] introduced a number of conceptual innovations with regard to the role of culture in psychiatric diagnosis and treatment. These included direct cross-referencing of multicultural explanations for clusters of symptoms within the descriptions of each DSM-5 disorder, more detailed and structured information about cultural concepts of distress, and expanded clinical interviewing tools to facilitate person-centered and culturally focused assessments. In addition, DSM-5 went further than any previous versions of the manual in its explicit assertion that "all forms of distress are locally shaped, including the DSM disorders."[7]

DSM-5 provides clinicians with two practical tools to help clinicians produce a nuanced cultural assessment: the Outline for Cultural Formulation (OCF), and the Cultural Formulation Interview (CFI), both of which bear further description here, given this chapter's focus on the role of culture in psychiatry.

The *Outline for Cultural Formulation* describes five distinct domains, as shown below, that can be used to describe an individual's ethnic and cultural context as related to psychiatric illness.

Cultural Identity of the Individual

Ethnic or cultural references and the degree to which an individual is involved with his or her culture of origin versus the host culture are all critical to understanding that individual's identity. Clinicians should delve into this topic using open-ended questions with reference to cultural and social context, recognition of the hybrid nature of cultures, and the possibility of change over time.[8] For instance, an Asian American man who grew up in the Southern United States may exhibit patterns, behaviors, and views of the world that are more consistent with those of a Caucasian Southerner. Attention to language abilities and preferences must also be addressed. Other important aspects of cultural identity may include religious affiliation, socioeconomic background, sexual orientation, gender identity, country of origin, and migration history.

Cultural Conceptualizations of Distress

How an individual understands and experiences his or her symptoms is often communicated through cultural syndromes and idioms of distress (e.g., *nervios*/"nerves," possession by spirits, somatic complaints, misfortune). Individuals may also make sense of their experience in terms of a specific sequence of events or prior episodes of illness.[8] Thus, the meaning and severity of an illness in relation to one's culture, family, community, and personal history should be elicited. The resultant explanatory model, in conjunction with past and current expectations of care, may prove extraordinarily helpful when developing an interpretation of symptoms, a diagnosis, and a treatment plan.

Psychosocial Stressors and Cultural Features of Vulnerability and Resilience

Culture exerts significant impacts at the level of the psychosocial environment—e.g., religion, family, social circle—and also significantly influences interpretations of stress, social support, and level of disability versus function. It is the physician's responsibility to determine a patient's level of functioning, resilience, and disability in the context of his or her cultural reference groups.[8]

Cultural Features of the Relationship Between the Individual and the Clinician

Clinicians should consider the cultural factors that affect both their relationship with the patient and the treatment itself. These could include difficulties with language (e.g., language discordance between treater and patient), establishing rapport, and eliciting symptoms or understanding their cultural significance. The consulting psychiatrist must also attend to the specific hospital environment in which the patient is receiving treatment. Interventions focused on these factors may improve the comfort of patients and providers alike as well as the quality of care more than any somatic therapy.

Overall Cultural Assessment

The formulation concludes with a summary of the implications of each component outlined above for psychiatric diagnosis, treatment, and other clinically relevant issues. This step directly acknowledges the fact that each society establishes its own criteria regarding which forms of behavior are acceptable or abnormal, and which behaviors represent a medical problem.

The DSM-5 also includes the *Cultural Formulation Interview* (CFI), which consists of 16 questions that physicians can use in a more structured manner to assess the impact of culture on an individual's clinical presentation and care. The CFI focuses on four domains: cultural definition of the problem; cultural perceptions of the cause, context, and support of the problem; cultural factors affecting self-coping and past help-seeking; and, cultural factors affecting current help seeking. The interview aims to avoid stereotyping, as it centers on the individual and incorporates the cultural knowledge of the patient as well as the social context of his or her illness experience. The CFI may be utilized when physicians experience difficulties in diagnostic assessment due to cultural differences, difficulties in determining illness severity or impairment, disagreements with patients regarding course of treatment, or difficulties engaging patients in treatment.

Cultural Concepts of Distress

The previous version of the DSM, DSM-IV-TR,[9] included a list of 25 "culture-bound syndromes" (also known as culture-specific syndromes or folk illnesses), defined as a combination of psychiatric and somatic symptoms considered to be a recognizable disease within a specific society or culture (i.e., not a voluntary behavior or false claim), not recognized as a disease in other cultures, and not associated with objective biochemical or structural alterations of body organs or functions. Examples of such syndromes included well-known entities such as *ataque de nervios*, *dhat* syndrome, and *shenjing shuairuo*.

The concept of culture-bound syndromes has been eliminated in DSM-5 and replaced with three related concepts: *cultural syndromes*, *cultural idioms of distress*, and *cultural explanations or perceived causes*.[7] The rationale for this change is that focusing on culture-bound syndromes "overemphasized the local particularity and limited distribution of cultural concepts of distress."[7] Additionally, the term "culture-bound syndrome" does not take into account that some "syndromes" are actually variations in ways people experience distress rather than distinct collections of symptoms (e.g., *nervios*), while others are causal explanations for a range of symptoms (e.g., *dhat* syndrome).

Cultural syndromes are clusters of symptoms that occur among individuals in specific cultural groups or communities. *Cultural idioms of distress* are shared ways of experiencing, communicating, and expressing personal or social concerns. *Cultural explanations or perceived causes* are labels, attributions, or features that indicate causation of symptoms, illness, or distress. As an example, depression fulfills the criteria for all three concepts. Western clinicians understand major depressive disorder as a "syndrome," or a cluster of symptoms that often appear together. Depression is also a cultural idiom of distress which is commonly used to talk about a certain clustering of physical and emotional symptoms. Finally, as a cultural explanation of distress or perceived cause, the term "depression" helps imbue a set of behaviors with meaning and associated etiology.

Despite these conceptual and semantic changes, DSM-5 continues to acknowledge the well-accepted place of culture-bound syndromes in psychiatric nosology and practice, and includes a glossary of some of the most well-recognized "cultural concepts of distress," summarized in Table 50-1.

Acculturation and Immigration

As described above, by 2060, nearly one in five of the nation's total population is projected to be foreign-born.[1] Recent

TABLE 50-1 Cultural Concepts of Distress

SYNDROME	POPULATIONS
Ataque de nervios	Caribbean, Latin American, and Latin Mediterranean groups
Dhat syndrome (*semen loss*)	South-east Asia
Khyâl cap	Cambodia
Kufungisisa	Shona of Zimbabwe
Maladi moun	Haiti
Nervios	Hispanics in the United States, Mexico, Central America, and South America
Shenjing shuairuo (neurasthenia)	China; Traditional Chinese Medicine
Susto (fright or soul loss)[17]	Hispanics in the United States, Mexico, Central America, and South America
Taijin kyofusho	Japan

immigrants or refugees often arrive in the United States with a host of psychosocial challenges. Clinicians should ask about, and make an effort to understand, the circumstances surrounding immigration. An individual may have been a political prisoner or a victim of trauma and torture, or he or she may have been separated suddenly from family members. Under these circumstances, the level of depression and PTSD symptoms may be high. There is abundant literature documenting the contribution of acculturative stresses to the emergence of mental symptoms and disorders, including depression, anxiety, "culture shock," and PTSD.[10]

The trauma and torture experienced by many refugees are unfamiliar to most American practitioners.[2] While limited research does exist on refugee trauma and trauma-related psychiatric disorders and social handicaps, along with numerous reports of the concentration camp experiences in Cambodia, the sexual abuse of Vietnamese boat women, and the serious emotional distress associated with escape, refugee camps, and resettlement experiences, much more research is needed in this area.[11,12]

Impact of Race/Ethnicity on Psychiatric Diagnosis and Treatment

In the United States, race and ethnicity have a significant impact on psychiatric diagnosis and treatment.[13,14] The need to reduce disparities in the mental health care of racial and ethnic minorities was vividly underscored by the Supplement on Culture, Race, and Ethnicity to the United States Surgeon General's landmark 2001 Report on Mental Health,[15] yet such disparities continue to persist. For example, African American and Latino patients are disproportionately diagnosed with psychotic disorders compared to their Caucasian counterparts, and parallel findings are documented in other countries globally when comparing immigrant minority patients to the majority race.[16]

The reasons for misdiagnosis are complicated. They include the fact that individuals from some ethnic or cultural backgrounds may present to the medical system later in the course of their illness than do Caucasian individuals, resulting in the perception of a more severe illness.[16] The late presentation itself may be related at least in part to mistrust of the healthcare system. Language barriers and unfamiliarity with cultural norms can contribute to misinterpretation and misattribution of patients' symptoms. Physician biases also play a major role in misdiagnosis. Psychiatric diagnoses are generally established by eliciting symptoms from patients that are then interpreted by a clinician. Different disorders have overlapping symptoms that can be used to support one diagnosis or disregard another, depending on the clinician's bias or initial impression. In the case of African Americans, affective symptoms are frequently ignored and psychotic symptoms are emphasized. This pattern has also been seen in other ethnic populations, including Hispanics, some Asian populations, and the Amish in the United States.[17]

Moreover, treatment decisions may also be affected by race. African American patients are more likely to receive higher doses of antipsychotic medications, to be prescribed depot preparations of antipsychotics, to have higher rates of involuntary psychiatric hospitalizations, and to undergo seclusion and physical restraint while in psychiatric hospitals.[14,18] One interpretation of these statistics is that medical practitioners have a tendency to over-sedate African American patients to reduce their perceived risk of violence despite, in some cases, little evidence that such a risk existed.

WORKING WITH INTERPRETERS

Miscommunication is common even between clinicians and patients who speak the same language and come from similar socioeconomic backgrounds. Therefore, it is not difficult to imagine the challenges and obstacles that arise when patients exhibit low or limited English proficiency (LEP) and exhibit some of the cultural variations in behavior and symptom expression described above. Misunderstandings may lead to misdiagnosis and result in unnecessary or inappropriate treatment.[19] Patients, in turn, may feel frustrated, discouraged, or dissatisfied, leading them to refuse treatment or avoid care altogether.[20] Fortunately, skillful use of an interpreter can help bridge at least some of the communication gap between doctors and non-English-speaking patients and is essential to providing high-quality care to patients from non-English-speaking backgrounds.[21,22]

Many states now have laws that require federally funded medical facilities to provide interpreters for their non-English-speaking patients. While most medical interpreters must be trained and certified to work with healthcare providers, interpreting within a psychiatric context poses a number of unique challenges. Some of the common issues include:[23]

- Clinicians may feel they have less control in their work because their direct contact with the patient is decreased by the presence of the interpreter.
- Clinicians may feel uncertain about their role when working with interpreters who are more active and involved in the treatment process.
- Clinicians may have transference issues toward the interpreter.
- Conflicts may arise when clinicians and interpreters hold opposing views on a patient's diagnosis and treatment plans.
- Clinicians may feel frustrated when they cannot verify what is being said to the patient.
- Clinicians may feel left out if the patient appears to have more of a connection with the interpreter.
- Interpreters may feel uncomfortable when asked to translate certain issues (e.g., sexual history or childhood abuse).

Recommendations When Working With Interpreters

Clinicians need to know the qualifications of interpreters. Does the interpreter have experience working with mental health clinicians? How much does he or she know about psychiatric disorders and their treatment? What are the interpreter's personal views about mental illness? Interpreters who come from cultures in which mental illness is highly stigmatized may bring those biases or beliefs into the therapeutic process. Clinicians should meet with the interpreter briefly before each session to discuss expectations and clarify any issues or points that the clinician would like to address during the session.[23,24]

Clinicians should avoid using family members or friends as interpreters.[24,25] Patients may be unwilling to disclose sensitive information in front of these individuals, and it may be too distressing for a young child to hear details about a parent's symptoms. Family members have been known to omit or alter information they feel is too embarrassing or inappropriate to reveal to a clinician. Janitors and clerical staff have been used as interpreters in the medical setting, a practice that is strongly discouraged due to concerns about the adequacy of their knowledge of medical or mental health terminology.

Trained interpreters should be treated as professional colleagues by clinicians.[24] Most interpreters can offer important cultural knowledge that can help promote the clinician–patient relationship and facilitate deeper understanding of the patient's culture, religion, and worldview. However, some clinicians prefer to use interpreters as word-for-word translation machines with no additional attempts to interpret or filter the meaning behind the patient's statements. Although such an approach allows the clinician to maintain his or her role as the primary caregiver and an illusion of control over what is being said to the patient, in reality, using direct translations can often lead to misunderstandings and confusion for both patients and clinicians alike. Literal translations from one language to another are often inaccurate and inappropriate. Certain words or concepts, such as depression and mental health, may not exist in the patient's native language. In addition, certain issues may be culturally inappropriate to discuss with a patient. For example, many women from Asian backgrounds feel uncomfortable when asked directly about topics such as sexual abuse or family discord. Interpreters can be used as cultural consultants to help clinicians navigate these more complex issues. Allowing interpreters the freedom and flexibility to re-phrase or summarize what is being said can help prevent misunderstandings and improve the exchange between the clinician and the patient.

Time is a crucial factor when interpreters are involved. Interpreters often have to explain psychiatric concepts to the patient, a process that may require much more time than expected. Clinicians must be patient, bearing in mind that it may take 10 minutes to translate a single word. Patients do not get as much time with the clinician when communication must be accomplished through an interpreter, and clinicians may feel frustrated by the relative inefficiency of the process. Clinicians should maximize their time with the patient by deferring any discussions with the interpreters that can wait until after the session.

Clinicians should always remember to introduce the interpreter to the patient at the start of the session if they have not met. This is also a good time to reaffirm issues of confidentiality.[23,24] Because many ethnic communities are small and close-knit, patients may fear that the interpreter will divulge their private information to others and therefore be less willing to speak candidly. If possible, clinicians should try to use the same interpreter over time to help build trust and ensure continuity of care for the patient.[25]

During the session, the clinician should face and speak directly to the patient rather than the interpreter to facilitate connection through eye contact, gestures of acknowledgment, and other non-verbal behaviors.[26] The clinician should speak slowly, pause often, and avoid long sentences and technical jargon. It is important for both the clinician and interpreter to feel comfortable asking for clarification. Two-way conversations should be avoided. Tension may arise when someone in the group feels left out.

After each session, the clinician should encourage the interpreter to give his or her impression of the session. The interpreter often can provide important observations and feedback about cultural and non-verbal factors that may not have been apparent based solely on the patient's spoken responses.[21] Clinicians can use this time to learn more from the interpreter about the patient's culture. In sum, good communication, trust, and teamwork between the clinician and interpreter are essential when caring for patients with low or limited English proficiency.

THE "MEDICAL OMBUDSMAN" ROLE

In 1988, Pasnau[27] enumerated six fundamental functions of the consultation–liaison psychiatrist, including the role of "medical ombudsman" for the patient. Although the use of this term did not catch on, it signified the sometimes important need of medical and surgical teams to be reminded of the unique human nature of each patient in their care. Racial, ethnic, and cultural factors are obviously important characteristics in this regard. Psychiatrists in the general hospital can pay attention to these factors in their consultations and, as a result, enrich patient care.

ETHNICITY, CULTURE, AND PSYCHIATRIC MEDICATIONS

There is a large and growing body of research on ethnopsychopharmacology, or the study of racial and ethnic differences in how individuals respond to medications. Additionally, a number of non-biological cultural factors are known to significantly affect minority patients' relationship to and use of psychotropic medications. A familiarity with the basic principles in both these areas is necessary for effectively treating diverse populations.

Cultural Factors in Psychotropic Medication Usage

Culturally shaped beliefs play a major role in determining whether a particular explanation about an illness and recommended treatment plan (explanatory model) will make sense to a patient; for example, Hispanics and Asians often expect rapid relief with treatment. Chinese and Vietnamese patients often express significant concerns about addictive and toxic potential of Western medications. Many immigrant East and South Asian populations prefer traditional approaches to address their symptoms (e.g., Traditional Chinese Medicine, Ayurvedic medicine, or *kampo*), all of which may rely on a mixture of different herbal medicines. Adherents to these traditions may believe that polypharmacy is more effective.

The use of herbal medicines carries with it the risk of drug interactions and medical or psychiatric side effects or toxicity. The Food and Drug Administration (FDA) has issued a number of warnings on herbal medicine products, including the most popular weight loss products containing

Ephedra sinica (*ma huang*), which is the main plant source of ephedrine and has been reported to cause mania, psychosis, and sudden death. The Japanese herbs *Swertia japonica* and *Kamikihi-to*, and the Cuban *Datura candida*, have anticholinergic properties that may interact with tricyclic antidepressants (TCAs) or with low-potency neuroleptics. South American holly, *Ilex guayusa*, has a high caffeine content. The Nigerian root extract of *Schumanniophyton problematicum* (used to treat psychosis) is sedating and may interact with neuroleptics and with benzodiazepines. The Chinese herbs *Fructose schisandrae*, *Corydalis bungeana*, *Kopsia officinalis*, *Clausena lansium*, *muscone*, ginseng, and *Glycyrrhiza* increase the clearance of many psychotropic medications by stimulation of cytochrome P450 (CYP) enzymes. Oleanolic acid in *Swertia mileensis* and *Ligustrum lucidum* inhibits CYP enzymes.

On the other hand, for some patients and for certain conditions, herbal remedies may produce significant benefits. The clinician should not foreclose discussion of complementary and alternative treatments through judgmental or disparaging comments, but rather use these topics to open up a discussion about the patient's illness explanatory model and preferred treatment. The Engagement Interview Protocol (EIP) is one tool for facilitating a culturally respectful negotiation when the patient's and clinician's explanatory models differ.[28] (See Chapter 42 for more information on herbal remedies.)

Communication difficulties and divergence between a patient's and a clinician's explanatory model play important roles in why a patient from an ethnic minority is significantly more likely to drop out of treatment. Exploring these beliefs will improve communication, adherence, and outcome.

Patient compliance may be affected by medication side effects, incorrect dosing due to differences in pharmacokinetics (see next section), and polypharmacy. Other factors include: a poor therapeutic alliance; a lack of community support, money, or transportation; and concerns about the addictiveness of a medication.

Understanding and addressing each patient's social support systems is crucial. The ways in which a family interacts and functions may have a significant impact on psychiatric treatment. For example, some Hispanic patients may be accustomed to relying on extended family for medical decision-making and may become demoralized if their relatives are not involved in their treatment. Hispanics and Asians have been described as relying on "closed networks" consisting of family members, kin, and intimate friends.

Biological Aspects of Psychopharmacology

Pharmacokinetics deal with absorption, distribution, metabolism, excretion, and blood levels of medications. Pharmacokinetics can be influenced by biochemical processes, such as conjugation, plasma protein-binding, and oxidation by the cytochrome [CYP]P450 isoenzymes, as well as by characteristics of the individual (including genetics, age, gender, total body weight, and medical co-morbidities). Environmental factors that affect pharmacokinetics include dietary factors, sex hormones, and use of caffeine, tobacco, alcohol, herbal medicines, steroids, as well as ingestion of other prescription or illicit drugs.

The baseline activity of CYP liver enzymes is determined genetically, although environmental factors can alter their activity. Understanding how pharmacokinetic and environmental factors interact in different populations can help the clinician predict side effects, blood levels, and potential drug–drug interactions. For example, CYP2D6 is the isoenzyme that metabolizes many antidepressants (including the tricyclic and heterocyclic antidepressants and the selective serotonin re-uptake inhibitors [SSRIs]); SSRIs can inhibit this enzyme, leading to accumulation of other substrates. CYP2D6 also plays a role in metabolizing antipsychotics such as clozapine, haloperidol, perphenazine, risperidone, thioridazine, and sertindole. Although much emphasis has been placed on CYP2D6's metabolism of psychotropic medications, it is also a major enzyme for the metabolism of numerous non-psychotropic medications as well. This fact, which is often ignored clinically, can have a significant effect on the tolerability or toxicity of a wide range of medications.

The incidence of poor metabolizers at the CYP2D6 isoenzyme ranges from 3% to 10% in Caucasians; 1.9% to 7.3% in African Americans; 2.2% to 6.6% in Hispanics; and approximately 0% to 4.8% in Asians.[29,30] Another genetic variation of the metabolizer gene leads to "intermediate metabolizers," or individuals who exhibit CYP 2D6 activity that is between that of poor (little or no CYP2D6 function) and extensive metabolizers (normal CYP2D6 function). Approximately 18% of Mexican Americans and 33% of Asian Americans and African Americans have this gene variation. This may help explain ethnic differences in the pharmacokinetics of neuroleptics and antidepressants. Although these individuals are not as likely to experience toxicity at extremely low doses (e.g., poor metabolizers), they are likely to experience significant side effects at lower doses. These individuals may be mistakenly classified as "difficult patients" because they complain of side effects at unexpectedly low doses.

CYP2D6*4 (CYP2D6B) appears to be responsible for poor metabolizers in Caucasians. CYP2D6*17 and CYP2D6*10 are found in individuals of African and Asian origin, respectively, and are responsible for lower enzyme activity (intermediate or slow metabolizers). Individuals from these backgrounds are at great risk for toxicity, even when medications are used at low doses. For instance, a woman who develops hypotension and a change in mental status several days after starting 20 mg of nortriptyline may be found to have toxic blood levels and require cardiac monitoring. Table 50-2 lists drugs that are metabolized through different CYP enzyme systems.

Finally, lithium appears to be a drug with significant differences in dosing and tolerability across populations. African Americans are more likely to experience lithium toxicity and delirium compared with Caucasians (likely related to a slower lithium–sodium pathway and connected to higher rates of hypertension). Individuals from East Asian backgrounds with bipolar disorder may respond to lower doses of lithium as compared with their Caucasian counterparts, with literature suggesting they can be successfully maintained at lower serum levels of 0.4 to 0.8 mEq/L.[31]

The choice of medications, particularly atypical antipsychotics, should be tempered by an understanding of

TABLE 50-2 Cytochrome P450 Isoenzymes, Substrates, Inhibitors, and Inducers

CYP	CYP1A2	CYP2C9/10	CYP2C19	CYP2D6	CYP2E1	CYP3A3/4
Inhibitors	Fluvoxamine Moclobemide Cimetidine Fluoroquinolones Ciprofloxacin Norfloxacin Naringenin (grapefruit) Ticlopidine	Fluvoxamine Disulfiram Amiodarone Azapropazone D-propoxyphene Fluconazole Fluvastatin Miconazole Phenylbutazone Stiripentol Sulfaphenazole Zafirlukast	Fluoxetine Fluvoxamine Imipramine Moclobemide Tranylcypromine Diazepam Felbamate Phenytoin Topiramate Cimetidine Omeprazole	Bupropion Fluoxetine Fluvoxamine Hydroxybupropion Paroxetine Sertraline Moclobemide Fluphenazine Haloperidol Perphenazine Thioridazine Amiodarone Cimetidine Methadone Quinidine Ritonavir	Diethylithio-carbamate (disulfiram)	Fluoxetine Fluvoxamine Nefazodone Sertraline Diltiazem Verapamil Dexamethasone Gestodene Clarithromycin Erythromycin Troleandomycin Fluconazole Itraconazole Ketoconazole Ritonavir Indinavir Amiodarone Cimetidine Mibefradil Naringenin (grapefruit) Isoniazid
Inducers	Tobacco Omeprazole	Barbiturates Phenytoin Rifampin		Rifampin		Ethanol Carbamazepine Barbiturates Phenobarbital Phenytoin Dexamethasone Rifampin Troglitazone

Table continued on next page

TABLE 50-2 Cytochrome P450 Isoenzymes, Substrates, Inhibitors, and Inducers—cont'd

CYP	CYP1A2	CYP2C9/10	CYP2C19	CYP2D6	CYP2E1	CYP3A3/4	
Substrates							
	Tertiary amine TCAs	THC	Citalopram	Fluoxetine	Ethanol	Carbamazepine	Amiodarone
	Clozapine	NSAIDs	Moclobemide	Mirtazapine	Acetaminophen	Alprazolam	Disopyramide
	Olanzapine	Phenytoin	Tertiary amine TCAs	Paroxetine	Chlorzoxazone	Diazepam	Lidocaine
	Caffeine	Tolbutamide	Diazepam	Venlafaxine	Halothane	Midazolam	Propafenone
	Methadone	Warfarin	Hexobarbital	Secondary and tertiary	Isoflurane	Triazolam	Quinidine
	Tacrine	Losartan	Mephobarbital	amine TCAs	Methoxyflurane	Buspirone	Erythromycin
	Acetaminophen	Irbesartan	Omeprazole	Trazodone	Sevoflurane	Citalopram	Androgens
	Phenacetin		Lansoprazole	Clozapine		Mirtazapine	Dexamethasone
	Propranolol		Phenytoin	Haloperidol		Nefazodone	Estrogens
	Theophylline		S-Mephenytoin	Fluphenazine		Reboxetine	Astemizole
	Warfarin		Nelfinavir	Perphenazine		Sertraline	Loratadine
			Warfarin	Risperidone		Tertiary amine TCAs	Terfenadine
				Sertindole		Sertindole	Lovastatin
				Thioridazine		Quetiapine	Simvastatin
				Codeine		Ziprasidone	Atorvastatin
				Dextromethorphan		Diltiazem	Cerivastatin
				Hydrocodone		Felodipine	Cyclophosphamide
				Oxycodone		Nimodipine	Tamoxifen
				Mexiletine		Nifedipine	Vincristine
				Propafenone (IC		Nisoldipine	Vinblastine
				antiarrhythmics)		Nitrendipine	Ifosfamide
				β-Blockers		Verapamil	Cyclosporine
				Donepezil		Acetaminophen	Tacrolimus
				D-Fenfluramine		Alfentanil	Cisapride
						Codeine	Donepezil
						Fentanyl	Lovastatin
						Sufentanil	Protease inhibitors
						Ethosuximide	Sildenafil
						Tiagabine	Disopyramide
						Warfarin	Losartan

NSAID, non-steroidal anti-inflammatory drug; TCA, tricyclic antidepressant; THC, tetrahydrocannabinol.

individual and population risk factors for medical morbidities (e.g., obesity, hypertension, diabetes mellitus, cardiovascular disease). For instance, many of the reports of diabetic ketoacidosis secondary to atypical antipsychotics have been in African Americans, who are at higher risk for diabetes.[32,33]

CASE 1

Mrs. E, a 30-year-old woman with obsessive–compulsive disorder originally from China, was recovering in the postpartum unit of a general hospital after giving birth to a healthy baby boy. She reported suicidal ideation and psychiatry was consulted. On interview, Mrs. E told the psychiatrist that ever since giving birth, she had experienced increasingly violent and ego-dystonic intrusive thoughts that she might harm her son and her husband, e.g., by stabbing them with a knife. These thoughts were so distressing that she felt she would be better off dead rather than expose her family to her potentially violent actions.

Recognizing the potential significance of cultural factors in this case, the psychiatrist made sure to request the same Mandarin-speaking interpreter whenever possible when interacting with the patient. She devoted some time to getting to know the interpreter, and learned that the interpreter had a good grasp of psychiatric illnesses and did not consider them shameful or representative of individual weakness. The psychiatrist also adopted an attitude of cultural humility and spent more time than she usually would have eliciting Mrs. E's own beliefs surrounding her symptoms and treatment. The psychiatrist learned that the patient had a long history of being bullied and treated as an outcast with regard to her long history of obsessive–compulsive disorder due to the stigmatization of mental illness in Chinese culture, and that she was reluctant to take psychiatric medications due to fears of addiction and toxicity. She also learned from the interpreter that suicide may be seen as a viable option to some Chinese patients when confronted with insurmountable odds or shameful feelings.

In her treatment plan, the psychiatrist focused on psychoeducation about obsessive–compulsive disorder and attempting to reduce feelings of stigma and shame. She allied with the patient's desire to be a good mother and convinced her to initiate treatment for her symptoms with a selective serotonin re-uptake inhibitor, taking extra time to address the patient's concerns about potential side effects. She also utilized cognitive-behavioral therapy techniques to gently challenge the patient's obsessions as well as her belief that suicide would result in a better future for her family. The patient felt understood and validated by the psychiatrist. Her suicidal ideation and obsessions gradually diminished with a combination of medications and psychotherapy, and she was ultimately discharged from the hospital with appointments for outpatient mental health follow-up.

RECOMMENDATIONS FOR OPTIMIZING CLINICAL CARE OF DIVERSE POPULATIONS

Helpful Techniques

Certain techniques may help to avoid misdiagnosis, mistreatment, and cultural clashes. The first moments of an encounter are often crucial. A clinician must be mindful of maintaining a respectful attitude, and may find it particularly useful to address patients from different ethnic backgrounds more formally (e.g., Mr., Ms., or Mrs.). In some cultures, an informal introduction is considered disrespectful and may have a lasting impact on the physician–patient relationship.

Forging an alliance with patients from diverse backgrounds may be more complex and require more time. It may also take extra time and effort to assure patients about confidentiality, to provide psychoeducation about mental illness to counteract cultural stigmas, and to work with interpreters. If the diagnosis is unclear or affected by ethnicity or culture, the clinician should consider utilizing a structured diagnostic interview (e.g., the tools from DSM-5, such as the OCF or the CFI) to reduce the possibility of misdiagnosis, and should consider seeking consultation from other members of the patient's community regarding which aspects of the presentation might be culturally influenced as opposed to representing pathology (taking care, of course, to protect the patient's privacy in the process). The services of a trained medical interpreter should be utilized whenever possible.

Moving Beyond "Cultural Competence" and Toward "Cultural Humility"

The idea of "cultural competence" has been challenged on both conceptual and semantic grounds. The term has been noted to be problematic in its implication that culture can be reduced to "a technical skill for which clinicians can be trained to develop expertise."[34] Further, a focus on attaining "cultural competence" has been criticized as reinforcing the notion of culture as a static and categorical "other" to be mastered, which may reduce a patient's ethnicity to a stereotyped core set of beliefs and values that may trivialize the role of culture in medical illness and treatment.[35]

Instead of striving for "competence," an alternative framework is that of "cultural respect" or "cultural humility." Cultural humility has been defined as the "ability to maintain an interpersonal stance that is open in relation to aspects of cultural identity that are most important to the patient."[36] The culturally humble physician is able to express respect and a lack of superiority with regard to the patient's culture, and does not assume competence in terms of working with a particular patient simply based on prior experience working with other patients from a similar population or cultural background.

REFERENCES

 Access the reference list online at https://expertconsult.inkling.com/.

Legal Aspects of Consultation

51

Ronald Schouten, M.D., J.D.
Rebecca Weintraub Brendel, M.D., J.D.

OVERVIEW

Legal issues are common and acknowledged, although rarely welcomed, aspects of modern medicine. Physicians respond to these issues in various ways, ranging from denial of their existence, to resentment at the perceived intrusion into the patient care they create, to obsessive concern that can ultimately interfere with good clinical care.

Although it is true that legal issues are ever-present, and at times are the dominant concerns of patients and providers, for the most part, they exist in the background of care. When specific legal issues do arise, medical and surgical physicians often turn to the consultation psychiatrist for assistance (perhaps because the most common legal issues that arise—decision-making capacity and treatment refusal—have to do with mental functions and abnormalities of behavior). Whatever the reason, the psychiatric consultant may be drawn into a turbulent atmosphere when medical and surgical staff are confronted with a legal issue. The well-prepared consultant can be invaluable in these matters.

The first and perhaps most important service provided by the consultant is to remind the consultee that the physician's safest havens within the law are the principles of good faith, common sense, and good clinical care. To be of maximum assistance, consultants should be familiar with relevant legal concepts, and use this knowledge to diminish consultees' anxiety and help them perform their jobs. The challenge for the psychiatric consultant is to ease the burden of the consultee by providing clinical insights and legal information and to know when and how to use the input of the hospital attorney.

Medicine advanced rapidly in the 20th century and continues to do so in the 21st, giving rise to an evolving array of medico-legal issues. These issues are reflected in questions asked by residents and staff alike. How do I determine whether a patient is incompetent? If the patient is competent and making an irrational decision, does that decision have to be honored? What is my liability exposure as a consultant? If a managed care organization refuses to pay for continued hospitalization or for a patient's admission to a psychiatric facility, can the physician be held liable if the patient commits suicide? If the patient has expressed a desire to hurt someone else, what are my obligations to that third party? What obligations do I have if my patient is human immunodeficiency virus (HIV)-positive and refuses to inform his or her sexual partner?

This chapter cannot provide definitive answers to these and all the other medico-legal questions faced by general hospital psychiatrists. Rather, this chapter outlines general principles that apply in almost all jurisdictions. Because state statutes and case law vary considerably on these medico-legal matters, hospital counsel and legal representatives of medical organizations and insurers should be consulted. They are excellent sources of information about legal aspects of general hospital psychiatry.

PHYSICIANS' RIGHTS AND OBLIGATIONS

Malpractice Liability

Malpractice, *negligence*, and *liability* are three terms that engender great concern and are often misunderstood. Malpractice law is a type of personal injury or tort law that concerns itself with injuries allegedly caused by the negligent treatment activities of professionals. To establish a claim of malpractice, a plaintiff (the complaining party) must prove four things. First, it must be proved that the defendant physician owed a duty to the injured party. Where the injured party is the patient, the duty is to perform up to the standards of the average physician in the community practicing in that specialty. Failure to practice in accordance with that standard, unless there is some justification, constitutes the second element: negligence. The third and fourth elements are closely tied to the first two: the negligent behavior has to be shown to have been the direct cause of actual damages. In the event that all four elements are proved, the defendant may be held liable (responsible for the damage) and ordered to pay compensation to the plaintiff, either directly or through his or her insurer.[1–5] The four elements of malpractice are often summarized as the four Ds: duty, dereliction of duty, direct causation, and damages.

Malpractice liability exposure can be a concern for psychiatric consultants as well as other clinicians. Treating clinicians have the primary duty of care for the patient. Consultants, who by definition are brought in to provide advice to the treating clinicians, do not have the same duty to the patient. The consultant's duty of reasonable care is owed to the consultee, not the patient. This rule does not hold, however, where the consultant steps out of the purely consultative role and assumes direct responsibility for some aspect of the treatment relationship. For example, the consultant who evaluates a patient and then advises the treating physician that a course of antidepressant treatment is appropriate is not liable for an adverse outcome from the treatment. If, however, the consultant writes the prescription and monitors the treatment course, he or she has assumed the status of the "treating physician" and may be held responsible for any adverse outcomes.[6,7]

Liability and Managed Care

Managed care and liability for injury when coverage is denied have been important issues ever since managed care arrived in force on the healthcare scene. The basic problem can be seen in this hypothetical example.

> **CASE 1**
>
> Mr. A was admitted to the trauma unit after leaping off a bridge into the river. After open reduction and internal fixation of his bilateral femoral fractures, the psychiatric consultant saw him. Mr. A was found to be suffering from major depression as well as alcohol abuse. He was believed to be at a moderate to high risk for suicide, and suicide precautions were instituted on the floor. Mr. A was started on a course of antidepressants, but these had not yet begun to work when he was deemed surgically ready for discharge. The consultant recommended transfer to an inpatient psychiatry unit where Mr. A could undergo treatment for both his depression and substance abuse. Mr. A's mental health coverage had been carved out from his medical–surgical coverage. The utilization reviewer for his medical–surgical coverage insisted that he be discharged from the hospital and scheduled for outpatient physical therapy with visiting nurse coverage. The mental health management company sent its own psychologist reviewer to evaluate Mr. A. The reviewer agreed that Mr. A was depressed but denied authorization for psychiatric hospitalization. The reviewer opined that Mr. A was not acutely suicidal, did not need inpatient substance abuse treatment, and could be managed as an outpatient. He was given the names of the three psychiatrists in his town who were authorized under his plan and was able to get an appointment scheduled for 2 weeks after discharge. Mr. A was discharged from the hospital, over the objections of the consultant. The consultant had found that the patient was still significantly depressed and at risk of drinking again but not committable because he was not imminently suicidal. Ten days later, the visiting nurse found him hanged in his apartment. The death was ruled a suicide. Mr. A's family brought a malpractice action against the hospital, the treating physicians, the consultant, and the managed care company.

What liability does the managed care company have in a case such as Case 1, in which the denial of care results in harm to the patient? Would the managed care company's liability supersede that of the physicians? The answers to these questions are still unclear. There have been a series of legal cases addressing these issues, and the law is still evolving. At present, there is a possibility that managed care companies may be held liable in these situations if the company exerted such control over the decision-making process that the physician's judgment was over-ridden. In other words, for the physician to avoid liability, he or she must protest the denial of care, appeal it to the highest level that the insurer provides, and take other reasonable steps to ensure the patient's safety. Depending on the facts, the liability may be assigned entirely to the managed care company, to the physician, or be shared.[8–11] At present, treating physicians are regarded as independent contractors and therefore bear separate and often sole responsibility. There are policy arguments against that model, which may lead to future changes.[12]

Whatever the policy arguments, under federal law, there are specific limits on managed care companies' liability for denial of care. Most often, decisions made by managed care organizations to limit care are subject only to limited legal remedies under the Employee Retirement Income Security Act (ERISA) of 1974. ERISA limits most employees of private companies to suing their health plans for the cost of the care denied by the managed care organization only, and not for recovery of losses that result from the denial of care or for punitive damages.[13] ERISA's protection of managed care plans from liability for the consequences of their decisions is increasingly seen as unfair given the level of control over treatment decisions exercised by some plans. As a result, several federal court cases have eroded the prohibition on damages under the law,[14] but these cases represent only small gains, the trend in cases has appeared to have come to a halt, there is no indication that lawmakers will amend ERISA to eliminate the preemption clause, and the Supreme Court continues to protect employer-sponsored plans from state requirements.[15] In addition, state law efforts to hold managed care companies liable for damages have been largely unsuccessful.[16] For the time being, in the face of bad outcomes, patients may try to shift liability to physicians and hospitals to recover losses.[17]

Confidentiality and Privacy

Confidentiality is the clinician's obligation to keep matters revealed by a patient from the ears of third parties.[2–4] It is usually demanded and protected by statute and custom. A variety of exceptions to confidentiality exist, usually where the courts or the legislature determine that maintenance of confidentiality will result in more harm than good from a societal standpoint. This rationale provided the basis for the California court's decision in *Tarasoff v. Board of Regents*,[18] in which the court held that psychotherapists have a duty to act to protect third parties where the therapist knows or should know that the patient poses a threat of serious risk of harm to the third party.[19,20] In looking at the public policy issue, the court stated:

> *The Court recognizes the public interest in supporting effective treatment of mental illness and in protecting the rights of patients to privacy. But this interest must be weighed against the public interest in safety from violent assault.*[18]

Although not all states have adopted this view, the majority have. A number of states have enacted statutes dealing with this fertile area of malpractice liability and either limited or eliminated the duty.[21] The consultant should be familiar with the relevant statutory and case law concerning this issue in his or her jurisdiction. The consultant should also be aware that liability can arise when medical or surgical colleagues fail to breach confidentiality and do not warn family members or other contacts about the potential for contagion from an infectious disease.[22] In fact, liability for such failure set the stage for the court's decision in *Tarasoff*.[18] Additionally, a small number of states, including Massachusetts, have held that a physician may be held liable for injuries to a third person that result from the failure to warn a patient about the side effects of medications, such as where a patient falls asleep at the wheel of a car and was not warned of the sedating effects of a medication.[23]

Although infectious disease has been the subject of duty to protect cases in the past, infection with HIV has been treated somewhat differently than other infectious diseases. Controversy persists about the obligation of a physician to warn the partner of an HIV-positive patient when the patient refuses to do so. Many states have statutes that address this issue, with varied approaches, adding to the confusion and highlighting the controversial nature of the issue. The psychiatric consultant should learn the requirements of the jurisdiction in which he or she practices. Several articles and book chapters have addressed this controversial issue, some of which are cited in the references for this chapter.[24–29]

In addition to situations in which disclosure is mandated to protect a third party, such as in *Tarasoff*[18] and infectious disease situations, other breaches of confidentiality may be mandated by statute or case law to protect vulnerable third parties. For example, all 50 states in the United States have statutes that require specific individuals, including physicians, to report suspected child abuse or neglect to state social service agencies.[30,31]

Many states also require that known or suspected abuse or neglect of the elderly or the disabled be reported.[31] Failure to comply with these requirements can result in substantial penalties. More recently, some states have begun requiring physicians and others to report known or suspected cases of domestic violence to law enforcement or to designated agencies. Mandatory reporting statutes serve an important societal purpose, but they are not without controversy. Every clinician should become aware of the specific requirements in his or her jurisdiction.[32]

Patient health information is also subject to regulation under a federal law known as the Health Insurance Portability and Accountability Act (HIPAA) of 1996. As of mid-2003, institutions and individual providers are required to comply with HIPAA rules. HIPAA has affected hospital practice by requiring distribution, in writing, of the institution's privacy policy to all patients and by mandating physicians to undergo training on privacy and disclosure provisions. The rules are too complex to review in full here; however, several salient points stand out for psychiatrists.

Among the most relevant provisions of HIPAA is the treatment of medical records and the distinction between general psychiatric records and psychotherapy notes. Patients are entitled to a copy of their medical records; they also have the explicit right to request changes in the record. Whether or not the applicable staff person amends the contested information, the involved correspondence becomes part of the record. Although HIPAA affords special status to psychotherapy notes and allows psychiatrists not to disclose these notes to patients, this exception is narrow. To qualify for protection under the psychotherapy notes provision, the notes must be kept separate from the patient's medical record. Specific types of information contained in psychotherapy notes are not subject to the psychotherapy notes exclusion; these include medications prescribed, test results, treatment plans, diagnoses, prognosis, and progress to date.[33–35] It should be noted, however, that notes falling within the HIPAA psychotherapy notes exception are considered to be part of the medical record in the event that a subpoena is received for medical records.

The practical implication of HIPAA regarding psychiatric record-keeping is that psychiatric records, whether in an outpatient clinic or contained in a medical chart from a non-psychiatric hospitalization, are broadly accessible to patients or anyone they authorize to access their records. Therefore, consulting psychiatrists should be careful in the documentation of sensitive therapy material because it will be treated like the rest of the medical record unless the psychotherapy notes are kept in a separate file.

As for patients, health insurance companies' access to psychotherapy records is restricted. Health insurance companies cannot demand access to information contained in psychotherapy notes as a requirement of payment for care. If, in a particular circumstance, psychotherapy notes are released to an insurance company, written consent from the patient is required under HIPAA. This consent requirement is in sharp contrast to the disclosure rules for the general medical and general psychiatric record for insurance purposes; HIPAA does not require consent for disclosure of this information to insurance companies for the purpose of obtaining payment for treatment—medical or psychiatric. HIPAA also does not require specific consent for the release of information for treatment or healthcare operations purposes. Operations purposes, for example, include quality assurance, licensing, and accreditation. There are 11 additional circumstances in which disclosure is permitted without patient consent, including emergencies and mandated reporting situations, such as child abuse—which are generally considered to be a part of current medical practice. But other situations, including exceptions for law enforcement and attorney requests, may be more concerning.[33,35]

Refusal to Treat Patients

Refusal to treat patients, in or out of the hospital, is a right that is rarely invoked by physicians. The physician–patient relationship is, at heart, contractual in nature. Both parties have the same right to enter, or to refuse to enter, the relationship as they do with other contracts. Once the physician offers to treat and the patient accepts, the contract is established and the physician's right to refuse or withdraw is limited in certain ways. For example, maintaining a walk-in clinic or Emergency Department (ED) can be construed as an implicit offer to treat on an emergent basis. The patient's presentation at the clinic or ED is an acceptance of the offer, creating a contract. It does not necessarily create an obligation to provide ongoing care, so long as the walk-in or emergency nature of the services is clear and appropriate information is provided regarding ongoing care. In a situation in which a prospective patient discusses his or her history with a physician, it may be difficult to assert that no relationship has been established, particularly if the patient is under the impression that a treatment relationship exists. Physicians should clarify at the outset of the treatment encounter that they may or may not accept a case. It is usually helpful to explain at the first visit that this is an initial evaluation to determine whether or not it is appropriate for the physician to take this particular individual as a patient. The terms of an individual physician's relationship with the employing clinic can make it difficult to exercise this option. Clearly, this principle does not include the emergent, or even urgent, medical problem, which imposes an obligation to provide care sufficient to stabilize the patient's condition. In the event that no physician–patient relationship has been created in the initial contact, referral of the patient to a healthcare facility, such as a walk-in clinic, demonstrates concern for the patient without necessarily creating an obligation to treat.[36–40]

When the physician elects not to treat an individual, the physician should make every effort to provide an alternative course to avoid claims of abandonment.[1–3] Abandonment is the unilateral severance of the relationship by the physician, leaving the patient without needed medical care. The optimal care of the patient is the first consideration. Whenever a physician desires to transfer the patient to another physician, the transferring physician must take steps to ensure continuity of care by specific arrangement with the physician who is going to treat the patient. The physician may terminate the treatment relationship with a patient for a variety of reasons, including non-payment, repeated failure to keep appointments, or threatening behavior. In such cases, the patient should be notified of the decision, the available treatment options (including a specific referral, if possible), and available sources of emergency care. The course pursued and the reasons and indications for the transfer or termination should be documented in the medical record.[2,3]

The physician's right to refuse to provide care for patients may be restricted where the refusal is based on the patient's specific illness or inherent characteristics. The refusal to care for patients of certain races, religions, ethnic origins, or disease type (e.g., acquired immunodeficiency syndrome) raises significant ethical concerns as well as potential liability under Title VII of the Civil Rights Act of 1964 and the Americans with Disabilities Act. These are beyond the scope of this chapter. The general rule, however, is that physicians and other clinicians may be charged with unethical conduct and in some situations with violation of patients' civil rights, when treatment is refused on a discriminatory basis.[39,40]

The issue of terminating the physician–patient relationship usually arises when some conflict has developed between physician and patient over the course of treatment or as a result of non-compliance.[41] Knowing about the physician's right not to treat is important for consultants. Often the knowledge that a physician can stop treating a particular patient allows enough "give" in a confrontation so that the consultee's anxiety diminishes and negotiation can begin.

End-of-Life Care and Advance Directives

Care of the dying and hopelessly ill patient continues to generate difficult questions, staff conflicts, and requests for help from physicians who find themselves faced with these clinical, ethical, and legal dilemmas.[42,43] Controversy and turmoil are generated when the patient loses the capacity to participate in the decision-making process. The decision of a competent patient to refuse life-sustaining treatment yields similar results. The general rule is that every competent adult has the right to make his or her own decisions about medical care, based on personal preference, even if that choice conflicts with what a majority of others would choose under similar circumstances. An important distinction must be drawn between the competent patient's request that treatment be withheld or withdrawn and requests that the physician take some active, independent step to terminate the patient's life. The former are generally regarded as being within the realm of the patient's right to make treatment decisions. The original illness, rather than the withholding or withdrawal of treatment, is regarded as the cause of death in such situations. Active steps taken to end a patient's life are considered euthanasia; in many states, the complying physician could be subjected to criminal prosecution.[43–45] In fact, in two 1997 cases, the Supreme Court of the United States upheld two state laws prohibiting physician-assisted suicide after physicians challenged the constitutionality of the laws.[45–47] However, the Supreme Court of the United States has also limited the ability of the federal government to prevent states from allowing physician-assisted suicide. Specifically, in 2006, the Court ruled against the federal government when it attempted to use federal law to block the ability of Oregon physicians to prescribe controlled substances for the purpose of physician-assisted suicide.[48] For more than a decade, Oregon was the only state that legalized physician-assisted suicide. As of this writing, Washington, Vermont, and California have joined Oregon in passing physician-assisted dying statutes.

The treatment requests of the dying patient have not always been taken seriously, especially when the patient's choice was to terminate care. Physicians struggle when faced with a patient who refuses further treatment, especially when there is some hope of improvement. Physicians often find it difficult to give up the fight even at the request of the patient. Consulting psychiatrists in such circumstances should be concerned with determining whether the patient's request to forego heroic efforts stems from a condition that can be reversed or mitigated, such as depression or pain, and whether or not the patient is capable of understanding the nature of the request. In other words, is the patient's refusal of further treatment informed? If it is, the next challenge is working with the treatment team so that they can accept the patient's decision.

When minor children suffer terminal conditions, in the absence of any over-riding legal requirements, parents are generally permitted to make decisions regarding continuation of extraordinary efforts.[32,49,50] The consulting psychiatrist is urged to seek the advice of the hospital's general counsel when confronted with these issues. The maze of governmental regulations, statutes, and case law in this area combined with the emotionally charged nature of the situation demand expert legal input. Nevertheless, the larger challenge for the consultant and the treatment team lies in helping the child's parents with the turmoil at hand and the grief ahead.

The psychiatrist should do what he or she can to ensure the comfort of the patient, such as seeing that treatment of clinical depression and alleviation of tractable pain are not overlooked in the anxiety that surrounds the dying patient. Development and documentation of written guidelines for the management of these difficult situations can be helpful in ensuring rational constancy in approach. Such attention to the relief of suffering decreases conflict between patient, family, and staff. In turn, this helps avoid legal involvement in the situation.

The status of the patient's right to refuse life-sustaining treatment varies among the states. In 1990, the Supreme Court of the United States handed down its opinion in *Cruzan v. Director, Missouri Department of Public Health*.[51] The Court held that all competent individuals have a constitutionally protected right to refuse life-sustaining treatment. When a patient lacks the capacity to make his or her own decisions, however, the court held that the state can assert its interest in preserving life and require clear and convincing evidence of the now-incapacitated patient's preferences in such matters before a surrogate decision-maker will be allowed to refuse the treatment on the patient's behalf. In most jurisdictions, surrogate decision-makers, whether family members or guardians, are allowed greater freedom in drawing conclusions about the patient's preference.

Many states have statutes that allow individuals to issue advance directives concerning future medical care in these situations. All states have statutes providing for durable powers of attorney, an instrument that can be used to delegate decision-making authority to another person in the event of incapacity. All physicians should be aware of what prior directives are valid in their jurisdictions and encourage their patients to explore these issues with them and with their legal representatives. Under the Patient Self-Determination Act of 1990, all healthcare facilities, nursing homes, and health maintenance organizations must inquire on admission or enrollment whether a patient has an advance directive. If not, the patient must be offered information on the subject and an opportunity to create a directive.[52–54] Notwithstanding nearly two decades of this legal requirement, it is estimated that only a minority of Americans (30% to <50%) have executed an advance directive.[29]

RIGHTS OF PATIENTS

It is no news that the relationship between physician and patient has changed considerably over the years. The pendulum has swung between the extremes of paternalism and total patient autonomy. More recently, the impact of restrictions on patient choice imposed by managed care has been added to the equation. Most physicians and their patients operate on some middle ground between the extremes of complete patient autonomy and medical paternalism. The fundamental principle is that it is the patient, not the physician, who makes the ultimate choice regarding treatment. This ethical concept has been operationalized by legal decisions and by legislation. Although some physicians still view these changes as dangerous to patient care and as intrusions into their domain of clinical judgment, they are part of an ever-shrinking minority, as more and more physicians have come to accept the idea of greater patient autonomy.

Informed Consent and Evaluation of Decision-Making Capacity

Informed consent issues and the evaluation of decision-making capacity (commonly referred to as competency) are major components of the medico-legal workload. Informed consent has been an essential feature of medical practice since the 1960s. It is a process by which the patient agrees to treatment, in which the consent is based on adequate information, and it is voluntarily given by a patient who is competent to do so.[55] The term *informed consent* is somewhat misleading; we are as concerned with informed refusal as we are with informed consent. Bowing to convention, the term *informed consent* is used with the understanding that the same standards apply to informed refusal.

Informed consent is required before the initiation of any medical treatment, but exceptions do exist. Informed consent need not be obtained in an emergency in which delay would seriously threaten the well-being of the patient. In such cases, the physician is under an obligation to use his or her best judgment and to act in good faith. Such behavior is unlikely to result in litigation, if the physician documents (immediately after the emergency passes) the events and the reasons for the steps taken, and that those steps were reasonable. Other exceptions to informed consent have been found where the patient waives the right to receive information, where the patient lacks the capacity to make decisions, or where providing the information needed for informed consent would cause the patient's physical or mental health to deteriorate (known as *therapeutic privilege*). The therapeutic privilege is problematic; it is mentioned here because it has been invoked in the past and was for many years a mainstay of medical paternalism (e.g., patients who were treated for carcinoma without being told the diagnosis for fear it "would just upset them" and worsen their overall condition). Situations in which the therapeutic privilege can be justifiably invoked are rare. The fact that providing the information might lead the patient to refuse treatment or would cause the patient considerable anxiety does not justify invoking therapeutic privilege. The situation must be one in which the informed consent process itself would cause risk of grave harm. The physician who forgoes the informed consent process under the name of therapeutic privilege does so at his or her own risk.[55–57]

An essential feature of modern consent is that it be informed. Simple consent, in which the patient gives the physician blanket permission to take care of medical problems, is not deemed adequate, unless the patient has made a specific decision to waive informed consent. The amount and type of information to be provided to the patient or the surrogate decision-maker vary somewhat among jurisdictions.[2] The two basic standards are the professional standard and the patient-oriented standard. In the former, the physician is required to give that amount of information that the average physician in that specialty would provide under the circumstances. In other words, it looks to the standard of care. In other states, the amount of information to be provided is determined by what the patient would require to make an informed decision. This is also known as the materiality standard. In some states, the materiality standard is applied on the basis of what the average patient would require to make a decision, whereas in other states it is assessed in terms of what the specific patient would require. In either case, the physician who covers the following information, taken from a leading Massachusetts case,[58] with the patient will generally be held to have provided adequate information:

- The diagnosis and condition to be treated
- The nature of the proposed treatment
- The nature and probability of the material risks of the treatment

- The benefits that may be expected from the treatment
- The inability of the physician to predict results
- The irreversibility of the procedure, if that is the case
- The likely results of forgoing treatment
- The likely results, risks, and benefits of alternative treatments.

The second requirement for informed consent is that the consent be given voluntarily. Coercion is often in the eye of the beholder; the fact that coercion ostensibly occurs in the service of the best interests of the patient does not justify it from the ethical standpoint or qualify it as an element of informed consent. The line between persuasion and coercion often appears both narrow and vague. Generally speaking, if some negative contingency (including an exaggerated prediction of a poor prognosis) is attached to the patient's refusal of treatment, there is coercion, and any subsequent consent is technically invalid.

The presence of decision-making capacity, commonly referred to as competency, is the threshold issue in the informed consent process. The term *competency* is familiar to all physicians, but it is used imprecisely in the clinical setting. Competency is defined as the legal capacity of an individual to perform either a specific function or a wide range of functions; before such a determination by a judge, all adults are presumed to be competent. Only a judge can declare a person incompetent for specific functions or for all activities (global incompetence). The psychiatric consultant can only make a clinical assessment of the patient's capacity to function in certain areas. That assessment is usually, but not always, accepted by the court in its determination of incompetence.[2,55] What then of the numerous requests received by the consultation psychiatrist to determine the competency of medical and surgical patients? The use of competency as a shorthand term is justifiable, so long as the consultant and the consultee are clear that the most the consultant can do is to assess the patient's capacity to engage in the decision-making process in question. The change in the patient's legal status must be left to a judge. Just to add to the semantic confusion, the modern trend in the law is to forego the term *competency*, and to instead refer to a person's *capacities*. A person who lacks capacity may be referred to by the court as "the incapacitated person" rather than "the incompetent individual." This trend is not yet complete, and we mention it here in anticipation that this change in terminology will spread.

Capacity is usually task-specific and defined in relation to a specified act: to make a will (testamentary capacity), to testify in court (testimonial capacity), to consent to or to refuse treatment (decision-making capacity), etc. Having the capacity to perform one act does not mean that one necessarily has the capacity to perform another. Hence, the consultant called to evaluate a patient's "competency" must first determine the specific type(s) of capacity in question and be aware of the applicable judgment criteria. Once the consultant has determined the type of capacity in question, the judgment hinges on how well the patient meets the criteria. For example, with regard to capacity to make treatment choices, we look to the patient's understanding of three things: the illness (that something is wrong and to some degree how wrong); the treatment (what is proposed and why it is relevant to what is wrong); and the consequences of the decision. Although a variety of means of assessing decision-making capacity have been proposed, Appelbaum[59] has suggested the following four criteria that are particularly useful and straightforward:

1. Does the patient manifest a preference? A patient who is unable or unwilling to express a preference presumably lacks the capacity to make a choice. It does not necessarily follow, however, that a patient who expresses a choice is competent.
2. Is the patient capable of attaining a factual understanding of the situation (nature of the illness, treatment options, prognosis with and without treatment, risks and benefits of treatment, and so on)? The patient need not possess this level of understanding at the time of admission; he or she need only be able to receive the factual information and retain it in some reasonable form during the decision-making process.
3. Does the patient have an appreciation of the significance of the facts presented? Appreciation, in contrast to factual understanding, indicates a broader level of understanding related to the significance of the facts presented and the implications these facts hold for the patient's future.
4. Is the patient able to use the information presented in a rational fashion to reach a decision, that is, to weigh the facts presented in a logical manner? The focus here is not on the rationality of the ultimate decision, but on the rationality of the thought processes leading to the decision.

When a substitute decision-maker is deciding on behalf of an incapacitated patient, the same elements of capacity to make a decision apply. The patient's healthcare agent has the responsibility to express the patient's choice, with an awareness of the facts and appreciation for their significance, thinking through the material in a logical fashion before making a decision.

Capacity is not an all-or-nothing proposition, and the same level of capacity is not required for all medical decisions. Most experts agree that the strictness of the capacity test should vary as the risk/benefit ratio changes. In essence, there is a sliding scale for the level of capacity needed to make informed medical decisions.[60–62] The more favorable the risk/benefit ratio, the lower the standard for capacity to consent and the higher the standard for capacity to refuse. For example, the patient who agrees to accept incision and drainage of an obvious wound abscess would not have his or her capacity subjected to rigorous assessment. Refusal could not be taken so lightly; the more serious the abscess, the more intense the examination of capacity would have to be. If the risk/benefit ratio were unfavorable to the patient (e.g., extensive surgery to remove a slow-growing brain tumor in a 94-year-old), refusal would not have to be examined as meticulously as would consent. Although some criticize this approach as being too open to manipulation by a paternalistic physician, it accurately reflects professional obligations to ensure that patients make a truly informed decision, based on a rational weighing of the risks and benefits involved. A similar approach was endorsed by the President's Commission for the Study of Ethical Problems in Medicine and Biomedical and Behavioral Research.[63,64]

Dementia, delirium, and psychosis are the conditions most often cited as causes of incapacity.[65–68] The consultant should always consider the possibility of a mood disorder as a basis for impaired competence to make medical decisions. The following example demonstrates some of the complexities of these evaluations.

CASE 2

A psychiatric consultant was asked to assess the decision-making capacity of Mr. B, a 62-year-old man who presented to the ED with a massive subdural hematoma that he had suffered in repeated falls owing to bradycardia. He had a profound expressive aphasia; despite the size of the subdural hematoma, Mr. B was medically stable and intermittently lucid. Nevertheless, neurosurgical staff were anxious to evacuate the subdural hematoma for fear of increased intracranial pressure. During his lucid intervals, the patient was verbally abusive to his physicians and to the consultant, stated clearly that he did not want surgery, and demanded to be discharged. The limited duration of his lucid intervals and his general irritability prevented the consultant from conducting a more complete mental status examination and determining the degree of his cognitive impairment, if any. An interview with his family members revealed that he had been drinking and becoming more depressed, with marked suicidal ideation, in the previous weeks. He had refused to see a physician about his bradycardia, stating that he would prefer to die. Based on this information, his mental status examination, and the risk/benefit ratio of the proposed treatment, the consultant determined that the patient lacked the capacity to give an informed refusal. An emergency court hearing was held with an "on-call" judge. The judge ruled that the patient lacked the capacity to refuse the planned procedure and appointed a family member to be his guardian. The guardian then consented to evacuation of the subdural. The patient tolerated the procedure well; on recovering from surgery and anesthesia, he informed the staff in a clear voice that he was going to sue all of them. The appointment of a guardian and his informed consent, along with the excellent clinical outcome, eliminated the basis for a malpractice action.

Although depression must be considered as a possible cause of impaired judgment and incapacity, caution must be exercised. Just as a patient with schizophrenia is not automatically considered to lack capacity, a patient with major depression may also retain the ability to make rational decisions. Studies have found that medical decision-making capacity is impaired by severe depression but not by depression of lesser severity.[69]

Patients may make decisions in one moment and change those decisions minutes or hours later. This can cause significant disruption of treatment for that patient and for others. Frequent shifts in patient choice can be the basis for questioning the patient's decision-making capacity. Ideally, the patient makes an informed choice with full capacity before suffering a shift in mental status. Family members should be included in this process so they can assist the treatment team in the event of a subsequent change in the patient's decision.

The cause of incapacity may be treatable. Intense pain may lead a patient to refuse a needed procedure; treatment with adequate doses of analgesics may resolve the problem. Treatment of depression, when it is a factor, may be attempted with psychostimulants, which may act within 1 to 2 days. This can restore the patient's perspective, so that the decision to refuse or accept is competently made. Delirium and agitation often interfere with treatment decisions and should be treated with a neuroleptic if no specific cause of the confusional state can be found. The consultant should not determine that the patient is permanently incapacitated until these medications have been given an adequate trial, and other potential causes of the confusional state have been addressed. It must be remembered that even psychotic patients may have clear, rational reasons for refusing a treatment. Conversely, the refusal may be the result of voices telling the patient to leave the hospital, that they do not deserve treatment, or that the surgeon is an FBI agent sent to spy on them.[70]

Occasionally, psychiatric consultants are asked to assess a patient's testamentary capacity, competency to execute a contract, financial competency, or the like. Such questions are unlikely to arise in the course of the usual medical consultation but instead are asked by an attorney or the courts, in anticipation, or as a result, of a challenge to the patient's competency to engage in these activities. In the case of testamentary capacity, for example, a psychiatrist may be asked to assess the mental status of a patient to determine whether he or she meets the legal standards for testamentary capacity and to provide documentation of this mental status in the event that the will is challenged after the patient's demise. To do so, the psychiatrist must possess both clinical skills and knowledge of the legal standards: The patient knows that he or she is executing a will, knows the extent of his or her estate, and knows the "natural objects of his or her bounty" (who would normally inherit). Because these assessments involve the application of specific legal requirements to clinical situations, the evaluation should be performed only after consultation with the referring attorney or court representative and with adequate knowledge of the legal standard. For this reason, many psychiatric consultants refer such consultations to colleagues who specialize in consultation to the legal system.[71]

To give consent, the patient must be able to make an informed judgment on the matter at hand. Patients with deficits in this area, owing to communication difficulties (e.g., foreign language, deafness, or aphasia) or ignorance of important aspects of their care, cannot technically give consent, whether or not they are competent. The physician who performs a procedure on a passive, confused, or fearfully mute patient who seems compliant or willing, does so at his or her own peril; the physician risks a suit for battery. There is little protection in the ancient maxim *Qui tacet consentire videtur* ("silence gives assent").

The patient's capacity to give consent, understanding, and judgment should be documented in the chart or in the office notes of the physician, along with the mental status examination and any specific questions asked about the proposed treatment. Impairment of intellect, memory, attention, or consciousness can limit the patient's understanding; impairment in reality testing, sense of reality, impulse control, and formal logic can influence judgment. The presence or absence of any or all of these should be documented clearly in the chart, along with their relationship to the illness and to the decision-making process. Many states provide standardized forms that must be completed by a physician or other clinicians when a medical guardianship is pursued in court.

The general rule in obtaining consent for treatment of minor children is that parents have both the obligation to provide care and the right to make treatment decisions. However, there are a number of complicating issues in this area. First, the age of majority varies by state. Second, minors' rights and the legal ability to consent vary according to the type of treatment being contemplated. Massachusetts, for example, permits minors to give consent for the treatment of drug addiction and sexually transmitted diseases without seeking parental authorization. Virginia allows minors to consent to psychotherapy without parental consent. Third, the law is open to examination of the reason for the parents' denial of consent, rather than upholding it automatically. Denial of life-saving treatment for a child because of the parents' religious beliefs will not be upheld by a court. Finally, the law recognizes the concept of the emancipated minor. This is a minor child who is free of parental control and dominance and is therefore deemed legally competent to consent in the eyes of the law, regardless of age. Informed consent by an emancipated minor, carefully documented in the record, usually protects the physician's action from criticism by the parent or guardian of that minor, so long as there is evidence of emancipation. Treating clinicians and consultants should learn the rules of their specific states concerning consent by minors.[49,50]

New drugs, treatments, and procedures should not be used without informed consent by patients (or the appropriate surrogate decision-maker) and proper authorization from hospital and government agencies. Although physicians have generally been given considerable freedom in prescribing medications and in doing procedures for off-label (not approved by Food and Drug Administration [FDA]) purposes, this freedom is constrained by federal and state regulations, the standard of care (enforced through malpractice actions), and the patient's right to be informed about the proposed treatment. Use of carbamazepine for treatment of bipolar disorder is a common example of this. As a matter of policy, patients should be informed that the medicine prescribed has not been given FDA-approval for that particular purpose and informed about the rationale for prescribing it.[36]

Civil Commitment and Restraint

Civil commitment and physical restraint are commonly encountered but poorly understood by patients and many non-psychiatric physicians. Civil commitment is a process by which the power of the state is used to remove an individual from society and place him or her in an institutional setting. Originally, the mentally ill were confined to institutions to protect the rest of society. As the approach toward the mentally ill became more enlightened, the goal of confinement was to provide treatment and protection. Under this approach, the state was fulfilling its role as protector of its citizens, much as a parent would act on behalf of a child. Hence, this is known as the state's *parens patriae* interest. With the blossoming of the civil liberties movement in the 1970s and the emphasis on individual autonomy, the individual's interest in personal freedom and privacy was given priority over the state's *parens patriae* interest. During the 1970s, the best interest or *parens patriae* approach to civil commitment was replaced by the dangerousness approach in most jurisdictions. This approach, based on the state's police powers, allows an individual to be involuntarily committed to a mental institution only if the individual poses a danger to himself or herself through direct injury, if there is a direct threat of physical harm to others, or if the individual is gravely disabled and unable to care for himself or herself in the community.[2,3,72]

In a general hospital, if a medical or surgical patient is psychiatrically committable but requires further medical or surgical treatment, the wisest course is to initiate commitment procedures and request that a local mental health facility accept the patient but allow the patient to remain in the general hospital for care. Budgetary concerns, insurance issues, and the general reluctance of both state and private psychiatric hospitals to take medically ill patients often make it difficult to place such patients. It behooves the consultation psychiatrist to learn how to anticipate the need for further psychiatric care and begin the search early. The need for commitment should be reassessed throughout this process and the process halted if appropriate.

The search for inpatient psychiatric placement increasingly requires negotiation with managed care companies to obtain permission for the hospitalization. Often, the interaction with health insurance companies occurs through the process of pre-certification, which requires the transferring hospital to gain approval for transfer and inpatient care from the insurer before the patient can be transferred and admitted to the receiving psychiatric facility. Because of frequent differences in general medical and psychiatric benefits within health plans, the same pre-certification process may be required even when a patient is transferred from a medical ward to a psychiatric unit in the same hospital. It is now commonplace for insurance plans to "carve out" or sub-contract mental health benefits to a subsidiary or a different company with procedures and guidelines distinct from those of the parent company.

The psychiatric consultant often encounters questions regarding the restraint of patients on medical and surgical floors. Delirium, dementia, acute or chronic psychosis, or severe anxiety or panic can lead a patient to assault staff, to wander off the ward, or to fall. The suicidal patient being treated on an unlocked medical floor poses the risk of elopement and successful fulfillment of suicidal urges. Many hospitals have policies that allow the patient to be restrained before the psychiatric consultant is called. When this occurs, the role of the consultant is to provide management recommendations and approval for the restraint. Usually, the psychiatric consultant is asked to decide whether the restraints can be discontinued.

The legal aspects of restraint of patients on a medical or surgical ward vary among jurisdictions.[4,36] Generally speaking, a patient may be restrained for the purpose of protecting the patient or other patients and staff, for the purpose of allowing examination during an emergency, or for the purpose of treatment in situations in which the patient appears to lack the capacity to make treatment decisions and is refusing care. In this latter situation, no forced treatment should be initiated in the absence of an emergency unless surrogate consent has been obtained. In handling these situations, physician and staff are required to use the least restrictive alternative available. For example, where a sitter or observer is available for a potentially suicidal patient, that option is more appropriate than four-point restraints. Family members often ask whether they can substitute for a sitter. Although this may be possible in some situations, it requires careful clinical judgment that takes into account the type of pathology, the degree of impulsivity, the overall degree of risk, and the relative ability of the sitter to act objectively. Restraint is uncomfortable for the staff, as well as for the patient and family, and there may be a tendency to avoid it whenever possible for some types of patients and a tendency to overuse it with others. Again, careful clinical assessment is essential so that protection is provided for those patients who need restraint without zealously over-protecting and restricting those who do not. The justification for restraint, including history and formal mental status examination, should be clearly documented in the medical record, along with the psychiatric differential diagnosis, treatment, and management recommendations.

The restraint of patients gives rise to two potential sources of liability: battery and false imprisonment.[1] A battery is defined as the touching of another person without his or her consent (expressed or implied) or justification. False imprisonment may be charged where an individual is denied the right to move about freely by real or perceived methods of confinement. Failure to restrain a patient with a tendency to wander, who is subsequently injured, may result in a charge of professional negligence.

Malpractice claims based on battery or false imprisonment are rarely successful if the use of restraint is reasonable under the circumstances, the reasons for the measures are documented in the medical record, proper technique is used, and hospital policies are followed. Failure to restrain when indicated and improper restraining techniques carry greater risks of harm to the patient and of malpractice claims.

Right to Refuse Treatment

The right to refuse a specific form of treatment or procedure has a long history and is firmly established in medicine. This right, based on the philosophical principle of autonomy, has been operationalized through the common law (case law), by legislation, and in state and U.S. constitutions.[73–76] Although widely acknowledged, the right to refuse treatment is not absolute. It may be limited when it is in conflict with legitimate state interests of preserving life, preventing suicide, protecting the interests of third parties, or protecting the integrity of the medical profession.[77] Generally, the decision of a patient who possesses decision-making capacity to end treatment presents a difficult dilemma for the treatment team. If the issue ever reaches court, the competent patient's preference is rarely over-ridden. With the advent of advance directives (e.g., healthcare proxies and durable powers of attorney), the wishes of the patient, expressed when competent, can be honored after the onset of incompetence. The path to this conclusion is not as smooth as this might suggest. Consider the following example.

CASE 3

Ms. C, a 22-year-old woman, was admitted to the hospital after sustaining severe head injuries in a motor vehicle accident. After emergency evacuation of a subdural hematoma, her condition stabilized. She was unresponsive to verbal stimuli, did not track, but did withdraw to pain. She showed decorticate posturing. The treatment team urged aggressive measures, arguing that the injury was recent and the ability to predict ultimate outcome was limited. Tube feedings were begun and an early pneumonia was treated with antibiotics. The patient's family told the treatment team that the patient would never want to be kept alive under such circumstances. The patient's mother explained that the patient's cousin had been in a motor vehicle accident 5 years earlier and had lingered in a persistent vegetative state for 3 years until her death. The family had to engage in a costly legal battle to get permission to terminate supportive care. When this occurred, the patient (who was a nursing student at the time) vowed that she would never allow this to happen to her or to her family. She told her family that she would want to be free of life-sustaining measures in the event of a serious injury if there was "no chance of recovery." In addition, she executed a healthcare proxy naming her mother as her agent for medical decision-making in the event of her incapacity. Her mother believed that the patient would have refused care if able to do so and insisted that the tube feedings be stopped. The treatment team resisted, arguing that there was hope for some recovery. After a series of meetings, the family acquiesced to the recommendations of the team and the patient was transferred to a rehabilitation facility, still posturing and not responding. Two weeks after transfer, she was returned to the hospital with septicemia. This time, the treatment team yielded to the family's preferences and the patient died peacefully.

As Case 3 suggests, there are often no perfect answers to these problems. Both the treatment team and the family were well-meaning and tried to do what they believed was right for the patient. Meetings between the treatment team and the family, facilitated by the consultants to the unit, allowed a process to develop that gave the patient some chance at early recovery and for nature to take its course. Although difficult, the decision-making process was conducted with dignity, with the aim of maintaining the patient's autonomy and ensuring that the decision was informed and with concern for the ethical integrity of her caretakers. In a more contentious setting, the family could have charged the treatment team with battery. Under the law in that state, the agent appointed by the healthcare proxy (the mother in this case) had the same authority to make decisions as the patient would have if competent, including refusal of permission for further treatment. The treatment team could have raised legal challenges to the exercise of the proxy, arguing that it was not evident that there was "no chance of recovery." In some states, an argument would be made that shutting off the life support constituted murder or assisted suicide or that the state's interest in preserving life and preventing suicide outweighed the individual's expressed wish. The likelihood of such arguments being made or succeeding is much less in light of the Cruzan decision.[51] Finally, if the physicians or the institution had been ethically opposed to the termination of treatment, the request might have been denied and the patient transferred to the care of another physician or facility. The best solution to these challenging problems lies in the sharing of information and concerns between the family and the treaters. Immediate resort to legal posturing hardens positions and shuts off communications in most cases, to the detriment of all concerned.

The requirement of informed consent and the right to refuse treatment do not automatically apply in emergencies. In emergencies that appear to endanger the patient, or in acute situations that threaten the safety of the staff and other patients, the physician who acts in good faith while administering a treatment or procedure is generally not liable for failure to obtain informed consent. Good faith is in doubt, however, when the patient has made his or her preferences regarding treatment in the event of an emergency clearly known before the emergency and the physician chooses to disregard these preferences. For example, the physician who agrees to perform surgery on a Jehovah's Witness with the stipulation that there be no transfusions, even in an emergency, is hard pressed to plead good faith should he or she violate that agreement in the event of a sudden hemorrhage. Some institutions have adopted policies specific to such situations. In the case of chronic medical conditions, ongoing situations, and prolonged heroic measures to sustain life, the emergency exception loses its applicability, and decisions regarding treatment must be returned to the competent patient or to an appropriate surrogate.

Leaving treatment against medical advice (AMA) is the prerogative of any competent, non-consenting patient.[78] The threat to leave AMA, similar to most other medico-legal conflicts, usually represents a clinical problem disguised as a legal dispute. The consultant called to evaluate the patient threatening to leave AMA must evaluate whether the patient has the capacity to make that decision. In the course of the evaluation, it is common to find that the patient is angry over a perceived lack of caring or dissatisfaction with the amount of information provided by the treating physician. The consultant who can restore communication between physician and patient may be successful in getting the patient to complete the course of treatment. If the patient does leave, the consultant may then have to calm the staff in preparation for the patient returning at a later date.

From a legal standpoint, if patients possess the capacity to make decisions and do not pose a risk of harm to themselves or others, they cannot be held against their will. A patient requesting to sign out AMA may be deemed to have the requisite capacity to do so if he or she understands the nature of the illness, the recommended treatment, the alternative treatments available, and the prognosis with or without treatment and is able to use this information in a rational manner to reach a decision. If the patient meets these criteria, he or she can leave against advice, whether or not the form is signed. The discussions before release and the fact that the patient refused to sign the form should be documented in the medical record. In the event that the patient refuses to sign the form, that documentation should suffice.

CONCLUSION

This chapter began with a discussion of the role of the psychiatric consultant in helping consultees deal with medico-legal issues. It is appropriate to close it with a few cautionary words about the temptations encountered by those who undertake this task. Consultants are often tempted to meet the needs of their consultees by telling them what they want to hear. Nowhere is this truer than in the assessment of a patient's capacity to consent to, or to refuse, treatment. This is compounded by the consultant's own bias, as a physician, to seek an outcome that is in the best clinical interests of the patient. In performing capacity assessments and other consultations on medico-legal issues, such temptations must be resisted. The role of the consultant is to be objective and focused on the issue at hand, rather than on what the consultant or consultee sees as the best overall clinical outcome. Such isolation of purpose is often difficult, but it is essential if the consultant is to serve the consultee and the patient. The consultant must also keep in mind that he or she is just that: a consultant whose job it is to advise, not to make treatment decisions. The treating physician may choose to disregard the consultant's assessment that a patient lacks the capacity to make treatment decisions and proceed with treatment. The treating physician assumes both the legal and moral liability of his or her own actions. The consultant can serve only as a guidepost and only then by being both knowledgeable and objective. This task is made easier by taking the following approach to consultation on these highly charged medico-legal issues:

1. Know what you are being asked to do. That is, understand both the overt request and any covert agenda that may exist.
2. Know the clinical facts of the consultation.
3. Know, or find out, the salient legal requirements involved.
4. Determine the presence of any apparent conflict between good clinical care and the law.
5. Get to know the hospital attorney; share information and attempt to develop a multidisciplinary team approach to patient care.
6. Try to move all parties away from a crisis mentality to gain some time to resolve conflicts and to encourage compromise. Avoid ultimatums. Pushing back deadlines for procedures, treatment, leaving the hospital AMA, etc., decrease time pressures and allow people to think more clearly.
7. Understand the personalities of the physician and the patient.
8. Know the patient's next of kin, their understanding, fears, biases, personalities, and the probabilities of obtaining informed consent from them.
9. Act as a go-between, so as to diminish anxiety and communication gaps among physician, patient, and family and try to find areas for compromise and agreement.
10. Search out covert disagreements and hidden fears in the physician and patient; try to find commonsense measures that would remedy these, and search for loopholes and areas in which conflicts can be mended or avoided.

11. Provide detailed documentation in the patient's medical record (or chart) of the patient's understanding, judgment, capacity to give consent, and clinical and psychiatric status, as well as the course pursued.
12. Maintain an objective point of view while remaining mindful that the consultant's responsibility is to assess as accurately as possible the patient's capacity to give an informed consent and that truth is a higher goal than scheduling concerns of the consultee and ward staff.
13. Use such consultations to teach physicians that they have little to fear from the law and to teach patients that they have little to fear from their physicians.

REFERENCES

Access the reference list online at https://expertconsult.inkling.com/.

Approaches to Collaborative Care and Behavioral Health Integration

52

Andrew D. Carlo, M.D.
BJ Beck, M.S.N., M.D.
Eric M. Weil, M.D.
Jonathan E. Alpert, M.D., Ph.D.

OVERVIEW

Historical trends in psychiatry[1] over the last century mirrored developments in the U.S. healthcare system more broadly[2] that promoted system re-design to provide safer and more personalized, cost-effective, and high-quality health care. Care re-design in the treatment of psychiatric disorders included innovative approaches to providing psychiatric care in the general medical setting, which is commonly the first site of presentation of mental illness, and is often the only resource available for patients. Advances in psychopharmacology greatly facilitated the development of such models, which were designed to address quality, cost-containment, and allocation of limited resources. Initially, psychiatric care provided to medically ill patients was primarily hospital-based, but ever-shorter inpatient stays increasingly drove those services to outpatient settings. This paralleled the trend for shorter inpatient psychiatric hospitalizations (often without the benefit of increased mental health resources in the ambulatory setting),[3] which left primary care providers (PCPs) responsible for treating more acute and complex psychiatric illness in their outpatient practices. Resourceful psychiatrists recognized the need to collaborate with their medical colleagues in developing and implementing pragmatic, cost-effective, outpatient models of high-quality psychiatric care that could be delivered in the primary care setting. One such model, known as collaborative care, is an evidence-based approach for integrating physical and behavioral health services that can be implemented within various primary care settings. Collaborative care includes: (1) care coordination and care management; (2) regular/pro-active monitoring and treatment to target using validated clinical rating scales; and (3) regular, systematic psychiatric caseload reviews and consultation for patients who do not show clinical improvement.[4] This and other models of care integration will be discussed below.

The realization of limited healthcare resources and rapid escalation of healthcare expenditures has forced a change in focus from patient- to population-based care, or from individualized to team-based strategies.[5] This change has, at times, been remarkably challenging for healthcare systems and providers, as it represents a fundamental organizational and philosophical shift in the traditional doctor–patient paradigm. Models of population health have long been applied to patients with chronic medical illness (e.g., diabetes, hypertension, medical complexity). It was not until relatively recently, however, that poor overall health outcomes and significant fiscal burden compelled healthcare systems to apply similar models to patients with psychiatric co-morbidities. Studies have consistently demonstrated that individuals with psychiatric disorders utilize physical health care resources more frequently and experience increased work absenteeism, unemployment, subjective disability, increased morbidity from chronic medical illness and premature mortality.[6–8] Though more difficult to demonstrate, there is also a cost-offset of appropriate and timely psychiatric treatment.[9–11]

Furthermore, changes in healthcare reimbursement have resulted in conflicted PCP incentives.[12] On the one hand, pre-paid, provider-risk plans (i.e., capitated programs), such as health maintenance organizations (HMOs), exposed the expensive use of general medical services by patients with untreated or poorly managed psychiatric illness, providing an incentive for the PCP to initiate treatment for the more common psychiatric problems seen in primary care. On the other hand, the PCP gatekeeper system of the 1990s, which evolved to manage the overall cost of care, including specialty care, created a potential incentive not to refer for psychiatric care, even conceivably in the setting of more severe mental illness. Limited formularies, varying by plan, with onerous, time-consuming prior authorization requirements, further complicated and deterred the initiation of appropriate treatment by all providers. Managed care organizations (MCOs) often carved-out substance use and mental health (collectively called behavioral health [BH]) benefits management to managed BH organizations (MBHOs),[13] some with limited referral networks not inclusive of the PCP's psychiatric colleagues. This not only resulted in a major referral disincentive, but also complicated future communication and collaboration between BH and physical health providers. While many MBHOs have spearheaded initiatives to promote primary care treatment of common psychiatric problems, most do not credential or contract with non-psychiatric physicians, so this essentially cost-shifts expense from the MBHO to the (medical) MCO.

Passage of the 2010 healthcare reform legislation (Patient Protection and Affordable Care Act [PPACA]) pushed the envelope to create more inclusive, accessible, coordinated, and integrated care systems,[14] and to achieve the "triple aim" (i.e., improved quality, improved outcomes, reduced total healthcare cost).[15] These initiatives include the patient-centered medical home, accountable care organizations, and integrated programs for the "dual eligible" populations (i.e., those eligible for both Medicare and Medicaid, either the elderly and indigent, or the disabled and poor).[16] To be successful in any of these initiatives, there is an important and recognized role for consultant psychiatrists[17] and an overall more robust strategy for the global management of patients with mental illness.

EPIDEMIOLOGY

Epidemiologic studies over the past several decades have underscored the scope and profound public health impact of psychiatric disorders in the community, as well as their widespread under-detection and under-treatment. The Epidemiologic Catchment Area (ECA) Study, conducted in the early 1980s, attempted to quantify the prevalence of psychiatric problems in community residents of the United States. Within a 6-month span, roughly 7% sought help for a BH problem. More than 60% never saw a BH professional, but sought care in a medical setting (e.g., emergency department, ED PCP's office).[18] Even among those who met full criteria for a diagnosable psychiatric disorder, 75% were seen only in the general medical (rather than the BH) setting.[19] It was inferred, therefore, that psychiatric distress was exceedingly common in the primary care population. About half of general medical outpatients had some psychiatric symptoms. The use of structured diagnostic interviews detected a prevalence of 25% to 35% for diagnosable psychiatric conditions in this patient population. However, roughly 10% of primary care patients had significant psychiatric distress without meeting diagnostic criteria for a psychiatric disorder.[20] The majority of diagnosable disorders were mood disorders (80%), with depression being the most prevalent (60%); anxiety disorders were a distant second (20%). The more severe disorders (e.g., psychotic disorders) were more likely to be treated by BH professionals.[19] The National Comorbidity Survey (NCS), conducted between 1990 and 1992, demonstrated a 50% life-time prevalence of one or more psychiatric disorders in US adults, with a 30% 1-year prevalence of at least one disorder.[21] Alcohol dependence and major depression were the most common disorders. A rigorous replication of the NCS (NCS-R), in 2001 to 2002, also measured severity, clinical significance, overall disability, and role impairment.[22] The NCS-R found the risk of major depression was relatively low until early adolescence, when it begins to rise in a linear fashion. The slope of that line has increased (i.e., becoming steeper) for each successive birth cohort since the Second World War. The life-time prevalence of significant depression was 16.2%; the 12-month prevalence was 6.6%. Two findings, however, were of particular interest. First, 55.1% of depressed community respondents seeking care received that care in the BH sector. The other significant finding, attributable to advances in pharmacotherapy and educational efforts, was that 90% of respondents treated for depression in any medical setting received psychotropic medication. While this suggested improved community depression treatment, it was tempered by the finding that only 21.6% of patients received what recent, evidence-based guidelines (American Psychiatric Association [APA]; Agency for Healthcare Research and Quality [AHRQ]) considered minimally adequate treatment (64.3% treated by BH providers, and 41.3% of those treated by general medical providers), and almost half (42.7%) of patients with depression still received no treatment.[22] Older studies documented PCPs' failure to diagnose over half of the full criteria mental disorders of their patients,[23,24] but later studies demonstrated that PCPs recognized their more seriously depressed[25] or anxious[26] patients. These studies also demonstrated that higher-functioning, less severely symptomatic primary care patients have relatively good outcomes, even with short courses of relatively low doses of medications. This highlights the diagnostic difficulty for PCPs—primary care patients are different from those who seek specialty care (i.e., the population in whom most psychiatric research is done). Primary care patients may seek treatment earlier in the course of their illness, since they have an established relationship with their PCP that is not dependent on their having a psychiatric disorder. They frequently present with somatic complaints, rather than psychiatric symptoms. Since the soma is often the primary focus of the PCP, this further obscures the diagnosis. Primary care patients often present acute psychiatric symptoms that clear quickly (i.e., before therapeutic medication levels are reached), suggesting they might benefit as much from watchful waiting and the empathic support of their PCP.

There is a high noise-to-signal ratio in psychiatrically distressed primary care patients. That is, as many as one-third of significantly distressed patients have sub-syndromal disorders not meeting criteria for diagnosable mental disorders. This diagnostic ambiguity, coupled with relatively good outcomes after brief trials of sub-therapeutic medication doses,[23,27] is cause to re-consider the significance of the PCP's "failure" to diagnose. Much primary care patient angst resolves spontaneously, either with resolution of an initiating event, expressed caregiver concern, or the placebo effect of a few days of medication. In such cases, the presenting symptoms may be attributable to an adjustment disorder.

BARRIERS TO TREATMENT

Symptom recognition is necessary but not sufficient to ensure primary care treatment of psychiatric problems.[28] Even when PCPs are informed of standardized screening results, they may not initiate treatment. PCP, patient, and system factors collude to inhibit the discussion necessary to promote treatment ("don't ask/don't tell").[29] Physician factors ("don't ask") include the failure to take a social history or to perform a mental status examination (MSE).[30] This may be attributed to deficits in training of medical students and residents,[31] to time and productivity pressures, and to personal defenses (e.g., identification, denial,[32] isolation of affect). Variation in skills and attitudes are broad across primary care. In general, PCPs tend to be more experienced and comfortable addressing physical complaints. Some PCPs fear their patients will leave the practice if asked about BH issues. Others may even question the benefit of treatment. More significantly, the absence of a ready response or approach, or the lack of a psychiatric referral source are major deterrents to screening and identification of a new problem within the context of a 15-minute primary care visit. Denial or avoidance may prevail when the time-pressured PCP feels unsure of how to treat, whether to refer, or whom to ask.

Stigma, prevalent among patients and providers, is a major patient deterrent to bringing up psychiatric symptoms. Often patients "don't tell" because of shame or embarrassment. Patients may not know they have a diagnosable or treatable BH disorder.[33] They may equate psychiatric problems with personal weakness, and assume their PCP shares that view. For these and other reasons, primary care patients frequently present with physical complaints, increasing diagnostic complexity substantially.[34] This is particularly confounding for physicians because medical disorders may simulate psychiatric disorders, psychiatric disorders may lead to physical symptoms, and psychiatric and medical disorders may co-exist.

System factors include the ever-changing healthcare finance and reimbursement climate (e.g., managed care, "carve-outs," provider risk, capitation, fee-for-service, coding nuances, differential formularies, prior authorization) that promotes financial imperatives to contain cost and to increase efficiency. This systemic instability, confusion, and administrative time-creep easily dwarfs the impulse to pursue the treatment of a possibly self-limited condition. BH carve-outs have complicated the possibility of reimbursing PCP treatment of BH disorders, while pre-paid plans (e.g., HMOs) decrease incentives to offer anything "extra."[35] The necessity to increase productivity has excessively shortened the "routine visit," now often less than 15 minutes, while the excessive burden of required documentation further erodes clinically available time. Although the electronic health record (EHR) has standardized and improved screening, documentation, and follow-up,[36] it is also a source of clinical time depletion. The care-promoting advent of new, safer, more tolerable psychotropic medications has been offset by soaring pharmacy costs and by restrictive (and possibly short-sighted[37]) formularies. The practice of primary care has reached a crisis point: the pressures are so overwhelming that few PCPs want to sustain full-time clinical practice.

THE GOALS OF COLLABORATION

Although effective, evidence-based treatments exist, access and quality of care remain significant issues that are best addressed through the collaboration of psychiatry and primary care. The four major goals of collaboration are to improve access, treatment, outcomes, and communication.

Access

Collaborative care in the primary care setting addresses both physician and patient factors that limit the patient's access to appropriate assessment and treatment. Most patients are familiar with the general medical practice and feel more comfortable and less stigmatized in that setting. Conversely, they may believe the mental health clinic is for "crazy people," not a (perceived) clientele with whom they identify. Even a defined BH unit in the primary care setting may be stigmatizing and thus a barrier to treatment access. Most patients do not know of a psychiatrist or how to access care from one and may not feel certain that they need one. The unaided decision to foray into the BH arena may be fraught with shame and anxiety, powerful deterrents to making that first call. Calling the PCP's office and making an appointment for fatigue, sleep problems, weight loss, or palpitations is infinitely less threatening.

An established relationship between the PCP and a trusted, accessible psychiatric consultant eases the burden of recognizing, treating, or referring patients with mental disorders. PCPs more readily identify psychiatric distress and initiate treatment when they have expert clinical back-up available.

Treatment

Historically, PCPs often prescribed insufficient doses of medications (e.g., amitriptyline 25 mg) for major depression.[38] Since the advent of safer, well-tolerated medications (e.g., selective serotonin re-uptake inhibitors [SSRIs]), PCPs' prescriptive choices have improved,[39,40] although practice largely remains inconsistent regarding dosing, augmentation, and the switching of medications when a drug trial has failed. Symptomatic and impaired patients may remain on ineffective medications for prolonged periods of time. Benzodiazepines has been prescribed by PCPs more frequently than any other class of psychotropic medication, even for major depression,[41] but they now are appropriately surpassed by antidepressant prescriptions.[40] Collaboration with the consultation psychiatrist can improve the choice, dose, and resourceful management of psychotropic medications. Collaboration is also helpful when the PCP's preferred medication is off-formulary for a given patient. Such a treatment deterrent may instead become an opportunity for brief, pragmatic education.

Outcomes

Several studies have demonstrated better outcomes for seriously depressed primary care patients treated collaboratively by their PCP and a psychiatrist.[42–44] Cost-offset, however, is difficult to demonstrate because of the hidden costs of psychiatric disability.[7,45,46] Nonetheless, there is evidence for decreased total healthcare spending when BH problems are adequately addressed.[11] Even if this were not so, the case for cost-effectiveness could be made.[9,47–49] That is, care for the patient's psychiatric problem is more cost-effective than spending the same amount of money addressing the often non-responsive, somatic complaints of high-utilizing medical patients.

Communication

Collaboration ends the PCP's justifiable complaint of the "black box" of psychiatry because communication is implicit in these care models. Information must flow in both directions to assist the psychiatrist and the PCP in the provision of quality care. Referrals by PCPs provide pertinent information and state the clinical question. In addition to the target psychiatric symptoms, the PCP has and provides important information about the medical history, allergies, treatments, and medications. The collaborating psychiatrist shares findings, diagnostic impressions, and treatment recommendations. Information about referrals and consultations should be written and, whenever possible, provided verbally to ensure an understanding between collaborating care providers. Secure e-mail, EHR staff messaging, or other IT approaches, may also provide nearly instantaneous feedback, and focus on pertinent details for the busy PCP. Patients, of course, must be aware of the collaborative relationship between the PCP and the psychiatrist, as well as their shared communication.

ROLES, RELATIONSHIPS, EXPECTATIONS, AND LIABILITY

Successful collaboration requires a clear understanding and definition of roles. All parties, including the patient, should recognize the PCP's responsibility for the patient's overall care. The PCP is the broker and overseer of all specialty services. The psychiatrist is a consultant to the PCP, and sometimes a co-treater, depending on the model. Collaboration does not breach patient confidentiality because the PCP and the psychiatrist are now within the circle of care, and the patient is informed of this relationship.

This free flow of communication and documentation has reasonable limitations. If a patient asks that particular details not be placed in his or her general medical record and these details do not directly affect the patient's medical care (e.g., a detailed description of childhood incest), it is reasonable to respect this wish. The pertinent information (e.g., the experience of childhood trauma) can be expressed in more general terms. If, however, information could affect medical treatment (e.g., current or past drug addiction) or safety (e.g., suicidal or homicidal intent, psychosis, or previous suicide attempt), such information cannot be withheld from the PCP, and the patient should be so informed.

When the PCP refers the patient to the psychiatrist, the patient should be given clear expectations for the visit. It is also the psychiatrist's responsibility to clearly describe the parameters of the contact (e.g., whether it will be a one-time consultation, with or without the possibility of medication follow-up, or possible referral for therapy). If the psychiatrist sees the patient more than once, the relationships (i.e., between the PCP and the psychiatrist, as well as between the patient and the psychiatrist) may need to be reiterated. The clarity of the providers' roles and relationship serves to spare the patient a sense of abandonment, either by the PCP when the patient is referred to the psychiatrist, or by the psychiatrist when the patient is returned to the PCP for ongoing psychiatric management.

In collaborative models of care, it is common for the psychiatric notes to be placed in the general medical record, which may raise issues of confidentiality and privacy. Most states require a specific release for mental health or substance use treatment records. With an EHR, there may be software coding solutions to avoid the inadvertent release of this information. As BH issues are increasingly treated by PCPs, the question of how to document and protect such information is a growing concern, preferably to be addressed in a way that does not further complicate and deter such treatment.

Finally, collaborative care raises several compelling legal questions about physician responsibility in the event of a poor outcome (e.g., completed suicide, catastrophic drug–drug interaction). In many collaborative care models, this malpractice liability is difficult to define (based on current legal precedent), as the psychiatrist is not the primary prescriber for the patient (and may never actually see the patient in person). To date, there have been no known cases of malpractice brought against collaborative care-related problems.[50] Since integrated and collaborative care are relatively new models of care, practice patterns differ widely among sites and physician roles are varying, it would seem that liability for alleged medical malpractice depends upon specific circumstances surrounding each case (and would be heavily influenced by state laws, regulations, and case-law).[50] Psychiatrists are strongly advised to be familiar with their state and local laws when practicing in integrated care settings. When questions arise, it is recommended that each provider seek legal counsel or a risk management professional.[50]

MODELS OF COLLABORATION

Collaborative models differ in terms of where the patient is seen, whether there is a single medical record, how providers communicate, whether the psychiatrist recommends or initiates treatment, and whether the psychiatrist sees the patient (at all, once, more than once) or serves as an ongoing treater. Another important variable is whether both providers belong to the same medical staff and how available (physically, electronically, or telephonically) the psychiatrist is to the PCP. Although the literature varies on the precise number of existing models, three core models appear to have emerged—coordinated care, co-located care, and collaborative care (also known as fully integrated care).[51] Table 52-1 summarizes these differences and Table 52-2 describes some of the advantages and limitations of each model.

COORDINATED CARE

Coordinated models of care are the least integrated of the three major models. Typically, the psychiatrist and PCP are in different care systems and do not communicate on a systematic or regular basis. Medical record systems and practice locations are typically separate (although there are exceptions). The following sections will describe various types of coordinated care models: longitudinal outpatient psychiatric care, specialty psychiatry clinics, and consultation psychiatrists (including consult-and-return models from off-site psychiatrists).

Longitudinal Outpatient Psychiatric Care

Longitudinal outpatient care describes scenarios in which the PCP refers a patient for specialty psychiatric care. Depending on the setting or the system, one medical record may be shared, or providers may maintain separate records and share pertinent information. However, under most circumstances, medical records are not shared and communication is facilitated by telephone, letters, or facsimile. This model is best exemplified by the practice of private psychiatrists with well-established referral sources in the primary care sector. In these consultation models, providers generally do not develop a truly collaborative relationship, communicate regularly, or share records. They treat in parallel, rather than in collaboration. Stigma is often problematic in these models, as patients may have a negative connotation associated with "seeing a psychiatrist."

TABLE 52-1 Integrated Care Models[49–58]

	COORDINATED CARE (LEAST INTEGRATED)	CO-LOCATED CARE	COLLABORATIVE CARE (MOST INTEGRATED)
Location of care	Separate	Shared	Shared
Medical record	Separate	Shared or separate	Shared
Communication	Not systematic—on an as-needed basis; often via telephone, letter, or fax, as secure e-mail communication is difficult among providers in different systems; sub-optimal understanding of each other's roles and cultures	Not systematic—on an as-needed basis; e-mail communication is typically available, as providers are in the same system; misunderstandings still may occur, as providers do not always understand each other's roles and cultures	Regular and systematic team collaboration and communication—staff share a panel of patients and understand each other's roles and cultures; e-mail and in-person communication are common; outcome registries are shared among providers
Where model is found	Most private practices and agencies	Common in HMO settings and community clinics.	In some large health systems, academic medical centers and hospice centers; increasingly seen in community clinics
Types of psychiatric diagnoses well-managed by care model	All psychiatric diagnoses can be managed in this model. However, those with few psychosocial stressors are most likely to have favorable outcomes	All psychiatric diagnoses can be managed in this model. However, this model is most successful in patients with moderate psychosocial stressors. Also assists with patients for whom stigma is a significant barrier	Mostly validated for treatment of depression (primarily). However, studies are ongoing for PTSD, anxiety, substance use, and other conditions. Patients with major psychosocial stressors benefit from this patient-centered, multidisciplinary team approach

TABLE 52-2 Pros and Cons of Integrated Care Models[51,52]

	PROS	CONS
Coordinated care	Privacy and autonomy for PCPs, patients and psychiatrists Practices do not have to adjust their operating structures Every patient sees a psychiatrist	Often a lack of coordination and understanding among providers Services may overlap or conflict due to lack of communication Referrals may fail due to barriers to care or stigma
Co-located care	May decrease stigma and lessen barriers Less risk of misdiagnosis (as patients are seen by psychiatrists) Expands access because psychiatrist does not expand panel (in models where psychiatrists do not continue to follow patients longitudinally) Allows for indirect consultation among providers and leads to new relationships among staff from different specialties Can successfully manage patients with serious mental illness (SMI) and multiple medical problems	Co-location does not guarantee integration and coordination Does not increase access to the same extent as the collaborative care model Patients may still experience stigma (e.g., going to the mental health floor of a health center) Potential for tension and conflicting agendas among providers as clinic boundaries dissolve
Collaborative care (fully integrated care)	Highest-quality care for diagnosis of depression (with an increasing body of evidence supporting anxiety and PTSD), increased patient and provider satisfaction, lowest cost Expands access to the greatest extent Best coordination and continuity	Possibility of misdiagnosis Must train additional staff High upfront financial and productivity costs Not ideal for managing serious mental illness (SMI) Not a desirable workflow for all providers

Specialty Psychiatric Clinics

Specialty psychiatric clinics (e.g., eating disorder or obsessive–compulsive disorder programs) are usually in teaching hospitals or tertiary care centers, but may also be free-standing specialty practices. These clinics generally maintain separate records, require the patient to be seen in the psychiatric clinic, and develop some means of ongoing, clinically relevant PCP communication. Patients typically need to have well-defined problems to be accepted into the clinic. Although stigma may interfere with patient adherence to such a referral, one major advantage of such clinics is the expert, multidisciplinary approach they provide for patients with complex psychiatric and medical problems, although some specialty clinics may provide overly narrow care for patients whose problems span multiple psychiatric (and other medical) diagnoses.

Consultation Psychiatry (Including Consult-and-Return Models)

Depending on the location of the consultation, these models may be classified as either coordinated or co-located (described in a subsequent section). In coordinated care outpatient consultation psychiatry models,[59,60] providers may follow the patient for a period of time or render a one-visit opinion in a separate office (similar to other specialty consultations). The one-visit opinions are often referred to as consult-and-return models. As in inpatient consultation work, the consultation request and report should be placed in the primary care record. Immediate verbal communication, whenever possible, by phone, e-mail, or voicemail, greatly enhances the utility of such consultations. However, given the presence of healthcare information privacy laws (requiring signed consent forms to be transmitted by facsimile prior to verbal or written communication), this is often a barrier in systems with limited integration. In these models, the consultant generally does not initiate treatment but makes practical recommendations. It is noteworthy that these models promote favorable opportunities for ongoing informal education between the PCP and the consultant.

CO-LOCATED CARE

Co-located care models often include a moderate degree of care integration, largely facilitated by the proximity of the psychiatrist to the primary care clinic staff. Although care integration is not inherent in co-located care, such models provide enhanced possibilities for shared care. The PCP–consultant proximity facilitates communication, formal and informal education, immediate access to curbside consultation, and heightened PCP awareness of psychiatric problems in their patients. This arrangement can also provide an excellent opportunity for training of both psychiatric and primary care residents. Patients appreciate being seen in the more familiar primary care setting, and they often feel less stigmatized. Several models of care have evolved or been developed to utilize the services of an in-house or staff psychiatrist. The psychiatrist may: (1) consult as a member of the medical team or evaluate, stabilize, and return the patient to the PCP with recommendations for continued care (including possible referral to outside psychiatric providers);[61] (2) evaluate and treat patients jointly and in parallel with the PCP; or (3) alternate visits with the PCP while treatment is initiated.[10,44,62] Co-located care models also include "reverse integration" (the placement of primary care clinicians into specialty psychiatry clinics), which is described below.

Staff Consultant/Stepped Care Models

Consultations, as above, are written in the general shared medical record. The permanency of the psychiatrist allows for a more finely tuned consultant–PCP relationship. For instance, with a previously established agreement, a staff consultant may initiate the recommended treatment and subsequently return the patient to the PCP for further care (a co-located consult-and-return model).[61] Furthermore, the consultation psychiatrist may offer clinically relevant suggestions during case conferences or discussions of more complex patients. The psychiatrist may also briefly see the patient with the PCP during a primary care visit to provide timely treatment recommendations or to perform a "warm hand-off,"[63] which gives the patient an opportunity to meet the psychiatric provider before a formal evaluation. This can increase patient and provider satisfaction, increase the chance of a successful consultation and reduce stigma and fear associated with mental health.

In some primary care settings, patients with major depressive disorder or an anxiety disorder are treated using a model called stepped care. In these settings, the staff psychiatrist is not consulted until a patient has shown an inadequate response to a 6–8-week course of at least one antidepressant medication.[64] Once behavioral health is requested, a patient will often have between two and four visits with a consulting psychiatrist in the PCP's office (depending on patient response). Stepped care has been shown to be superior to usual care with regard to medication adherence, satisfaction with treatment, and depression outcomes.[64] Similarly to the consultation models described above, patients are returned to the PCP for further management once stabilized from a psychiatric perspective.

Re-evaluation of patients previously seen occurs when there is a change, such as roughening (the re-emergence of symptoms short of full syndromic relapse while on previously effective treatment), the development of new psychiatric symptoms, medication side effects, or a change in medical condition or medications that affect psychiatric symptoms or medications. It is noteworthy that a premise of this model is that not all patients are appropriate for PCP management. The psychiatrist should help the PCP recognize which patients are better served by longitudinal follow-up (either by a staff psychiatrist or in a specialty care clinic) and assist with appropriate referral. Patients not recommended for PCP management include those with significant suicidal ideation (or high-risk factors for suicide such as near lethal previous attempts), severe personality disorders, treatment refractory depression or anxiety, inherently unstable conditions (e.g., psychotic disorders, bipolar disorder), or complicated medication regimens that require close monitoring. Other in-house behavioral health services available on a consultation basis may include focused, short-term, goal-oriented individual or group therapy (with master's-level clinicians located within the primary care clinical area).

Parallel Care

In these systems, psychiatrists assume the ongoing psychiatric care of patients in parallel with the PCP (usually within the same building or clinic space). If the psychiatric area is an identifiable, geographical locus within the clinic, it may be fraught with the same stigma that occurs when the clinics are truly separate. Although still within the circle of care, the larger the clinic and more separate the clinical services, the greater the diligence required on the part of each provider to meet the challenge of continued communication. When medical records are not shared between the PCP and psychiatrist, parallel care requires some overt means of communication to keep all providers informed. In clinics with an EHR, a single up-to-date medication list will at least keep both providers aware of current medications and medication changes.

Depending on staffing and space, the psychiatric capacity of primary care clinics that offer these services may be inadequate to meet the needs of the total clinic patient population. This situation can be problematic and delay access because most patients would like to be treated in this setting. Uniform criteria may facilitate the triage of patients for in-house treatment or outside referral. These criteria may include diagnosis and measures of acuity and complexity and take into account relevant community resources and specialty centers, language requirements, and payment sources. Certain unstable or less common psychiatric problems may be better served in the behavioral health sector, either in community clinics with "wrap-around" services or in specific subspecialty clinics. In most communities, English-speaking patients have more options for treatment. Depending on the location and availability of appropriate, non-English-speaking services, patients may be preferentially kept in-house, or referred out. Patients with insurance will generally have more options outside the primary care setting than those who are uninsured, and some insurance plans with behavioral health carve-outs may not cover psychiatric care in the same setting in which they cover medical services.

Joint (or Collaborative) Patient Management

In joint (or collaborative) management,[44] which is not to be confused with collaborative (or fully integrated) care, the patient alternates visits between the psychiatrist and the PCP in the primary care setting during initiation of treatment (i.e., the first 4 to 6 weeks). The PCP then assumes responsibility for the patient's continued psychopharmacological treatment. This model was developed as a research protocol for the treatment of depressed, primary care patients (and has been extended to the treatment of panic disorder).[9] Patients are referred by the PCP, usually after an initial ineffective trial of medication. This intensive program of care has been cost-effective for more severely depressed primary care patients. Implicit in this model are certain underlying assumptions. Joint (or collaborative) management assumes that PCPs can initiate appropriate treatment for depression, manage the care of patients stabilized on antidepressant medications and improve behavioral health care for more seriously depressed patients with the assistance of an in-house psychiatric consultant.[65] This model also assumes that such collaborative relationships begin with PCP education and training. As would be the case in learning to manage any chronic illness, PCPs participate in regular teaching conferences. A psychoeducational module for patients is also an integral part of the treatment.

Primary Care in Psychiatry ("Reverse Integration")

Multiple studies have examined the effectiveness of co-located primary care clinicians in psychiatric clinic settings. These models are ideal for patients with SMI and chronic medical conditions who are best managed in psychiatry specialty clinics (e.g., clozapine clinics). It is well-known and described in the literature that psychiatric patients are more likely than age-matched controls to have medical disorders.[66] This is particularly true in individuals with SMI conditions, such as schizophrenia, schizoaffective disorder and bipolar disorder. For example, patients with schizophrenia have a higher prevalence of HIV infection, osteoporosis, obesity, diabetes mellitus, and cardiovascular disease than those in the general population.[66] Therefore, these patients often require higher level medical care. When this care is integrated into the psychiatric setting, improvements have been identified in health maintenance, care coordination, and satisfaction with care. Furthermore, when care managers are utilized, additional patient education and management services are provided, which may improve adherence with outpatient treatment.[66]

COLLABORATIVE (FULLY INTEGRATED) CARE

Collaborative care management employs the highest level of care integration by working to broker and coordinate the care of patients with complicated medical or mental health problems who use services in multiple (otherwise discontinuous) settings. It bridges the communication needs when patients access services outside of the primary care setting. After a comprehensive diagnostic and functional assessment (often by a care manager, as opposed to the team psychiatrist), necessary releases are signed to allow the care manager to serve as a liaison between the PCP and all other care providers. The care manager involves the patient and all treaters in the development of a comprehensive treatment plan within a network of services, and tracks the patient from site to site throughout this plan. As a member of the discharge planning team, the care manager also ensures that the patient returns to the appropriate network of services after care in a hospital, a detoxification program, or another residential/institutional setting. Of note, as stated above, psychiatrists often do not see patients themselves in collaborative care models. Instead, the care manager interacts with the patient on a regular basis and receives systematic supervision from the team psychiatrist. Patients' medical and behavioral health outcomes are tracked together in care registries maintained by the care manager. If a particular patient does not meet objective outcomes of successful treatment (e.g., reduction of PHQ-9 score, a 10-item, 1-page, self-administered tool that quantifies the patient's mood and neurovegetative symptoms of depression,[67] by 50%), the psychiatrist may elect to see that patient for a brief series of visits for diagnostic clarification and further treatment planning.

The IMPACT Model

Spearheaded by researchers at the University of Washington, the IMPACT (Improving Mood-Promoting Access to Collaborative Treatment) collaborative care management model was designed to improve the management of late-life depression. In this model, patients were encouraged to see a care manager designated as a depression clinical specialist (DCS) in the primary care setting. In the initial study, the

DCS was a licensed healthcare professional (clinical social worker, psychologist, psychiatric nurse). Later models have employed non-licensed healthcare professionals. During the initial interaction with the patient, the DCS conducted a history, provided psychosocial education, and discussed patient preference for treatment (pharmacotherapy versus psychotherapy versus both). New cases and challenging follow-ups were discussed in a weekly team meeting with the PCP, psychiatrist, and care manager. The patient's PCP and care manager then worked with the patient to develop a comprehensive treatment plan, which often included an antidepressant and a short course of evidence-based psychotherapy (e.g., Problem-Solving Treatment in Primary Care [PST-PC]).[62] For 12 months, patients' depression scores (measured with the SCL-20) were recorded in an electronic data registry. Patients who responded (defined as >50% reduction in SCL-20 score and fewer than 3 of 9 symptoms of major depression) were engaged in relapse prevention. For those who did not respond, a subsequent care plan was developed by the IMPACT team. According to the published IMPACT results, intervention patients had lower depression severity (as measured with the SCL-20) than usual care (with the difference between usual care and intervention increasing from the 3- to 12-month follow-up points). The intervention group also had higher rates of treatment response and complete remission of symptoms.[62] The IMPACT model has now been adapted for various other diagnoses in multiple healthcare systems nationwide.

Three-Component Model

Supported by the MacArthur Initiative on Depression in Primary Care, the three-component model (TCM)[68] is a formalized system of consultative care that promotes the primary care treatment of depression as a chronic disease, with regular measures of adherence and outcome to guide the evidence-based protocol of medication and other treatment adjustments. Educational modules exist for PCPs, consultant psychiatrists, phone-based care managers, and patients. The PHQ-9 is repeatedly used to track the patient's progress. Multiple measures of symptoms and treatment adherence are recorded on a standard form that facilitates consultation, communication, and organized treatment review, planning, and adjustment. Dissemination of the TCM and its standardized materials, manuals, and educational modules addresses the need to improve care for this large population (i.e., patients receiving depression treatment in primary care) while also providing data to inform policy (and payment) decisions. A similar evidence-based endeavor is the Health Disparities Collaborative, which is the combined effort of the Department of Health and Human Services, the Health Resources and Services Administration, and the Bureau of Primary Health Care.

CHOOSING THE RIGHT MODEL

The choice of model depends on a variety of practice factors, such as patient population, payer mix, range of available community resources, as well as the location, type, and size of the practice. Patients with higher educational or socioeconomic status may feel less stigmatized and be more willing to seek and to pay for outside psychiatric services.[69] Some patients feel more comfortable in private practice settings that allow the greatest possible privacy, albeit at the cost of less integrated care. Behavioral health problems are less acceptable or even shameful in some cultures. These patient populations will favor a more integrated and "invisible" system within the primary care setting. It is noteworthy that collaborative care models require adequate community resources to refer patients not considered appropriate for primary care management. Suburban or rural areas that lack these resources are better served by parallel, or shared, care models. Small groups or solo practitioners may favor consultation models, either with a part-time but regularly scheduled consultant or through access to an outside consultant, as needed. Large practices, and especially training facilities, will benefit most from the full range of in-house consultative and collaborative services that include formal education, case conferences, curbside consultation, and collaborative care management. The Affordable Care Act promoted integrated care models and provided funding opportunities to help make these services sustainable. At present, the impact of potential changes to the health care system at the state and federal levels is yet to be determined.

CONCLUSIONS

PCPs have held (and will continue to hold) an important front-line position in total health care, population-based care, and all levels of prevention.[70] Although at least in part driven by changes in the healthcare system, collaborative models serve to increase access and improve treatment for patients who would otherwise be unable or unlikely to receive psychiatric care outside of the primary care setting. A number of considerations determine the best model for a given practice setting. Such factors include size, patient population, available community resources, payer mix, and other reimbursement sources. To remain viable, high-quality and cost-effective models will need to adapt and evolve with the changing healthcare system and emerging value-based models for healthcare financing. Psychiatrists and PCPs will need to be flexible and innovative in their approaches to patient care and rigorous demonstration of cost-offsets will be needed to encourage allocation of adequate resources to reimburse their services.[71,72] Medical,[73] psychiatric, and patient education will need to reflect these changes in caregiver roles and expectations.

CASE 1

Ms. T, a 26-year-old single woman moved to the area to start a post-doctoral fellowship. On her first visit with her new PCP, a screening PHQ-9 was elevated (16) suggesting moderate depressive symptoms. Although records sent to her new PCP from her prior PCP had not described a history of mental health treatment, Ms. T explained that she had received psychiatric care and psychotherapy at a separate clinic whose records were not accessible to or routinely shared with her PCP. Indeed, Ms. T acknowledged previous reluctance to have her mental health treaters communicate with her other medical treaters. Her new PCP discussed some of the advantages to greater integration of her psychiatric and general health care, took a careful history of depressive symptoms and an initial history that suggested prior trauma, and excluded imminent safety concerns. She recommended re-starting citalopram, which the patient endorsed as having been helpful in the past, and suggested that Ms. T meet with the practice's care manager who would also work closely with a consulting psychiatrist. The practice care manager reviewed plans for medication dose escalation, created a safety plan in the event of worsening symptoms or suicidality, and introduced Ms. T to an on-line cognitive-behavior therapy (CBT) resource. The practice care manager subsequently reviewed Ms. T's history and presentation with the consulting psychiatrist who agreed with the plan.

During a scheduled follow-up call with the care manager one week later, Ms. T endorsed increasing, but passive, suicidal thoughts. The PCP consulted with the practice psychiatrist and contacted the patient with the recommendation that she be evaluated in the Psychiatry Urgent Care Clinic the following day. The evaluation confirmed the diagnosis of major depressive disorder with a history of prior trauma, and the PHQ-9 remained high, at 18. An initial safety plan was developed with Ms. T's input. Along with the recommendation to continue titration of citalopram from 20 to 40 mg, the previously effective dose, the Urgent Care psychiatrist determined that Ms. T had not accessed the on-line CBT resource as suggested. Given this finding, and her long-standing difficulties with distress tolerance and struggles with self-injurious urges, the Urgent Care psychiatrist conferred with the PCP and referred Ms. T to group and individual dialectical behavior therapy (DBT). During the 2-week interim for these appointments, Ms. T had a weekly visit with the Urgent Care social worker and phone check-ins with the care manager.

Over the ensuing weeks, Ms. T continued to maintain regular contact with the care manager and PCP and worked closely with her DBT team whose EHR records were readily available to the PCP, care manager, and psychiatrist. When she was feeling better but still suffering some residual symptoms, the consultant psychiatrist recommended the addition of low-dose aripiprazole, which had been effective for her in the past. The PCP prescribed the atypical antipsychotic and initiated enhanced metabolic screening while she was on the medicine. By the third month of treatment, Ms. T was feeling substantially better (back to herself) and was thriving in her post-doctoral program. With the help of the care manager, a plan for follow-up was coordinated with the PCP, psychiatrist, DBT therapists, and Ms. T.

REFERENCES

Access the reference list online at https://expertconsult.inkling.com/.

Physician Well-Being and Coping With the Rigors of Psychiatric Practice

53

Deanna C. Chaukos, M.D.
Abigail L. Donovan, M.D.
Theodore A. Stern, M.D.

This chapter is dedicated to Dr. Edward Messner, whose commitment to resident well-being was unparalleled. He taught us not only how to heal our patients but also how to heal ourselves.

OVERVIEW

The practice of medicine is focused on disease, not health, and on treatment, not primary prevention. Therefore, it is not surprising that physicians have difficulty maintaining their own health, minimizing stress, and preventing burnout in their own lives. The very same character traits that make physicians successful (e.g., perfectionism, an exaggerated sense of responsibility, selflessness) also make physicians vulnerable to chronic stress.

Stress can be defined as the physiologic, emotional, and cognitive response to adverse external influences; chronic stress is capable of affecting both physical and psychological health. The daily stressors of the medical practice environment, when left unmanaged, can progress over time to burnout. Burnout is a pathologic syndrome in which prolonged occupational stress leads to emotional and physical depletion and ultimately to the development of maladaptive behaviors (e.g., cynicism, depersonalization, hostility, detachment). Understanding the root causes of stress and burnout, exploring ways to reduce vulnerability to burnout, and learning skills to cope with the stresses inherent in psychiatric practice are important factors in building and maintaining a successful career and establishing a fulfilling life.

EPIDEMIOLOGY

Despite their academic, vocational, and societal success, physicians are immune to neither disease nor suffering. The practice of medicine is inherently stressful, and physicians are at high risk for burnout. Reported rates of physician burnout range between 22%[1] and 60%;[2] these rates are even higher for residents (as high as 75% in one study[3]). Physicians are also at risk for experiencing high levels of emotional distress, given the nature of their work, and studies have identified high rates of depression and suicide among physicians. Whereas physicians have lower mortality rates from several diseases (e.g., chronic obstructive pulmonary disease [COPD] and liver disease), they have higher rates of suicide than other professionals and members of the general population[4] (Figure 53-1); for male physicians, the relative risk ranges from 1.1 to 3.4, and for female physicians, the relative risk ranges from 2.5 to 5.7.[5] In the general population, the suicide rate is four times higher for men than women; in physicians, the rate of suicide for women is equal to men.[6] Up to 12% of physicians report increased use of substances during residency;[7] psychiatrists have particularly high rates of substance use compared to those in other medical specialties.

ETIOLOGIES FOR STRESS AND BURNOUT

The practice of psychiatry is challenging and rewarding. Several aspects of psychiatric practice leave the psychiatrist vulnerable to stress and, ultimately, to burnout (Figure 53-2).

Frequent Encounters With Distress

Psychiatrists encounter human suffering every day. The nature of psychiatric practice is that clinicians witness countless stories of sadness, anger, and betrayal. Although moments of joy and happiness arise, they often seem few and far between. The chronic and devastating nature of many psychiatric diseases increases the emotional burden on the clinician. Psychiatrists must remain emotionally available to their patients to experience and express the empathy that is necessary for forming an alliance—this emotional availability can make psychiatrists particularly vulnerable to suffering alongside their patients. Psychiatrists must strike a critical balance between emotional availability, while still maintaining enough distance to remain objective.

While encounters with suffering may increase stress, interpersonal connections with patients may also be protective. Bearing witness to distress, maintaining empathy, and establishing humanistic connections may even be protective against depersonalization, a characteristic of burnout. Depersonalization describes a dehumanization and detachment from our patients, which in the short term might be protective for the physician, but in the long run may detract from the rewards of the profession.

Ethical Dilemmas

The patient's reliance on the psychiatrist for guidance can raise a host of ethical conflicts. Psychiatrists can find themselves watching their patients make unwise, and even

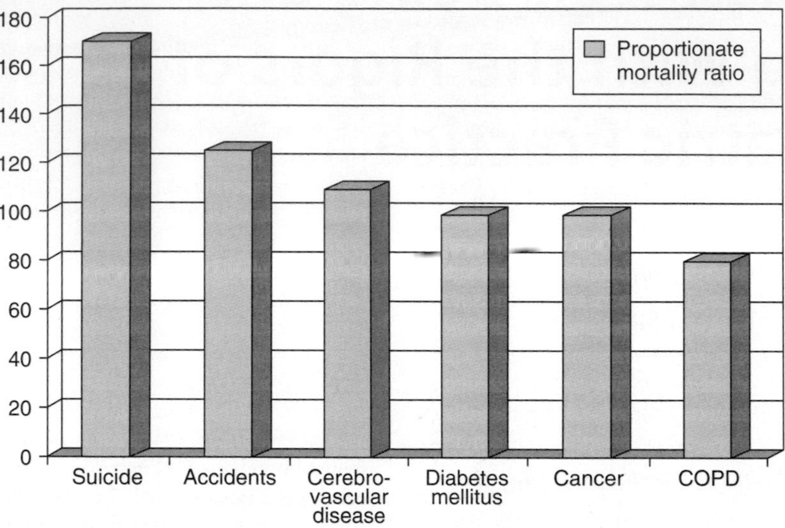

Figure 53-1. Proportionate mortality ratio for causes of death among white male physicians. The proportionate mortality ratio compares the proportion of deaths due to a specific cause in white male physicians with the proportion of that cause of death in all white male professionals. COPD, chronic obstructive pulmonary disease. *(From Linzer M, Visser MR, Oort FJ, et al: Predicting and preventing physician burnout: results from the United States and the Netherlands,* Am J Med *2001; 111(2):170–175.)*

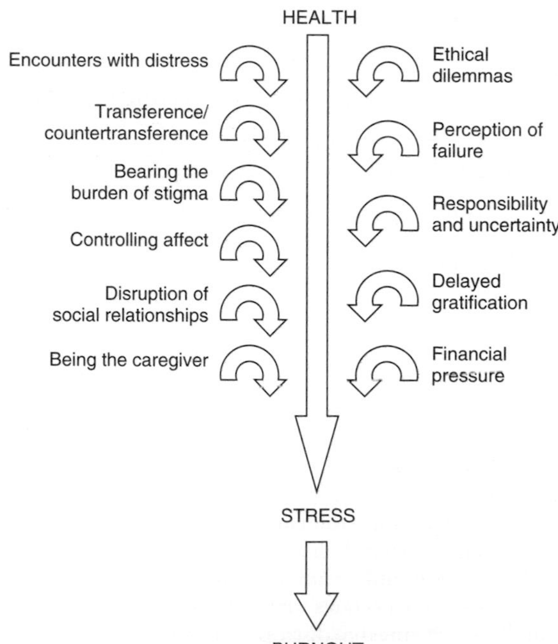

Figure 53-2. Etiologies of stress.

dangerous, decisions and being unable to curtail this destructive behavior. Psychiatrists might have to enforce mandated treatment regimens, to hospitalize patients against their will, or even to physically restrain violent patients. There may even be times when psychiatrists must intentionally break patients' confidentiality for their safety or for the safety of others. None of these decisions is made lightly, and each requires a great deal of reflection and emotional energy.

Transference and Countertransference

The daily practice of psychiatry is filled with issues of transference and countertransference, leading to the development of intense emotions (e.g., hostility, aggression, love) in the patient and the clinician. Furthermore, several psychiatric illnesses have, as core symptoms, difficulty with interpersonal interactions. Afflicted patients, including those with borderline personality disorder and narcissistic personality disorder, can pose a special challenge. Coping with intense transference, while monitoring one's own countertransference, can be exhausting; it is a daily challenge for most psychiatrists.

The Perception of Failure

Psychiatrists treat chronic illnesses, which are subject to relapse and carry significant morbidity and mortality; thus, the very nature of psychiatric disease can lead the psychiatrist to experience feelings of failure as a doctor and a healer. Despite knowledge of treatment–response rates, psychiatrists might believe that if they could only find the right medication or say the right words, the patient would be healed. Failure to respond to treatment can be, and often is, viewed as a failure of not only the medical intervention, but also the treater. Vulnerable psychiatrists may then question the purpose and meaning of their work.

Bearing the Burden of Stigma

Psychiatry and its practitioners are under intense public scrutiny. Psychiatric treatment, medications, and research have been called into question by the media, the government, and even popular culture icons. Whereas psychiatric successes take place behind closed doors, treatment failures have grown increasingly public and fuel stigma of mental illness. This public criticism can be disheartening and can make it difficult to maintain meaning in one's work.

Controlling Affect

Despite the intensely emotional nature of psychiatric work, psychiatrists must consistently control their affect to do their jobs well. Although this control is necessary for the practice of psychiatry, it can ultimately lead to increased stress and vulnerability to burnout. Instead, informal processing with colleagues, or formal supervision, can encourage the necessary expression of what is controlled during patient encounters.

Responsibility and Uncertainty

The practice of psychiatry is multi-dimensional, and it incorporates interpersonal and individual dynamics, sociology, biology, and pharmacology. The complex nature of psychiatry makes it an exhilarating, yet uncertain field. Although the breadth and depth of psychiatric research are growing exponentially, there is still a dearth of research to guide many clinical decisions; psychiatrists must often base clinical decisions on biased, incomplete, or ambiguous data. These challenges are further compounded by the added stress of answering to institutions, insurers, patients, and their families. Health insurance organizations often establish standards of care without involvement of psychiatrists, which can undermine the self-determination of practitioners. Psychiatrists can find themselves in the difficult position of not being able to provide the treatment they believe is best, due to systems' limitations.

Disruption of Social Relationships

Psychiatrists often work in isolation, leaving them alone to face the effects of psychopathology and disease. Furthermore, rules regarding confidentiality inhibit sharing the details of one's day with family and friends. Social engagements and family time can be interrupted (without warning) by emergencies. These factors can fracture social relationships, decrease social support, and increase the risk of burnout. Thus, it is important for psychiatrists to develop robust and diverse support systems—professionally, for the necessary debriefing of clinical challenges, and personally, for the maintenance of well-being outside of the practice environment.

Delayed Gratification

The ability to delay gratification is an important developmental milestone. The practice of medicine raises it to an art form. But this skill, when taken to an extreme, can lead to burnout. Physicians may be tempted to put personal goals on hold, in the service of career success (e.g., "I can't get married, have children, or buy a house until I have a stable practice."). Such rationalizations can be extended indefinitely and lead to a life lacking balance and devoid of non-vocational success.

Being the Caregiver

Physicians have a strong need to be needed and to care for others. These traits are part of what initially draws individuals to the practice of medicine. At the same time, the dependence some patients develop on their psychiatrists can be overwhelming in its intensity. Focusing intently on the needs of others can lead to denial of one's own need to be cared for.

Financial Stress

Although the popular perception is that doctors make copious amounts of money, the reality is quite different. The cost of medical education can be exorbitant, and it continues to rise each year; however, physician salaries do not enjoy the same growth, and the increases in earnings over time might not even match the rate of inflation. Many young doctors finish residency with enormous debt and have limited options for repayment and deferment of loans. Furthermore, the practical options for improving one's financial situation are limited to working longer hours or seeing more patients (for shorter periods of time). Either option is likely to increase, rather than to decrease, vocational stress; this pressure may be especially intense for physicians early in their careers.

SPECIAL SITUATIONS IN PSYCHIATRY

Coping With Patient Suicide

A Profound and Enduring Effect

Half of all psychiatrists have had one (or more) of their patients commit suicide;[8,9] approximately one-third of those psychiatrists experienced this loss while still in residency.[8] One-fourth of psychiatrists who experienced patient suicide stated that it had "a profound and enduring effect" on them throughout their careers.[8] Because one of the primary treatment tools in psychiatry is the individual practitioner, when the treatment fails, it can feel as if the treater has failed. Furthermore, whereas death from cancer can be seen as inevitable, death from suicide can be viewed as a choice.[10] When coping with a patient's suicide, it is important to remember that "a patient suicide is neither a unique event nor a personal failure."[11]

Reactions to Suicide

A psychiatrist's reactions to a patient's suicide can be varied and intense. In addition, psychiatrists must cope not only with their own reactions but also with the reactions of the patient's family and friends. The psychiatrist can experience grief, guilt, inadequacy, anxiety, depression, shock, shame, betrayal, and anger. The experience of anger and hostility toward the patient who committed suicide can further trigger guilt and self-blame. A sense of rejection can also be particularly poignant; although the psychiatrist was working to the best of his or her ability and trying all available therapies, the patient has said, through suicide, "You just weren't good enough." Younger clinicians may be especially vulnerable to this intense distress.

Coping

To cope effectively with a patient's suicide, clinicians must give themselves permission to experience a variety of emotions. While difficult, experiencing anger and hostility toward the patient is a necessary component of healing. Clinicians might find themselves ruminating over treatment decisions, asking, "What if …?" Although it is important to review the treatment course to learn from the unfortunate outcome, obsessive ruminations are likely to diminish one's confidence in decision-making and to impair coping. Shame and embarrassment can prevent a psychiatrist from reaching out to colleagues.

Treating Dying Patients

In extreme situations, clinicians may find themselves refusing to care for suicidal (or terminally ill) patients or wanting to leave the practice of psychiatry altogether. These wishes defend against the fear of future traumatic experiences with at-risk patients. Yet, as a seasoned therapist said about treating suicidal patients, "If we do not treat dying patients, our patients will die alone." (A. Alonso 2005, personal communication.)

Coping With Boundary Crossings and Violations

Boundary Violations

The practice of psychiatry is filled with intense emotions (encouraged by regular, frequent, and lengthy patient contact). The intensity of these emotions, combined with disruption of personal and romantic relationships, can be a setup for boundary crossings and violations.[12] Boundary crossings are considered harmless deviations from clinical practice or from the therapeutic frame; however, boundary violations are deviations that are harmful and exploitive of the patient's emotional, financial, or sexual needs.

Decreasing Vulnerability

All clinicians must recognize that they are at risk for boundary violations; denial of this vulnerability prevents introspection and analysis of motives, as well as early consultation for difficult dilemmas. Other factors (including crises at work, at home, or in physical or psychological health) can increase risk for boundary violations. In such situations, the clinician may be tempted to confide personal problems to the patient; such self-disclosure should be a warning that the clinician is on the rim of the proverbial slippery slope. Other warning signs include idealizing the patient, and thus believing that he or she is deserving of special treatment; holding sessions at the end of the day or even "after hours"; allowing sessions to go on longer than the allotted time; allowing the patient to maintain a large, unpaid bill;[13] and, most important, a reluctance to discuss the case with colleagues or supervisors. Any of these signs should immediately prompt the clinician to seek objective consultation to examine these issues in depth.

Coping With Malpractice Litigation

Practicing medicine in today's society leads many doctors to fear litigation, regardless of actual negligence. This fear can be paralyzing and lead to the desire to treat only "low-risk" patients. Unfortunately, there are no reliable methods to predict which patients will be litigious. Thus, the practitioner must cope effectively with the continuous risk of malpractice litigation.

Protecting Yourself

All practitioners can take steps to protect themselves against potential litigation. Appropriate documentation is critically important. The most common malpractice claim against psychiatrists occurs in cases where a patient has committed suicide; thus, documentation of both the risks and the protective factors, in addition to the rationalizations behind clinical decisions, is crucial.

Perhaps the most protective factor is a strong alliance with the patient (which is also a key component of effective treatment). Similarly, it may be beneficial for the clinician to maintain an alliance with the patient's family. This may be difficult to accomplish because of patient confidentiality. Even if the patient refuses contact, it may be helpful simply to convey one's desire to speak with the family, in the present or in the future.

Coping With a Lawsuit

What if a clinician is actually faced with a lawsuit?[14] Unfortunately, the very same traits that constitute careful and competent doctors (e.g., responsibility, perfectionism, high standards) also subject them to self-doubt and unearned guilt when confronted with a lawsuit. It may be reassuring that only a small percentage of malpractice lawsuits go to trial, and those usually find in favor of the physician. Regardless of whether negligence actually occurred, it is normal to feel shame, guilt, and anger during (and even after) a lawsuit.

Coping With Residency Training

The rigors of a psychiatric practice are demanding, and psychiatric residency training is often especially challenging (given a lack of control over daily schedules, sleep deprivation, a caseload filled with difficult-to-treat patients, responsibility without authority, and the need to balance autonomy and dependence). Internship is perhaps the culmination of these stressors, with the largest expertise–responsibility gap. In training, there is also a desire to appear strong and competent to both colleagues and supervisors, leading some residents to view asking for help as a sign of weakness. These factors and multiple role conflicts conspire to make residents especially vulnerable to burnout (see Case 1).[15]

CASE 1

Sarah, a first-year psychiatry resident at a large, urban, teaching hospital, went into medicine because she valued taking care of people, especially those with serious mental illness. During medical school, she worked at a local food bank, cared for the homeless, and volunteered abroad with refugee populations. She managed the stress associated with being in medical school by running daily, hiking on weekends, and decompressing with friends. Sarah moved to Boston from Wyoming so that she could pursue opportunities in public psychiatry and global mental health.

During her first rotation on the inpatient psychiatry unit, Sarah worked long hours and, for the first time, felt like her patients were truly her responsibility. She felt like a vital member of the team, and that her work was making a difference; as a result, most of the time, she did not mind spending long hours at the hospital. However, her work schedule made it difficult for her to run every day, and she struggled to make new friends.

When Sarah switched rotations to an off-campus internal medicine clinic, she struggled to understand her role on the team. She was responsible for covering the after-hours pager, yet felt ill-prepared to respond to the calls she received, and she wasn't sure whom she could turn to for help. There was a different attending on call each day, and none seemed particularly interested in assisting trainees. As a result, Sarah felt intimidated and ashamed by her lack of knowledge. Sarah increasingly found herself disengaging from the patients, hoping that they wouldn't have complicated issues, so she wouldn't need to bother anyone in the clinic. She found herself becoming dismissive of patient complaints. By her third month on this rotation, Sarah felt fatigued, alienated, and bitter. She wondered why she had chosen medicine in the first place.

Sarah confided to a friend in her residency class, who suggested that she enter psychotherapy. Sarah found a therapist who could see her after work, and she learned to understand the roots of her dissatisfaction. She also re-incorporated coping skills, like running and connecting with nature, back into her life, although briefer than before. Over time, she came to feel more confident in her role as a resident and grew to enjoy medicine once again.

WHEN THE COBBLER'S CHILDREN HAVE NO SHOES

The cobbler was so busy making shoes for everyone else that he neglected to make them for his own children. Similarly, it is easy, in days filled with caring for the needs of others, to neglect one's own needs. Yet, to be good doctors, physicians must care for themselves. Several factors contribute to this type of self-neglect and burnout (Figure 53-3).

Denial of Vulnerability

Many doctors treat themselves as if they were superhuman. Although others need to sleep, eat regular meals, and take vacations, physicians often deny their own basic needs. Moreover, psychiatrists wish to see themselves as consummate copers, immune to emotional impairment. When placed under stress, it is common for them to work harder and longer, which ends up compounding the initial problem.

Negation of Personal and Familial Concerns

Personal and family concerns can be misjudged as being less critical than relieving pain and suffering at work. It can seem easy, if not important, to spend 1 more hour at work to see a patient in crisis; however, this practice can rapidly expand and become a pattern of working longer and sacrificing personal time. After long and stressful days, clinicians may be too emotionally exhausted for empathic listening, even-handed conversation, or recreation. As a result, clinicians can turn inward, internalizing their concerns and cutting themselves off from family and friends. This behavior compromises the strength of family relationships and decreases the support available for the clinician.

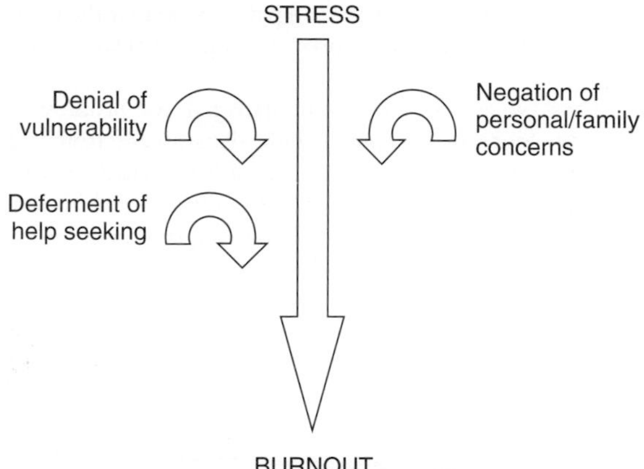

Figure 53-3. Factors contributing to self-neglect.

Deferment of Seeking Help

It is common to view seeking help for personal problems as a sign of frailty or failure. Some physicians are reluctant to seek help because of the stigma of mental illness. Although psychiatrists may be more open to psychotherapy for themselves, the possibility of a formal diagnosis and breaches of confidentiality, or having to report a problem to a licensing board, can make seeking help difficult. These challenges—concerns about confidentiality, financial burden, scarcity of personal time and perceived weakness—are often compounded in residency training.[16] The intense pressure of a doctor's work can foster the creation of unachievable expectations. However, the physician's well-being is only undermined by this intolerance for human vulnerability.

How to Recognize Stress in Oneself

Psychiatrists are good at recognizing stress in others; however, recognizing stress in oneself requires a different skill set. Unrecognized and unmanaged stress can lead to anxiety or depression, and it can have long-lasting effects for clinicians, patients, and families. Signs of stress include fatigue, apathy, anhedonia, and despair, as well as somatic manifestations (including headaches and gastrointestinal disturbances). Further warning signs include disrupted sleep, conflict in family relationships, and changes in memory, concentration, and problem-solving ability. Perhaps the most important warning sign is the suggestion from friends, family, and colleagues that help is needed.

Stress can also affect attitudes toward patients. Clinicians may develop reactive misanthropy when they frequently encounter patients' pain and suffering, especially when expressed as hostility or devaluation. Clinicians might then find that warmth and concern are replaced with apathy, or even defensiveness and contempt. This depersonalization can progress and carry over to all patients, so that the clinician is no longer able to appreciate fulfilling relationships with patients.

Stress, when prolonged or unmanaged, can progress to burnout. Signs of burnout include detachment from the meaning of one's work, open hostility, cynicism, and overwhelming occupational dissatisfaction. In addition, reactive misanthropy can progress to malignant misanthropy in the burned-out clinician. In this malignant form, the misanthropy toward a patient extends to other relationships, including those with staff, colleagues, other health professionals, and even friends or family. The unfortunate result is then a conflict with one's social values and intentions, leading to feelings of self-punishment and guilt.

HEALING THE WOUNDED HEALER

Be Your Own Most Important Patient

Maintaining a caring and empathic attitude toward one's patients requires treating oneself with kindness and concern. The medical learning and practice environment is known to cause physician burnout.[17] Though all doctors have strong coping skills and exhibit many resilient traits, these skills can always be expanded and refined, especially given the stressors of the practice environment. Anticipating and preparing for difficulty can prevent emotional overload. Some useful coping strategies are outlined here and in Figure 53-4.

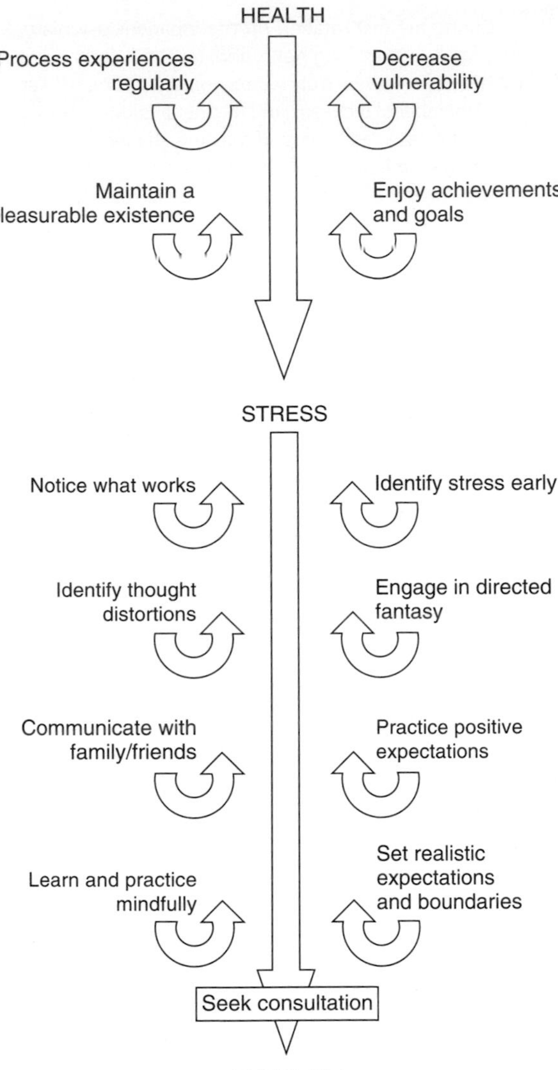

Figure 53-4. Coping with stress and preventing burnout.

Process Experiences Regularly

One should talk with colleagues and supervisors regularly about difficult interactions, even when it means revealing personal vulnerability. Residents, in particular, may be tempted to use supervision as a time to discuss only therapeutic successes, in order to project a sense of competence; however, supervision can be even more valuable when used to discuss difficult patient encounters or conflicted reactions to a patient. It is also possible to process experiences independently, perhaps reserving the commute home as a time for reflecting on the day's events. Coping with stress on a daily basis, and processing emotions before one arrives home, makes it less likely that the strain of the day will be taken out on family or friends. Furthermore, learning important lessons from difficult events can mitigate some of the distress they cause.

Set Realistic Expectations and Boundaries

It can be gratifying when a patient professes the need to communicate between sessions, or when a patient forgets an appointment but feels he or she cannot possibly wait until the following week to see the treater. Being needed in this way can seem like an affirmation of why one became a doctor: to help those who cannot help themselves. However, speaking with patients frequently between encounters, or for extended periods, not only dilutes the therapeutic process but also adds a time-consuming burden for the physician. Re-scheduling appointments again and again when a patient has forgotten the original appointment simply reinforces poor planning and adds additional stress to the physician's already crowded schedule. Although emergencies should be treated as such, physicians who maintain boundaries around phone calls and missed appointments for non-emergency issues protect the therapeutic frame and their own need for a manageable schedule, including time free from responsibilities of patient care.

Review Your Own History

Psychiatrists can identify useful coping strategies from the past and eliminate maladaptive ones. It is also helpful to identify prior manifestations of stress, so that one can recognize them early and intervene before they reach a caustic level.

Notice What Works

Here, we review a number of coping strategies, including those that have been studied in physician populations.

However, one should also reflect on individual coping strategies that have previously worked. In training, a typical realization is that residents no longer have the time for past effective coping strategies (e.g., training with a sports team, daily yoga practice). This may be true to some extent, however, it is important to find ways (though abbreviated) to integrate important health-maintenance behaviors. During moments of extreme distress or crisis, it can be difficult to recall adaptive strategies. As a result, it is important to integrate adaptive strategies during relatively calm periods, to ensure easy access during times of adversity.

Decrease Vulnerability to Stress

There are many aspects of clinical practice (such as long hours and copious amounts of paperwork) over which clinicians have no control, but there are factors (e.g., treating physical illness, eating a balanced diet, exercising, getting enough sleep) that the individual can control that can reduce vulnerability to emotional stress.

Doctors are often poor patients. Despite access to health care, many physicians rarely visit their primary care physician, even when they are ill. Unfortunately, untreated illness only compounds stress.

Hectic schedules sometimes dictate meals on-the-go, or no meals at all, but proper nutrition is crucial for a healthy body and a healthy mind.

Exercise releases endorphins, and it can improve mood and energy. Enjoying exercise is an excellent way to relieve stress. Regular physical exercise contributes to physical health and an overall sense of well-being.

Sleeping at least 8 hours every night has benefits; fatigue can leave one vulnerable to emotional stress and dysregulation.

Identify Thought Distortions and Practice Positive Expectations

When a potentially difficult meeting or conversation is anticipated, it is helpful to rehearse statements and responses to questions. Resiliency training programs for residents and physicians integrate behavioral strategies to identify typical thought distortions, which are part of the stress response. Recognizing the impact of thought distortions (e.g., "I am a terrible public-speaker; this presentation will be an embarrassment.") on stress is the first step to counteracting them. Mental rehearsal before a stressful event or practicing other positive adaptive strategies (like gratitude, self-compassion, and meaning-finding) can make it more likely that one will stay calm in a tense situation. These techniques foster a sense of control over the unexpected.

Engage in Directed Fantasy

One can also imagine expressing intense feelings (such as anger, sadness, or fear) as a means of decompression. Fantasizing in this way is most useful when one recognizes that the fantasy is distinct from real action; fantasies need not be enacted. One can imagine scenarios that are affectively intense (e.g., hitting a frustrating patient with a fire axe or duct-taping his mouth closed). The more outrageous the fantasies are, the more effective they will be at discharging emotion. The more unrealistic and outlandish, the easier it will be to distinguish between fantasy and a corresponding reality.

Communicate With Family and Friends About Anticipated Unavailability

Communication about one's unavailability will help others prepare and thereby lessen the likelihood that they will respond with anger and withdrawal. As one communicates about future work commitments, one can also make future social commitments. This action allows family and friends to know they are still held in high regard and sets a framework for ongoing relationships. Above all else, open communication and a sense of togetherness should be maintained; hardship experienced as a team can deepen intimacy and mutual respect.

Enjoy Your Achievements and Your Goals

Previous triumphs should be pondered and joyful moments recalled. Original goals should be remembered (perhaps even written down), the progress made toward achieving them noted, and new goals for the future set. Being mindful of the progress toward life goals can instill a sense of pride and mastery. The strength gathered from memories of life's high points can facilitate coping with everyday stresses.

Learn and Practice Mindfulness

Mindfulness is thought to enhance the ability to find meaning in one's work through self-awareness; thus, it may be that mindfulness helps to counter the depersonalization and emotional exhaustion that contribute to burnout. Interestingly, many coping strategies directed at physician well-being emphasize self-awareness, or autognosis (literally "self-knowledge"). Mindful practice and meditation have been shown to positively impact physician well-being: formal curricula have been correlated with improvements in mood disturbance, physician empathy, and decreased burnout.[18] Mindfulness-based stress reduction programs for physicians and trainees have been shown to significantly lower levels of perceived stress and improve confidence in the ability to cope, with effects sustained over time.[19–21] Other strategies, like self-hypnosis, behavioral strategies for stress awareness, and positive psychology skills (practicing gratitude and positive-perspective-taking) can also help physicians keep well in the midst of stressful careers.

Autognosis Rounds

Attendance at *autognosis* rounds allows psychiatrists to share common experiences and to identify individual reactions to clinical situations. This knowledge can then be used to inform diagnoses and to minimize potentially harmful reactions to patients (e.g., managing hostility toward a patient so that it will not interfere with treatment). Autognosis rounds have proved valuable for psychiatric resident groups at the Massachusetts General Hospital for the past four decades.[22]

Maintain a Pleasurable Existence

It is often helpful to make a commitment to yourself to have one pleasurable experience each day. A pleasurable event can be something as simple as having a cup of tea, taking a short walk outside, reading a favorite poem, or speaking with a friend on the telephone. Even taking a few minutes between patients to stretch, chat with a colleague, or have a favorite snack can be rejuvenating. Keeping balance between stress and pleasure on a daily basis prevents burnout and promotes a positive mindset.

WHEN TO SEEK CONSULTATION

Consultation offers an objective point of view; it can be the first step in seeking help for the overwhelmed clinician. Consultation is not a sign of weakness; rather, it is the sign of a wise physician who recognizes that to help patients, one must first help oneself. Consultation should be considered for a variety of problems: symptoms of depression, disabling anxiety, self-prescription, escalating use of alcohol, inappropriate expressions of anger, impulsive behavior, trouble in significant relationships or impaired clinical judgment.

TYPES OF PROFESSIONAL HELP

It is not easy to acknowledge that one needs professional help. It can be extremely difficult to surrender control when one is used to being in complete control. But it can also be a wise decision, especially to halt a downward spiral.

Psychotherapy

Psychotherapy provides the psychiatrist a valuable opportunity to experience the other side of the therapeutic relationship. Psychotherapy can be a rich, life-enhancing experience, it can improve coping skills, and it provides much-needed support for the overwhelmed clinician.

Psychopharmacology

Many physicians might see the need for medication as a sign of weakness. However, doctors would not fail to use chemotherapy to treat a patient with cancer or insulin to treat a patient with diabetes. So too should medication be used to treat a biologically based psychiatric illness.

Couples Therapy

Strong family relationships are crucial for stress resilience. Unfortunately, family relationships are often among the first victims of vocational burnout. Couples therapy or family therapy can heal wounded relationships and restore lines of open communication, ultimately building protection against future stresses.

Group Therapy

Group therapy allows individuals to recognize that they are not alone in their suffering. Professional support groups can facilitate sharing common experiences, promoting connections between people who have similar strengths and difficulties. More general groups promote understanding the difficulties inherent to all lifestyles.

CONCLUSION

The practice of psychiatry, with all its inherent stresses, is an honor and a fulfilling calling.

> *When we find ways to cope ..., we move toward the equanimity that can enable us to serve our patients with greater effectiveness and compassion. We also progress toward greater satisfaction in this noble profession of medicine and in our personal lives.*
>
> — Dr. Edward Messner[23]

REFERENCES

Access the reference list online at https://expertconsult.inkling.com/.

Management of a Psychiatric Consultation Service

54

John B. Taylor, M.D., M.B.A.
Felicia A. Smith, M.D.
Theodore A. Stern, M.D.

OVERVIEW

The purpose of this chapter is to give psychiatric providers of consultation-liaison (C-L) services an understanding of the complex business aspects of their work. Understanding that appropriately adhering to the often-confusing guidelines for reimbursement can be stressful to clinicians and expose them to time-consuming and stressful audits and substantial penalties, both personally and for their institutions. In this atmosphere, providing ethical, legal, and clinically astute services can be a daunting task. A fuller understanding of coding and billing will also help psychiatrists, C-L hospital-based programs, and hospital administrators to collect the appropriate reimbursement for services rendered. In this chapter, we will address principles of coding, billing, and documentation that will improve medical documentation by C-L clinicians, as well as address improvements in clinical outcomes and economic benefits accrued by the general hospital due to a smoothly run C-L service. Assessment, assurance, and improvement of the C-L service's quality will also be discussed.

CASE 1

Mr. D, a 50-year-old man was admitted to the medical service for pneumonia. He reported to the medical team that he drinks "from time to time," and that his last drink was 2 weeks ago. His alcohol level in the Emergency Department was undetectable. On hospital day 2, he developed a coarse tremor, an elevated blood pressure and heart rate, and on hospital day 3, he became disoriented and started to experience visual hallucinations, which prompted a psychiatric consultation. In looking thoroughly through the electronic medical record, the psychiatric consultant noted that Mr. D had a prior admission for alcohol withdrawal and that he had been to a detox facility on numerous occasions.

DOCUMENTATION SHOULD REFLECT THE SERVICE PERFORMED

Successful C-L services rely on the establishment of cooperative and collaborative relationships with medical colleagues. Hospital-based physicians are exposed to psychiatric co-morbidity on a daily basis. Consultations may be requested for guidance regarding the creation of a differential diagnosis, recommendations for evaluation and treatment, as well as assistance with their approach to inpatient care. The needs of a physician do not always mirror the severity of the patient's medical condition. *Billing, however, is always geared to the patient's illness.* Although a medical service may purchase a psychiatrist's time and involvement due to their expertise or to guarantee a readily available psychiatrist, the insurance company or other third-party payer is paying solely for a service for an individual patient (rather than purchasing the expertise of a clinician).

BILL ONLY FOR SERVICES DOCUMENTED IN THE MEDICAL RECORD

The overriding principle for third-party reimbursement is to bill only for those services documented in the medical record. The charge for service and the reimbursement available for the service are guided by definitions established by Current Procedure Terminology (CPT) codes. A brilliant, life-saving consultation that goes undocumented is not billable. The effectiveness and expertise of the consultant is not an issue for the collection of a reasonable fee. Moreover, significant pressure may be placed on clinicians to "maximize revenue" for the services they provide. Efforts to "game" the system, by "up-coding" (i.e., charging for a more intensive service than delivered) are illegal and unethical. On the other hand, inadvertent "down-coding" on account of the sometimes Kafkaesque documentation and billing rules is also unfair and ultimately damages the ability of hospitals and providers to care for patients.

FOLLOW THE MEDICARE GUIDELINES FOR ALL ENTRIES IN THE MEDICAL RECORD

Medicare is the predominant insurance coverage in the general hospital. This is especially true for a psychiatric consultation on an elderly or disabled patient. CPT codes were developed by the American Medical Association (AMA) and adopted by the Health Care Financing Administration (HFCA) in the early 1990s. Current guidelines dictate that Evaluation and Management (E&M) CPT codes, which are not specific to psychiatry but cover all psychiatric hospital-based and outpatient encounters, along with the 10th revision of the International Statistical Classification of Diseases and Related Health Problems (ICD-10), are to be used for billing. These guidelines, established as mandatory for Medicare and Medicaid billing, are essentially universal, in that they apply to most insurance plans. More important, Medicare guidelines for reimbursement are the strictest among insurance plans. *Adhering to the Medicare guidelines ensures that the provider will be in compliance with all insurance plans for appropriate coding and reimbursement purposes.*

Documentation requirements for inpatient psychiatric and consultation services are different in form and content from the documentation that might be employed in outpatient practices. Codes for billing inpatients reflect the need for the consultant to be aware of the physical status of the patient as well as the patient's psychiatric state. A premium is paid for thoroughness and attention to "process of care." Thus *documentation for inpatient consultative psychiatric services requires documentation of co-morbid medical problems, laboratory studies, and imaging*. An extensive psychiatric examination, including recommendations for treatment and medication without the inclusion of elements of the review of systems, for example, can be billed only for the lowest consultation service code. The critical ingredients of an appropriate note congruent with an appropriate billing code will be addressed in the section on documentation and coding.

OBTAIN PREAUTHORIZATION FOR SERVICES WHENEVER NECESSARY

Although mental health parity was mandated in the 2010 Patient Protection and Affordable Care Act, mental health coverage largely remains governed by insurance carve-outs and frequently requires prior authorization. Health insurance companies vary in their requirements for precertification (i.e., permission for providing a consultation before the delivery of the service to enable payment for that service). Medicare does not require precertification, while most carve-out behavioral health organizations do. A patient may be authorized by the primary insurance carrier for the medical admission, authorizing payment for all physicians performing medical consultations save for the psychiatrist who requires specific and separate authorization from the carve-out company for payment for the psychiatric consultation. Critical to the financial viability of C-L services is the management and monitoring of the billing and collection of third-party claims, and the understanding that the billing and authorization process for each payer is essential to receive payment for services rendered.

IDENTIFY THE PAYER

During the admission process, most hospitals will have identified the primary, secondary, and supplementary insurance coverage. It is critical for the managers of a C-L service to understand how each type of insurance adjudicates claims for professional services. Health insurance claims for hospital services are separated into two components: the technical or hospital charges, and the professional or physician charges. For some insurers these charges are billed together, whereas for others they are billed separately.

Medicare, non-managed Medicaid, Blue Cross, and commercial indemnity plans will each pay for both the technical (hospital) and professional (physician) components. Payments for each component are based on a previously negotiated fee schedule or percentage of charges submitted. Managed care plans will typically negotiate an all-inclusive fee for services rendered and will not pay for the professional charges separately, unless they are specifically contracted for, apart from the day-rate for hospital charge.

When a patient is insured by a managed care plan, C-L services must be contracted for separately to be reimbursed beyond the all-inclusive rate the hospital receives through the day-rate. If the insurer carves out the management of its mental health and substance abuse benefit to a behavioral health subcontractor, separate professional bills must be submitted to the carve-out behavioral health subcontractor. A common error for C-L services is the sending of the C-L consultation claim to the primary insurance carrier rather than the behavioral health subcontractor and receiving rejection for "service not covered" or "bill to carve-out." Too often, these rejected claims are written off, which engenders increased irritation with the primary carrier or blaming of the C-L service for not obtaining prior authorization. The best method for ensuring that the correct payer is billed is to confirm with the medical insurer, usually by telephone, in advance of the treatment, to determine whether the mental health benefit is carved out and, if so, to what organization. Then, one should contact the carve-out company to obtain prior authorization for the service. The critical request should be for both the initial consultation and follow-up visits, if necessary. Ideally, a systematic method for navigating this system should be built into the consultation process through departmental or hospital-level billing/reimbursement staff with at least initial guidance, and periodic review, by the C-L administrator.

DEVELOP A STANDARD FORMAT FOR WRITING THE CONSULTATION NOTE

Several standards and guidelines collide when writing an efficient and effective consultation note. Standards established by the American Psychiatric Association (APA) Practice Guidelines for the Psychiatric Evaluation of Adults, 3rd edition,[1] address the content of an appropriate psychiatric examination; these standards should then be adapted to the special conditions of the consultative examination. As noted by the Academy of Psychosomatic Medicine (APM) Practice Guidelines for Psychiatric Consultation in the General Medical Setting,[2] the psychiatric consultation should also address the consultee-stated versus the consultant-assessed reason for referral, the extent to which the patient's psychiatric disturbance was caused by the medical or surgical illness, the adequacy of pain management, the extent of the psychiatric disturbance caused by medications or substance abuse, disturbances in cognition, the patient's character style, thoughts of dying, and psychiatric symptomatology. At the same time, those same APM guidelines state that the "note is best if brief and focused on the referring physician's concerns."[2]

The consultation note should include the chief complaint, history of present illness, medical and psychiatric history, social and family history, review of systems, mental status examination, and an impression and treatment plan. It should also include data to support the billing code for reimbursement; documentation should reflect the appropriate level of care provided. Given the proliferation of electronic medical record (EMR) systems, the creation of an electronic template that meets Medicare guidelines for billing and the practice guidelines outlined by the APA and APM will allow for quick, routinized documentation without worry about meeting billing and compliance standards. In addition, a template can facilitate more complete consultations, serve as a teaching tool for trainees, and catalyze research or internal review projects. Templates also lend themselves to inclusion in computerized medical records, prevent loss of critical observations and recommendations resulting from illegible notes, and decrease medical errors. With the developing capacity to import computerized (observational and laboratory) results, vital signs, recent laboratory values, medication orders, and drug administration, data can be more easily included in the consultation note. At the same time, care must be taken to keep computerized notes focused and helpful.[3] The ability, conferred by technology, to import information easily or cut and paste text can be more a hindrance than a help if not coupled with actual human attention to what is pertinent and accurate.

BILL THE APPROPRIATE CODE

Inpatient consultations are reimbursable under the Inpatient Hospital Care (IHC) codes (99221–99223 for initial consults, 99231–99233 for follow-up visits). The Psychiatric Diagnostic Interview Evaluation with Medical Services (90792) can also be used for an initial consult or Emergency Department evaluation.

To use consultation codes properly, it must be clear that the consultation is a service requested by another physician or another provider rather than by the patient or the patient's family. The requesting physician must enter a written or digital request for psychiatric consultation; a statement in a progress note indicating the desire for psychiatric input is insufficient for reimbursement purposes. The content of the history, comprehensiveness of the examination, complexity of medical decision-making, and average time required to complete the consultation determine the reimbursement that will be provided. Engaging the assistance of a professional coder to perform periodic audits and training sessions for physicians is essential to remain abreast of changes in federal auditing guidelines. Additionally, providing psychiatrists with simplified pocket billing guidelines and definitions of terms selecting the appropriate CPT code can be helpful.

EVALUATE THE COSTS AND BENEFITS OF THE CONSULTATION SERVICE

C-L services are rarely lucrative cost centers.[4] Moreover, providing fee-for-service psychiatric consultation by independent practitioners rarely leads to a financially viable service or career. Meaningful consultation requires that clinicians expend significant time away from the bedside. Necessary tasks include the review of the medical record and case discussion before and after the consultation with the referring physician, nursing staff, and social service. Ancillary meetings with family members are often necessary to collect critical information unobtainable from a medically compromised patient. A cost–benefit analysis that sees cost as the psychiatrists' salary and the benefit as the lowest expenditure of finances to provide the service without severely compromising the service is far too common.

In contrast to the preceding scenario, a "value accounting" methodology approaches the consultation service in a broader systematic manner.[5] This methodology looks at cost, clinical outcome, and consumer satisfaction as interrelated domains. With a broader view, we can examine the impact of a C-L service on the care of the patient, the educational or academic mission of the hospital, and the financial function of the hospital. From a fiscal perspective, the availability of C-L services results in decreased length of stay (LOS)[6] and recidivism rates, outcomes especially critical in a capitated, managed care environment. Decreasing LOS lowers overall hospital costs; there is also evidence that effective consultation reduces the use of other medical services as well.[7] This additional revenue is separate from the financial savings in staff time expended while managing aggressive, confused, uncooperative, or "undesirable" patients; the costs of security; and the use of restraints and secondary problems of injuries and infections.

There is an emerging literature on proactive consultation services, in which a mental health professional reviews all admissions to a service and facilitates early consultation rather than waiting for the primary team to identify the need.[8] In one study, this resulted in a significant reduction in length of stay (0.64 days in patients admitted for fewer than 31 days). This study also noted high satisfaction rates and expansion to units beyond those designated in the study. If C-L services are able to concretely demonstrate their worth using LOS as an indicator, the cost/benefit analysis may continue to tip in psychiatry's favor.

From a public health perspective, the involvement of the C-L psychiatrist may lead to improved disease-management protocols and best practices, helping patients understand and cope with chronic illness. Enrolling patients in smoking-cessation or weight-control programs may initiate or support their general health and wellness. Consider that 25% to 40% of patients in the general hospital are being treated for ailments secondary to alcoholism and that the societal losses secondary to alcoholism may exceed US$115 billion per year.[7,9]

For hospitals and healthcare systems, there is an increasing focus on assigned populations of patients through structures such as accountable care organizations (ACOs). In this model, the individual patient and the assigned population of patients become simultaneous priorities, requiring resources to be allocated so that all of the assigned patients receive the necessary care. Although this can be done creatively (e.g., using electronic "virtual visits," via telepsychiatry, and others), reimbursement has not caught up, leaving many innovative care delivery methods uncompensated, and therefore, undervalued as tools. Value-based purchasing has increasingly become a strategy for the buyers of care (e.g., government and insurers) to ensure that the care being provided is high-quality and efficient with the insurers' and hospitals' goals aligned; as C-L psychiatry demonstrates its ability to decrease LOS and improve care in the hospital, its inclusion in value-based purchasing may be an area of future growth.

PROVIDE QUALITY ASSURANCE AND QUALITY IMPROVEMENT ON THE PSYCHIATRIC CONSULTATION SERVICE

Consensus has emerged that the overarching goals of health care, from provider-to-department-to-system, are "the triple aim": improving the health of populations, improving the experience of care, and reducing healthcare costs.[10] The cost of health care, and the rate of its growth as a percentage of gross domestic product (GDP), is widely thought to be unsustainable. The government and insurers are increasingly demanding proof that the money being spent on health care is actually improving the outcomes of the patients they are responsible for insuring. Transparency about outcomes has led to public reporting of success rates for some procedures, allowing patients to make better-informed decisions about where they will receive their health care. Measures of quality are increasingly being tied to reimbursement, whether as part of pay-for-performance (i.e., increased reimbursement for better outcomes) or non-payment for so-called "never events" (e.g., medical errors, the development of decubitus ulcers, rapid readmission after discharge).

Interestingly, though the care provided by proceduralists (e.g., surgeons) and hospitalists (e.g., internists) has come under the most scrutiny, the care provided by consultants has to date been off the radar. This is likely only temporary. Given the prevalence of co-morbid medical/surgical and psychiatric illness, the percentage of hospitalized patients who are seen by a psychiatric consultation service (as high as 13% in some hospitals), and the role consultants have in either reducing or increasing the cost of care (through their ordering of diagnostic tests as well as their impact on LOS and readmissions), there will be increased emphasis on defining, measuring, and reporting the quality of consultants across medical disciplines, including psychiatry.

UNDERSTAND DONABEDIAN'S MODEL

Donabedian was an epidemiologist and health services researcher who many consider to be the father of the modern healthcare quality movement. Among his contributions was a simplified model that identified three types of interconnected pieces of information (structure, process, and outcome) from which one could draw inferences about the quality of care delivered.[11]

By structure, he referred to both the material and human resources required to provide healthcare. By process, he referred to the actual activities that comprised care delivery. By outcome, he referred to a wide-ranging set of changes (positive or negative) in patients that could be attributed to the processes of care delivered. These three components are not attributes of quality *per se*, but rather they are windows through which the quality of care can be viewed and assessed.

The model is elegant in its simplicity; it has stood the test of time as a framework for the assessment of healthcare quality in a number of settings. Defining exactly how these general concepts apply to a specific aspect of health care (e.g., general hospital psychiatry) has proven more difficult. In addition, the hypothesized linkages between structure, process, and outcome may not always be robust causal connections. Nevertheless, this provides a reasonable frame for thinking about quality in any practice setting.

USE STRUCTURAL MEASURES OF CONSULTING QUALITY

A consultation service is only as good as the consultants who comprise it. Unlike other technical areas of medicine, psychiatric consultation is knowledge work, and, as such, the key measure of structural quality relates to human resources (consultation psychiatrists) that form the team. In this regard, two questions need to be asked: (1) Is the team well-staffed? and (2) Is the team well-trained?

Staffing refers to the quantity of psychiatrists who provide coverage to the general hospital (based on recruitment, retention, and full-time equivalents). The size of the roster will depend on multiple factors (e.g., the size of the hospital, the prevailing patient mix, the presence of trainees, the full-time/part-time status of staff, and the referral frequency). Defining "adequate coverage" is certainly up for discussion; no doubt there is a minimum threshold, below which the timeliness of consultations becomes an issue and the burden on individual practitioners so substantial as to promote burnout. Beyond the raw number of staff on the service, the turnover rate of psychiatric consultants is another important structural measure of quality. One cannot underestimate the value of in-depth knowledge of the structure and culture of the specific setting in which one is employed; high rates of turnover make it difficult to develop this inside knowledge that is so critical to the framing of recommendations that are actually accepted.

Training refers both to the formal educational and training background of the psychiatrist and his or her actual clinical experience within general hospital psychiatry. The former would include measures such as the percentage of board-certified staff, the percentage of staff with subspecialty training in psychosomatic medicine, or the percentage of staff with formal subspecialty certification. The latter refers more to the years of experience, numbers of total cases seen, and markers of expertise in specific domains (such as publication of peer-reviewed articles and chapters). There is evidence that both physician certification[12] and volume of cases seen[13] can be associated with clinical outcome, though to our knowledge these relationships have not yet been established for psychiatry.

One final structural indicator relates to the degree of organizational learning that occurs with experience. This concept, sometimes referred to as "knowledge management," is an important aspect of major management consulting firms. How can the consultation service use the combined wisdom and experience of thousands of cases seen over time and bring this to bear on the next consult request? Can the service itself have value beyond the sum of the individuals that comprise it? The answer is likely yes, but methods of knowledge management within hospital-based consultation services are at present rudimentary when compared with those used in business. This may improve with the more widespread use of electronic medical records for inpatient care. Until then, services might consider other aspects of knowledge management, such as the use of daily team rounding, the creation of an anonymous consult registry with "lessons learned," and publication of important observations in peer-reviewed literature.

APPLY PROCESS MEASURES OF CONSULTING QUALITY

As outlined in Chapter 2, there is a core set of processes that make up the actual practice of "consultation psychiatry." These processes can be broadly construed under the categories of data gathering (speaking with the referring clinician, reviewing the chart, interviewing and examining the patient); data integration (formulating a diagnosis and crafting a plan); and communication (writing and discussing impressions and recommendations). The skill with which these activities are carried out likely influences the patient outcomes. It will also influence the service's reputation within the general hospital, in turn influencing the volume of referrals or high-performing consultation services; this can set up a positive reinforcement loop in which a high-quality consult leads to high perceived value, which leads to increasing consultation requests, which leads to increased experience, which when captured leads to greater process skill, and so forth. Despite the widely acknowledged importance of process excellence in these three domains, they are only rarely, if ever, assessed once a physician has completed his or her postgraduate training. Unlike many other areas of the general hospital, there are no national standards for process quality in consultation psychiatry.

CONSIDER OUTCOME MEASURES OF THE CONSULTANT'S QUALITY

When a well-staffed and -trained service implements high-quality processes, good outcomes are bound to occur. Donabedian identified seven domains of outcomes (Clinical, Physiological, Physical/Functional, Psychological, Social, Mortality/Longevity, and Patient Satisfaction) that ran the gamut from enhanced patient understanding of their condition to prolongation of life. Even a cursory glance at these items makes it clear that high-quality psychiatric consultation can have a substantial impact on many, if not all, of these outcomes.

In addition, there are a number of patient-safety issues that could be addressed by timely and effective psychiatric consultation. Within-hospital suicides, suicide attempts, and staff assaults are a few dramatic and important examples. Other events may include removal of intravenous lines, tubes, or wires by delirious patients. Tracking the frequency of these events on a hospital-wide basis may be a useful marker of the effectiveness of care implemented as a result of a psychiatric consultation. This requires a robust and reliable event reporting system, so that bad outcomes and "near misses" can be tallied and used as the basis for discussion.

FOLLOW THE GUIDING PRINCIPLES OF QUALITY MEASUREMENT

There is benefit in measuring the structure, processes, and outcomes associated with a psychiatric consultation service. Through measurement, value can be identified that contributes to the mission of the general hospital, serving to justify the expense of maintaining this type of internal consultancy to hospital leadership. It may also enhance the standing of knowledge-based specialties in the eyes of healthcare purchasers and payers, while working toward equilibrating reimbursement disparities that have long favored procedure-based specialties. Most of all, this type of measurement can provide the type of feedback needed to continually improve overall quality.

That said, attempts at measurement in and of themselves are potentially costly and time-consuming. All too many measurement efforts in today's healthcare landscape seem to be nothing more than costly box-checking exercises that do little to create actual practice change. There follow three suggestions to avoid a similar fate:

1. Measurements should be devised, conducted, and reviewed by those on the front lines of care, sometimes called *clinical microsystems*.[14] In this way, those with the greatest knowledge of the care delivery processes and expected outcomes can play the central role in the measurement effort. This type of bottom-up effort is critical in the change process, because it engenders "buy-in" from the beginning, rather than pushing mandates down the throats of providers in a top-down fashion.
2. Measurement cannot be considered a stand-alone process. It must be integrated with quality assurance and quality improvement activities. A quarterly report on the frequency of in-house suicide attempts is meaningless unless it is linked with careful efforts to reduce the rate of occurrence through root cause analysis of reported adverse events[15] and the implementation of rapid cycle change. In addition to formal quality assurance review and specific project-based quality improvement efforts, a wide variety of tools are available to promote change within the hospital setting. These include presentations at grand rounds, discussions at case conferences, systematic surveillance for complex cases with early intervention, and supervision with feedback for both trainees and staff.
3. The actual cost of measurement (in time and dollars) should be accounted for, and measurement efforts reassessed periodically to determine whether they are providing an adequate return on this investment. In this way, the hospital (or hospital microsystem, such as the consultation psychiatry service) can make certain that quality assessment actually enhances, rather than detracts from, the core capacity of the institution: to provide excellent clinical care.

CONCLUSION

Running a psychiatric consultation service simultaneously requires adherence to strict billing and documentation guidelines and maintenance of nebulous quality standards.

Proving the service's worth to the general hospital can be challenging, but may require demonstrating cost offset and indirect means of value.

Over the past half-century psychiatric consultation in the general hospital has advanced from a novelty to a full-fledged medical subspecialty. As part of this coming of age the time has come to not simply ask, "Do you have a psychiatric consultation service?," but rather "How good is the psychiatric consultation service at your institution?" This question is posed to initiate introspection by all who are involved in this field. Continuous examination of the consultation service's functioning is necessary to ensure that its practices are up-to-date and optimal.

REFERENCES

Access the reference list online at https://expertconsult.inkling.com/.

Index

Page numbers followed by "*f*" indicate figures, "*t*" indicate tables, and "*b*" indicate boxes.

A

AACAP. *See* American Academy of Child and Adolescent Psychiatry.
A-β fibers, 189
Ablative limbic surgery, 411
Abnormal Involuntary Movement Scale (AIMS), 60, 237–238
Abnormal movements, patients with, 231–239
  drug-induced movement disorders, 235–238
    acute dystonic reaction, 236
    akathisia, 236, 237*b*
    antipsychotic-induced extrapyramidal symptoms, 236, 236*f*
    parkinsonism, 237
    tardive dyskinesia, 237–238, 238*f*
    tremors, 235–236
  functional movement disorders, 238–239
  idiopathic movement disorders, 232–235
    Huntington's disease, 233–234, 234*b*
    Parkinson's disease, 232–233, 232*b*
    restless legs syndrome, 235
    Tourette's syndrome, 234
    Wilson's disease, 234–235
  patient history and physical examination for, 231–232, 232*b*
  tremors, 235
Absence seizures (petit mal), 214
Absorption, of drugs, 418–419
Abulia, 233, 376
Abuse, medical, in children, 534–535
Academy of Psychosomatic Medicine (APM), 1
"A CALM VISAGE" mnemonic, 102
Accidents, pediatric, 530–531
Accountability, setting of, 466
Accountable care organizations (ACOs), 601–602
Accreditation Council for Graduate Medical Education, 4
Acculturation, immigration and, 561–562
Acoustic nerve, 40
Acquired immunodeficiency syndrome (AIDS)
  See also Human immunodeficiency virus (HIV) infection and acquired immunodeficiency syndrome (AIDS).
  depression and, 74
  suicide and, 493
Acronyms CATIE, CUtLASS, and EUFEST clinical trials, 115–116
Action tremor, in motor symptoms, 232*b*
Activities of Daily Living (ADL)
  neurocognitive disorder and, 100, 100*t*
  post-stroke depression and, 223*b*–224*b*, 226
Acupuncture, 474
Acute alcohol intoxication, signs and symptoms associated with, 142–143
Acute dystonic reaction, 236
Acute intermittent porphyria, 393
Acute intoxication, in alcohol use disorder, 142–143
Acute kidney injury (AKI), 303–304
Acute pain, 191
Acute stress disorder, 133
  burn injuries and, 364
Acute tubular necrosis (ATN), 303–304
A-δ fibers, 189
Addiction, in opioids, 203
ADHD. *See* Attention-deficit/hyperactivity disorder.
ADHD Rating Scale-IV (ADHD RS-IV), 61
Adherence, for HIV infection, 343–344
Adjustment disorder with depressed mood, 79
Administration, of opioids, 201–202
Adolescents
  See also Children and adolescents.
  anorexia nervosa in, 177
  burn injuries in, 363, 363*b*
  eating disorders in, 177
  in end-of-life care, 525
  evaluation of, in emergency psychiatry, 511
  interview techniques for, 523
  key points and parenting tips in, 537*t*
  pediatric consultation for, 525
  psychiatric interview of, 34
α_2-Adrenergic agonists, 435
α-Adrenergic agonists, for ADHD, in children and adolescents, 444–445
α_1-Adrenergic antagonists, 435
Adrenocorticotropic hormone (ACTH), 456
Adrenoleukodystrophy, X-linked, 394
Adult ADHD Self-Report Scale (ASRS), 61
Adult burn patients, 366
Advance directives, 572–573
Advanced sleep phase disorder, 272
Affect, controlling of, psychiatrists and, 593
Affective blunting, 112–113
Affective illness, parents with, pediatric consultation for, 524
Against Medical Advice (AMA), 578
Agency for Healthcare Research and Quality (AHRQ), 582
Aggressive dissonance, 481*t*

Aging patients
  See also Elder abuse; Elder care.
  burn injuries in, 363
  depression and falls in, 69–70
  laboratory test for, 64
  memory difficulties in, 96
  psychosis in, 115
  sexual dysfunction in, 280
Agitated Behavior Scale (ABS), 374–375
Agitation
  in geriatric patients, 541
  management of, in emergency psychiatry, 508–509, 508*b*–509*b*
  psychosis and, 118
  during rehabilitation, 374–375
  treatment strategies for, 377–378
AGNA (SOX1) antigen, associated with autoimmune encephalitides, 244*t*–245*t*
Agnosia, 102
Agranulocytosis, antipsychotic drugs and, 424–425
AIDS Clinical Trials Groups (ACTG), 338
AIMS. *See* Abnormal Involuntary Movement Scale.
Akathisia, 236, 237*b*
  in children and adolescents, 440
  in psychosis, 116
Akinesia, in motor symptoms, 232*b*
Al-Anon, 414–415
Albee, George, 458
Alcohol, in emergency psychiatry, 505–506
Alcohol dependence, 582
  epidemiology of, 386*t*
  suicide and, 492
Alcohol problems screening
  AUDIT-C questionnaire for, 142*b*
  CAGE Questionnaire for, 142*b*
Alcohol use disorder (AUD)
  acute intoxication and psychiatric sequelae of, 142–143
  alcohol withdrawal syndrome in, 143–146
  patients with, 141–148, 141*b*
  pharmacotherapy for, 146–147
  psychosocial treatment of, 147–148
  screening for, 142
  Wernicke-Korsakoff syndrome and, 146
Alcohol Use Disorders Identification Test (AUDIT), 61
Alcohol withdrawal delirium (AWD), 145
Alcohol withdrawal seizures, 144
Alcohol withdrawal syndrome, 143–146
  clusters, receptors and recommended treatment options, 144*t*
  neurotransmitters affected in, 143*f*
  treatment of, 145–146
  types of, 144–145
Alcoholic hallucinosis, 144–145
Alcoholics Anonymous (AA), 414–415
Alcohol-induced persisting amnestic disorder, 146
Alcoholism, in geriatric patient, 543
Alexander, Franz, 1
Allodynia, 191
Allograft rejection, 327
Allostasis, 457–458
Allostatic loading, 457–458
Alogia, 112–113
Alpha waves, in polysomnography, 267
Alprazolam, for anxiety disorders, 135*t*, 136
Alprostadil (Caverject and Edex), for erectile dysfunction, 288*t*
Alternative anticonvulsants, for bipolar disorder, in children and adolescents, 450
Alzheimer's disease
  clinical features of, 96*t*
  dementia and, 58
  depression and, 74
  in Down syndrome, 390
  in geriatric patients, 539
  neurocognitive disorders due to, 96–97
Amantadine
  for catatonia, 261
  for neuroleptic malignant syndrome, 263
Amenorrhea, anorexia nervosa and, 182
American Academy of Child and Adolescent Psychiatry (AACAP), 437
American Board of Medical Specialties, 1
American Board of Psychiatry and Neurology (ABPN), 1
American Cancer Society (ACS), 537*b*
American College of Neuropsychopharmacology, 498
American Psychiatric Association (APA), 1–2
  on collaborative care, 582
  Practice Guidelines for the Psychiatric Evaluation of Adults, 600
  on suicidal behaviors, 496
American Psychosocial Oncology Society (APOS), 537*b*
American Psychosomatic Society, 1–2
Amisulpride, for anorexia nervosa, 184
Amitriptyline, 74
Amnesia, anterograde, after electroconvulsive therapy, 408
Amotivation cluster, negative symptoms of schizophrenia, 112–113
AMPAR antigen, associated with autoimmune encephalitides, 244*t*–245*t*
Amphetamines
  for ADHD, in children and adolescents, 442
  psychosis and, 115
  use of, 152–153
Amphiphysin, associated with autoimmune encephalitides, 244*t*–245*t*
Amygdala, 47–48
Analgesic adjuvants, for pain, 204, 205*t*–206*t*
Andragogy, 466
Anesthesia, for anxiety disorder, 127
Angelman syndrome, 390
Anger, depression and, 72–73
Anhedonia, 112–113
  in cancer patients, 354
  during rehabilitation, 376
ANNA-1 antigen, associated with autoimmune encephalitides, 244*t*–245*t*
Anorexia nervosa, 178
  See also Eating disorders.
  cardiac consequences of, 182
  hospitalization for, 183

Anorexia nervosa *(Continued)*
nutritional rehabilitation for, 182–183
onset of, 177
pediatric consultation for, 528
pharmacologic management of, 184
prevalence of, 177
psychological therapies for, 183–184
treatment of patients with, 182–184
Anosognosia
in post-stroke depression, 225
during rehabilitation, 376
Anterior cingulate cortex (ACC), 257–258
Anterograde amnesia, after electroconvulsive therapy, 408
Anticholinergics
for catatonia, 261
for parkinsonism, 237
tricyclic antidepressants, 76
Anticipatory anxiety, 124
Anticonvulsant agents
for anxiety disorder, 294
for binge eating disorder, 186
drug interactions of, 428
for generalized anxiety, 138
for pain, 207
for pregnancy, 551
for seizure disorders, 216
Antidepressant agents
anticholinergic effects of, 76
antipsychotic drugs and, 424
for anxiety disorder, 135–136, 293
cardiac conduction effects of, 76–78
for depression in cardiac disease, 299
discontinuation syndrome, 79
drug interactions of, 428–432, 429*t*, 431*t*
for kidney disease, 309–311
liquid and orally-disintegrating formulations of, 324*t*
for medically ill, 74–79, 75*t*
for myocardial depression, 78
non-oral preparations of, 323*t*
for orthostatic hypotension, 76, 77*t*
for pain, 204–207
for post-stroke depression, 225
for pregnancy, 548–549
for seizure disorders, 216
for sexual dysfunction, 285–286
for suicide risk, 498
Antiepileptic drugs. *See* Anticonvulsant agents.
Antihistamines, for sleep disorders, 270
Anti-Ma2 (Ta) antigen, associated with autoimmune encephalitides, 244*t*–245*t*
Antipsychotic agents
for anxiety disorder, 293–294
for delirious cardiac patients, 300
for difficult patients, 485
for elderly patients, 107
first-generation, 116–117
for geriatric patients, 541, 542*t*
for HIV infection, 346
for kidney disease, 311–312
liquid and orally-disintegrating formulations of, 324*t*
non-oral preparations of, 323*t*
Antipsychotic agents *(Continued)*
psychopharmacology of, 423–425
drug interactions of, 424*t*
second-generation, 117–118
for sexual dysfunction, 286
for sleep disorders, 270
Antipsychotic-induced extrapyramidal symptoms, 236, 236*f*
Antisocial behaviors, 47
XYY disorder and, 390–391
Antisocial personality disorder, 478
Anxiety disorders
brain tumors and, 356
in cancer patients, 353
in cardiac patients, 291–295
approach to, 294–295
differential diagnosis of, 293
psychopharmacologic issues in, 293–294
diagnostic rating scales for, 60–61
in emergency psychiatry, 504–505
in end-of-life care, 514–515
in geriatric patients, 543
in HIV infection, 341, 346
in kidney disease, 306
in medical settings, 125–132
failure to cope, 126, 126*b*
interferes with evaluation/treatment, 127–128, 127*b*
mimics of medical illness, 128–132, 129*b*–132*b*
traumatic procedures, 126–127, 126*b*
nature and origin of, 123–125
in pain, 196
physical signs and symptoms of, 124*b*
during pregnancy, 553
primary, 132–134
generalized anxiety disorder as, 133
obsessive-compulsive disorder as, 134
panic disorder as, 132–133
post-traumatic stress disorder as, 133–134
social phobia as, 133
specific phobias as, 133
seizure disorders and, 217
sleep disorders and, 274
somatic symptoms and, 165
suicide and, 492–493
in traumatic brain injury, 228–229
treatment of, 134–139
cognitive-behavioral therapy for, 139
pharmacologic, 135–137, 135*t*
strategies for, 377
Anxiolytic antidepressants, for HIV infection, 346
Anxiolytics
as complementary medicine, 473
liquid and orally-disintegrating formulations of, 324*t*
non-oral preparations of, 323*t*
Anxious patients, 123–139
Apathy, in Alzheimer's disease, 106, 106*t*
Apathy, post-stroke, 225–226
Aphasia, during rehabilitation, 374
Apnea
diagnosis of, 270
treatment of, 270–271
Appearance, in neurocognitive disorder, 102
Appraisal, stress and, 457

Appreciative inquiry (AI), 466
Apraxia, 102
Aprosodia, during rehabilitation, 375
Arachidonic acid, in pain signal, 189
Architecture, sleep cycle and, 268
Aripiprazole
for bipolar disorder, in children and adolescents, 450
for difficult patients, 485
for psychosis, 117
Armodafinil
for ADHD, in children and adolescents, 445
drug interactions of, 433
Arousal disorders, 272
Arrhythmias, ECT risk of, 409
Ascending reticular activating system (RAS), in delirium, 84
Asenapine, for bipolar disorder, in children and adolescents, 450
Aspirin, properties of, 201*t*
ASRS. *See* Adult ADHD Self-Report Scale.
Asterixis, in motor symptoms, 231, 232*b*
Asthma
pediatric consultation for, 530
sleep disorders in, 274
Asymptomatic neurocognitive impairment, HIV infection and, 339
Ataque de nervios, 561
Athetosis, in motor symptoms, 232*b*
Atomoxetine
for ADHD, in children and adolescents, 444
for binge eating disorder, 186
Atonic seizures ("drop attacks"), 214
Attention
in neurocognitive disorder, 102
in neurologic examination, 41
neuropsychological assessment for, 56
Attention disorders, diagnostic rating scale for, 61
Attention-deficit/hyperactivity disorder (ADHD)
in children and adolescents, 440–445
α-adrenergic agonists for, 444–445
alternative treatments for, 444–445
amphetamines for, 442–443
atomoxetine for, 444
bupropion hydrochloride for, 444
clonidine for, 444–445
FDA-approved treatments for, 441–444, 441*t*
guanfacine (Tenex) for, 445
methylphenidate for, 442
modafinil/armodafinil for, 445
novel treatments for, 445
stimulants for, 441–443
epidemiology of, 386*t*
neuropsychological assessment for, 57–58
rating scale for, 61
Atypical antipsychotics, for bipolar disorder, in children and adolescents, 449
Atypical Parkinsonian syndromes, 232
AUDIT. *See* Alcohol Use Disorders Identification Test.
AUDIT-C questionnaire, for alcohol problems screening, 142*b*
Autism, epidemiology of, 386*t*
Autism spectrum disorder (ASD)
behavioral plans for, 532
in children and adolescents, 451
parents with, 532
Autobiographic memory, after electroconvulsive therapy, 408
Autognosis rounds, 597
Autoimmune encephalitides, remaining questions on, 250–251
antibody subtypes in, 251
Hashimoto's encephalitis, 250
late diagnoses of, 250
low-titer autoantibodies in, 250
Autoimmune encephalitis
clinical features of, 242–243
treatment of, 249–250, 249*t*
Automatisms, 214
Autonomic nervous system
distress and, 455
stress and, 456
Autosomal dominant single-gene disorders. *See* Genetics, of psychiatric disorders.
Avanafil (Stendra), for erectile dysfunction, 287*t*
Aversion disorder, sexual, 284
Aviptadil (Senatek), for erectile dysfunction, 288*t*
Avoidance, 582–583
Avoidant/Restrictive Food Intake Disorder (ARFID), 528
Avolition, 112–113
Axons
diffuse injury, in traumatic brain injury, 227
in pathophysiology of pain, 189

B

Baclofen
for alcohol use disorder, 147
causing catatonia, 255
Bacterial meningitis, 248
Barbiturates
abuse of, 159
in emergency psychiatry, 506
Barnes Akathisia Rating Scale, 60
Basal ganglia, 37
BDI. *See* Beck Depression Inventory.
BDRS. *See* Bipolar Depression Rating Scale.
Beck Depression Inventory (BDI), 60, 60*t*
Bedside examination, in diagnostic evaluation of psychotic patients, 109–111
Behavior modification counseling, 5 As of, 463–464
advice, 464
agree, 464
arrange, 464
assess, 464
assist, 464
Behavioral difficulties
in children, 530
hospitalization and, 532
Behavioral health integration, approaches to, 581–589, 588*b*–589*b*
Behavioral medicine. *See* Behavioral therapy.
Behavioral observation, 29

Behavioral therapy
  interventions
    for anxiety, 294
    for cancer patients, 355
    for neurocognitive disorders, 105, 105*b*
    in traumatic brain injury, 230
  for pain, 210–211
Behavioral weight loss (BWL) treatment, for binge eating disorder, 186
Behaviorally-induced insufficient sleep syndrome, 271
Benign essential tremor, 235
Benzodiazepines, 143, 145, 583
  for anxiety disorder, 135*t*, 136–137
  for anxiety in cardiac patients, 293
  breast-feeding and, 554
  for burn injuries, 366
  in children and adolescents, 440
  for delirium, 90, 92
  drug interactions of, 433–434
  in emergency psychiatry, 506, 509
  for generalized anxiety, 137–138, 138*t*
  for HIV infection, 346
  for kidney disease, 311
  liquid and orally-disintegrating formulations of, 324*t*
  for neurocognitive disorders, 107
  for neuroleptic malignant syndrome, 263
  for pain, 207–208
  for post-traumatic stress disorder, 133–134
  pregnancy and, 553
  for sleep disorders, 270
  use of, 157–158
Bereavement, 79
  in HIV infection, 340–341
  suicide and, 494
Bibring, Edward and Grete, 2–3
Bill, for psychiatric consultation
  code, 601
  for services documented in medical records, 599
Billing for C-L services, 599
  See also Psychiatric consultation services.
Binge eating disorder (BED), 179
  See also Eating disorders.
  co-morbidities of, 182
  pharmacologic management of, 186
  prevalence of, 177
  psychological therapies of, 186
  treatment of patients with, 185–186
Binger, Carl, 3
Bioavailability, of drugs, 418
Biological clock, 268
Biological model, in clinical formulation, 19
Bipolar Depression Rating Scale (BDRS), 60
Bipolar disorder, 134
  burn injuries and, 361
  in children and adolescents, 448–450
    alternative anticonvulsants for, 450
    aripiprazole for, 450
    asenapine for, 450
    atypical antipsychotics for, 449
    carbamazepine for, 449
Bipolar disorder *(Continued)*
    lithium for, 448–449
    olanzapine for, 450
    oxcarbazepine for, 449
    pharmacotherapy for, 448
    quetiapine for, 450
    risperidone for, 449–450
    valproic acid for, 449
    ziprasidone for, 450
  epidemiology of, 386*t*
  in geriatric patients, 540
  heritability of, 385–386
  in HIV infection, 346–347
  during pregnancy, 550–552, 550*b*–551*b*
  suicide and, 492
Bispectral index, for anxiety disorder, 127
Black box warning, in antidepressants and suicide risk, 498
Black cohosh, 474
Blessed Dementia Scale, 103
β-Blockers
  for generalized anxiety, 138
  psychopharmacology of, 435–436
Blood-brain barrier, in HIV infection, 338
Body dysmorphic disorder, suicide and, 493
Body image surgery, for burn injuries, 367–368
Body mass index (BMI), in eating disorders, 179
Borderline personality disorder, 478–480
  See also Difficult patients.
  psychotherapies for, 489*t*–490*t*
  sleep disorders and, 272
  substance abuse and, 486
  suicide assessment for, 486
Boston Naming Test, 56
BPRS. *See* Brief Psychiatric Rating Scale.
Bradykinesia, in motor symptoms, 232*b*
Bradykinin, in pain signal, 189
Brain
  neuroanatomy of, 37, 37*b*–38*b*, 38*f*
  in sexual dysfunction, 280
  sleep-wake cycle and, 268
  trauma. *See* Traumatic brain injury.
Brain tumors, in cancer patients, 356
Breast Cancer.org, 537*b*
Breast-feeding, psychotropic drug use and, 554–555
Breathing disorders, sleep-related, 270–271
Brief Psychiatric Rating Scale (BPRS), 60, 414
Brief Symptom Inventory (BSI), 352
British Medical Journal, 499
Broaden-and-build model, 466
Bromocriptine, for neuroleptic malignant syndrome, 263
Bulimia nervosa, 178–179
  See also Eating disorders.
  cardiac consequences of, 182
  cognitive-behavioral therapy for, 184
  pharmacologic management of, 185
  prevalence of, 177
  psychological therapies of, 184–185
  treatment of patients with, 184–185
Buprenorphine, for opioid use disorder, 156–157

Bupropion
for ADHD, in children and adolescents, 444–445
anticholinergic effects of, 76
for binge eating disorder, 186
bulimia nervosa and, 185
for HIV infection, 345
during pregnancy, 548
side effects of, 78
for smoking cessation, 468–469
Burn injuries, 359
end-of-life care for, 370
epidemiology of, 359–360
ethical considerations for, 370
history of, 359, 360*b*
intermediate phase of, 367–368
body image and plastic and reconstructive surgery, 367–368
massive burns, 368
psychological interventions, 367
long-term phase and outcomes of, 368–370
chronic pain in, 370
depression in, 369
general, 368–369
post-traumatic stress disorder in, 369
management of, 361–364
acute phase in, 363–364
developmental stage and burns in, 362–363
adolescence, 363
elderly, 363
infancy, 362
pre-school age, 362
school-age, 362
young adulthood, 363
diagnosis and developmental assessment in, 361–362
pain assessment for, 364–368
drug side effects, toxicity, and adverse interactions in, 366–367
pharmacologic treatment of, 365–366
benzodiazepines, 366
neuroleptics, 366
opiates, 366–367
psychological treatment of, 365
pre-burn psychopathology of, 361
risk factors for, 360–361, 361*b*
staff support, staff stress in, 370
types of, 360
Burn patients, 359–370
Burnout, of physicians, 591
signs of, 596
Bush-Francis Catatonia Rating Scale, Modified, 254*t*
Business aspects. *See* Billing for C-L services.
Buspirone
for anxiety disorders, 135*t*
for generalized anxiety, 138–139
for HIV infection, 346
Butalbital, 159

C

Café au lait spot, 391
CAGE Questionnaire, 61, 61*b*
for alcohol problems screening, 142*b*
Calcium channel blockers, for catatonia, 261
Caloric requirements, for anorexia nervosa, 183
Canadian Cardiac Randomized Evaluation of Antidepressant and Psychotherapy Efficacy (CREATE), 297
Cancer
end-of-life care for, 517
gastrointestinal, 319
in geriatric patients, 539
pancreatic, 321–322, 321*b*–322*b*
patients with, 349–358
anxiety syndromes in, 353
brain tumors, 356
chemotherapy-related cognitive impairment and, 357
childhood, survivors of, 358
confusion and cognitive impairment in, 355–358
Cushing's syndrome in, 357
denial and "middle knowledge" in, 349
depression in, 353–354
distress in, 349–352
drugs of, neuropsychiatric side effects of, 350*b*–351*b*
effect of hormonal therapy on, 357–358
fatigue in, 354–355
hope and doctor-patient relationship in, 349
hypercalcemia in, 355–356
hyperviscosity syndrome in, 356–357
hyponatremia in, 356
idiopathic hyperammonemia in, 357
leptomeningeal disease in, 356
medical choices for, 349
nausea and vomiting in, 353
paraneoplastic limbic encephalitis in, 357
psychosocial interventions for, 353
screening for, 352
types of, concerns of, 352*t*
suicide and, 493
CancerCare, 537*b*
Candidate Gene Approach, 387
Cannabis, use of, 154–155
Cannon, Walter B., 1
Carbamazepine
adverse effects of, 64
antipsychotic drugs and, 425
for bipolar disorder, in children and adolescents, 449
breast feeding and, 555
for catatonia, 261
drug interactions of, 427–428
for HIV infection, 346
for neurocognitive disorders, 107
for pain, 207–209
Cardiac disease
anxiety disorder in, 291–295, 293*b*
approach to, 294–295
differential diagnosis of, 293
epidemiology of, 291–295
psychopharmacologic issues in, 293–294
delirium in, 299–302, 300*b*
differential diagnosis of, 299–300
epidemiology of, 299
management of, 301–302
psychopharmacologic issues in, 300–302

Cardiac disease *(Continued)*
depression in, 295–299
differential diagnosis of, 296–297, 297*b*
management of, 298–299
psychopharmacologic issues in, 297–298
risk factors for, 295–296
treatment modalities for, 298
ECT risk of, 409
in geriatric patients, 539
psychiatric management of patients with, 291–302
Cardiopulmonary disease, suicide and, 493
Care providers, challenges for, in end-of-life care, 516
Caregiver fabricated illness, 534
Caregivers
in end-of-life care, 516
for geriatric patients, 545
psychiatrists as, 593
CARF. *See* Commission on Accreditation of Rehabilitation Facilities.
Carisoprodol, 159
Case studies
in anxiety disorders, in cardiac patients, 295*b*
in burn injuries, 362*b*–363*b*
in cancer, 354*b*
in coping mechanisms, 402*b*
in delirium in cardiac disease, 302*b*
in depression in cardiac disease, 299*b*
in electroconvulsive therapy and neurotherapeutics, 411*b*
in genetic disorders, 388*b*
in HIV infection and AIDS, 342*b*
in metabolic disease, 392*b*–393*b*
in pain, 199*b*
for psychopharmacology, 413*b*
in substance use disorders, 149*b*–150*b*
in suicide, 499*b*–500*b*
CASPR2 antigen, associated with autoimmune encephalitides, 244*t*–245*t*
Cassem, Edwin (Ned), 2–3
Cataplexy, 271
Catastrophic reactions, 226
Catatonia, 253–261, 253*b*
clinical features and diagnosis of, 254*t*, 256, 257*b*–258*b*
definition of, 253–254
ECT indication for, 408
in emergency psychiatry, 505
epidemiology of, 254–255, 254*t*
management and treatment of, 259–261, 260*b*–261*b*
neuropathophysiology of, 256–259, 259*f*
potential etiologies of, 254–255, 254*t*, 260*b*
prognosis and complications of, 261
risk factors of, 254–255, 254*t*
subtypes of, 255–256
Central nervous system
adverse effects of ECT in, 408–409
complications of, in kidney disease, 307–308, 308*b*
HIV infection and, 338
Cerebellar dysmetria, in motor symptoms, 232*b*
Cerebrospinal fluid (CSF), in psychiatric consultations, 11*b*, 12
Cerebrovascular disease, 223–227, 223*b*–224*b*
cognitive impairment in, 224
delirium in, 224
neuropsychiatric symptoms, 224*t*
other post-stroke psychiatric phenomena, 226–227
patients with, 223–230
post-stroke depression (PSD) in, 224–225, 226*b*
CGI. *See* Clinical Global Impression.
Chemotherapy-related cognitive impairment (CRCI), in cancer patients, 357
Children and adolescents
See also Psychiatric consultation, pediatric.
abuse
confidentiality of, 571
medical, 534–535
agitation or aggression in, 439
akathisia in, 440
anorexia nervosa in, 177
anxiety disorders in, 439–440
attention deficit hyperactivity disorder in, 440–445
α-adrenergic agonists for, 444–445
alternative treatments for, 444–445
amphetamines for, 442–443
atomoxetine for, 444
bupropion hydrochloride for, 444
clonidine for, 444–445
FDA-approved treatments for, 441–444, 441*t*
guanfacine (Tenex) for, 445
methylphenidate for, 442
modafinil/armodafinil for, 445
novel treatments for, 445
bipolar disorder in, 448–450
alternative anticonvulsants for, 450
aripiprazole for, 450
asenapine for, 450
atypical antipsychotics for, 449
carbamazepine for, 449
lithium for, 448–449
olanzapine for, 450
oxcarbazepine for, 449
pharmacotherapy for, 448
quetiapine for, 450
risperidone for, 449–450
valproic acid for, 449
ziprasidone for, 450
combined agents for, 453
delirium in, 439
depression in, 527
developmental disorders in, 450–451
mental retardation, 450
emergency interventions in, 439
in emergency psychiatry, 510–511
basic principles of, 510
demographics of, 510
evaluation of, 510–511
management of, 511
HIV infection and AIDS in, 335–336
informed consent in, 576
maltreatment in, 532–535
medical precautions and contraindications for, 438–439, 438*b*

Children and adolescents *(Continued)*
mood disorders in, 445–450
antidepressant-associated suicidality and, 446–447
depression in, 445–446
pharmacotherapy of, 446
obsessive-compulsive disorder in, 439
pharmacokinetics of antidepressants in, 447
psychiatric consultation in, interview techniques for, 522–523
psychiatric interview of, 34
psychoactive medications for, 438*b*
psychotic disorders in, 451–453, 452*t*
SSRIs for, 447–448
stimulants for, 441–443
guidelines on the use of, 443
medication interactions with, 443–444
side effects of, 443, 443*t*
suicide in, 527–528
survivors of cancer, 358
tic disorders in, 439
Children's Hospital of Eastern Ontario Pain Scale (CHEOPS), 365
Chlorpromazine
for delirium, 91–92
for psychosis, 116
Choline magnesium trisalicylate, for pain, 200
Cholinesterase inhibitors (ChE-Is)
liquid and orally-disintegrating formulations of, 324*t*
for neurocognitive disorders, 105, 105*t*
Chorea, in motor symptoms, 232*b*
Chorea Huntington, 233
Choreoathetosis, in motor symptoms, 232*b*
Chromosomes, abnormalities and microdeletions. *See* Genetics, of psychiatric disorders.
Chronic disease, behavioral management of, 461–469, 467*b*
Chronic medical illness, rehabilitation and, 371–379
diagnostic considerations for, 371–376
developmental factors in, 374–376
phases of rehabilitation, 371–373, 372*b*–373*b*, 372*f*
psychiatric look-alikes, 374–376
somatic symptom disorder in, 376
symptom interfering goals of rehabilitation as, 374
symptom type and intensity as, 374
treatment strategies for, 376–379
addressing denial, 376–377
agitation in, 377–378
anxiety and depression in, 377
co-morbid medical and psychiatric conditions, 378–379
sexual dysfunction after spinal cord injury, 378
Chronic pain, 191, 192*t*
in burn injuries, 370
Cigarette smoking
antipsychotic drugs and, 425
in schizophrenia, 120
Circadian rhythm, 268
sleep disorders and, 271–272
Citalopram
for anorexia nervosa, 184
for anxiety disorders, 135*t*
for HIV infection, 345
Civil commitment, 504, 512
legal aspects of, 576–577
Civil Rights Act of 1964, 572
Claustrophobia, during MRI, 353
Clinical Anxiety Scale, 60–61
Clinical formulation, 19–20
Clinical Global Impression (CGI), scale, 59, 414
Clinical microsystems, 603
Clinical staff, in pediatric consultation, 523–524
Clock drawing test, 41, 61
for delirium, 87–88, 88*f*
Clomipramine, for anxiety disorders, 135*t*
Clonazepam
for anxiety disorders, 135*t*, 137
for pain, 207–208
Clonidine
for ADHD, in children and adolescents, 444–445
for benzodiazepine withdrawal, 159
for opioid withdrawal, 156
Clozapine
for burn injuries, 366
for HIV infection, 347
for Parkinson's disease, 107
for psychosis, 115–116
Club drugs, 149
Cobb, Stanley, 2–3
Cocaine, 115
in emergency psychiatry, 506
sleep disorder and, 275
use of, 150–152
Cocoanut Grove fire, 359
Codes (Current Procedure Terminology), 599
Cognitive changes, in end-of-life care, 515
Cognitive disorders, diagnostic rating scale for, 61–62
Cognitive function
complementary medicine for, 474
neurocognitive disorders and, 100
Cognitive impairment
in cancer patients, 355–358
in traumatic brain injury, 228
Cognitive intervention, for traumatic brain injury, 230
Cognitive testing, standardized, for neurocognitive disorders, 103
Cognitive-behavioral therapy (CBT)
for anxiety disorders, 139
for binge eating disorder, 186
for bulimia nervosa, 184
for cancer patients, 353
for coping, 403
for HIV infection, 344
for pain, 210–211
for post-stroke depression, 225
rehabilitation and, 377
for smoking, 468
for somatic symptom disorders, 169
Collaboration, for HIV infection, 343
Collaborative care, 587–588
approaches to, 581–589, 588*b*–589*b*
barriers to treatment, 582–583
co-located care, 586–587
joint patient management, 587
parallel care, 586–587

Collaborative care *(Continued)*
primary care, 587
staff consultant/stepped care models, 586
coordinated care, 584–586
consultation psychiatry, 586
longitudinal outpatient psychiatric care, 584
specialty psychiatric clinics, 585–586
epidemiology of, 582
expectations and, 584
goals of, 583–584
access, 583
communication, 583–584
outcomes, 583
treatment, 583
IMPACT model, 587–588
liability and, 584
models of collaboration, 584, 585*t*
relationships and, 584
right model, choosing of, 588
roles and, 584
three-component model, 588
Collateral information, in psychiatric interview, 32
Co-located care, 586–587
Combined therapy, in treatment failure, 417
Commission on Accreditation of Rehabilitation Facilities (CARF), 209–210
Communication, in doctor-patient relationship, 17
Communion, 400–401
Co-morbid illnesses, in geriatric patient, 543
Co-morbid medical and psychiatric conditions, 8, 8*b*
treatment strategies for, 378–379
Compassion fatigue, 536
Complementary medicine, 471–475, 475*b*
anxiolytics and hypnotics in, 473
for cognition and dementia, 474
efficacy and safety of, 471
for mood disorders, 471–473
non-medication therapies in, 474
for premenstrual and menopausal symptoms, 474
Complex partial seizures, 214
Complex regional pain syndrome (CRPS), 191–192
Compliance, in cultural differences, 564
Computed tomography (CT)
for psychiatric symptoms, 67
for traumatic brain injury, 227
Confabulatory psychosis, 146
Confidentiality, 512
interpreters and, 563
in pediatric consultation, 538
physicians' rights and, 570–571
Confrontational visual fields, in visual examination, 40
Confrontations, with difficult patients, 482*b*, 483
Confusion, in cancer patients, 355–358
Confusion Assessment Protocol (CAP), 374–375
Confusional arousal, 272
Congestive heart failure (CHF), ECT risk of, 409
Consciousness, 41
delirium and, 87
in traumatic brain injury, 227
Constipation, 316
Consultation, legal aspects of, 569–579
advance directives in, 572–573
civil commitment and restraint in, 576–577
end-of-life care and, 572–573
physicians' rights and obligation in, 569–573
confidentiality and privacy in, 570–571
liability and managed care in, 570–571, 570*b*
malpractice liability in, 569–570
refusal to treat patient and, 571–572
refuse treatment and, 577–578, 577*b*
rights of patients in, 573–578
competency in, 573–574
decision-making capacity in, 573–576, 575*b*
informed consent in, 573–576
Consultation-Liaison (C-L) psychiatrist
billing for. *See* Billing for C-L services.
coping skills. *See* Coping mechanisms.
for medically ill, 397
role of religion in, 399
Containment, of difficult patients, 487
Continuous pain, in terminally ill, 191
Conversion disorder, 164
differential diagnosis of, 8
prognosis and treatment of, 169
Coordinated care, 584–586
Coordination, in neurologic examination, 42
Coping mechanisms
adaptation of illness as, 398–399
in anxiety, 294
assessment of, 400–402, 401*t*
courage for, 400
definition of, 397–399
in eating disorder, 180
good, 398, 398*b*
with illness, 397–403
medical predicament in, 399
for pain, 211
of physician with rigors of psychiatric practice, 591–598, 594*b*–595*b*
with boundary crossings and violations, 594
countertransference and, 592
epidemiology of, 591
etiologies for, 591–593, 592*f*
with a lawsuit, 594
with malpractice litigation, 594
with patient suicide, 593–594
effect of, 593
reactions to, 593
professional help for, 598
couples therapy and, 598
group therapy and, 598
psychopharmacology and, 598
psychotherapy and, 598
with residency training, 594
self-neglect and, 595, 595*f*
autognosis rounds for, 597
being your own most important patient, 596, 596*f*
communication about one's unavailability for, 597
decreasing vulnerability to stress for, 597
directed fantasy for, 597
enjoyment of achievements and goals for, 597
identification of thought distortions for, 597

Coping mechanisms *(Continued)*
mindfulness for, 597
pleasurable existence for, 597–598
practice of positive expectations for, 597
process experiences for, 596
realistic expectations and boundaries for, 596
reviewing own history for, 596
strategies for, 596–597
stigma and, bearing the burden of, 592–593
treating dying patients and, 594
poor, 398, 398*b*
resilience and, 400–401, 402*t*
role of religion in, 399
social support for, 399–400
techniques for better, 402
vulnerability and, 400–401, 401*t*–402*t*
Copper-transporting adenosine triphosphatase, 393–394
Copy number variants (CNVs), 387
Coronary artery disease (CAD)
anxiety and, 291
ECT risk of, 409
Cortex, of brain, 37
Corticosteroids
for catatonia, 261
psychiatric side effects of, 332*t*
Cortico-striato-pallido-thalamo-cortical (CSPTC) loop, 37
Cortisol, 456
Corydalis bungeana, 563–564
Cost-offset, 583
Counseling, nutritional, for anorexia nervosa, 182
Couples therapy, for psychiatrist, 598
COX-2 inhibitors, for pain, 200
Crack, 150
Cranial nerves, 39*t*
motor (III, IV, VI, XI, XII) and sensorimotor (V, VII, IX, X), 41–42
sensory, 39–40
Creatinine clearance (CrCl), for renal disease, 309
Creutzfeldt-Jakob disease, 99
Criminality, 47
XYY disorder and, 390–391
CRMP-5 antigen, associated with autoimmune encephalitides, 244*t*–245*t*
CRPS. *See* Complex regional pain syndrome.
CT. *See* Computed tomography.
Cultural Formulation Interview (CFI), 561
Cultural syndromes, 561
Culture and psychiatry, 559–567, 567*b*
acculturation and immigration in, 561–562
assessment of, 560–561
cultural identity in, 560
culture-bound syndromes, 561
distress in, 561, 561*t*
in end-of-life care, 516
ethnicity on, 562
psychiatric medications and, 563–567, 565*t*–566*t*
in illness presentation, 559–560
individual, and clinician, relationship between, 561
interpreters and, 562–563
"medical ombudsman" role in, 563
misdiagnosis, and cultural clashes, 567
psychosocial stressors and, 561
Cup Push, 45*t*
Cushing's syndrome, 296
in cancer patients, 357
Cyclic guanosine monophosphate (cGMP), in sexual dysfunction, 280
2',3' -Cyclic nucleotide 3'-phosphodiesterase (CNP) gene, in catatonia, 255
Cyclosporine, psychiatric side effects of, 331, 332*t*
Cystathionine β-synthase (CBS) gene, 393
Cytochrome p450 1A, drug interactions of, 430
Cytochrome p450 2C, drug interactions of, 430
Cytochrome p450 2D6, drug interactions of, 430
Cytochrome p450 3A4, drug interactions of, 430
Cytochrome P450 enzymes
isoenzymes, 65, 65*t*, 420, 421*t*
pharmacodynamic effects of, 430

D

Dacrystic seizure, 215
Dantrolene, for neuroleptic malignant syndrome, 118
DAST. *See* Drug Abuse Screening Test.
Datura candida, 563–564
Davanloo, Habib, 45–46
Daytime sleepiness, excessive, 270
Death, desire to hasten, in end-of-life care, 514
Deception, microexpressions and, 48
Deception syndromes, 170–173
factitious disorder, 165, 170–172
clinical presentation of, 171*t*
imposed on another, 171
malingering and, 172–173
management of, 173
Decision-making capacity, legal aspects of, 573–576, 575*b*
Deep brain stimulation (DBS), 410–411
indications of, 410–411
safety of, 411
technique in, 410
Deep tendon reflexes, 40–41
Defense mechanisms, in pediatric consultation, 524
Defibrillator, automatic implantable cardioverter, ECT risk in, 409
Dehydroepiandrosterone (DHEA), 474
Delayed ejaculation, 282–283
Delirious mania, 255–256
Delirious patients, 83–93, 83*b*
Delirium, 83, 115
after electroconvulsive therapy, 408
burn-induced, 364
in cardiac disease, 299–302, 300*b*
differential diagnosis of, 299–300
epidemiology of, 299
management of, 301–302
psychopharmacologic issues in, 300–302
in children and adolescents, 439
clinical features of, 96*t*
diagnosis of, 83–84, 85*t*
differential diagnosis of, 84–87, 85*b*, 85*t*–86*t*, 87*b*
drug management of, 89–92, 91*t*
in emergency psychiatry, 507, 507*t*
end-of-life care for, 515
examination of patient with, 87–89, 88*f*, 88*t*

Delirium *(Continued)*
in geriatric patients, 540–541
in hematopoietic stem cell transplantation, 356
in HIV infection, 340
management strategies for, 89
in specific diseases, 92
suicide and, 493
Delirium tremens (DTs), 89–90, 92, 144–145
Delta (δ)-receptors, in pain, 191
Delta waves, in polysomnography, 268
Delusional misidentification syndromes, 102
Delusions, 109
in geriatric patients, 542
Dementia
complementary medicine for, 474
in delirious cardiac patients, 293
depression and, 74
in emergency psychiatry, 507
in geriatric patients, 540–541
HIV-associated, 338–339
sleep disorders and, 274
subcortical, 74
Dementia Rating Scale (2nd edition; DRS-2), 57
Denial, 582–583
addressing, treatment strategies for, 376–377
by difficult patients, 482*b*
Dental erosion, eating disorders and, 182
Dependency, by difficult patients, 483
Depersonalization, 591, 595–596
Depression
adjustment disorder with depressed mood and, 79
antidepressant treatment for
anticholinergic effects of, 76
cardiac conduction effects of, 76–78
choice of, 74–79
discontinuation syndrome, 79
myocardial depression, 78
orthostatic hypotension, 76, 77*t*
prescribing of, 74–79, 75*t*
anxiety and, 134
assessment in intensive care unit, 382
bereavement and, 79
burn injuries and, 361, 369
in cancer patients, 353–354
in cardiac disease, 295–299
differential diagnosis of, 296–297, 297*b*
management of, 298–299
psychopharmacologic issues in, 297–298
risk factors for, 295–296
treatment modalities for, 298
in children and adolescents, 445–446
clinical use of SSRIs for, 447–448
in chronic medical illness, 371
clinical features of, 96*t*
despondency consequent to serious illness and, 79–81
diagnosis of, 70–74
differential diagnosis of, 71
major depression, 70–72, 71*b*–72*b*
diagnostic rating scale for, 59–60
in emergency psychiatry, 504
in end-of-life care, 514
in geriatric patients, 539–540, 541*t*
Depression *(Continued)*
hepatic metabolism and, 79
in HIV infection, 340, 344–346
in kidney disease, 306
organic causes of, exclusion of, 73–74
in pain, 194–195
pediatric consultation for, 527
persistent depressive disorder, 79
post-ictal, 216
post-stroke, 224–225, 226*b*
during pregnancy, 549–550
seizure disorders and, 214
sleep disorder and, 273
somatic symptoms and, 165
states commonly mislabeled as, 72–73
suicide and, 492
symptoms of, 298
thioridazine and, 79
transcranial magnetic stimulation for, 406
treatment strategies for, 377
Dermatomes, in pathophysiology of pain, 191, 193*f*
Desipramine, orthostatic hypotension and, 76
Despair, as phases of separation anxiety, 524
Despondency
acute phase of, management of, 80
consequent to serious illness, 79–81
post-acute, management of, 80–81
Desynchrony, 45
Detachment, as phases of separation anxiety, 524
Deutsch, Felix and Helene, 1–3
Devaluation, by difficult patients, 480–481, 482*b*
Developmental approach, to pediatric consultation, 524–526
Developmental disorders, in children and adolescents, 450–451
Developmental history, in psychiatric interview, 32
Dexmedetomidine, for delirium, 92
Dextroamphetamine
for ADHD, in children and adolescents, 442–443
for depression, 78
Dextromethorphan (DXM), 153
Dhat syndrome, 561
Diabetes
depression and, 69, 74
eating disorders and, 178–179
type 1, pediatric consultation for, 529–530
Diadochokinesia, 42
Diagnosis, 19
See also Diagnostic and Statistical Manual, 5th edition (DSM-5).
of delirium, 83–84, 85*t*
of neurocognitive disorders, 96–99, 97*b*, 98*f*
in treatment failure, 416
Diagnostic and Statistical Manual, 5th edition (DSM-5), 527
for acute stress disorder, in burn injuries, 364
in cultural assessment, 560
for delirium, 83
for depression, 70–72, 79
in cancer patients, 353–354
differential diagnosis of, 31
for eating disorder, 528

Diagnostic and Statistical Manual, 5th edition (DSM-5) *(Continued)*
- in general psychiatric diagnostic instrument, 59
- for HIV infection, 339
- for post-stroke depression, 225
- in routine clinical use, 414
- for sexual dysfunction, 280
- for sleep disorders, 269

Diagnostic rating scales, 59
- for anxiety disorders, 60–61
- for attention disorders, 61
- for cognitive disorders, 61–62
- general psychiatric diagnostic instrument in, 59–62
- for mood disorders, 59–60, 60*t*
- for psychotic disorders and related symptoms, 60
- for substance abuse disorders, 61, 61*b*

Dialectical behavior therapy, 489*t*–490*t*
Dialysis, for kidney disease, 305
Diarrhea, 316–317
Diazepam, for anxiety disorders, 135*t*
Dietary plan, for eating disorders, 182
Difficult patients, 477–490, 477*b*
- antisocial and narcissistic personality disorders in, 478
- borderline personality disorder in, 478–480
- consultation management for, 481*t*
- consultee and, 480–485, 480*f*
  - consultant's role in, 483–484, 483*b*–484*b*
  - helping, 481–483, 481*t*, 482*b*
- differential diagnosis of, 485–486
- medication for, 484–485
- psychiatrist's work with, 485–488
- substance abuse by, 486–487
- suicide assessment for, 486
- tactical psychotherapy for, 487–488, 489*t*–490*t*
- termination of, 488
- types of, 477–480
- violence in, assessment of potential for, 486

DiGeorge syndrome, 388
Digital technology, evaluating adherence, 531
Disorganization, 113
Disrupted-in-Schizophrenia-1 (DISC-1) gene, 387–388
Disruptions, in treatment failure, 417
Dissociative states
- by difficult patients, 480
- in pain, 197–198

Dissonance, 481*t*
Dissonant reality, 481*t*
Distress
- broad differential diagnosis for patient's, 294
- in cancer patients, 349–352
- conceptualizations of, 560–561
- cultural concept of, 561, 561*t*
- definition of, 455
- frequent encounters with, psychiatrist and, 591

Distress Assessment and Response Tool (DART) program, 352
Disulfiram
- for alcohol use disorder, 147
- causing catatonia, 255

"Do not resuscitate" orders, 536–538
Doctor-patient relationship, 15–22, 16*f*
- in cancer, 349

Doctor-patient relationship *(Continued)*
- in clinical formulation, 19–20
- communication in, 17
- empathy in, 17
- in general hospital, 15–16, 16*f*
- in history-taking, 17–19
- interview and, 17–19
- mindfulness in, 17
- obstacles and difficulties in, 21–22
- outcomes in psychiatry and, 15
- in treatment planning, 20–21, 20*b*–21*b*

Documentation, of psychiatric consultation, 599
Donabedian's model, 602
Donepezil, for neurocognitive disorders, 105, 105*t*
Dopamine antagonist medications, causing catatonia, 255
Dopamine-depleting medications, causing catatonia, 255
Dopaminergic agents, for neuroleptic malignant syndrome, 263
Dosing
- of opioids, 203
- in treatment failure, 416

Double effect, principle of, in end-of-life care, 517
Down's syndrome, genetic factors in, 390
DPPX antigen, associated with autoimmune encephalitides, 244*t*–245*t*
Drawings, performance, 54
Dronabinol, for anorexia nervosa, 184
DRS. *see* Mattis Dementia Rating Scale.
Drug Abuse Screening Test (DAST), 61
Drug Abuse Warning Network (DAWN), 149
Drug delivery, of opioids, 203
Drug dependence, suicide and, 492
Drug interactions, in psychopharmacology, 422–434
- antidepressants, 428–432, 429*t*, 431*t*
- antipsychotic drugs, 423–425, 424*t*
- benzodiazepines, 433–434
- mood stabilizers, 425–428, 426*t*–427*t*
- psychostimulants and modafinil, 433

Drug-drug interactions
- in HIV infection, 344, 345*t*
- in psychiatric consultation, 13

Drugs
- reduction, for neurocognitive disorders, 103
- in treatment failure, 416–417

Duloxetine
- for binge eating disorder, 186
- for kidney disease, 309

Dunbar, Helen Flanders, 1
DXA scanning, for eating disorders, 182
Dying patients, psychiatrists coping with, 594
Dyskinesia, in motor symptoms, 232*b*
Dysmetria, 235
Dyspareunia, 284
Dysphagia, 313
Dysphoric disorder, inter-ictal, 216–217
Dystonia, 116
- in motor symptoms, 232*b*

E

Early/uncomplicated withdrawal syndrome, 144
Eating Disorder Inventory, 184

Eating disorders, patients with, 177–187, 178*b*
anorexia nervosa, 182–184
binge-eating disorder, 185–186
bulimia nervosa, 184–185
complications of, 181
differential diagnosis for, 178–179
clinical detection of, 178
weight assessment for, 179
epidemiology of, 177
heritability of, 177
initial assessment of, 178–179
interventions for, 179–182
hospitalization, 180–181, 181*t*
medical, 181–182
reluctant patients, 179–180
laboratory tests for, 64–65
onset and course of, 177
other specified feeding or eating disorder (OSFED), 177, 179
pediatric consultation for, 528
in specialty psychiatric clinics, 585–586
Eaton, James, 2
Echolalia, 234
E-cigs, 467–468
Ecstasy, 152
ECT. *See* Electroconvulsive therapy.
Education
of clinical staff, eating disorders and, 179
for pain, 210
Efavirenz, for HIV infection, 337
Ego defenses, by difficult patients, 479, 482*b*
Elder abuse, 545
confidentiality of, 571
Elder care, 414–415
Elderly
burn injuries in, 363, 363*b*
depression and risk of falls in, 69–70
Electrocardiogram (ECG)
baseline, 63
polysomnography and, 267
Electroconvulsive therapy (ECT), 406–409
bilateral, 407
for geriatric patients, 539–540
indications of, 407–408
for post-stroke depression, 225
during pregnancy, 409, 550, 553–554
psychotropic medications with, 407
right unilateral, 407
safety of, 408–409
cardiovascular, 409
cognitive, 408
other CNS adverse effects in, 408–409
respiratory, 409
for suicide, 499
technique in, 407
Electroencephalography (EEG), 66–67, 66*t*
of delirium, 89
polysomnography and, 267
in psychiatric consultations, 11*b*, 12
for psychotic patients, 109–111
Electrolytes, in eating disorders, 181
Electromyogram (EMG), in polysomnography, 267
Electronic health record (EHR), 583
Electro-oculogram (EOG), in polysomnography, 267
Emergency Department care, in geriatric patient, 544–545
Emergency psychiatry, 501–512
acute symptoms, management of, 507–510
disposition, 510
environmental interventions, 508
pharmacologic interventions, 508, 509*t*
psychological interventions, 508
restraint and seclusion, 509–510
children in, 510–511
basic principles, 510
demographics, 510
evaluation, 510–511
management, 511
delivery models in, 501–502
demographics of, 501
legal responsibilities in, 511–512
capacity evaluation, 511–512
civil commitment, 512
confidentiality and release of information, 512
mandatory reporting, 512
medical evaluation in, 503*b*
outpatient treatment in, 510
psychiatric interview in, 502–503, 502*b*
safety evaluation in, 504
symptoms and presentations of, 504–507
anxiety, 504–505
catatonia, 505
depression, 504
intoxication or withdrawal, 505–507
alcohol, 505–506
barbiturates, 506
benzodiazepines, 506
cocaine, 506
marijuana, 506
methamphetamine, crystal, 506
opiates, 506
phencyclidine, 506
mania, 504
mental status, change in, 507
personality disorders, 505
psychosis, 505
trauma, 505
Emotional function, neuropsychological assessment for, 55
Empathy, 17
expression of, 464–466
Employee Retirement Income Security Act (ERISA), 570
Encephalitic neuropsychiatric impairment, 242–246, 242*t*
work-up for infectious and inflammatory causes of, 243–245
bloodwork, 243
intracellular *versus* cell surface-targeted neural autoantibodies, 243–245
neural autoantibody testing, 243, 244*t*–245*t*
Encephalitis, 241
paraneoplastic limbic, in cancer patients, 357
vs. delirium, 84

Encephalopathy, 241
hepatic, 321
hypertensive, *vs.* delirium, 84
Wernicke's, 146
Endocrine function, of kidney, 303
End-of-life care, 513–519, *516b–517b*
anxiety in, 514–515
burn injuries for, 370
challenges for care providers in, 516
cognitive changes in, 515
delirium in, 515
depression in, 514
desire to hasten death in, 514
ethics and, 517–518
goals of treatment for, 513–514
legal aspects of, 572–573
life-sustaining treatment, limitations of, 517–518
pain in, 515
in pediatric consultation, 535–536
personality considerations of, 515
physician-assisted suicide in, 518
psychosocial considerations in, 515–516
role of psychiatrists in, 514–516
"Endophenotypes", 388
End-stage renal disease (ESRD)
cognitive impairment in, 306
psychiatric disorders in, 306
Enemas, in eating disorders, 178–179
Enfuvirtide, for HIV infection, 338
Engagement Interview Protocol (EIP), 564
Enhanced CBT (CBT-E), for anorexia nervosa, 184–185
Enkephalins, in pathophysiology of pain, 191
Entry inhibitors, for HIV infection, 337–338
Environmental factors
in circadian rhythm, 268
doctor-patient relationship and, 16–17
gene interactions with, 386
of psychiatric consultations, 9
Enzymes
biological aspects of psychopharmacology, 564, *565t–566t*
cytochrome P450 isoenzymes, 420, *421t*
in gastrointestinal tract, 418
hepatic, 418
inhibitors and inducers, 419, *420t*
Epidemiological Catchment Area (ECA) study
collaborative care in, 582
depression and, 69
Epidemiology
of anxiety in cardiac patients, 291–295
of burn injuries, 359–360
of burnout, in physicians, 591
of delirium in cardiac patients, 299
of eating disorders, 177
in genetics of psychiatric disorders, 385–386, *386t*
of HIV infection and AIDS, 335–336, *336t*
of kidney disease, 304
of neurocognitive disorders, 95–96
of sexual dysfunction, 279
of suicide, 491
of traumatic brain injury, 227
Epilepsy
pediatric consultation for, 530
sleep disorders and, 274
suicide and, 493
temporal lobe, 214
vagus nerve stimulation for, 410
Epithelial sodium channels (ENaK), 303
Epworth Sleepiness Scale, 275, *276t*
Erectile disorder, 282
Erectile dysfunction, 286–288
first-line treatment for, *287t*
risk factors associated with, *283b*
second-line treatment for, *288t*
EROS-CTD, for female sexual dysfunction, 288
Erythrocyte sedimentation rate (ESR), elevated, in infectious or inflammatory encephalitis, 243
Escitalopram
for anxiety disorders, *135t*
for HIV infection, 345
Esgic, 159
Estimated glomerular filtration rate (eGFR), *310t*
Ethanol. *See* Alcoholism.
Ethical issues
for burn injuries, 370
end-of-life care and, 517–518
in pediatric consultation, 536–538
psychiatrists and, 591–592
Ethnicity
psychiatric diagnosis and, 562
psychiatric medications and, 563–567, *565t–566t*
Eustress, 455
Euthanasia, 518
Excretion, of drugs, 420–422
Executive function
in neurologic examination, 41
neuropsychological assessment for, 56
Exercise
for cancer patients, 355
efficacy of, 462

F

Faces Scale, 365
Facial nerve, 40
FACIT-F. *See* Functional Assessment of Chronic Illness Therapy-Fatigue Scale.
Factitious disorder, 165
clinical presentation of, *171t*
in deception syndromes, 170–172
with physical symptoms, in pain, 197
by proxy, 534
Failure, perception of, psychiatrists and, 592
Failure of treatment, 416–417
Falls, in elderly, depression and, 69–70, 76
Family
in end-of-life care, 536
of geriatric patients, 545
in pediatric consultation, 523, 526
of psychiatrists
communication of anticipated unavailability to, for self-neglect, 597
concerns in, 595

Family history
neurocognitive disorders and, 101
in psychiatric interview, 32
Family members
in end-of-life care, 515
as interpreters, 563
neurocognitive disorders and, 99–100
Family-based treatment (FBT), for anorexia nervosa, 183–184
Family-centered approach, to pediatric consultation, 524–526
Family-centered care, in pediatric consultation, 524–526
Fasciculations, in motor symptoms, 232*b*
Fatigue
in cancer patients, 354–355
in HIV infection, 340
Fatty acids, omega-3, 471
Fear, 128
anxiety and, 123
pediatric consultation and, 530
Feeding disorders, pediatric consultation for, 528
Female sexual dysfunction, 288–289
See also Sexual dysfunction.
Fetal alcohol syndrome, genetic factors of, 395–396
Fetal anomalies, during pregnancy, anticonvulsants and, 551
Fibromyalgia, 167–168
Financial stress, psychiatrists and, 593
Finger Localization Test, 57
Finger-Tapping Test, 57
Fiorinal, 159
Firearms, suicide and, 494
First-generation antipsychotics, 116–117
Flumazenil, for benzodiazepine overdose, 158
Fluorescence in situ hybridization (FISH), 387
Fluoxetine
for anorexia nervosa, 184
anticholinergic effects of, 76
for anxiety disorders, 135*t*
for binge eating disorder, 186
for bulimia nervosa, 185
for children and adolescents, 447
Fluphenazine, for delirium, 91
Fluvoxamine, 118
for anxiety disorders, 135*t*
for binge eating disorder, 186
for bulimia nervosa, 185
Focal seizures, 214
in motor symptoms, 232*b*
Focal unaware seizures, 214
Folic acid, for mood disorders, 471
Folstein Mini-Mental State Examination (MMSE), 61
for delirium, 87–88
for emergency psychiatry, 507
in psychiatric consultation, 11
Formal thought disorder, 109
Fractional absorption, 418
Fragile X syndrome, 391
Fricchione, Gregory, 3
Frontal lobe function, in delirium, 88
Frontal lobe syndrome, 72–73, 228
Frontotemporal neurocognitive disorder, 98–99
Functional Assessment of Chronic Illness Therapy-Fatigue Scale (FACIT-F), in cancer patients, 355
Functional neurologic symptom disorder(FND), in pain, 196–197
Functional somatic syndromes, 166–168, 167*t*
anxiety disorders and, 165
depressive disorders and, 165
fibromyalgia and, 167–168
irritable bowel syndrome and, 168
organic mental disorders and, 166
personality disorders and, 166
psychotic disorders and, 165–166
substance use disorders and, 165
systemic exertion intolerance disease and, 167
Funduscopy, in visual examination, 39
Fusion inhibitors, for HIV infection, 338

G

$GABA_BR$ antigen, associated with autoimmune encephalitides, 244*t*–245*t*
Gabapentin, 331
for alcohol use disorder, 147
drug interactions of, 428
for kidney disease, 311
GAD-65 antigen, associated with autoimmune encephalitides, 244*t*–245*t*
Gait, observation of, 42
Gait syndromes, 232*b*
Galantamine, for neurocognitive disorders, 105, 105*t*
Gaslight phenomenon, 9
Gastric bypass, 315–316, 315*b*
Gastroesophageal reflux disease, 313–314
Gastrointestinal bleeding, SSRI-related, 323–324
Gastrointestinal cancer, 319
Gastrointestinal disease, patients with, 313–326
cases of, 315*b*, 317*b*–318*b*, 321*b*–322*b*
liver disorders, 320–321
lower, 316–319
constipation, 316
diarrhea, 316–317
inflammatory bowel disease, 318–319, 318*b*
irritable bowel syndrome, 317–318, 317*b*
medication considerations in, 322–324, 323*t*–324*t*
oropharyngeal and upper, 313–316
dysphagia, 313
gastric bypass, 315–316, 315*b*
gastroesophageal reflux disease, 313–314
gastroparesis, 315
globus hystericus, 313
nausea and vomiting, 314–315
xerostomia, 313
pancreas, disorders of, 321–322
Gastrointestinal (GI) drug absorption, 418
Gastroparesis, 315
Gender dysphoria, 280, 284–285, 289
Gender identity disorder, 285
Gene expression
epigenetic pathways of, mind-body therapies and, 457–458
lifestyle and, 462

Gene-by-environment interactions, 386
Generalized anxiety disorder (GAD), 133
pharmacologic treatment of, 137–139
post-stroke depression and, 226
somatic symptoms of, 165
Generalized tonic-clonic convulsions (grand mal), 214
Generalized tonic-clonic (GTC) seizures, 214
Genetic syndromes, patients with, 385–396
Genetics
of metabolic disease, 392–396
assessment for, 392, 392*t*
questions for, 389*b*
autosomal dominant disorders, 393
porphyria/acute intermittent porphyria in, 393
autosomal recessive disorders, 393–394
homocystinuria, 393
metachromatic leukodystrophy in, 394
Niemann-Pick disease, Type C in, 394
Wilson's disease in, 393–394
selected, with psychiatric features, 392–395
X-linked disorders, 394–395
adrenoleukodystrophy, 394
ornithine transcarbamylase deficiency, 395
urea cycle defects in, 395
of mitochondrial disorders, 395–396
fetal alcohol syndrome in, 395–396
teratogen exposure causing, 395–396
of psychiatric disorders, 385–391
assessment of, 388, 389*b*
questions for, 388, 389*b*
autosomal dominant single-gene disorders in, 391
Huntington's disease, 391
neurofibromatosis type I, 391
tuberous sclerosis, 391
due to chromosomal abnormalities and microdeletions, 388–391
Down's syndrome, 390
Klinefelter's syndrome, 390
Prader-Willi syndrome, 390
Smith-Magenis syndrome, 389
Turner's syndrome, 390
velocardiofacial syndrome/Di George syndrome, 388
Williams syndrome, 389–390
47, XYY, 390–391
epidemiology of, 385–386, 386*t*
gene-by-environment interactions in, 386
genes and genomic regions linked to, 386–388
selected, 388–391, 389*t*
X-linked dominant disorders, 391
fragile X syndrome, 391
Rett syndrome, 391
suicide and, 494
Genito-pelvic pain/penetration disorder, 284
Genome-wide association studies (GWAS), 387
Geriatric Depression Scale, 539, 540*b*
Geriatric patient, care of, 539–545, 543*b*–544*b*
See also Aging patients.
anxiety in, 543
bipolar disorder in, 540
delirium in, 540–541
dementia in, 540–541
Geriatric patient, care of *(Continued)*
depression in, 539–540, 541*t*
elder abuse in, 545
Emergency Department care in, 544–545
families and caregivers for, 545
health care decision-making in, 544
pharmacotherapy for, 544
psychosis in, 542–543
substance abuse and withdrawal in, 543
GFAP antigen, associated with autoimmune encephalitides, 244*t*–245*t*
Ginkgo biloba, 474
Ginseng, 563–564
Glasgow Coma Scale (GCS), 87, 88*t*
for traumatic brain injury, 228, 228*b*
Global Assessment of Function Scale, 414
Globus hystericus, 313
Globus pallidus, 37
Glossopharyngeal nerve, 40
GlyαR antigen, associated with autoimmune encephalitides, 244*t*–245*t*
GM2 gangliosidosis, 394
Grafenberg spot (G-spot), 284
Graphesthesia, 39
Gratification, delayed, in psychiatrists, 593
Grief, depression and, 79
Group therapy, for psychiatrist, 598
Guanfacine, for ADHD, in children and adolescents, 445
Guidelines, for pain management, 209–210

H

HAART. *See* Highly active antiretroviral therapy.
Habit-reversal training, 234
Hackett, Thomas, 2
Hallucinations, 109
cultural differences and, 560
by geriatric patients, 542
hypnagogic, 271
in neurocognitive disorders, 102, 106
seizure disorders and, 214
Hallucinogens, use of, 153–154
Haloperidol, 331
for delirious cardiac patients, 300
for delirium, 90
for difficult patients, 485
in intensive care unit, 384
intravenous, 143
for neurocognitive disorders, 106
HAM-A. *See* Hamilton Anxiety Rating Scale.
Hamilton Anxiety Rating Scale (HAM-A), 60–61
Hamilton Depression Scale (HDS), 376
Hamilton Rating Scale for Anxiety, 414
Hamilton Rating Scale for Depression (HAM-D), 59–60, 60*t*, 414
Hashimoto's encephalitis, 250
Head trauma, suicide and, 493
Healing, in rehabilitation, brain pathways involved, 374, 375*f*
Health care decision-making, for geriatric patients, 544
Health Care Financing Administration, 599–600

Health Insurance Portability and Accountability Act (HIPAA), 571
Health maintenance organizations (HMOs). *See* Collaborative care.
Healthy habits
  adoption of, five-step cycle for, 464–466, 465*f*
  disease prevention and management of, 461–462
Healthy habits index, 461
Heinroth, Johann, 1
Hematomas, in traumatic brain injury, 227
Hematopoietic stem cell transplantation (HSCT), delirium in, 356
Hemiballism, in motor symptoms, 232*b*
Hemodialysis (HD), 305, 305*b*
Hepatic encephalopathy, 321
Hepatitis C, 320–321
Herman, William, 2
Heroin, use of, 155–157
Highly active antiretroviral therapy (HAART), for HIV infection and AIDS, 335
Hip fractures, in geriatric patient, 541
HIPAA. *See* Health Insurance Portability and Accountability Act.
Hippocampus, 47
Hippocrates, 1
Histamine, in pain signal, 189
HIV-1, depression and, 74
Home pregnancy tests, 552
"Homecoming depression", 80
Homeless patients, with burn injuries, 360–361
Homeostasis, clearance of, 303
Homocystinuria, genetic factors of, 393
Hooper Visual Organization Test, 56
Hopelessness, suicide and, 495
Hormonal therapy, effect on cancer patients, 357–358
Hospice, 513–514
Hospital Anxiety and Depression Scale, 374
Hospitalization
  for anorexia nervosa, 183
  behavioral difficulties during, 532
  for burn injuries, 367
  of children, 530
  for eating disorders, goals of, 180
  for suicidal behavior, 498
House staff, pediatric consultation and, 524
Human immunodeficiency virus (HIV) infection and acquired immunodeficiency syndrome (AIDS), patients with, 335–348
  central nervous system and, 338
  delirium in, 92
  dementia associated, 338–339
  epidemiology of, 335–336, 336*t*
  medications for, 336–338, 337*t*
    entry inhibitors, 337–338
    fusion inhibitors, 338
    integrase inhibitors, 337
    non-nucleoside reverse transcriptase inhibitors, 337
    nucleoside (and nucleotide) reverse transcriptase inhibitors, 337
    protease inhibitors, 337
  mild neurocognitive disorder associated, 339
Human immunodeficiency virus (HIV) infection and acquired immunodeficiency syndrome (AIDS), patients with *(Continued)*
  neurocognitive disorders associated, 338–339
  psychiatric care for, approach to, 342–344
    adherence in, 343–344
    collaboration in, 343
    screening and prevention in, 342–343
  treatment for, 344–348
    non-pharmacologic, 344
    pharmacologic, 344–348, 345*t*
Human sexual response, 280
Hunter Serotonin Toxicity Criteria, for serotonin syndrome, 263–264
Huntington's disease, 233–234, 234*b*
  depression and, 74
  genetic factors of, 391
  in psychotic patients, 111
  suicide and, 493
Hurricane Voices Breast Cancer Foundation, 537*b*
Hydrocephalus, normal pressure, 99
Hydrocortisone, for post-traumatic stress disorder, 133–134
Hydroxymethylbilane synthase (HMBS) gene, 393
Hydroxyzine, causing catatonia, 255
Hyperactivity, from sensory deprivation, 375–376
Hyperalgesia, 191
Hypercalcemia, in cancer patients, 355–356
Hypercholesterolemia, antidepressants and, 74
Hyperesthesia, 191
Hyper-or hypothermia, delirium *vs.*, 84
Hyperpathia, 191
Hyperphosphatemia, eating disorders and, 181
"Hypersexual disorder", 281
Hypersomnias, of central origin, 271
Hypertension
  ECT risk of, 409
  suicide and, 493–494
Hypertensive crisis, 432
Hyperviscosity syndrome, in cancer patients, 356–357
Hypnosis
  for burn injuries, 365
  as complementary medicine, 474
  for pain, 210
Hypnotics
  as complementary medicine, 473
  non-oral preparations of, 323*t*
Hypoactive sexual desire disorder, male, 284
Hypochondriasis, in pain, 196
Hypocretin, in narcolepsy, 271
Hypoglycemia, delirium *vs.*, 84
Hypomania, in geriatric patients, 540
Hyponatremia, 308
  in cancer patients, 356
Hypothalamic-pituitary-adrenal (HPA) axis activity
  stress and, 456
  suicide and, 495
Hypoxanthine-guanine phosphoribosyltransferase, deficiency of, 395
Hypoxia, delirium *vs.*, 84
Hysterical seizures, 218

I

IASP. *See* International Association for the Study of Pain.
Ibuprofen, for pain, 200
Ictal psychosis, 214–215
  treatment of, 215
ICU psychosis, 83–84
Idealization, by difficult patients, 480–481, 482*b*
Idiopathic hyperammonemia (IHA), in cancer patients, 357
Idiopathic hypersomnia, 271
Idiopathic insomnia, 269
Idiopathic pain, 192
Idiosyncratic speech, 113
Ilex guayusa, 563–564
Illness anxiety disorder, 163–164
  prognosis and treatment of, 169–170
Illusions
  in neurocognitive disorder, 102
  in psychiatric interview, 33
IM formulation (Vivitrol), for alcohol use disorder, 147
Imaging, for pain, 189–190
Imipramine
  for anxiety disorders, 135*t*, 136
  orthostatic hypotension and, 76
Immigration, acculturation and, 561–562
Immune system, stress and, 457
Immunosuppressive medications, psychiatric side effects of, 331, 332*t*
IMPACT model, of collaborative care, 587–588
Impairments, verbal and non-verbal, after electroconvulsive therapy, 408
Implicit bias, 48–49
Inborn errors of metabolism. *See* Genetics, of psychiatric disorders.
Incubus, 272
Infancy
  burn injuries in, 362, 362*b*
  key points and parenting tips in, 537*t*
  in pediatric consultation, 524–525
Infectious encephalitis
  clinical features of, 242
  treatment strategies for patients with, 248
Infectious or inflammatory neuropsychiatric impairment, patients with, 241–251
  illustrative autoimmune encephalitic syndromes manifesting with, 246–248
  potential etiologies of acute and sub-acute, 241–246
    encephalitic, 242–246, 242*t*
    encephalitis *versus* encephalopathy, 241–242
  psychiatric considerations in treatment of, 250
  treatment strategies for patients with, 248–250
Inflammatory bowel disease, 318–319, 318*b*
  pediatric consultation for, 530
Information
  gathering, in pain patients, 194, 195*t*
  release of, in emergency psychiatry, 512
Informed consent, in psychotropic medications, 415
Inositol, for mood disorders, 473
Inpatient Hospital Care (IHC), codes, 601
Insomnia, 269–270
  diagnosis of, 269
  treatment of, 269–270
Institute of Medicine Report on Preventing Medication Errors, 545
Instrumental activities of daily living (IADL), neurocognitive disorder and, 100, 100*t*
Insurance plans. *See* Billing for C-L services
Integrase inhibitors, for HIV infection, 337
Intellectual disability, in children and adolescents, 450–451
Intellectual functioning, assessment of, 52–53
Intensity, of anxiety, 123
Intensive care unit
  capacity evaluation in, 383
  depression assessment in, 382
  patients in, 381–384
  psychiatrists in, 381–384, 382*b*
  setting of, 381
Intensive Short Term Dynamic Psychotherapy, 45–46
Intention tremor, 235
Inter-ictal anxiety disorders, 217
Inter-ictal dysphoric disorder, 216–217
Inter-ictal psychosis, 217
  treatment of, 218
Internal pulse generator (IPG)
  in deep brain stimulation, 410
  in vagus nerve stimulation, 409
International Association for the Study of Pain (IASP), 189
International Classification of Sleep Disorders, 269
International Statistical Classification of Diseases and Related Health Problems, 599–600
Interpreters, 562–563
Interview, psychiatric, 23–35, 23*b*–24*b*
  assessment and treatment in, disagreements about, 35
  attachment theory in, lessons from, 24–25, 24*b*
  children and adolescents in, evaluation of, 34
  context of, 25–27
    setting, 25–26
    significance, 27
    situation, 26
    subject, 26–27
  data collection in, 29–33
    behavioral observation, 29
    medical and psychiatric history, 29–32, 30*b*
    mental status examination, 32–33, 32*b*–33*b*
  dealing with sensitive subjects during, 34–35
  difficulties in, 34–35
  doctor-patient relationship and, 17
  effective communication in, 27–28
  errors in, 35, 35*b*
  establishing alliance in, 27–28, 28*b*
  mindful practice in, 24–25
  narrative medicine in, 24–25
  presenting problems in, 29–31
  purpose of, 23
  relationship and therapeutic alliance in, building, 28–29
  treatment preparation during, 33–34
Intoxication, in emergency psychiatry, 505–507

Intracavernosal injection, for erectile dysfunction, 288*t*
Intraurethral suppository, for erectile dysfunction, 288*t*
Intubated patients, communication of, 384
Ipecac, syrup of, eating disorders and, 178–179
Irritable bowel syndrome, 168, 317–318, 317*b*
Ischemic heart disease, ECT risk of, 409
"I WATCH DEATH" mnemonic, 84, 85*t*

J

JCAHO. *See* Joint Commission on Accreditation of Healthcare Organizations.
Jefferson Scale of Empathy, 464–465
Jehovah's Witness, right to refuse treatment of, 578
Jet lag, 272
Joint Commission on Accreditation of Healthcare Organizations (JCAHO), in pain management, 209–210
Joint Commission Sentinel Event Alert, 496
Joint patient management, 587
Jurisigenic pain, 192

K

Kahlbaum, Karl, 253
Kaplan model, in sexual dysfunction, 280
Kappa (κ)-receptors, in pain, 190
Kava, 473
Kayser-Fleischer rings, 111, 393–394
Ketamine, 154
  for post-traumatic stress disorder, 133–134
Ketoprofen, for pain, 200
Ketorolac, for pain, 200
Kidney disease, 303–307
  advanced, therapeutic options for, 304–305
  cognitive impairment in, 306–307
  complications of, 304
  depression and anxiety in, 306
  dialysis for, 305
  epidemiology and risk factors of, 304
  lithium and, 304
  transplantation for, 305–306
Kidney function
  patients with normal, 303
  psychopharmacologic considerations of, 309–312
  treatment considerations of, 307–309
Kleine-Levin syndrome, 271
Klinefelter's syndrome, 390
Korsakoff's psychosis, 146
Kübler-Ross, Elizabeth, 513

L

La belle indifference, 238
Laboratory test, 62–66, 62*t*, 66*b*
  for anxiety, 64
  for eating disorders, 64–65, 178
  electroencephalogram for, 66–67, 66*t*
  for geriatric population, 64
  for metabolic disease, 392, 392*t*
  for mood disorders and affective symptoms, 63–64
  for neurocognitive disorders, 101, 101*b*
Laboratory test *(Continued)*
  neuroimaging, 67–68
    computed tomography in, 67
    magnetic resonance imaging in, 67–68
    positron emission tomography/single photon emission computed tomography in, 68
  pharmacogenomic, 65–66, 65*t*
  in psychiatric consultations, 11, 11*b*
  for psychosis and delirium, 62–63, 63*b*
  routine screening in, 62
  for substance abuse, 64, 65*t*
Lamotrigine
  breast feeding and, 554
  for difficult patients, 485
  drug interactions of, 427
  for kidney disease, 311
  for pain, 208
  during pregnancy, 551
Lance Armstrong Foundation (LAF), 537*b*
Language
  cultural differences and, 559–560
  in neurocognitive disorder, 102
  in neurologic examination, 41
  neuropsychological assessment for, 56
  use of, in psychiatric consultations, 9–10, 9*b*
Late paraphrenia, 115
Latency-age children
  evaluation of, in emergency psychiatry, 511
  interview techniques for, 523
  key points and parenting tips in, 537*t*
Lawsuit, psychiatrist coping with, 594
Laxatives, in eating disorders, 178–179, 182
Lead-pipe rigidity, in motor symptoms, 232*b*
Learning, neuropsychological assessment for, 56–57
Left ventricular assist devices (LVADs), anxiety and, 291
Legal aspects, of consultation, 569–579
  advance directives in, 572–573
  civil commitment and restraint in, 576–577
  end-of-life care and, 572–573
  physicians' rights and obligation in, 569–573
    confidentiality and privacy in, 570–571
    liability and managed care in, 570–571, 570*b*
    malpractice liability in, 569–570
    refusal to treat patients and, 571–572
  refuse treatment and, 577–578, 577*b*
  rights of patients in, 573–578
    competency in, 573–574
    decision-making capacity in, 573–576, 575*b*
    informed consent in, 573–576
Legal guardian, in emergency psychiatry, 510
Legal responsibilities, in emergency psychiatry, 511–512
  capacity evaluation, 511–512
  civil commitment, 512
  confidentiality, 512
  information, release of, 512
  mandatory reporting, 512
Leptomeningeal disease, in cancer patients, 356
Lesch-Nyhan syndrome, genetic factors of, 395
Leukodystrophy, metachromatic, 394
Lewy bodies
  in dementia, 232
  neurocognitive disorders with, 98

LGI-1 antigen, associated with autoimmune encephalitides, 244*t*–245*t*
LGI-1 encephalitis, 247–248, 248*b*
Liability, battery and false imprisonment and, 577
Liaison, 1
Life span, sleep across, 268
Lifestyle medicine, 462
Life-sustaining treatment, for end-of-life care, 517–518
Lignoceroyl-CoA ligase, deficiency of, 394
Limbic encephalitis, 247
  paraneoplastic, in cancer patients, 357
Limbic music, 43–49, 44*f*
  clinical examples of, 49, 49*b*
  definition of, 44–46
  implicit bias in, 48–49
  microexpressions in, 48
  polyvagal theory in, 47–48
Limbic probes, 44, 45*t*
Limbic system, 47
  anatomic expansion of, 46*t*
  in pathophysiology of pain, 189
Linkage studies, 388
Lisdexamfetamine, for ADHD, in children and adolescents, 443
Listening, in pain patients, 199
Lithium
  adverse effects of, 64
  for bipolar disorder, in children and adolescents, 448–449
  and breast feeding, 554
  for catatonia, 261
  drug interactions of, 425–426, 426*t*
  for HIV infection, 346
  kidney disease and, 304
  for neurocognitive disorders, 107
  during pregnancy, 551
Liver, transplantation, parent-to-child, 328
Liver disease, 320–321
  medication considerations in, 324–326
Living Beyond Breast Cancer, 537*b*
Locus ceruleus (LC), 124
Long-acting injectable antipsychotics, 116
Longitudinal outpatient psychiatric care, 584
Long-term memory, 41
Lorazepam
  for catatonia, 260
  for neurocognitive disorders, 107
Lorenzo's oil, 394
Low-titer autoantibodies, in autoimmune encephalitides, 250
Lung Allocation Score (LAS), 327, 328*b*
Lung disease, end-stage, 330
  Model for End-stage Liver Disease (MELD) for, 327, 328*b*
Lurasidone, 117
Lysergic acid diethylamine (LSD), 153

M

MacLean, Paul, 44
MADRS. *See* Montgomery-Asberg Depression Rating Scale.
Magnetic resonance imaging (MRI)
  anxiety during, 127–128
  claustrophobia during, 353
  in psychiatric consultation, 11–12
  for psychiatric symptoms, 67–68
  for traumatic brain injury, 227
Magnetic resonance spectroscopy (MRS), 68
Major depressive disorder (MDD), 69, 295
  ECT indication for, 407
  epidemiology of, 386*t*
  suicide and, 492
  vagus nerve stimulation for, 410
Malingering, 172–173
  in pain, 197
Malpractice, 569
  liability, 569–570
  litigation of, psychiatrists coping with, 594
Maltreatment, child, 532–535
Managed Behavioral Health organizations (MBHOs). *See* Collaborative care.
Managed care
  See also Collaborative care.
  liability and, 570–571, 570*b*
Managed care organizations (MCOs), 581
Mandatory reporting, confidentiality and, 571
Mania
  in emergency psychiatry, 504
  in geriatric patients, 540
  in HIV infection, 341
  post-stroke, 226
  in traumatic brain injury, 229
Manic State Rating Scale (MSRS), 60
MAOIs. *See* Monoamine oxidase inhibitors.
Maprotiline
  anticholinergic effects of, 76
  cardiac conduction effects of, 78
Maraviroc, for HIV infection, 337–338
Marijuana, in emergency psychiatry, 506
Mattis Dementia Rating Scale (DRS), 62
Meaning-centered group psychotherapy, 403
Medial orbitofrontal cortex (MOFC), 257–258
Medical child abuse, 534–535
Medical conditions or treatment
  psychiatric complications of, 7, 7*b*
  psychiatric presentations of, 7, 7*b*
  psychological reactions to, 8, 8*b*
Medical history
  neurocognitive disorders and, 100
  in psychiatric interview, 29–32, 30*b*
    past, 31
Medical illness
  anxiety mimic of, 130–132, 131*b*–132*b*
  chronic, in children, 535
  mimic of anxiety disorder, 128–130, 129*b*–130*b*
  psychiatric factors affecting, 529–530
Medical interventions, for neurocognitive disorders, 103–105
Medical records
  confidentiality of, 571
  Medicare guidelines for, 599–600
  reviewing current and pertinent, in psychiatric consultations, 10
  services documented in, bill for, 599

Medical team, pediatric consultation and, 523–524
Medical-psychiatric team approach, 529
Medicare and Medicaid
  guidelines of
    for medical record, 599–600
    for pain management, 209–210
  in health care decisions, 544
Medications
  discontinuation of, 417–418
  for psychotropic drug side effects, 434–435
  selection and administration of, 415–416
Melanosis coli, 182
Melatonin, 473
Memantine, for neurocognitive disorders, 105–106
Memory
  in Alzheimer's disease, 96
  in elderly individuals, 96
  long-term, 41
  in neurologic examination, 41
  in neuropsychological assessment, 56–57
  short-term, 41
Memory deficit, agitation and, 377–378
Memory loss, after electroconvulsive therapy, 408
Meningitis
  delirium *vs.*, 84
  treatment strategies for patients with, 248
Menopausal symptoms, complementary medicine for, 474
Mental status examination (MSE), 582–583
  in history-taking, 19
  for neurocognitive disorder, 101–102
  in neurologic examination, 41
  in psychiatric interview, 32–33, 32*b*–33*b*
  for suicidal behavior, 497
Mentalization-based therapy, 489*t*–490*t*
Meperidine
  delirium and, 87*b*
  for HIV infection, 348
Mescaline, 153
Mesolimbic system, 258
Mesostriatum, 258
Mesulam's olfactocentric paralimbic belt, limbic system and, 47
Metabolic disorders. *See* Genetics, of psychiatric disorders.
Metabolism
  of benzodiazepines, 158
  of drugs, 419–420, 420*t*–421*t*
Metachromatic leukodystrophy, 394
Methadone, 156–157
Methamphetamine, crystal, in emergency psychiatry, 506
Methyl-CpG-binding protein 2 (MeCP2), in Rett syndrome, 386–387, 391
Methylphenidate
  for ADHD, in children and adolescents, 442
  for depression, 78
Methylxanthines, lithium and, 426
Metoclopramide, causing catatonia, 255
Micotrol beads, for ADHD, in children and adolescents, 442
Microexpressions, 48
Mild neurocognitive disorder, HIV-associated, 339
Millon Clinical Multiaxial Inventory-III (MCMI-III), 53
Mind-body medicine, 455–460, 456*t*, 459*b*
  allostatic loading and, 457–458
  defined, 455
  hypotheses for, 458–459
  use and efficacy of, 459–460
Mind-Body Medicine Equation, 458, 458*f*
Mindfulness, 17
  for self-neglect, 597
MINI. *See* Mini International Neuropsychiatric Interview.
Mini International Neuropsychiatric Interview (MINI), 59
Mini-Mental State Examination (MMSE)
  for abnormal movements, 233
  for autoimmune encephalitis, 249
  for neurocognitive disorders, 103
  in psychiatric interview, 33
  for psychosis, 109–111
Minnesota Multiphasic Personality Inventory (MMPI)
  in non-epileptic seizure, 219
  in psychiatric consultation, 12
Minnesota Multiphasic Personality Inventory-2 (MMPI-2), 53, 173
Mirtazapine
  drug interactions of, 430
  hepatic metabolism of, 79
  for HIV infection, 345
  orthostatic hypotension and, 76
  for pregnancy, 549
  side effects of, 78–79
Misanthropy, 596
Misconceptions, by geriatric patients, 542
Misoprostol, for pain, 200
Mitochondrial disorders, 395–396
  fetal alcohol syndrome in, 395–396
  teratogen exposure causing, 395–396
MMSE. *See* Folstein Mini-Mental State Examination.
Mnemonics
  "A CALM VISAGE", 102
  "I WATCH DEATH", 84, 85*t*
  "VICTIMS DIE", 62*t*
  "WHHHHIMPS", 84, 85*b*
  "WWHHHHIMPS", 63*b*
MoCA. *See* Montreal Cognitive Assessment.
Modafinil
  for ADHD, in children and adolescents, 445
  drug interactions of, 433
Model for End-stage Liver Disease (MELD), 327, 328*b*
Molindone, for delirium, 92
Monoamine oxidase A (MAO_A) gene promoter, 386
Monoamine oxidase inhibitors (MAOIs)
  for anxiety disorders, 135*t*
  cardiac conduction effects of, 78
  drug interactions of, 431–432
  for HIV infection, 346
  seizure disorders and, 217
Montgomery-Asberg Depression Rating Scale (MADRS), 60, 376
Montreal Cognitive Assessment (MoCA)
  for autoimmune encephalitis, 249
  for delirium, 87–88
  for neurocognitive disorder, 103, 104*f*

Mood disorders
  in children and adolescents, 445–450
    antidepressant-associated suicidality and, 446–447
    depression in, 445–446
    pharmacotherapy of, 446
  complementary medicine for, 471–473
  depression. *See* Depression.
  diagnostic rating scales for, 59–60
  during pregnancy, 547–550
  sleep disorder and, 273–274
  suicide and, 492
  in traumatic brain injury, 228–229
Mood stabilizers
  for bipolar disorder, 551
  drug interactions of, 425–428, 426*t*–427*t*
  for HIV infection, 347
  for kidney disease, 311
  liquid and orally-disintegrating formulations of, 324*t*
  non-oral preparations of, 323*t*
Morbidity, of traumatic brain injury, 227
Morgellons disease, 165
Morphine, for post-traumatic stress disorder, 133–134
Mortality rate, in eating disorders, 177
Motivational interviewing
  in five-step cycle, 465
  goals of, 465
  principles of, 465
Motor examination, 42
Motor functions, neuropsychological assessment for, 57
Movement disorders
  deep brain stimulation for, 410
  sleep-related, 273
MRI. *See* Magnetic resonance imaging.
MRS. *See* Magnetic resonance spectroscopy.
MSRS. *See* Manic State Rating Scale.
Mu (μ) receptors, in pain, 190
Multicenter AIDS Cohort Study, 338
Multi-center Sertraline AntiDepressant Heart Attack Randomized Trial (SADHART), 297
Multiple chemical sensitivity (MCS), 168
Multiple ligation dependent probe amplification (MLPA), 388
Multiple Risk Factor Intervention Trial, 462
Multiple sclerosis, suicide and, 493
Multisystem atrophy (MSA), 232
Munchausen syndrome, 171, 534
Muromonab-CD3, psychiatric side effects of, 332*t*
Murray, George, 2–3, 8, 43
Muscle atrophy, in neurologic examination, 42
Muscle bulk, in motor examination, 42
Muscle paralysis, lithium and, 425–426
Muscle strength, in motor examination, 42
Muscle tone, in motor examination, 42
MUSE (alprostadil), for erectile dysfunction, 288*t*
Mycophenolate, psychiatric side effects of, 332*t*
Myocardial infarction
  depression and, 69
  ECT risk of, 409
Myocardial Infarction Depression Intervention Trial (MIND-IT), 297–298
Myoclonic seizures, 214
Myoclonus
  in motor symptoms, 231, 232*b*
  nocturnal, 273
Myofascial pain, 193

N

Naltrexone
  for alcohol use disorder, 147
  for bulimia nervosa, 185
  for cocaine use disorder, 151–152
  as opioid antagonist, 157
Naproxen, for pain, 200
Narcissistic personality disorder, 478
Narcolepsy, 271
Narcotics Anonymous, 414–415
National Burn Repository, 359–360
National Child Abuse and Neglect Data System (NCANDS), 532–533
National Comorbidity Survey (NCS), 582
  depression and, 69
National Comprehensive Cancer Network (NCCN), 349–352, 355
National Institute of Mental Health (NIMH), 2
National Institute on Alcohol Abuse, 543
Natural medications, 471–475, 475*b*
  See also Complementary medicine.
Nausea and vomiting, in cancer patients, 314–315, 353
NCANDS. *See* National Child Abuse and Neglect Data System.
Negative symptoms, of psychosis, 113
Neglect, pediatric consultation and, 533
Nephrogenic diabetes insipidus (NDI), 304
Nephrons, 303
"Nervous laugh", 45
Neural autoantibody testing, for encephalitic neuropsychiatric impairment, 243, 244*t*–245*t*
Neurexin-3α antigen, associated with autoimmune encephalitides, 244*t*–245*t*
Neuroanatomy, functional, 37, 37*b*–38*b*, 38*f*
Neurocognitive assessment, bedside, of neurocognitive disorder, 102
Neurocognitive disorders
  bedside neurocognitive assessment for, 102
  case of, 95*b*
  Creutzfeldt-Jakob disease, 99
  diagnosis of, 96–99, 97*b*, 98*f*
  due to Alzheimer's disease, 96–97
  epidemiology of, 95–96
  evaluation of, 99–103
  frontotemporal, 98–99
  history of, 99–101, 100*t*
  HIV-associated, 338–339
  laboratory examination for, 101, 101*b*
  with Lewy bodies, 98
  medical and neurologic examination for, 101
  mental status examination for, 101–102
  multiple etiologies of, 99
  normal pressure hydrocephalus (NPH) and, 99
  patients with, 95–107

Neurocognitive disorders *(Continued)*
pharmacotherapy for, 105–107
for cognitive symptoms, 105–106, 105*t*
for neuropsychiatric symptoms, 106–107, 106*t*
standardized cognitive testing for, 103, 104*f*
substance/medication-induced, 99
treatment considerations for, 103–107
behavioral, 105, 105*b*
medical and surgical, 103–105
vascular, 97–98
Neurofibromatosis type I, 391
Neurogenic neuroinflammation, 457
Neuroimaging
for psychiatric symptoms, 67–68, 67*b*
for psychotic patients, 109–111
Neuroleptic malignant syndrome (NMS), 118, 261–263, 261*b*
clinical features of, 262–263, 262*t*
delirium in, 92
diagnosis of, 262–263, 262*t*
epidemiology of, 262
risk factors of, 262
Neuroleptics
for burn injuries, 366
for delirium, 90
for pregnancy, 552
Neurologic conditions. *See* Cerebrovascular disease; Movement disorders; Multiple sclerosis; Seizure disorders; Traumatic brain injury.
Neurologic diseases, in geriatric patient, 539
Neurologic examination, 37*b*–38*b*, 38–42
input in, 38–40
mental status examination in, 41
peripheral sensory examination in, 39
sensory (I, II, VIII) and sensorimotor (V, VII, IX, X) cranial nerves in, 39–40, 39*t*
integration and evaluation in, 40–41
output in, 41–42
coordination in, 42
motor examination in, 42
motor (III, IV, VI, XI, XII) and sensorimotor (V, VII, IX, X) cranial nerves in, 41–42
Neuromyelitis optica, 242–243
Neuropathic pain, 191
Neuropsychiatric side effects, of cancer drugs, 350*b*–351*b*
Neuropsychological assessment, 54–58
case of, 54*b*–55*b*
methods of, 55–57
referral questions for, 57–58
statistical analysis and interpretation of, 57
test reports in, 58
Neuropsychological tests
in HIV infection, 338
for non-epileptic seizure, 219
Neurotherapeutics, 405–411
Neurotransmitters, anxiety and, 124
Nevirapine, for HIV infection, 337
NF-κB, 457–458
Nicotine-replacement therapy, for smoking cessation, 468–469
Niemann-Pick disease, type C, 394
Night terrors, 272
Nightmare disorder, 272
Nitric oxide (NO), for sexual dysfunction, 280
NMDAR antigen, associated with autoimmune encephalitides, 244*t*–245*t*
NMDAR encephalitis, 246–247
Nociception. *See* Pain.
Nociceptive reflexes, 40
Nocturnal leg cramps, 273
Non-24-hour day syndrome, 272
Non-adherence, pediatric, 531–532
Non-benzodiazepine sedative-hypnotics, for kidney disease, 311
Non-epileptic seizures (NES), 218–219, 218*b*–219*b*, 220*t*
Non-interpretive intervention, 484
Non-medication therapies, in complementary medicine, 474
Non-nucleoside reverse transcriptase inhibitors (NNRTIs), for HIV infection, 337
Non-pharmacologic strategies, for delirious cardiac patient, 301
Non-rapid eye movement (NREM), 267
Non-steroidal anti-inflammatory drugs (NSAIDs)
lithium and, 426
for pain, 200, 200*f*, 201*t*
Norepinephrine (NE), distress and, 455
Normal pressure hydrocephalus (NPH), 231
Nortriptyline, for post-stroke depression, 225
NSAIDs. *See* Non-steroidal anti-inflammatory drugs.
Nucleoside and nucleotide reverse transcriptase inhibitors (NRTIs), for HIV infection, 337
Nucleus tractus solitarius (NTS), 409–410
Nutritional counseling, for anorexia nervosa, 182
Nutritional rehabilitation, for anorexia nervosa, 182–184

O

Obesity
antidepressants and, 74
binge eating disorder and, 179, 186
Obsessive-compulsive disorder (OCD), 134
in children and adolescents, 439
deep brain stimulation for, 410
sleep disorder and, 273*b*
in specialty psychiatric clinics, 585–586
suicidal behavior and, 492–493
Occupational therapy, in pediatric consultation, 532
Oculogyric crisis, 236
Olanzapine
for anorexia nervosa, 184
for bipolar disorder, in children and adolescents, 450
for burn injuries, 366
for delirious cardiac patients, 300
for delirium, 91
for psychosis, 117
Oleanolic acid, 563–564
Olfactory hallucinations, 144–145
Olfactory nerve, 39
Omnipotence, by difficult patients, 480–481, 482*b*
Ondansetron, for alcohol use disorder, 147

One-time consultation, 584
Opiates, 155
  for burn injuries, 364–365
  in emergency psychiatry, 506
Opioid adjuvants, 203
Opioids, for pain, 201–204
  administration of, 201–202
  maintenance of, guidelines for, 203–204
  potencies, 201, 202*t*
  toxicity, 202
  use of, 155–157
Opisthotonus, 236
Optic nerve, 39–40
Oregon Death with Dignity Act (DWDA), 518
Organ failure and transplantation, 327–334
  long-term care of, 332–333
  pediatric, 333–334, 333*b*
  psychiatric care of
    post-transplant patients, 331
    pre-transplant patients, 330–331
  psychiatric considerations of, 330–333, 330*b*
  short-term care of, 331–332, 332*t*
Organ Procurement and Transplant Network (OPTN), 327
Organic brain syndromes, suicide and, 493
Organic mental disorders, somatic symptoms and, 166
Organic personality syndrome, 228
Orgasmic disorder, female, 284
Orlistat, for binge eating disorder, 186
Ornithine transcarbamylase deficiency, 395
Orthostatic hypotension, antidepressants and, 76, 77*t*
Osteopenia, anorexia nervosa and, 182
Osteoporosis, anorexia nervosa and, 182
Oucher Scale, for pain assessment, 365
Outline for Cultural Formulation, 560
Overdose, with benzodiazepines, 158
Oxcarbazepine
  for bipolar disorder, in children and adolescents, 449
  drug interactions of, 427–428
  for kidney disease, 311
  for pain, 208
Oxycodone, 155

P

Pacemakers, cardiac, ECT risk with, 409
Pain
  assessment of, in burn injuries, 364–368
  diagnosis of
    anxiety, 196
    depression, 194–195
    dissociative states, 197–198
    factitious disorder with physical symptoms, 197
    functional neurologic symptom disorder(FND), 196–197
    hypochondriasis, 196
    malingering, 197
    pain disorder, 196, 196*t*
    psychosis, 196
    somatic symptom disorders, 196, 197*t*
Pain *(Continued)*
  in HIV infection, 342, 347–348
  measurement of, 193–194
  medication for, 199–208
    analgesic adjuvants, 204, 205*t*–206*t*
    antidepressants, 204–207
    antiepileptic drugs, 207–208
    non-steroidal antiinflammatory drugs, 200, 200*f*, 201*t*
    opioids, 201–204, 202*t*
    sympathetically-maintained pain (SMP), 208
  pathophysiology of, 189–191, 190*f*–191*f*
  patients with, 189–211
  in peripheral sensory examination, 39
  psychiatry consultant and, 194–198
  sleep disorders and, 274
  terminology of, 191–193, 192*t*, 193*f*
  treatment of
    central neuropathic pain states, 208–209, 209*t*
    multidisciplinary pain clinics, 209–211
    principles of, 198–199
Paliperidone, for burn injuries, 366
Pancreas
  carcinoma of, depression and, 73
  disorders of, 321–322
Pancreatic cancer, 321–322, 321*b*–322*b*
Pancreatitis, 322
Panic attacks, 124
  during pregnancy, 553
Panic disorder, 132–133
  associated with medical illness, 132
  cultural differences and, 560
  epidemiology of, 386*t*
Panic mechanism, 124
PANSS. *See* Positive and Negative Syndrome Scale.
Papez circuit, 47
Parabrachial nucleus, 409–410
Paradoxical insomnia, 269
Paradoxical sleep, 267–268
Parainfectious autoimmune encephalitis, 245–246
  brain imaging for, 246
  CSF analysis of, 245
  electroencephalography for, 245–246
  malignancy screening for, 246, 247*f*
Parallel care, 586–587
Paralysis, sleep, 271
Paraneoplastic disorders, 242
Paraneoplastic limbic encephalitis (PLE), in cancer patients, 357
Paranoid, 113–114
Paraphilias, 282, 285*b*
Paraphilic disorders, 280, 284, 289
Parasomnias, 272–275
Parasympathetic nervous system, 456
Paratonia, 231
Parent
  anxiety of, in pediatric consultation, 526
  with ASD, 532
Parenting at a Challenging Time (PACT) Model, 536, 537*b*
Parenting classes, 414–415
Parkinsonism, 237

Parkinson's disease, 232–233, 232*b*
antipsychotic drugs in, 424
delirium in, 92
depression and, 74
ECT indication for, 408
in geriatric patients, 539
Lewy bodies in, 98
in psychotic patients, 111
sleep disorders and, 274
Paroxetine
anticholinergic effects of, 76
for anxiety disorders, 135*t*
Paroxetine-CR, for anxiety disorders, 135*t*
Pathogenic stress, 455
Pathologic anxiety, 123
Patient. *See* Doctor-patient relationship.
Patient education, in psychotropic medications, 415
Patient examination, in psychiatric consultation, 11
Patient Protection and Affordable Care Act (PPACA), 581–582
Patient Self-Determination Act of 1990, 544, 573
Patient-centered care, 16–17, 17*b*
physician practice in, 17
Patient's medication, review of, in psychiatric consultations, 10–11
Patients' rights, 573–578
competency in, 574
decision-making capacity in, 573–576, 575*b*
in end-of-life care, 517
informed consent in, 573–576
Pavor nocturnus, 272
Pediatric symptom falsification, 534
Pediatric transplantation, 333–334, 333*b*
post-transplant care in, 334
pre-transplant evaluation in, 333–334
Peer interactions, pediatric, 536
Penile self-injection, for erectile dysfunction, 288*t*
Peptic ulcer disease, suicide and, 493
Periodic limb movement disorder (PLMD), 273
in HIV infection, 341
Peripheral nervous system complications, in kidney disease, 308–309
Peripheral sensory examination, 39
Perphenazine
for delirium, 91–92
for neurocognitive disorders, 106
Persecutory delusions, 115
Persistent depressive disorder, 79
Persistent pulmonary hypertension of newborn (PPHN), 549
Personality Assessment Inventory (PAI), 53
in psychiatric consultation, 12
Personality disorders, 477–478
See also Difficult patients.
antisocial, 478
borderline, 478–480
coping skills and, 398–399
in emergency psychiatry, 505
in end-of-life care, 515
narcissistic, 478
somatic symptoms and, 166
suicide and, 492
Personality tests, 53–54
PET. *See* Positron emission tomography.
P-glycoprotein (Pgp), in drug absorption, 419
Phantom-limb pain, 192–193
Pharmacogenomic testing, 65–66, 65*t*
Pharmacokinetics
See also Psychopharmacology.
biological aspect and, 564
in psychiatric consultation, 12–13
Pharmacology, for traumatic brain injury, 229–230
Pharmacotherapy. *See* Psychopharmacology.
Phencyclidine, in emergency psychiatry, 506
Phenelzine, for anxiety disorders, 135*t*, 136
Phenobarbital, 145
Phenytoin, for pain, 207
Phobias, 133
in traumatic brain injury, 229
Phobic disorders, 125
Physical abuse, pediatric consultation and, 533
Physical examination, in pain patients, 194, 196*t*
Physician, mortality of, 591, 592*f*
Physician practice, in patient-centered care, 17
Physician-assisted suicide, 572
in end-of-life care, 518
Physicians' Desk Reference (PDR)
in drug interactions, 427
in psychopharmacologic management of children and adolescents, 438–439
Physostigmine, for delirium, 89
Placebos, in pain, 198
Plaques, neuritic, in Alzheimer's disease, 96
Plastic surgery, in burn injuries, 367–368
Poisoning, delirium *vs.*, 84
Polymorphisms, 387
Polypharmacy, in geriatric patients, 544
Polysomnography, 267–268
Polyvagal theory, 47–48
Porphobilinogen (PBG) deaminase, 393
Porphyria/acute intermittent porphyria, 393
Positive and Negative Syndrome Scale (PANSS), 60
Positron emission tomography (PET), 68
Post-ictal agitation (PIA), 408
Post-ictal depression, 216
Post-partum psychiatric illness, 555–557
depression, 555–556
obsessive-compulsive disorder, 556
panic attacks, 556
prevention of, 556–557
psychosis, 556
Post-stroke apathy, 225–226
Post-stroke depression (PSD), 224–225, 226*b*
Post-stroke mania, 226
Post-stroke psychosis, 226
Post-traumatic stress disorder (PTSD), 133–134
burn injuries and, 364, 369
in cancer patients, 353
in children and adolescents, 439
cultural differences and, 560
resulting from traumatic procedures, 126–127, 126*b*
Postural tremor, in motor symptoms, 232*b*
Potency, of opioids, 201
Prader-Willi syndrome, 390

Prefrontal cortex (PFC)
  appraisal and, 457
  stress response and, 456
Pregabalin
  drug interactions of, 428
  for pain, 208
Pregnancy, psychiatric illness during, 547–557
  antidepressant use for, 548–549
  anxiety disorders, 553
  bipolar disorder, 550–552, 550*b*–551*b*
  breast-feeding and psychotropic drug use, 554–555
  depression, pharmacologic treatment of, 549–550
  electroconvulsive therapy for, 550, 553–554
  mood disorders, 547–550
  perinatal psychiatry, 557
  post-partum period and, 555–557
    depression, 555–556
    obsessive-compulsive disorder, 556
    panic attacks, 556
    prevention of, 556–557
    psychosis, 556
  psychotic disorders, 552–553
  suicide and, 494
  treatment of, 547
Premature ejaculation, 283, 286
Premenstrual symptoms, complementary medicine for, 474
Preoptic anterior hypothalamus, 258
Pre-school age
  burn injuries in, 362, 362*b*
  evaluation of, in emergency psychiatry, 510–511
  key points and parenting tips in, 537*t*
  in pediatric consultation, 525
President's Commission for the Study of Ethical Problems in Medicine and Biomedical and Behavioral Research, 574
Primary anxiety disorder, 132–134
Primary care, 587
Primary care providers. *See* Collaborative care.
Primary catatonia, 254
Primary generalized seizure, 214
Primitive denial, by difficult patients, 482*b*
Primitive ego defenses, by difficult patients, 479, 482*b*
Primitive idealization, by difficult patients, 480–481, 482*b*
Primitive reflexes, 40–41
Proactive consultation services, 601
Prochaska, James, 462
Profanity, 45*t*
Projective identification, by difficult patients, 481, 482*b*
Prolactin
  antipsychotic drugs in, 424
  in non-epileptic seizure, 219
Propofol, for delirium, 92
Propranolol, 235
  for anxiety disorders, 135*t*
  for post-traumatic stress disorder, 133–134
Proprioceptive reflexes, 40–41
Prosody, depression and, 73–74
Prostaglandins, in pain signal, 189
Protease inhibitors (PIs), for HIV infection, 337
Protriptyline, anticholinergic effects of, 76
Pseudo-Bartter's syndrome, 181
Pseudobulbar affect (PBA), 226
  during rehabilitation, 375
Pseudobulbar palsy, 226
Pseudologia fantastica, 171, 197
Pseudoseizures, 213, 218
Psychiatric care, for HIV infection, 342–344
Psychiatric conditions or treatment
  co-morbid medical and, 8, 8*b*
  medical complications of, 8, 8*b*
  medical presentations of, 8, 8*b*
  principles of, 12–14
Psychiatric consultation
  See also Difficult patients.
  in emergencies. *See* Emergency psychiatry.
  in general hospital
    adverse effects of, 14
    approach to, 7–14
    art of, 8–10
    biological management of, 12–14
    clinical approach of, 8–9
    collateral data, gathering of, 11
    diagnosis and management plan in, 11–12
    differential diagnosis in, 7–8, 8*f*
    environment of, 9
    laboratory tests in, 11, 11*b*
    language, use of, 9–10, 9*b*
    personality assessment and management in, 13*t*, 14
    process of, 10–12, 10*b*
    providing periodic follow up in, 12
    psychological management of, 13*t*, 14
    social management of, 14
    speaking with referring clinician during, 10, 12
    style of interaction in, 9
    writing a note in, 12
  pediatric, 521–538, 521*b*–522*b* *See also* Children.
    for anorexia nervosa, 528
    for behavioral difficulties, 530
    for child maltreatment, 532–535
    for chronic illness, 535
    consultation requests in, 526–532
    for depression, 527
    developmental approach to, 524–526
      adolescent, 525
      infancy, 524–525
      pre-school age, 525
      school age, 525
    end-of-life care in, 535–536
    ethical issues in, 536–538
    for factitious disorder by proxy, 534
    family-centered approach to, 524–526
    family-centered care in, 524–526
    future considerations of, 538
    interview techniques for, 522–523
    medical team and, 523–524
    Parenting at a Challenging Time (PACT) Model for, 536, 537*b*
    physical abuse and neglect in, 533
    process of, 522–526
    psychiatric factors affecting medical illness in, 529–530
    sexual abuse in, 533–534

Psychiatric consultation *(Continued)*
for somatic symptoms, 528–529
for suicide, 527–528
for post-partum psychiatric illness, 547, 555–557
Psychiatric consultation services
bill for, 599
consultation note in, standard format for, 600–601
costs and benefits of, 601–602
documentation of, 599
Donabedian's model in, 602
guiding principles of quality measurement of, 603
management of, 599–604, 599*b*
outcome measures of consultant's quality of, 603
payer of, 600
preauthorization for, 600
process measures of consulting quality of, 603
quality assurance and quality improvement on, 602
structural measures of consulting quality of, 602–603
Psychiatric Diagnostic Interview Evaluation with Medical Services, 601
Psychiatric disorders, suicide and, 492, 492*t*
Psychiatric distress, 582
differential diagnosis of, 339–342, 340*b*
anxiety in, 341
bereavement in, 340–341
delirium in, 340
depression in, 340
fatigue in, 340
mania in, 341
mental disorder, due to another medical condition, 339
pain in, 342
psychosis in, 341
sleep in, 341
substance use in, 341–342
suicide in, 341
Psychiatric evaluation
pre-transplant, 329–330, 329*b*
of transplant patients, 328–330
Psychiatric examination, in pain patients, 194
Psychiatric history, in psychiatric interview, 29–32, 30*b*
past, 31
Psychiatric illnesses, pediatric consultation for, 527–528
Psychiatric interview, 23–35, 23*b*–24*b*
assessment and treatment in, disagreements about, 35
attachment theory in, lessons from, 24–25, 24*b*
children and adolescents in, evaluation of, 34
context of, 25–27
setting, 25–26
significance, 27
situation, 26
subject, 26–27
data collection in, 29–33
behavioral observation, 29
medical and psychiatric history, 29–32, 30*b*
mental status examination, 32–33, 32*b*–33*b*
dealing with sensitive subjects during, 34–35
difficulties in, 34–35
effective communication in, 27–28
errors in, 35, 35*b*
establishing alliance in, 27–28, 28*b*
mindful practice in, 24–25
Psychiatric interview *(Continued)*
narrative medicine in, 24–25
presenting problems in, 29–31
purpose of, 23
relationship and therapeutic alliance in, building, 28–29
treatment preparation during, 33–34
Psychiatric look-alikes, 374–376
Psychiatric management, of patients with cardiac disease, 291–302
Psychiatric medications
for anxiety in cardiac patients, 294–295
for psychiatric and medical differential diagnoses, 298
Psychiatric sequelae, in alcohol use disorder, 142–143
Psychiatrist
in intensive care unit, 381–384, 382*b*
in pain patients, 194
role of, in end-of-life care, 514–516
Psychogenic non-epileptic seizures (PNESs), 218
Psychogenic polydipsia, 119–120
Psychological assessment, 51–54
case of, 51*b*–52*b*
of intellectual functioning, 52–53
of personality, psychopathology, and psychological function, 53–54
test reports in, 58
Psychological therapies
for anorexia nervosa, 183–184
for binge eating disorder, 186
for bulimia nervosa, 184–185
Psychological unconscious, 45
Psychomotor agitation, in emergency psychiatry, 507
Psychomotor seizures, 214
Psychopathology tests, 53–54
Psychopharmacologic management, in children and adolescents, 437–453, 437*b*–438*b*
issues in, 437
medical precautions and contraindications of, 438–439
Psychopharmacology
for anxiety in cardiac patients, 293–294
for depression in cardiac disease, 297–298
drug interactions in, 422–434
antidepressants, 428–432, 429*t*, 431*t*
antipsychotic drugs, 423–425, 424*t*
benzodiazepines, 433–434
mood stabilizers, 425–428, 426*t*–427*t*
psychostimulants and modafinil, 433
ethnicity and, 564–567
in medical setting, 413–436
non-psychiatric medications in, 434–436
α_2-adrenergic agonists, 435
α_1-adrenergic antagonists, 435
β-blockers, 435–436
for psychotropic drug side effects, 434–435
pharmacokinetics in, 418–422
absorption, 418–419
distribution, 419
excretion, 420–422
metabolism, 419–420, 420*t*–421*t*
principles of, 413–418
discontinuing medications, 417–418
initiating treatment, 414–415

Psychopharmacology *(Continued)*
selecting and administering medication, 415–416
treatment failure, 416–417
for psychiatrists, 598
Psychophysiologic insomnia, 269
Psychosis, 109
See also Schizophrenia.
acute, during pregnancy, 552
clinical pictures and corresponding problems on medical ward of, 113–115
depressed, 115
disorganized patients, 114
elderly, 115
manic patients, 114–115
with negative symptoms, or neurocognitive deficits, 114
paranoid, or delusional patient, 113–114
from cocaine, 150
diagnostic evaluation of, 109–113, 110*b*–112*b*
in emergency psychiatry, 505
extrapyramidal side effects of, 116–117
in geriatric patients, 542–543
in HIV infection, 341, 347
management of, 115–118
drug interactions with antipsychotic agents, 118
drug selection, 115–116
first-generation antipsychotics, 116–117
general considerations, 115
neuroleptic malignant syndrome, 118
second-generation antipsychotics, 117–118
treating agitation, 118
medication adherence and insight into, 120–121
in neurocognitive disorder, 102
in pain, 196
patient and family, working with, 119
post-stroke, 226
problems in care of, 119–120
assessment of dangerousness, 119
cigarette smoking, 120
medical co-morbidities, 120
pain threshold in schizophrenia, 119
psychogenic polydipsia, 119–120
seizure disorders and, 216
sleep disorders and, 274
in traumatic brain injury, 229
Psychosocial considerations, in end-of-life care, 515–516
Psychosocial interventions, for cancer, 353
"Psychosomatic conditions", 161–175, 162*b*
gratification of, 175
manifestations of, 174
parameters of, 173–175, 174*f*
production of, 174–175
Psychosomatic medicine, 1
consultation service in, 3–4
history of, 1–3
patient care in, 3
recent direction of, 4–5
research in, 4
residency training programs, 1–2
teaching of, 3–4
Psychostimulants
drug interactions of, 433
for HIV infection, 346
for post-stroke depression, 225
Psychotherapy
for bulimia nervosa, 184
for difficult patients, 487–488, 489*t*–490*t*
for HIV infection, 344
for medically ill, 403
for non-adherence, 531–532
for pain, 211
for psychiatrists, 598
for suicidal behavior, 499
Psychotic disorders
in children and adolescents, 451–453, 452*t*
diagnostic rating scales for, 60
during pregnancy, 552–553
sleep disorders and, 274
somatic symptoms and, 165–166
Psychotic patients, 109–121, 109*b*
Psychotic symptoms, in delirious cardiac patient, 301–302, 302*b*
Psychotropic drug use, breast-feeding and, 554–555
Psychotropic medications
liquid and orally-disintegrating formulations of, 324*t*
non-oral preparations of, 323*t*
usage, cultural factors in, 563–564
PTSD. *See* Post-traumatic stress disorder.
Pulse oximetry, polysomnography and, 267
Pupillary measurement, in visual examination, 40
Putnam, James Jackson, 2

Q

QT interval, prolonged, 383
Quetiapine
for bipolar disorder, in children and adolescents, 450
for burn injuries, 366
for delirious cardiac patients, 300
for difficult patients, 485
for psychosis, 117
Quick Inventory for Depressive Symptomatology, 414

R

Rabbit tremor, 237
Ramelteon, for sleep disorders, 270
Rapid eye movement (REM), 267
in sleep disorders, 267
Rating scale. *See* Diagnostic Rating Scales.
Reality distortion, 113
Rebound effects, 417
Receptors
for antipsychotic drugs, 423
in pathophysiology of pain, 190
sites, in drug distribution, 419
Reconstructive surgery, for burn injuries, 367–368
Recurrence, 417
Re-feeding syndrome, 183
Reflexes, 40–41
Refusal to treat patients, 571–572

Rehabilitation
  See also Chronic medical illness.
  healing in, brain pathways involved, 374, 375*f*
  for pain, 210
  phases of, 371–373
  psychiatric symptoms in, questions for, 372, 372*b*
  in psychopharmacology, 414–415
  settings of, 372, 372*f*
Reimbursement climate, 583
Relapse, 417
Relationship-centered care, 16
Relaxation response (RR), 455
Release reflexes, 40–41
Religion
  coping skills and, 399
  in end-of-life care, 515
REM
  See also Rapid eye movement.
  in sleep disorder, 267
Renal disease
  end-stage, 328
    cognitive impairment in, 306
    psychiatric disorders in, 306
  patients with, 303–312
Renal failure
  neurologic complications in, 307
  suicide and, 493
Residency training
  programs, in psychosomatic medicine, 1–2
  psychiatrists coping with, 594
Resilience, 458
  coping and, 400–401
  vulnerability *versus*, 400–401, 402*t*
Respiration, in polysomnography, 267
Responsibility, psychiatrists and, 593
Rest tremor, in motor symptoms, 232*b*
Restless legs syndrome (RLS), 235, 273, 308
Restraint
  in emergency psychiatry, 509–510
  for geriatric patients, 541
  legal aspects of, 576–577
"Retarded ejaculation", 282–283
Rett syndrome, 386–387, 391
Review of systems, in psychiatric interview, 31–32
Rey-Osterrieth Complex Figure, 56
Rheumatoid arthritis, suicide and, 493
Right to refuse treatment, 577–578, 577*b*
Risk factors
  for burn injuries, 360–361
    in adults, 361*b*
    in child and adolescents, 361*b*
  of depression in cardiac disease, 295–296
  of kidney function, 304
  for sexual dysfunction, 279
Risperidone
  for anorexia nervosa, 184
  for bipolar disorder, in children and adolescents, 449–450
  for burn injuries, 366
  for delirious cardiac patients, 300
  for delirium, 91–92
  for psychosis, 117
Rivastigmine, for neurocognitive disorders, 105, 105*t*
Rorschach inkblot test, 53
Roux-en-Y gastric bypass, 316
Russell's sign, 178

S

Sachs, Hans, 2
S-adenosylmethionine (SAMe), for mood disorders, 472
Safety issues, in emergency psychiatry, 501
SANS. *See* Scale for the Assessment of Negative Symptoms.
SAPS. *See* Scale for the Assessment of Positive Symptoms.
Scale for the Assessment of Negative Symptoms (SANS), 60
Scale for the Assessment of Positive Symptoms (SAPS), 60
Schema focused therapy, 489*t*–490*t*
Schizophrenia
  See also Psychosis.
  burn injuries and, 361
  diagnostic rating scales for, 60
  ECT indication for, 408
  genes involved, 387
  in geriatric patient, 542–543
  suicide and, 492
Schneiderian first-rank symptoms, 112–113
School-age children
  burn injuries in, 362, 362*b*
  in pediatric consultation, 525
Screening
  for cancer patients, 352
  for delirium, 84
  for depression in cardiac disease, 298
  for HIV infection, 342–343
  perinatal, 557
  prenatal, for congenital malformations, 551
  for sexual dysfunction, 282
Seclusion, in emergency psychiatry, 509–510
Secondary gain, 172
Secondary generalization, 214
Second-generation antipsychotics, 117–118
Security guards, for difficult patients, 486
Sedation, opioids and, 203
Sedative-hypnotics, use of, 159
Seizure disorders, patients with, 213–221, 213*b*
  after ECT, 409
  psychiatric symptoms in, management of, 213–218
    ictal neuropsychiatric phenomena, 214–215, 215*t*
    inter-ictal (chronic) neuropsychiatric phenomena, 216–218
    non-epileptic, 218–219, 218*b*–219*b*, 220*t*
    peri-ictal neuropsychiatric phenomena, 215–216
Self-efficacy, 465
Self-reflection, in psychiatric interview, 25
Self-report tests, 53
Sensory abnormalities, during rehabilitation, 375–376
Separation anxiety, in children and adolescents, 439
Serotonin, 263
  suicide and, 495
  transporter gene, 386

Serotonin selective re-uptake inhibitors (SSRIs), 583
for alcohol use disorder, 147
for anorexia nervosa, 184
for anxiety disorders, 135–136, 135*t*
for binge eating disorder, 186
for depression, in children and adolescents, 447–448
for depression and anxiety, 377
for difficult patients, 485
drug interactions of, 429–430, 429*t*
for HIV infection, 344–345
liquid and orally-disintegrating formulations of, 324*t*
lithium and, 426
for neurocognitive disorders, 106
for post-traumatic stress disorder, 133–134
precautions in, 64
during pregnancy, 548
for pseudobulbar affect, 375
for suicidal behavior, 498
upper GI bleeding due to, 323–324
Serotonin syndrome, 263–265, 263*b*
clinical features and diagnosis of, 263–264, 264*t*, 265*b*
definition of, 263
drug interactions in, 430, 432
epidemiology of, 263
management and treatment of, 264–265
pathophysiology of, 264
prognosis and complications of, 265
Serotonin-norepinephrine re-uptake inhibitors (SNRIs)
for anxiety disorders, 135*t*
for HIV infection, 345
Sertraline
for anxiety disorders, 135*t*
for binge eating disorder, 186
for bulimia nervosa, 185
Sexual abuse, of children, 533–534
Sexual arousal disorder, female, 284
Sexual dysfunction, 279–290, 281*b*
affecting both genders, 284
after spinal cord injury, 378
classification of, 280*t*
clinical features and diagnosis of, 280, 281*t*–283*t*, 283*b*
diagnostic criteria of, 282–285
differential diagnosis of, 285
epidemiology and risk factors of, 279
female disorders of, 284
gender identity disorder and, 285
history-taking of, 280–282
male disorders of, 282–284
paraphilias and, 282, 285*b*
pathophysiology of, 279–280
physical examination and laboratory investigation of, 282
psychotropic medication-induced, 285–286
specified and unspecified, 284
treatment of
organically-based, 285–289, 285*t*
psychologically-based, 289, 290*t*
Sexual interest/arousal disorder, female, 284
Shift-work sleep disorder, 272
Short-term memory, 41
Siblings, in pediatric consultation, 526
Sibutramine, for binge eating disorder, 186
Sickness, conceptualization of, 399
Sildenafil (Viagra), for erectile dysfunction, 287*t*
Simultaneous Extinction Test, 57
Single nucleotide polymorphisms (SNPs), 387
Single photon emission computed tomography (SPECT), 68
Sleep, in HIV infection, 341
Sleep attacks, 271
Sleep disorders
antidepressants and, 74–76
breathing disorders related to, 270–271
circadian rhythm and, 271–272
classification systems for, 269
hypersomnias of central origin, 271
insomnia, 269–270
in medical condition, 273–275
narcolepsy, 271
neuroanatomic basis for, 268–269
parasomnias, 272–275
patients with, 267–277, 268*b*
approach to, 275–277
REM, 272–273
sleep stages and normal sleep in, 267–268
substance-induced, 274–275
treatment options for, 276*t*–277*t*
Sleep hygiene, 269*b*
Sleep latency, 268
Sleep logs, 414
Sleep onset, in polysomnography, 267
Sleep-wake cycle, in delirious cardiac patients, 301–302, 302*b*
Sleepwalking disorder, 272
SMART goals, co-creation of, 466
Smith-Magenis syndrome, 389
Smokers, characteristics of, 467–469
Smoking
cessation of
behavioral treatments for, 468
medications for, 468–469
cognitive-behavioral therapy approaches to, 468
prevalence of, 467–469
quitting from, 468
Snore monitor, in polysomnography, 267
Social anxiety disorder, 133
Social history, in psychiatric interview, 32
Social intervention, for traumatic brain injury, 230
Social model, in clinical formulation, 19
Social phobia, 133
Social relationships, of psychiatrists, disruption of, 593
Social support
for coping with illness, 399–400
for depression in cardiac disease, 298
Soldiers, suicide among, 494
Soma, 159
Somatic symptom and related disorders, 162–165, 163*f*
conversion disorder in, 164
diagnostic considerations for, 376
differential diagnosis of, 165–168, 166*b*
factitious disorder in, 165
clinical presentation of, 171*t*
in deception syndromes, 170–172
imposed on another, 171

Somatic symptom and related disorders *(Continued)*
  functional somatic syndromes in, 166–168, 167*t*
    anxiety disorders and, 165
    depressive disorders and, 165
    fibromyalgia and, 167–168
    irritable bowel syndrome and, 168
    organic mental disorders and, 166
    personality disorders and, 166
    psychotic disorders and, 165–166
    substance use disorders and, 165
    systemic exertion intolerance disease and, 167
  gratification of, 175
  illness anxiety disorder in, 163–164
  manifestation of, 174
  in pain, 196, 197*t*
  pediatric consultation for, 528–529
  production of, 174–175
  prognosis and treatment of, 168–169
  psychological factors affecting medical illness in, 164
  treatment of, 168–170
Somatization disorder, 130
South American holly, 563–564
Specialty psychiatric clinics, 585–586
SPECT. *See* Single photon emission computed tomography.
Spinal cord injuries
  depression and anxiety in, 377
  sexual dysfunction after, 378
  suicide and, 493
Spinoreticular tract, 189
Spiritual model, in clinical formulation, 19
Splitting, by difficult patients, 481, 482*b*
SSRI-induced sexual dysfunction, treatment strategies for, 286*t*
SSRIs. *See* Serotonin selective re-uptake inhibitors.
St. John's wort
  drug interactions of, 432
  for mood disorders, 472
Staff consultant/stepped care models, 586
Staff support, for burn injuries, 370
Staffing, in psychiatric consultation, 602
Stanford Integrated Psychosocial Assessment for Transplant (SIPAT), 329
Status epilepticus, delirium *vs.*, 84
Stereognosis, 39
Stereotypies, in motor symptoms, 232*b*
Stern, Theodore, 2–3
Sternbach criteria, for serotonin syndrome, 263–264
Steroid-resistant nephrotic syndrome (SRNS), 304
Stevens-Johnson syndrome, 554
Stimulants
  for ADHD, in children and adolescents, 441–443
    guidelines on the use of, 443
    medication interactions with, 443–444
    side effects of, 443, 443*t*
  for cancer patients, 355
  liquid and orally-disintegrating formulations of, 324*t*
Stress
  appraisal and, 457
  autonomic nervous system and, 456
  decrease in vulnerability to, for self-neglect, 597
  definition of, 455
Stress *(Continued)*
  financial, psychiatrists and, 593
  hypothalamic-pituitary-adrenal axis and, 456
  immune system and, 457
  pathogenic, 455
  physiology of, 455–457
  recognition of, in oneself, 595–596
  response to, 455
    activation of, 456
    specificity of, 457
  system for, 455
  unhealthy behaviors and, 461
Stress disorder
  burn injuries and, 364
  in children and adolescents, 439
Stroke, depression and, 73–74
Stroop Color Word Interference Test, 56
Structured Clinical Interview, 59
Substance abuse
  diagnostic rating scales for, 61, 61*b*
  by difficult patients, 486–487
  in emergency psychiatry, 503*b*
  in geriatric patients, 543
  laboratory tests for, 64
Substance Abuse and Mental Health Service Administration (SAMHSA), 149
Substance P, in pain signal, 189
Substance use disorders (SUDs)
  in HIV infection, 341–342, 347
  patients with, 149–159, 149*b*–150*b*
    amphetamines in, 152–153
    benzodiazepines in, 157–158
    cannabis in, 154–155
    CNS stimulants in, 152–153
    cocaine in, 150–152
    hallucinogens in, 153–154
    heroin in, 155–157
    opioids in, 155–157
    sedative hypnotics in, 159
    stimulants of, 150–153
    synthetic cannabinoids in, 154–155
  somatic symptoms and, 165
Substance/medication induced-sexual dysfunction, 284
Substance/medication-induced neurocognitive disorder, 99
Suicidal patient, care of, 491–500
Suicide
  burn injuries and, 361
  in chronic medical illness, 371
  clinical features and diagnosis of, 495–497, 496*b*
  by difficult patients, 486
  difficulties in assessment of risk, 500
  ECT indication for, 407–408
  in emergency psychiatry, 504
  epidemiology of, 491
  evidence-based clinical approaches to, 496
  in HIV infection, 341
  pathophysiology of, 495
  of patient
    effect of, 593
    psychiatrists coping with, 593–594
    reactions to, 593

Suicide *(Continued)*
pediatric consultation for, 527–528
physician-assisted, 572
rates of, 491
risk factors of, 491–495, 492*b*
familial and genetic, 494
medical, 493–494
past and present suicidality in, 494–495
physician contract in, 495
psychiatric, 492–493, 492*t*
social, 494
treatment of risk in, 497–499, 497*b*
Supplements, for anorexia nervosa, 183
Support groups, 414–415
Suprachiasmatic nuclei (SCN), 268
Surgery
for burn injuries, 367–368
deafferentation, in pain, 198–199
for neurocognitive disorders, 103–105
suicide and, 494
Sympathetic nervous system, 456
distress and, 455
Sympathetically-maintained pain (SMP), 208
Symptom amplification, 161
Syndrome of inappropriate antidiuretic hormone (SIADH), 356
Synthetic cannabinoids
in psychotic patients, 109–111
use of, 154–155
Systemic exertion intolerance disease, 167

T

Tacrolimus, psychiatric side effects of, 331, 332*t*
Tactical intervention, for difficult patients, 488
Tactical psychotherapy, for difficult patients, 487–488, 489*t*–490*t*
Tactile hallucinations, 144–145
Tadalafil (Cialis), for erectile dysfunction, 287*t*
Talking, in pain patients, 199
Tangles, neurofibrillary, in Alzheimer's disease, 96
Tardive dyskinesia, 116–117
Tay-Sachs disease, late-onset type, 394
TBI. *See* Traumatic brain injury.
TCAs. *See* Tricyclic antidepressants.
Temporal lobe, 37
Temporal lobe epilepsy (TLE), 214
Temporal lobe symptomatology, during rehabilitation, 376
Tenofovir alafenamide, for HIV infection, 337
Teratogen exposure, 395–396
Teratogenesis
anticonvulsant effects, 551
of antidepressant drugs, 548
lithium effects, 551
valproic acid effects, 551
Terrors, sleep, 272
Test for Severe Impairment (TSI), for neurocognitive disorder, 103
Tetrabenazine, 117
Thalamus, 37
brain response and, 37
The Life Institute, 537*b*
The Station nightclub fire, 359
The Wellness Community, 537*b*
Thematic Apperception Test (TAT), 54
Therapeutic interventions, for anxiety, 294
Theta waves, in polysomnography, 267–268
Thiazide diuretics, lithium and, 425
Thioridazine, 79
Thiothixene
for delirium, 91
for neurocognitive disorders, 106
Thought disorders, in psychiatric interview, 33, 33*b*
Thought distortions, identification of, for self-neglect, 597
"Thought-as-language", 44–45
Three-component model, 588
Three-legged stool, 455
Thyroid hormones, lithium and, 426
Tic disorders, in children and adolescents, 439
Tics, in motor symptoms, 232*b*
T-lymphocytes, CD4 subpopulation of, in HIV infection and AIDS, 335
Tolerance, in opioids, 203
Topiramate
for alcohol use disorder, 147
for binge eating disorder, 186
for bulimia nervosa, 185
for difficult patients, 485
drug interactions of, 428
for pain, 208
Torsades de pointes (TDP), 297
in burn injuries, 366
Torticollis, 236
Tourette's syndrome, 234
Toxic leukoencephalopathy, in cancer patients, 357
Toxicity, of drugs, in burn injuries, 366–367
Toxins, clearance of, 303
Trail Making Test, 56
Training, psychiatric, 602
Transactional Model for Stress Management, 397
Transcranial magnetic stimulation (TMS), 405–406
high frequency rTMS, 406
indications of, 406
low frequency rTMS, 406
repetitive, 405–406
safety of, 406
technique for, 405–406
Transference, psychiatrists and, 592
Transference focused psychotherapy, 489*t*–490*t*
Transplantation. *See* Organ failure and transplantation.
Transtheoretical model of change, 462–463
action in, 463
contemplation in, 463
maintenance in, 463
pre-contemplation in, 463
preparation of, 463
Trauma, in emergency psychiatry, 505
Traumatic brain injury (TBI)
patients with, 223–230
management of, 227–230
behavioral, cognitive, and social intervention, 230

Traumatic brain injury (TBI) *(Continued)*
clinical presentation of, 228–229, 228*b*
epidemiology of, 227
mood and anxiety disorders, 228–229
pathophysiology of, 227–228
pharmacology for, 229–230
treatment of, 229–230
personality changes due to, 228
Trazodone
anticholinergic effect of, 76
for delirious cardiac patients, 301
for HIV infection, 345
for neurocognitive disorders, 107
orthostatic hypotension and, 76
side effects of, 79
for sleep disorders, 269–270
Tricyclic antidepressants (TCAs)
for ADHD, in children and adolescents, 444
anticholinergic effects of, 76
cardiac conduction effects of, 76–78
discontinuation syndrome, 79
drug interactions of, 430–431, 431*t*
for HIV infection, 346
for medically ill, 74–79, 75*t*
for myocardial depression, 78
for neurocognitive disorders, 106
for orthostatic hypotension, 76, 77*t*
for pregnancy, 548
side effects of, 63–64
for suicidal behavior, 499
Trifluoperazine
for delirium, 91
for neurocognitive disorders, 106
Trigeminal nerve, 40
Trismus, 236
Triune brain, 44
Tuberous sclerosis, 391
Turner's syndrome, 390
Two-Point Discrimination, 57

U

Uncertainty, psychiatrists and, 593
Unemployment, suicide and, 494
Unhealthy habits, behavioral management of, 461–469, 467*b*
Unipolar depressive disorders, 70, 71*b*
United Network for Organ Sharing (UNOS), 327
Uniting Couples (in the treatment of) Anorexia Nervosa (UCAN), for anorexia nervosa, 184
UNOS. *See* United Network for Organ Sharing.
Urea cycle defects, 395
Urine toxicologic screening test, diagnostic evaluation of, in psychotic patients, 109–111
Uvulopalatopharyngoplasty (UPPP), 270–271

V

Vacuum constriction device, for erectile dysfunction, 288*t*
Vaginismus, 284
Vagus nerve, 40
Vagus nerve stimulation (VNS), 409–410
indications of, 410
management in, 410
safety of, 410
stimulation parameters of, 410
technique in, 409–410
Valerian, 473
Valeriana officinalis, 473
Valproate
for catatonia, 261
for difficult patients, 485
Valproic acid (VPA)
adverse effects of, 64
for bipolar disorder, in children and adolescents, 449
breast feeding and, 555
drug interactions of, 426–427, 427*t*
for neurocognitive disorders, 107
for pain, 207
teratogenic effects of, 551
Vaptans, 119–120
Vardenafil (Levitra), for erectile dysfunction, 287*t*
Varenicline, 120
for smoking cessation, 468–469
Vascular neurocognitive disorder, 97–98
Vasoactive intestinal polypeptide (VIP) + phentolamine, for erectile dysfunction, 288*t*
Vegetative state, 517–518
Velocardiofacial syndrome/DiGeorge syndrome, 388
Venlafaxine
anticholinergic effects of, 76
for anxiety disorders, 135*t*, 136
for post-stroke depression, 225
during pregnancy, 549
side effects of, 78
VGCC (N-type) antigen, associated with autoimmune encephalitides, 244*t*–245*t*
VGKC complex antigen, associated with autoimmune encephalitides, 244*t*–245*t*
Vibration sense, in peripheral sensory examination, 39
"VICTIMS DIE" mnemonic, 62, 62*t*
Video-EEG monitoring, for non-epileptic seizure, 219
Vigilance, 124
Violence
assessment of, 504
by difficult patients, 486
domestic, confidentiality of, 571
"Visceral brain", 44
Visual acuity, in visual examination, 40
Visual Analog Scale, for pain assessment, 193–194, 365
Visual-spatial skills
in neurologic examination, 41
neuropsychological assessment for, 55
Vitamin B_{12}, for mood disorders, 472
Vocational assessment, 414–415
Vocational identity, in end-of-life care, 515
Voltage-gated calcium channel (VGCC), in encephalitic neuropsychiatric impairment, 243
Volume control, of kidney, 303
Vomiting, as purging method, 178–179

Vulnerability
  conceptualization of, 399
  coping and, 400–401, 401*t*–402*t*
  of psychiatrist
    decrease in, 594
    denial of, 595
  resilience *versus*, 400–401, 402*t*

W

Wakefulness, 268
Waking state, 267
Warm hand-off, 586
Water intoxication, 119–120
Wechsler Abbreviated Scale of Intelligence (WASI), 52–53
Wechsler Adult Intelligence Scale-IV, 52–53
Wechsler Preschool and Primary Scale of Intelligence-IV, 52–53
Weight assessment, for eating disorder, 179
Weight gain, for anorexia nervosa, 183
Weisman, Avery, 2
Wernicke-Korsakoff syndrome, 146
Wernicke's disease, delirium *vs.*, 84
Wernicke's encephalopathy, 146
"WHHHHIMPS" mnemonic, 84, 85*b*
Williams syndrome, genetic factors of, 389–390
Wilson's disease, 234–235
  genetic factors of, 393–394
  in psychotic patients, 111
Wisconsin Card Sorting Test, 56
Withdrawal syndrome, in emergency psychiatry, 505–507
World Health Organization Disability Assessment Schedule (WHODAS 2.0), 414
"WWHHHHIMPS" mnemonic, 63*b*

X

Xerostomia, 313
X-linked dominant disorders. *See* Genetics, of psychiatric disorders.
47, XYY disorder, 390–391

Y

Yale-Brown Obsessive Compulsive Scale (Y-BOCS), 60–61, 410–411
Y-BOCS. *See* Yale-Brown Obsessive Compulsive Scale.
Y-MRS. *See* Young Mania Rating Scale.
Young adulthood, burn injuries in, 363, 363*b*
Young Mania Rating Scale (Y-MRS), 60
Young Survival Coalition, 537*b*

Z

Zidovudine, in HIV infection, 341
Ziprasidone
  for bipolar disorder, in children and adolescents, 450
  for burn injuries, 366
  for delirium, 91
  for psychosis, 117
Zonisamide
  for binge eating disorder, 186
  drug interactions of, 428